MEDICAL RADIOLOGY
Radiation Oncology

Editors:
L. W. Brady, Philadelphia
H.-P. Heilmann, Hamburg
M. Molls, Munich

Springer

Berlin
Heidelberg
New York
Barcelona
Hong Kong
London
Milan
Paris
Singapore
Tokyo

Z. Petrovich · L.W. Brady · M.L. Apuzzo
M. Bamberg (Eds.)

Combined Modality Therapy of Central Nervous System Tumors

With Contributions by

R. Atkinson · J. R. Adler · A. P. Amar · M. L. J. Apuzzo · M. Bamberg · A. Bettini · B. D. Birch
L. W. Brady · S. D. Chang · J. Chen · R. Class · P. Conti · J. L. Daigle · J. D. Day · B. Dykes
J. Flagel · S. C. Formenti · R. A. Freidman · B. George · S. Ghosh · S. L. Giannotta · J. L. Go
A.-L. Grosu · G. Harsh · G. Hsu · D. Huang · D. J. Hyder · B. Jeremic · G. Jozsef · M. G. Kaiser
L. T. Khoo · P. Kim · M. Kocher · R. D. Kortmann · M. D. Krieger · J. E. Lahaniatis
R. S. Lavey · M. L. Levy · M. Liker · D. P. Martin · W. H. McBride · J. G. McComb
P. C. McCormick · C. T. Miyamoto · M. Molls · R.-P. Müller · M. J. Murphy · S. O'Day
A. T. Parsa · Z. Petrovich · S. Preston-Martin · M. Salcman · R. Sawaya · M. Selch
E. M. Thomson · V. C.-K. Tse · J. Voges · M. H. Weiss · H. R. Withers · C. Yu · C.-S. Zee

Foreword by

L. W. Brady, H.-P. Heilmann, and M. Molls

With 226 Figures in 391 Separate Illustrations, 25 in Color and 80 Tables

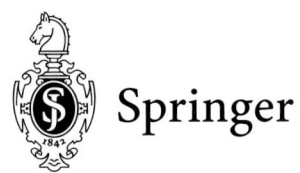

Springer

ZBIGNIEW PETROVICH, MD, FACR
Professor and Chairman
Department of Radiation Oncology, University of Southern California
Keck School of Medicine
1441 Eastlake Avenue, Room G356
Los Angeles, CA 90033-0804, USA

LUTHER W. BRADY, MD
Hylda Cohn/ American Cancer Society
Professor of Clinical Oncology and Professor
Department of Radiation Oncology, Hahnemann University Hospital
Broad & Vine Sts., Mail Stop 200
Philadelphia, PA 19102, USA

MICHAEL L.J. APUZZO, MD
Edwin M. Todd/Trent H. Wells, Jr.
Professor of Neurological Surgery and Professor of Radiation Oncology
Keck School of Medicine of the University of Southern California
Los Angeles, CA 90033, USA

MICHAEL BAMBERG, MD
Professor
Department of Radiotherapy, Eberhard-Karls-Universität
Hoppe-Seyler-Strasse 3
72076 Tübingen, Germany

Medical Radiology · Diagnostic Imaging and Radiation Oncology

Continuation of
Handbuch der medizinischen Radiologie
Encyclopedia of Medical Radiology

ISBN 3-540-66053-4 Springer-Verlag Berlin Heidelberg New York

Library of Congress Cataloging-in-Publication Data
Combined modality of central nervous system tumors / Z. Petrovich ... [et al.] (eds.);
with contributions by R. Adkinson ... [et al.]; foreword by L. W. Brady and H.-P. Heilmann.
    p. ; cm. -- (Medical radiology)
    Spine title: Combined modality therapy of central nervous system tumors.
    Includes bibliographical references and index.
    ISBN 3540660534 (alk. paper)
    1. Central nervous system--Cancer--Treatment. I. Title: Combined modality therapy of
central nervous system tumors. II. Petrovich, Zbigniew. III. Series.
    [DNLM: 1. Central Nervous System Neoplasms--therapy. 2. Combined Modality
Therapy. WL 358 C731 2000]
    RC280.N43 C66 2000
    616.99'4806--dc21   00-055628

Springer-Verlag Berlin Heidelberg New York
a member of BertelsmannSpringer Science+Business Media GmbH

© Springer-Verlag Berlin Heidelberg 2001
Printed in Germany

Cover-Design and Typesetting: Verlagsservice Teichmann, 69256 Mauer

SPIN: 107 309 08   21/3130 – 5 4 3 2 1 0 – Printed on acid-free paper

Foreword

The Surveillance Research Program of the American Cancer Society's Department of Epidemiology and Surveillance Research reported in *CA – A Cancer Journal for Clinicans* in January/February 2000 that the estimated number of new primary malignant tumors involving the central nervous system in the year 2000 was 16,500 patients: 9,500 males and 7,000 females. The cancer deaths in 2000 for brain and other nervous system primary tumors were estimated at 13,000: 7,100 males and 5,900 females. Input into this data also came from the National Cancer Institute: SEER Cancer Incidence Public-Use Database, 1973–1996, August 1998 Submission to the United States Department of Health and Human Services of the Public Health Service, Bethesda, Md, 1999.

With the advances that have been made in the treatment of solid tumors by combined integrated multimodal programs of management including surgery, radiation therapy and chemotherapy, more patients are now being diagnosed with metastatic disease involving the brain. It has been estimated that more than 150,000 patients per year in the USA have brain metastasis as a part of their primary presentation or identified in subsequent follow-up. More than 50% of all patients with primary malignant tumors of the brain have high-grade gliomas of the brain. With the increase in primary malignant tumors among older patients over the past decade, there have been major developments and increased interest in new technologies in the treatment of these tumors. In general, primary brain neoplasms spred invasively without forming a natural capsule and present symptoms based on expansion of the tumor and surrounding edema within the skull.

The management of primary malignant tumors of the brain remains a very significant and difficult problem in clinical practice. The lack of major response to treatment by the high-grade gliomas of the brain has been discouraging and clearly indicates the need for innovative new approaches in the management of these tumors.

The present volume represents a concerted effort on the part of the authors to present data with regard to basic science evaluation and translation into clinical practice of techniques based on combined, integrated multimodal programs of management. The data brought together in this book clearly indicate the progress that has been made but, also, clearly indicate the need for additional innovative efforts in terms of management.

It is the Editors' firm belief that this volume represents the first publication of new innovative programs for combined treatment of primary malignant tumors of the brain as well as addressing the issues of the growing incidence of brain metastasis from solid tumors that are better controlled now by combined, integrated programs of management.

Philadelphia

Hamburg

Munich

L. W. BRADY

H.-P. HEILMANN

M. MOLLS

Preface

Respice, Adspice, Prospice:
Consider the Past, the Present, the Future

Neoplastic involvement of the nervous system presents unique problems to the specialist therapeutic community. No other neoplasms have the capability of functional disruption with relatively small tumor burdens or challenge traditional surgical or oncologic principles more. There has been a natural evolution toward application of combined therapies which has been particularly evident with increasing sophistication in the closing decades of the twentieth century. In surgery, the specialty of *neurological surgery* has been completely reinvented thanks to the introduction of the operating microscope, modern imaging, novel stereotactic principles, and the computer as a functional and practical operative tool. Similar refinements have been seen in the field of *radiation oncology,* with computerized planning and the introduction of stereotactic imaging-directed radiosurgery by rotational and fixed beam methods. Concurrently, the practical emergence of *cellular and molecular biology* as a diagnostic probe and therapeutic companion to more traditional treatment methods is offering exciting new possibilities for the management of problems that have been persistently enigmatic. More information is available regarding the efficacy and application of *chemotherapeutic* methods to a broad spectrum of these neoplasms.

Therefore, in general overview the remarkable escalation in technical ability, information base and knowledge within the past two decades allows new capabilities and possibilities in management protocols. This is particularly exciting regarding central nervous system neoplasms, which in general lend themselves to combined, multimodality management for optimization of outcome and the satisfying of the all-important requirement for functional preservation.

Given these considerations, this multidimensional text has been composed and carefully assembled to present a view of the past, present, and future in the management of central nervous system neoplasms. It also has an international perspective presented in order to convey the current body of knowledge related to epidemiology, pathology, molecular biology, and therapeutic principles as a basis for individual attention to the principal categories of neoplastic problems affecting the nervous system – extraaxial, and intraaxial, cranial and spinal, adult and pediatric, primary and metastatic. Sophisticated perspectives of the surgeon, radiation oncologist, oncologist, and oncology nurse are presented in an effort to define modernity in the field for those desiring a succinct but substantive overall view.

Los Angeles   Z. Petrovich
                                                              M. L. Apuzzo
Philadelphia   L. W. Brady
Tübingen   M. Bamberg

Contents

1 Epidemiology of Primary Brain Tumors

Susan Preston-Martin

CONTENTS

1.1 Introduction

It was estimated that in 1999, 16,800 individuals in the United States would be diagnosed with a malignant primary nervous system tumor and 13,100 of these would die from the disease (LANDIS 1999). When benign as well as malignant brain tumors are included, the incidence is over twice that for malignant brain tumors alone [34,345 individuals were newly diagnosed with a benign or malignant nervous system tumor in 1998 (CBTRUS 1998)]. Only about half of the patients with malignant brain tumors are still alive 1 year after diagnosis (DAVIS 1999). Although the incidence of brain tumors, particularly the more lethal subtypes, increased in recent decades (GREIG et al. 1990; MODAN et al. 1992; DESMEULES et al. 1992), it appears that trends in childhood brain tumors (SMITH 1998; BLACK 1998) and adult tumors (LEGLER et al. 1999) increased due to the introduction of diagnostic improvements, including computerized tomography (CT) scans in the mid-1970s and magnetic resonance imaging (MRI) in the mid-1980s. This issue and the recent explosion of epidemiologic and molecular genetic studies of brain tumors has focused attention on this important human cancer, which up until only a few decades ago was relatively little studied. Despite this surge of interest, the etiology of the majority of nervous system tumors remains unknown. Inherited syndromes that predispose affected individuals to brain tumor development and/or the presence of nervous system tumors in other family members appear to be present in fewer than 5% of brain tumor patients. Some environmental agents, in particular ionizing radiation, are clearly implicated in the etiology of brain tumors, but also appear to account for few cases. Numerous other physical, chemical, and infectious agents that have long been suspected risk factors have not yet been established as etiologically relevant.

This review will focus on tumors of the brain, cranial nerves, and cranial meninges, which account for 95% of all central nervous system (CNS) tumors. These tumors are unique because of their location within the bony structure of the cranium. Symptoms depend on location of the tumor. Furthermore, histologically benign tumors can result in similar symptomatology and outcome as malignant tumors because growth of both normal and tumor tissue is confined to the cranial space. For this reason, some cancer registries voluntarily include both benign and malignant intracranial tumors. For simplicity, this group of tumors will be called "brain tumors" or,

S. PRESTON-MARTIN, PhD
Professor, Department of Preventive Medicine, University of Southern California School of Medicine, 1441 Eastlake Avenue, MS #44, Los Angeles, CA 90089, USA

when benign tumors are excluded, "brain cancer." The term "central nervous system tumors " (or cancer) indicates that tumors of the spinal cord and spinal meninges are included along with brain tumors, and "nervous system tumors" indicates that tumors of the peripheral nerves are also included. This review will first discuss the descriptive epidemiology of CNS tumors including the change of incidence rates in different age groups over time – patterns of occurrence by gender, race, geography, and social class – and median survival. Evidence relating to a number of other suggested risk factors will be summarized and prospects for future research explored. For each topic, reference will be made only to a few of the numerous relevant papers but will include a recent paper with a comprehensive bibliography.

1.2
Descriptive Epidemiology

1.2.1
Variation in Inclusion Criteria

The descriptive epidemiology of CNS tumors has been difficult to study because of the wide variation in specific tumors included in published rates. Quantitatively, the most important variation is estimated to be approximately 50% and relates to the inclusion or exclusion of benign tumors (DAVIS 1996). This critical difference has often been ignored in comparisons across geographic areas. Although reporting of malignant tumors alone eases geographical comparisons, it is unfortunate that incidence rates for benign nervous system tumors are not also reported. For this reason, benign tumors will not be excluded from descriptive data shown here for Los Angeles County. It should be noted that pineal and pituitary tumors, included in some standard definitions of brain and central nervous system tumors, are not included. In fact, as will become clear from discussions of analytic studies below, more is known about the etiology of benign histologic types such as meningiomas than about the etiology of neuroepithelial tumors which are more common than meningiomas and are usually malignant.

Another variation relates to whether or not clinically diagnosed tumors are included. The microscopic confirmation rate of brain and nervous system cancers included in the latest edition of *Cancer Incidence in Five Continents* varies widely across geographic areas from a high of 99% (e.g., Los Ange-

les County Japanese and Koreans) to a low of 0% (in Setifi, Algeria; PARKIN et al. 1992). Rates vary considerably across registries as well as across specific population groups within a country. For example, the rates of histologic verification range from 76 to 95% in Switzerland, 27 to 91% in Canada, 45 to 87% in Brazil, 52 to 98% in Japan, and 63 to 99% in the United States (PARKIN et al. 1992). Such wide variation suggests that caution in the interpretation of these rates is warranted. In general, for relatively inaccessible cancer sites, a higher rate of microscopic confirmation increases the likelihood that a neoplasm actually existed and that it was correctly classified. In some registries, however, a high rate of microscopic confirmation of brain tumors may indicate that clinically or radiologically diagnosed tumors may have been missed. With the advent of radiosurgery, this is an increasing limitation.

1.2.2
Pathologic Classification

The histologic groups of tumors which occur within the central nervous system and their corresponding ICD-O codes are shown in Table 1.1. A modification of this scheme is proposed for classification of pediatric brain tumors (RORKE et al. 1985). In both children and adults, neuroepithelial tumors (still more commonly called gliomas) are the most common major histologic type; these are predominantly malignant tumors that arise in the glial cells which comprise the supporting structure for the brain. In Los Angeles, neuroepithelial tumors account for 59% of primary tumors of the brain and cranial meninges among men and 42% among women. Over 80% of neuroepithelial tumors are astrocytic gliomas (i.e., astrocytomas and glioblastoma multiforme). Astrocytic tumors that are grades I and II are generally classified as astrocytomas, those that are grade III are classified as anaplastic astrocytomas, and those with grade IV are classified as glioblastomas. The possibility that this practice is not followed consistently is suggested, however, by the considerable geographic variation in the relative proportions of astrocytic tumors that are classified as glioblastomas. This variation is seen, for example, among the various United States registries in the SEER Program. In comparison with the other SEER registries, Connecticut has a considerably higher proportion of tumors classified as glioblastomas, and a correspondingly lower proportion of astrocytomas (VELEMA and PERCY 1987).

Table 1.1. Anatomic and pathologic classification of tumors of the central nervous system

Subsite	ICD-O codes, 1976	ICD-O codes, 1991
Brain	191.0–191.9	C-71.1 – C-71.9
Cranial nerve	192.0	C-72.2 – C-72.5
Cerebral meninges	192.1	C-70.0
Spinal cord	192.2	C-72.0
Spinal meninges	192.3	C-70.1<?13>

Histologic type	ICD-O codes
Neuroepithelial tumors	9380–9481
Astrocytoma	9384, 9400–21
Glioblastoma multiforme	9440–42
Ependymoma	9391–94
Primitive neuroectodermal tumor (PNET)	9470–73
Oligodendroglioma	9450–60
Other neuroepithelial tumors	9380–83, 9390, 9422–30, 9443, 9472–81
Meningioma	9530–39
Nerve sheath tumors	9540–60
Other	9120–61
Unspecified	8000–02
No microscopic confirmation	9990

The other two most common major histologic types are both predominantly benign. Meningiomas arise in the cranial meninges and account for 20% of all primary brain tumors in men and 36% in women. Nerve sheath tumors, called neuromas, neurilemmomas, or schwannomas arise in the Schwann cells of the nerve sheath. About 8% of brain tumors in both men and women are nerve sheath tumors. It is curious that approximately 90% arise in the eighth cranial nerve, also known as acoustic neuromas.

Now that improved diagnostic technology is available in many general hospitals in the United States and other industrialized countries, the differential diagnosis of intracranial masses is often made by physicians who are not specialists in neurological disease. The heterogeneous nature of many CNS tumors makes the assignment of histologic class difficult. In a recent survey in the United Kingdom, fewer than half of the patients with CT diagnoses were referred to neurosurgeons for histologic confirmation by surgery or biopsy; the positive predictive value of the CT diagnosis was around 90% for neuroepithelial tumors and meningiomas but only 50% for metastatic tumors (Todd et al. 1987). The introduction of CT imaging technology in the United States in the mid-1970s and MR imaging in the mid-1980s appears to have resulted in increases in brain tumor incidence rates, without parallel increases in mortality, and rates have stabilized in all age groups in the most recent period (Smith et al. 1998; Black 1998; Legler et al.1999). Accuracy of clinical diagnosis of primary brain tumors will continue to vary by geographical region and hospital, even though CT and MR imaging is now available to a greater proportion of regions in the United States, due to variation in how the equipment is used and the degree of training of individuals who interpret the films.

1.2.3
Distribution by Age and Changes in Age Incidence Curves Over Time

The average annual age-specific incidence of brain tumors is shown in Fig. 1.1. In both males and females, rates decline after a peak in childhood (under the age of 10 years), increase after 25 years of age and level off after 75 years of age. Comparisons of data from different areas of the United States have shown that the shape of the age-incidence curve after age 60 is highly dependent on the autopsy rate (Percy et al. 1972). Prior to 1955, rates among those over 55 years old increased steeply with age in data from Rochester, Minnesota (location of the Mayo Clinic), but decreased in data from other areas (e.g., the Second National Cancer Survey, Connecticut and Iowa). Subsequent analyses showed that the proportion of cases first diagnosed at death was considerably higher in

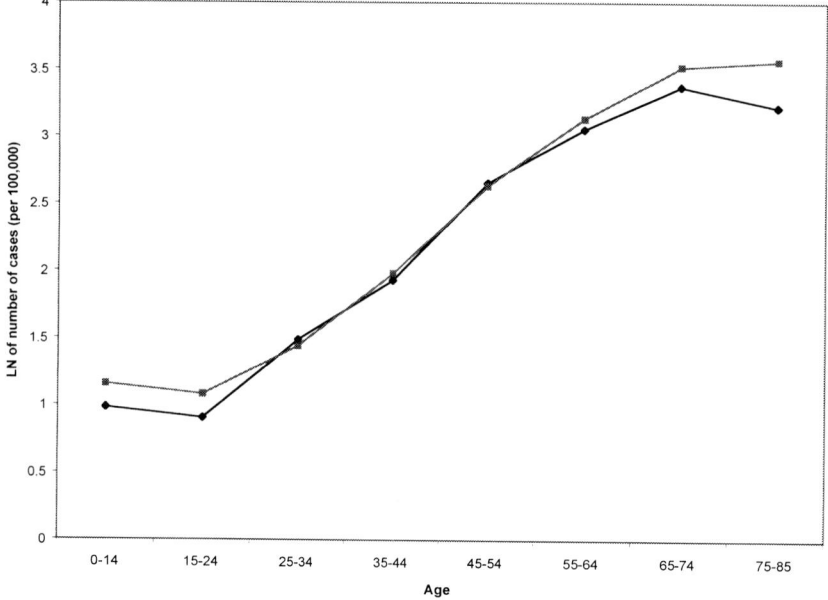

Fig. 1.1. Average annual age-specific incidence of tumors of the brain, cranial nerves, and cranial meninges (benign and malignant combined) in males and females, Los Angeles County, 1972–1997, whites (excluding Spanish-surnamed). Total cases, 5724 in males and 6180 in females

Rochester than in Connecticut and that when these cases were excluded from the Rochester data, rates declined after 65 years of age rather than continuing to rise sharply (SCHOENBERG et al. 1978; ANNEGERS et al. 1981). These comparisons suggest that brain tumor incidence continues to increase with age throughout life, but that there is, or at least there was, often a significant under-ascertainment of cases in the oldest age groups. Therefore, historical comparisons of brain tumor rates from different registries might be more meaningful if restricted to groups under 65 years of age. The dramatic increases in brain tumor incidence rates in the elderly in recent decades indicates that this under-ascertainment has become less pronounced.

1.2.4
Distribution by Gender, Race, and Geography

In Fig. 1.1 we see that for all types of brain tumors combined, rates are higher in males than in females. Table 1.2 shows the age-adjusted annual incidence rates for the major histologic groups of primary brain tumors by sex and ethnic group in Los Angeles County, 1972–1997. For all histologic types and races combined, the rate is higher in men than in women. For most ethnic groups, male rates for all histologic types combined are higher than female rates. The male:female sex ratio (SR) varies considerably, however, by histologic type. In each ethnic group, neu-roepithelial rates are higher in males than in females (SR for all races combined=1.5), and meningioma rates are higher in women (SR=0.6). The SR in children under 15 years of age is 1.2 for all tumor types combined. In contrast, primitive neuroectodermal tumors (PNET, formerly called medulloblastoma), which occur almost exclusively in children, have an SR of around 2 (PRESTON-MARTIN 1985; CRUZ 1958), but no male excess is seen among black children in the United States (BUNIN 1987).

SRs for specific histologic types also vary by anatomic subsite and by age group. One of the most interesting examples of this relates to meningiomas. Among non-Spanish-surnamed whites in Los Angeles County, spinal meningiomas are 3.5 times more common in women than in men (SR=0.3), whereas cerebral meningiomas are only 1.5 times more common in women (SR=0.7). Similar patterns are seen for meningiomas in Norway (HELSETH et al. 1989b). Also, the female:male ratio for spinal meningiomas increases with age, whereas for cerebral meningiomas the female excess is greatest during the female reproductive years and declines after 55 years of age. The sex differential for spinal meningiomas suggests the etiologic relevance of some factor related to aging in women. We hypothesized that this factor may be vertebral osteoporosis, and a series of three epidemiologic studies designed to test this hypothesis do provide it with some, although limited, support (PRESTON-MARTIN et al. 1995).

Incidence rates in the CBTRUS registries are 12.07 and 10.97 per 100,000 for males and females respectively, and overall rates are lower among blacks than among whites (7.72 and 11.6 per 100,000, respectively) (SURAWICZ et al. 1999). Some of these racial differences vary, however, from one histologic type of brain tumor to another. For example, the rate of neuroepithelial tumors is lower among black males and females than among whites but the reverse is true for meningiomas (Table 1.2).

In general, rates among whites in Canada, the United States, Europe, the United Kingdom, and Australia are relatively similar although rates are lower in certain Eastern European countries and former Soviet republics (Russia, Belarus, Kyrgystan). Rates are lowest in Asian populations in Japan, India, and among the Chinese in Singapore. Rates are also lower in Puerto Rico, Costa Rica, and Brazil. Among each racial group, rates are usually higher in migrant populations than in native populations, which remain in their country of origin. These differences between migrant and native populations suggest that some change in lifestyle may be occurring in migrant populations which places them at higher risk for brain tumors, although an increase in diagnostic efficiency may be an alternate explanation for these differences.

1.2.5
Social Class

Table 1.3 shows the proportional incidence ratios (PIRs) for primary tumors of the brain and cranial meninges by social class (as determined by census tract of residence) for Los Angeles County non-Spanish-surnamed whites. These age-adjusted PIRs represent the ratio of the number of cases observed to that expected in a subgroup; a PIR of 100 indicates that the number observed is the same as the expected number which was calculated for each 5-year age group by assuming that the distribution of brain tumors by social class was the same as that for all other cancer sites combined. There is a clear trend of increasing incidence with increasing social class. For males, this trend is evident for neuroepithelial tumors and nerve sheath tumors. For females, this trend is only clearly evident for nerve sheath tumors. The exception to this is meningiomas, which show the inverse relationship among both males and females. A similar trend of increasing overall brain cancer rates with increasing social class (as determined by occupation) was reported for men in England and Wales a few decades ago (BUELL et al. 1960) and more recently in Washington State

Table 1.2. Average annual age-adjusted incidence rates (per 100,000) by major histologic type of primary brain tumor by sex and ethnic group, Los Angeles County, 1972–1997

	Neuroepithelial	Meningiomas	Nerve sheath tumors	All histologic types	Number
Males					
Black	3.9	2.1	0.4	7.0	679
Spanish surnamed	4.3	1.3	0.4	6.6	1200
Other whites	6.4	1.7	1.0	9.8	5724
Chinese	2.6	0.7	0.3	4.3	85
Japanese	1.7	0.8	0.9	3.6	59
Filipino	2.0	1.6	0.7	4.9	81
Korean	2.4	0.4	0.1	3.2	39
Other races	1.6	1.2	0.7	3.8	111
All races	5.3	1.6	0.8	8.4	7978
Females					
Black	2.6	3.0	0.4	6.7	789
Spanish surnamed	3.4	2.4	0.4	6.7	1295
Other whites	4.3	2.9	1.0	8.9	6180
Chinese	1.5	1.6	0.4	3.9	77
Japanese	1.1	1.4	0.7	3.5	68
Filipino	1.9	1.9	0.6	4.7	100
Korean	1.7	1.1	0.3	3.7	47
Other races	1.5	1.9	0.8	4.3	146
All races	3.6	2.7	0.8	7.8	8702

Table 1.3. Proportional incidence ratios for primary brain tumors by social class and total number of cases, Los Angeles County, 1972–1997, non-Latino whites

SES	Proportional incidence ratios		
	Neuro-epithelial	Meningiomas	Nerve sheath tumors
Males			
1 (high)	104.5	93.5	154.1
2	110.6	96.1	113.2
3	106.9	99.2	87.0
4	103.7	100.4	72.9
5 (low)	68.7	114.5	58.8
Females			
1	92.7	96.4	119.0
2	112.7	87.7	121.7
3	108.8	99.1	90.5
4	106.8	114.7	87.0
5	73.7	106.1	70.3

(DEMERS et al. 1991) and New Zealand (PRESTON-MARTIN et al. 1993a). Because this trend occurs more strikingly among males than among females, it seems unlikely that it might relate to factors such as diagnostic efficiency or exposure to diagnostic radiography of the head (e.g., dental X-rays), both of which might be expected to be greater among those in higher social classes.

1.2.6
Survival

Recent relative 5-year survival rates for brain and nervous system cancer are around 25%(24% for whites and 32% for blacks among United States cases diagnosed from 1981 to 1986) compared to just under 20% 20 years earlier (18% for whites and 19% for blacks diagnosed from 1960 to 1963) (BORING et al. 1991). Survival rates for all tumors vary considerably by location, behavior, histologic type, and age (SURAWICZ et al. 1998). For example, astrocytomas that occur in the cerebrum have a much lower 5-year survival rate than those that occur in the frontal lobe (13.3 versus 28.1, respectively) and for malignant versus nonmalignant tumors (21.6% and 72.4%, respectively) (SURAWICZ et al. 1998). The relative 5-year survival rate in children 0–14 years of age is now 59% compared to 35% 20 years ago (SURAWICZ et al. 1998; CRIST AND KUN 1991), although the health status of survivors often remains poor (FORMAN et

al.1999). Clinically significant improvements in survival rates are not apparent in patients over the age of 65 years (DAVIS 1998).

A study in Victoria, Australia, found that 52% of female compared to 37% of male brain tumor patients are alive 5 years after diagnosis (PRESTON-MARTIN et al. 1993b). As might be expected, nerve sheath tumors, tumors in the "other" category (mostly hemangiomas and gangliogliomas not classified as malignant), and meningiomas, all of which are predominantly benign, have the best prognosis; 100%, 96%, and 92% of patients with tumors of these three types survived 5 years. Patients with glioblastoma multiforme have the poorest prognosis (5% survive 5 years), although aggressive treatment can make long-term survival possible among patients whose performance status is high at diagnosis (SCOTT et al. 1999). The proportion who survive 5 years is also low for patients with unspecified tumors (20%) and those whose tumors were not confirmed microscopically (28%). Survival varies considerably for the other subtypes of neuroepithelial tumors. The proportion who are alive 5 years after diagnosis is considerably greater for patients with ependymoma (65%) and oligodendroglioma (61%) than for those with medulloblastoma (43%) or astrocytoma (44%). For most individual histologic types, survival curves for the two sexes are similar. However, females who develop meningioma are more likely to have benign tumors and survive significantly longer than males with meningiomas (94% versus 87% 5-year survival in women and men).

1.2.7
Summary of Descriptive Epidemiology

Perhaps the most important finding from our review of the descriptive epidemiology of brain tumors is that both the pattern of occurrence and survival vary considerably by histologic type, age, and tumor location. For neuroepithelial tumors: (a) the sex ratio is greater than one; (b) incidence declines after an early peak under 10 years of age and continues to rise again after 25 years of age; (c) rates are higher in whites than non-whites and are lowest in Asians; and (d) incidence increases with increasing social class, particularly in males. For meningiomas: (a) the sex ratio is less than one; (b) the female excess is greatest from ages 25–54; and (d) rates in United States populations are commonly higher in blacks than in whites.

1.3
Suggested Causes
of Human Brain Tumors

1.3.1
Ionizing Radiation

The occurrence of excess brain tumors after high-dose exposure to ionizing radiation is well established. An updated follow-up of the Israeli cohort who received scalp irradiation as a treatment for ringworm showed the relative risk (RR) is greatest for nerve sheath tumors of the head and neck (RR=33.1), intermediate for meningiomas (RR=9.5), and lowest for neuroepithelial tumors (RR=2.6; RON et al. 1988). Case-control studies of meningiomas and nerve sheath tumors in adults have found elevated risks associated with exposure to full-mouth dental X-rays decades ago when doses were relatively high as well as with prior radiation treatment to the head (PRESTON-MARTIN et al. 1980, 1983, 1989a; RYAN et al. 1992b). The association with low-dose exposure is more controversial. Prenatal exposure to diagnostic radiography has been related to excess pediatric brain tumors in several studies since this association was first reported in 1958 (STEWART et al. 1958), including a study of Swedish twins which found abdominal X-rays of the mother during pregnancy were associated with increased CNS tumor incidence. The findings appeared not to be confounded by the mother's age, obstetrical complications, or other factors (RODVALL et al. 1990). Exposure to low levels of ionizing radiation during infancy was associated with an elevated risk of intracranial tumors (SIR 1.42; 1.13, 1.75) in a pooled analysis of two Swedish hemangioma cohorts and was highest among infants exposed before 5 months of age (KARLSSON et al. 1998).

1.3.2
Nonionizing Radiation

1.3.2.1
Electromagnetic Fields

Much controversy in the last 15 years has surrounded the suggestion that exposure to nonionizing electromagnetic radiation, such as power frequency (50–60 Hz) magnetic fields, might contribute to the development of CNS tumors. These fields have not been shown experimentally to be either genotoxic or carcinogenic, but there is some suggestion that they

may act as a tumor promoter (MCCANN et al. 1997). Epidemiologic evidence is puzzlingly inconsistent both in studies of residential exposures and pediatric CNS tumors (TOMENIUS 1986; PRESTON-MARTIN et al. 1996) and in studies of CNS cancer in relation to high levels of job exposure (RODVALL et al. 1996; FLODERUS et al. 1994; SAVITZ et al. 1995; KHEIFETS et al. 1999a). Two recent studies showed no evidence of a link between residential exposure and brain tumors in children (PRESTON-MARTIN et al. 1996; GURNEY et al. 1996), and a recent review article concludes that overall there is little evidence for an association (KHEIFETS et al. 1999b). A comparative analysis of studies of electric utility workers suggests a small increase in brain tumor risk, but notes that findings vary across studies as do exposure measurements (KHEIFETS et al. 1999c). A Swedish study finds a stronger association with brain tumor risk in analyses in which exposure is based on magnetic field measurements rather than job titles or the assessment of an electrical engineer (RODVALL et al. 1998).

1.3.2.2
Radiofrequency Radiation

Studies of the effect of radiofrequency (RF) exposure in humans have included microwave exposures, the use of radar equipment (occupational and handheld), and direct occupational exposures such as RF heaters, sealers and plastic welders, medical exposures, amateur radio operator exposures, and telecommunication worker exposures. While some studies suggest a possible effect of RF on all cancers, brain cancer, or other types of cancers, a recent review found that relative risks are small, not statistically significant, and inconsistent across studies (BLETTNER and SCHLEHOFER 1999). An association with cellular telephone usage and the development of brain tumors has been raised in the legal arena. The rapid increase in the use of cellular telephones combined with their direct exposure to selected regions of the brain have stimulated ongoing epidemiologic studies.

1.3.3
Occupational Exposures

Numerous epidemiologic studies have investigated the variation in brain tumor occurrence as it relates to employment, which have been summarized previously (THOMAS and WAXWEILER 1986). Repeated studies in various geographic areas have been completed for only a few groups of workers, including those employed in agricultural (VIEL 1998; PRESTON-MARTIN et al. 1993a; DALY et al. 1994 KHUDER et al. 1998) or health professions (McLAUGHLIN et al. 1987a; PRESTON-MARTIN, 1989c), and for rubber (SORAHAN et al. 1989), petrochemical (TETA et al. 1991; MARSH et al. 1991), and electrical (FLODERUS et al. 1994; SAVITZ and LOOMIS 1995) workers. A recent meta-analysis of 33 studies of brain cancer and farming found an increased risk of 1.25 among farmers in the central United States (KHUDER et al. 1998). For the most part, however, various studies of each occupational group have shown conflicting findings and no specific chemical or other exposure has been implicated. Even when a particular chemical exposure was investigated, results have been inconclusive as in studies of job exposure to vinyl chloride which were prompted by experimental findings (WONG et al. 1991; SIMONATO et al. 1991).

Similarly, several studies have investigated possible associations between occupational exposures of parents and the development of brain tumors in their children, but many associations have been suggested by only one study. Multiple studies have suggested an increase in pediatric brain tumor risk among children with a parent employed in paint-related, aircraft, electricity-related, agricultural, metal, and construction industries, although these studies too have failed to implicate any particular exposure (SAVITZ and CHEN 1990).

The marked inconsistency of these occupational studies may be partially attributed to the often small sample sizes (leading to imprecise risk estimates); the different geographic areas (with different major industries) studied; and the variation across studies in tumor types, ages at diagnosis, years of diagnosis, and presumed latent period from exposure to tumor diagnosis. The exposure periods of interest also vary, and thus for many industries in which procedures changed over time, the exposures vary as well. Variation also relates to the sources of data about, and the criteria used for classifying, occupations and nervous system tumors. All studies are limited by the fact that occupation acts as a surrogate for often unidentified specific environmental agents, the true exposures of interest.

1.3.4
Pesticides

Several epidemiologic studies have investigated home and occupational use of pesticides, insecticides, or

herbicides as possible etiologic factors for brain tumors, which have been reviewed (DANIELS 1997; ZAHM 1998). Excess risk of brain cancer was found in a study of licensed pesticide applicators (SMR=200; BLAIR et al. 1983) and occupational exposure to pesticides (RR=1.8; 95%CI 0.6–5.1) (RODVALL 1996). Some case-control studies have linked household use or pest exterminations to the development of childhood brain tumors (DAVIS et al. 1993), but few associations were seen in a recent study of pesticide exposure during gestation and childhood and pediatric brain tumors (POGODA and PRESTON-MARTIN 1998). Associations of CNS tumors with either household or occupational exposures to pesticides are not well established and require confirmation.

1.3.5
Nitroso Compounds

Although various chemical, physical, and biological agents can cause nervous system tumors in experimental animals, N-nitroso compounds (NOC), in particular the nitrosoureas, are by far the most effective and the most studied (LIJINSKY 1992). These carcinogens show a striking nervous system selectivity in some species including various primates, and tumors can be produced by relatively low levels of NOC precursors in the animals' food and drinking water. If exposure is transplacental, only 1/50 of the dose of ENU required in adult animals is sufficient to cause 100% tumor induction (IVANKOVIC 1979), however, no tumors develop if ascorbate (vitamin C) is also added to the pregnant dam's diet (MIRVISH 1981). Because there is no reason to think that man is less susceptible to these compounds, it is likely that NOC cause cancer in humans as well. Although NOC exposures in some occupational settings (e.g., machine shops, tire and rubber factories) can be substantial, most people have low level, but virtually continuous, exposure to NOC throughout life. But, because NOC are the most potent of carcinogens in animals (and likely in humans as well) only small doses are needed to cause cancer.

1.3.5.1
Population Exposure to NOC

Human exposure to NOC is estimated to derive half from exogenously and half from endogenously formed compounds (NATIONAL RESEARCH COUNCIL 1981). Only levels of nitrosamines (not nitrosamides) have been widely measured in human environments and consumer products, even though many of these exposures probably involve both nitrosamines and nitrosamides. Endogenous formation in the stomach or bladder when both an amino compound and a nitrosating agent are present simultaneously is likely to be the primary source of human exposure to nitrosamides. Food is a primary source of both highly concentrated nitrite solutions (e.g., from cured meats) and amino compounds (e.g., in fish and other foods, but also in many drugs). Another source of nitrite is reduction (e.g., in the saliva) from nitrate which comes predominantly from vegetables in the diet. This source is likely to be a far less important contributor to the NOC formed endogenously because it is highly diluted (and, therefore, less readily reactive) and because vegetables also contain vitamins which inhibit the nitrosation reaction. Drinking water also contains nitrate (in the absence of vitamins), but this is a minor source unless levels are extraordinarily high (CHILVERS et al. 1984). The level of NOC in the human body is also influenced by other factors such as which amino compounds are present, presence of nitrosation inhibitors (e.g., vitamins C or E), presence of bacteria or other nitrosation catalysts, gastric pH, and other physiologic factors. Uncertainty as to the simultaneous presence of NOC precursors and of inhibitors and/or catalysts of nitrosation make this hypothesis difficult to study epidemiologically. This difficulty is compounded by further uncertainty about which exposure period (during a person's life) is most likely to be etiologically relevant.

1.3.5.2
Epidemiologic Evidence

Epidemiologic studies of pediatric (PRESTON-MARTIN 1996; BUNIN 1994; PRESTON-MARTIN et al. 1982a; BUNIN et al. 1993) and adult (LEE 1997; BLOWERS 1997; GILES 1994; PRESTON-MARTIN and MACK 1991; BOEING et al. 1993) brain tumor patients have provided limited support for the hypothesis that NOC exposure is related to the development of CNS tumors. Findings that use of vitamin supplements and/or high intake of fresh fruit or vegetables protect against brain tumor development might also be interpreted as supportive of the *N*-nitroso hypothesis, although this effect may be due to another mechanism (BUNIN et al. 1994). The experimental model and its potential relevance to humans are sufficiently compelling to encourage further investigation of this hypothesis despite the fact that it is a difficult one to test epidemiologically. Future studies must include

more complete dietary histories if they hope to differentiate between findings supportive of the NOC/brain tumor hypothesis and those suggestive of other mechanisms for dietary effects.

1.3.6
Other Dietary Factors

The majority of dietary investigations among CNS tumor patients have only collected data on dietary sources of NOC exposures, rather than complete dietary histories. Nonetheless, these studies have attempted to evaluate the association between certain dietary micronutrients and brain tumor risk; adequate evaluation of micronutrient intake will require investigation of complete dietary histories. Use of vitamin supplements, particularly vitamins C, E, and multivitamins, has been found to reduce brain tumor risk in adults in some studies (PRESTON-MARTIN and MACK 1991), but not others (RYAN et al. 1992a; BOEING et al. 1993). In children, risk may be reduced by their personal vitamin use (CORDIER 1994; MCCREDIE et al. 1994b), by their mother's vitamin use during pregnancy (PRESTON-MARTIN et al. 1982b, 1998; BUNIN et al. 1993), or by her intake of fruit, fruit juice, and vegetables (BUNIN et al. 1993, 1994; MCCREDIE et al. 1994b).

Although the findings of reduced risk of brain tumors in children and adults associated with increased intake of vitamin supplements, fruits, and vegetables may be related to the *N*-nitroso hypothesis by inhibiting endogenous formation of nitrosamines, it is important to consider other potential mechanisms of effect. In this respect, it is interesting that a study of childhood brain tumors reported higher relative risks associated with the child's consumption of cured meats when the child did not take multivitamins than when they did take multivitamins (SARASUA and SAVITZ 1994).

Recent studies have investigated the possible associations of brain tumors with other dietary micronutrients (BUNIN et al. 1993, 1994). In particular, a case-control study of childhood PNET found significant protective trends with increasing levels of dietary vitamins A and C, betacarotene, and folate by the mother during pregnancy (BUNIN et al. 1993). In a related study of childhood astrocytoma, reduced risks were evident for dietary vitamins A and C, however, these trends were not significant (BUNIN et al. 1994). There was no relationship of childhood astrocytoma to dietary betacarotene or folate. Although these preliminary results suggest exciting prospects for the possible prevention of childhood brain tumors, interpretation is difficult because both studies were primarily focused on the evaluation of dietary NOCs. Thus, evaluation of other micronutrients was limited to the micronutrient composition of NOC-related food items. These results highlight the need to incorporate complete dietary evaluations in future epidemiologic studies.

Two recent studies suggest an association of brain cancer with household drinking water. A study in England found an elevated risk in geographic areas with the highest levels of nitrate in the water compared to areas with the lowest levels, which were more than ten times lower (BARRETT et al. 1998). A study in Iowa found an increase in risk related to level of intake of chlorinated water and average levels of trihalomethanes, with a stronger association among men who drank an above average amount of tap water (CANTOR et al. 1999). Caution is urged in the interpretation of such studies, however, because of assumptions made in exposure assessment.

1.3.7
Prior Head Trauma, Infection, or Other Medical Conditions

1.3.7.1
Head Trauma

The epidemiologic evidence associating head trauma and brain tumors is strongest for meningiomas. Numerous case reports present convincing circumstantial evidence, and case-control studies have found an excess risk of meningiomas in women with histories of head trauma treated medically, in men who boxed as a sport, and in men with histories of serious head injuries (PRESTON-MARTIN et al. 1980, 1983, 1989a, 1998). Limited experimental evidence suggests that trauma may act as a co-carcinogen in the induction of neuroepithelial tumors as well as meningiomas (MORANTZ and SHAIN 1978). Childhood brain tumors, which are predominantly neuroepithelial tumors, have sometimes been associated with birth trauma (prolonged labor, forceps delivery, cesarean section; PRESTON-MARTIN et al. 1982b; MC-CREDIE et al. 1994b; GURNEY et al. 1996). Because trauma is often regarded by laypersons as related to tumor development, an attempt must be made to limit reporting of trauma to injuries of a certain minimum severity (such as those requiring medical attention or hospitalization) and thereby limit recall bias.

1.3.7.2
Acoustic Trauma and Acoustic Neuromas

The observation that over 90% of all nerve sheath tumors arise in the eighth cranial nerve (the acoustic nerve) suggests an exposure unique to this nerve. A case-control study of acoustic neuromas in Los Angeles County residents supports the hypothesis that acoustic trauma may relate to the development of these tumors (PRESTON-MARTIN et al. 1990). A dose-response analysis showed an increase in risk related to number of years of job exposure to extremely loud noise (P for trend=0.02) with an OR of 13.2 (CI=2.01, 86.98) for exposure of 20 or more years accumulated up to 10 years before diagnosis. These findings may support the more general hypothesis that mechanical trauma may contribute to tumorigenesis (PRESTON-MARTIN et al. 1990).

1.3.7.3
Viruses and Infectious Agents

Astrocytomas, but not other histologic types of brain tumors, were previously associated with positive antibody titers to *Toxoplasma gondii,* but a recent study failed to confirm this (RYAN et al. 1993). There are numerous reports of the isolation of viruses or virus-like particles from human cerebral tumors or tumor cell lines in the literature, but whether these findings may have etiologic implications is uncertain (CORALLINI et al. 1987). In general, excess brain tumors have not been found among those who received polio vaccines contaminated with SV40 and those whose mothers had influenza or various other infections while they were in utero (PRESTON-MARTIN and MACK 1996), although a recent study found an elevated risk of neuroblastoma and other pediatric nervous system tumors among children whose mothers had influenza during pregnancy (LINOS et al. 1998). Reanalyses of those exposed to SV40-contaminated vaccines have had conflicting findings (STRICKLER et al. 1998; FISHER et al. 1999). Recently, a reduced risk was reported between patients with neuroepithelial tumors and chicken pox, shingles, and the associated immunoglobulin G antibodies to varicella-zoster virus, a novel finding requiring replication (WRESCSH et al. 1997).

1.3.7.4
Chronic Diseases

Brain tumors have been associated with various chronic diseases, but none of these associations has been investigated in more than one or two studies. Neuroepithelial tumors, but not meningiomas, occur much less frequently in diabetics (SCHLEHOFER et al. 1992), who have a lower frequency of all cancers at autopsy (HERDAN 1960). Excesses of brain tumors reported in various cohorts of epileptics most likely occur because seizures are a common early brain tumor symptom (OLSEN et al. 1989), and studies have found no increase in risk related to in utero or childhood exposure to barbiturates after a history of epilepsy was considered (GOLDHABER et al. 1990). Serum cholesterol has been positively related to brain cancer in some, but not all, studies (KNECT et al. 1991), however, because none has evaluated dietary intake, the possibility that an existing brain tumor might cause a spurious rise in serum cholesterol has not been excluded. A deficit of allergic conditions has been found in case-control studies of neuroepithelial tumors alone (RYAN et al. 1992a) and of all brain tumors (SCHLEHOFER et al. 1992, 1999).

Clinicians should be aware that an association between meningiomas and breast cancer has been observed (HELSETH et al. 1989a) so that they will not assume that CNS lesions which are discovered after breast cancer diagnosis and treatment are necessarily metastatic. Tissues from meningiomas have been shown to contain hormone receptors but it is unclear whether or not this finding has etiologic implications (HALPER et al. 1989).

1.3.8
Predisposing Genetic Syndromes and Familial Occurrence

Some central nervous system tumors have a relatively clear genetic character, particularly those which occur in association with neurofibromatosis and other phakomatoses that often display an autosomal dominant pattern of inheritance with varying degrees of penetrance. The occurrence of multiple primary brain tumors of either similar or different histologic types are associated with the phakomatoses, but also occur in the absence of such syndromes (DEEN and LAWS 1981).

Data from registries of families with multiple members diagnosed with primary brain tumors are hard to evaluate in that they are not population-based (GROSSMAN et al. 1999). There are few population-based studies of familial aggregation of CNS tumors. One study found that Connecticut children with CNS tumors more often had relatives with nervous system tumors than did control children, but

this familial occurrence, although statistically significant, was observed for fewer than 2% of the children with CNS tumors (FARWELL and FLANNERY 1984). Medulloblastoma and glioblastoma were over represented among children whose relatives had nervous system tumors (FARWELL and FLANNERY 1984). What needs to be kept in mind is that population-based studies that have investigated associations of brain tumors with recognized predisposing genetic syndromes and/or with familial aggregations suggest that the proportion of brain tumors attributable to inheritance is no more than 4% (BONDY et al. 1991; WRENSCH et al. 1990).

1.3.9
Other Suggested Risk Factors

A number of other factors have been suggested as related to brain tumor risk including barbiturates and other drugs, alcohol, tobacco smoke, and reproductive and hormonal factors (PRESTON-MARTIN and MACK 1996). For the most part, these possible associations have not been studied often or very thoroughly. The few brain tumor studies that have investigated some factors (e.g., alcohol, tobacco) have had conflicting findings. The best one can do in attempting to evaluate their etiologic relevance is to keep them in mind and hope that future brain tumor studies will also investigate possible associations with these factors.

1.4
Pathogenesis of Nervous System Tumors

Various physical, infectious, and chemical agents appear to relate to the development of cancer because they increase cell proliferation (PRESTON-MARTIN et al. 1990); for example, this may explain why acoustic trauma can lead to the development of acoustic neuromas (PRESTON-MARTIN et al. 1989b). Replication may perpetuate a DNA mutation before it can be corrected in the cell in which it arises. Apparently, various genetic pathways can be involved in the pathogenesis of CNS tumors, and this may be true even for tumors of the same phenotype. Although many of the inherited syndromes that predispose to CNS tumors were described decades ago, the chromosomal locus of the affected gene has now been identified for most. In the past decade, hundreds of investigators have described molecular events that they have observed in tumor tissue from patients with various types of CNS tumors. A few of the most common of these mutations are summarized below.

1.4.1
Molecular Genetic Characteristics

Studies of the molecular biology and cytogenetics of CNS tumors suggest that specific types of tumors have characteristic genetic abnormalities which are summarized in review papers (BLACK 1991a,b; LEON et al. 1994; BEIGEL 1999). Such characterization contributes importantly to our understanding of the pathogenesis of CNS tumors. Glioblastomas, for example, commonly show losses of chromosome 9p, 10 or 17p; gains of chromosome 7; and p53 mutations. Loss of alleles at 17p appear to be the earliest abnormalities that occur in the genesis of these tumors. Most of these tumors express the c-*sis* oncogene, and some express other oncogenes as well. Related characteristics include the synthesis and secretion of growth factors which influence mitotic activity (JENNINGS et al. 1991).

Various CNS tumors, but in particular those of astrocytic origin, have been associated with loss or mutation of the p53 gene located on the short arm of chromosome 17 (KLEIHUES et al. 1994). p53 is a tumor suppressor gene, and mutations in this gene appear to play a role in the development of a number of human cancers (NIGRO et al. 1989). p53 mutations have been observed in glioblastoma multiforme as noted above (NIGRO et al. 1989), in neurofibrosarcoma occurring in association with neurofibromatosis 1 (NIGRO et al. 1989; MENON et al. 1990), and in patients with Li-Fraumeni syndrome (MALKIN et al. 1990). Li-Fraumeni syndrome is a rare autosomal dominant genetic syndrome that predisposes those affected to cancers of the brain and other sites (GARBER et al. 1990). This predisposition may relate to germ cell mutations in the tumor suppressor gene p53 (MALKIN et al. 1990). Because benign tumors from patients with neurofibromatosis 1 appear not to have p53 mutations, it is thought that inactivation of this gene may be associated with the malignant transformation of these tumors (MENON et al. 1990).

Other tumor types show distinct pathophysiologic features, for example, loss of regions on chromosome 22 is the characteristic feature of meningiomas. Also, pediatric CNS tumors show different genetic patterns from adult tumors (GRIFFIN et al. 1988; CRIST AND KUN 1991; BIEGEL 1999). For example, as-

trocytomas (WHO grade II–IV) of children and young adults may demonstrate loss of heterozygosity for chromosome 17p and/or mutations in p53 (LOUIS 1994; GRIFFIN 1988; LOUIS 1993; LANG 1994), while astrocytomas of older adults often have mutations in chromosome 10, amplification of the epidermal growth factor receptor (EGFR), and no mutations in p53 (LOUIS et al. 1993; LOUIS 1994). Characterization of the various types is still in progress and the etiologic, prognostic, and other implications of specific characteristics remain to be defined. It is anticipated that molecular markers may help reduce the known misclassification in the diagnosis of some tumor subtypes.

1.4.2
Possible Interactions of Genetic and Environmental Factors

For a number of other reasons, epidemiologic studies of the hypothesis that nitrosamide exposures relate to brain tumors are very difficult. For this reason, it is appealing to be able to rely on some biomarker of exposure. Unfortunately, finding a biomarker of *N*-nitroso exposure for use in brain tumor patients or their mothers when the relevant exposures occurred years earlier has not proved easy. Adduct formation by *N*-nitrosoureas in vivo is beginning to be studied, but the extent of damage induced in various tissues does not seem to correlate well with tumorigenicity (Eisenbrand et al. 1994). What seems more promising is to identify a genetic polymorphism (one that could easily be assayed in epidemiologic studies) for an enzyme or other system that regulates *N'*-nitroso metabolism or detoxification or the repair of the molecular damage caused by nitroso compounds. One interesting candidate might be alkyltransferase, an enzyme involved in the repair of O^6-alkylguanine which is formed and persists in brain DNA after exposure to alkylating agents such as the nitrosoureas (Pegg 1990). Study of genetic polymorphisms of human O^6-alkylguanine DNA alkyltransferase (AGT) may prove helpful in defining susceptibility to the development of nervous system tumors (Deng et al. 1999). Nitrosoureas produce different types of nervous system tumors in different species; identifying those histologic types in humans will also make future studies of nitrosamide exposures more efficient.

Many of the problems confronted by epidemiologic studies of brain tumors and nitrosamides also apply to studies of other suspected brain carcinogens such as several investigated in occupational studies. Although a number of industries have long been noted to have an apparent excess of brain tumors among workers, it has proved difficult to implicate specific exposures (DELZELL et al, 1999). Simultaneous evaluation both of exposures to specific chemicals and of individual susceptibility to insult from those chemical may be the direction of the future.

1.5
Prospects

We simply have no idea what causes most nervous system tumors. Certain inherited syndromes can predispose individuals to the development of brain and other nervous system tumors. However, at most, only a small percentage of patients with nervous system tumors have one of these rare phakomatoses or a family member with a nervous system tumor. Studies of such patients and their families have described genetic events that are correlates of nervous system tumor pathogenesis, but the etiologic implications of these findings are unclear.

Ionizing radiation, the only well-established environmental risk factor for nervous system tumors, can cause all three major histologic types of brain tumors – neuroepithelial tumors, meningiomas, and nerve sheath tumors – but only a small percentage of incident CNS tumors are likely to relate to such exposure, and the association appears weakest for gliomas. Nonetheless, minimizing population exposure to X-rays of the head is, at this point, the best prospect for prevention of all three types of tumors. Beyond this, the etiology of neuroepithelial tumors remains largely unknown. More is known about the etiology of meningiomas and nerve sheath tumors. Ionizing radiation and trauma appear to be important risk factors for both.

Because nitrosamides, especially the nitrosoureas, are the most potent nervous system carcinogens used experimentally, it seems likely that these compounds may also cause nervous system tumors in humans. To date, most epidemiologic investigations of a possible association of brain tumors with N-nitroso exposures have focused on the other major group of these compounds, nitrosamines. Nitrosamines are easier to study because reliable assays exist for nitrosamines, unlike nitrosamides, and monitoring of human environments and consumer products for levels of nitrosamines has been done. But, nitrosamines have not caused nervous system

tumors in any of the many experimental species tested. Field and laboratory investigations of potential environmental sources of human exposure to nitrosamides and of their precursors, such as alkylamides, are needed.

Incorporating assays of relevant genetic polymorphism, such as AGT, into epidemiologic studies of nervous system tumors is one potentially promising new direction. Diet will be an important focus of the next generation of epidemiologic investigations on neuroepithelial tumors. Studies to date have included some questions about a limited number of dietary variables, such as those that looked at foods thought likely to be relevant to the N-nitroso hypothesis. A number of intriguing associations are emerging from these and other studies including the suggestion that intake of cured meats, fruit, and vitamin supplements all relate to neuroepithelial tumor risk, with fruit and vitamins being protective. Future studies must include relatively complete dietary surveys in order to evaluate adequately associations with various micronutrients, cholesterol, nitrite from cured meats, and other suggested associations.

Are there additional etiologic clues to be gleaned from the descriptive epidemiology of brain tumors? The increase in incidence and mortality rates in recent decades was initially thought by some to suggest the effect of an environmental exposure, but on further consideration appears to be largely an artifact of improved diagnosis. Compared to other cancer sites, brain tumor rates show relatively little international variation. This suggests that either the relevant environmental exposures are ubiquitous or that endogenous factors are important. The gender differences in distribution by histologic type of brain tumor, namely the male predominance of neuroepithelial tumors and the female predominance of meningioma, have long been noted and although evidence suggesting the importance of hormonal factors is weak, any compelling hypotheses related to this difference would be worth investigating. Most brain tumors in children are neuroepithelial tumors, and some types such as PNET occur predominantly in children under 5 years of age. The observation that PNET rates, unlike rates of other pediatric brain tumors which are similar in the two genders, are up to two times higher in boys than in girls also remains unexplained. For neuroepithelial tumors as a major group as well as for specific glioma subtypes, it seems possible that some of the crucial etiologic questions have not yet been posed.

The etiology of the majority of nervous system tumors remains unexplained. Genetic predisposition, ionizing radiation, and the other suggested risk factors each seem to account for only a small proportion of total cases. It may be that there are numerous nervous system carcinogens, as there are known animal neurocarcinogens which have not been fully evaluated in human studies, each with low attributable risk. Our continued investigation of suspected brain carcinogens needs to identify and focus on histology-specific associations and use improved methods of exposure assessment. In addition, we need to simultaneously consider host factors, in particular detectable polymorphisms that influence susceptibility.

References

Annegers JF, Schoenberg BS, Okazaki H, et al. (1981) Epidemiologic study of primary intracranial neoplasms. Arch Neurol 38:217–219

Barrett JH, Parslow RC, McKinney PA, et al. (1998) Nitrate in drinking water and the incidence of gastric, esophageal, and brain cancer in Yorkshire, England. Cancer Causes and Control 9(2):153–159

Biegel JA (1999) Cytogenetics and molecular genetics of childhood brain tumors. Neuro-Oncology 1:139–151

Black WC (1998) Increasing incidence of childhood primary malignant brain tumors – enigma or no-brainer? J Natl Cancer Inst 90(17):1269–1277

Black PM (1991a) Brain tumors (Part 1). N Engl J Med 324:1471–1476

Black PM (1991b) Brain tumors (Part 2). N Engl J Med 324:1555–1564

Blair A, Grauman DJ, Lubin JH, et al. (1983) Lung cancer and other causes of death among licensed pesticide applicators. JNCI 71:31–37

Blettner M, Schlehofer B (1999) [Is there an increased risk of leukemia, brain tumors or breast cancer after exposure to high-frequency radiation? Review of methods and results of epidemiologic studies]. [Review] [41 refs] [German] Medizinische Klinik. 94(3):150–8

Blowers L, Preston-Martin S, Mack WJ (1997) Dietary and other lifestyle factors of women with brain gliomas in Los Angeles County. Cancer Causes Control 8(1):5–12

Boeing H, Schlehofer B, Blettner M, et al. (1993) Dietary carcinogens and the risk for glioma and meningioma in Germany. Int J Cancer 53:561–565

Bondy ML, Lustbader ED, Buffler PA, et al. (1991) Genetic epidemiology of childhood brain tumors. Genet Epidemiol 8:253–267

Boring CC, Squires TS, Tong T (1991) Cancer statistics, 1991. Ca-A Cancer J Clin 41:19–36

Bunin G (1987) Racial patterns of childhood brain cancer by histologic type. JNCI 78:875–880

Bunin GR, Kuitjen RR, Boesel CP, et al. (1994) Maternal diet and risk of astrocytic glioma in children: a report from the Childrens Cancer Group (United States and Canada). Cancer Causes Control 5:177–187

Bunin GR, Kuitjen RR, Rorke LB, et al. (1993) Evidence for a role of maternal diet in the etiology of primitive neuroectodermal tumor of brain in young children. N Engl J Med 329:536–541

Cantor KP, Lynch CF, Hildesheim ME, et al. (1999) Drinking water source and chlorination byproducts in Iowa. III. Risk of brain cancer. Am J Epidemiology 150(6):552–560

CBTRUS (1998) 1997 Annual Report. Published by the Central Brain Tumor Registry of the United States

Chilvers C, Inskip H, Caygill C, et al. (1984) A survey of dietary nitrate in well-water users. Int J Epidemiol 13:324–331

Corallini A, Pagnani M, Viadana P, et al. (1987) Association of BK virus with human brain tumors and tumors of pancreatic islets. Int J Cancer 39:60–67

Cordier S, Iglesias MJ, Le Goaster C, et al. (1994) Incidence and risk factors for childhood brain tumors in the Ile de France. Int J Cancer 59(6):776–782

Crist WM, Kun LE (1991) Common solid tumors of childhood. N Engl J Med 324:461–471

Cruz BL (1958) Medulloblastoma. Springfield, Charles C. Thomas

Daly L, Herity B, Bourke GJ (1994) An investigation of brain tumours and other malignancies in an agricultural research institute. Occup Environ Med 51:295–298

Daniels JL, Olshan AF, Savitz DA (1997) Pesticides and childhood cancer. Environ Health Perspect 105(10):1068–1077

Davis JR, Brownson RC, Garcia R, et al. (1993) Family pesticide use and childhood brain cancer. Arch Environ Contam Toxicol 24:87–92

Davis FG, McCarthy BJ, Freels S, et al. (1999) The conditional probability of survival of patients with primary malignant brain tumors Surveillance, Epidemiology, and End Results (SEER) data. Cancer 85(2):485–491

Davis FG, Freels S, Grutsch J, et al. (1998) Survival rates in patients with primary malignant brain tumors stratified by patient age and tumor histological type: an analysis based on Surveillance, Epidemiology, and End Results (SEER) data, 1973–1991. J Neurosurg 88:1–10

Davis FG, Malinski N, Haenszel W, et al. (1996) Primary brain tumor incidence rates in four United States regions, 1985–1989: a pilot study. Neuroepidemiology 15:103–112

Deen HG, Laws ER (1981) Multiple primary brain tumors of different cell types. Neurosurgery 8:20–25

Delzell E, Beall C, Rodu B, et al. (1999) Case-series investigation of intracranial neoplasms at a petrochemical research facility. Am J Indust Med 36:450–458

Demers PA, Vaughan TL, Schommer RR (1991) Occupation, socioeconomic status, and brain tumor mortality: a death certificate-based case-control study. J Occup Med 33:1001–1006

Deng C, Xie D, Capasso H, et al. (1999) Genitic polymorphism of human 0^6-alkylguanine-DNA alkyltransferase: identification of a missense variation in the active site region. Pharmacogenetics 9:81–87

Desmeules M, Mikkelsen T, Mao Y (1992) Increasing incidence of primary brain tumors: influence of diagnostic methods. JNCI 84:442–445

Eisenbrand G, Pfeiffer C, Tang W (1994) DNA adducts of N-nitrosoureas. In: Hemminki K, Dipple A, Shuker DEG, et al. (eds) DNA adducts: Identification and biological significance. IARC Scientific Publications, No. 125, Lyon, IARC, pp 277–293

Farwell J, Flannery JT (1984) Cancer in relatives of children with central-nervous-system neoplasms. N Engl J Med 311:749–753

Fisher SG, Weber L, Carbone M (1999) Cancer risk associated with simian virus 40 contaminated polio vaccine. Anticancer Research 19:2173–2180

Floderus B, Tornquist S, Stenlund C (1994) Incidence of selected cancers in Swedish railway workers, 1961–79. Cancer Causes Control 5:189–194

Foreman NK, Faestel PM, Pearson J, et al. (1999) Health status in 52 long-term survivors of pediatric brain tumors. J Neuro-Oncology 41(1):47–53

Garber JE, Dreyfus MG, Kantor AF, et al. (1990) Cancer occurrence on follow-up of 24 kindreds with the Li-Fraumeni syndrome (Abstract). Proc Am Assoc Cancer Res 31:210

Giles GG, McNeil JJ, Donnan G, et al. (1994) Dietary factors and the risk of glioma in adults: results of a case-control study in Melbourne, Australia. Int J Cancer 59:357–362

Goldhaber MK, Selby JV, Hiatt RA, et al. (1990) Exposure to barbiturates in utero and during childhood and risk of intracranial and spinal cord tumors. Cancer Res 50:4600–4603

Greig NH, Ries LG, Yancik R, et al. (1990) Increasing annual incidence of primary malignant brain tumors in the elderly. JNCI 82:1621–1624

Griffin CA, Hawkins AL, Packer RJ, et al. (1988) Chromosome abnormalities in pediatric brain tumors. Cancer Res 48:175–180

Grossman SA, Osman M, Hruban R, et al. (1999) Central nervous system cancers in first-degree relatives and spouses. Cancer Invest 17(5):299–308

Gurney JG, Schwartz SM, Davis S, et al. (1996) Reply to "Evolution of epidemiologic evidence on magnetic fields and childhood cancers." Am J Epid 143(2):137–143

Hagmar L, Akesson B, Nielsen J, et al. (1990) Mortality and cancer morbidity in workers exposed to low levels of vinyl chloride monomer at a polyvinyl chloride processing plant. Am J Indust Med 17:553–565

Halper J, Colvard DS, Scheithauer BW, et al. (1989) Estrogen and progesterone receptors in meningiomas: comparison of nuclear binding, dextran-coated charcoal, and immunoperoxidase staining assays. Neurosurgery 25:546–553

Helseth A, Mork SJ, Glattre E (1989a) Neoplasms of the central nervous system in Norway. V. Meningioma and cancer of other sites. An analysis of the occurrence of multiple primary neoplasms in meningioma patients in Norway from 1955 through 1986. APMIS 97:738–744

Helseth A, Mork SJ, Johansen A, et al. (1989b) Neoplasms of the central nervous system in Norway. A population-based epidemiological study of meningiomas. APMIS 97:646–654

Herdan G (1960) Frequency of cancer in diabetes mellitus. Br J Cancer 14:449–456

Jennings MT, Maciunas RJ, Carver R, et al. (1991) TGFb1 and TGFb2 are potential growth regulators for low-grade and malignant gliomas in vitro: evidence of an autocrine hypothesis. Int J Cancer 49:129–139

Karlsson P, Holmberg E, Lundell M, et al. (1998) Intracranial tumors after exposure to ionizing radiation during infancy: a pooled analysis of two Swedish cohorts of 28,008 infants with skin hemangioma. Radiat Res 150(3):357–364

Kheifets LI, Gilbert ES, Sussman SS, et al. (1999) Comparative analyses of the studies of magnetic fields and cancer in electric utility workers: studies from France, Canada, and the United States. Occup Environ Med 56:567–574

Kleihues P, Ohgaki H, Eibl RH, et al. (1994) Type and frequency of p53 mutations in tumors of the nervous system and its coverings. Recent Results Cancer Res 135:25–31

Khuder SA, Mutgi AB, Schaub EA (1998) Meta-analyses of brain cancer and farming. Am J Indust Med 34:252–260

Knekt P, Reunanen A, Teppo L (1991) Serum cholesterol concentration and risk of primary brain tumours. Br Med J 302: 90

Landis SH, Murray T, Bolden S, et al. (1999) Cancer Statistics, 1999. CA-A cancer journal for clinicians 49(1):8–31

Lange FF, Miller DC, Pisharody S, et al. (1994) High frequency of p53 protein accumulation without p53 gene mutation in human juvenile pilocytic, low grade and anaplastic astrocytomas. Oncogene 9:949–954

Lee M, Wrensch M, Miike R (1997) Dietary and tobacco risk factors for adult onset glioma in the San Francisco Bay Area. Cancer Causes Control 8(1):13–24

Legler JM, Gloeckler Ries LA, Smith MA, et al. (1999) Brain and other central nervous system cancers: Recent trends in incidence and mortality. J Nat Cancer Inst 91(16):1382–90

Leon SP, Zhu J, Black PM (1994) Genetic aberrations in human brain tumors. Neurosurgery 34:708–722

Lijinsky W (1992) Chemistry and Biology of N-Nitroso Compounds. Cambridge University Press

Linos A, Kardara M, Kosmidis H, et al. (1998) Reported influenza in pregnancy and childhood tumour. Euro J Epid 14:471–475

Louis DN (1994) The p53 gene and protein in human brain tumors. J Neuropathol Exp Neurol 53(1):11–21

Louis DN, Rubio MP, Correa KM, et al. (1993) Molecular genetics of pediatric brain stem gliomas. Application of PCR techniques to small and archival brain tumor specimens. J Neuropathol Exp Neurol 52(5):507–515

Malkin D, Li FP, Strong LC, et al. (1990) Germ line p53 mutations in a familial syndrome of breast cancer, sarcomas and other neoplasms. Science 250:1233–1238

Marsh GM, Enterline PE, McCraw D (1991) Mortality patterns among petroleum refinery and chemical plant workers. Am J Indus Med 19:29–42

McCann J, Kavet R, Rafferty CN (1997) Testing electromagnetic fields for potential carcinogenic activity: A critical review of animal models. Environ Health Perspect 105(Suppl 1):81–103

McCredie M, Maisonneuve P, Boyle P (1994b) Perinatal and early postnatal risk factors for malignant brain tumours in New South Wales children. Int J Cancer 56:11–15

McLaughlin JK, Malker HSR, Blot W, et al. (1987a) Occupational risks for intracranial gliomas in Sweden. JNCI 78:253–257

Menon AG, Anderson KM, Riccardi VM, et al. (1990) Chromosome 17p deletions and p53 gene mutations associated with the formation of malignant neurofibrosarcomas in von Recklinghausen neurofibromatosis. Proc Natl Acad Sci USA 87:5435–5439

Mirvish SS (1981) Inhibition of the formation of carcinogenic N-nitroso compounds by ascorbic acid and other compounds. In: Burchenal JH, et al. (eds). Cancer: achievements, challenges and prospects for the 1980's. New York, Grune & Stratton

Modan B, Wagener DK, Feldman JJ, et al. (1992) Increased mortality from brain tumors: a combined outcome of diagnostic technology and change of attitude toward the elderly. Am J Epidemiol 135:1349–1357

Morantz RA, Shain W (1978) Trauma and brain tumors: an experimental study. Neurosurgery 3:181–186

National Research Council (1981) Committee on Diet Nutrition and Cancer Diet Nutrition and Cancer. Washington, D.C., National Academy Press

Nigro JM, Baker SJ, Preisinger AC, et al. (1989) Mutations in the p53 gene occur in diverse tumor types. Nature 342:705–708

Olsen JH, Boice JD Jr, Jensen JPA, et al. (1989) Cancer among epileptic patients exposed to anticonvulsant drugs. JNCI 81:803–808

Parkin DM, Muir CS, Whelan SL, et al. (1992) Cancer Incidence in Five Continents, Volume VI. IARC Scientific Publications, No. 120, Lyon, IARC

Pegg AE (1990) Mammalian 0^6-Alkylguanine-DNA Alkyltransferase: Regulation and importance in response to alkylating carcinogenic and therapeutic agents. Cancer Res 50:6119–6129

Percy AK, Elveback LR, Okazaki H, et al. (1972) Neoplasms of the central nervous system. Neurology 22:40–48

Pogoda J, Preston-Martin S (1998) Pesticide exposure and development of brain tumors in children in Los Angeles County. Environ Health Perspect 105:1214–1220

Preston-Martin S, Pogoda JM, Mueller BA, et al. (1996) Maternal consumption of cured meats and vitamins in relation to pediatric tumors. Cancer Epidemiol Biomarkers Prev 5(8):599–605

Preston-Martin S (1985) Epidemiology of childhood brain tumors. Italian J Neurol Sciences 6:403–409

Preston-Martin S (1989c) Descriptive epidemiology of primary tumors of the brain, cranial nerves and cranial meninges in Los Angeles County. Neuroepidemiology 8:283–295

Preston-Martin S, Henderson BE, Peters JM (1982a) Descriptive epidemiology of central nervous system neoplasms in Los Angeles County. Ann NY Acad Sci 381:202–208

Preston-Martin S, Lewis S, Winkelmann R, et al. (1993a) Descriptive epidemiology of primary cancer of the brain, cranial nerves, and cranial meninges in New Zealand, 1948–88. Cancer Causes Control 4:529–538

Preston-Martin S, Mack W (1991) Gliomas and meningiomas in men in Los Angeles County: investigation of exposures to n-nitroso compounds. In: O'Neill IK, et al. (eds) Relevance to human cancer of n-nitroso compounds, tobacco smoke and mycotoxins. IARC Scientific Publications, No. 105, Lyon, IARC, pp 197–203

Preston-Martin S, Mack W (1996) Neoplasms of the nervous system. In: Schottenfeld D, Fraumeni JF, Jr (Eds.). Cancer Epidemiology and Prevention, Second Edition, Chapter 58. New York, NY, Oxford University Press

Preston-Martin S, Mack W, Henderson BE (1989a) Risk factors for gliomas and meningiomas in males in Los Angeles County. Cancer Res 49:6137–6143

Preston-Martin S, Monroe K, Lee P, et al. (1995) Spinal meningiomas in women in Los Angeles County: investigation of an etiologic hypothesis. Cancer Epidemiol Biomarkers Prev 4:333–339

Preston-Martin S, Paganini-Hill A, Henderson BE, et al. (1980) Case-control study of intracranial meningiomas in women in Los Angeles County. JNCI 75:67–73

Preston-Martin S, Pike MC, Ross RK, et al. (1990) Increased cell division as a cause of human cancer. Cancer Res 50:7413–7419

Preston-Martin S, Staples M, Farrugia H, et al. (1993b) Primary tumors of the brain, cranial nerves and cranial meninges in Victoria Australia, 1982–1990: patterns of incidence and survival. Neuroepidemiology 12:270–279

Preston-Martin S, Thomas DC, Wright WE, et al. (1989b) Noise trauma in the aetiology of acoustic neuromas in men in Los Angeles County, 1978–1985. Br J Cancer 59:783–786

Preston-Martin S, Yu MC, Benton B, et al. (1982b) N-nitroso compounds and childhood brain tumors: a case-control study. Cancer Res 42:5240–5245

Preston-Martin S, Yu MC, Henderson BE, et al. (1983) Risk factors for meningiomas in men in Los Angeles County. JNCI 70:863–866

Rodvall Y, Ahlbom A, Spannare B, et al. (1996) Glioma and occupational exposure in Sweden, a case-control study. Occup Environ Med 53(8):526–37

Rodvall Y, Ahlbom A, Stenlund C, et al. (1998) Occupational exposure to magnetic fields and brain tumours in central Sweden. Euro J Epid 14(6):563–9

Rodvall Y, Pershagen G, Hrubec Z, et al. (1990) Prenatal x-ray exposure and childhood cancer in Swedish twins. Int J Cancer 46:362–365

Ron E, Modan B, Boice J, et al. (1988) Tumors of the brain and nervous system following radiotherapy in childhood. N Engl J Med 319:1033–1039

Rorke LB, Gilles FH, Davis RL, et al. (1985) Revision of the World Health Organization classification of brain tumors for childhood brain tumors. Cancer 56:1869–1886

Ryan P, Hurley SF, Johnson AM, et al. (1993) Tumors of the brain and presence of antibodies to *Toxoplasma gondii*. Int J Epidemiol 22:412–419

Ryan P, Lee MW, North B, et al. (1992a) Risk factors for tumors of the brain and meninges: Results from the Adelaide Adult Brain Tumor Study. Int J Cancer 51:20–27

Ryan P, Lee MW, North B, et al. (1992b) Analgam fillings, diagnostic dental x-rays and tumors of the brain and meninges. Eur J Cancer 28B:91–95

Sarasua S, Savitz DA (1994) Cured and broiled meat consumption in relation to childhood cancer: Denver, Colorado (United States). Cancer Causes Control 5:141–148

Savitz DA, John EM, Kleckner RC (1990) Magnetic field exposure from electric appliances and childhood cancer. Am J Epidemiol 131:763–773

Savitz DA, Loomis DP (1995) Magnetic field exposure in relation to leukemia and brain cancer mortality among electric utility workers. Am J Epidemiol 141:123–134

Schlehofer B, Blettner M, Becker N, et al. (1992) Medical risk factors and the development of brain tumors. Cancer 69:2541–2547

Schlehofer B, Blettner M, Preston-Martin S, et al. (1999) The role of medical history in brain tumor development: results from the international adult brain tumor study. Int J Cancer 82:155–160

Schoenberg BS, Christine BW, Whisnant JP (1978) The resolution of discrepancies in the reported incidence of primary brain tumors. Neurology 28:817–823

Scott JN, Rewcastle NB, Brasher PM, et al. (1999) Which glioblastoma multiforme patient will become a long-term survivor? A population based study. Ann Neurol 46(2):183–8

Simonato L, L'Abbe KA, Andersen A, et al. (1991) A collaborative study of cancer incidence and mortality among vinyl chloride workers. Scand J Work Environ Health 17:156–169

Smith MA, Freidlin B, Ries LA, et al. (1998) Trends in reported incidence of primary malignant brain tumors in children in the United States. J Natl Cancer Inst 90(17):1249–1251

Sorahan T, Parkes HG, Veys CA, et al. (1989) Mortality in the British rubber industry, 1946–85. Br J Ind Med 46:1–11

Stewart A, Webb J, Hewitt D (1958) A survey of childhood malignancies. Br Med J 1:1495–1508

Strickler HD, Rosenburg PS, Devesa SS, et al. (1998) Contamination of poliovirus vaccines with simian virus 40 (1955–1963) and subsequent cancer rates. JAMA 279(4):292–5

Surawicz TS, McCarthy BJ, Kupelian V, et al. (1998) Descriptive epidemiology of primary brain and CNS tumors: Results from the Central Brain Tumor Registry of the United States, 1990–1994. Neuro-Oncology January 14–25

Surawicz TS, Davis F, Freels S, et al. (1998) Brain tumor survival: results from the National Cancer Data Base. J Neuro-Oncol 40(2):151–60

Teta MJ, Ott MG, Schnatter AR (1991) An update of mortality due to brain neoplasms and other causes among employees of a petrochemical facility. J Occup Med 33:45–51

Todd NV, McDonagh T, Miller JD (1987) What follows diagnosis by computed tomography of solitary brain tumour? Lancet 1:611–612

Tomenius L (1986) 50-Hz electromagnetic environment and the incidence of childhood tumors in Stockholm County. Bioelectromagnetics 7:191–207

Velema JP, Percy CL (1987) Age curves of central nervous system tumor incidence in adults: variation of shape by histologic type. JNCI 79:623–629

WHO, ICD-O (1976) International Classification of Diseases for Oncology, First Edition, Geneva, Switzerland

WHO, ICD-O (1990) International Classification of Diseases for Oncology, Second Edition, Geneva, Switzerland

Wong O, Whorton MD, Foliart DE, et al. (1991) An industry-wide epidemiologic study of vinyl chloride workers. Am J Ind Med 20:317–334

Wrensch M, Barger GR (1990) Familial factors associated with malignant gliomas. Genet Epidemiol 7:291–301

Wrensch M, Weignerg A, Wiencke J, et al. (1997) Does prior infection with Varicella-Zoster virus influence risk of adult glioma? Am J Epidemiol 145(7):594–597

Zahm SH, Ward MH (1998) Pesticides and childhood cancer. Environ Health Perspect 106 (Suppl 3):893–908

2 Pathology of CNS Tumors

Roscoe Atkinson

Contents

2.1 Introduction

The incidence of CNS tumors is 7–10 per 100,000 (Parkin and Muir 1992). These include parenchymal tumors as well as other non-CNS intracranial lesions like meningioma. CNS tumors can be organized according to the cell of origin, location, or behavior. Consideration of metastatic lesions provides an additional criterion for organization into primary and secondary lesions. Most presentations and classifications are based on the cell of origin, including the recent classification protocols established by the World Health Organization (WHO) (Kleihues et al. 1993; Burger 1995). The bulk of this chapter is organized according to the cell of

R. Atkinson, MD
Assistant Professor, Clinical Medicine, Pathology and Neurology, USC Keck School of Medicine, McKibben Annex 346, 2011 Zonal Avenue, Los Angeles, CA 90033, USA

origin. The cell of origin is not known for all CNS tumors. The identity of the hemangioblastoma stromal cell, for example, is not known. The bulk of the mature central nervous system cellular population consists of neurons, astrocytes, oligodendrocytes, and ependymal cells. These are all derivatives of the primitive embryonal neuroectoderm. The most common intraparenchymal neoplasms arise from the astrocyte and will be discussed first.

2.2 Astrocytic Neoplasms

The astrocyte is a glial derivative of the neuroectoderm. Its functions include supportive, reactive, and metabolic activity. The astrocyte provides support for other cells in the CNS and can react during injury by providing an intertwining meshwork of long cytoplasmic processes, a procedure known as gliosis. This characteristic gives the astrocyte a star-like appearance, resulting in its name. The astrocyte is also thought to play an important role in microenvironment potassium levels (Paulson et al. 1987), neurotransmitter uptake (Norenberg and Martinez-Hernandez 1979), and ion exchange (Langley 1990). It may also play an important role in blood–brain barrier formation (Abbott et al. 1992). Neoplastic transformation of an astrocyte results in the formation of an astrocytoma. Astrocytomas occur throughout the CNS and are associated with a progressive spectrum of biological activity and aggressiveness. This spectrum has been dealt with in a number of ways. A four-tiered grading protocol has become standard although other grading systems still exist (Coons and Johnson 1991; Daumas-Duport et al. 1988). The grade I astrocytoma refers to a benign astrocytic neoplasm that does not show significant pleomorphism, mitotic activity, endothelial proliferation, or necrosis. From a behavioral perspective, a grade I astrocytoma should not recur if completely resected and implies a corresponding lack of tumor infiltration. The grade II, III, and IV astrocytomas are more infiltrative and will show varying combinations of pleomorphism, mitotic activity, endothelial proliferation, and necrosis. Beginning with a baseline grade of I, one additional grading unit is added for the presence of each additional criterion. For example, an astrocytoma (one point) demonstrating pleomorphism (second point) and mitotic activity (third point) is considered to be grade III. This grading system roughly corresponds to the older three-tiered nomenclature of "low grade astrocytoma", "anaplastic astrocytoma", and "glioblastoma multiforme". In most cases these correspond to astrocytoma grades II, III, and IV, respectively. Small sample sizes such as those provided during stereotactic biopsy can provide significant problematic sampling error and result in undergrading. Effective communication between the surgeon, radiologist, and pathologist is important in providing a diagnosis in problematic cases.

The grade II or low-grade astrocytoma is very infiltrative as seen by the lack of grossly identifiable margins. This tumor is typically solid although degeneration can result in cyst formation. The consistency and color will vary. The microscopic features can be subtle with cellularity only minimally above that seen in the normal brain (Fig. 2.1). The pleomorphism may also overlap that seen in reactive gliosis, the nemesis of the surgical neuropathologist. Intraoperative cytologic preparations yield a mild to moderately dense population of neoplastic astrocytes with prominent but delicate cytoplasmic processes. Reactive gliosis around a high-grade lesion can mimic the histology of a low-grade astrocytoma.

Non-neoplastic gliotic processes can be similarly misdiagnosed. Helpful criteria seen in paraffin sections include microcystic change, irregular cell distribution, perineuronal satellitosis, and linear filling. Some low-grade astrocytomas show more extensive pleomorphism and are easier to diagnose (Fig. 2.2A). A moderate degree of variation in nuclear size and shape is a welcome feature.

An immunohistochemical stain for the glial-fibrillary acidic protein (GFAP), an intermediate filament protein specific for astrocytes, delineates the cytoplasm of both neoplastic and non-neoplastic astrocytes. The presence of reactivity within the cytoplasm of tumor cells confirms the astrocytic nature of the lesion. Immunostains specific for the proliferation associated antigen Ki-67 (MIB-1) can be helpful in distinguishing between a low-grade astrocytoma and reactive gliosis. It can also be helpful in determining whether a higher-grade lesion is present in a small biopsy specimen with prominent pleomorphism but no additional grading criteria (Hsa et al. 1997). Some grade II astrocytomas contain sufficient components of other glial elements (Cooper 1935; Hart 1974) and justify a diagnosis of mixed glioma. The oligoastrocytoma is a common example. The use of this mixed terminology should only be reserved for clear examples of mixed lesions. A long survival is possible if a low-grade astrocytoma retains its low grade. They can, however, undergo malignant transformation and become a more aggressive higher-grade lesion.

The grade III astrocytoma is usually analogous to an anaplastic astrocytoma. The cerebral hemispheres are the usual site of occurrence. The gross appearance is soft and it shows moderate delinea-

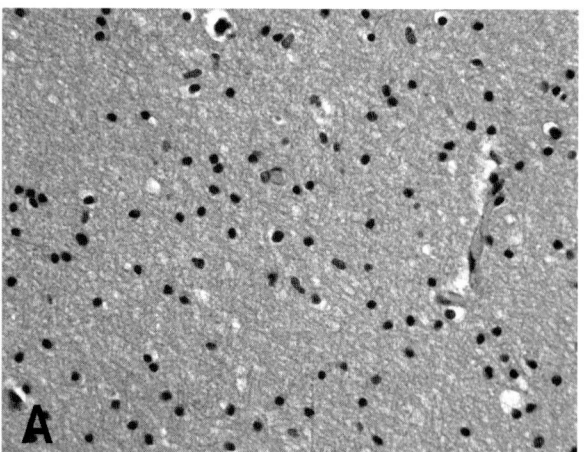 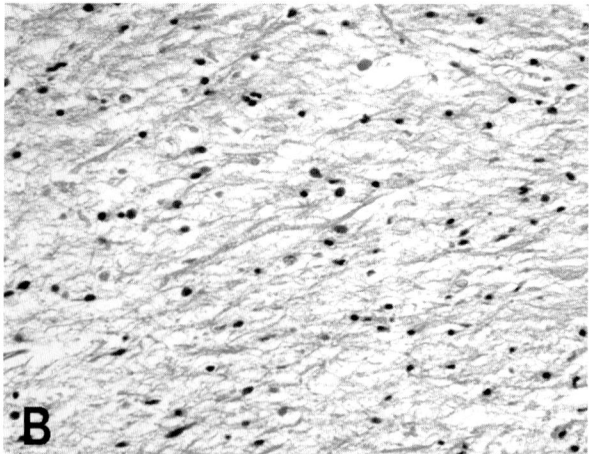

Fig. 2.1A,B. Normal cerebral white matter (A). +100. Note the glial density compared to that of a paucicellular low-grade (grade II) astrocytoma (B) +100

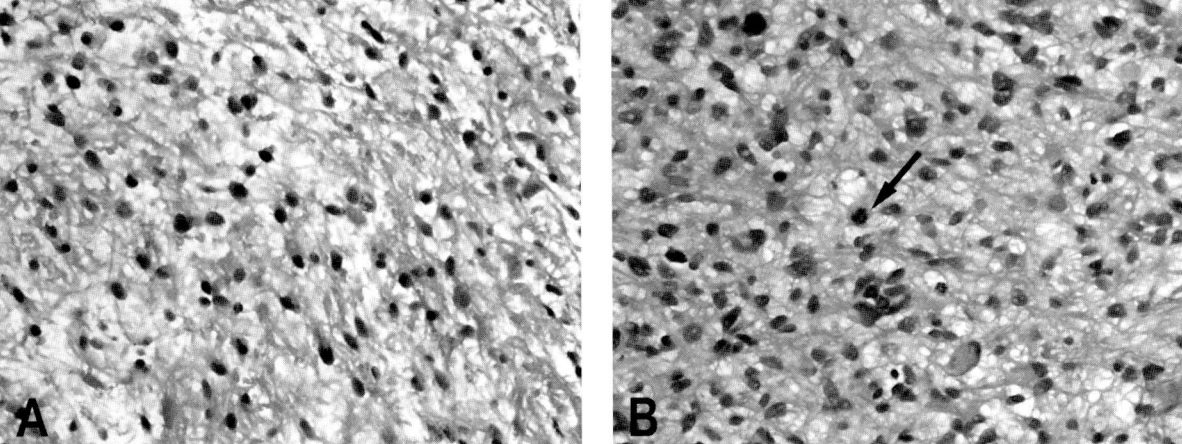

Fig. 2.2. **A** A low-grade astrocytoma (grade II) showing significant cellularity and nuclear pleomorphism. +100. **B** An anaplastic astrocytoma (grade III). Note the extensive nuclear pleomorphism and mitotic figure (*arrow*).+100

tion. Pleomorphism is more extensive than that seen in a grade II lesion and mitotic activity is usually apparent (Fig. 2.2B).

A thorough search for mitotic activity may be required in a small stereotactic biopsy specimen. The tumor cell density is also substantially greater and the nuclear:cytoplasmic ratio is increased. Cellular processes are often still present as demonstrated with the GFAP immunostain (Fig. 2.4B). The Ki-67 proliferation fraction ranges from 5 to 10%. As with the low-grade mixed gliomas, a significant component of more than one glial element can lead to a diagnosis of an anaplastic mixed glioma.

At the far end of the behavioral spectrum of astrocytoma is the glioblastoma multiforme (GBM) and is analogous to the WHO grade IV astrocytoma. The nosology of this tumor is old but effective. The high-grade malignant nature of the lesion is implicated in its "-blastoma" suffix while the glial derivation is clear in its prefix. Its variable coloration, texture, and shape with intervening areas of necrosis and hemorrhage had once been an inspiration for the term "multiforme". Of the astrocytomas, GBM is the most common. It can arise de novo or begin by a transformation of a preexisting lower grade astrocytoma. It peaks in the fifth and sixth decades of life and usually occurs in the cerebral hemispheres. The GBM is very infiltrative and will follow fiber tracts as well as the subpial space. This ability to tract is exemplified by the classic extension across the corpus callosum to provide a "butter-

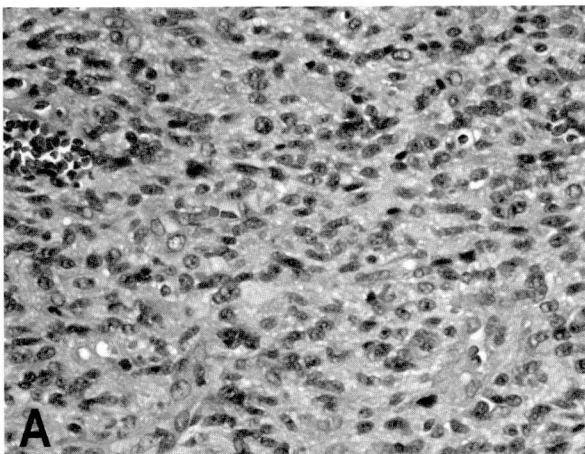
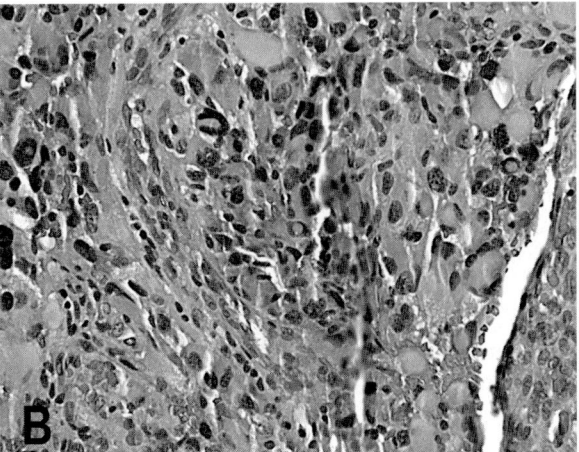

Fig. 2.3A,B. Numerous small malignant cells (**A**) and scattered larger cells (**B**) seen in a glioblastoma. +100

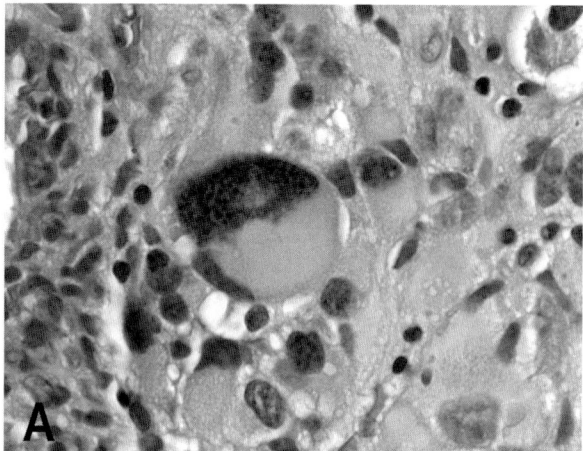 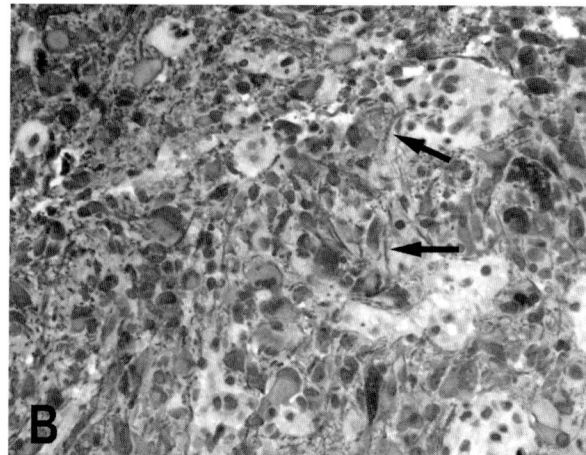

Fig. 2.4. A Glioblastomas can demonstrate large bizarre cells. +400. **B** Cytoplasmic processes immunoreactive for GFAP are often associated with astrocytomas. DAB, +100

fly" appearance. The neoplastic astrocytes of a GBM show a spectrum of morphology. Some lesions consist of numerous small malignant cells (Fig. 2.3A) while others may demonstrate scattered larger cells (Fig. 2.3B). Bizarre cells and strange mitotic figures are often present (Fig. 2.4A). GFAP immunoreactivity by immunohistochemistry is usually present but not invariably. Endothelial proliferation or tumor necrosis is required for the assignment of a grade IV classification. Endothelial proliferation is a hypertrophic and hyperplastic reaction of the endothelial cells of capillaries, venules, and arterioles (Fig. 2.5A). The capillary reaction can result in small tufts of twisted proliferated capillaries known as glomeruli, a result of their resemblance to renal glomeruli. Endothelial prolifera-

tion is not confined to the GBM and can be seen in other lesions. Tumor necrosis may be in the form of irregular isolated islands. There is often a very characteristic "palisading" or "pseudopalisading" type of necrosis characterized by an alignment of neoplastic cells along small oblong necrotic foci. The presence of necrosis must be carefully examined in patients having undergone radiation therapy as this is an alternate etiology of necrosis in a tumor. Radionecrosis should not produce a pseudopalisading pattern.

Should the presence of extensive pleomorphism, mitotic figures, necrosis, and endothelial proliferation not provide convincing evidence regarding the lesions aggressiveness, the Ki-67 (MIB-1) immunostain will show a proliferation fraction of up to 25% (5–25%)

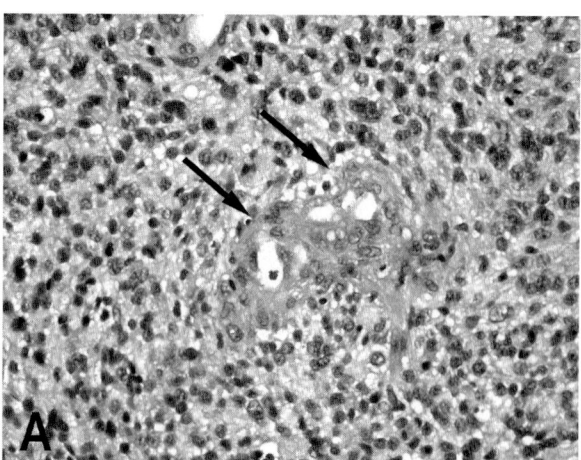 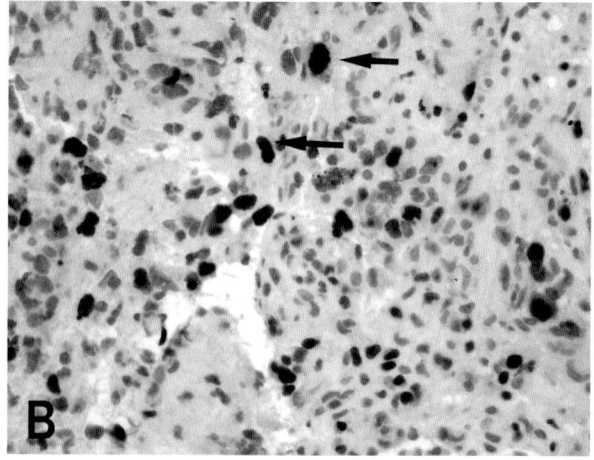

Fig. 2.5. A Endothelial proliferation in a glioblastoma (*arrow*). +100. **B** The proliferation-associated antigen Ki-67 (MIB-1) visualized by immunohistochemistry (*arrows*). DAB, +100

(Fig. 2.5B). Diagnostic pitfalls include the risk of undergrading the tumor due to sampling error. An entire biopsy showing only necrosis is possible. Although radiotherapy can eradicate the bulk of the lesion, recurrence and short survival is the rule. The differential diagnosis of a GBM includes metastatic carcinoma and high-grade cerebral lymphoma.

Grade II and III astrocytomas may retain sufficient differentiation to distinguish among different astrocyte subtypes. This distinction can provide additional classification. Most astrocytomas are of the "fibrillary astrocytoma" variety. The cell of origin is the fibrillary astrocyte, the primary astrocyte of the brain's white matter. This astrocyte contains minimal perinuclear cytoplasm and possesses numerous GFAP positive cytoplasmic processes that emanate from the cell body in a radial fashion. This fibrillarity is responsible for the fibrillar background seen in fibrillar astrocytomas. The neoplastic cells of some astrocytomas are "gemistocytic" and contain abundant eosinophilic cytoplasm (Fig. 2.6A). The term "gemistocytic astrocytoma" is appropriate if this type of astrocyte makes up the bulk of an lesion. Gemistocytic astrocytomas provide a poorer prognosis for a given grade. The protoplasmic astrocytoma is a rare lesion composed of astrocytes with small cell bodies, few cell processes, and low GFAP density (PRAYSON and ESTES 1995). This type of astrocyte is seen in the gray matter and is called the "protoplasmic" astrocyte. It arises from the gray matter as opposed to fibrillar astrocytes that begin in the white matter.

The giant cell glioblastoma is a variant of glioblastoma that is characterized by large bizarre malignant astrocytes. Bizarre mitotic figures may also be present. These lesions usually show a better circumscription when compared to other high-grade astrocytomas but the prognosis is poor in spite of this circumscription.

The gliosarcoma is composed of a glioblastomatous component alongside a second, sarcomatous component. The sarcomatous component is found in fascicles that weave through the gliomatous areas, dividing them into discreet regions (Fig. 2.6B). The immunohistochemistry of the gliomatous component is similar to that seen in other glioblastomas. The origin of the sarcomatous component is debated. Popular theories include the presence of extensively severe endothelial proliferation or the coincidental formation of a separate sarcoma. The lack of consensus is strengthened by the sarcoma immunoreactivity to endothelial, histiocytic, and astrocytic markers (KOCHI and BUDKA 1987; SLOWIK et al. 1985).

The grade I astrocytomas are considered benign and should not demonstrate mitotic activity. The remaining criteria (endothelial proliferation, etc.) are not relevant in grading these benign astrocytomas. A grade I astrocytoma that demonstrates endothelial proliferation retains its grade I status. Necrosis may also be present, although pseudopalisading necrosis is not expected. It is not infiltrative and, if completely resected, will not recur. The juvenile pilocytic astrocytoma (JPA) is a classic example of the grade I astrocytoma and is discussed in the cerebellar lesion section.

The pleomorphic xanthoastrocytoma (PXA) is a recently described lesion of the young (KEPES et al. 1979). It usually arises in the temporal or parietal lobes. The classic presentation consists of a cyst with

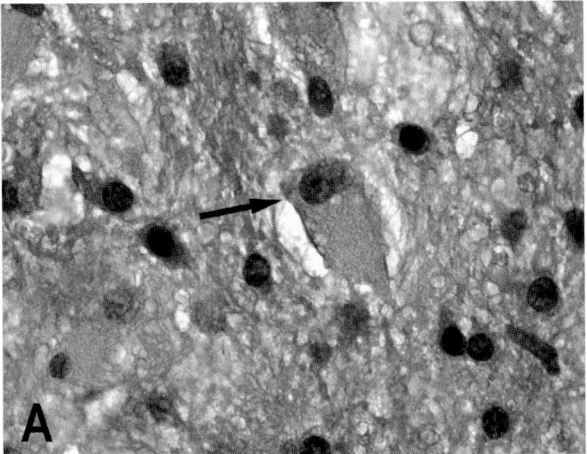
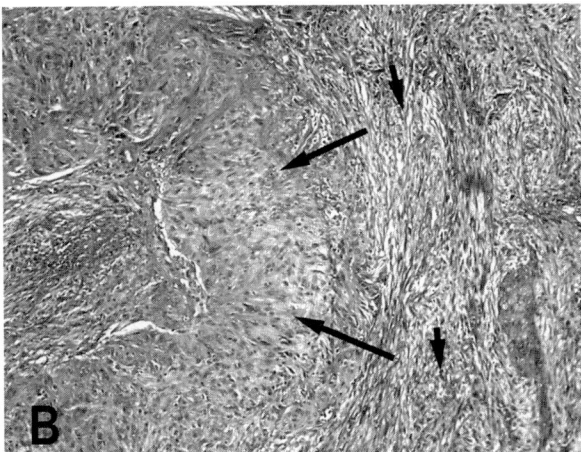

Fig. 2.6. A A gemistocytic astrocyte or "gemistocyte" shows plump cytoplasm and an ex-centric nucleus. +400. **B** A gliosarcoma demonstrates both gliomatous elements (*long arrows*) and sarcomatous elements (*short arrows*). +100

a mural nodule that is superficial and in communication with the leptomeninges. Microscopically, the PXA is cellular with large pleomorphic, even bizarre astrocytes. Many of the lesion's neoplastic astrocytes possess vacuoles of lipid (xanthomatous). The background consists of a fibrillar matrix and areas of perivascular lymphocytes are usually seen. Reticulin staining reveals a prominent pattern that may extend around individual cells. Mitotic activity, endothelial proliferation, and necrosis are usually absent but can be seen. Local infiltration is variable. The PXA presents a spectrum of biological behavior, although most are associated with a favorable prognosis or even cure (WELDON-LINNE et al. 1983). They occasionally present as aggressive lesions with high rates of recurrence (ALLEGRANZA et al. 1991).

2.3
Oligodendrogliomas

As the name implies, oligodendrogliomas arise from the oligodendrocyte, the myelin-producing cell of the CNS white matter. Oligodendroglioma is a low-grade neoplasm that is usually seen in the fourth and fifth decades of life. It occurs in the cerebral hemispheres and consist of a white matter mass with overlying cortical infiltration. The mass is soft and moderately well demarcated although demarcation may be lost in the overlying infiltrated cortex. There may also be subpial spread and cyst formation. Scattered calcifications produce a gritty consistency. Microscopically, the lesion shows a dense population of

small cells with round monomorphic nuclei and small nucleoli (Fig. 2.7A). Characteristic artifactual perinuclear halos are usually seen in fixed specimens but may be absent in intraoperative frozen section preparations. Oligodendrogliomas possess a characteristic pattern of small winding capillaries that has been described as "chicken wire" (Fig. 2.7B). Significant pleomorphism and mitotic activity are absent. The calcification seen grossly is associated with numerous microscopic calcifications scattered within the lesion and in the surrounding tissue. There is no commercially accepted stain or antibody that will specifically identify the neoplastic oligodendrocyte. Immunostudies are, therefore, confined to the exclusion of other entities like the GFAP positive astrocytoma. The classic low-grade (grade II) oligodendroglioma is associated with a 5–10-year survival. Some lesions show a significant astrocytic component and are given the popular diagnosis of "oligoastrocytoma" already mentioned above. The presence of malignant features supports a diagnosis of anaplastic oligodendroglioma. This anaplastic variety will show increased cellularity, mitotic activity, and significant nuclear pleomorphism. Examples of endothelial proliferation and necrosis may also be present.

2.4.
Ependymomas

The ependymal lining of the CNS ventricular system is composed of a delicate single-layered epithelial lining composed of ciliated columnar-cuboidal

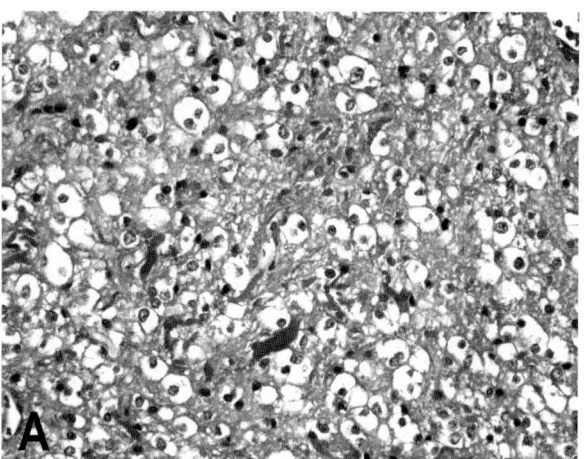
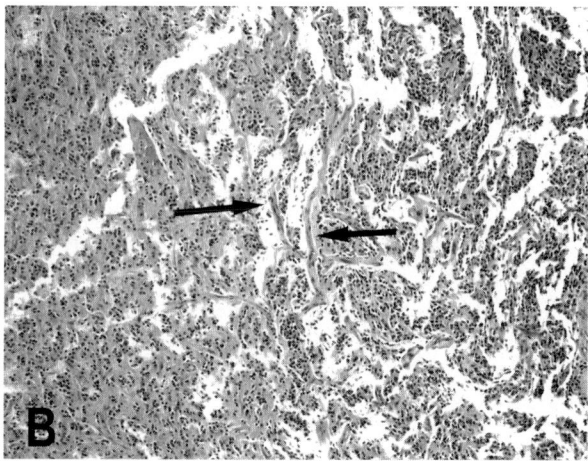

Fig. 2.7. A A classic grade II oligodendroglioma demonstrates small round nuclei and perinuclear halos. +100. **B** Narrow winding "chicken wire" vasculature (*arrow*) is often seen in oligodendrogliomas. +40

cells. This epithelium at first glance seems to lack a basement membrane as its basement membrane equivalent is found lining the intraparenchymal vascularity and the pial surface. All intervening tissue between the ependymal layer and the subpial/perivascular basement membrane comprises the embryological equivalent of the neuroectodermal epithelium. Neoplasms of the ependyma naturally arise from the ependymal lining of the ventricular system and are usually seen in children and young adults. Many of these are associated with the fourth ventricle. A rare ependymoma arises in areas of the nervous system not associated with the ventricular system or its ependymal lining (LITTLE et al. 1994). Rare cases are even found in non-neural tissues (GUERRIERI and JARLSFELT 1993; KING et al. 1993). Most ependymomas develop in children and young adults. The classic posterior fossa lesion characteristically arises as an exophytic mass from the floor of the fourth ventricle. Resulting obstruction of CSF flow will result in hydrocephalus. The tumors are slow-growing low-grade lesions that show local invasion. There is a high rate of local recurrence. A rare lesion may also show metastasis outside of the CNS.

Ependymomas are moderately well-circumscribed solid gray masses that may contain calcification, cyst formation, or hemorrhage. Microscopically, they are composed of a neoplastic ependymal cells with mild nuclear pleomorphism (Fig. 2.8A). Cellular processes provide a fibrillar background that in some areas projects around small vascular structures in a radial fashion. The term perivascular pseudorosette is given to well-formed examples of

these structures (Fig. 2.8B). The "true" ependymal rosette, in contrast, consists of similar rosette formation around small ependymal lumena, canals, or cavities. These seem to mimic the embryonal formation of the CNS ventricular system. Mitotic activity and endothelial proliferation are rare. Necrosis may accompany larger specimens.

There are four categories of ependymoma: the classic ependymoma and three subtypes – cellular, papillary, and clear cell. The cellular ependymoma shows a greater relative cell density and fewer rosettes. Papillary ependymomas consist of numerous papillary structures that resemble the choroid plexus. The clear cell ependymoma is composed of round cells with clear cytoplasm and distinct cell membranes. The immunohistochemistry (below) is similar among the different types of ependymoma. Misdiagnosis is the primary significance of these subtypes, with potential overlapping histology with choroid plexus papillomas, oligodendrogliomas, central neurocytomas, and clear cell carcinomas.

Immunoreactivity of ependymomas to GFAP is most intense within the perivascular pseudorosettes. The epithelial membrane antigen (EMA) shows a curious focal intracytoplasmic immunostaining pattern that probably represents a vestigial intracytoplasmic ependymal lining. EMA immunoreactivity is also prominent within the lumena of true ependymal rosettes.

The classic ependymoma corresponds to a grade of II. Occasional ependymomas show increased pleomorphism, increased cellularity, high mitotic activity, endothelial proliferation, and necrosis and corresponds to a grade of III (anaplastic ependy-

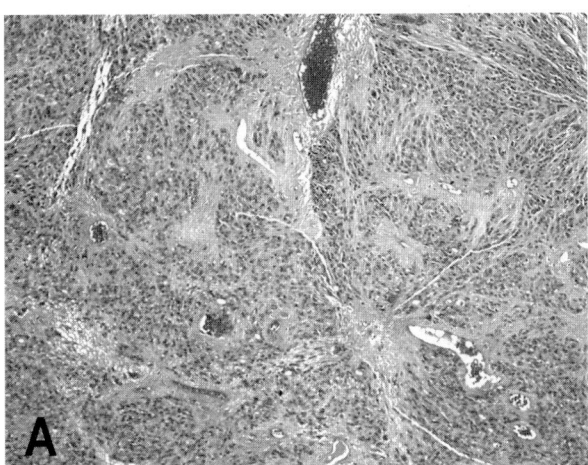
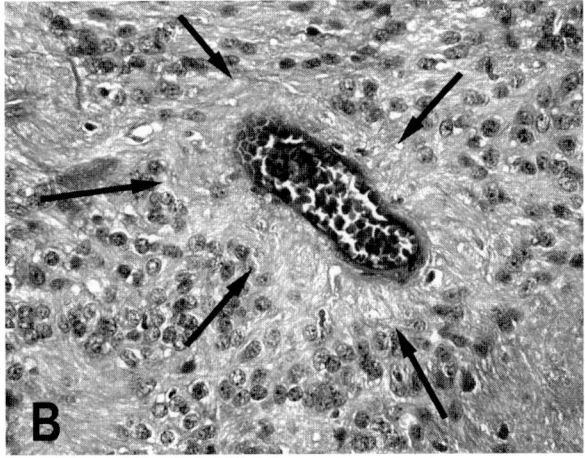

Fig. 2.8. A An ependymoma with a classic perivascular pseudorosetting pattern. +40. **B** High magnification of a single perivascular ependymal pseudorosette (*arrows*). +400

momas). These are less well circumscribed and more aggressive.

2.5
Neoplasms with Neuronal Differentiation

2.5.1
Central Neurocytoma

The central neurocytoma is a relatively unusual tumor that shows proclivity for the central supratentorial structures, especially the septum pellucidum or the medial aspect of the lateral ventricles. It is a slow-growing lesion occurring in young adults. A relatively good prognosis is characteristic but not the rule. Grossly, the lesion is a grayish well-circumscribed mass attached to adjacent structures. Significant calcification is often present. Microscopic features consist of a monomorphic population of small or medium-sized cells containing minimally pleomorphic nuclei with speckled chromatin (Fig. 2.9A). Mitotic activity is rare and the KI-67 proliferation fraction is usually about 2%. Perinuclear halos, if present, can mimic the histology of an oligodendroglioma. Evidence of neuronal differentiation is required for the diagnosis. Additional histologic evidence includes the presence of Homer-Wright rosettes similar to those seen in medulloblastomas. More specific and consistent evidence for neuronal differentiation is the immunoreactivity for neuronal markers including neuron specific enolase (NSE) and synaptophysin.

2.5.2
Ganglioglioma

The ganglioglioma is a glioneuronal neoplasm consisting of two separate neoplastic populations (Fig. 2.9B). One population is composed of low-grade neoplastic astrocytes similar to those found in a grade II astrocytomas. The second population consists of large neuronal forms similar in appearance to the cell bodies of the pseudounipolar neurons in the dorsal root ganglia and other sensory ganglia. These large neurons, or ganglion cells, contain very large conspicuous vesicular nuclei and prominent nucleoli. Atypical features like binucleation may be seen. The astrocytic component is expected to stain with GFAP while the ganglion cells show reactivity for neuronal markers (NSE, synaptophysin). Other characteristic microscopic features include microcalcification and perivascular cuffing by benign reactive lymphocytes. Grossly, the ganglioglioma may be solid or cystic. Formation of mural nodules and multiple cysts is common. The lesion is usually seen as a temporal lobe lesion in the young adult population.

2.6
Tumors Resembling Primitive Neuroectoderm

There are a number of lesions that have very similar morphology and immunoreactivity. They all consist of dense populations of round, small to medium-

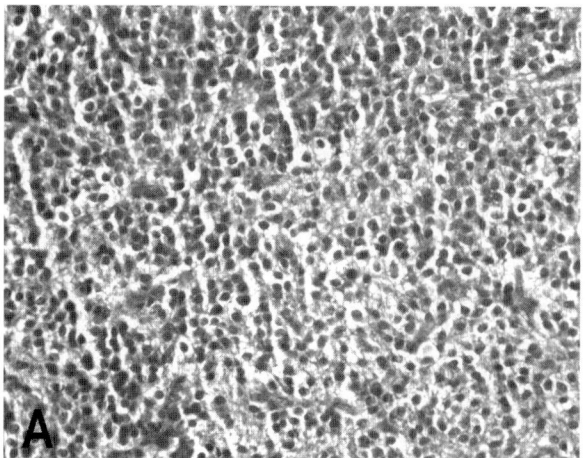 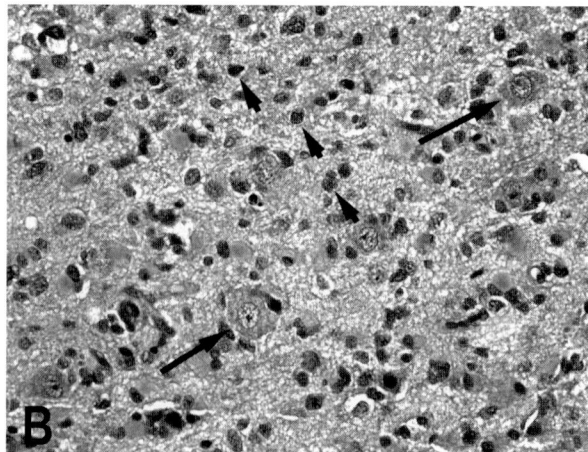

Fig. 2.9. A Central neurocytoma showing a monomorphic population of small to medium-sized cells with minimal nuclear pleomorphism. +100. **B** A ganglioglioma showing a population of small low-grade neoplastic astrocytes (*short arrows*) and large neoplastic ganglion cells (*long arrows*). +100

sized cells with scanty cytoplasm and dark blue hyperchromatic nuclei (Fig. 2.10A). Various types of rosette formation may be present including the Homer-Wright rosette (Fig. 2.10B) and the larger Flexner-Wintersteiner rosette. The cells are very discohesive as demonstrated by cytological preparations. This lack of cellular cohesiveness is responsible for the proclivity for CSF seeding seen in lesions involving the ventricular system. Although the neoplastic cells are undifferentiated, they maintain an immunoreactive profile consistent with neuronal differentiation and will stain with markers for NSE and synaptophysin. Other markers may be positive but are less useful. The dedifferentiated nature of these tumors is seen in their potential for differentiation along non-neuronal cell lines including astrocytic, ependymal, and pigmented tissues.

Peripheral versions of the lesion are called neuroblastomas and usually arise in the adrenal medulla. Cerebellar medulloblastomas are relatively common brain tumors in children, second only to the pilocytic astrocytoma. Medulloblastomas commonly arise in the medial aspect of the cerebellum adjacent to the roof of the fourth ventricle. Expansion of the mass will lead to ventricular obstruction and hydrocephalus. Medulloblastomas, as mentioned above, show a tendency to seed the CSF and produce distant metastasis. Similar lesions are occasionally seen supratentorially. A relatively recent term, "primitive neuroectodermal tumor" (PNET) encompasses both supratentorial and posterior fossa medulloblastomas (BECKER and HINTON 1983; RORKE 1983). Other site-specific lesions resembling the primitive neuro-

ectoderm include the olfactory neuroblastoma and the pineoblastoma.

2.7
Cerebral Lymphoma

Cerebral lymphoma is invariably primary. Secondary lymphomatous spread is confined to the meninges or other non-neural intracranial structures. Cerebral lymphoma is relatively unusual although its incidence is increasing in the immunosuppressed population including those with acquired immune deficiency syndrome (AIDS). CNS lymphoma usually occurs after the fifth decade of life in non-immunosuppressed individuals. The average age is much younger in high-risk individuals. The lesion can begin anywhere in the CNS and can take on a number of macroscopic forms with varying levels of demarcation, infiltration, necrosis, hemorrhage, and multifocality. By far the most common type of CNS lymphoma is the high-grade B-cell lymphoma with histology similar to that seen in non-CNS sites. Areas with dense populations of malignant lymphocytes are interspersed among areas of necrosis, gliosis, or normal tissue (Fig. 2.11). Perivascular cuffing or spread is a characteristic pattern seen in the CNS lymphoma. Although immunohistochemistry is expected to show a dominant population of B lymphocytes, a significant amount of associated reactive inflammatory lymphocytes can introduce a potentially confusing number of T lymphocytes. This in-

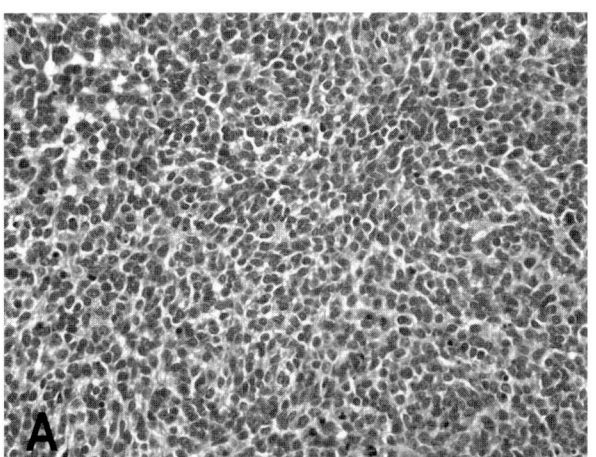 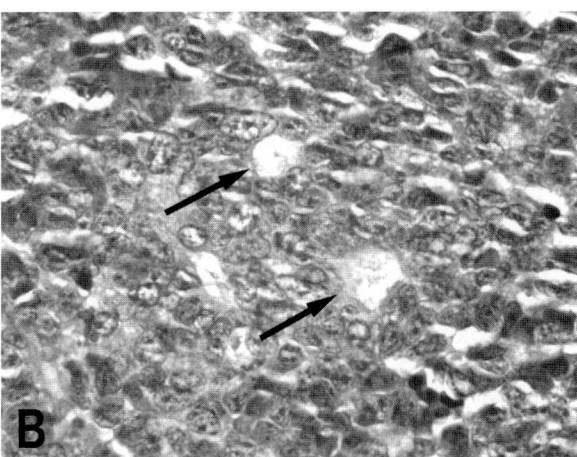

Fig. 2.10A,B. A medulloblastoma composed of numerous small to medium-sized cells with scanty cytoplasm and dark blue hyperchromatic nuclei (**A**). Homer-Wright rosettes (*arrows*) typical of many tumors with neuroblastic differentiation. +100

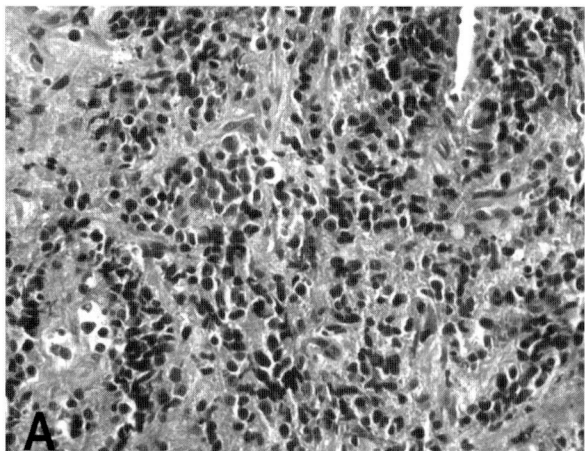 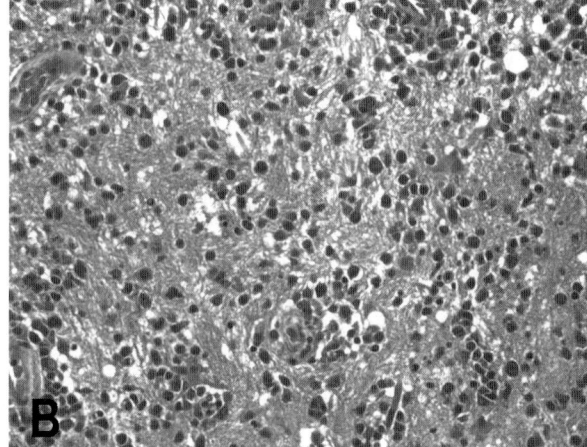

Fig. 2.11. Cerebral lymphomas composed of varying densities of malignant B lymphocytes (**A, B**). +100

flammatory component may even predominate in lymphomas following steroid treatment. The CNS lymphoma (also known as the disappearing tumor) will shrink as its malignant component responds to therapy. The inflammatory component, albeit also sensitive to such therapy, will persist. This can provide difficulty during the diagnosis of surgical or autopsy tissue.

2.8
Choroid Plexus Lesions

Atrial meningiomas arising in the ventricular trigone may develop in association with the choroid plexus. Metastatic carcinoma may also be found in the choroid plexus. The only significant lesions arising from the actual choroid plexus epithelium are the choroid plexus papilloma and carcinoma. Both are uncommon and seen mainly in children. The papilloma can cause hydrocephalus as a result of obstruction or increased CSF production. The papilloma has a well-circumscribed cauliflower appearance. Histologically, it is a grade I lesion comprised of numerous vascularized papillary fronds covered by a single-layered choroid plexus epithelium (Fig. 2.12). There may be microcalcifications scattered throughout the mass. The presence of nuclear pleomorphism, mitotic activity, and necrosis support a diagnosis of choroid plexus carcinoma. The differential diagnosis includes the papillary ependymoma and a papillary metastatic carcinoma. Immunoreactivity for transthyretin supports the diagnosis of a choroid plexus lesion.

2.9
Meningeal Neoplasms

Meningioma is the primary tumor of the meninges. The meningioma cell of origin is the arachnoid cap cell found in incidental nests throughout the leptomeninges (KEPES 1986). A young meningioma will eventually grow to considerable size and adhere to the adjacent dura with which it forms a wide physical connection. This connection can provide the deceptive appearance that the meningioma arose from the dura. Meningiomas can form wherever the leptomeninges and their associated arachnoid cap cells are found. They are typically seen in the cerebrum along the cerebral convexities and parasagittal areas. Spinal meningiomas are seen mostly in female patients. Meningiomas are usually slow-growing tumors that are exceedingly well demarcated. There is very little propensity for invasion and complete resection usually constitutes a cure.

Meningiomas are divided into a number of subtypes with similar clinical behavior, the most common being the meningothelial meningioma (Fig. 2.13A). This type is composed of small sheets and whorls of cells with pale oval nuclei and indistinct cytoplasm. The whorls often surround small vascular structures or spherical laminated concretions known as psammoma bodies. An occasional lesion will be composed almost entirely of psammoma bodies at the exclusion of other cellular components (psammomatous meningiomas) (Fig. 2.13B). The fibroblastic meningioma (Fig. 2.14A) is composed of fascicles and winding bundles of elongated spindle cells that resemble fibroblasts. Some meningiomas, known as transitional meningiomas, contain a more

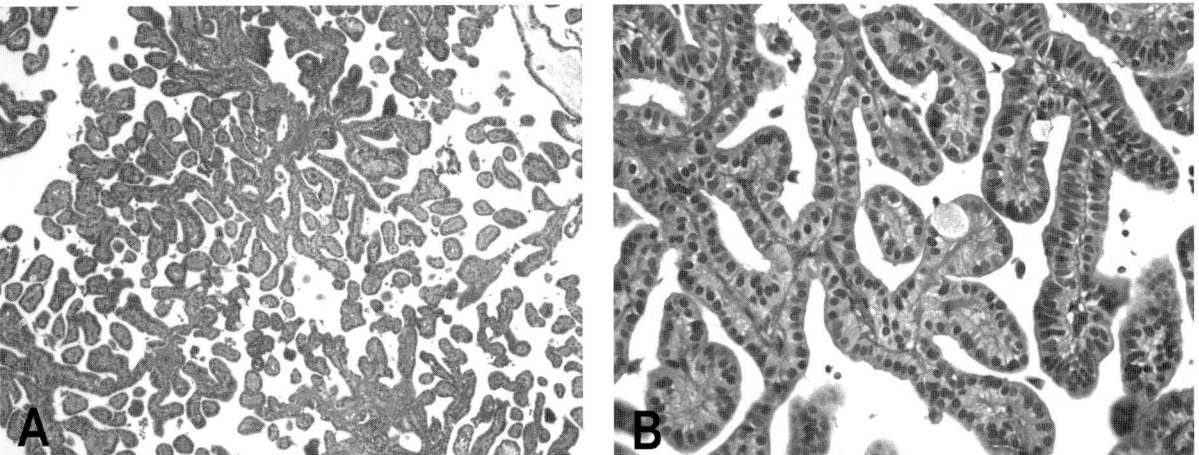

Fig. 2.12A,B. Low (**A**, +40) and high (**B**, +100) magnification photomicrographs of a choroid plexus papilloma. Note the single simple epithelium covering a delicate fibrovascular core

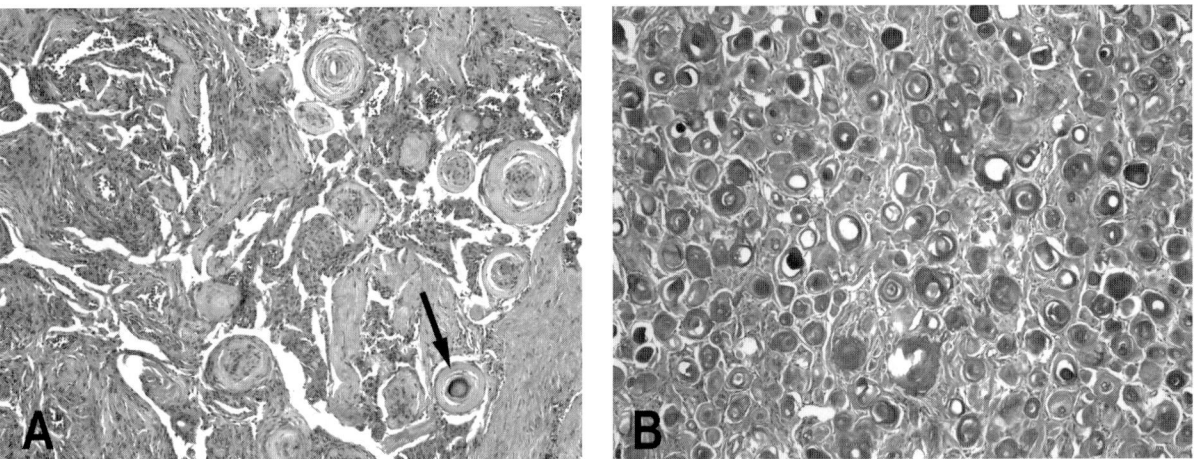

Fig. 2.13. A A meningothelial meningioma with scattered psammoma bodies (*arrow*). +100. **B** A psammomatous meningioma consists of numerous psammoma bodies at the expense of the meningothelial architecture. +100

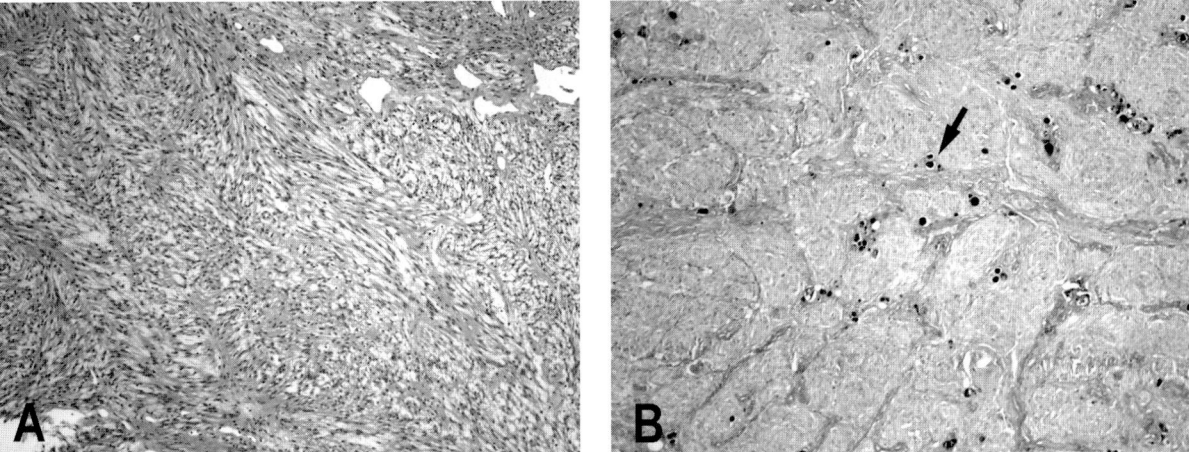

Fig. 2.14. A The fibroblastic meningioma is composed of fascicles and winding bundles of elongated spindle cells that resemble fibroblasts. +100. **B** A secretory meningioma with classic droplets of PAS positive secretory product (*arrow*). PAS, +100

or less even component of fibroblastic and meningothelial components. Some meningothelial or fibroblastic meningiomas demonstrate increased epithelial differentiation by the formation of glandular elements that contain a secreted PAS positive material (Fig. 2.14B) and are appropriately named "secretory meningiomas" (ALGUACIL-GARCIA et al. 1986). Meningiomas are classically immunoreactive for EMA. Many meningiomas also express estrogen and progesterone receptors. The role of either has been debated but it is clear that such expression may be associated with increased incidence of meningioma in female patients, its association with breast cancer (BURNS et al. 1986; SCHOENBERG et al. 1975), and with its explosive growth seen in pregnant patients (CIOFFI et al. 1996).

A few meningiomas will demonstrate more aggressive or atypical features along with a correspondingly less favorable clinical behavior. Atypical features include the presence of mitotic activity, increased cellularity, tumor necrosis, and increased pleomorphism (Fig. 2.15A). Loss of the classic histologic features (whorls, psammoma bodies) and replacement by monotonous sheets of cells is also seen. Atypical meningiomas correspond to a grade of II and show a greater risk of recurrence. The definition of a malignant meningioma is debated, although most agree that clear brain invasion in the presence of aggressive features above that seen in atypical meningiomas is sufficient enough to warrant the diagnosis.

The hemangiopericytoma is not a meningioma although it has historically been classified as a subtype, known as the "angioblastic meningioma" (BAILEY et al. 1928). Sufficient differences exist to define it as a separate unique entity. The hemangiopericytoma is typically a dural-based vascular mass that can occur in any age group. The exact cell of origin is debated. Its histology is nearly identical to that of non-CNS hemangiopericytomas arising in other somatic soft tissues. Crowded cells with scanty cytoplasm and oval nuclei cluster to form sheets, nests, and lobules that are separated by narrow sinusoidal structures (staghorn vessels) (Fig. 2.15B). Mitotic activity varies. In contrast to the meningioma, hemangiopericytomas are aggressive lesions with a high rate of recurrence. There is also significant metastatic potential.

2.10 Notochordal Neoplasms (Chordoma)

The chordoma cell of origin is found in the remnants of the embryonal notochord. These remnants are concentrated at the ends of the axial skeleton and thus dictate its clival and sacral location. It is usually seen in the middle aged and presents as a locally invasive mass with the potential to metastasis. Grossly, the lesion consists of clear mucinous gray tissue. The classic microscopic appearance is that of trabeculae composed of neoplastic cells with eosinophilic cytoplasm in a background of fibrous tissue with varying amounts of mucin (Fig. 2.16A). The cell cytoplasm may show vacuolization which, when extreme, results in a bubbly appearance (physaliphorous cells)(Fig. 2.16B).

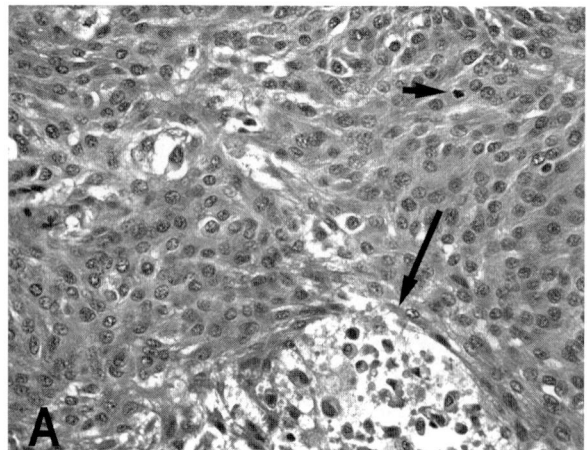
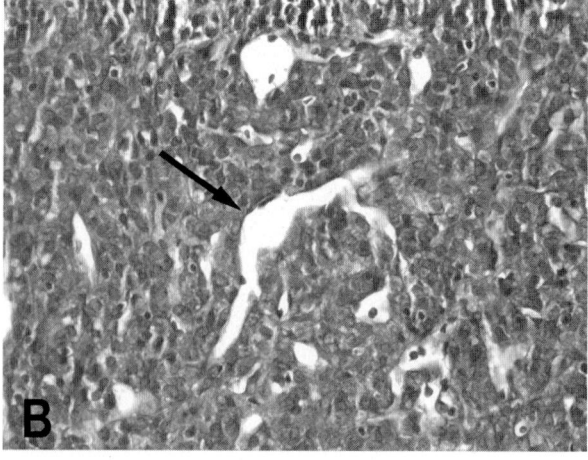

Fig. 2.15. A An atypical meningioma with necrosis (*long arrow*) and mitotic activity (*short arrow*). +100. **B** A hemangiopericytoma with classic "staghorn" vasculature (*arrow*). +100

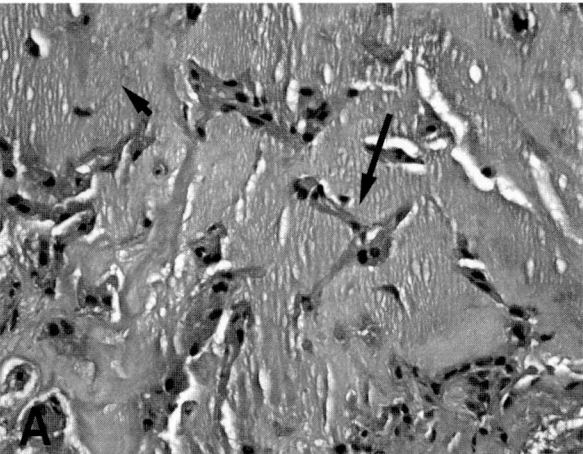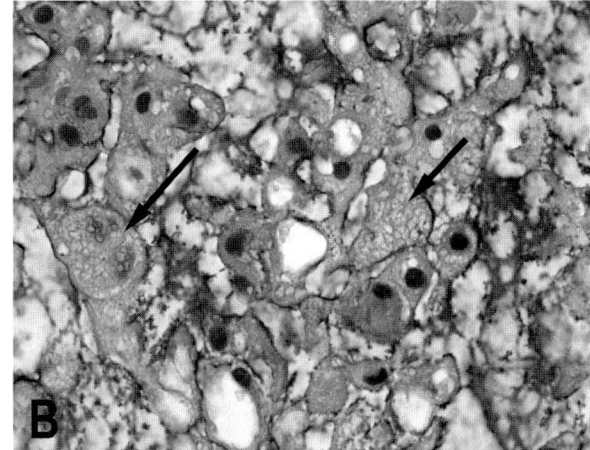

Fig. 2.16. A Chordoma with trabeculae of neoplastic cells (*arrow*) in a mucinous background. +100. **B** A high-magnification micrograph of a chordoma showing the bubbly "physaliphorous" cell. +400

2.11
Metastatic Carcinoma

Common metastatic lesions affecting the CNS include those originating in the lung, breast, kidney, gastrointestinal tract, and skin (melanoma). Many other types of cancer have also been observed to metastasize to the CNS. Metastatic carcinoma in the CNS will usually possess the histology of the parent primary lesion (Fig. 2.17A). Undifferentiated lesions may require immunohistochemistry or electron microscopy for identification. A patient will occasionally succumb to a metastatic cerebral lesion for which the corresponding primary lesion could not be found (unknown primary). Cerebral metastatic lesions usually begin at the junction between the gray and white matter. Similar filtration-like behavior of this junctional area is seen in bacterial abscess formation and fatty emboli. The metastatic lesion is well demarcated from the surrounding brain tissue. The growing lesion, in conjunction with associated peritumoral edema, will produce a mass effect. Intratumoral hemorrhage will result in an acute increase in such mass effect. Metastatic carcinoma is usually easy to diagnose microscopically, although the occasional lesion will resemble a glioma and require further investigation (Fig. 2.17B).

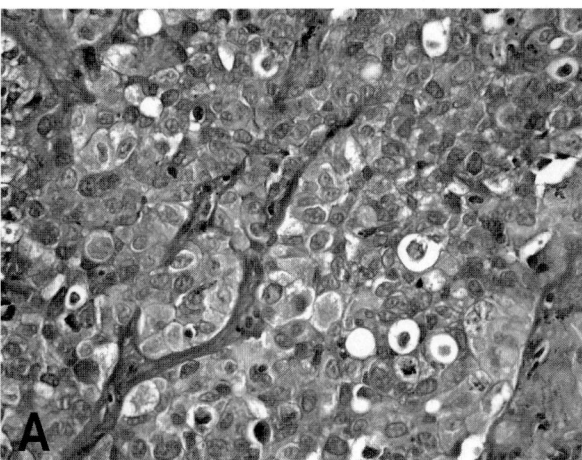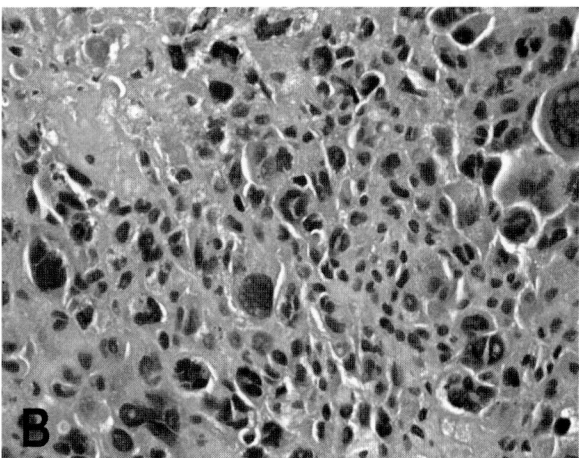

Fig. 2.17. A Metastatic adenocarcinoma showing a typical glandular appearance. +100. **B** Metastatic melanoma with histology similar to that of a glioblastoma. +100

2.12
Tumors of the Cerebellopontine Angle

The numerous types of tissue found in or near the cerebellopontine (CP) angle is reflected in the various types of lesions that can occur in this location. By far, the most common lesion is the schwannoma, a neoplasm arising from Schwann cells found at the oligodendrocyte/Schwann cell junction of the eighth cranial nerve near the opening of the internal auditory meatus. The schwannoma is a slow-growing well-circumscribed mass that usually grows away from the nerve to produce an adjacent perineuronal mass which extends into and fills the CP angle with resulting auditory or vestibular dysfunction. CP angle schwannomas are usually seen in adults before or during middle age. They have a benign behavior although complete resection may be challenging. Schwannomas of the eighth cranial nerve are also called acoustic neuromas. Bilateral acoustic neuroma is a classic finding in patients with neurofibromatosis type 2. Histologically, the schwannoma consists of a combination of two types of histology. The first type is named "Antoni type A" architecture and consists of fascicles and bundles of eosinophilic cells with elongated nuclei (Fig. 2.18A). Cytoplasmic borders are not apparent and the cells often form a linear palisading arrangement called the "Varocay body" (Fig. 2.18A). The second type of architecture is called "Antoni type B" architecture and consists of smaller cells with round hyperchromatic nuclei in a vacuolated background (Fig. 2.18B). Antoni type B histology is thought to represent degenerative changes. The neoplastic Schwann cell shows immu-

noreactivity for the S-100 protein. Schwannomas may show significant pleomorphism although this is not related to aggressive behavior. Rare schwannomas show additional more worrisome malignant features. Other lesions seen in the CP angle include the meningioma, astrocytoma, and metastatic carcinoma. Rarely, a fourth ventricular ependymoma will project through the lateral foramen and into the CP angle.

2.13
Cerebellar Neoplasms

Many neoplasms of the cerebellum have already been discussed. The medulloblastoma and ependymoma are typically seen in this location. In addition, the metastatic carcinoma, astrocytoma, glioblastoma, and lymphoma also occur in the cerebellum. Two additional cerebellar lesions will be discussed: the pilocytic astrocytoma and the hemangioblastoma. The pilocytic astrocytoma is a grade I astrocytic neoplasm seen in the cerebellar hemispheres, hypothalamic region, or optic nerve. Most cases occur in the posterior fossa of young patients and are called juvenile pilocytic astrocytomas. This lesion is not infiltrative and if completely resected will not recur. The term "pilocytic" infers the state of being hairlike and derives from the lesion's possession of bipolar cytoplasmic processes arranged in a vacuolated or even microcystic background (Fig. 2.19A). Mitotic figures should not be found although nuclear pleomorphism may be marked. Acellular refractile eosi-

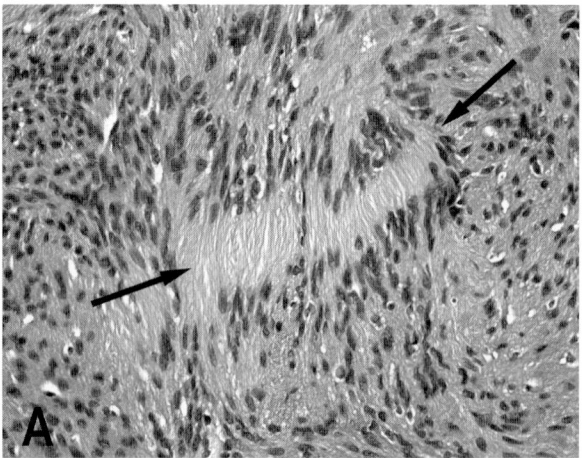
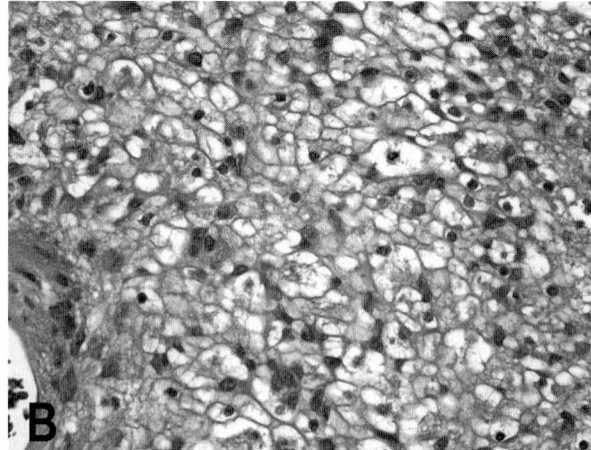

Fig. 2.18A,B. A schwannoma showing "Antoni A" (**A**) and "Antoni B" (**B**) architecture. Note the Verocay body in **A** (*arrows*) and the vacuolated degenerated appearance in **B**. +100

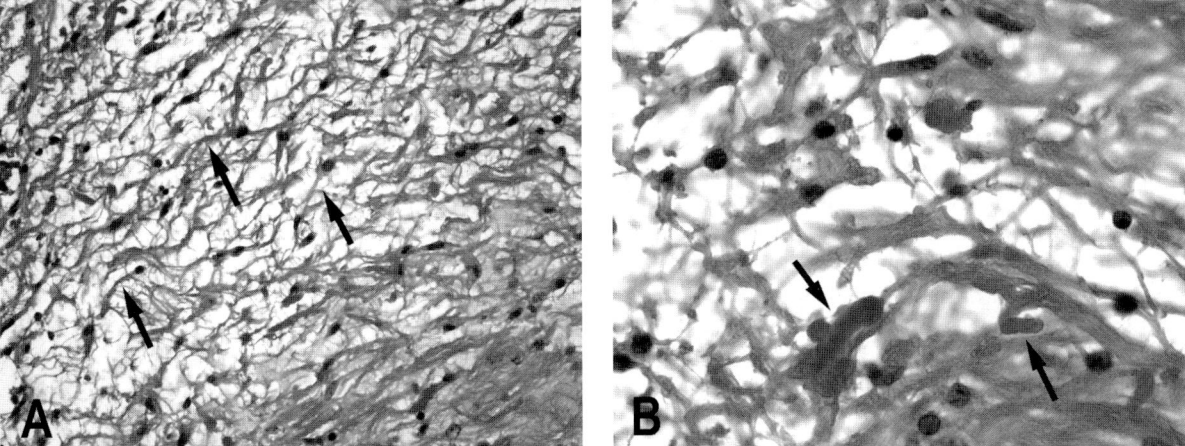

Fig. 2.19. A A pilocytic astrocytoma demonstrating the classic hair-like astrocytes with long bipolar processes (*arrows*). +100. **B** Rosenthal fibers are appreciated at high magnification. +400

nophilic bundles of alpha-B-crystallin, called Rosenthal fibers, are the hallmark of this lesion (Fig. 2.19B). The juvenile pilocytic astrocytoma can be associated with long survival, or even cure, depending on location and the completeness of resection.

The hemangioblastoma is a lesion with an unknown cell of origin. Like other cerebellar lesions, it is not confined to the cerebellum. Lesions outside of the cerebellum should prompt a search for further evidence of von Hippel-Lindau syndrome, an inherited condition associated with, among other things, multiple hemangioblastomas. Hemangioblastomas occur in adults through middle ages and are rarely seen in the young. They arise in the midline or hemispheres of the cerebellum. Growth of the mass leads to ventricular obstruction and hydrocephalus. The lesions are grossly vascular, cystic, and well demarcated. Numerous vascular structures may be present. Some lesions form cysts with solid neural nodules. Microscopically, there are two cell populations that show variable ratios from lesion to lesion. One population consists of endothelial cells and associated pericytes that contribute to the formation of numerous small vascular structures (Fig. 2.20A). The second population consists of stromal cells that are often laden with lipid (Fig. 2.20B). Paraffin embedding during the preparation of microscope sections dissolves the stromal cell intracytoplasmic lipid. An unstained intraoperative frozen section can be submitted for the oil red O histochemical stain for lipids.

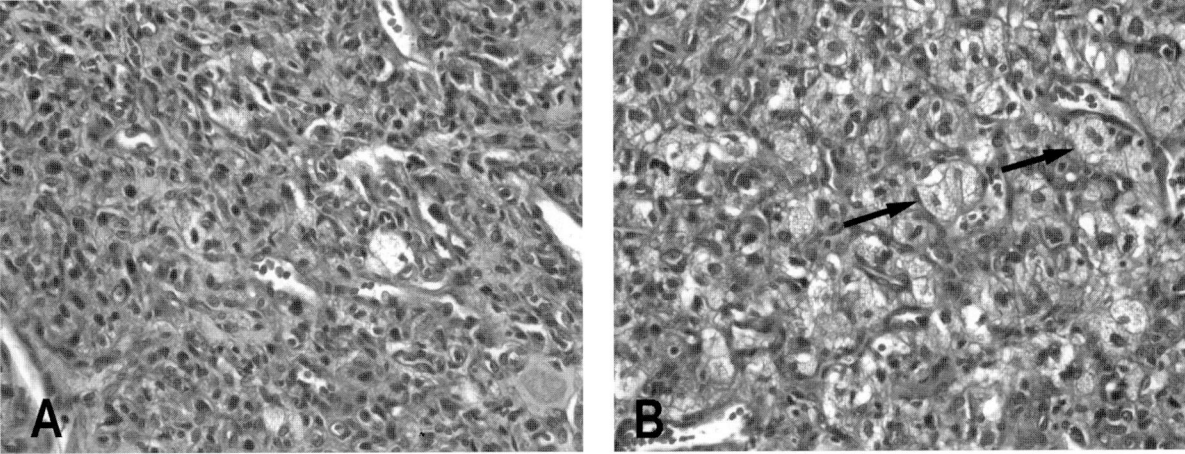

Fig. 2.20A,B. A hemangioblastoma with an endothelial and pericytic component (**A**) and a stromal cell component (**B**). Note the vacuolated stromal cells in **B** (*arrows*). +100

This, in conjunction with appropriate histology and a factor VIII immunostain for confirmation of the endothelial component, is sufficient to make the diagnosis. A helpful, but not required feature, is the presence of mast cells. The origin of the stromal cell is not known (Ho 1984; SHIMURA et al. 1985; BECKER et al. 1989) . On a hematoxylin and eosin (H&E) stained paraffin section, they will appear foamy or vacuolated and may show significant nuclear pleomorphism. Mitotic activity is minimal. Some hemangioblastomas produce erythropoietin and even demonstrate intratumoral hematopoiesis (CHISTI and BANNISTER 1992). The prognosis after total resection is usually favorable for patients without von Hippel-Lindau syndrome.

2.14
Neoplasms of the Pineal Region

Pineal region neoplasia is divided into three categories. One category includes tumors arising from the adjacent neural tissue and includes the astrocytoma and glioblastoma. The second category consists of tumors of the pineal parenchyma and includes the rare pineocytoma and the higher grade pineoblastoma. The pineoblastoma is an undifferentiated neuroblastic tumor and has much in common with the other primitive neuroectodermal tumors described above. This lesion is seen in children and has a poor prognosis. This is in contrast to the more differentiated pineocytoma that affects young adults and provides a much more favorable prognosis. The histology of the pineocytoma is similar to that of normal pineal tissue.

Germ cell neoplasms comprise the third group. These are grossly and microscopically similar to their counterparts arising in gonadal tissue. The germinoma, which is the most common variety, is analogous to the male gonadal seminoma in both histology and response to radiotherapy. Other pineal germ cell tumors are the yolk sac tumor, choriocarcinoma, and teratoma.

2.15
Sellar Neoplasms

Like the CP angle, the list of potential neoplasms in the sella is extensive and includes the germinoma, lymphoma, metastatic carcinoma, meningioma, and astrocytoma. The most common sellar neoplasm is the pituitary adenoma of the anterior pituitary. A comprehensive discussion of the different types of pituitary adenoma is beyond the scope of the chapter. Suffice it to say that such adenomas can arise from any of the endocrine cell types found in the anterior pituitary. Their histology is that of a neuroendocrine tumor and consists of a monomorphic population of cells with salt and pepper chromatin and moderate amounts of cytoplasm (Fig. 2.21A). Prolactinomas are the most common. Coinciding supraphysiological levels of hormone production may produce galactorrhea and amenorrhea in female patients with prolactinomas. Spared from the hormonal effects of prolactin, the prolactinoma of a male patient may grow large enough to compress the central aspects of the overlying optic chiasm and produce a gradual bilateral hemianopsia. Other adenomas may produce growth hormone, adrenocorticotropic hormone (ACTH), thyroid-stimulating hormone (TSH), follicle-stimulating hormone (FSH), or luteinizing hormone (LH). Clinical symptoms depend on the level of hormone production and the local effects of tumor growth. Some adenomas do not produce elevated levels of circulating hormone but may still react with immunohistochemical stains for the pituitary hormones. Classification of pituitary adenomas is done using immunohistochemical criteria. Many adenomas show reactivity for more than one hormone. Common combinations include prolactin/growth hormone and FSH/LH. ACTH-secreting adenomas usually do not show reactivity for other pituitary hormones. These ACTH-producing pituitary adenomas are often small microadenomas that may prove difficult to find during intraoperative frozen section examination. The differential diagnosis during frozen section diagnosis is usually confined to adenoma and non-adenomatous anterior pituitary tissue. Further classification is done after processing.

Small non-neoplastic cysts lined by columnar epithelium can arise in the sella, usually in the intermediate lobe of the pituitary gland. Such cysts, called Rathke's cleft cysts, impinge on the adjacent pituitary or even supracellar structures. Surgical removal is curative.

The craniopharyngioma is a suprasellar lesion seen in children and young adults. Although benign, it demonstrates significant local invasion in an area of complex anatomy. Complete excision is often impossible. The tumor consists of a mass with irregular-shaped cysts filled with viscid cholesterol-laden "crank case oil". The most common histol-

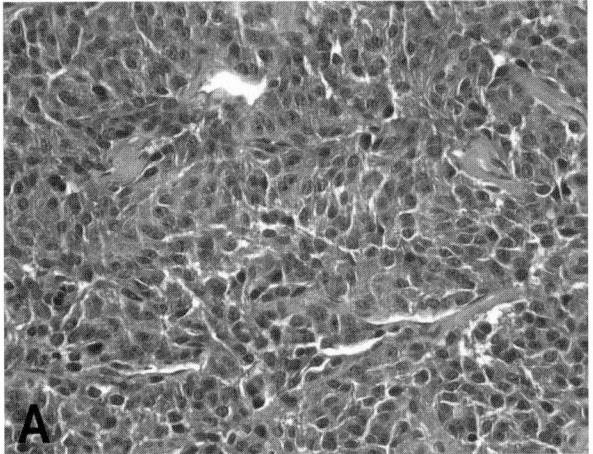 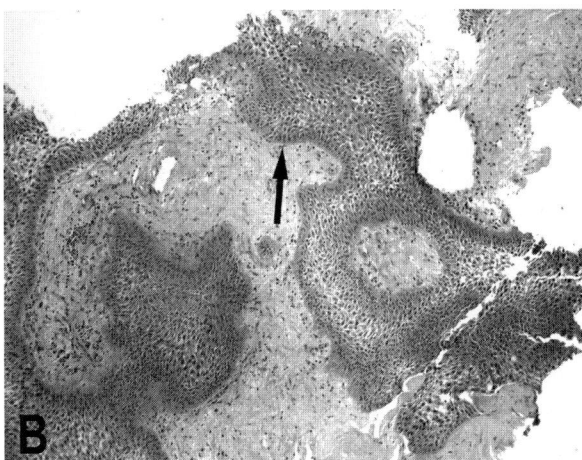

Fig. 2.21. A A pituitary adenoma composed of a monomorphic population of neuroendocrine-like cells. +100. **B** A typical craniopharyngioma with sheets of squamous epithelium and an underlying fibrous stroma. Note that the squamous epithelium lacks an apical surface. +100

ogy is that of squamous epithelial nodules and trabeculae that overlie a fibrous stroma (Fig. 2.21B). Calcification, cholesterol spaces, and degenerative changes are frequent. The surrounding reactive neural tissue may show gliosis with Rosenthal fibers and may resemble a pilocytic astrocytoma if biopsied.

2.16
Spinal Neoplasms

Spinal cord neoplasms are relatively infrequent when compared to intracranial neoplasms. Neoplasms of the spinal cord include many of those that we have already discussed and include the astrocytoma, medulloblastoma, schwannoma, meningioma, metastatic carcinoma, central neurocytoma, ependymoma, oligodendroglioma, hemangioblastoma, and lymphoma. The spinal meningioma is usually confined to female patients. A special variety of ependymoma, called the myxopapillary ependymoma, is confined to the filum terminale or conus medullaris of the spinal cord. This tumor forms a nodular vertically oriented oblong mass among the nerve roots of the cauda equina. Microscopically, it is characterized by papillary structures that are scattered in a mucinous vascular background. It is usually seen in the third and fourth decades of life and will not recur if completely resected. Incomplete resection will result in a slow-growing recurrent lesion associated with a long survival.

2.17
Conclusion

The morphology of CNS tumors is complex with extensive overlap in the appearance of many different lesions. Close teamwork between the surgeon, radiologist, and pathologist is necessary in order to provide the most appropriate environment for accurate diagnostic results. Ultimately, the diagnosis, classification, and grading of CNS neoplasia depends on the information that the pathologist acquires through light microscopic examination of H&E stained sections of neoplastic tissue, a method that has not significantly changed over the last 100 years. The relationship between surgeon, radiologist, and pathologist may soon change as the new millenium progresses with quantum jumps that will radically change the process of CNS tumor analysis. Relevant technological advances include those related to molecular pathology, image analysis, and robotics.

References

Abbott NJ, Reverst PA, Romero IA (1992) Astrocyte endothelial interaction: physiology and pathology. Neuropath Appl Neurobiol 18:424–433

Alguacil Garcia A, Pettigrew NM, Sima AA (1986) Secretory meningioma. A distinct subtype of meningioma. Am J Surg Pathol 10: 102–111

Allegranza A, Ferraresi S, Bruzzone M, et al. (1991) Cerebromeningothelial pleomorphic xanthoastrocytoma. Report on four cases: clinical, radiologic and pathologic features. (Including a case with malignant evolution). Neurosurg Rev 14:43–49

Bailey P, Cushing H, Eisenhardt L (1928) Angioblastic meningiomas. Arch Pathol 6: 953–990

Becker LE, Hinton D (1983) Primitive neuroectodermal tumors of the central nervous system. Hum Pathol 14:538–550

Becker I, Paulus W, Roggendorf W (1989) Histogenesis of stromal cells in cerebellar hemangioblastomas: an immunohistochemical study. Am J Pathol 134:271–275

Burns PE, Jha N, Bain GO (1986) Association of breast cancer with meningioma. A report of five cases. Cancer 58:1537–1539

Burger PC (1995) Revising the World Health Organization (WHO) blue-histological typing of tumors of the central nervous system. J Neurooncol 24:3–7

Chisti MK, Bannister CM (1992) Foci of extramedullary hematopoiesis in a cerebellar hemangioblastoma. Br J Neurosurg 6:157–162

Cioffi F, Buric J, Carnesecchi S, et al. (1996) Spinal meningiomas in pregnancy: report of two cases and review of the literature. Eur J Gynecol Oncol 17:384–388

Coons SW, Johnson PC (1991) Histopathology of astrocytomas: grading, patterns of spread, and correlation with modern imaging modalities. Sem Radiat Oncol 1:2–9

Cooper ERA (1935) The relation of oligocytes and astrocytes in cerebral tumors. J Pathol 41:259–266

Daumas-Duport C, Scheithauer BW, OFallon J, et al. (1988) Grading of astrocytomas. A simple and reproducible method. Cancer 62:2152–2165

Guerrieri C, Jarlsfelt I (1993) Ependymoma of the ovary. A case report with immunohistochemical, ultrastructural, and DNA cytometric findings, as well as histogenetic considerations. Am J Surg Pathol 17:623–632

Hart MN, Petito CK, Earle KM (1974) Mixed gliomas. Cancer 33:134–140

Ho K-L (1984) Ultrastructure of cerebellar capillary hemangioblastoma. I. Weibel-Palade bodies and stromal cell histogenesis. J Neuropathol Exp Neurol 43:592–608

Hsa DW, Louis DN, Efird JT, et al. (1997) Use of MIB-1 (Ki-67) immunoreactivity in differentiating grade II and grade III gliomas. J Neuropathol Exp Neurol 56:857–865

Kepes JJ, Rubinstein LJ, Eng LF (1979) Pleomorphic xanthoastrocytoma: a distinctive meningiocerebral glioma of young subjects with relatively favorable prognosis. A study of 12 cases. Cancer 44:1839–1852

Kepes JJ (1986) Presidential address: the histopathology of meningiomas. A reflection of origins and expected behavior? J Neuropathol Exp Neurol 45:95–107

King P, Cooper PN, Malcolm AJ (1993) Soft tissue ependymoma: a report of three cases. Histopathology 22:394–396

Kleihues P, Burger PC, Scheithauer BW (1993) The new WHO classification of brain tumors. Brain Pathol 3:255–268

Kochi N, Budka H (1987) Contribution of histiocytic cells to sarcomatous development of the gliosarcoma. An immunohistochemical study. Acta Neuropathol (Berl) 73:124–130

Langley OK (1990) Ion exchange at the node of Ranvier. Histochem J 100:113–123

Little NS, Morgan MK, Eckstein RP (1994) Primary ependymoma of a cranial nerve: Case report. J Neurosurg 81:792–794

Norenberg MD, Martinez-Hernandez A (1979) Fine structural localization of glutamine synthetase in astrocytes of the rat brain. Brain Res 161:303–310

Parkin DM, Muir CS (1992) Cancer incidence in five continents. Comparability and quality of data. International Agency for Research on Cancer (IARC) Scientific Publications 120:45–173

Paulson OB, Newman EA (1987) Does the release of potassium from astrocyte end-feet regulate cerebral blood flow? Science 237:896–898

Prayson RA, Estes ML (1995) Protoplasmic astrocytoma. A clinicopathological study of 16 tumors. Am J Clin Pathol 103:705–709

Rorke LB (1983) The cerebellar medulloblastoma and its relationship to primitive neuroectodermal tumors. J Neuropath Exp Neurol 42:1–15

Schoenberg BS, Christine BW, Whisnant JP (1975) Nervous system neoplasms and primary malignancies of other sites. The unique association between meningiomas and breast cancer. Neurol 25:705–712

Shimura T, Hirano A, Llena JF (1985) Ultrastructure of cerebellar hemangioblastoma: some new observations on the stromal cells. Acta Neuropathol (Berl) 67:6–12

Slowik F, Jellinger K, Gaszo L, et al. (1985) Gliosarcomas: histological, immunohistochemical, ultrastructural, and tissue culture studies. Acta Neuropathol (Berl) 67:201–210

Weldon-Linne CM, Victor TA, Groothuis DR, et al. (1983) Pleomorphic xanthoastrocytoma. Ultrastructural and immunohistochemical study of a case with a rapidly fatal outcome following surgery. Cancer 52:2055–2063

3 Molecular Biology

REINER CLASS

CONTENTS

3.1 Introduction

The initial event in the generation of all central nervous system (CNS) tumors is the transformation of a normal cell into a cancer cell. The biological processes associated with this development eventually lead to the survival of cancer cells and to the formation of a solid tumor. Steps involved in this tumorigenic process include the cell's escape from the immune system surveillance (i.e., antitumor response), aberrant proliferation and multiplication, tumor cell invasion, and angiogenesis. Over the past decade, much has been learned about the basic genetic events and the molecular biology underlying the development of CNS cancers. This review attempts to describe the molecular biology of CNS tumors, highlighting potential targets for therapeutic interventions.

The initial step in tumorigenesis is undoubtedly of genetic nature (e.g., mutation, deletion, amplification). However, it is not the gene that ultimately carries the burden of a cell's life, it is the protein coded by the gene. Even if an aberrant gene expresses a protein with an abnormal biological activity, a tumor cell can only develop if that particular event results in a survival advantage. Most mutations, however, remain silent and will not result in the generation of a tumor. Paying tribute to the cellular workhorses, the proteins, the focus of this review will be less on the genomics and more on the proteomics of CNS tumors. It should be emphasized that none of the areas outlined below should be viewed as isolated and independent events but rather as one link in an enormous network of intertwined pathways, subject to control and regulation at multiple levels. It is unrealistic to believe that targeting one structure with therapeutic regimens will by all means result in the eradication of the tumor.

3.2 Proteomics of CNS Tumorigenesis

3.2.1 Proliferation and Multiplication

Successful tumor growth is a consequence of the imbalance of the host's antitumor defense and tumor growth kinetics. Regarding proliferation, a pathological situation can arise by either increasing the cell's multiplication rate and/or by extending its biological lifetime. Both events will inevitably result in a net increase of the tumor mass. The four areas with major importance in this regard are cell cycle control, tumor suppressor proteins, growth factors and their receptors, and apoptosis.

R. CLASS, PhD
Assistant Professor, Department of Radiation Oncology, MCP Hahnemann University, Broad and Vine Street, Philadelphia, PA 19102-1192, USA

3.2.2
Cell Cycle Control

The field of cell cycle control has grown rapidly over the past few years with the discovery of regulatory proteins that work on "checkpoints" at the transition from one cell cycle stage into the next. These proteins ultimately decide whether or not, and how fast, the cell can pass through the different cell cycle stages towards mitosis, or whether a suicide process termed apoptosis is activated to remove a damaged and potentially harmful cell from the organism. The importance of checkpoints in CNS tumors is underscored by the fact that at least one tumorigenic change associated with the G_1 checkpoint has been reported for the majority (85%) of glioblastomas (UEKI et al. 1996; ICHIMURA et al. 1996; HE et al. 1995).

Cyclin-dependent kinases (cdk) are specialized cell cycle proteins that are constitutively expressed within the cell. Cdk can form heterodimeric complexes with their binding partners, the cyclins, which are generally synthesized only upon stimulation. The cyclin–cdk complex represents the biologically active component, the monomers are inactive. Each progression from one cell cycle stage into the next is positively and/or negatively regulated by the coordinated activity (e.g., activation or repression) of these cell cycle proteins. The central regulatory events are the phosphorylation of downstream effector proteins and/or the transcriptional control of protein expression. Together, they control cell progress throughout the cell cycle into mitosis.

The complexity of this system can best be demonstrated with molecular events occurring at the G_1 cell cycle checkpoint (Fig. 3.1): Mitotic stimuli (e.g., growth factors) force the quiescent cell to leave the G_0 stage, enter G_1 stage and progress through S, G_2, and M phase. This positive stimulation results in the synthesis of the cyclins D1, -2, -3, which in turn activate cdk4, -6. The cyclin D/cdk heterodimer forms a heterotrimer with the proliferating cell nuclear antigen (PCNA). This complex phosphorylates its target protein, the retinoblastoma protein (rb), the transcriptional product of the Rb tumor suppressor gene. In its hypophosphorylated form, rb is usually tightly bound to its natural ligand, the transcription

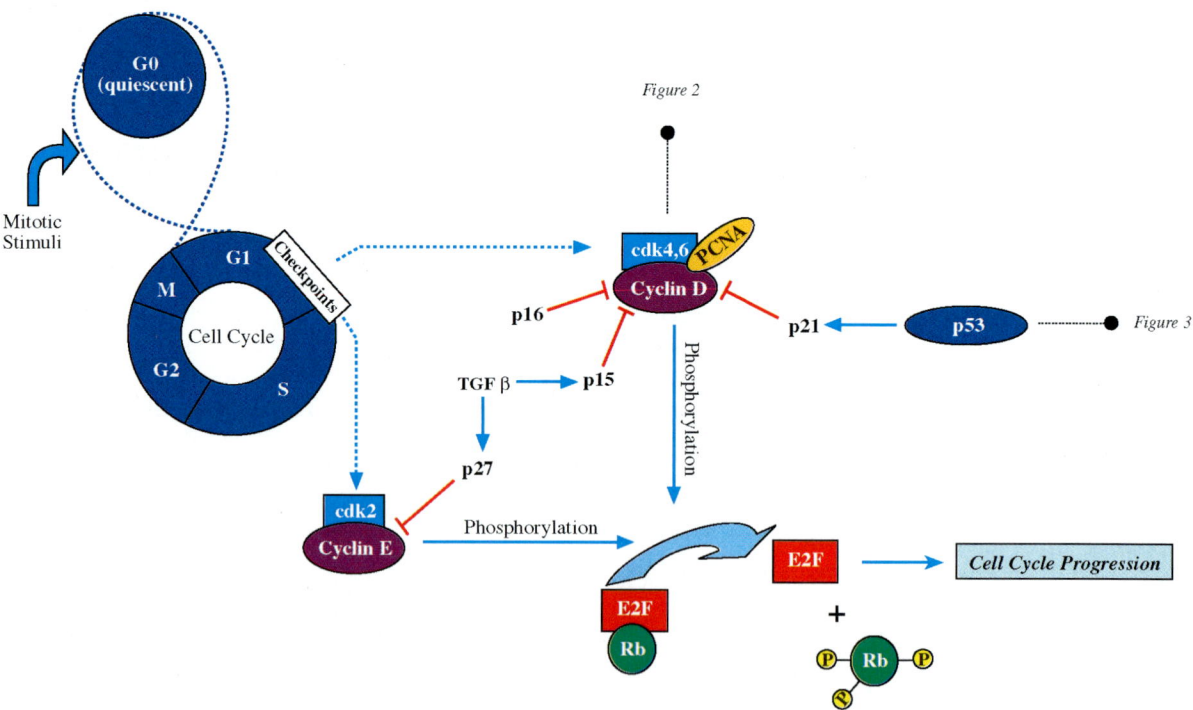

Fig. 3.1. G_1 cell cycle checkpoint. The transition from G_1 to S phase is tightly controlled at the G_1 checkpoint. Cyclin D and cyclin E form a complex with cdk4,-6 and cdk2, respectively. PCNA is additionally required for cyclin D/cdk3, -4. The active cyclin–ckd complex phosphorylates rb, which in turn releases the transcription factor E2F. Deliberated E2F binds to promoter regions of proteins necessary for cell cycle progression. Cki inhibits the formation of an active cdk-cyclin complex by binding to cyclin. P15, p16, and p21 bind to cyclin D, p27 binds to cyclin E. p21 is induced by wild-type p53

factor E2F. In its hyperphosphorylated form, rb is not able to maintain this binding and subsequently releases E2F from the complex. The free E2F immediately binds to the promoter region of a selected group of genes and induces the transcription of downstream proteins needed to cross the G_1 cell cycle restriction point into S phase.

If cyclins are already synthesized, cells have another, posttranslational, mechanism to control cell cycle progression. Cdk4, -6 are also negatively regulated by p15 and p16, two small proteins found on chromosome 9p21. They belong to a group of well-characterized cdk-inhibitory proteins (cki) that prevent activation of cdk by binding to cdk4 in competition with already synthesized cyclin D (SERRANO et al. 1993) (Fig. 3.2). Tampering with the inhibitory activity of cki results in the loss of control to attenuate cell cycle progression.

Although p15 and p16 are rarely mutated in CNS tumors, loss by homozygous deletion has been reported (UEKI et al. 1996; SATO et al. 1996; ICHIMURA et al. 1996; TSUZUKI et al. 1996; SCHMIDT et al. 1997). Deletions of p16, however, have not been found in primary medulloblastomas or meningiomas, restricting the p16 loss to tumors of glial origin (BARKER et al. 1997). In the absence of cki, observed

in 40% of glioblastomas (SCHMIDT et al. 1994) and 20% of anaplastic astrocytomas (ICHIMURA et al. 1996), the uninhibited cdk–cyclin complex maintains a hyperphosphorylated rb. This in turn keeps E2F in its released form, always allowing the cell to proceed through the G_1 checkpoint. Besides cki, cdk are subject to regulation on multiple levels (Fig. 3.2) and their expression is altered in many CNS tumors.

Some gliomas have been found to contain the P15 and P16 genes but still do not possess active forms of the proteins. Here, the biological activity of p15/16 is regulated on the transcriptional level by gene repression. These tumor cells guarantee proliferation through silencing the gene by hypermethylation and chromatin condensation (COSTELLO et al. 1996), thus preventing the synthesis of the two cki.

In contrast to above-mentioned loss of negative regulation of the cell cycle by p15/16, a constitutive expression of positive regulators has been seen in a subset of glioma cells where cdk4 is highly overexpressed due to gene amplification (HE et al. 1995). This event leaves rb phosphorylated and dissociated from E2F, pushing the cell past the G_1 checkpoint into S phase.

Another important regulatory protein with relevance in CNS tumors is the cyclin D/cdk inhibitor

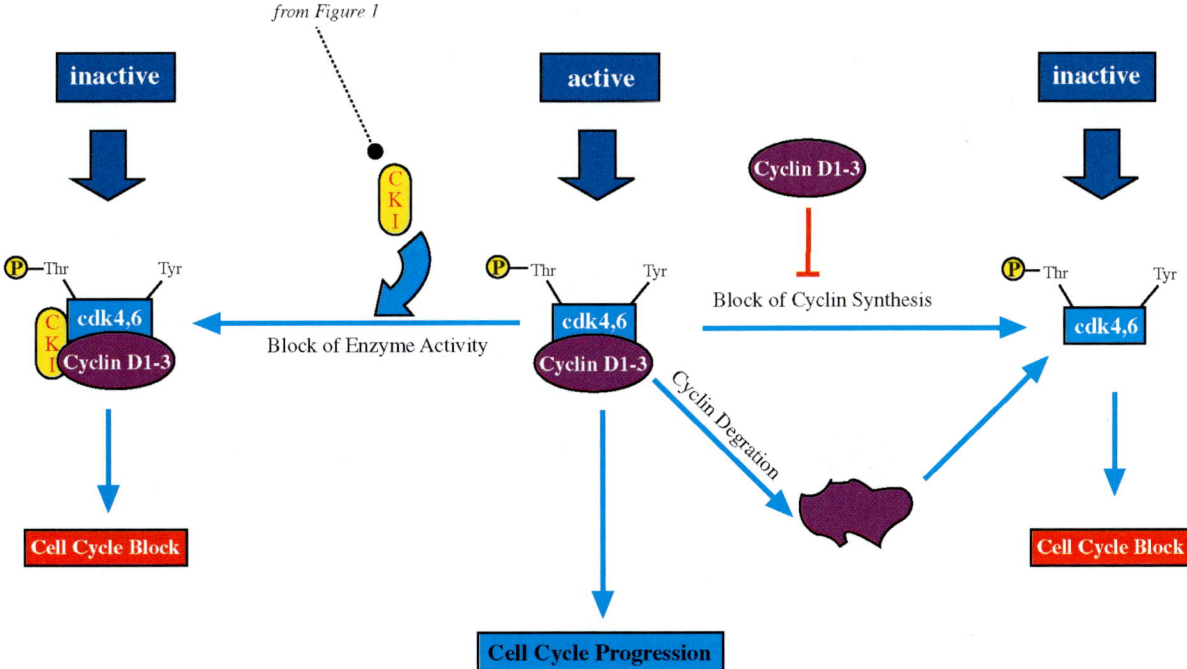

Fig. 3.2. Regulation of the biological activity of cdk. Cdk in complex with cyclin represents the enzymatically active form of the protein. The complex is capable of phosphorylating target proteins such as rb, causing cell cycle progression. Inactive forms can be induced by proteolytic cyclin degradation, block of cyclin synthesis, or the production of specific inhibitors, cki

p21 (also known as SDI1, WAF1, CIP1, CAP20, MDA6, or PIC1). The P21 promoter contains two elements recognizable by the tumor suppressor protein p53 (see below). Binding of wild-type p53 to these elements upregulates transcription of p21 (EL-DEIRY et al. 1994). Apparently, p21 blocks cell cycle progression in normal cells by inactivating several cdk at the G_1 cell cycle checkpoint (Fig. 3.1). Although mutations or deletions are rarely observed in glial tumors, p21 is a major downstream target of p53, which is mutated in 50% of all cancer cells and approximately 60% of astrocytomas (REMPEL 1998). Besides being a direct downstream target of p53, p21 is also regulated by transcription factors other than p53, since it can be induced in p53-negative cells (MICHIELI et al. 1994) and its expression level is independent of the p53 mutational status (DIRKS et al. 1997). Although the exact contribution of p21 in cell cycle disturbances of CNS tumors is not exactly known, it seems to have a more important role than previously believed.

The last cell-cycle-related protein with relevance in CNS tumors is the cki p27, first identified in transforming growth factor (TGF)-b-induced growth arrested cells (KOFF et al. 1993). This protein shares significant homology with p21 above described and is also functionally related, sharing high affinity to a wide range of cdk. p27 (as well as p15) transcription is induced by TGF-b and inhibits cell cycle progression after the onset of the S phase by binding to cdk2/cyclin E complex (Fig. 3.1), similar to other cki described above.

3.2.3
Tumor Suppressor Protein p53

The p53 protein has been termed the cellular gatekeeper for growth and division (LEVINE 1997). It plays a central role in cell cycle control, cell differentiation, apoptosis, and angiogenesis of CNS tumors either by interacting with other proteins or as a transcription factor. The p53 protein arrests the cell cycle both at the G_1 checkpoint and the G_2/M phase transition (AGARWAL et al. 1995)(Fig. 3.3). The loss of p53-mediated cell cycle control is believed to contribute to the development of many CNS tumors (FULCI and VAN MEIR 1999).

P53 gene mutations have been described in 67% of anaplastic astrocytomas and 41% of glioblastoma multiforme (TADA et al. 1997) but only in 13% of oligodendrogliomas, 11% medulloblastomas, and none in other CNS tumors (NOZAKI et al. 1998). The importance of wild-type p53 is underscored by the finding that an adenovirus-mediated overexpression of wild-type p53 induces rapid cell death in glioma cells, accomplished by apoptosis (GOMEZ-MANZANO et al. 1996).

One of the major functions of the p53 protein is to stop the cell cycle in case of DNA damage (e.g., by ionizing radiation or drugs). This allows the cellular DNA repair machinery to fix the damage. However, if the damage is beyond the repair capabilities of the cell, p53 triggers apoptosis to remove the potentially harmful cell from the organism. A mutated p53 will not be able to accomplish this task, thus allowing damaged (as well as cancer) cells to remain within the organism, eventually resulting in a pathological situation.

The 20-kb P53 gene contains a pax-5 binding site within the untranslated first exon (STUART et al. 1995a) and is translated to a 53-kDa nuclear phosphoprotein. The pax-5 protein is believed to act as a downregulator of P53 transcription, keeping p53 protein levels low. STUART et al. reported a significant overexpression of pax-5 in high-grade gliomas, effectively bypassing p53-induced cell cycle block (STUART et al. 1995a). High pax-5 levels have been correlated with increased malignancy in astrocytomas and also with overexpression of the epidermal growth factor receptor (EGFR) gene (STUART et al. 1995b).

P53 transcription is also important from a therapeutic point of view since it can be induced by DNA-damaging agents including chemotherapeutics (KASTAN et al. 1991) and ionizing radiation (MALTZMAN and CZYZYK 1984). Unfortunately, such therapeutic approaches occasionally favor the expansion of cancer cells with vital p53 mutations thus inducing progression to a more malignant cell type (VAN MEIR 1996).

The transcription of the P53 gene itself is regulated by mdm2 in an autoregulatory feedback loop: p53 induces transcription of the MDM2 gene and its translation to the mdm2 oncoprotein, which in turn suppresses the P53 gene by binding to and concealing the P53 DNA binding domain, thus preventing further transcription(KUBBUTAT et al. 1997). Since the biological half-life of p53 is only 20–30 min, the cellular p53 protein level is rapidly reduced (HAUPT et al. 1997). MDM2 gene amplifications and mdm2 overexpression have been found in 48% of astrocytomas (KORKOLOPOULOU et al. 1997) and in the majority of primary glioblastomas, but far less frequently in progressing glioblastomas (HAUPT et al. 1997).

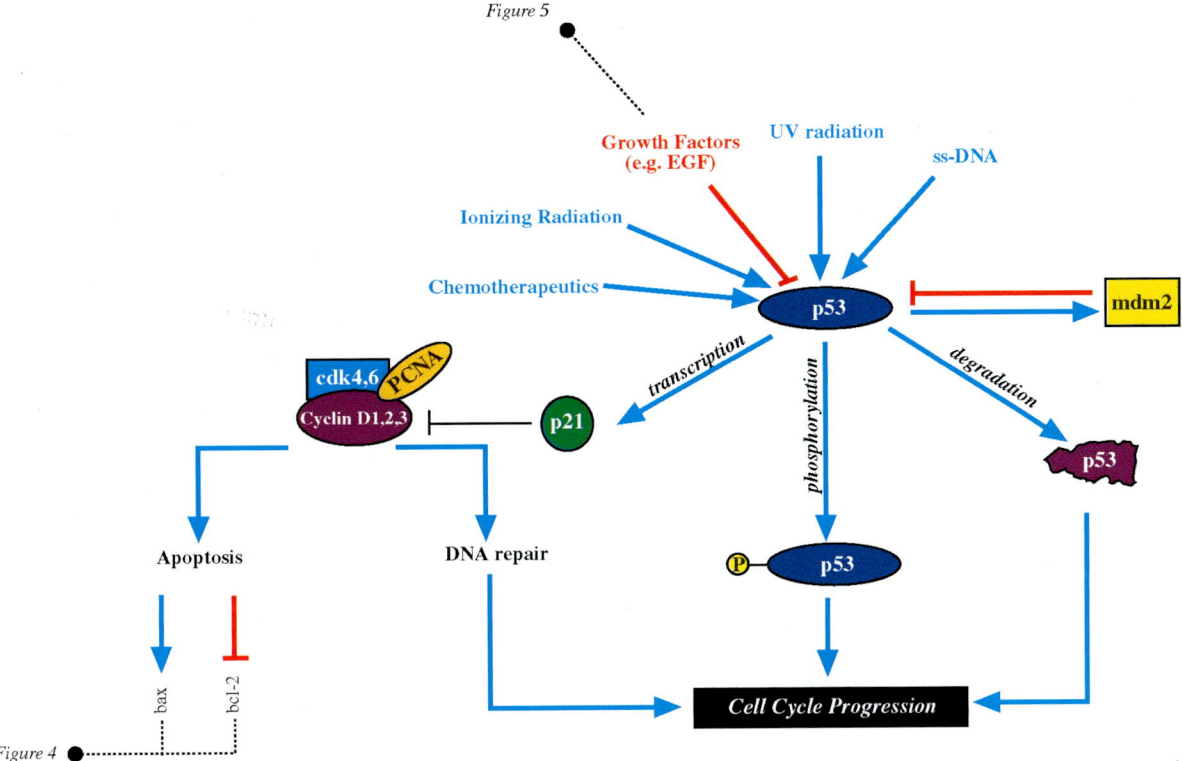

Fig. 3.3. Tumor suppressor protein p53. Wild-type p53 induces transcription of the p53 inhibitor mdm2 and the cki p21. p21 blocks cell cycle progression by binding to cyclin D. Transcription of p53 is induced by chemotherapeutics, ionizing radiation, UV-radiation, and ss-DNA. Growth factors such as EGF are major inhibitors of p53 transcription. P53 can be inactivated posttranslationally by phosphorylation or by proteolytic degradation. After a p21-induced cell cycle block, p53 triggers either DNA repair or apoptosis depending on the amount of DNA damage sustained. Apoptosis is mediated through members of the bcl-2 protein family

Despite the undoubtedly pivotal role of p53 in tumorigenesis, recent studies revealed discrepancies between the proposed function of p53 and the situation in vivo: cells with a functional wild-type p53 unexpectedly failed to respond to cancer therapy, whereas cells lacking wild-type p53 could be killed easily. Many oncologists have recently challenged the early theory that anticancer drugs and radiation treatment cause a p53-dependent apoptotic death of cancer cells, especially in solid tumors (FINKEL 1999). Again, as already alluded to, no single molecule can be viewed as an isolated component that is not subject to regulation. The vast cross-linking of the network enables the cell in specific stress situations to activate alternative pathways, to bypass faulty proteins (such as mutated p53), to functionally substitute proteins, to silence aberrant proteins, or to stimulate backup mechanisms. Only if all of these solutions fail and the cell runs out of options, apoptosis might be initiated. The p53 inactivation often seen in gliomas and its dominant position in cell cy-

cle control make it a crucial factor in most tumorigenic processes and an attractive tool for therapeutic approaches (FUEYO et al. 1998).

3.2.4
Apoptosis

Apoptosis or programmed cell death is made possible by an intrinsic network of proteins. Once activated, apoptosis is supposed to eliminate potentially dangerous cells from the host system. Cells may opt for this pathway when their DNA is damaged beyond repair by radiation or cytotoxic drugs. In the past few years, much information on regulatory proteins, their function and connection within the apoptosis machinery has become available (for an excellent review on apoptosis, see WHITE 1996). Growth factor withdrawal, Rb inactivation, and c-myc induction (KO and PRIVES 1996) are all known to induce apoptosis. The potential of drugs and radiation to trigger apoptosis in cancer cells has recently been debated by oncologists (FINKEL 1999). Due to the complexity of the topic, the focus of this chapter will be on those apoptotic processes that are known to be involved in CNS tumors.

As already mentioned earlier, p53 is considered the key molecule in the decision whether a cell holds the cell cycle progression and allows for DNA repair or whether it activates the apoptosis machinery, ultimately resulting in the fragmentation of the DNA and cell death.

In general, apoptosis can be triggered in a p53-dependent or p53-independent way.

3.2.4.1
p53-Dependent Induction of Apoptosis

Although many members of the p53-initiated apoptotic cascade are still unknown, the pathway involves the activation of pro-apoptotic signaling proteins (e.g., bax), or the repression of contra-apoptotic proteins (e.g., bcl-2, bak, bcl-X_L, and NF-B) on the transcriptional level (MIYASHITA and REED 1995; OWEN-SCHAUB et al. 1995) (Figs. 3.3, 3.4).

As outlined earlier, glioma cells with wild-type p53 are generally capable of making a p53-dependent decision between cell cycle arrest followed by DNA damage repair, cell cycle progression, or apoptosis (LI et al. 1997a). Studies on brain tumor specimens demonstrated that apoptotic cells can be readily detected (PATSOURIS et al. 1996) and that malignant gliomas are susceptible to apoptosis induced by antibody stimulation of Fas-L (WELLER et al. 1995). Unfortunately, although many human gliomas that have been treated with ionizing radiation show a p53-mediated G_1 cell cycle arrest, they do not induce apoptosis (YOUNT et al. 1996), pointing at critical changes in the apoptosis machinery. A possible explanation for this phenomenon was found in three human GBM cell lines that, upon irradiation, failed to induce p53-dependent bax expression (SHU et al. 1998). Alterations like these obviously have the potential to silence the ability of a tumor cell to induce programmed cell death, eventually resulting in the formation of a tumor mass.

3.2.4.2
p53-Independent Induction of Apoptosis

Besides p53-dependent apoptosis induction, several p53-independent pathways exist with major implications in CNS tumors. Here, apoptosis can be triggered either by positive signals such as activation of Fas-R (by Fas-L), TNF-R (by TNF), and perforin-secreting CTL, or by negative signals such as lack of growth factor receptor activation (ASHKENAZI and DIXIT 1998). The following events are summarized in Fig. 3.4.

3.2.4.2.1
CELL DEATH FOLLOWING POSITIVE SIGNALS
Fas (Apo-1, CD95) and tumor necrosis factor receptor-1 (TNF-R1) belong to the family of NGF/TNF-R superfamily (BEUTLER and VAN HUFFEL 1994) and stimulate apoptosis upon binding of effector ligands (Fas-L, TNF-a, and antibodies). The binding of such ligands is transmitted to the carboxy-terminal part of the receptor containing a cytoplasmic "death domain" (DD). Upon activation, the DD interacts with cytosolic adapter proteins that also contain DDs of their own (FRASER et al. 1996): Fas-R interacts with the "Fas-associated protein with death domain" (FADD, MORT1) and the "receptor interacting protein" (RIP), whereas TNF-R interacts with the "TNF-R1-associated death domain protein" (TRADD) and RIP (CHINNAIYAN et al. 1996). FADD and TRADD contain an N-terminal domain needed for signal transduction called "death effector domain" (DED), which activates procaspase 8. From this point on downstream, the activation pathways of TRADD and FADD converge in the activation of further procaspases. Caspases are *cysteinyl as*partate-specific *protein*ases that are synthesized as inactive procaspases called zymogens. The latter require proteolytic cleavage to convert to an active proteolytic enzyme. At this stage, the apoptosis pathway lacks additional downstream regulatory elements and reaches the "point of no return". The subsequent cascade of events culminates in chromatin condensation, the activation of an endonuclease that generates short DNA fragments, cytoplasmic boiling, the generation of apoptotic bodies, and, ultimately, cell death (Fig. 3.5).

There is sufficient evidence that alterations in the apoptotic network, which would result in prolonged cell survival and a net increase in tumor cell numbers, are implicated in the formation of most CNS tumors. Several in vitro studies proved that malignant glioma cells generally express CD95 (Fas) and that apoptosis can be induced by anti-CD95 antibodies (WELLER et al. 1994). Although many tumor cells contain a functioning cascade required for Fas-mediated apoptosis, RT-PCR studies on 34 astrocytic tumors have demonstrated a strong correlation between Fas mRNA expression and the malignancy

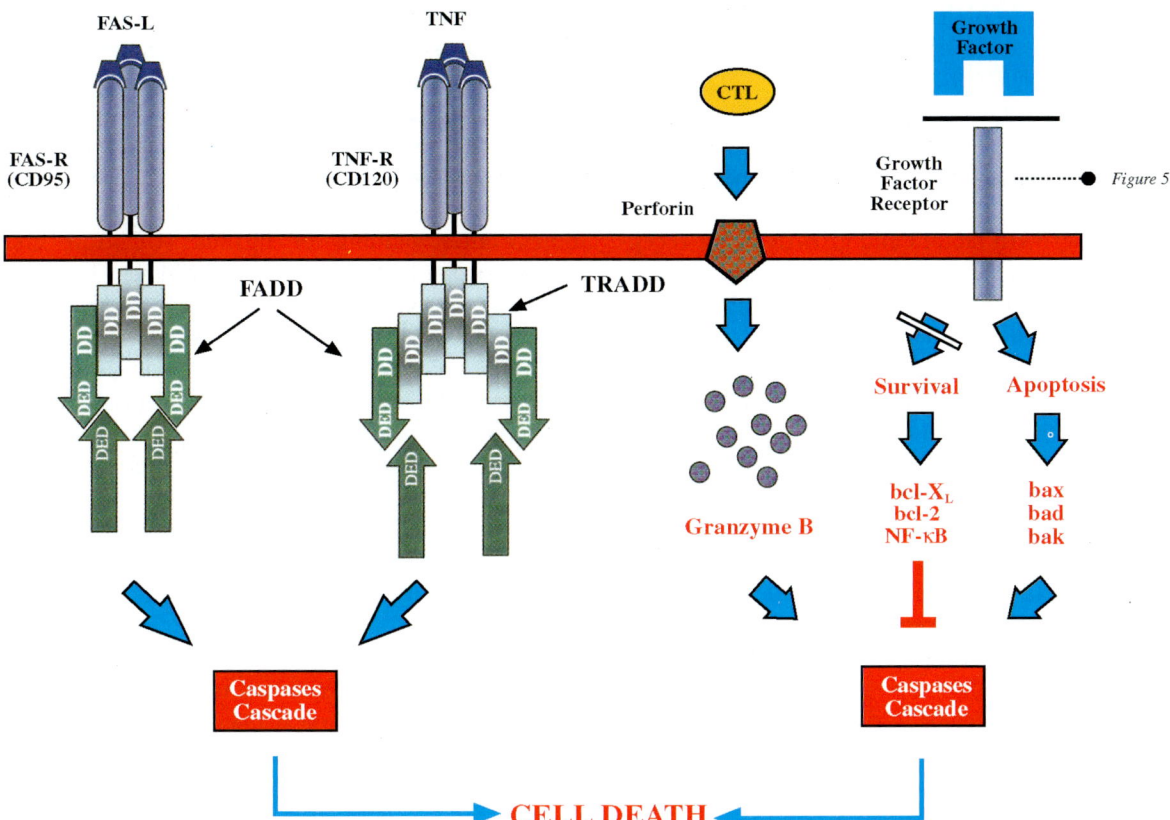

Fig. 3.4. Apoptosis network. Apoptosis is induced by positive signals such as binding of Fas-L or TNF to their receptors CD95 or TNF-R, respectively. The binding signal is transmitted to a cytoplasmic death domain (*DD*), which recruits the DD containing FADD or TRADD, respectively. The death effector domain (*DED*) of FADD and TRADD interact with DED-containing proteins that induce the activation of the caspases cascade. The cascade ends in the activation of a DNA endonuclease that cleaves the DNA in distinct fragments, causing cell death. CTL can induce apoptosis by inserting the perforin membrane channel in the membrane of target cells and by inducing the secretion of granzyme B, a caspase cascade-inducing protease. The lack of positive, growth-stimulating signals (e.g., EGF) causes a shift from the survival to the apoptosis signals, executed by members of the bcl-2 protein family. Pro-apoptotic proteins (e.g., bax, bad, bak) activate the caspases cascade and induce cell death

grade of tumors (TACHIBANA et al. 1995). Apparently, high-grade glioma cells avoid the induction of apoptosis by inhibiting the expression of pro-apoptosis proteins on the translational level. It is also possible that pro-apoptotic proteins are expressed but that this event is compensated by expression of even more pro-survival proteins. In both cases, the glioma cells continue to proliferate by making sure that the survival signals outnumber the death signals.

3.2.4.2.2
Cᴇʟʟ Dᴇᴀᴛʜ Fᴏʟʟᴏᴡɪɴɢ Lᴀᴄᴋ ᴏꜰ Pᴏꜱɪᴛɪᴠᴇ Sɪɢɴᴀʟꜱ
In order to survive, a cell has to maintain a supercritical level of pro-survival proteins (e.g., bcl-2, bcl-X_L) that are in constant battle with death-promoting proteins (e.g., bax, bak, and bad). Survival proteins het-

erodimerize with their death partner thereby preventing them from inducing the death cascade (OLTVAI et al. 1993). Tumor cells can prevent apoptotic cell death by overexpression of growth factors such as EGF, PDGF, IGF, and FGF and their respective receptors (see Sect. 3.2.5), effectively tipping the balance in favor of pro-survival proteins. A lack of such growth factors induces cell death through a cascade of events that involve the proteolytic activation of several caspases and ultimately results in DNA fragmentation (Fig. 3.4).

Instead of overexpressing growth factor receptors, tumor cells can mimic their function by overexpressing one of their downstream second messengers. Bcl-2, for example, a pro-survival protein that is induced upon growth factor receptor activation, is more abundant in high-grade (III, IV) gliomas than low-grade gliomas (I, II).

3.2.5
Growth Factors and Growth Factor Receptors

Numerous growth factors and growth factor receptors have been implicated in growth stimulation of CNS tumors (REMPEL 1998). Gliomas and meningiomas are known to upregulate expression of fibroblast growth factor (FGF) and insulin-like growth factor (IGF), whereas platelet-derived growth factor (PDGF) is upregulated in many gliomas, meningiomas and ependymomas (the same accounts for their respective receptors). Vascular epithelial growth factor (VEGF), which also plays a critical role in angiogenesis (see Sect. 3.5), is overexpressed in glioblastomas. All growth factor receptors implicated in CNS tumors are transmembrane proteins and belong to the same family of receptor tyrosine kinases (COHEN et al. 1982) (Fig. 3.5).

Since the EGFR seems to play a major role in the generation of malignant forms of CNS tumors, espe-

cially glioblastoma multiforme (GBM), a more detailed analysis of its molecular biology seems warranted. Other growth factor receptors use similar activation cascades.

EGFR is a member of the class I receptor tyrosine kinase family with a cysteine-rich extracellular domain, which is important for stabilization of receptor dimers after binding of ligands (ULLRICH and SCHLESSINGER 1990). The human EGFR gene has been localized to chromosome 17p11–12 and appears to play a major role in proliferation as well as transformation. The initial event in the activation of the EGFR leading to cell proliferation is the binding of EGF or other agonists (e.g., monoclonal antibodies). The signal transduction is accomplished by receptor oligomerization on the cell surface (SCHLESSINGER 1988) and subsequently through the shc-grb2-*ras* pathway (PRIGENT et al. 1996). The oncogene v-*erbB* encodes for a truncated EGFR that is missing most of the extracellular domain and 32 C-terminal amino acids. Although this mutated EGFR has lost its EGF-binding capabilities, it retains the tyrosine kinase activity that is pivotal for growth stimulation (YAMAMOTO et al. 1983), rendering it a constitutively activated growth factor receptor.

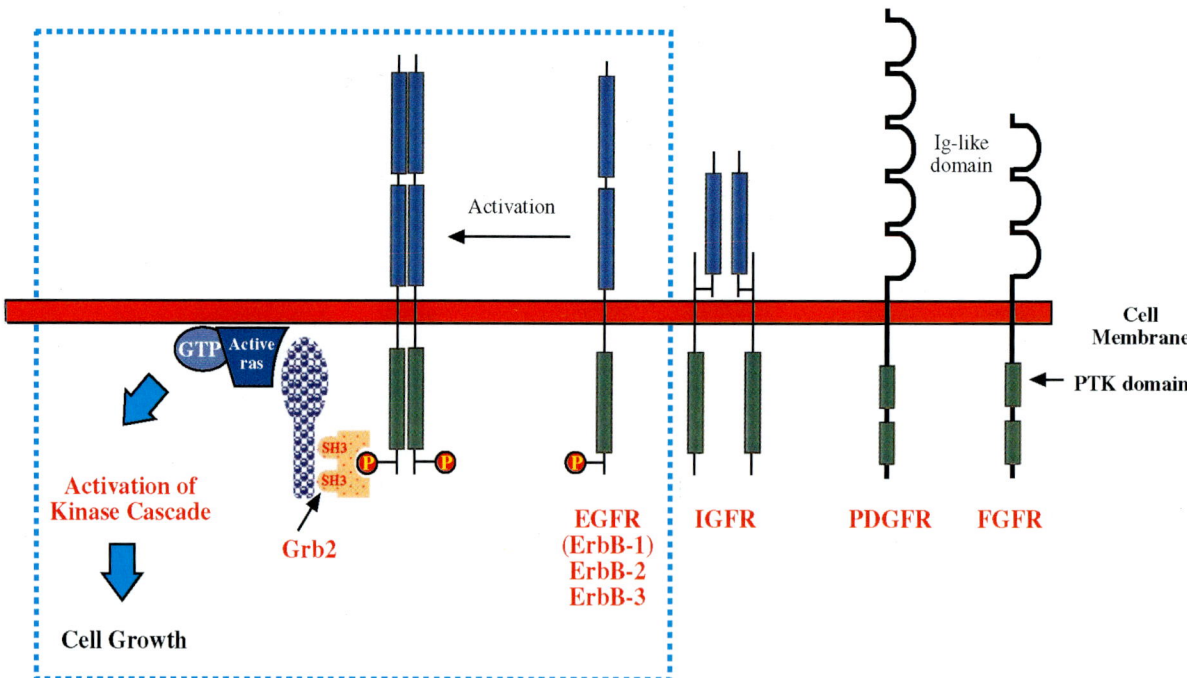

Fig. 3.5. Growth factor receptors. FGFR, PDGFR, IGFR. and EGFR belong to the family of tyrosine kinase receptors that translate the binding of their respective ligands into a phosphorylation of a target protein. A phosphorylated EGFR attracts the SH3-domain of Grb2 that has high affinity to the EGFR-receptor phosphotyrosine. The grb2-SH3 complex is translocated to the cell membrane and comes in close proximity of the inactive membrane standing ras-oncoprotein. Cell growth is induced by ras through activation of a kinase cascade

Glioblastomas and some malignant astrocytomas often show two types of EGFR abnormalities: gene amplification of the wild-type EGFR (40–50% of all glioblastomas) and expression of the mutated EGFR, termed DEGFR or EGFRvIII. The former usually translates into overexpression of the EGFR protein on the cell surface whereas the latter is characterized by a lack of the extracellular EGF-binding domain (NISHIKAWA et al. 1994) and a constitutively activated tyrosine kinase. Interestingly, overexpression of EGFR is usually not accompanied by p53 mutations, indicating that both events represent independent mechanisms to bypass growth control (REMPEL 1998). It has been suggested that secondary GBMs are characterized by PDGF overexpression, CDK4 gene amplification, and loss of heterozygosity (LOH) for P53, Rb, P15 and P16, whereas primary glioblastomas exhibit MDM2 and EGFR gene amplification (WATANABE et al. 1996). The increased proliferation rate of EGFR mutants is often accompanied by a marked decrease in apoptotic cell death mediated by the death protein bcl-X_L (NAGANE et al. 1996).

The EGFR overexpression and the mutant EGFR have been viewed as the Achilles' heel of GBM. Several clinical trials use monoclonal antibodies linked to toxins or radioactive isotopes to specifically target the malignant cell population, some of them with great success (see Chap. 25 of this volume).

Besides EGF and EGFR, PDGF and their respective receptors are also overexpressed in all grades of gliomas, indicating the presence of an autocrine self-stimulatory loop similar to the one described for EGFR (HERMANSON et al. 1996).

The following chapters will highlight events that occur post transformation and are a prerequisite for a successful establishment of a CNS tumor.

3.3
Antitumor Immune Responses and Immune Escape

Under normal circumstances, a potent cellular antitumor response is activated by the host immune system once a sufficient number of tumor cells has been generated. In CNS tumors, however, this immune response is inept to efficiently fight off the cancer cells. Currently, only limited patient information is available on this topic, but a number of promising studies in cell culture and animals have been performed that help us understand the molecular biology involved in these processes.

Although the CNS is known as an immune-privileged organ that possesses an immunosuppressive microenvironment, cellular antitumor responses have repeatedly been documented. Antigen-specific cytotoxic T cells (CTL), lymphokine-activated killer (LAK) cells, or natural killer (NK) cells usually mediate these responses. Antigen-specific CTL that show cytotoxicity towards allogeneic GBM cell lines are frequently detected in anaplastic astrocytomas and glioblastomas (TSURUSHIMA et al. 1996). The fact that these tumors are rarely controlled by CTL led to the assumption that these patients have a T helper cell activity that is insufficient to provide adequate help to the CTL (PERRIN et al. 1999). BHONDELEY et al. (1988) indeed reported a significant decrease both in the absolute number of circulating $CD3^+$ T cells and $CD4^+$ T helper cells in 39 glioma patient. $CD8^+$ suppressor T cell and B cell numbers remained unchanged (BHONDELEY et al. 1988). Other researchers found a significantly expanded population of immature, nonkilling CTL precursor cells instead of fully activated tumor-specific CTL. They hypothesized that the CNS microenvironment suppressed the normal CTL development thereby preventing an efficient antitumor response (GORDON et al. 1997). In another study, CTL have been sensitized in vivo against glioma cells and subsequently expanded in vitro. Systemically administered CTL eradicated or slowed down the progression of an intracerebral glioma demonstrating the clinical potential of adoptive CTL transfer (MERCHANT et al. 1997).

There is also some evidence that signals required to stimulate T cells such as costimulatory molecules (B7-1, B7-2), human lymphocyte antigens (HLA), and intercellular adhesion molecules (ICAM-1) are downregulated in critical stages of tumor development. Experiments with genetically altered glioma cells expressing these antigens led to a substantial growth inhibition of subcutaneously transplanted tumor cells. Unfortunately, those located in the brain remained unharmed (JOKI et al. 1999). Another study compared major histocompatibility complex (MHC)-I positive with negative glioma cells and found that only the MHC-I positive cells could be rejected by the host, whereas the MHC-I negative cells escaped the T-cell-mediated immunosurveillance and grew progressively in the brain (YAMASAKI et al. 1996).

Several attempts have been undertaken to enhance host antitumor responses by using tumor antigen-pulsed dendritic cells (DC), the most potent professional antigen-presenting cells (APC). In an animal model, perilesional and intratumoral infiltration of CD8[+] and CD4[+] T cells could be significantly increased by DC-based vaccines (ASHLEY et al. 1997). Furthermore, the DC vaccination also resulted in the generation of mature tumor-killing CTL (LIAU et al. 1999).

The above experiments suggest that antitumor responses, especially the generation of antigen-specific CTL, are indeed elicited in vivo. Due to circumstances not completely understood, however, CNS tumors are not receptive to their activity. The limited accessibility of the immune privileged CNS, the suppressive microenvironment of CNS tumors, and the downregulation of costimulatory molecules in the tumor cells have been made responsible for this effect.

3.4
Invasion

The process of invasion renders most CNS tumors difficult to cure. Better understanding of the molecular biology underlying this process might lead to improved therapeutic approaches (GIESE and WESTPHAL 1996). In order to invade a tissue, cells have to degrade a physical barrier formed by the extracellular matrix (ECM) of cells, which consists mainly of laminin, fibronectin, vitronectin, collagen I–IV, heparin sulfate, hyaluronate, and glycosaminoglycans. A functional ECM is important in the regulation of cell behavior, tissue formation, and homeostasis. Proteolytic disassembly of the ECM has been implicated in several diseases including tumors (LUKASHEV and WERB 1998). The process of invasion appears not to be random in nature; rather, CNS tumor cells seem to migrate along the path of blood vessels and myelinated axons (GIESE and WESTPHAL 1996). The cascade of events encompassing tumor cell invasion can be defined as a three-step process: receptor-mediated tumor cell adhesion to ECM, proteolytic digestion of the ECM by tumor-cell-secreted metalloproteinases (MMP), and locomotion of the tumor cells into the newly-created space (LIOTTA 1986).

3.4.1
Receptor-Mediated Adhesion to ECM

Cell adhesion or cell–cell contact is mediated by the receptor proteins cadherins, Ig superfamily proteins such as intracellular adhesion molecule (ICAM) or nerve cell adhesion molecule (NCAM), selectins, and integrins. The latter play a critical role in the recognition process between tumor cells and ECM by mediating cell attachment to the ECM (HYNES 1987). The binding of glioma cells to integrins does not only confer ECM adhesion, it also triggers several second messengers, including Ca^{2+} influx and activation of protein kinases (GUAN and SHALLOWAY 1992), which are directly linked to the subsequently required dissemination steps (i.e., proliferation, migration and proteinase secretion). In addition to the already existing ECM in the CNS, glial tumor cells are capable of creating their own permissive environment by secreting an autologous ECM that greatly facilitates tumor cell adherence and locomotion. It has been shown that glioma cells deposit tenascin, vitronectin, several collagen types, fibronectin, and laminin in their immediate surrounding (BOURDON and RUOSLAHTI 1989; GLADSON and CHERESH 1991; LIESI et al. 1983). The expression of these proteins is believed to play an important role in glioma cell invasion and has been positively correlated with tumor grade (HIGUCHI et al. 1993). In vitro experiments with tumor-derived ECM as artificial matrices demonstrated that glioma cells can render their immediate neighborhood more favorable for tumor spread by secreting appropriate ECM proteins (GIESE et al. 1995).

3.4.2
ECM Degradation by Tumor-Secreted Proteinases

Once tumor cells have gained access to tissues by means of ECM adhesion, specific ECM-degrading proteinases are synthesized and secreted into the immediate vicinity of the cells in preparation of an invasion into the tissue. Tumor cells are capable of producing several classes of ECM-specific proteinases such as matrix metalloproteinase (MMP), serine proteinase, cysteine proteinase, aspartic proteinase, and endoglycosidase (ENNIS and MATRISIAN 1994; ROMANIC and MADRI 1994). MMPs such as gelatinase and collagenase (APODACA et al. 1990), and more recently, matrilysin and stromelysin (NAKANO et al. 1993), have been described to be secreted by glioma cells. Within the family of serine proteases, the plasminogen activators (PA) urokinase-type (u-PA) and tissue-type PA (t-PA) have been implicated in glioma cell invasion (GROSS et al. 1988; SAWAYA et al. 1991). Cathepsin B, a member of the cysteine proteinases, has also been found in glioblastomas, but its role remains unclear (REMPEL et al. 1994).

The specific inhibitors TIMP-1, -2, and -3, can block the ECM-degrading activity of MMPs. TIPMs have been found to be expressed at high levels in the periphery of brain tumors compared to a low expression in their center regions, and have also been inversely correlated with tumor cell invasiveness (HALAKA et al. 1983). Ultimately, the balance between ECM-degrading enzymes and their inhibitors will determine the invasiveness of the particular tumor cells.

3.4.3
Locomotion

Numerous studies have shown that malignant glioma cells are inherently capable of migration to remote areas of the brain. Single glioma cells were observed to migrate in culture system at a speed of 12 μm/h (CHICOINE and SILBERGELD 1995), whereas the dissemination speed could be increased fivefold by using a culture surface that was coated with suitable (see above) ECM proteins (GIESE et al. 1995). As outlined previously (Sect. 3.4.1), glial tumor cells synthesize a variety of ECM proteins that support their dissemination.

Cell motility in general also requires a sharp reduction in intracellular adhesion factors that would slow down or even arrest a cell on its migratory path. The "deleted in colorectal cancer" (DCC) protein, coded by a putative tumor suppressor gene on chromosome 18q21, belongs to the family of neural cell adhesion molecules. Immunohistochemical analysis of 57 human resected astrocytic tumors revealed that 94% of the low-grade astrocytomas were positive for this protein compared to only 66% of the high-grade glioblastomas (REYES-MUGICA et al. 1997), indicating a correlation between protein expression, reduced cell–cell contact, and tumor cell motility.

Another factor that enhances tumor cell locomotion by reducing cell–cell contacts has been found in PTEN, the product of a putative tumor suppressor gene located on chromosome 10q23 (LI et al. 1997b). PTEN has a high degree of homology to tensin, a protein that interacts with actin filaments at focal adhesions. Mutations in the PTEN gene, resulting in increased cell motility, have been detected in 31% (13/42) of glioblastoma cell lines (LI et al. 1997b).

The neurofibromatosis 2 (NF2) gene product, merlin, is another tumor suppressor protein that affects cell motility, adhesion, and dissemination (GUTMANN et al. 1999). The NF2 gene has been mapped to chromosome 22q, a region known for frequent LOH in sporadic meningiomas, ependymomas, and schwannomas (GUTMANN et al. 1997, 1999). The loss of merlin causes reduced cell–cell contact and has been associated with the pathogenesis of these cells. Regarding locomotion, however, merlin alterations do not appear to play a critical role in neoplastic astrocytes since astrocytomas express much higher levels of this protein than normal astrocytes (GUTMANN et al. 1997).

A protein has recently been identified that is involved in tumor cell dissemination. This "secreted protein acidic and rich in cysteine" (SPARC) is a secreted ECM protein implicated in cell adhesion and, more importantly, migration (SAGE 1997). SPARC is absent in virtually all noninvasive glial tumors but highly expressed in invasive tumors, regardless of differentiation grade (REMPEL et al. 1999).

Dissemination of glioma cells preferentially occurs along myelinated fiber tracts and ECM-containing structures such as basement membranes of blood vessels without disruption of the adjacent tissue (GIESE et al. 1998). Besides previously mentioned ECM glycoproteins, glioma cells also express high levels of chondroitin sulfate, heparan sulfate, and hyaluronate (BERTOLOTTO et al. 1986). Hyaluronate has several charged groups that can bind many water molecules thus occupying a space that is larger than expected from its molecular mass. The molecular function of this molecule is, once secreted into the extracellular lumen, to create a water-filled space that can be occupied by migratory cells (e.g., glioma cells). Cells are attracted to this area by cell surface receptors for hyaluronate, CD44 (or H-CAM) and RHAMM (ARUFFO et al. 1990; SHERMAN et al. 1994). Glioma cells synthesize hyaluronate, hyaluronate receptors (i.e., CD44), and other hyaluronate-binding proteins (DELPECH et al. 1993; KUPPNER et al. 1992), which allows them not only to create their own space but also to direct themselves (and other disseminating glioma cells) into that newly created space. The phenomenon of migration is characteristic for the embryonic development of tissues including the CNS. Malignant cells seem to activate this primitive feature as a consequence of their tumorigenic transformation. The genetic events that trigger this dedifferentiation to a more immature phenotype are still poorly understood. In view of the above summarized intrinsically high mobility of the majority of glial tumor cells, the efficacy of locoregional therapy as the sole treatment approach should be reevaluated.

3.5
Angiogenesis

If a CNS tumor mass continues to grow, it will eventually reach a point where macromolecular nutrients cannot reach all cells by diffusion. A capillary transport system is needed providing nutrients even to the innermost tumor cells. Angiogenesis plays an important role in the progression of gliomas into more malignant stages (PLATE and RISAU 1995). CNS tumors trigger this neovascularization process by stimulating neighboring endothelial cells to produce angiogenesis inducers and/or by downregulating inhibitors thereof (HANAHAN and FOLKMAN 1996). One of the most potent angiogenesis-promoting factors is VEGF, whereas thrombospondin-1 is a potent angiogenesis inhibitor. VEGF, a growth factor highly specific for endothelial cells (GUERIN and LATERRA 1997), is significantly upregulated in gliomas and GBMs. Immunohistochemical staining of tumor biopsies showed that the VEGF protein localized to the cytoplasm of tumor cells (TAKANO et al. 1996), the peripheral microvessels, and around necrotic areas of the tumor (PLATE and RISAU 1995; TAKANO et al. 1996). To complete the paracrine VEGF loop, receptors for VEGF (also called flt-1), have been found in large numbers on endothelial cells of high-grade gliomas (PLATE and RISAU 1995). Recently, investigators could stop glioblastoma angiogenicity by using an antisense VEGF expression construct (CHENG et al. 1996). Additionally, the positive angiogenesis effectors, EGFR and the basic fibroblast growth factor (bFGF), have been found upregulated in glial tumors.

Besides the upregulation of angiogenesis-promoting factors such as VEGF, flt-1, EGFR, and bFGF, the potent angiogenesis inhibitor thrombospondin-1 is often downregulated in glial tumors. This protein is coded on chromosome 10 and is victim of the LOH of chromosome 10 (see Sect. 3.2.5), often seen in primary and secondary GMB (HSU et al. 1996). These data clearly show the consequences of the molecular defects occurring in CNS tumors, contributing to solid tumor angiogenesis.

3.6
Conclusion

This chapter outlines in great detail the most important characteristics of CNS tumors regarding their proteomics, proliferation and multiplication, cell cycle control, the function of tumor suppressor proteins, apoptosis, growth factor and growth factor receptors, antitumor immune responses, immune escape, invasion, adhesion to ECM and its degradation by tumor-secreted proteinases, locomotion, and finally, angiogenesis. Identification of the molecular changes that result in the formation of a pathological situation will undoubtedly help to customize future treatment options. Nevertheless, one should always keep in mind that none of the areas outlined above should be viewed as isolated and independent events, but rather as one member of a vast network of interconnected pathways with multiple levels of regulations and feedback loops. Therefore, targeting one single entity in the network is unlikely to cure the cancer. Future developments in the diagnosis and molecular fingerprinting of the tumor have great potential to enhance therapeutic regimens.

References

Agarwal M L, Agarwal A, Taylor W R and Stark G R (1995) p53 controls both the G2/M and the G1 cell cycle checkpoints and mediates reversible growth arrest in human fibroblasts. Proc Natl Acad Sci U S A 92: 8493–8497

Apodaca G, Rutka J T, Bouhana K, Berens M E, Giblin J R, Rosenblum M L, McKerrow J H and Banda M J (1990) Expression of metalloproteinases and metalloproteinase inhibitors by fetal astrocytes and glioma cells. Cancer Res 50: 2322–2329

Aruffo A, Stamenkovic I, Melnick M, Underhill C B and Seed B (1990) CD44 is the principal cell surface receptor for hyaluronate. Cell 61: 1303–1313

Ashkenazi A and Dixit V M (1998) Death receptors: signaling and modulation. Science 281: 1305–1308

Ashley D M, Faiola B, Nair S, Hale L P, Bigner D D and Gilboa E (1997) Bone marrow-generated dendritic cells pulsed with tumor extracts or tumor RNA induce antitumor immunity against central nervous system tumors. J Exp Med 186: 1177–1182

Barker F G, Chen P, Furman F, Aldape K D, Edwards M S and Israel M A (1997) P16 deletion and mutation analysis in human brain tumors. J Neurooncol 31: 17–23

Bertolotto A, Magrassi M L, Orsi L, Sitia C and Schiffer D (1986) Glycosaminoglycan changes in human gliomas. A biochemical study. J Neurooncol 4: 43–48

Beutler B and van Huffel C (1994) Unraveling function in the TNF ligand and receptor families [comment]. Science 264: 667–668

Bhondeley M K, Mehra R D, Mehra N K, Mohapatra A K, Tandon P N, Roy S and Bijlani V (1988) Imbalances in T cell subpopulations in human gliomas. J Neurosurg 68: 589–593

Bourdon M A and Ruoslahti E (1989) Tenascin mediates cell attachment through an RGD-dependent receptor. J Cell Biol 108: 1149–1155

Cheng S Y, Huang H J, Nagane M, Ji X D, Wang D, Shih C C, Arap W, Huang C M and Cavenee W K (1996) Suppression of glioblastoma angiogenicity and tumorigenicity by inhibition of endogenous expression of vascular endothelial growth factor. Proc Natl Acad Sci U S A 93: 8502–8507

Chicoine M R and Silbergeld D L (1995) Assessment of brain tumor cell motility in vivo and in vitro. J Neurosurg 82: 615–622

Chinnaiyan A M, Tepper C G, Seldin M F, O'Rourke K, Kischkel F C, Hellbardt S, Krammer P H, Peter M E and Dixit V M (1996) FADD/MORT1 is a common mediator of CD95 (Fas/APO-1) and tumor necrosis factor receptor-induced apoptosis. J Biol Chem 271: 4961–4965

Cohen S, Ushiro H, Stoscheck C and Chinkers M (1982) A native 170,000 epidermal growth factor receptor-kinase complex from shed plasma membrane vesicles. J Biol Chem 257: 1523–1531

Costello J F, Berger M S, Huang H S and Cavenee W K (1996) Silencing of p16/CDKN2 expression in human gliomas by methylation and chromatin condensation. Cancer Res 56: 2405–2410

Delpech B, Maingonnat C, Girard N, Chauzy C, Maunoury R, Olivier A, Tayot J and Creissard P (1993) Hyaluronan and hyaluronectin in the extracellular matrix of human brain tumour stroma. Eur J Cancer 7: 1012–1017

Dirks P B, Hubbard S L, Murakami M and Rutka J T (1997) Cyclin and cyclin-dependent kinase expression in human astrocytoma cell lines. J Neuropathol Exp Neurol 56: 291–300

El-Deiry W S, Harper J W, O'Connor P M, Velculescu V E, Canman C E, Jackman J, Pietenpol J A, Burrell M, Hill D E, Wang Y and et al. (1994) WAF1/CIP1 is induced in p53-mediated G1 arrest and apoptosis. Cancer Res 54: 1169–1174

Ennis B W and Matrisian L M (1994) Matrix degrading metalloproteinases. J Neurooncol 18: 105–109

Finkel E (1999) Does cancer therapy trigger cell suicide? [news]. Science 286: 2256–8

Fraser A, McCarthy N and Evan G I (1996) Biochemistry of cell death. Curr Opin Neurobiol 6: 71–80

Fueyo J, Gomez-Manzano C, Yung W K and Kyritsis A P (1998) The functional role of tumor suppressor genes in gliomas: clues for future therapeutic strategies. Neurology 51: 1250–1255

Fulci G and Van Meir E G (1999) p53 and the CNS: tumors and developmental abnormalities. Mol Neurobiol 19: 61–77

Giese A, Laube B, Zapf S, Mangold U and Westphal M (1998) Glioma cell adhesion and migration on human brain sections. Anticancer Res 18: 2435–2447

Giese A, Loo M A, Rief M D, Tran N and Berens M E (1995) Substrates for astrocytoma invasion. Neurosurgery 37: 294–301; discussion 301–302

Giese A and Westphal M (1996) Glioma invasion in the central nervous system. Neurosurgery 39: 235–50; discussion 250–252

Gladson C L and Cheresh D A (1991) Glioblastoma expression of vitronectin and the alpha v beta 3 integrin. Adhesion mechanism for transformed glial cells. J Clin Invest 88: 1924–1932

Gomez-Manzano C, Fueyo J, Kyritsis A P, Steck P A, Roth J A, McDonnell T J, Steck K D, Levin V A and Yung W K (1996) Adenovirus-mediated transfer of the p53 gene produces rapid and generalized death of human glioma cells via apoptosis. Cancer Res 56: 694–699

Gordon L B, Nolan S C, Cserr H F, Knopf P M and Harling-Berg C J (1997) Growth of P511 mastocytoma cells in BALB/c mouse brain elicits CTL response without tumor elimination: a new tumor model for regional central nervous system immunity. J Immunol 159: 2399–2408

Gross J L, Behrens D L, Mullins D E, Kornblith P L and Dexter D L (1988) Plasminogen activator and inhibitor activity in human glioma cells and modulation by sodium butyrate. Cancer Res 48: 291–296

Guan J L and Shalloway D (1992) Regulation of focal adhesion-associated protein tyrosine kinase by both cellular adhesion and oncogenic transformation. Nature 358: 690–692

Guerin C and Laterra J (1997) Regulation of angiogenesis in malignant gliomas. Exs 79: 47–64

Gutmann D H, Giordano M J, Fishback A S and Guha A (1997) Loss of merlin expression in sporadic meningiomas, ependymomas and schwannomas. Neurology 49: 267–270

Gutmann D H, Sherman L, Seftor L, Haipek C, Hoang Lu K and Hendrix M (1999) Increased expression of the NF2 tumor suppressor gene product, merlin, impairs cell motility, adhesionand spreading. Hum Mol Genet 8: 267–275

Halaka A N, Bunning R A, Bird C C, Gibson M and Reynolds J J (1983) Production of collagenase and inhibitor (TIMP) by intracranial tumors and dura in vitro. J Neurosurg 59: 461–466

Hanahan D and Folkman J (1996) Patterns and emerging mechanisms of the angiogenic switch during tumorigenesis. Cell 86: 353–364

Haupt Y, Maya R, Kazaz A and Oren M (1997) Mdm2 promotes the rapid degradation of p53. Nature 387: 296–299

He J, Olson J J and James C D (1995) Lack of p16INK4 or retinoblastoma protein (pRb), or amplification- associated overexpression of cdk4 is observed in distinct subsets of malignant glial tumors and cell lines. Cancer Res 55: 4833–4836

Hermanson M, Funa K, Koopmann J, Maintz D, Waha A, Westermark B, Heldin C H, Wiestler O D, Louis D N, von Deimling A and Nister M (1996) Association of loss of heterozygosity on chromosome 17p with high platelet-derived growth factor alpha receptor expression in human malignant gliomas. Cancer Res 56: 164–171

Higuchi M, Ohnishi T, Arita N, Hiraga S and Hayakawa T (1993) Expression of tenascin in human gliomas: its relation to histological malignancy, tumor dedifferentiation and angiogenesis. Acta Neuropathol 85: 481–487

Hsu S C, Volpert O V, Steck P A, Mikkelsen T, Polverini P J, Rao S, Chou P and Bouck N P (1996) Inhibition of angiogenesis in human glioblastomas by chromosome 10 induction of thrombospondin-1. Cancer Res 56: 5684–5691

Hynes R O (1987) Integrins: a family of cell surface receptors. Cell 48: 549–554

Ichimura K, Schmidt E E, Goike H M and Collins V P (1996) Human glioblastomas with no alterations of the CDKN2 A (p16INK4 A, MTS1) and CDK4 genes have frequent mutations of the retinoblastoma gene. Oncogene 13: 1065–1072

Joki T, Kikuchi T, Akasaki Y, Saitoh S, Abe T and Ohno T (1999) Induction of effective antitumor immunity in a mouse brain tumor model using B7-1 (CD80) and intercellular adhesive molecule 1 (ICAM-1; CD54) transfection and recombinant interleukin 12. Int J Cancer 82: 714–720

Kastan M B, Onyekwere O, Sidransky D, Vogelstein B and Craig R W (1991) Participation of p53 protein in the cellular response to DNA damage. Cancer Res 51: 6304–6311

Ko L J and Prives C (1996) p53: puzzle and paradigm. Genes Dev 10: 1054–1072

Koff A, Ohtsuki M, Polyak K, Roberts J M and Massague J (1993) Negative regulation of G1 in mammalian cells: inhibition of cyclin E- dependent kinase by TGF-beta. Science 260: 536–539

Korkolopoulou P, Christodoulou P, Kouzelis K, Hadjiyannakis M, Priftis A, Stamoulis G, Seretis A and Thomas-Tsagli E (1997) MDM 2 and p53 expression in gliomas: a multivariate survival analysis including proliferation markers and epidermal growth factor receptor. Br J Cancer 75: 1269–1278

Kubbutat M H, Jones S N and Vousden K H (1997) Regulation of p53 stability by Mdm2. Nature 387: 299–303

Kuppner M C, Van Meir E, Gauthier T, Hamou M F and de Tribolet N (1992) Differential expression of the CD44 molecule in human brain tumours. Int J Cancer 50: 572–577

Levine A J (1997) p53, the cellular gatekeeper for growth and division. Cell 88: 323–331

Li H, Lochmuller H, Yong V W, Karpati G and Nalbantoglu J (1997a) Adenovirus-mediated wild-type p53 gene transfer and overexpression induces apoptosis of human glioma cells independent of endogenous p53 status. J Neuropathol Exp Neurol 56: 872--878

Li J, Yen C, Liaw D, Podsypanina K, Bose S, Wang S I, Puc J, Miliaresis C, Rodgers L, McCombie R, Bigner S H, Giovanella B C, Ittmann M, Tycko B, Hibshoosh H, Wigler M H and Parsons R (1997b) PTEN, a putative protein tyrosine phosphatase gene mutated in human brain, breast, and prostate cancer [see comments]. Science 275: 1943–1947

Liau L M, Black K L, Prins R M, Sykes S N, DiPatre P L, Cloughesy T F, Becker D P and Bronstein J M (1999) Treatment of intracranial gliomas with bone marrow-derived dendritic cells pulsed with tumor antigens. J Neurosurg 90: 1115–1124

Liesi P, Dahl D and Vaheri A (1983) Laminin is produced by early rat astrocytes in primary culture. J Cell Biol 96: 920–924

Liotta L A (1986) Tumor invasion and metastases–role of the extracellular matrix: Rhoads Memorial Award lecture. Cancer Res 46: 1–7

Lukashev M E and Werb Z (1998) ECM signalling: orchestrating cell behaviour and misbehaviour. Trends Cell Biol 8: 437–441

Maltzman W and Czyzyk L (1984) UV irradiation stimulates levels of p53 cellular tumor antigen in nontransformed mouse cells. Mol Cell Biol 4: 1689–1694

Merchant R E, Baldwin N G, Rice C D and Bear H D (1997) Adoptive immunotherapy of malignant glioma using tumor-sensitized T lymphocytes. Neurol Res 19: 145–152

Michieli P, Chedid M, Lin D, Pierce J H, Mercer W E and Givol D (1994) Induction of WAF1/CIP1 by a p53-independent pathway. Cancer Res 54: 3391–3395

Miyashita T and Reed J C (1995) Tumor suppressor p53 is a direct transcriptional activator of the human bax gene. Cell 80: 293–299

Nagane M, Coufal F, Lin H, Bogler O, Cavenee W K and Huang H J (1996) A common mutant epidermal growth factor receptor confers enhanced tumorigenicity on human glioblastoma cells by increasing proliferation and reducing apoptosis. Cancer Res 56: 5079–5086

Nakano A, Tani E, Miyazaki K, Furuyama J and Matsumoto T (1993) Expressions of matrilysin and stromelysin in human glioma cells. Biochem Biophys Res Commun 192: 999–1003

Nishikawa R, Ji X D, Harmon R C, Lazar C S, Gill G N, Cavenee W K and Huang H J (1994) A mutant epidermal growth factor receptor common in human glioma confers enhanced tumorigenicity. Proc Natl Acad Sci U S A 91: 7727–7731

Nozaki M, Tada M, Matsumoto R, Sawamura Y, Abe H and Iggo R D (1998) Rare occurrence of inactivating p53 gene mutations in primary non- astrocytic tumors of the central nervous system: reappraisal by yeast functional assay. Acta Neuropathol (Berl) 95: 291–296

Oltvai Z N, Milliman C L and Korsmeyer S J (1993) Bcl-2 heterodimerizes in vivo with a conserved homolog, Bax, that accelerates programmed cell death. Cell 74: 609–619

Owen-Schaub L B, Zhang W, Cusack J C, Angelo L S, Santee S M, Fujiwara T, Roth J A, Deisseroth A B, Zhang W W, Kruzel E and et al. (1995) Wild-type human p53 and a temperature-sensitive mutant induce Fas/APO-1 expression. Mol Cell Biol 15: 3032–3040

Patsouris E, Davaki P, Kapranos N, Davaris P and Papageorgiou K (1996) A study of apoptosis in brain tumors by in situ end-labeling method. Clin Neuropathol 15: 337–341

Perrin G, Schnuriger V, Quiquerez A L, Saas P, Pannetier C, de Tribolet N, Tiercy J M, Aubry J P, Dietrich P Y and Walker P R (1999) Astrocytoma infiltrating lymphocytes include major T cell clonal expansions confined to the CD8 subset. Int Immunol 11: 1337–1350

Plate K H and Risau W (1995) Angiogenesis in malignant gliomas. Glia 15: 339–347

Prigent S A, Nagane M, Lin H, Huvar I, Boss G R, Feramisco J R, Cavenee W K and Huang H S (1996) Enhanced tumorigenic behavior of glioblastoma cells expressing a truncated epidermal growth factor receptor is mediated through the Ras- Shc-Grb2 pathway. J Biol Chem 271: 25639–25645

Rempel S A (1998) Molecular biology of central nervous system tumors. Curr Opin Oncol 10: 179–185

Rempel S A, Ge S and Gutierrez J A (1999) SPARC: a potential diagnostic marker of invasive meningiomas. Clin Cancer Res 5: 237–241

Rempel S A, Rosenblum M L, Mikkelsen T, Yan P S, Ellis K D, Golembieski W A, Sameni M, Rozhin J, Ziegler G and Sloane B F (1994) Cathepsin B expression and localization in glioma progression and invasion. Cancer Res 54: 6027–6031

Reyes-Mugica M, Rieger-Christ K, Ohgaki H, Ekstrand B C, Helie M, Kleinman G, Yahanda A, Fearon E R, Kleihues P and Reale M A (1997) Loss of DCC expression and glioma progression. Cancer Res 57: 382–386

Romanic A M and Madri J A (1994) Extracellular matrix-degrading proteinases in the nervous system. Brain Pathol 4: 145–156

Sage E H (1997) Terms of attachment: SPARC and tumorigenesis [news]. Nat Med 3: 144–146

Sato K, Schauble B, Kleihues P and Ohgaki H (1996) Infrequent alterations of the p15, p16, CDK4 and cyclin D1 genes in non- astrocytic human brain tumors. Int J Cancer 66: 305–308

Sawaya R, Ramo O J, Shi M L and Mandybur G (1991) Biological significance of tissue plasminogen activator content in brain tumors. J Neurosurg 74: 480–486

Schlessinger J (1988) Signal transduction by allosteric receptor oligomerization. Trends Biochem Sci 13: 443–447

Schmidt E E, Ichimura K, Messerle K R, Goike H M and Collins V P (1997) Infrequent methylation of CDKN2 A(MTS1/p16) and rare mutation of both CDKN2 A and CDKN2B(MTS2/p15) in primary astrocytic tumours. Br J Cancer 75: 2–8

Schmidt E E, Ichimura K, Reifenberger G and Collins V P (1994) CDKN2 (p16/MTS1) gene deletion or CDK4 amplification occurs in the majority of glioblastomas. Cancer Res 54: 6321–6324

Serrano M, Hannon G J and Beach D (1993) A new regulatory motif in cell-cycle control causing specific inhibition of cyclin D/CDK4 [see comments]. Nature 366: 704–707

Sherman L, Sleeman J, Herrlich P and Ponta H (1994) Hyaluronate receptors: key players in growth, differentiation, migration and tumor progression. Curr Opin Cell Biol 6: 726–733

Shu H K, Kim M M, Chen P, Furman F, Julin C M and Israel M A (1998) The intrinsic radioresistance of glioblastoma-derived cell lines is associated with a failure of p53 to induce p21(BAX) expression. Proc Natl Acad Sci USA 95: 14453–14458

Stuart E T, Haffner R, Oren M and Gruss P (1995a) Loss of p53 function through PAX-mediated transcriptional repression. Embo J 14: 5638–5645

Stuart E T, Kioussi C, Aguzzi A and Gruss P (1995b) PAX5 expression correlates with increasing malignancy in human astrocytomas. Clin Cancer Res 1: 207–214

Tachibana O, Nakazawa H, Lampe J, Watanabe K, Kleihues P and Ohgaki H (1995) Expression of Fas/APO-1 during the progression of astrocytomas. Cancer Res 55: 5528–5530

Tada M, Iggo R D, Waridel F, Nozaki M, Matsumoto R, Sawamura Y, Shinohe Y, Ikeda J and Abe H (1997) Reappraisal of p53 mutations in human malignant astrocytic neoplasms by p53 functional assay: comparison with conventional structural analyses. Mol Carcinog 18: 171–176

Takano S, Yoshii Y, Kondo S, Suzuki H, Maruno T, Shirai S and Nose T (1996) Concentration of vascular endothelial growth factor in the serum and tumor tissue of brain tumor patients. Cancer Res 56: 2185–2190

Tsurushima H, Liu S Q, Tsuboi K, Yoshii Y, Nose T and Ohno T (1996) Induction of human autologous cytotoxic T lymphocytes against minced tissues of glioblastoma multiforme. J Neurosurg 84: 258–263

Tsuzuki T, Tsunoda S, Sakaki T, Konishi N, Hiasa Y and Nakamura M (1996) Alterations of retinoblastoma, p53, p16(CDKN2), and p15 genes in human astrocytomas. Cancer 78: 287–293

Ueki K, Ono Y, Henson J W, Efird J T, von Deimling A and Louis D N (1996) CDKN2/p16 or RB alterations occur in the majority of glioblastomas and are inversely correlated. Cancer Res 56: 150–153

Ullrich A and Schlessinger J (1990) Signal transduction by receptors with tyrosine kinase activity. Cell 61: 203–212

Van Meir E (1996) Hypoxia-mediated selection of cells with diminished apoptotic potential to solid tumours [letter]. Neurosurgery 39: 878–879

Watanabe K, Tachibana O, Sata K, Yonekawa Y, Kleihues P and Ohgaki H (1996) Overexpression of the EGF receptor and p53 mutations are mutually exclusive in the evolution of primary and secondary glioblastomas. Brain Pathol 6: 217–223; discussion 23–4

Weller M, Frei K, Groscurth P, Krammer P H, Yonekawa Y and Fontana A (1994) Anti-Fas/APO-1 antibody-mediated apoptosis of cultured human glioma cells. Induction and modulation of sensitivity by cytokines. J Clin Invest 94: 954–964

Weller M, Malipiero U, Rensing-Ehl A, Barr P J and Fontana A (1995) Fas/APO-1 gene transfer for human malignant glioma. Cancer Res 55: 2936–2944

White E (1996) Life, death, and the pursuit of apoptosis. Genes Dev 10: 1–15

Yamamoto T, Nishida T, Miyajima N, Kawai S, Ooi T and Toyoshima K (1983) The erbB gene of avian erythroblastosis virus is a member of the src gene family. Cell 35: 71–78

Yamasaki T, Akiyama Y, Fukuda M, Kimura Y, Moritake K, Kikuchi H, Ljunggren H G, Karre K and Klein G (1996) Natural resistance against tumors grafted into the brain in association with histocompatibility-class-I-antigen expression. Int J Cancer 67: 365–771

Yount G L, Haas-Kogan D A, Vidair C A, Haas M, Dewey W C and Israel M A (1996) Cell cycle synchrony unmasks the influence of p53 function on radiosensitivity of human glioblastoma cells. Cancer Res 56: 500–506

4 Biological Principles of Radiotherapy in the Central Nervous System

Jennifer L. Daigle, William H. McBride, and H. Rodney Withers

CONTENTS

4.1 Introduction

Responses of the central nervous system (CNS) to irradiation may be broadly classified as acute, subacute, and late, and occur in a similar manner for a conventional course of treatment or single-dose stereotactic radiotherapy (Plowman 1999). Acute effects of brain irradiation are transient and occur 6–48 h after therapy. They are characterized by edema and drowsiness. These effects do not necessarily predict that later complications will occur. Drowsiness is claimed to be more pronounced in children than in

J. L. Daigle, SB
Roy E. Coats Research Laboratories and Department of Radiation Oncology, University of California, Los Angeles, 10833 Le Conte Avenue, Los Angeles, CA 90095-1714, USA
W. H. McBride, DSc
Roy E. Coats Research Laboratories and Department of Radiation Oncology, University of California, Los Angeles, 10833 Le Conte Avenue, Los Angeles, CA 90095-1714, USA
H. R. Withers, MD, DSc
Roy E. Coats Research Laboratories and Department of Radiation Oncology, University of California, Los Angeles, 10833 Le Conte Avenue, Los Angeles, CA 90095-1714, USA

adults. Irradiation of the nucleus tractus solitarius and area postrema can stimulate brain stem emetic mechanisms. Subacute effects of brain irradiation have an insidious onset beginning 6-10 weeks after the start of a course of radiation therapy, with somnolence and fatigability being the predominant symptoms. They are fully or partially reversible. In the spinal cord, radiation-induced meningeal changes can lead to a positive Lhermitte's sign, but this is not a precursor of effects in the cord itself. If late sequelae develop, they do so most commonly between about 5 months and 2 years, with the onset of symptoms occurring earlier with higher doses. (Lo et al. 1992; Chiang et al. 1997). However, injury may not become apparent for many years after exposure (Million and Parsons 1999).

Most dose–response data and measurements of the kinetics of development of late CNS injury are derived from irradiation of the spinal cord in animal studies using paresis or paralysis as the end point (Nieder et al. 1999). The limited human data are derived mostly from misadventures before the radiobiology of CNS responses became better understood. However, in general, the pattern of responses of the spinal cord is similar in humans and animals, but because of the lack of human data, the commonly used human spinal cord dose limit of 45 Gy in 22–25 fractions may be conservative (Schultheiss et al. 1995).

The response of the brain to irradiation can be studied in experimental animals, but only by assessing motor dysfunction after relatively high doses. Reversible subacute and irreversible late effects have been observed in mice after brain irradiation (Chiang et al. 1993). High doses to the human brain in excess of 60 Gy conventional fractionation can produce white matter degeneration and, over months and years, a decline in cerebral function. Certain cognitive functions, including memory, may be more vulnerable than others, although this requires further investigation (Komaki et al. 1995; Roman and Sperduto 1995). The neurocognitive defects from lower radiation doses given to the brains of children as part of the treatment of acute lympho-blastic leukemia have been better studied. These treatments can cause leukoencephalopathy with modest decrements in test scores for intellectual function (CHRISTIE et al. 1995; ROMAN and SPERDU-TO 1995; SMIBERT et al. 1996). After doses of up to 18 Gy in 1.5–1.8 Gy fractions, with or without intrathe-cal methotrexate, there is no detectable drop in intel-ligence scores, but after 24 Gy there is a significant, although not large, decrement (HALBERG et al. 1992). Since intrathecal methotrexate was commonly used to supplement radiation therapy, the dose for a 10-point fall in tests of cognitive function after radia-tion therapy alone may be greater than 24 Gy in 1.5–1.8 Gy fractions. Data gathered from treatment of younger children (less than 5 years old) were also predictive of poor long-term outcome for cognitive and education ability (HALBERG et al. 1992; SMIBERT et al. 1996). This observation is supported by find-ings from animal studies (RUIFROK et al. 1994), such as the spinal cord being more radiosensitive in young guinea pigs than in older animals (MASON et al. 1993).

4.2
Cellular Response to Radiotherapy in the CNS

Most of the histopathologic reports on specimens from patients with radiation-induced complications following CNS irradiation, as well as data gathered from experimental animal studies, are concerned with the events associated with severe late radionecrosis. Lesions have been described that are mainly in the white matter but vary in their cardinal features (SCHULTHEISS et al. 1995). Selective coagulative ne-crosis is frequently reported. Focal and diffuse demy-elination with accompanying gliosis are often domi-nant features. Chronic vascular injury and generalized atrophy appear as very late effects (HOPEWELL and VAN DER KOGEL 1999). In experimental animals, the time and dose dependency of these different lesions has been documented (ANG 1999; HOPEWELL and VAN DER KOGEL 1999). It is important to recognize the diversity of responses when considering possible in-volvement of different cell populations, since multiple mechanisms probably operate to result in the different manifestations of late damage.

4.3
Radiation-Induced Apoptosis in the CNS

Within the brain, different regions may manifest damage at different times. One of the earliest man-ifestations of cellular damage, occurring within 6 h of brain irradiation in experimental animals, is ap-optosis. Irradiation of developing brain leads to rapid and massive apoptosis in immature cells of both the neuronal and glial lineages (FERRER et al. 1995). Apoptosis is essential for the normal devel-opment of CNS tissues, and perhaps because of this necessity, these immature cells may have a predis-position towards an apoptotic response when irra-diated. Irradiation of young adult rat brain with single doses of 5 or 30 Gy were reported to cause an increase in apoptosis predominantly in the putative stem cell areas of the subependyma, corpus callo-sum (BELLINZOA et al. 1996; SHINOHARA et al. 1997), and dentate gyrus (PEISSNER et al. 1999). In the latter study, this was associated with a decrease in cell proliferation. In addition, oligodendrocytes have been found to be particularly susceptible to apoptosis following in vitro irradiation (BAR-BARESE 1989; VRJOLJAK et al. 1992) and biochemical studies of the mouse brain 1–2 days after in vivo irradiation show a rapid decrease in oligodendro-cyte markers (MCBRIDE et al. 1997). In the rat spinal cord, apoptosis after high-dose irradiation was also associated with a loss of oligodendrocytes (LI et al. 1996). Endothelial cells have also been reported to be susceptible to rapid radiation-induced apoptosis (BILLIS et al. 1998), although this was not observed in the rat spinal cord following irradiation (LI and WONG 1996).

The significance of radiation-induced apoptosis following CNS irradiation is still not clear. The loss of oligodendrocytes is attenuated on subsequent ex-posure (LI and WONG 1997), and their loss may sim-ply represent a radiation-induced acceleration of a natural process of cell loss during turnover of this population. On the other hand, it may precipitate the subsequent cell proliferation that occurs in the CNS within weeks of irradiation (HORNSEY et al. 1981; CHIANG et al. 1993; LI and WONG 1998). Perhaps more controversial is the significance of the rapid radiation-induced apoptosis that occurs in the puta-tive stem cell areas within the brain since this may be depleted in the long term, with currently unknown consequences (TADA et al. 1999).

4.4
Stem Cells in the CNS

In the mammalian brain, the area within the walls of the lateral ventricles, known as the subventricular zone (SVZ), remains mitotically active well into adulthood. This observation led to speculation that these areas may contain a multipotent stem cell that could give rise to both glial cells and neurons. Studies have shown that two distinct regions of the SVZ, the ependyma and the subependyma, contain cells that show characteristics of stem cells, including self-renewal capability (DOETSCH et al. 1997).

Cells in the SVZ have been shown to divide in response to various types of brain injury, and the resulting progeny may migrate to the site of injury. Little is known about the capacity of these cells to participate in tissue recovery. In rodents, it is suggested that cells that eventually differentiate into neurons migrate to the olfactory bulb, which may be a default pathway. However, cells that could differentiate into glia appear to radiate from the SVZ throughout the brain and even down to the spinal cord depending on the site of injury (HOPEWELL and CAVANAGH 1972; TADA et al. 1999). The extent of migration may depend upon the age of the animal and the nature of the injury. Recently, CHIASSON et. al. (CHIASSON et al. 1999) have shown that these two types of migrating progenitors may originate from different regions within the SVZ, with the glial precursors occurring mainly in the ependyma and the neural stem cells residing within the subependyma; however, JOHANSSON et. al. (JOHANSSON et al. 1999a,b) reported that the ependyma can also contain neural stem cells.

A cardinal feature of brain radionecrosis is loss of oligodendrocytes with subsequent demyelination. Therefore, there is much interest in determining if the decrease in these cells could be caused in part by the loss of this stem cell population or loss of its ability to repopulate areas in the brain that have been damaged by radiation. HOPEWELL and CAVANAGH were the first to show that the mitotic count in the rat subependyma was drastically reduced in the first 24 h after irradiation, only to recover by 3 months after doses of 20 Gy. No recovery was seen at higher doses (40 Gy) even at 6 months post-irradiation (HOPEWELL and CAVANAGH 1972). HOPEWELL and CAVANAGH also suggested that the eventual occurrence of delayed white matter necrosis might be due to loss of this cell population. More recently, TADA et. al. (TADA et al. 1999) have used immunohistochemical techniques to measure the number of proliferating cells, immature neurons and astrocytes, and undifferentiated components present in the subependyma after various doses of ionizing radiation in the rat brain. They found progressively more stem cell damage with increasing doses of radiation. Like HOPEWELL and CAVANAGH, they found that after higher doses, these stem cells were unable to repopulate the subependyma. The suggestion is that the stem cell population of the subependyma is involved in the radioresponse of the brain, but more experimentation is needed to confirm that this is not simply a rudimentary population with a small role in preventing long-term damage.

4.5
Acute Cellular Responses
to CNS Irradiation

Amelioration of the symptoms associated with radiation-induced CNS tissue damage requires understanding of the underlying cellular processes that produce these symptoms. The transient acute effects may be attributable to rapid cell loss, but are more likely mediated by the release of pro-inflammatory cytokines that are induced over the first 24-h period after irradiation. Experimental studies have shown increases in tumor necrosis factor (TNF-a), interleukin-1 (IL-1), cell adhesion molecules such as ICAM-1, proteases and anti-proteases (HONG et al. 1995), and glutathione and glutathione synthesis-related proteins (KOJIMA et al. 1998). ICAM-1 is primarily expressed on endothelial cells and microglia (KYRKANIDES et al. 1999), but also on astrocytes (OLSCHOWAKA et al. 1997). This acute phase pro-inflammatory response promotes interactions between leukocytes and blood vessel walls, as well as other vascular changes that can lead to the edema observed soon after irradiation (NAKATA et al. 1995; ACKER et al. 1998). Furthermore, pro-inflammatory cytokines are known to stimulate the hypothalamus-pituitary-adrenal axis and through this pathway mediate effects such as fever, fatigue, and neurological effects (BERCZI et al. 1998). Anti-inflammatory drugs, including steroids (HONG et al. 1995), can block this pathway, although high doses might be needed for complete suppression. It is not clear what effect administering these drugs might have on later responses, but steroids are an important part of the management of radiation-induced symptoms in the CNS.

4.6
Subacute and Late Cellular Responses to CNS Irradiation

Cellular responses following the acute changes seen after mouse brain irradiation are of a cyclical nature. In rat brain, imaging studies described cyclical fluctuations ascribed to edema formation with peaks at 2–6 weeks, 8–12 weeks, and 16–24 weeks (RUBIN et al. 1994). Imaging studies in humans variably indicate the presence of edema, white matter changes, cerebral atrophy, and/or necrosis, generally at doses above 50 Gy given in a conventional fractionation scheme. Transient changes have been observed during the so-called latent period and late after irradiation, but these changes are not necessarily associated with symptoms (CORN et al. 1994; ESTEVE et al. 1998; KIHLSTROM and KARLSSON 1999; RUSSO et al. 1999).

Following mouse brain (CHIANG et al. 1993) or guinea pig spinal cord irradiation (CHIANG et al. 1992), biochemical markers of oligodendrocytes and myelin fall at 1–2 months and again at 6 months, indicative of attempted replenishment from precursor pools or division of mature cells (CHIANG et al. 1992, 1993; MCBRIDE et al. 1997). Loss of oligodendrocytes and related demyelination preceded and correlated in a dose-dependent fashion with lethality. In contrast to this, protein levels of glial fibrillary acidic protein (GFAP) increased by 2 weeks after irradiation and were re-elevated over the subacute to late time period, with a peak around 1 month after doses of 20–60 Gy. This reflects gliosis with astrocyte and microglia activation. The role of this response is uncertain, but it is possible that excessive gliosis is detrimental to the healing process. Irradiation has been reported to have a beneficial effect on the healing of lesioned central nervous tissue, presumably by inhibiting cell proliferation (KALDERON 1990).

The cyclical changes in cellular markers following CNS irradiation are paralleled by cyclical changes in pro-inflammatory molecules (CHIANG et al. 1997) The expression of neurological symptoms correlates with peaks seen in this cyclical process. However, the only marker found to be elevated at 6 months postirradiation was TNF-a. We have recently shown that TNF-R2 knockout mice are more sensitive to the effects of brain irradiation, indicating that this may serve as a radioprotective pathway (DAIGLE et al. 1999). Given the known properties of TNF-a, it seems highly likely that this molecule plays a role in the expression, if not the pathogenesis, of subacute and late radiation damage. Recently, an association between cytokine expression and radiation injury in clinical specimens has been noted (KURESHI et al. 1994).

Studies in the rat brain have emphasized the importance of loss of vascular endothelial cells in the development of late radionecrosis after 22.5 and 25 Gy irradiation (CALVO et al. 1987, 1988). Loss of endothelial cells and a decrease in blood vessel number in the fimbria preceded demyelination and necrosis. In these studies, no loss of oligodendrocytes was noted histopathologically. A vascular/astrocytic "tissue injury unit" (TIU) was postulated as being the critical target for radiation. The TIU was defined as the combination of four highly correlated changes in vasculature: blood vessel dilation, thickening of vessel walls, enlargement of the nuclei of the endothelial cells lining these vessels, and hypertrophy of the astrocytes surrounding the blood vessels (CALVO et al. 1988).

Recent experiments using boron neutron capture confirm that radiation damage to vasculature can lead to late radionecrosis in rat spinal cord (HOPEWELL and VAN DER KOGEL 1999). The experiments used two different boronated compounds, p-boronophenylalanine (BPA), which crosses the blood–brain barrier, and boracaptate sodium (BSH), which does not. Most of the dose from the boron capture reaction using BSH was to the vasculature, while the dose resulting from the reaction in BPA was distributed throughout both the vasculature and brain parenchyma. With BSH-mediated BNCT, more rats developed paralysis than with BPA-mediated BNCT. Surprisingly, the latent period to paralysis differed significantly for the different exposure conditions, perhaps indicating different pathogenetic mechanisms. These experiments confirm that vasculature injury may play a role in the progression of radiation-induced damage, although they do not rule out direct radiation damage to glial cells as an alternate mechanism.

What is clear is that a predictable sequence of multiple cellular events follows irradiation of the CNS and is associated with attempts at healing and recovery. Failure of critical elements in this response may vary with the radiation dose, fractionation scheme, site within the CNS, as well as with genetic background and environmental influences. Understanding the cascadic responses that follow irradiation has, however, allowed identification of possible targets for intervention aimed at improving the therapeutic ratio in CNS radiotherapy (ANG 1999; NIEDER et al. 1999; NOEL et al. 1999).

4.7
Tolerance Doses

Tolerance is a very elastic concept, being loosely defined as the severity of injury prospectively deemed tolerable by the patient (and others involved) given an approximate understanding of the risk:benefit ratio and the consequences of the projected possible outcomes. Since the brain is most commonly irradiated when it harbors primary or metastatic cancer, the "tolerance" dose is usually accepted to be higher than for the spinal cord, where irradiation is usually only coincidental to treatment of a cancer at some other site (e.g., lung, esophagus, or head and neck), and it should be technically possible to avoid high doses to the cord. This difference in tolerance doses does not reflect differences in the radiobiology of different parts of the CNS: the pathogenesis of injury, and the dose responses are similar, although, of course, the clinical sequelae vary, depending upon the site of injury.

4.8
Dose Responses

The incidence of a radiation effect on the spinal cord or brain can be described by a threshold-sigmoid dose–response curve (Fig. 4.1). The magnitude of the threshold depends upon the effect being studied. In animal studies, the most commonly used end point has been paresis or paralysis from demyelination of the spinal cord, although it is also possible to quan-tify motor disturbances from brain irradiation (ALAOUI et al. 1995; JUSTINO et al. 1997). The threshold for these effects is quite large, corresponding to doses in excess of 50 Gy in 2-Gy fractions. The pattern is similar in all animals studied (HOPEWELL et al. 1987; KNOWLES 1983; LO et al. 1992; MASON et al. 1993; VAN DER AARDWEG et al. 1995; VAN DER KOGEL 1991a; WONG et al. 1992). In rhesus monkeys, the doses for a 5% and 50% incidence of myelitis are approximately 60 Gy and 70 Gy for doses given in approximately 2-Gy fractions (ANG et al. 1993). The incidence after 50 Gy in 2-Gy fractions is too low to be measured using practical numbers of animals. Likewise, the dose response for myelitis in humans as a result of radiation therapy is difficult to determine because the incidence is low. However, the available data indicate that the results from animal studies are relevant to humans (ANG 1999; LEIBEL and SHELINE 1991; SCHULTHEISS et al. 1995).

4.9
Dose Fractionation Effects

The effectiveness of a course of fractionated x-irradiation in causing injury to the CNS is highly dependent on the dose size per fraction. This fractionation effect is greater in the CNS than in any other tissue (ANG et al. 1995; MASON et al. 1993; SCHULTHEISS et al. 1990, 1994, 1995; VAN DER KOGEL 1991a,b; WONG et al. 1992). The total injury is a summation of "single-hit" non-repairable damage, and accumulative or interactive "multiple-hit" damage, with the propor-

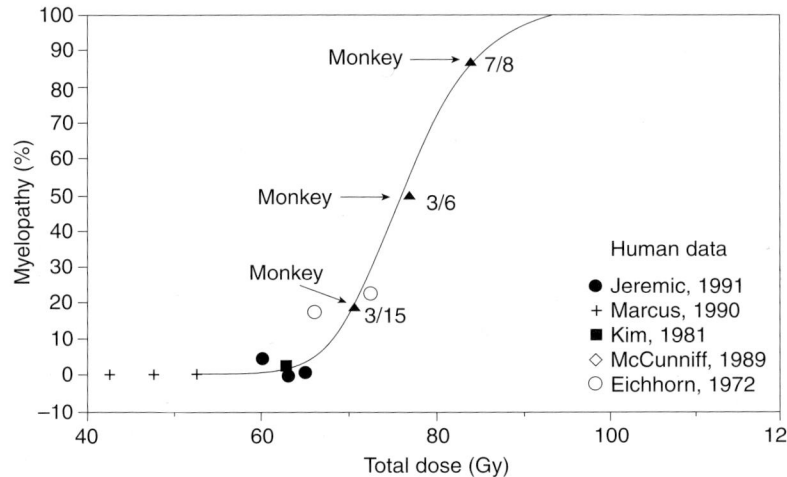

Fig. 4.1. Threshold sigmoid dose–response curve for myelitis in monkeys treated with 2.2-Gy fractions, and some data points estimated from clinical reports. These data justify the use of experimental animals to investigate responses of the human spinal cord. (Reprinted with permission from ANG 1999a, and Karger)

tion of injury resulting from multi-hit damage being greater than that seen in other organs. Thus, an increase in dose per fraction causes a steep increase in injury, and conversely, reduction in dose per fraction yields a large "sparing" effect. In terms of a linear quadratic dose–response equation, the a:b ratio is low, where a is the coefficient for single-hit injury, which increases linearly with dose, and b is the coefficient for multi-hit injury, which increases in proportion to dose-squared. The actual value for a/b is uncertain, but is probably less than 2 Gy, perhaps as low as 1 Gy.

4.10
Interfraction Intervals

The large sparing effect which can be derived from using multiple small fractions depends upon the repair of sublethal (b-type) injury between dose fractions. The CNS continues to repair sublethal injury over a longer time period than other tissues, and this time period is longer than would be expected from in vitro studies of repair kinetics (Ang et al. 1992). It is likely that, although largely complete by 8 h, some repair continues thereafter. This is an important consideration in regimens requiring more than one fraction per day, e.g., in hyperfractionated or accelerated fractionation regimens. The increased tolerance associated with lowering the dose per fraction can be offset by the diminished tolerance resulting from incomplete repair between fractions in twice-a-day treatment with a shortened interfraction interval (Lavey et al. 1994). For instance, during the development of the CHART regimen for head and neck cancer, which delivered three fractions per day with two 6-h intervals and one 12-h interval per 24 h, there was a small but unexpected incidence of myelitis (Dische 1987). When the technique was modified such that the spinal cord was treated twice per day, at 12-h intervals, there were no further cases of myelitis.

4.11
Retreatment Tolerance: Decay of Remembered Dose

Experiments with animals have shown that, after months or years, the residual injury in irradiated spinal cord diminishes (Hornsey et al. 1982; Knowles 1983; Ang et al. 1993; Mason et al. 1993;

Ruifrok et al 1992; Wong et al. 1993b). There is also some evidence that the same type of recovery can occur in humans (Dritschilo et al. 1981; Ryu et al. 2000). Whereas the dose from a second course of irradiation is additive to the first if given soon after the first course, there is recovery of some or all of the tolerance of the cord if months or years elapse before re-irradiation. The extent of the recovery (that is, of the loss of remembered dose) depends upon both the magnitude of injury from the first dose and the interval elapsing before re-irradiation (Wong et al. 1993a,b). Unfortunately, there is little information on the kinetics of recovery, and the dose the irradiated cord will tolerate in a retreatment is still a difficult guess. This is especially true in humans, where the necessary data do not, and never will, exist. In rhesus monkeys, there is extensive recovery from a dose of 44 Gy in 2-Gy fractions by 2 years (Ang et al. 1993). Rats irradiated with a single dose of 10 Gy as newborns showed complete recovery by 12 months (Knowles 1983). In guinea pigs, recovery from nine fractions of 4.5 Gy was complete within months (Mason et al. 1993), and in adult rats it was extensive by 6 months (van der Kogel 1991b).

The effect of the retreatment dose required to produce injury months or years after a first dose is a measure of long-term recovery in the spinal cord. Figure 4.2 presents a review of some data for "remembered" dose as a function of size of the dose given in a first course (Mason et al. 1993). It is not surprising that the magnitude of the first dose is important since it will determine the ability of the cord to reestablish a functional tissue architecture.

There are as yet no useful data on remembered dose in brain. However, in principle, the processes of recovery should be similar throughout all the white matter of the CNS.

4.12
Effect of Length of Treatment Field

The risk of myelitis increases with the length of spinal cord irradiated (Hopewell et al. 1994; Powers et al. 1998; Schultheiss et al. 1994; van den Aardweg et al. 1995; van der Kogel 1993) because the functional subunits are arranged in series, and, like links in a chain, must all retain their functional capacity if overt injury is to be avoided (Schultheiss et al. 1983; Withers et al. 1987). The greater the number of functional subunits in the chain, the greater the probability of a break. Increasing the

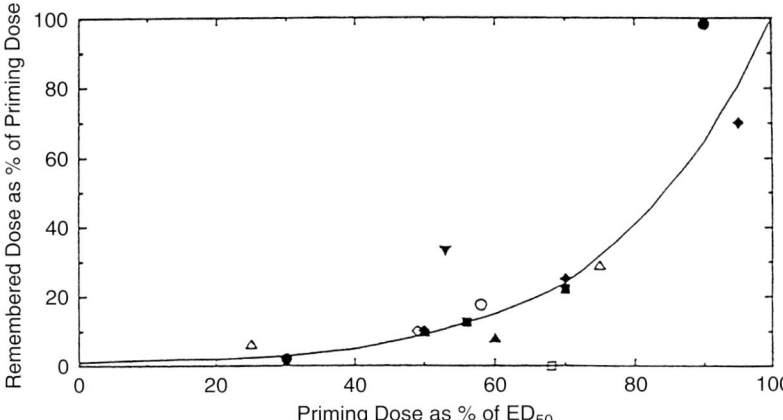

Fig. 4.2. Estimates of the percentage of the first dose "remembered" at the time of re-irradiation, as a function of the size of the first dose (expressed as a % of the ED_{50}). The interval between treatments varied in the different experiments but was months or years. A variety of experimental animals was used. Higher initial doses reduce the tolerance for re-irradiation. (Reprinted with permission from MASON et al. 1993, and Elsevier)

length of nerve tracts included in the radiation field decreases the threshold for injury but increases the slope for incidence of, e.g., myelitis, once the threshold is exceeded.

The divergence of dose–response curves at higher incidences of myelitis affects experimental animal studies (VAN DER KOGEL 1993) but is less significant in humans where doses are prescribed with a view to remaining below the threshold (POWERS et al. 1992). Although the "probability" model deals with the phenomenon of increasing incidence of myelitis traditionally linked to a volume effect, there are two effects of the length of cord irradiated which are of more clinical relevance.

A factor which could masquerade as a volume effect in the treatment of long fields is dose heterogeneity. For example, the lesser thickness of the thoracic inlet could lead to a higher dose to that part of the spinal cord than to the thoracic cord in the middle of a chest field used to treat lung cancer. Left uncorrected, the biological dose in the relatively overdosed length of cord at the inlet would be further amplified by the "double trouble" of the higher physical dose being also delivered in larger doses per fraction (WITHERS and McBRIDE 1997).

A second volume effect may occur when very small lengths (e.g., millimeters) are included in, for example, a tightly conformal stereotactic and/or intensity modulated treatment plan for a tumor at the base of the skull or in a vertebral body. It seems likely that surviving oligodendrocytes (or Schwann cells) at the margins of such a small "clip" of the cord, brain stem, optic or other cranial nerves etc., could either remyelinate the nerve fibers from the margins, or, more likely, migrate into the irradiated segment and maintain or reestablish neuron function after doses which would

be destructive of longer lengths. Experimental data do show a steep increase in the ED_{50} when irradiation is restricted to very short lengths (HOPEWELL et al. 1987; VAN DER KOGEL 1993). Endothelial responses are different from glial responses and show less change in tolerance as the field size is changed (HOPEWELL et al. 1987). This volume (or length) influence on tolerance of subvolumes of a structure such as the base of the brain, spinal cord, or cranial and other nerves is clearly an area which will require detailed analysis of clinical (rather than experimental animal) results of tightly conformal irradiation.

4.13
Conclusion

The potentially serious and even fatal late consequences of irradiation delivered to the CNS drives clinicians to err on the side of safety even at the expense of tumor control. Experimental studies have therefore been a primary source of information about tolerance doses, effects of altered fractionation schedules, interfraction interval, retreatment tolerance, and volume effects. These factors determine the magnitude of the cyclical changes in different subpopulations of cells that are set in motion by radiation and that proceed to an inevitable conclusion of recovery of tissue function or irretrievable damage. Recent developments in neurobiology give insight into how these processes might be manipulated with benefit. Understanding the contribution of these cellular changes to the pathogenesis of radiation-induced CNS injury and how they might be altered is crucial for the development of new therapeutic strategies aimed at increasing the therapeutic benefit of radiotherapy involving the CNS.

Acknowledgements. This investigation was supported by PHS grant numbers CA-31612 (Withers) and CA-66605 (McBride) awarded by the National Cancer Institute, DHHS.

References

Acker JC, Marks LB, Spencer DP, Yang W, Avery MA, Dodge RK, Rosner GL, Dewhirst MW (1998) Serial in vivo observations of cerebral vasculature after treatment with a large single fraction of radiation. Radiat Res 149:350–359

Alaoui F, Pratt J, Trocherie S, Court L, Stutzmann JM (1995) Acute effects of irradiation on the rat brain: protection by glutamate blockade. Europ J Pharmacol 276:55–60

Ang KK (1999a) Radiation injury to the central nervous system: clinical features and prevention. In: Meyer JL (ed) Radiation Injury. Advances in Management and Prevention, Krager Basel, Front Radiat Ther Oncol 32:145–154

Ang K (1999b) Clinical application of laboratory data on neurotoxicity. Front Radiat Ther Oncol 33:253–264

Ang KK, Jiang GL, Guttenberger R, Thames HD, Stephens LC, Smith CD, Feng Y (1992) Impact of spinal cord repair kinetics on the practice of altered fractionation schedules. Radiother Oncol 25:287–294

Ang KK, Price RE, Stephens LC, Jiang GL, Feng Y, Schultheiss TE, Peters LJ (1993) The tolerance of primate spinal cord to re-irradiation. Int J Radiat Oncol Biol Phys 25:459–464

Ang KK, Xu FX, Landuyt W (1985) The kinetics and capacity of repair of sublethal damage in mouse lip mucosa during fractionated irradiations. Int J Radiat Oncol Biol Phys 11:1977–1985

Barbarese E, Barry C (1989) Radiation sensitivity of glial cells in primary culture. J Neurol Sci 91:97–107

Bellinzona M, Gobbel GT, Shinohara C, Fike JR (1996) Apoptosis is induced in the subependyma of young adult rats by ionizing irradiation. Neuroscience Letters 208:163–166

Berczi I, Chow DA, Sabbadini ER (1998) Neuroimmunoregulation and natural immunity. Domestic Animal Endocrinology 15:273–281

Billis W, Fuks Z, Kolesnick R (1998) Signaling in and regulation of ionizing radiation-induced apoptosis in endothelial cells. Recent Progress in Hormone Research 53:85–92

Calvo W, Hopewell JW, Reinhold HS, van den Berg AP, Yeung TK (1987) Dose-dependent and time-dependent changes in the choroid plexus of the irradiated rat brain. Br J Radiol 60:1109–1117

Calvo W, Hopewell JW, Reinhold HS, Yeung TK (1988) Time- and dose-related changes in the white matter of the rat brain after single doses of X rays. Br J Radiol 61:1043–1052

Chiang CS, Hong JH, Stalder A, Sun JR, Withers HR, McBride WH (1997) Delayed molecular responses to brain irradiation. Int J Radiat Biol 72:45–53

Chiang CS, Mason KA, Withers HR, McBride WH (1992) Alteration in myelin-associated proteins following spinal cord irradiation in guinea pigs. Int J Radiat Oncol Biol Phys 24:929–937

Chiang CS, Mason KA, Withers HR, McBride WH (1992) Alteration in myelin-associated proteins following spinal cord irradiation in guinea pigs. Int J Radiat Oncol Biol Phys 24:929–937

Chiang CS, McBride WH, Withers HR (1993) Myelin-associated changes in mouse brain following irradiation. Radiother Oncol 27:229–236

Chiang CS, McBride WH, Withers HR (1993) Radiation-induced astrocytic and microglial responses in mouse brain. Radiother Oncol 29:60–68

Chiang CS, McBride WH, Withers HR (1993) Radiation-induced astrocytic and microglial responses in mouse brain. Radiother Oncol 29:60–68

Chiasson BJ, Tropepe V, Morshead CM, van der Kooy D (1999) Adult mammalian forebrain ependymal and subependymal cells demonstrate proliferative potential, but only subependymal cells have neural stem cell characteristics. J Neurosci 19:4462–4471

Christie D, Leiper AD, Chessells JM, Vargha-Khadem F (1995) Intellectual performance after presymptomatic cranial radiotherapy for leukaemia: effects of age and sex. Archives of Disease in Childhood 73:136–140

Corn BW, Yousem DM, Scott CB, Rotman M, Asbell SO, Nelson DF, Martin L, Curran WJ, Jr. (1994) White matter changes are correlated significantly with radiation dose. Observations from a randomized dose-escalation trial for malignant glioma (Radiation Therapy Oncology Group 83–02). Cancer 74:2828–2835

Daigle JL, Chiang CS, Withers HR, McBride WH (1999) Molecular and cellular responses of TNF receptor knock-out mice to brain irradiation. Proceedings of the American Association for Cancer Research Annual Meeting 40:199.

Dische S (1991) Accelerated treatment and radiation myelitis (editorial). Radiother Oncol 20:1–2.

Doetsch F, García-Verdugo JM and Alvarez-Buylla A (1997) Cellular composition and three-dimensional organization of the subventricular germinal zone in the adult mammalian brain. J Neurosci 17:5046–5061

Dritschilo A, Bruckman JE, Cassady JR, Belli JA (1981) Tolerance of brain to multiple courses of radiation therapy. I. Clinical experiences. Brit J Radiol 54:782–786

Estève F, Rubin C, Grand S, Kolodié H, Le Bas JF (1998) Transient metabolic changes observed with proton MR spectroscopy in normal human brain after radiation therapy. Int J Radiat Oncol Biol Phys 40:279–286

Ferrer I, Macaya A, Blanco R, Olivé M, Cinós C, Munell F, Planas AM (1995) Evidence of internucleosomal DNA fragmentation and identification of dying cells in X-ray-induced cell death in the developing brain. Int J Develop Neurosci 13:21–28

Halberg FE, Kramer JH, Moore IM, Wara WM, Matthay KK, Ablin AR (1992) Prophylactic cranial irradiation dose effects on late cognitive function in children treated for acute lymphoblastic leukemia. Int J Radiat Oncol Biol Phys 22:13–16

Hong JH, Chiang CS, Campbell IL, Sun JR, Withers HR, McBride WH (1995) Induction of acute phase gene expression by brain irradiation. Int J Radiat Oncol Biol Phys 33:619–626

Hopewell JW, Cavanagh JB (1972) Effects of X irradiation on the mitotic activity of the subependymal plate of rats. Brit J Radiol 45:461–465

Hopewell JW, Morris AD, Dixon-Brown A (1987) The influence of field size on the late tolerance of the rat spinal cord to single doses of X-rays. Brit J Radiol 60:1099–1108

Hopewell JW, van der Kogel AJ (1999) Pathophysiological mechanisms leading to the development of late radiation-induced damage to the central nervous system. Front of Radiat Ther Oncol 33:265–275

Hornsey S, Myers R, Coultas PG, Rogers MA, White A (1981) Turnover of proliferative cells in the spinal cord after X irradiation and its relation to time-dependent repair of radiation damage. Brit J Radiol 54:1081–1085

Hornsey S, Myers R, Warren P (1982) Residual injury in the spinal cord after treatment with X rays or neutrons. Brit J of Radiol 55:516–519

Jannoun K (1983) Are cognitive and educational development affected by age at which prophylactic therapy is given in acute lymphoglastic leukemia? Arch Dis Child 58:953–958

Johansson CB, Momma S, Clarke DL, Risling M, Lendahl U, Frisén J (1999a) Identification of a neural stem cell in the adult mammalian central nervous system. Cell 96:25–34

Johansson CB, Svensson M, Wallstedt L, Janson AM, Frisén J (1999b) Neural stem cells in the adult human brain. Exp Cell Res 253:733–736

Justino L, Welner SA, Tannenbaum GS, Schipper HM (1997) Long-term effects of cysteamine on cognitive and locomotor behavior in rats: relationship to hippocampal glial pathology and somatostatin levels. Brain Res 761:127–134

Kalderon N, Alfieri AA, Fuks, Z (1990) Benefical effects of x-irradiation on recovery of lesioned mammalian central nervous tissue. Proc Natl Acad Sci USA 87:10058–10062

Kihlström L, Karlsson B (1999) Imaging changes after radiosurgery for vascular malformations, functional targets, and tumors. Neurosurg Clinics No Amer 10:167–180

Knowles JF (1983) The radiosensitivity of the guinea-pig spinal cord to X-rays: the effect of retreatment at one year and the effect of age at the time of irradiation. Int J Radiat Biol and Related Studies in Physics, Chemistry and Medicine 44:433–442

Kojima S, Matsuki O, Nomura T, Shimura N, Kubodera A, Yamaoka K, Tanooka H, Wakasugi H, Honda Y, Honda S, Sasaki T (1998) Localization of glutathione and induction of glutathione synthesis-related proteins in mouse brain by low doses of gamma-rays. Brain Res 808:262–269

Komaki R, Meyers CA, Shin DM, Garden AS, Byrne K, Nickens JA, Cox JD (1995) Evaluation of cognitive function in patients with limited small cell lung cancer prior to and shortly following prophylactic cranial irradiation. Int J Radiat Oncol Biol Phys 33:179–182

Kureshi SA, Hofman FM, Schneider JH, Chin LS, Apuzzo ML, Hinton DR (1994) Cytokine expression in radiation-induced delayed cerebral injury. Neurosurg 35:822–829; discussion 829–830

Kyrkanides S, Olschowka JA, Williams JP, Hansen JT, O'Banion MK (1999) TNF alpha and IL-1beta mediate intercellular adhesion molecule-1 induction via microglia-astrocyte interaction in CNS radiation injury. J Neuroimmunol 95:95–106

Lavey RS, Taylor JM, Tward JD, Li LT, Nguyen AA, Chon Y, McBride WH (1994) The extent, time course, and fraction size dependence of mouse spinal cord recovery from radiation injury. Int J Radiat Oncol Biol Phys 30:609–617

Leibel SA, Sheline GE (1991) Tolerance of the brain and spinal cord to conventional irradiation. In: Gutin PH, Leibel SA, Sheline GE (eds) Radiation Injury to the Nervous System, Raven Press, New York, pp. 239–256

Li YQ, Jay V, Wong CS (1996) Oligodendrocytes in the adult rat spinal cord undergo radiation-induced apoptosis. Cancer Res 56:5417–5422

Li YQ, Wong CS (1997) Radiation-induced apoptosis in the rat spinal cord: lack of equal effect per fraction. Int J Radiat Biol 71:413–420

Li YQ, Wong CS (1998) Apoptosis and its relationship with cell proliferation in the irradiated rat spinal cord. Int J Radiat Biol 74:405–417

Lo YC, McBride WH, Withers HR (1992) The effect of single doses of radiation on mouse spinal cord. Int J Radiat Oncol Biol Phys 22:57–63

Mason KA, Withers HR, Chiang CS (1993) Late effects of radiation on the lumbar spinal cord of guinea pigs: re-treatment tolerance. Int J Radiat Oncol Biol Phys 26:643–648

McBride WH, Chiang CS, Hong JH, Withers HR (1997). Molecular and cellular responses of the brain to radiotherapy. In: Khayat D, Hortobagyi G (eds) Current Clinical Topics in Cancer Chemotherapy. Blackwell Science, Inc, Cambridge, MA, pp 91–101

Million RR, Parsons JT (1999) Radiation-induced eye injury from head and neck therapy. In: Meyer JL (ed) Radiation Injury. Advances in Management and Prevention, Karger, Basel. Front Radiat Ther Oncol 32:21–33

Nakata H, Yoshimine T, Murasawa A, Kumura E, Harada K, Ushio Y, Hayakawa T (1995) Early blood-brain barrier disruption after high-dose single-fraction irradiation in rats. Acta Neurochirurgica 136:82–86; discussion 86–87

Nieder C, Ataman F, Price RE, Ang KK (1999) Radiation myelopathy: new perspective on an old problem. Radiat Oncol Invest 7:193–203

Noel F, Raju U, Happel E, Marchionni MA, Tofilon PJ (1999) X-irradiation-induced loss of O-2 A progenitor cells in rat spinal cord is inhibited by implants of cells engineered to secrete glial growth factor 2. Neuroreport 10:535–540

Olschowka JA, Kyrkanides S, Harvey BK, O'Banion MK, Williams JP, Rubin P, Hansen JT (1997) ICAM-1 induction in the mouse CNS following irradiation. Brain, Behavior, and Immunity 11:273–285

Peissner W, Kocher M, Treuer H, Gillardon F (1999) Ionizing radiation-induced apoptosis of proliferating stem cells in the dentate gyrus of the adult rat hippocampus. Mol Brain Res 71:61–68

Plowman PN (1999) Stereotactic radiosurgery. VIII. The classification of postradiation reactions. Brit J Neurosurg 13:256–264

Powers BE, Thames HD, Gillette SM, Smith, C, Beck ER, Gillette EL (1998) Volume effects in the irradiated canine spinal cord: do they exist when the probability of injury is low? Radiother Oncol 46:297–306

Roman DD, Sperduto PW (1995) Neuropsychological effects of cranial radiation: current knowledge and future directions. Int J Radiat Oncol Biol Phys 31:983–998

Rubin P, Gash DM, Hansen JT, Nelson DF, Williams JP (1994) Disruption of the blood-brain barrier as the primary effect of CNS irradiation. Radiother Oncol 31:51–60

Ruifrok ACC, Kleiboer BJ, van der Kogel AJ (1992) Fractionation sensitivity of the rat cervical spinal cord during radiation retreatment. Radiother Oncol 25:295–300

Ruifrok ACC, Stephens LC, van der Kogel AJ (1994) Radiation

response of the rat cervical cord after irradiation at different ages: tolerance, latency and pathology. Int J Radiat Oncol Biol Phys 29:73–79

Russo C, Fischbein N, Grant E, Prados MD (1999) Late radiation injury following hyperfractionated craniospinal radiotherapy for primitive neuroectodermal tumor. Int J Radiat Oncol Biol Phys 44:85–90

Ryu S, Gorty S, Kazee AM, Bogart J, Hahn SS, Dalal PS, Chung CT, Sagerman RH (2000) "Full dose" reirradiation of human cervical spinal cord. Am J Clin Oncol (CCT) 23:29–31

Schultheiss TE, Kun LE, Ang KK, Stephens LC (1995) Radiation response of the central nervous system. Int J Radiat Oncol Biol Phys 31:1093–1112

Schultheiss TE, Orton CG, Peck RA (1983) Models in radiotherapy: volume effects. Med Phys 10:410–415

Schultheiss TE, Stephens LC (1992) Pathology of radiation myelopathy, widening the circle. Int J Radiat Oncol Biol Phys 23:1089–1091

Schultheiss TE, Stephens LC, Ang KK, Price RE, Peters LJ (1994) Volume effects in rhesus monkey spinal cord. Int J Radiat Oncol Biol Phys 29:67–72

Schultheiss TE, Stephens LC, Jiang GL, Ang KK, Peters LJ (1990) Radiation myelopathy in primates treated with conventional fractionation. Int J Radiat Oncol Biol Phys 19:935–940

Shinohara C, Gobbel GT, Lamborn KR, Tada E, Fike JR (1997) Apoptosis in the subependyma of young adult rats after single and fractionated doses of X-rays. Cancer Res 57:2694–2702

Smibert E, Anderson V, Godber T, Ekert H (1996) Risk factors for intellectual and educational sequelae of cranial irradiation in childhood acute lymphoblastic leukaemia. Brit J Cancer 73:825–830

Tada E, Yang C, Gobbel GT, Lamborn KR, Fike JR (1999) Long-term impairment of subependymal repopulation following damage by ionizing irradiation. Exper Neurol 160:66–77

van den Aardweg GJMJ, Hopewell JW, Whitehouse EM (1995) The radiation response of the cervical spinal cord of the pig: effect s of changing the irradiated volume. Int J Radiat Oncol Biol Phys 31:51–55

van der Kogel AJ (1991a) Central nervous system radiation injury in small animal models. . In: Gutin PH, Leibel SA, Sheline GE (eds) Radiation Injury to the Nervous System, Raven Press, New York, pp. 91–111

van der Kogel AJ (1991b) The nervous system: Radiobiology and experimental pathology. In: Scherer E, Streffer C, Trott, KR (eds) Medical Radiology. Diagnostic Imaging and Radiation Oncology Radiopathology of Organs and Tissues, Springer, Heidelberg, pp. 191–212

van der Kogel AJ (1993) Dose volume effects in the spinal cord. Radiother Oncol 29:105–109

Vrdoljak E, Bill CA, Stephens LC, van der Kogel AJ, Ang KK, Tofilon PJ (1992) Radiation-induced apoptosis of oligodendrocytes in vitro. Int J of Radiat Biol 62:475–480

Withers HR, McBride WH (1997) Biologic basis of radiation therapy. In: Perez CA, Brady LW (eds) Principles and Practice of Radiation Oncology, 3rd Edition. JP Lippincott-Raven, New York, pp 79–118

Withers HR, Taylor JMG, Maciejewski B (1988) Treatment volume and tissue tolerance. Int J Radiat Oncol Biol Phys 14:751–759

Wong CS, Minkin S, Hill RP (1992) Linear-quadratic model underestimates sparing effect of small doses per fraction in rat spinal cord. Radiother Oncol 23:176–184

Wong CS, Minkin S, Hill RP (1993a) Re-irradiation tolerance of rat spinal cord to fractionated X-ray doses. Radiother Oncol 28:197–202

Wong CS, Poon JK, Hill RP (1993b) Re-irradiation tolerance in the rat spinal cord: influence of level of initial damage. Radiother Oncol 26:132–138

5 Principles of Physics of External Beam Radiotherapy

Gabor Jozsef

CONTENTS

5.1
Introduction

The overall goal of radiation therapy is to inflict maximum radiation damage in the volume to be treated (target) and to minimize that damage to any non-target tissue. This chapter is a short overview of the principles of physics and technology that are employed in external beam radiation therapy to achieve a high degree of conformity between the total irradiated volume and the target volume. These principles are described in the context of treating tumors of the central nervous system.

Radiation beams originating from external sources must pass through normal tissue before they reach the target and continue irradiating the tissue beyond the target. Therefore, it is unavoidable that a significant dose from any beam is delivered to non-

G. Jozsef, PhD
University of Southern California, Keck School of Medicine, Department of Radiation Oncology, 1441 Eastlake Avenue, Room G350, Los Angeles, CA 90033-0804, USA

target tissue and an elaborate treatment planning process is required to deliver a tumoricidal dose to the target while keeping the dose to the non-target tissue to the lowest possible, generally acceptable limits. A number of physical and technological principles can be utilized – alone or combined – to achieve that goal. These general principles are:

1. Choice of radiation beam (photon or particle beams of various energy)
2. Use of multiple beams (fields) overlapping in the target volume
3. Adjusting the field shape to the shape of the projection of the target volume as seen from the source of the radiation beam
4. Varying the intensity of the beam within one field

The International Commission on Radiation Units and Measurements (ICRU) issued a recommendation (ICRU Report 50) to clarify the concept "target volume". The Clinical Target Volume (CTV) is defined as the union of the tumor as demonstrated by diagnostic procedures and the supposed microscopic involvement or spread-out routes around the tumor. Planning Target Volume (PTV) includes the CTV plus a margin to allow for limitations of the treatment technique, such as machine setup accuracy, patient movement, etc. This is the volume which should be irradiated to a prescribed dose. Irradiated Volume is a volume which receives a significant dose, such as 50% of the prescribed dose, during the treatment. In the following discussions "target volume" will mean PTV.

An "optimal" treatment plan is developed based on the above principles. The word optimal does not necessarily involve any mathematical optimization (see Sect. 5.6) The plan, however, is only as good as can be accurately executed. This accuracy depends on the mechanical features of the treatment machine and the accuracy of target localization and patient setup. While mechanical accuracy of setting up the treatment machine (e.g., gantry angles, beam shapes, table motions etc. for a linear accelerator) is typically within ±1 mm, patient immobilization and patient position reproducibility is still a problem. This is especially true in the trunk where the target can move due to breathing, the circulation cycle, changing fullness of bladder and rectum etc. Not surprisingly, the first beneficiaries of the technological advance of radiation treatment delivery systems were patients with CNS tumors, since the rigid skull can be immobilized and repositioned accurately with relatively simple devices (frames and/or plastic masks etc.) (see Sect. 5.7).

The following sections will concentrate on the physical and technological implications of the four principles mentioned above, and briefly describe techniques for immobilization and repositioning. Basic interactions between radiation and tissue are discussed in Chap. 4 of this volume.

5.2
Choice of Radiation Beam

5.2.1
Photons

The sources of photons in external beam therapy are either radioisotopes, emitting high-energy photons in their decay process, or X-rays generated by hitting a dense metal target with a focused beam of electrons accelerated to very high energy. The acceleration of electrons can be achieved by a static electric field (conventional X-ray machines), a slowly oscillating (50–180 Hz) magnetic field in a circular accelerating tube (betatrons), or a high frequency (~3000 MHz) electromagnetic field in a linear tube (linear accelerators). Some other types of electron accelerators (e.g., microtrons, "racetrack" accelerators) have also been built, but they did not find their way into the mainstream of radiation therapy.

The energy of X-ray beams is expressed in accelerating potential. For orthovoltage X-ray machines, it is up to about 250 kV, for linear accelerators in radiation therapy it is between 4 and 25 MV, and some betatrons can go above 40 MV. Betatrons, however, are no longer widely used, as the low-dose rate they produce requires long treatment times. The average photon energy in an X-ray beam is about 1/2 of the accelerating potential.

The photon-emitting radioisotope of choice in teletherapy is Cobalt-60. It emits high-energy photons (1.17 and 1.33 MeV), its half-life (5.26 years) is long enough to operate an irradiator for several years before the decreasing strength of the source results in long treatment times and has to be replaced. Its specific activity (decays/mass) is high, therefore a 2×2×2 cm source can have enough activity [~185 TBq (5000 Ci)] to provide about 100 cGy/min dose rate at 1 m distance. Most units operate with 80 cm of source-skin distance (SSD) or source to axis of gantry rotation distance (SAD).

Presently, the overwhelming majority of external beam treatments of CNS tumors are performed with linear accelerators. Telecobalt units in the United States are still in use in some medical centers. Cobalt-60 sources are also used in the gamma knife, a special device, designed for radiosurgical treatment of intracranial CNS lesions (for details, see Chap. 6 of this volume).

Photon beams of various energy differ in their ability to penetrate the tissue. Fig. 5.1 shows depth

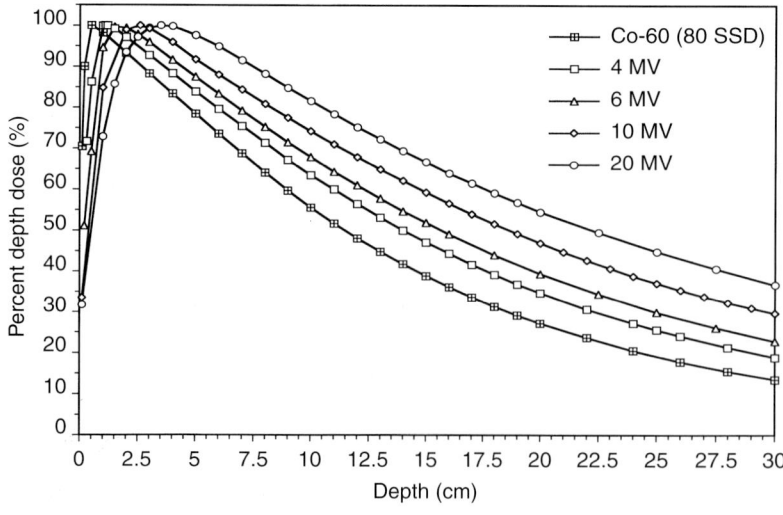

Fig. 5.1. Percent depth dose curves for several photon energies. Field size 10×10 cm, focus skin distance (FSD) 100 cm. (The Co-60 data were taken from BRJ Suppl. 11, 1978)

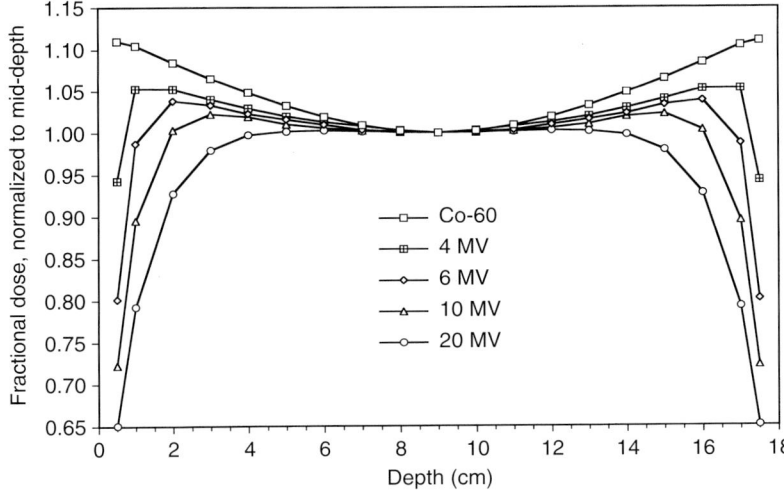

Fig. 5.2. Depth dose curves of parallel opposed fields with several photon energies. Field size 10×10 cm, tissue thickness 18 cm

dose curves of a 10×10 cm field of a cobalt unit, and 4, 6, 10, and 20 MV photon beams. The curves show a "build-up" region between the entry point and the depth of the maximum dose, where the dose gradually grows from a low superficial value to the maximum. The maximum dose depth increases with increasing photon energy. This phenomenon provides a "skin-sparing effect": the skin receives a much lower dose than the tissue below it.

The curves also indicate that any of these beams are capable of penetrating deep enough to treat brain tumors (maximum depth 8–9 cm) according to two criteria: (1) crossing as few as two beams already gives a higher dose in the intersecting volume than at the maximum dose depth below the entry points of each individual field (see Sect. 5.3); and (2) opposing two beams results in a more homogeneous dose

distribution (±10%) between the two entry points (Fig. 5.2).

5.2.2
Electron Beams

Electrons accelerated by linear accelerators (and betatrons) can be used directly to form a therapeutic beam. Depth dose curves for several electron energies are presented in Fig. 5.3. The maximum treatable depth, as defined by the 80% isodose line, is about 6 cm for the 18 MeV electrons, and the dose decreases sharply beyond that point. For a single beam treatment, therefore, a tumor in the brain cannot extend more than about 4 cm from the skull. The sharp dose fall-off beyond the 80% depth makes crossing elec-

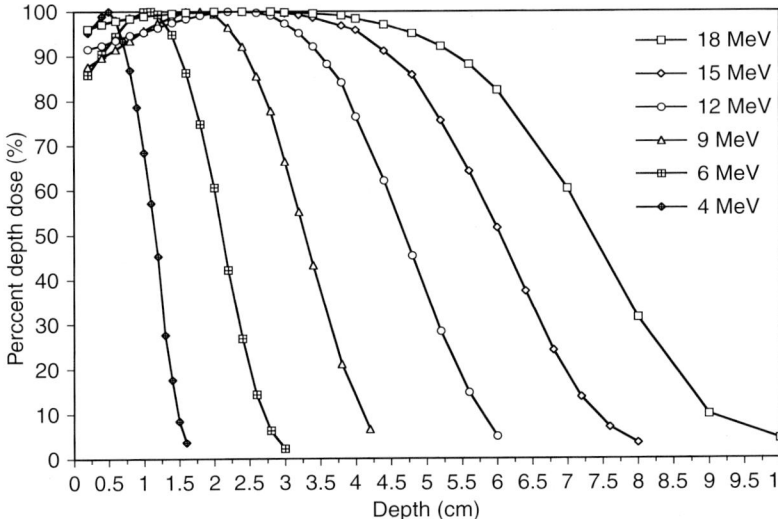

Fig. 5.3. Percent depth dose curves for several electron energies. Field size 10×10 cm, FSD=100 cm

tron fields impractical. A further disadvantage of this modality is that the gradual dose build-up at shallow depth, as seen in the photon beam depth dose curves, is missing. Hence, the skin dose is about the same as the tumor dose, which might cause serious skin reaction. However, electron beams combined with photon beams can be used, giving up some of the benefit of the sharp dose fall-off of the electron beams for the skin-sparing effect of the photons.

5.2.3
Charged Particles (protons, heavy ions)

Charged particle beams would be the most suitable for external beam radiation therapy if technological complexity of producing and controlling them would not drive the price of their application to over $40 million for installation in addition to a high operational cost. This is due to a phenomenon called the Bragg peak. Charged particles produce more ionization (and therefore dose) per centimeter at the end of their track as they slow down due to multiple collisions with electrons. The depth dose curve of a He^{2+} ion beam is shown in Fig. 5.4. The Bragg peak itself is too narrow to treat most clinical targets, but by placing an absorber of variable thickness into the beam, the width of the peak can be extended to meet the needs of clinical applications.

A further advantage of charged particle beams is that their relative biological effect per unit dose (RBE) is greater than that of photon and electron beams. Furthermore, the RBE is higher in the Bragg peak region than in the plateau. Therefore, the target in the Bragg peak not only receives more radiation dose, but also a biologically more effective one than

the tissue outside that region. The RBE of a certain type of radiation is defined as the ratio of the doses delivered by a 250-kV(p) X-ray beam and by the beam of that type, causing the same biological effect. An RBE value greater than 1 means biologically more effective radiation than a photon beam. For proton beams, an RBE value of 1.1–1.2 is employed in most treatment centers, but recent research indicates that this value is probably too low, especially in the Bragg peak region and in CNS tissue. Values of about 1.4–2 were reported for a dose of 2 Gy (WOUTERS et al. 1996; BELLI et al. 1997; GERWECK and KOZIN 1999). For ion beams, the difference of RBEs in the Bragg peak and the plateau region is greater than for protons, up to about the C^{6+} ion (RBE ~1.7–1.8) (HALL 1988). For heavier ions, this benefit decreases (KJELLBERG 1988).

Ion beams can intersect and be shaped like photon beams with a very sharp fall-off region around the field edges, further advancing their dosimetric advantage.

Despite the extreme costs of installing and operating a cyclotron (a circular type accelerator for positively charged particles), the number of proton and ion therapy facilities is rapidly growing and application of these beams is the subject of many exciting research papers (e.g., CARLSSON 1997; LOMAX et al. 1999; KARGER 1999). However, it is still limited to major research-oriented institutions with abundant resources (see Chap. 6).

5.2.4
Neutrons

Neutrons can be produced with several nuclear reactions. Early attempts at producing neutron beams

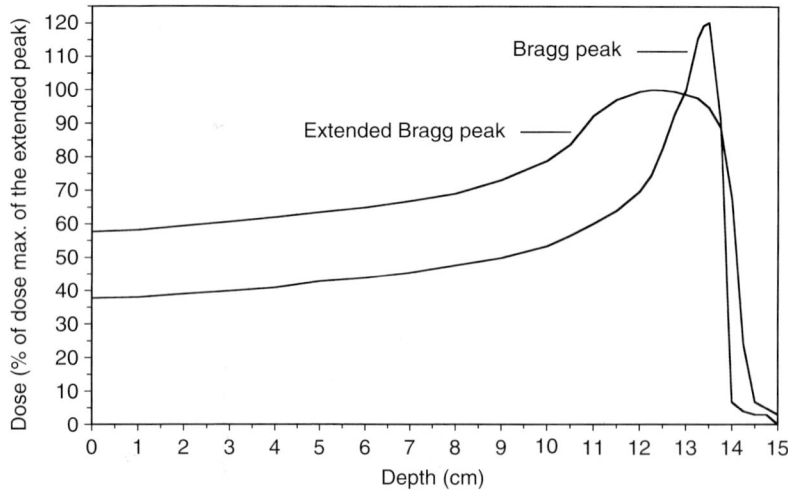

Fig. 5.4. Percent depth dose curve of a 230-MeV He^{2+} beam with and without extending the Bragg peak. (LYMAN et al. 1986)

employed accelerated deuterium nuclei bombarding tritium targets, yielding helium nuclei and 14-MeV neutrons. However, the neutron yield from this reaction is very low, and it is very difficult to build adequate tritium targets. The depth dose curve of these neutrons is about the same as that of a Co-60 beam. Proton or deuterium bombardment of a beryllium target can also produce neutrons. However, in order to produce high-energy neutrons, a cyclotron with accelerating potential of ~50–70 MeV is needed. The depth dose curves are similar to those of the 4- and 6-MV photon beams (HALL 1988; HOVER 1991).

Although neutrons have much higher biological effectiveness than photons (by a factor of 3–10), clinical trials so far fail to prove definite superiority over radiation therapy with photons. This fact, combined with the technical difficulties of producing and controlling the beam, reduced the original enthusiasm of employing neutrons in external beam radiation therapy (SCHMITT and WAMBERSIE 1990).

5.3
Use of Multiple Beams Overlapping in the Target Volume

5.3.1
General Remarks

In the following sections, only photon beams generated by linear accelerators will be considered (except Sect. 5.3.3.1 on the gamma knife).

The isodose line values in figures showing dose distributions are percentages of the dose maximums (except in Fig. 5.13). The lines are alternately black and white; white numbers indicate the values of black isodose lines and vice versa.

Intersecting beams is the oldest and most natural method to increase the dose in the treatment volume while decreasing irradiation to normal tissue. The use of multiple beams means a compromise: it decreases the dose to the non-target tissue, but increases the volume receiving that lower dose. This compromise is demonstrated in Fig. 5.5a and 5.5d. In Fig. 5.5a, the whole irradiated volume is between the two portals of the parallel opposed fields, delivering the full tumor dose to that entire volume. In Fig. 5.5d, two pairs of parallel opposed beams are crossed, the total volume receiving radiation outside the intersecting volume is doubled, but the dose to that volume is only about half of the dose delivered to the target.

The number of fields to be used is determined by the anatomic location, size and shape of the target, the available beam energies, the prescribed total dose and dose per treatment fractions, and often the preference of the treating team. These preferences might be different as there are not always clear-cut criteria to decide the superiority of one treatment plan over others (Sects. 5.5, 5.6).

About 10–15 years ago, most of radiation treatments, with the exception of stereotactic radiosurgery, were co-axial, i.e., the central rays of the beams were in the axial plane. With the advent of three-dimensional image reconstruction techniques and relocatable and reliable fixation devices for fractionated treatments, non-axial plane coplanar or non-coplanar treatments of brain lesions have become more common.

The relative dose delivered by each field to the target (more specifically to the isocenter or the depth of the dose maximum of each beam), i.e., the "weight", can be varied. The weight should be adjusted to homogenize the dose within the target or to increase/decrease the dose along the path of a particular field. Single field applications of photon beams are practically limited to a palliative treatment of the spine or the spinal cord (Fig. 5.6a).

5.3.2
Coplanar Treatments

5.3.2.1
Parallel Opposed Fields

A pair of lateral parallel opposed fields is used for whole-brain irradiation to deliver a homogeneous dose to the entire intracranial volume (Fig. 5.7). The beam energy is usually < 10 MV, to avoid underdosing brain tissue close to the surface which is within the dose build-up region. Higher energy (20 MV) lateral parallel opposed fields might be used for centrally located smaller targets if the distance between the entry points is small (Fig. 5.5b), exploiting the lower dose in the build-up region. However, for almost any smaller volume than whole brain, irradiation intersecting beams are regarded to be better than parallel opposed fields. The exception is for spinal lesions, which are frequently treated with a single posterior field. Sometimes, posteriorly weighted anterior/posterior parallel opposed fields are used for the treatment of lesions of the lumbar spine (Fig. 5.6b).

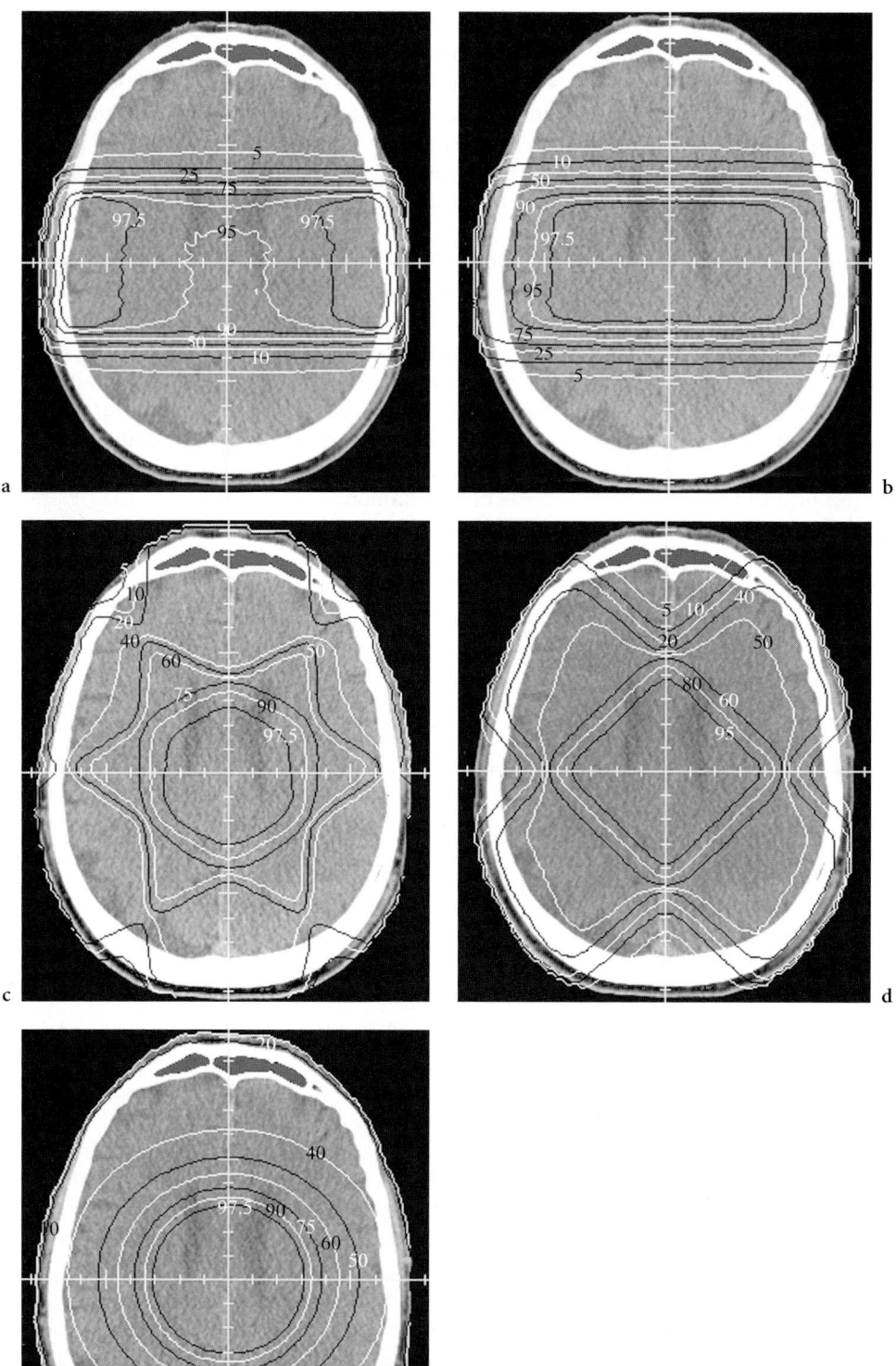

Fig. 5.5a–e. Dose distributions of several typical field arrangements in the axial plane. **a** 7×7-cm parallel opposed fields with 6-MV X-ray. **b** 7×7-cm parallel opposed fields with 20-MV X-ray. **c** Three 7×7-cm fields with 20-MV X-ray. **d** Four (two pairs of parallel opposed) 7×7-cm fields with 20-MV X-ray. **e** Full 360° arc with 7×7-cm field size and 6-MV X-ray

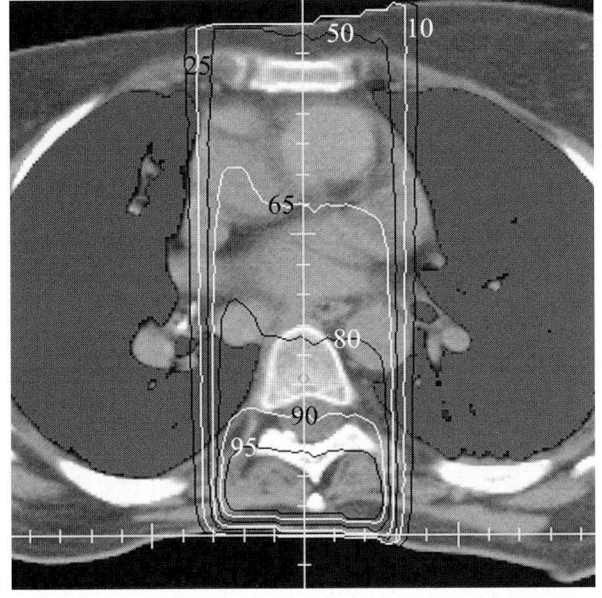

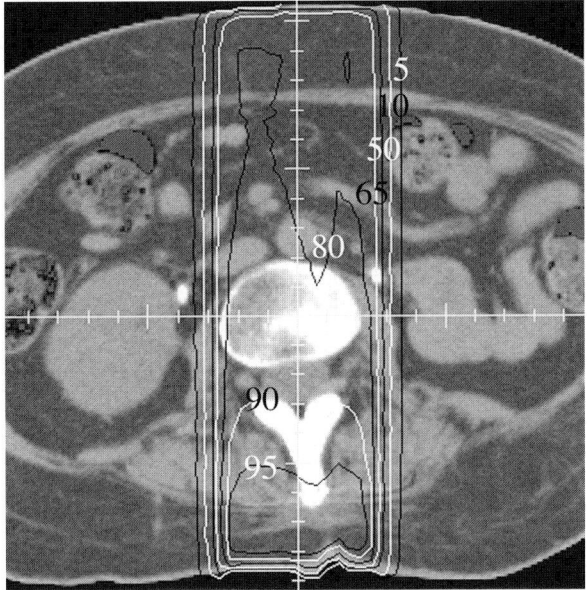

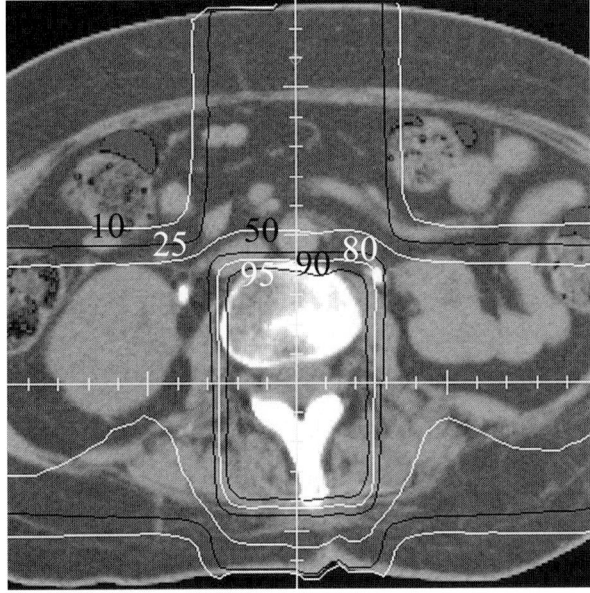

Fig. 5.6. Dose distributions for typical spine treatments. **a** Single posterior field with 6-MV X-ray. **b** Posteriorly weighted parallel opposed fields with 20-MV X-ray. **c** One posterior and two lateral opposed fields with 20-MV X-ray

5.3.2.2
Crossing Beams

Several typical coplanar beam arrangements are shown in Figs. 5.5 and 5.8, in an axial and a coronal plane, respectively. The two-field plan (Fig. 5.8a) can be used for targets near the surface; for more centrally located lesions, usually three- or four-field arrangements are used (Figs. 5.5c, 5.5d, 5.8b). The beam angles can be modified to avoid direct beams to especially sensitive organs, like the eye, optic nerves, and chiasm. Targets near the surface are equally often treated with a two-field plan in the axial plane, containing an anterior (or posterior) and lateral field, resulting in a dose distribution similar to that shown in Fig. 5.8a.

Spinal lesions may also be treated with posterior and lateral parallel opposed fields (Fig. 5.6c). This technique is limited to those vertebrae where only a small volume of the kidneys and lungs receives a dose from the lateral fields (e.g., lower lumbar spine).

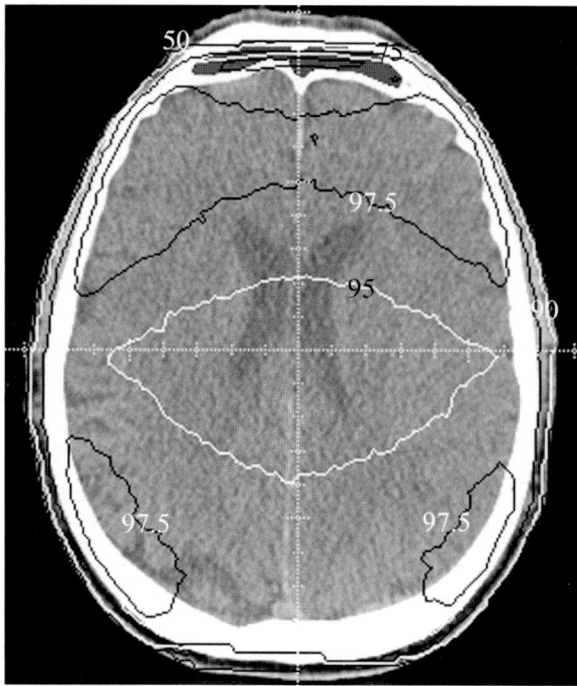

Fig. 5.7. Dose distribution for a whole-brain irradiation with 6-MV X-ray

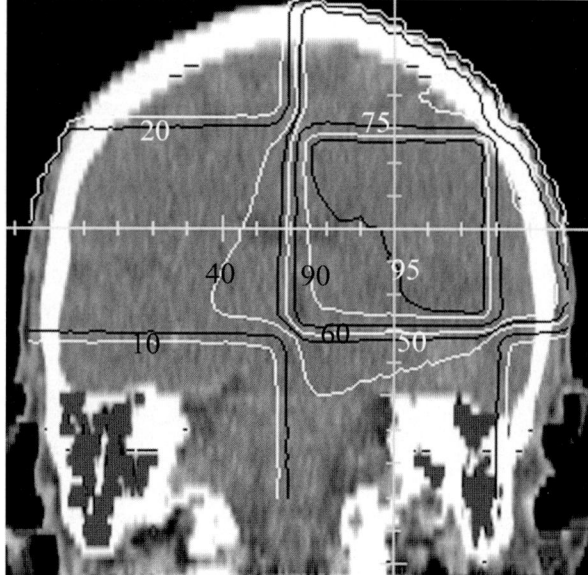

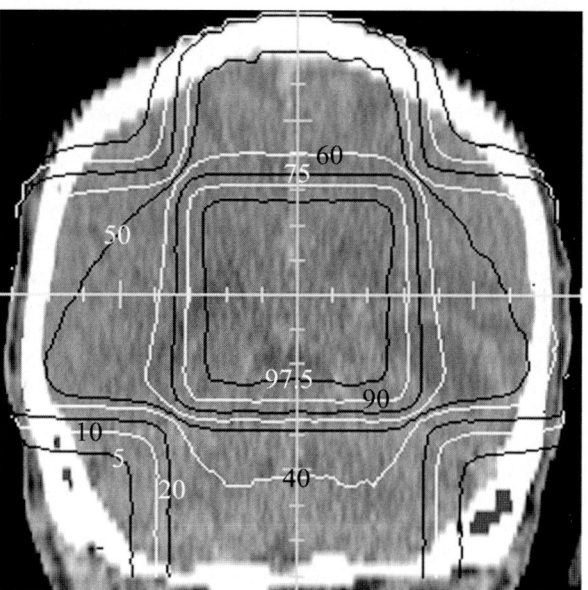

Fig. 5.8a,b. Dose distributions in the coronal plane. **a** Cephalo-caudal and lateral fields with 45° wedges and 6-MV X-ray. **b** Cephalo-caudal and a pair of lateral fields with 20-MV X-ray. The lateral fields are wedged (45°)

The penultimate use of intersecting beams is a continuous arc. Figure 5.5e shows a dose distribution with a continuous 360° rotation of the beam. As a rule of thumb, a circle (a cylinder in 3-D space) with a diameter 1.4–1.5 times the width of the field receives more than 50% of the dose to the center of the rotation. Therefore, the use of a single arc should be limited to treatment of small targets.

5.3.3
Non-Coplanar Treatments

The anatomy of the head – the nearly spherical shape and the size of the skull – the deep penetrating ability of high-energy photon beams, and the mechanics of radiation delivery systems allow aiming for the target from any direction in a spherical section. This section is somewhat larger than the half-sphere, superior to the center of the lesion. Beams that are not in an axial plane can be set by rotating the treatment couch and the gantry to the desired position. Straightforward non-coplanar treatments are, for example, an anterior, a lateral, and a vertex field for lateral lesions; a pair of parallel opposed fields augmented by a vertex field for medial lesions; or a combination of two fields in the coronal and two

fields in the sagittal plane for lesions near the top of the skull. The possibilities are simply too numerous to list. Some examples are shown in SHAW et al. (1998).

The most prominent non-coplanar techniques for brain lesions, however, are stereotactic radiosurgery or radiotherapy (SRS or SRT, respectively). SRS is a single fraction high-dose treatment for a small target (diameter < 4 cm), SRT is a multi-fractionated treatment where the dose per fraction is frequently much larger than 180–200 cGy used in traditional external beam radiation therapy (see Chap. 6 of this volume). Treatments are performed with the use of: multiple (7–12) fixed fields or multiple arcs (4–11) using linear accelerators (or cobalt units); a gamma knife, a special device designed for SRS; or with proton or heavy ion beams (KOOY 1993; LUTZ 1993; LUXTON et al. 1993).

5.3.3.1
Gamma Knife

This device contains 201 cylindrical Cobalt-60 sources; each is 20 mm long and 1 mm in diameter. Their activity is approximately 25–30 Ci at installation (see Chap. 6 for relevant details). The central source in the U-type gamma knife (Elekta Instrument AB) shown in Fig. 5.9, installed at the University of Southern California, is 55° above the horizontal plane. The sources are distributed evenly on a spherical surface extending ±48° from the central source in the vertical and ±55° in the horizontal plane. The radius of the sphere is 40.5 cm. Four "helmets" with very precisely aligned holes direct the 201 beams to the center of the sphere (isocenter) and collimate them to 4, 8, 14, and 18 mm in diameter, measured at the center. A special frame holds the patient's head rigid and a positioning device attached to that frame can move practically any point in the brain to the isocenter. The dose distribution of a single isocenter ("shot") is spherical; the 50% isodose surface (relative to the maximum dose) is very close to a sphere with a diameter of the helmet size.

For larger and/or irregular targets, multiple isocenters are applied. The isocenter is set to different locations inside the target. The helmet size, location, and dose delivered to the isocenter by each shot can be adjusted to match the 50% isodose surface of the combined dose distribution to the shape of the target (see Chap. 6).

5.3.3.2
Linear Accelerator-Based Radiosurgery or Radiotherapy

Linear accelerator-based radiosurgery or radiotherapy is mostly performed with the use of multiple arcs. The plane of the arcs is vertical and the arcs are of equal angular distance from each other (Fig. 5.10). The arc lengths are about 100°. Usually, a set of circular secondary collimators (cones) are used to produce small circular field sizes. Their diameter can be much larger (up to about 4 cm) than the gamma knife collimator sizes. Therefore, it is not necessary to use multiple isocenters for large spherical targets. Even targets with elliptical shape can be treated with a single isocenter by carefully adjusting the field sizes, arc lengths and planes, and doses delivered to the isocenter by each arc (LUXTON and JOZSEF 1994). Irregularly shaped targets, however, might require multiple isocenter treatments. For single isocenter treatments, the goal is usually to define the dose of the 80% isodose surface (relative to the maximum) to the prescribed dose. For multiple isocenter treatments, the dose prescription is given to the highest isodose surface covering the target. The dose distribution over the target, therefore, is usually more

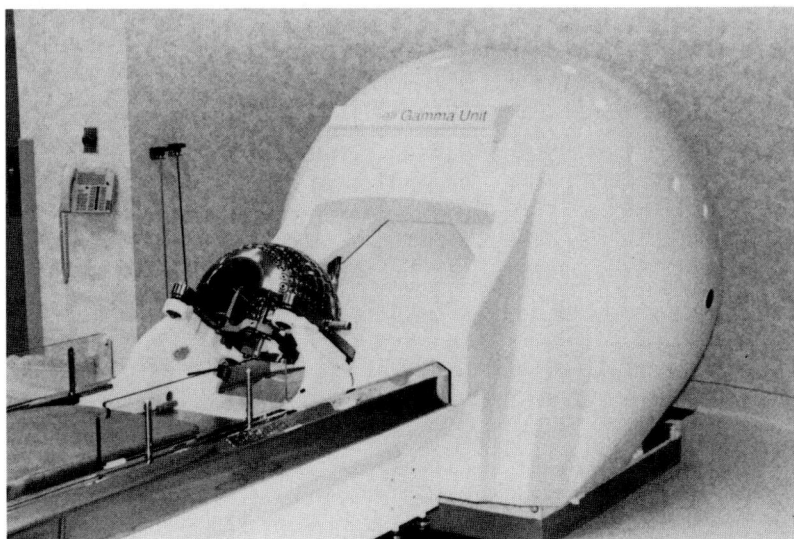

Fig. 5.9. The gamma knife (Leksell Gamma Unit, Elekta Instrument AB)

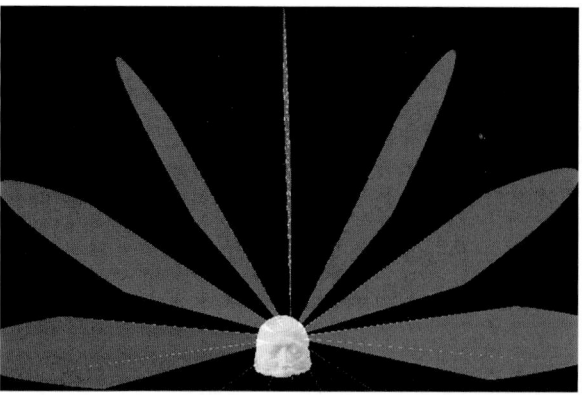

Fig. 5.10. Seven arc arrangement for linear-accelerator-based radiosurgery

Dose distributions calculated for gamma knife and multi-arc linear accelerator treatment for the same lesion are presented in Fig. 5.11. The gamma knife is able to match the "boomerang" shape of the lesion with a fairly inhomogeneous distribution since only the 50% isodose surface covers the target. The linear accelerator plan is more homogeneous over the target – the 90% isodose surface covers it – but it also encompasses a larger elliptical volume around the lesion. The isodose lines representing the volumes receiving half of the prescription dose are also marked. There is still ongoing debate between "believers" of the gamma knife and the linear-accelerator-based SRS and SRT (Yu C et al. 1999).

homogeneous than in the case of gamma knife treatments (see Chap. 6).

Although SRS and SRT can be performed on standard radiotherapy linear accelerators, specialized linear accelerators are designed for radiosurgery (e.g., Novalis System, BrainLAB GmbH). These systems allow an increase in setup accuracy and have frame holders and collimator sets. Recently, a special "miniature" linear accelerator appeared on the market which is so compact that the whole accelerator can be moved and set to any direction in the 3-D space (Cyberknife, Accuray Inc.) (see Chap. 20 of this volume).

5.4 Field Shaping

Tumors frequently are of irregular shape. In practice, most fields in the radiation therapy, especially for brain lesions, should be "blocked", i.e., the fields are shaped by high-density metal blocks according to the projection of the target as viewed from the direction of the beam. Doing so minimizes radiation exposure of non-target tissue. Traditional blocking was made by manually cutting a cast to the desired shape and pouring hot liquid Cerrobend (a low melting point alloy containing bismuth, lead, tin, and cadmi-

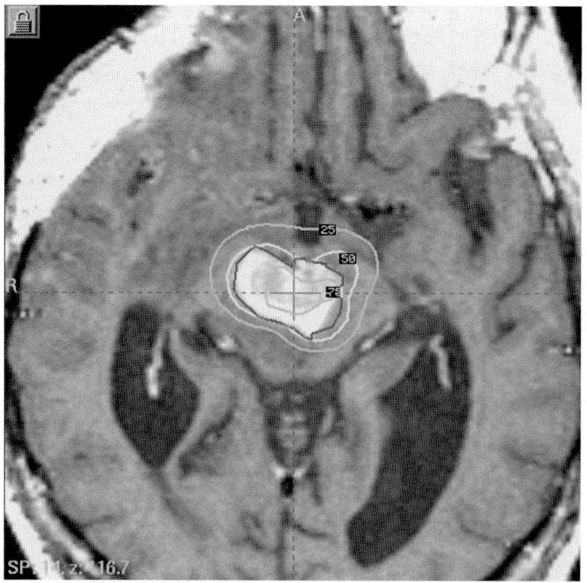
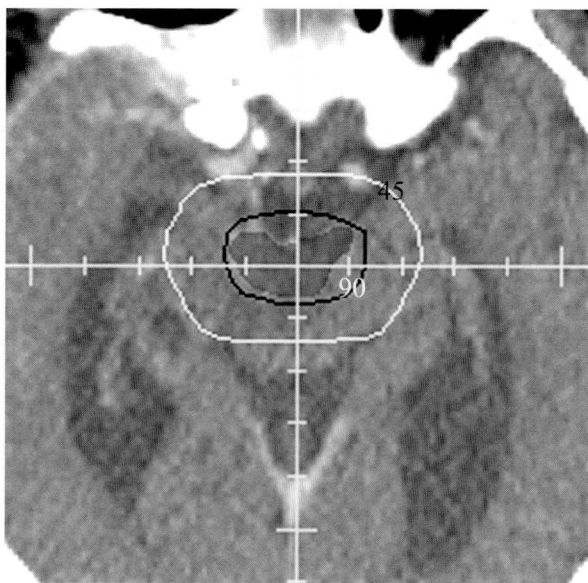

Fig. 5.11. Dose distributions for the same lesion with (a) gamma knife and (b) seven arc linear accelerator radiosurgery. The rectangular field sizes in the linear accelerator treatment are adjusted to the largest projection of the lesion along each rotation

um) into the cast. The "desired shape" is obtained by outlining the target by hand on a radiograph taken from the same direction as the intended radiation therapy field. Obviously, this film cannot be taken for vertex or for most caudal-oblique fields. This is one of the main reasons that radiation treatments until recently used only co-axial planar fields.

With advanced computer technology and rapid progress in imaging software, virtual three-dimensional reconstruction of the anatomy can be built from CT (or MR) scans. With this capability, the projection of the target from any view or beam direction can also be reconstructed and displayed (i.e., beam's eye view or digital radiograph displays). Blocking any fixed beam to conform the shape of the field to the target has now become possible. Traditional block cutting, however, is fairly labor intensive and not very accurate. The need for manual block cutting had been largely eliminated with the introduction of multi-leaf collimators. These are two sets of thin plates (vanes or leaves) made of high-density material, usually tungsten, on two sides of the field, set parallel to the beam direction. The thickness of the plates is less than 1 cm as projected from the source to the accelerator axis of rotation (usually 100 cm). Each of the vanes can be moved separately into the beam with computer control blocking part of the field. Thus, the opening between the two sets of vanes defines the radiation field (Fig. 5.12).

Multileaf collimators can also be used for blocking in arc therapy. Obviously, the shape of the target as viewed from the beam direction changes as the beam rotates, hence the leaves must be continually readjusted. The multileaf technique allows a quasi-continuous arc, as it divides the arc into a number of intervals. Rotation of the gantry stops at the end point of each interval, adjusts the leaves, delivers the dose appropriate for that interval, and moves to the next position (stop and shoot). A dynamic multileaf system even allows leaf motion while the beam is on. The extensive use of field shaping to conform the beam shape to the target in a multiple – mostly non-coplanar – beam setup is called *conformal therapy*.

5.5
Intensity Modifiers

Besides adjusting the dose delivered by a field as a whole (weighting), there is often a need to modify the dose delivered within the field to homogenize the dose over the target volume. Inhomogeneous dose distribution in the target volume is due to the fact that the patient surface is not flat and perpendicular to the central ray under the area of the field. Additionally, for larger targets, the dose delivered to points distal to the skin can be significantly less than to proximal points along the field. The first kind of inhomogeneity can be compensated by a tissue compensator. It is a block with zero thickness along the ray in the field which intersects the patient surface nearest to the source and different thicknesses along any other rays to absorb the same amount of radiation as the "missing tissue" would absorb (Djordjevich et al. 1990) (Fig. 5.13). Constructing compensators is time consuming and they are not used very often in treatments of CNS tumors.

The second kind of dose inhomogeneity is compensated by placing so-called wedge filters in the beam. They are wedge-shaped metal (lead, steel, or copper) blocks, decreasing the beam's intensity more along the rays going through the thicker parts of the wedge. The wedges are characterized by the angle shown in Fig. 5.14. The dose distribution in Fig. 5.8a was calculated using wedges, while Fig. 5.15 shows the same field arrangements without wedges. The increased inhomogeneity in the high-dose region when not using wedges is clearly demonstrated. Cobalt units and linear accelerators are usually equipped with 15°, 30°, 45°, and 60° wedges. Lately,

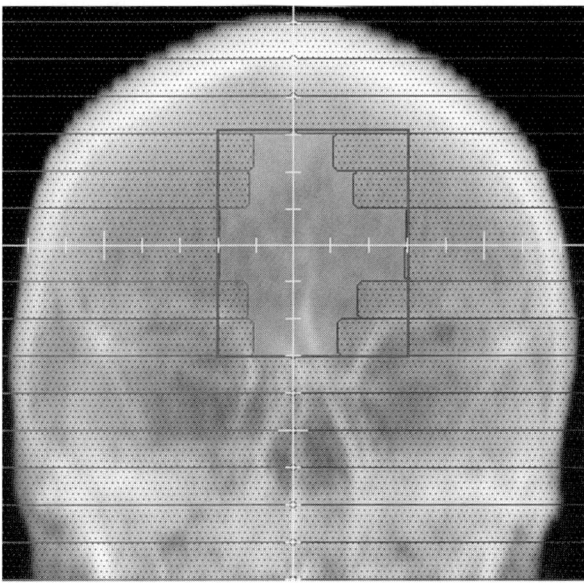

Fig. 5.12. Creating an irregularly shaped field with 1-cm multileaf collimators

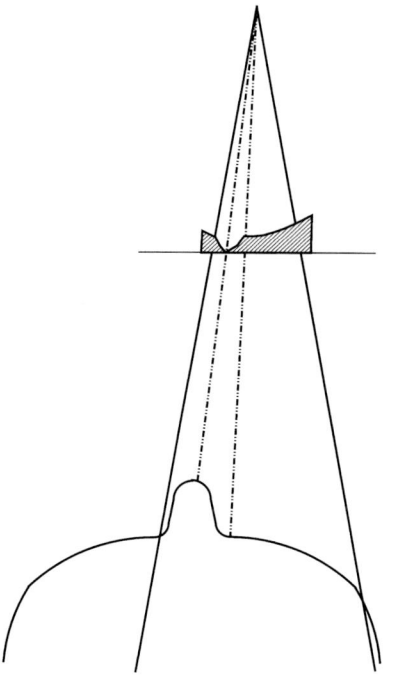

Fig. 5.13. The principle and design of a compensator

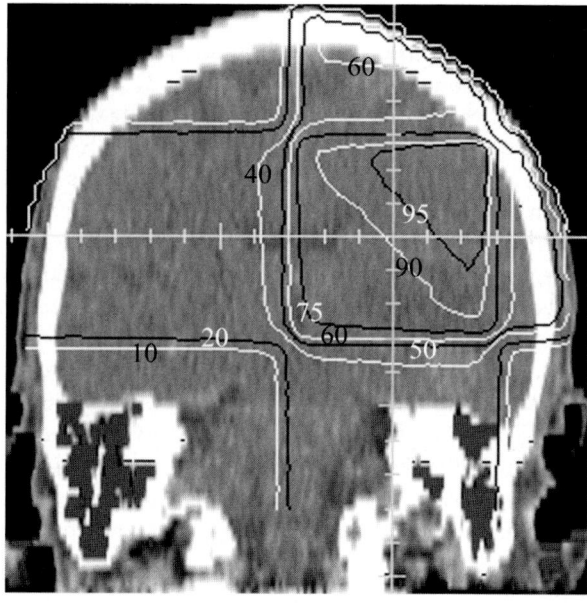

Fig. 5.15. Dose distribution of the same field arrangement as Fig. 5.8a, without wedges

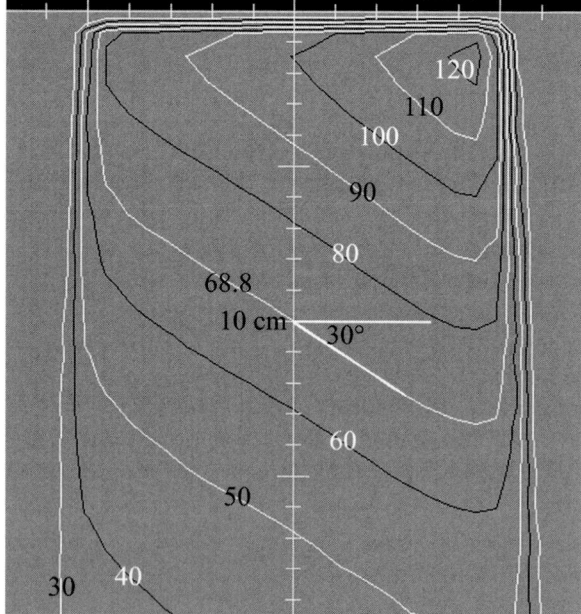

Fig. 5.14. Dose distribution of a 10×10-cm 6-MV X-ray beam with a 30° wedge. The wedge angle measured as the complement of the angle between the isodose line and the central axis at 10 cm depth

however, the concept of the dynamic wedge had been introduced. One of the field-size-defining collimator blades moves into the field while the beam is on. A computer controls the speed of the blade moving in or out of the beam. The field edge, which during most of the beam-on time is blocked by the blade, receives less dose than the opposite side, creating the desired wedge effect. Dynamic wedge software usually has blade motion control tables built in for a large number of wedge angles, e.g., from 5° to 75° in 5° intervals.

If the blades can be moved with computer control during irradiation, why not the leaves of the multileaf collimator? Indeed, they can be moved and their motion can be programmed in a very complex way. As an example, the two opposite leaves produce only a 1-cm open space between them. By moving these vanes simultaneously and spending a different amount of time at each position, the dose delivered through these openings can be varied. By doing the same with the other pairs of vanes at the same time, arbitrary predetermined doses can be delivered to any location within the field. This is the basic principle of *Intensity Modulated Radiotherapy* (IMRT). Certainly, there are more optimal leaf positioning methods than the simultaneous motion of the leaf with constant openings.

IMRT is a complex system. First, an optimum intensity modulation is calculated for multiple fields by an optimization software, the leaf positions are then calculated to achieve intensity modulation, and finally, the leaf positions are downloaded to the multileaf control computer. The first commercially available product using the IMRT principle was the Peacock system (Nomos Corp., Sewickley, Pa., USA).

Since its introduction, IMRT has been the subject of intense research, and newer treatment planning software and linear accelerators are equipped with IMRT capability. Figure 5.16 demonstrates the level of conformity achievable by using conformal therapy and IMRT principles, even by a relatively simple "intensity modulation" without mathematical optimization. A spine lesion threatening with spinal cord compression can be treated by a high dose while the cord receives less than 50% of the target dose. Figure 5.16a shows a treatment plan with a U-shaped distribution covering the spine anterior and lateral from the spinal cord with the 70% isodose line. The dose distribution in Fig. 5.16b forms a ring around the spinal cord. The center of the cord in each case receives less than 10% of the maximum dose.

The dose distributions were achieved by 12 coplanar beams in 30° intervals with the spinal cord blocked from every direction. In the case of U-shaped distribution, the processes are also blocked. The posterior and posterior oblique fields are closer to the surface, and therefore, are treated with a 6-MV X-ray while the rest of the fields are treated with the better penetrating 20-MV beam. Additionally, the posterior beams are weighted more but no intensity modulation is applied within the fields.

For ring-shaped distribution, the fields treat the entire vertebral body, including pedicle and lamina (the spinal cord is blocked), and all fields are treated with a 20-MV X-ray beam. As a simple intensity modulation, the parts of the fields treating either the processes or the vertebral body can now be given different weights. Several papers on all aspects of the IMRT technique can be found in PURDY et al. (1997).

5.6
Optimization

For any optimization – mathematical or not – there must be criteria by which the superiority of one treatment plan over another can be decided. In case of manual optimization, these criteria should be easy to calculate, intuitive, and of obvious physical meaning. Some of the quantities used for analyzing dose distributions are the dose homogeneity over the target (can be measured, for example, as the ratio of the maximum and minimum dose within the target), the maximum and/or average doses to sensitive organs, or some special points outside the target. A more complex tool, but still relatively easy to use in manual treatment planning, is the (cumulative) dose-volume histogram which is a graph or table showing the

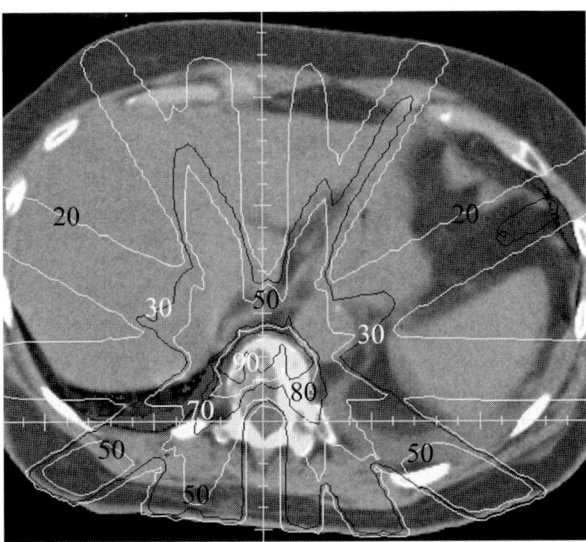 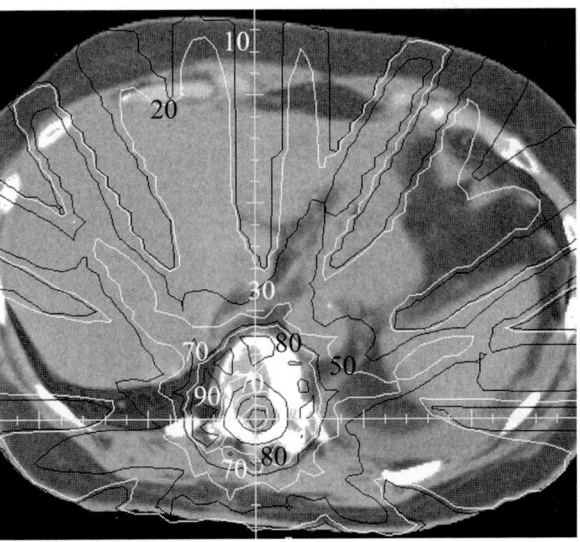

a   b

Fig. 5.16. Dose distribution of conformal treatment of the vertebra, minimizing the dose to the spinal cord. **a** Treatment of the vertebral body and the pedicles. **b** Treatment of the whole vertebra

volume (vertical axis) receiving more than a certain dose (horizontal axis). It can be calculated for any region of interest or for the whole volume of dose calculation. Dose–volume histograms for the entire volume of several treatment plans are presented in Fig. 5.17. They demonstrate the compromise mentioned in Sect. 5.3.1. The parallel opposed beams irradiate a larger volume with high doses (>50%), but less volume with lower doses, than the pair of parallel opposed fields or the arc. The arc irradiates less volume with mid-range (25–55%) doses, but treats a larger volume below 25% than the other two techniques.

As the 3-D treatment planning process becomes more complex, manual optimization may not be able to fully exploit the potential of any future technological developments. Automated optimization procedures are needed. Mathematical optimization (or programming) is a procedure to find the extreme value of a quantity, called the score function, by varying its dependent variables, with or without imposing constraints on the values of these variables.

As early as the 1960s, attempts were made to mathematically optimize dose distributions for radiation therapy treatments, but none of them have become routinely and widely employed (e.g., HOPE et al. 1967; REDPATH et al. 1967; JOZSEF 1982). These attempts differed in the choice of the quantity to be optimized, e.g., homogeneity over the target; large dose gradient around the target; theoretical tumor control and normal tissue complication probabilities; or best fit to a desired, ideal dose distribution (NIEMERKO et al. 1992). Sometimes even the mathematical form of the score functions based on the

same quantities, e.g., beam weights, beam entry points and angles, field sizes, and even wedge angles.

One of the early optimization criteria was recently revived and given the name of "inverse programming"; fitting the real dose distribution to an ideal one. This is the criterion used by most IMRT systems. The underlying mathematical problem in the first IMRT systems has been solved by the so-called back-projection method, practically an inverse of the method by which CT scans are created. In the CT scan, an absorption pattern (therefore, an electron density map) is generated from knowledge of the intensity changes along a ray. Here, the intensity of a ray is determined from the absorption pattern, as defined by the desired dose distribution (BORTFELD et al. 1990, 1994). Different optimization schemes, however, can also be used. Generally, there are two families of methods of solving a mathematical optimization problem: direct search, used by most earlier optimization attempts; or stochastic methods. The search for a minimum of a score function can be visualized as a skier trying to get to the deepest point of the deepest valley. In a search, skiers can look for the direction of the steepest slope (if they can measure the slope) and slide down along that direction for a while and repeat the procedure. If the slopes cannot be measured, they can select points around them and slide to the deepest one among them. The skiers, however, can never be sure whether or not they could get into a deeper valley if they made a less lucrative choice along the path. They will find the locally deepest point but not necessarily the deepest one.

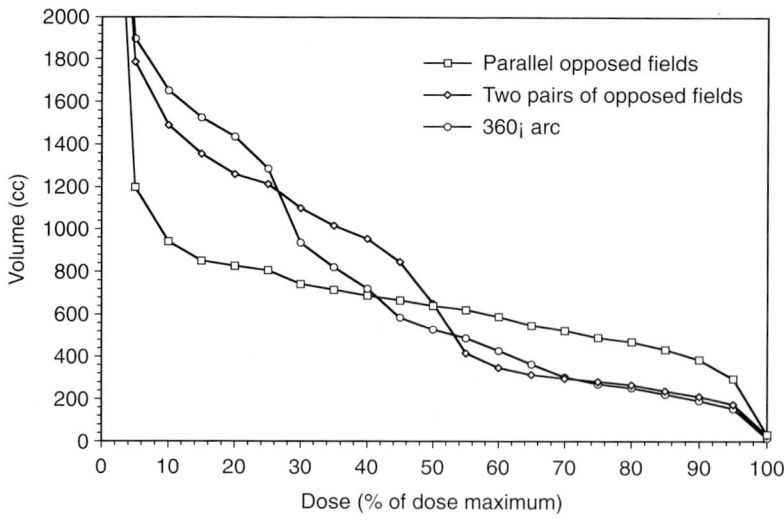

Fig. 5.17. Cumulative dose volume histograms for dose distributions in Fig. 5.5a,d,e

The stochastic methods, in principle, can overcome this difficulty. The skiers are allowed to choose points with certain probability which do not necessarily provide the deepest descent at each step, they might sometimes even go uphill. It is proven that a method with certain kind of probability assignment to each direction can lead to the absolute minimum. The two most popular optimization algorithms of this kind are the genetic (Langer et al. 1996; Yu Y et al. 1997) and the simulated annealing methods (Webb 1989, 1991; Morrill et al. 1991).

It should be emphasized that the choice of the optimum criteria (and the score function) reflects the preferences and treatment philosophies of the treating team. For example, some groups might accept more inhomogeneous dose distribution over the target volume than others and they might differ in their preferences of the maximum doses to certain organs etc. Therefore, optimized plans from different centers are not necessarily the same.

5.7
Machine and Patient Setup Accuracy

The manufacturer's specification of new treatment machines on most mechanical parameters is ±1 mm. For example, in the case of linear accelerators and Co-60 units these include: (a) coincidence of the physical isocenter with a built-in light source projected crosshair and the center of an external system of laser localization, (b) coincidence of the radiation field with a light field obtained by the same built-in light source, (c) stability of the isocenter when rotating the field defining collimator and/or the gantry, and (d) the read-out of positions, distances, and field sizes. An elaborate quality assurance protocol, as in Kutcher et al. (1994), must be followed to regularly check and keep mechanical accuracy within the required limits. In newer machines, further tests are needed to verify the accuracy of the multileaf collimators (static and dynamic mode) and the dynamic wedges.

The output of the machines and the energy of the beams must also be checked regularly (usually monthly) with calibrated radiation measurement systems (an ionization chamber and an electrometer), following recommended measurement protocols, such as the American Association of Physics in Medicine Task Group 21 (1983) protocol.

Since even the simplest treatment procedure (patient setup, initiating the beam, etc.) can take several minutes, immobilization devices should be applied in order to maintain setup accuracy. For traditional spine treatments a "vacuum bag" will usually suffice. This is like a slightly inflated cushion filled with small beads. As the patient lies down, it conforms to his/her shape. The air is then quickly pumped out, the beads are pushed together, and the bag becomes firm, preserving the shape of the patient. Conformal treatment of the spine, however, requires more accurate positioning. It can be achieved by using a thermoplastic sheet attached to a mounting tray under the patient and the vacuum bag. The thermoplastic sheet, while hot, can be stretched around the patient's body, and attached to the mounting tray. When it cools down, it becomes rigid again, preserving the shape of the patient's head and face (Fig. 5.18a).

Thermoplastic masks or strips, the same kind as described above, are practically always used for brain treatments (Fig. 5.18b). For increased accuracy, the mask can be attached to rigid frames mountable to the treatment couch (Fig. 5.18c). Some repositioning and immobilization systems use bite blocks or ear plugs attached to the frame, further increasing the reproducibility of the head's position. Fiduciary markers can be placed on the surface of the mask. In more advanced systems, the frame itself has built-in markers and rulers. The isocenter can be set up by obtaining the relative position of the planned isocenter to these markers from the treatment planning process and moving the mask and/or frame to that position.

The above systems are noninvasive and are used for multiple fraction treatments. Invasive positioning and immobilization devices are used in single fraction treatments like radiosurgery (either with a gamma knife or linear accelerator). A head frame is rigidly attached to the skull with screws (Fig. 5.18d). A good summary of patient positioning and immobilization techniques has been provided by Reinstein (1998).

A new technology, called gating, is emerging to eliminate inaccuracies caused by intrinsic motion of the patient. A detector determines whether some markers or specially assigned points are out of their originally planned positions by a preset limit. If they are, the beam is shut down. When the points are back in their correct positions, the beam is turned on again. Since time periods when the beam is on might be brief, the accelerator must have a high dose rate mode and very short transition period between zero and maximum dose rate (Ramsey et al. 1999).

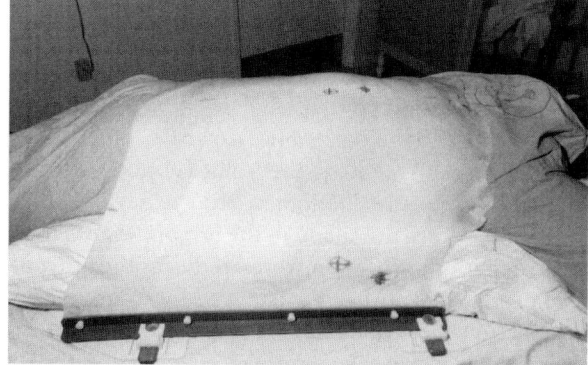

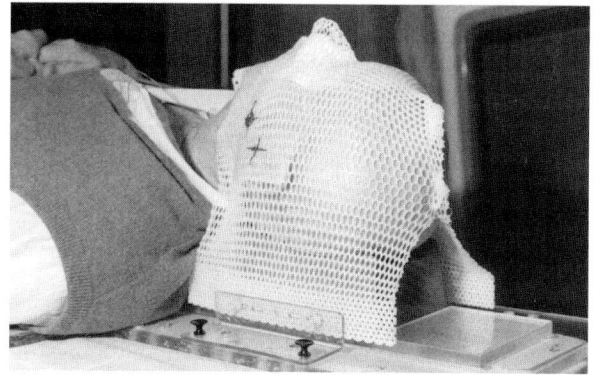

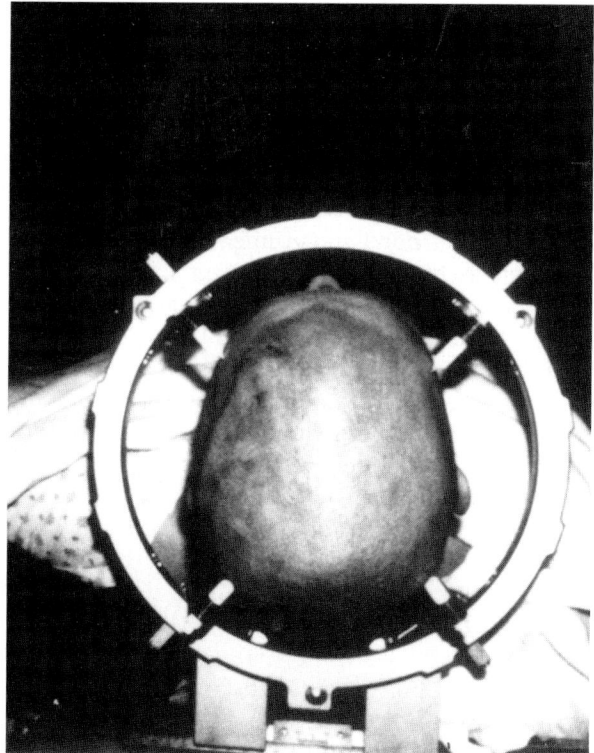

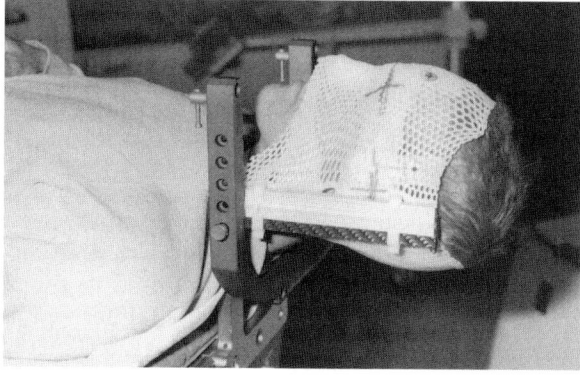

Fig. 5.18a–d. Frequently used positioning and immobilization devices. **a** Immobilization of the torso with vacuum bag and thermoplastic body mask. **b** Simple thermoplastic head mask. **c** Two-part thermoplastic mask on a rigid frame attachable to the treatment couch. **d** Invasive head frame (BRW) for single fraction stereotactic radiosurgery

5.8
Practical Examples

In the previous sections, we briefly discussed methods of improving dose distributions from conventional to the newest techniques. In this section, a few examples are given to demonstrate the benefit of these efforts:

1. Conventional fractionation (180–200 cGy/fraction)

   It is known from experience that the brain and spinal cord tissue can tolerate about 4500 cGy given in 180–200-cGy fractions. It is also known, however, that some tumors of the CNS require doses of about 6000 cGy to respond to this fractionation regimen. In Fig. 5.17 the dose volume histograms of three coplanar beam arrangements are compared. It is clear that the parallel opposed beam arrangement cannot be used, since a very large volume of normal brain tissue receives a high dose. The multiple beam arrangements and arc therapy (Sect. 5.3.2.2) decrease the dose outside the target to about half of that within the target, therefore, the higher dose can now be safely delivered to the target volume. Applying blocked or conformal fields or more non-coplanar fields can further increase the ratio between target dose and normal tissue dose.

2. Non-conventional fractionation (twice a day or < 250 cGy/fraction)

   In the case of smaller target volumes or relatively radioresistant lesions (e.g., melanoma or sarcoma) higher doses per fraction can be more effective. Normal tissue, however, is more sensitive to these accelerated regimens. An example of when a spine should be treated with a regimen of 5×500 cGy, while the cord has to be protected, is shown in Fig. 16. By delivering that dose to the 70% isodose surface, the cord receives between 70–150 cGy, which is well within the tolerance range. The dose per fraction to the tissue around the vertebra is about 300–350 cGy, higher than the conventional 200 cGy, but being given only five times, it is still well tolerated. Conformal therapy and IMRT methods are employed in this modality (Sect. 5.5).

3. Radiosurgery (1200–2500 cGy in a single fraction)

   For very small lesions (diameter <3.5–4 cm), a large tumoricidal dose can be delivered in a single fraction without complication. If the volume is that small, even large dose inhomogeneity within that volume (as in the gamma knife treatments) does not seem to cause complications. The dose fall-off around the lesion, however, must be very steep. As shown in Fig. 5.11, 50% of the tumor dose (600–1250 cGy) is delivered to a volume which is roughly 1.5 times the diameter of the tumor. The brain tolerance for single fraction whole-brain irradiation is about 1000 cGy, therefore a small volume receiving this amount of dose is tolerable (Sect. 5.3.3).

5.9
Conclusion

External beam radiation therapy has undergone major changes in the last decade mostly due to the introduction of computer control technology into radiation delivery systems (dynamic wedges, dynamic multileaf collimators, preprogrammed treatment sequences etc.). Faster computers allow real 3-D treatment planning based on full 3-D modeling of the patient's anatomy and allow one to perform dose optimization algorithms in reasonable time. Treatment planning computers can download full treatment sequences to the delivery device, allowing the running of very complex field setups.

The first beneficiaries of most of these technological advancements were patients with brain lesions. The increased accuracy and conformity of the treatment enabled the physicians to apply more radical treatment regimens with decreased incidence of treatment toxicity. Stereotactic radiosurgery and radiotherapy are now performed routinely, and special devices, like the gamma knife, were introduced to specifically treat brain lesions.

Despite some arch-conservative views questioning the value of further improving dose distributions (Schulz 1999), research efforts continue to explore the limit of existing technologies and introduce newer ways of treatment delivery. As an old Chinese proverb says: "If something is not moving forward, it is moving backward". In the interest of our patients, we do not want this to happen to radiation therapy.

References

American Association of Physics in Medicine Task Group 21 (1983) A protocol for determination of absorbed dose from high energy photon and electron beams. Med Phys 10:741–771

Belli M, Campa A, Ermolli I (1997) A semi-empirical approach to the evaluation of the relative biological effectiveness of therapeutic proton beams: the methodological framework. Radiat Res 148: 592–598

Bortfeld T, Bürkelbach J, Boesecke R, et al. (1990) Methods of image reconstruction from projections applied to conformation radiotherapy. Phys Med Biol 35:1423–1434

Bortfeld T, Boyer AL, Schlegel W, et al. (1994) Realization and verification of three dimensional conformal radiotherapy with modulated fields. Inter J Radiat Oncol Biol Phys 30:899–908

Carlsson AK, Andreo P, Brahme A (1997) Monte-Carlo and analytical calculation of proton pencil beams for computerized treatment plan optimization. Phys Med Biol 42:1033–1053

Djordjevich A, Bonham DJ, Hussein EMA, et al. (1990) Optimal design of radiation compensators. Med Phys 17:397–404

Gerweck LE, Kozin SV (1999) Relative biological effectiveness of proton beams in clinical therapy. Radiother Oncol 50: 135–142

Hall EJ (1988) Radiobiology for the radiologist. 3rd edn. J.B. Lippincott Co, (ed) New Radiation Modalities, Philadelphia, PA pp 261–292

Hope CS, Laurie J, Orr JS, et al. (1967) Optimization of X-ray treatment planning by computer judgment. Phys Med Biol 12:531–542

Hover KH, Hesse BM, Oetzel D, et al. (1991) Comparison of dosimetric properties of 15 MV photons and 14 MeV neutrons in external stereotactic convergence therapy (in German). Strahlenther Onkol 167:651–657

International Commission on Radiation Units and Measurements (1993) Prescribing, recording and reporting photon beam therapy. Report 50, Bethesda, MD

Jozsef G (1982) Computerized optimization of the dose distribution of telecobalt treatments (in Hungarian). Magyar Onkologia 26:171–180

Karger CP, Jäkel O, Hartmann GH (1999) A system for three dimensional dosimetric verification of treatment plans in intensity modulated radiotherapy with heavy ions. Med Phys 26:2125–2132

Kjellberg RN, Abe M (1988) Stereotactic Bragg-peak proton beam therapy. In: Lunsford LD (ed) Modern stereotactic neurosurgery. Martinus Nijhoff, Boston, MA, pp 463–470

Kooy H (1993) Three dimensional treatment planning for stereotactic radiosurgery. In: Alexander E, Loeffler JS, Lunsford LD (eds) Stereotactic radiosurgery. McGraw-Hill, Inc., New York, pp 17–30

Kutcher GJ, Coia L, Gillin M, et al. (1994) Comprehensive quality assurance for radiation oncology: report of AAPM Radiation Therapy Committee Task Group 40. Med Phys 21:581–618

Langer M, Brown R, Morrill S, et al. (1996) A generic genetic algorithm for generating beam weights. Med Phys 23:965–971

Lomax AJ, Bortfeld T, Gotein G, et al. (1999) A treatment planning intercomparison of proton and intensity modulated photon radiotherapy. Radiother Oncol 51:257–271

Lutz W (1993) Radiation physics for radiosurgery. In: Alexander E, Loeffler JS, Lunsford LD (eds) Stereotactic radiosurgery. McGraw-Hill, Inc., New York, pp 7–16

Luxton G, Jozsef G (1994) Single isocenter treatment planning for homogeneous dose delivery to non-spherical targets in multi-arc linear accelerator radiosurgery. Inter J Radiat Oncol Biol Phys 31:635–543

Luxton G, Petrovich Z, Jozsef G, et al. (1993) Stereotactic radiosurgery: principles and comparison of treatment methods. Neurosurg 32:241–259

Lyman JT, Kanstein L, Yeater F, et al. (1986) A helium ion beam for stereotactic radiosurgery of central nervous system disorders. Med Phys 13:695–699

Morrill SM, Lane RG, Jacobson G, et al. (1991) Treatment planning optimization using constrained simulated annealing. Phys Med Biol 36:1341–1361

Niemerko A, Urie M, Goitein M (1992) Optimization of 3D radiation therapy with both physical and biological end points and constraints. Inter J Radiat Oncol Biol Phys 23:99–108

Purdy JA, Carol MP, Rosen II, et al. (1997) The theory and practice of intensity modulated radiation therapy. Sternick ES (ed) Advanced Medical Publishing, Madison, WI

Ramsey CR, Cordrey IL, Oliver AL (1999) A comparison of beam characteristics for gated and nongated clinical X-ray beams. Med Phys 26:2086–2091

Redpath AT, Vickery BL, Wright DH (1967) A new technique for radiotherapy planning using quadratic programming. Phys Med Biol 21:781–791

Reinstein LE (1998) Patient positioning and immobilization. In: Khan FM, Potish AR (eds) Treatment planning in radiation oncology. Williams and Wilkins, Baltimore, MD, pp 55–88

Schmitt G, Wambersie A (1990) Review of the clinical results of fast neutron therapy. Radiother Oncol 17:47–56

Schultz RJ (1999) Further improvement in dose distributions are unlikely to affect cure rates. Med Phys 26:1007–1009

Shaw EG, Bourland JD, Marshall MG (1998) Cancers of the central nervous system. In: Khan FM, Potish AR (eds) Treatment planning in radiation oncology. Williams and Wilkins, Baltimore, MD, pp 491–543

Webb S (1989) Optimization of conformal radiotherapy dose distributions by simulated annealing. Phys Med Biol 34:1359–1370

Webb S (1991) Optimization by simulated annealing of three dimensional conformal treatment planning for radiation fields defined by a multileaf collimator. Phys Med Biol 36:1201–1226

Wouters BG, Lam GK, Oelfke U, et al. (1996) Measurements of relative biological effectiveness of the 70 MeV proton beam at TRIUMF using Chinese hamster V79 cells and the high-precision cell sorter assay. Radiation Research 146: 159–170

Yu C, Luxton G, Jozsef G, et al. (1999) Dosimetric comparison of three photon radiosurgery techniques for an elongated target. Inter J Radiat Oncol Biol Phys 45:817–826

Yu Y, Schell MC, Zhang JB (1997) Decision theoretic steering and genetic algorithm optimization: application to stereotactic radiosurgery treatment planning. Med Phys 24:1742–1750

6 Principles of Physics of Stereotactic Radiosurgery

Cheng Yu

CONTENTS

6.1 Introduction

6.1.1 Development of the Gamma Knife

Stereotactic radiosurgery was first introduced by Leksell in 1951 as an application of precise delivery of a single high dose of photon irradiation to destroy an intracranial lesion (LEKSELL 1951). Leksell initially proposed radiosurgery as a noninvasive method for functional neurosurgery, directed at small lesions of only a few millimeters. The method initially used many collimated 300-kV stationary X-ray beams convergent on a common focus (LEKSELL 1971a,b,c). He and his colleagues experimented with different types of radiation. In the late1960s, Leksell developed the first gamma knife, using collimated Co-60 beams to

C. YU, PhD
Assistant Professor, Department of Radiation Oncology, University of Southern California School of Medicine, 1441 Eastlake Ave., Los Angeles, CA 90033-0804, USA

deliver radiation to a common focus (LEKSELL 1968, 1983). The success of this first unit led to the construction of a second unit at the Karolinska Institute in Stockholm, Sweden in 1975. The second gamma knife containing 179 Co-60 sources was designed to produce spherical dose distribution to treat brain tumors and intracranial arteriovenous malformations. The instrument was subsequently modified and evolved into the commercially available Leksell gamma knife which contains 201 collimated Co-60 sources located in a hemisphere and convergent upon a common focal point (WALTON et al. 1987; WU et al. 1990).

Recently, a novel, rotating gamma unit for stereotactic radiosurgery has been developed in China and distributed to 15 hospitals there (GOETSCH et al. 1999). The first unit was installed in September 1996. Today, about 1000 patients have been treated with the Rotating Gamma System. The unit contains 30 Co-60 gamma radiation sources with initial activity of 200 Ci each, equivalent to the total strength of the Leksell gamma knife. The sources are positioned along 30 arcs, and rotate continuously as a group in an axis orthogonal to the patient's body. Radiation-absorbed dose rates and profiles measured for this unit are comparable to those previously measured with the same techniques for the Leksell gamma knife units.

6.1.2 Development of Particle Beam Radiosurgery

In a parallel development, clinical uses of heavy charged particle beams began to draw extensive attentions because of their unique characteristics. In 1946, Wilson, a physicist who had worked on developing particle accelerators, first proposed the clinical use of charged particle beams (WILSON 1946). In the late 1950s and early 1960s, the Lawrence group at Berkeley began to use the cyclotron's Bragg peak to irradiate pituitary adenomas (LAWRENCE et al. 1957, 1962; TOBIAS et al. 1958). Due to the limitations of the low-energy X-rays, the Leksell group proceeded to investigate the use of high-energy proton beams

(LARSSON et al. 1958). Using the Uppsala University cyclotron, Larsson and Leksell used a cross-fired proton beam in initial experiments in animals and in the first treatments of patients. In 1968, Kjellberg began treating patients using the Bragg peak of proton beams from the Harvard Cyclotron Laboratory (KJELLBERG et al. 1968). As a result of earlier achievements of patient treatment with high-energy proton beams, the search of new modalities for stereotactic radiosurgery was carried over to other heavy charged particle beams, such as helium, carbon, and neon from synchrocyclotron (LYMAN et al. 1977, 1986; CHEN et al. 1987; FABRIKANT et al. 1984, 1985, 1988; LUDEWIGT et al. 1991), and even to neutrons from an isocentrically mounted cyclotron (GRIFFIN et al. 1988). Today, radiosurgery or therapy with particle beams plays a very important role in the management of various brain tumors and other diseases (KJELLBERG et al. 1979, 1980, 1983, 1986, 1988; LAWRENCE 1985; LYMAN et al. 1985, 1992; LEVY et al. 1989, 1999; SLATER et al. 1988; STEINBERG et al. 1990). Worldwide, more than 25,000

patients have been treated alone with proton beams (*Particles*, a newsletter sponsored by the Proton Therapy Cooperative Group). The number of operating proton facilities increased from 10 in 1990 to 19 in 1999, as shown in Table 6.1. It has been predicted that there will be about 30 proton facilities operating worldwide early this century, as more facilities have been proposed (Table 6.2).

6.1.3.
Development of Clinical Linear Accelerator

In the late 1970s, Barcia-Salorio et al. adapted a conventional Co-60 teleradiotherapy unit for the stereotactic radiosurgery technique (BARCIA-SALORIO et al. 1977, 1982). Radiosurgery was performed by the attachment of a collimator to the teleradiotherapy unit, followed by irradiation of the target through 35 fixed portals. Following the theoretical proposal for the use of linear accelerators in stereotactic radio-

Table 6.1. Existing particle beam facilities, up to July 1999[a]

Institution	Location	Particle	No. of patients
Berkeley	California, USA	p	30
Berkeley	California USA	He	2054
Uppsala	Sweden	p	73
Harvard	Massachusetts, USA	p	8160
Dubna	Russia	p	84
Moscow	Russia	p	3100
Los Alamos	New Mexico, USA	p$^-$	230
St. Petersburg	Russia	p	1029
Berkeley	California, USA	heavy ion	433
Chiba	Japan	p	96
TRIUMF	Canada	p$^-$	367
PSI	Switzerland	p$^-$	503
PMRC	Tsukuba, Japan	p	606
PSI	Switzerland	p	2753
Dubna	Russia	p	41
Uppsala	Sweden	p	147
Clatterbridge	UK	p	817
Loma Linda	California, USA	p	4330
Louvain-la-Neuve	Belgium	p	21
Nice	France	p	1350
Orsay	France	p	1219
NAC	South Africa	p	310
MPRI	Indiana, USA	p	9
UCSF – CNL	California, USA	p	214
HIMAC	Chiba, Japan	heavy ion	473
TRIUMF	Canada	p	47
PSI	Switzerland	p	20
GSI Darmstadt	Germany	heavy ion	20
Berlin	Germany	p	30
NCC	Kashiwa, Japan	p	8

[a] Based on *Particles*, a newsletter sponsored by the Proton Therapy Cooperative Group.

Table 6.2. Proposed particle beam facilities, up to July 1999*

Institution	Location	Particle	First treatment
INFN-LNS	Catania, Italy	p	1999
NPTC (Harvard)	Massachusetts, USA	p	2000
Hyogo	Japan	p, ion	2001
NAC, Faure	South Africa	p	2001
Tsukuba	Japan	p	2001
CGMH	Taiwan	p	2001?
Wakasa Bay	Japan		2002
Bratislava	Slovakia	p, ion	2003
IMP, Lanzhou	PR China	C-Ar ion	2003
Shizuoka	Japan		2002?
Erlangen	Germany	p	2002?
CNAO	Italy	p, ion	2004?
AUSTRON	Austria	p, ion	?
Beijing	China	p	?
Central Italy	Italy	p	?
Clatterbridge	UK	p	?
TOP project ISS	Italy	p	?
Moscow	Russia	p	?
Krakow	Poland	p	?
PDNA Inc.	Illinois, USA	p	?

* Based on *Particles*, a newsletter sponsored by the Proton Therapy Cooperative Group.

surgery by Larsson (LARSSON et al. 1974), the clinical uses of radiosurgery on modified linear accelerators were pioneered by Betti and Derechinsky (BETTI et al. 1983, 1984), and others (COLOMBO et al. 1985a,b, 1986, 1989; HARTMANN et al. 1985; HOUDEK et al. 1985; LUTZ et al. 1988; PODGORSAK et al. 1988; LOEFFLER et al. 1989). These clinical applications were all based on a technique referred to as the multiple non-coplanar converging arcs radiosurgical technique. The center of the target is placed stereotactically at the machine isocenter and multiple non-coplanar arcs, each with a different stationary treatment couch position, are used for each treatment.

More recently, a new portable, low-power miniature X-ray source was developed for stereotactic interstitial radiosurgery by Photoelectron (BIGGS et al. 1993; DINSMORE et al. 1996; BEATTY et al. 1996). The device generates low-energy X-rays at the tip of a 10-cm long, 3-mm diameter needle-like probe. Electrons from a small thermionic gun are accelerated to a final energy of up to 40 keV and directed along a 3-mm outside diameter drift tube to a thin Au target, where the beam size is approximately 0.3 mm. The irradiation field is similar to that of a localized, low-energy brachytherapy source, but is electronically controllable and has the dose delivery of 0.6 Gy/min to the periphery of a 30-mm diameter lesion.

Today, numerous particle beam facilities and linear accelerator-based stereotactic radiosurgery centers have been established. In addition, more than 120 Leksell gamma unit facilities have been established for stereotactic radiosurgery, as seen in Table 6.3. The number of patients treated annually worldwide with stereotactic radiosurgery using Leksell gamma unit alone has increased from 500 in 1988 to 21,520 in 1998 (Survey of the Leksell Gamma Knife Society, December, 1998). Stereotactic radiosurgery has gained great importance in the management of many types of intracranial lesions, including benign and malignant neoplasms and arterial venous malformations (BACKLUND 1974, 1979; WALTON et al. 1987; APUZZO et al. 1988; BETTI et al. 1989; LUN-

Table 6.3. Leksell gamma unit geographic sites, up to 1999

Region/country	No. of sites	No. of patients*
USA	49	24,966
Japan	27	20,324
China	12	26,974
Europe and Middle East	18	21,258
Far East	14	5,370
Latin America	3	1,089

* Based on the survey of the Leksell Gamma Knife Society, December, 1998, reported from 91 sites.

SFORD et al. 1989, 1991, 1993; FLICKINGER et al. 1990a,b, 1993; STERNER et al. 1972, 1984, 1988, 1992; LUXTON et al. 1993).

6.2
Radiation Beams

6.2.1
Particle Beams

The early recognition that X-rays could produce local tumor control in some patients and not in others led to the search for other ionizing radiations. The uses of heavy particle beams, such as neutrons, protons, negative p-mesons, and other heavy ions were all based on an advantage of either physical dose distribution or radiobiological properties.

Neutrons posses no electric charge. When interacted with matter, they give up their energy to produce recoil protons, alpha particles, and other nuclear fragments. The earlier rationale for the use of neutrons in radiotherapy was based on the reduced oxygen enhancement ratio (OER) to overcome the problem of hypoxic cells. The revised rationale for neutrons was their higher relative biological effectiveness (RBE) for slow-growing tumors, which has clinically been proved in the treatment of salivary gland and prostate tumors and soft tissue sarcoma. Protons have radiobiological properties similar to X-rays, plus the superiority of the physical dose distribution. Negative p-mesons and heavy ions were introduced with the hope of combining the radiobiological advantages for neutrons and the dose distribution characteristics for protons. However, controlled clinical trials have shown that radiotherapy with heavy particle beams has limited advantages compared to conventional X-rays in a few circumstances, specifically for the treatment of prostate cancer and salivary gland tumors for the neutrons, and uveal melanoma and certain chordomas for the protons, where a sharp fall-off of dose is important (HALL 1994). So far, only a few institutions in the world have been able to acquire the particle beams for clinical trials because of the enormous cost involved to establish such a facility. In this chapter, our discussion will be limited to proton beam radiosurgery, the most widely used charged particle technique in the clinic. Proton beams for therapeutic application range in energy from 150 to 250 MeV, corresponding to a range in tissue of 15–35 cm. These beams can be produced by a cyclotron or a linear accelerator.

Charged particle beams can be divided into two groups: (1) electrons, including positrons and beta particles, Auger electrons, and internal conversion electrons; and (2) heavy charged particles such as alpha particles, protons, fission fragments, deuterons, mesons. The charged particles have special advantages with regard to doses localization and therapeutic gain (WILSON 1946; BARENDSEN 1968; CURTIS 1977; HALL 1994). The characteristics of the charged particles include their finite range and sharp beam edges, which make them superior to X-rays for stereotactic radiosurgery. The finite range, determined by the energy of the charged particles being accelerated, can be used to spare normal structures distal to the radiosurgical target. In addition, when collimated by metallic apertures, the charged particle beams show very little lateral broadening from multiple scattering, which results in sharp beam edges.

The accelerated charged particles interact with matter primarily through the Coulomb force between the electric field of the traveling particle and electric fields of orbital electrons, and nuclei of atoms of the medium. The first interaction results in ionization and excitation of the atoms, while the second results in radiative energy loss or bremsstrahlung. Differences in the mass determine differences in the energy deposition between the two types of charged particles. The rate of energy loss or stopping power caused by ionization interactions for charged particles is proportional to the square of the particle charge and inversely proportional to the square of its velocity, i.e.:

$$dE/dx \propto Q^2/v^2 \qquad (1)$$

where dE/dx is the rate of kinetic energy loss per unit path length of the particle, Q and v are the electric charge and the speed of the particle, respectively. Thus, as a particle slows down because of the loss of kinetic energy through the numerous electronic collisions to the medium, its rate of energy loss increases. At low velocities, the particles capture electrons, the individual particle's effective charge is reduced, and the rate of energy loss decreases. The particles continue to slow down until their energy is reduced to the thermal energy of atoms in the medium. As the combination of these effects, the dose deposition in water increases at first relatively slowly with depth, referred to as the plateau region, and very sharply near the end of the particle range, before dropping to almost zero as the particle comes to rest. This peaking of the dose near the end of the particle range is

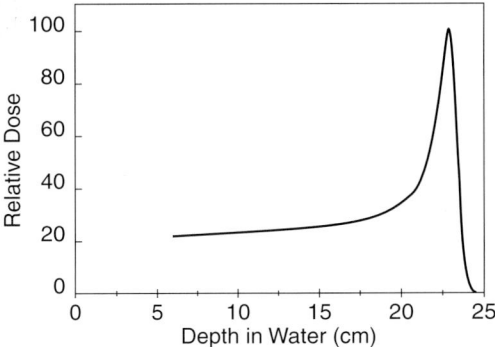

Fig. 6.1.. A typical depth dose distribution for charged particle beams with a sharp peak, i.e., Bragg peak at the depth of about 23 cm

called the Bragg peak, as seen in Fig. 6.1. The dose beyond the Bragg peak is virtually zero for protons, and relatively small for heavier ions due to the contribution of secondary ions produced by nuclear fragmentation of some of the incident primary ions (Tobias et al. 1971).

The physical characteristics of charged particle beams offer unique dosimetric properties that are potentially advantageous for stereotactic radiosurgery. When incident on a uniform tissue-like medium, a monoenergetic beam of charged particles provides a dose distribution characterized by a precise range and a dose build-up, or Bragg peak, near the end of the range. The range or distance that a monoenergetic beam of charged particles travels in the medium before stopping is a function of the charge and kinetic energy or speed of the particle and the physical characteristic of the absorbing medium. The peak is due to the increase in ionization per unit length traversed by the charged particle as its velocity decreases with loss of energy due to multiple ion–electron collisions. The ranges of monoenergetic charged particle beams produced by particle accelerators can be modified or modulated to specific initial energy by interposing absorbing filters of appropriate thickness in the beam path.

Another advantage of charged particle beams for radiosurgery is their minimal lateral spreading in the tissue of scattered radiation. In the other words, collimated beams can be produced with relatively sharp edges as compared with photon beams, particularly at the lower-percentage dose levels. When a beam of parallel charged particles passes through a medium, the particles are scattered due to Coulomb-force interactions between the incident particles and the nuclei of the medium. As a result of the interac-

tion, the beam profile is gradually expanded with increasing depth. This scattering consists of two parts: a single large deflection of relatively few particles (single scattering) and many small deflections (multiple scattering). The multiple scattering predominates over single scattering. Heavier ions are scattered less than lighter ions. A beam of low-energy charged particles that undergoes final collimation at the medium surface is scattered less than high-energy charged particles.

6.2.2
Co-60 Gamma Rays

The Co-60 source has several advantages over other radionuclides, such as radium and cesium, as radiation beams for stereotactic radiosurgery. These advantages include higher possible specific activity (curies per gram), greater radiation output per curie, and higher average photon energy. The Co-60 source with the half-life of 5.26 years is produced by placing the stable Co-59 in a nuclear reactor, where the stable Co-59 becomes activated by neutron bombardment. The actual disintegration scheme of the excited Co-60 source is illustrated in Fig. 6.2. Most of the disintegrations (99.8%) are an allowed transition to an excited state of Ni-60 with the emission of a β^- with maximum energy of 0.32 MeV. The excited Ni-60 quickly gives up its energy by the emission of two gamma rays in cascade, with energies of 1.17 and 1.33 MeV, respectively. In a few of the disintegrations (0.12%), a β^- particle with a maximum energy of 1.49 MeV is emitted, leading to the lowest excited state of Ni-60, followed by the emission of gamma rays with energy of 1.33 MeV. The two gamma rays provide the

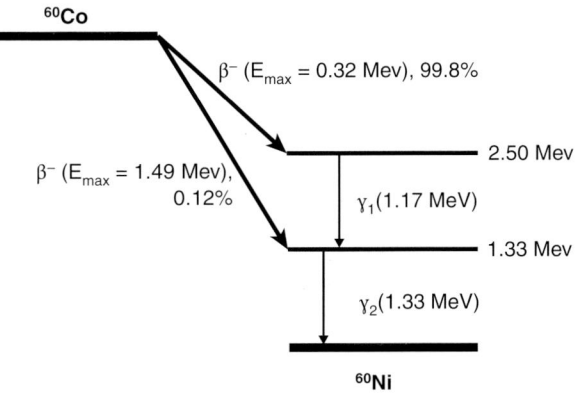

Fig. 6.2. Disintegration scheme for Co-60 nucleus

useful radiation in radiosurgery. The beta particles are absorbed in the cobalt material itself and the steel capsules resulting in the emission of bremsstrahlung X-rays and a small amount of characteristic X-ray. However, these X-rays of average energy around 0.1 MeV are strongly attenuated in the material of the source and the capsules. Their contributions to dose in the patient are insignificant. In the meantime, the primary gamma beams generate the secondary gamma rays with lower energies when they interact with the source itself, the capsule, the source housing, and the collimator system. In addition, electrons are also produced by these interactions and constitute what is usually referred to as the electron contamination of the photon, or gamma beam. All these secondary interactions thus result in heterogeneity of the beam. The scattered components of the beam contribute approximately 10% to the total intensity of the beam. As the beam penetrating the medium, the absorbed dose changes with depth, as seen in Fig. 6.3. The percent depth dose (PDD) is referred to as the absorbed dose versus the depth on the beam central axis in a medium, normalized to 100 at a depth of a maximum dose.

6.2.3
Linear Accelerator X-Rays

In 1895, Roentgen discovered X-rays while studying cathode rays in a vacuum tube. Following this historic discovery, the characteristics of X-rays was extensively studied. In the meantime, the applications of

X-rays have been involved in almost every medical field. In the early 1950s, the first stationary linear accelerator for radiotherapy was developed by collaboration of three groups, led by Miller (MILLER 1954, 1956; KARZMARK et al. 1992). The machine was installed at Hammersmith Hospital, London, in June 1952. The first patient was treated on August 19, 1953. The first orientable linear accelerators for radiotherapy were independently developed in the United Kingdom and the United States, and then were installed in 1954 at Manchester and Stanford University, respectively (GINZTON et al. 1957; WEISSBLUTH et al. 1959; KARZMARK et al. 1992).

In medical electron linear accelerators, electrons, boiled out of a hot cathode, are accelerated in a linear tube or gun by high-frequency electromagnetic waves. When the high-energy electron beam strikes a target of a high Z material such as tungsten, the electron energy is converted into a spectrum of X-ray energies with maximum energy equal to the incident electron energy. The average photon energy of the beam is approximately one-third of the maximum energy. In other words, the beam quality of the 4-MeV X-rays from a linear accelerator is approximately equivalent to that of the gamma rays from Co-60. As the photon beam is incident on a medium, the absorbed dose in the patient varies with depth. This variation depends on other conditions, such as beam energy, depth in the medium, field size, distance from source, and beam collimation system. The energy of X-rays for radiosurgery ranges from 4 to 20 MeV.

In the therapeutic range X-rays, the percent depth dose grows with the increase in beam energy, i.e., higher-energy beams have greater penetrating power. Generally, as a photon beam (X- or gamma rays) penetrates a medium, the dose at first rises rapidly from a relatively low value on the surface toward a maximum dose, and then decreases beyond that point (Fig. 6.3). The maximum dose reaches a depth normally referred to as the depth of dose maximum (d_{max}). The region between the surface of the medium and the point of the maximum dose is called the dose build-up region for the higher-energy beams, which gives rise to what is clinically known as the skin-sparing effect. As the high-energy beam of X-rays enters the medium, it sets electrons in motion with high speed along its path in the medium. The high-speed electrons deposit their energy a definite distance away from their site of origin. Combination of the two results in the rapid increase of the electron fluence and hence the absorbed dose and a dose maximum at depth. In the meantime, the production

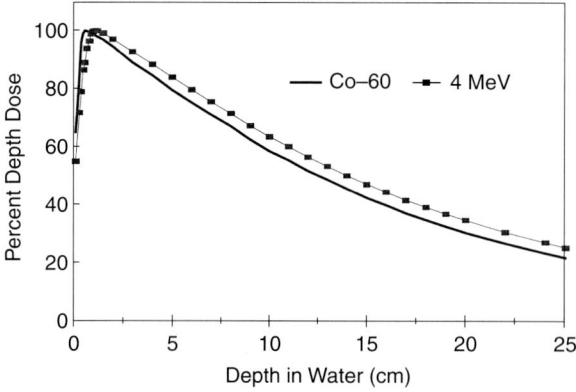

Fig. 6.3. Depth dose distributions for Co-60 gamma rays and linear accelerator 4-MeV X-rays. The percent depth dose exhibits an initial build-up region of approximately 0.5 cm and 1 cm for gamma rays and X-rays, respectively, then falls exponentially

of electrons also decreases with depth as a result of continuous decreases of the photon energy fluence with depth. The resulting effect is that beyond a certain depth, the dose decreases with depth gradually.

A plot of dose distributions for points off the central axis at a certain depth is referred to as a dose profile or off-axis ratio (OAR). The dose profile for a stationary radiation beam is obtained by measuring the dose distributions at a given depth in a tissue-equivalent phantom, along a line perpendicular to the beam central axis. Usually, the results are normalized to the dose measured on the central axis at the same depth in the phantom. The dose profiles are functions of the dimensions of the radiation source, the shape of the collimators, the distance between the source and the surface of the phantom, and the depth in the phantom. The width of the dose profile increases with the depth in the medium as a result of the beam divergence with an increasing distance from the source and the changes in scattering conditions with depth. Figure 6.4 shows a typical profile of a collimator of 1-cm diameter measured at d_{max} in water for a beam of 4-MeV linear accelerator X-rays.

For radiosurgery treatment, a dose at any point in a medium can be determined by knowing the percentage depth dose distribution for the beam, the dose profile for the point, and the dose rates and output factors for collimators. Generally, a three-dimensional treatment plan is calculated by using tabulated data for percentage depth doses and dose profiles. Data for intermediate points not found in the table are obtained through a simple interpolation of appropriate tabulated data. The dose distributions are then superimposed onto the magnetic resonance (MR) images or computed tomography (CT) images, readily appreciated in either two or three dimensions.

6.3
Stereotactic Radiosurgery Techniques

In stereotactic radiosurgery, a large dose in a single session is normally delivery to the relatively small target volumes, which may be surrounded by sensitive brain structures, such as in the treatment of pituitary adenoma and trigeminal neuralgia. In these cases, deviations of dose delivery as small as a few millimeters could result in significant complications. Thus, the requirement for accuracy of dose delivery to the target is very stringent in the management of radiosurgery, not only for the linear accelerator-based but also charged particle beam and gam-

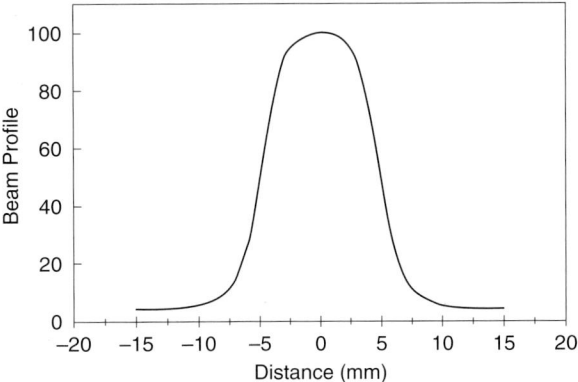

Fig. 6.4. A radiation dose profile for a 10-mm circular collimator. The measurement was taken with linear accelerator 4-MeV X-rays at the 1-cm depth of a water phantom

ma knife surgery. Rigorous quality assurance (QA) is necessarily a multidisciplinary program involving radiation oncology, neuroradiology, neurosurgery, and medical physics (TSAI et al. 1991; SCHELL et al. 1994, 1995). For a large medical center, a dedicated clinical medical physicist with board certification or eligible for board certification is recommended to perform all tasks involved in stereotactic radiosurgery. Some of these tasks include the following:
1. Stereotactic equipment (hardware) evaluation
2. Treatment planning system (software) evaluation
3. Dosimetry measurements
4. Routine quality assurances
5. Treatment planning and delivery for each case
6. Regulatory issues
7. Stereotactic system design and improvement

6.3.1
Proton Beam Radiosurgery

Due to insufficient energy of the particle beams, initial medical applications used only the plateau portion of the dose distribution of the particle beam (LAWRENCE 1957; TOBIAS et al. 1958). The plateau corresponds to minimum-ionizing particles traveling at speeds close to the speed of light. In the early 1960s, a group leaded by KJELLBERG at the Harvard Cyclotron Laboratory first used the Bragg peak of a proton beam to irradiate intracranial lesions (KJELLBERG et al. 1962). The Bragg peak of a monoenergetic charged particle beam is very sharp, and the dose in the peak region is much higher than that in the plateau region. In charged particle radiosurgery, the precise location of the Bragg peak region within an intracranial target becomes extremely important for achieving optimal dose localization and an acceptable dose distribution throughout the entire radiosurgical lesion.

For most radiosurgical lesions, multiple beam ports (three to five) are needed for achieving a well-localized dose distribution. Each beam port can be collimated by a metallic aperture to conform to the cross-sectional size and shape of the lesion in a projection along the direction of the beam.

A monoenergetic particle beam extracted from an accelerator has a narrow profile or a small cross-sectional area, normally too small to cover the lesion. The desired dose coverage is achieved by modifying the beam to dimensions which are larger than that of the original beam from the accelerator. There are basically two methods: static beam delivery methods and active methods. In static beam methods, the beam can be modified by either the insertion of a dynamically variable absorber in the beam path (KOEHLER et al. 1975, 1977) or the magnetic defocus of the beam. The absorber increases the beam divergence by multiple scattering. For a small field size like one used in the radiosurgery, beam uniformity can be accomplished by simply scattering or defocusing the beams using collimators to sharpen the beam edges and to remove the unwanted portions of the beam. On the other hand, the beam uniformity for larger field sizes can be obtained by using a flattening beam technique (KOEHLER et al. 1977). It is an extension of usual multiple-scattering techniques, a combination of blocking out some of the central peak and rescattering to fill in the profile, resulting in flat distributions up to 30 cm in diameter. In active methods, the particle beams are modulated by scanning the beam magnetically in either a single Lissajous pattern or multiple Lissajous patterns.

The dose delivery for a charged particle beam, particularly for the Bragg peak, requires precise knowledge of the water-equivalent depth of the tissues along each beam direction. The dose to a homogeneous tissue or medium at a specified depth is straightforward with the unmodulated Bragg peak. However, it is more complicated to heterogeneous mediums such as the skull and brain. Dose prescription and other treatment planning calculations require detailed information on tissue inhomogeneities, such as bone. The range of the charged particle beam depends strongly on tissue type, primarily on the electron density of the tissue (CHEN et al. 1979). In general, tissues with higher density, such as bone, slow down the incident beam of charged particles more per unit length of tissues than less dense tissues. In other words, the Bragg peak of a beam traversing denser tissue is moved to shallower depth than that of a beam traversing less dense tissue. Due to the sharpness at the distal end of the Bragg peak, incorrect evaluation of the water-equivalent depth can cause a significant underdose in the lesion or overdose beyond the lesion. Digital CT data provide electron density information (X-ray absorption coefficients) that can be converted into a water-equivalent thickness for each pixel. The density information is used to identify and to compensate for tissue inhomogeneities traversed by the charged particle beams and to calculate the dose distribution throughout the entire targeted volume in each patient.

A beam of monoenergetic charged particles entering the tissue deposits much of its energy at a depth determined by the energy of the entrant beam particles and by the energy-absorption characteristics of the tissue. The depth of the Bragg peak can be decreased by placing absorbing material in the beam line upstream of the point of entry into the tissue. Although a region of a single Bragg peak is too narrow to cover most lesions, the range of the beam can be modulated to produce a high-dose region at the desired depth (LARSSON 1961; GOITEIN 1983). By means of beam stacking, i.e., adding or subtracting material from a range-adjusting absorber which results in changes of the energy spectrum of the incident particles, the high dose region of the Bragg peak can be broadened in the direction of beam propagation.

In particle beam radiosurgery, multiple beam directions with different entry angles and coplanar or non-coplanar beam ports are commonly used for most radiosurgical lesions. Each beam is stereotactically directed to achieve an individually shaped three-dimensional high-dose region precisely within the target volume and a much lower dose distribution to surrounding normal brain tissue. These three-dimensional conformal dose distributions are accomplished by adjusting the range, spreading the Bragg peak, introducing tissue-equivalent compensators, and using an appropriately shaped aperture for each beam. As a result of virtually zero exit dose for protons, and relatively very small exit for heavier ions beyond the Bragg peak, large portions of normal brain tissue surrounding the lesion can be completely protected (LYMAN et al. 1985, 1992, HOSOBUCHI et al. 1987).

6.3.2
Linear Accelerator-Based Radiosurgery

Most of clinical linear accelerator-based radiosurgi-cal techniques involve rotations of the gantry and the treatment couch, except for the frameless stereotac-tic technique (ADLER et al. 1994; BOVA et al. 1997) or the image-guided robotic radiosurgery frequently referred to as Cyberknife (ADLER et al 1994, 1996, 1999). The Cyberknife is designed to accomplish pre-cisely localized irradiation of focal lesions anywhere in the body. In this image-guided robotic system, treatment planning, real-time imaging, and delivery components are all integrated by a powerful computer workstation. Details on the Cyberknife are discussed in Chap. 20 of this volume. The discussion in this section will be limited to the conventional linear accel-erator-based isocentric radiosurgery techniques.

Linear accelerator-based radiosurgery techniques are based on the modification of standard linear ac-celerators with the addition of tertiary collimation and a stereotactic frame system. These systems are mostly built by an individual institute through a manufacturer, although complete systems such as Xknife (Radionics, Burlington, Mass., USA), Brain-Lab (Heimstetien, Germany), and Peacock system (Nomos, Sewickley, Pa., USA) are commercially available. The basic system includes image-based treatment plan software, a stereotactic head frame system, a set of secondary collimators (i.e., circular or miniature multileaf collimators), a remote-con-trolled motorized couch, and brackets or a floor stand for mounting the stereotactic frame.

Most linear accelerator-based radiosurgical tech-niques use circular collimators, which are attached to the head of the linear accelerator. Circular colli-mators offer several advantages over rectangular collimators, such as more precise dose delivery, easi-er calculation of the three-dimensional dose distri-bution, plus better and more reliable field definition for the small fields used in radiosurgery. Usually, cir-cular collimators range from 5 mm to 40 mm in di-ameter at the linear accelerator isocenter. The iso-center is the point of intersection between the gantry rotation axis and the rotation axes of the treatment couch. Each circular collimator is attached to the head of the linear accelerator, which is set to its pri-mary rectangular collimators or jaws to a filed size of 5×5 cm at the isocenter. The secondary collimators are typically made of lead or tungsten in the cylinder shape with a thickness of about 10 cm. However, shapes other than circular have been suggested for collimators for the treatment of irregular targets

with a single isocenter, such as the use of elliptical apertures (SERAGO et al. 1991), an adjustable colli-mator (McGINLEY et al. 1992), and a dynamically ad-justable collimator (LEAVITT et al. 1991; CARON et al. 1992). The ellipsoidal isodose surfaces can also be obtained by computer-controlled couch rotation combined with different fixed gantry angles and dif-ferent rectangular field sizes (COLOMBO et al. 1990). In addition, conforming dose distributions for elon-gated targets of different orientations can be achieved by shaping the dose distribution through the use of different sizes of circular collimators, arc lengths, and doses for the different arcs (LUXTON et al. 1994). On the other hand, the large and irregularly shaped targets can be covered by placing different isocenters within the target volume and appropriate collimator sizes for each isocenter. The technique of multiple isocenters will result in dose inhomogene-ity in the target and relatively complicated treatment planning and dose delivery.

Several techniques have currently been used in the linear accelerator-based radiosurgery, such as single-plane rotation, multiple noncoplanar con-verging arcs, dynamic rotation (PODGORSAK et al. 1988, 1990), and conical rotation (PODGORSAK 1992). Dosimetrically, these four approaches are approxi-mately equivalent (PHILLIPS et al. 1990, 1994; SCHELL et al. 1991; SERAGO et al. 1992). However, lin-ear accelerator-based radiosurgery is frequently per-formed by the gantry rotation or arc in a vertical plane about the isocenter with a stationary treat-ment couch, as seen in Fig. 6.5. The patient, placed

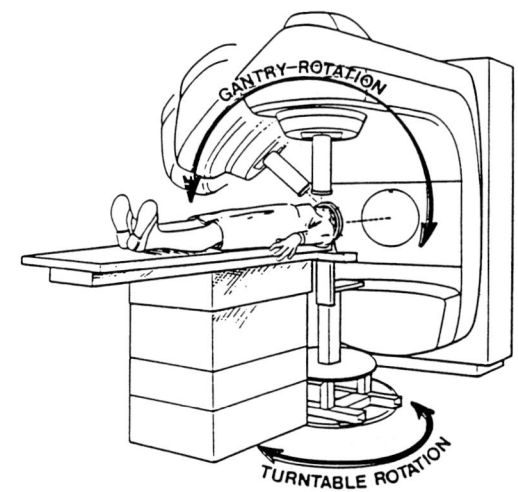

Fig. 6.5. Illustration of the linear accelerator-based multiple arc technique. Each arc is achieved by rotating the gantry in the vertical plane about the isocenter while keeping the treat-ment couch stationary

supine on the treatment couch, is usually stationary during irradiation, and the full dose of each arc is delivered in several segments of arc. On completion of the arc, the couch is moved to a new position and a new arc is executed. This procedure is repeated for all arcs. Typically, four to seven non-coplanar arcs are used for the treatment of patients with a single isocenter plan. All the non-coplanar arcs intersect at the isocenter within the target volume, resulting in a high radiation dose to the selected target and a relatively low dose to the adjacent normal tissue. A radiation dose to the adjacent normal tissue rises from an entrance dose of a single arc and exit doses of other arcs. However, for patients with irregularly shaped targets, multiple isocenters can be used to provide sufficient tumor volume coverage.

An alternative technique, commonly referred as conformal stereotactic radiosurgery, has been proposed to implement field shaping for a larger and irregularly shaped target, such as the static field shaping (SERAGO et al. 1991; OTTO-OELSCHLAGER et al. 1994) and dynamic field shaping (LEAVITT et al. 1991; NEDZI et al. 1993; SIXEL et al. 1993). The technique uses an adjustable collimator or jaw to conform the beam profile to the target cross-section in the beam eye view (BEV), which is analogous to the collimation of the charged particle beam to the BEV of the target for each beam port. Another approach uses the static field with individually or custom-shaped apertures for radiosurgery (LAING et al. 1993; BOURLAND et al. 1994; YU et al. 1999b). It has advantages over the traditional circular field treatment approach; but it is difficult to manufacture a custom-shaped aperture and to measure the dosimetry accurately. Currently, most commercial multileaf collimator systems are designed for larger field treatments up to 40×40 cm and have leaf widths of about 1.0 cm at the isocenter, which are too coarse for radiosurgery. On the other hand, the miniature multileaf collimator system has the ability to conform the dose distribution to an irregularly shaped target volume (COSGROVE et al. 1999). The single isocenter treatment with the miniature multileaf collimator is preferable to both single and multiple isocenter treatment with the circular collimator (SHIU et al. 1997).

Standard mechanical tolerances for a linear accelerator are ±1 mm over the full 360-deg range of gantry rotations. The same rotation accuracy can be obtained for the couch rotations. Total isocenter accuracy can be improved to about ±0.5 mm by adding some relatively minor modifications to the linear accelerator. Achieving such an improved tolerance may require precise mechanical adjustment of the equipment on the day of treatment. These mechanical inaccuracies of rotation, however, represent only a minor problem compared to the inherent inaccuracies of the imaging systems used for target localization.

Several systems for target localization and fixation have been developed and used for linear accelerator-based radiosurgery. These localization techniques include the most widely used Brown-Roberts-Wells (BRW) stereotactic apparatus (Radionics, Burlington, Mass.) (HEILBRUN et al. 1983; SAUNDERS et al. 1988; WINSTON et al. 1988), the Talairach stereotactic system (BETTI et al. 1983), and other designs (COLOMBO et al. 1984; HARTMANN et al. 1985, STURM et al. 1983; 1987). Figure 6.6 shows the BRW stereotactic apparatus used at the University of Southern California School of Medicine (USC).

Currently, there are two methods to immobilize the stereotactic apparatus or head frame during patient treatment. The frame can be immobilized by attaching it to a special floor stand (PETROVICH et al. 1997), as seen in Fig. 6.7. This technique is more popular in that it provides better immobilization of the patient. In the other method, the head frame is attached directly to the treatment couch, which is properly locked with special brackets. This technique with an appropriate design can sufficiently immobilize the stereotactic frame. In addition, the direct couch mounting method may prevent injury to a patient under treatment in the case of accidental vertical motion of the couch. Patient setup is also easier, and gantry rotation below the patient is unrestrained (PODGORSAK et al. 1988, 1989, 1992).

The accuracy of a radiosurgical target with CT or MR images depends on several factors, such as the resolution of the image, the relationship of the macroscopic image with the microscopic extent of the disease, and image artifacts and distortions, especially for MR images. The image resolution is a result of the uncertainty of the image voxel. The pixel dimensions are typically 0.7×0.7 mm, and the separation between slices ranges from 1 mm to 2 mm. Therefore, the location of the target cannot be known better than within 1.4–2.2 mm. The net uncertainty in target localization and treatment delivery is approximately 2–3 mm when summing all factors in quadrature.

The dose distributions for radiosurgery are generally based on stereotactic three-dimensional information obtained from CT or MR images, the patient's anatomic contours, and the appropriate depth in tissue. The depth for each point of interest on the dose calculation matrix is an important factor for achieving an accurate calculation of dose for each radiation beam.

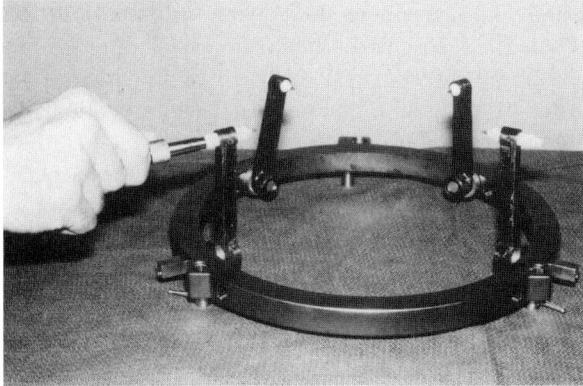

Fig. 6.6. The Brown-Roberts-Wells (BRW) stereotactic apparatus

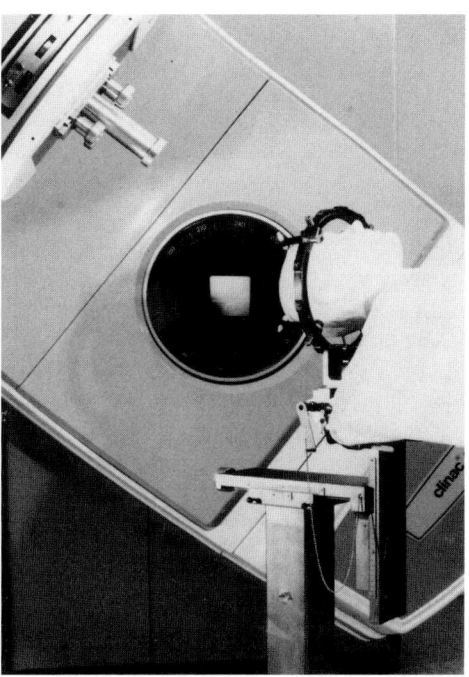

Fig. 6.7. Illustration of the BRW floor stand immobilization system. A phantom patient lies in supine position with the BRW ring attached to the floor stand. The stand, equipped with three-dimensional rectilinear positioning capability, is directly locked to the linear accelerator turntable assembly

In linear accelerator-based multiarc radiosurgery, the treatment plan is defined by selections of arcs, the extent of each arc, the size of the collimator aperture, and the relative weighting. Target and surrounding tissue anatomy are identified on CT or MR images by the neuroradiologist, neurosurgeon, and radiation oncologist. The dose distributions are then directly superimposed onto the CT or MR images to provide information on doses not only within the target but also to sensitive structures outside the target (Fig. 6.8). In addition, dose–volume histograms are another important factor in determining the suitability of a particular radiosurgical treatment plan.

The aim of a stereotactic radiosurgery treatment plan is to achieve a high dose of radiation within a defined target volume while depositing the least possible dose to the surrounding non-target tissue. Theoretically, the optimal dose distribution can be achieved when all of the beams are focused to the target through a large number of surface points distributed uniformly over the upper hemisphere of the patient's skull. It has been suggested that parallel-opposed beams should be avoided in radiosurgery because of the possibility of degrading the dose fall-off outside the target in the plane containing the beams (PODGORSAK 1992). In parallel-opposed beams, the dose to a given point outside the target represents a superposition of contributions from the entrance dose of one beam and the exit dose of the other beam.

6.3.3
Gamma Knife Radiosurgery

The dedicated radioisotope radiosurgery unit, the Leksell gamma unit, was originally developed for radiosurgery at the Karolinska Institute in 1968 (LEKSELL 1968, 1983). In the mid-1970s, it was replaced with a second gamma unit that produced more spherically shaped isodose distributions using 179 Co-60 sources for treatment of tumors and AVM (STEINER et al. 1972, 1984). Due to good clinical outcomes, the remodified device was installed in the other parts of the world (WALTON et al. 1987; LUNSFORD et al. 1987, 1989; MAITZ et al. 1990; WU et al. 1990). Presently, there are more than 125 operational Leksell gamma units worldwide (Survey of the Leksell Gamma Knife Society, December, 1998). The current models (B and U) contain 201 Co-60 sources located in a hemisphere around a common focal point. These two models only differ in the arrangement of Co-60 sources and the angle of the collimation helmet. The new computerized gamma unit (model C) is to be installed in the United States early

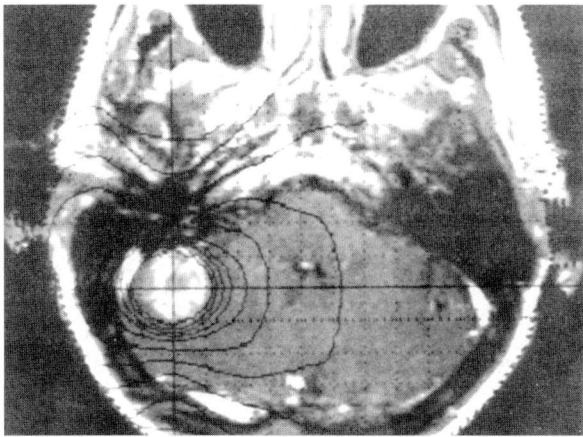

Fig. 6.8. The isodose distribution in the transverse plan for a regularly shaped lesion of 2.5 cm in diameter. The treatment plan was developed from seven arcs with the same size of the secondary collimator. The prescribed 80% isodose surface covered the entire lesion with a margin

in 2000. In this section, discussions will be limited to model U only.

The radiation unit contains a radially convergent set of 201 Co-60 sources located in a hemispherical central body. The radiation unit with treatment table is shown in Fig. 6.9. The radiation beam from each individual source is collimated and all beams converge precisely to a common focal point or isocenter at the center of the spherical radiation unit. At the time of loading of the radiation unit, the activity of the radioactive material is normally 6000 Ci (222×10^{12} Bq), which delivers a dose rate of approxi-

mately 3.5 Gy/min to the 18-mm collimator at the center of a 16-cm diameter spherical polystyrene phantom. The radiation unit is heavily shielded in order to provide adequate radiation protection for the patient under the treatment and hospital staff.

The units come with four different collimator sizes of the helmet, i.e., 4 mm, 8 mm, 14 mm, and 18 mm, with 201 collimators for each helmet. The size is referred to a full width at the 50% isodose line for the beam profile of a single collimator. Because of the limitation of the radiation source distribution, the isodose surfaces are not exactly like a sphere although the aperture is circular for each collimator. The actual width at the 50% isodose line from all 201 sources is approximately 5.5, 10.2, 17.3, and 21.8 mm along the x-axis or lateral direction for the 4-, 8-, 14-, and 18-mm collimator helmets, respectively. Figure 6.10 shows a beam profile from the 8-mm collimator helmet. Only one size of collimator is used for each helmet. The treatment volume for an individual shot or isocenter is determined by the choice of helmet. The radiation dose distribution for an individual shot can be further varied by replacing some of the collimators with solid tungsten plugs, for example, to protect the optic chiasm.

The dose calculation algorithm used in the Leksell GammaPlan (Elekta Instrument AB, Sweden) computes the total dose received at any nominated point within the three-dimensional stereotactic space defined by the frame coordinates. Within its system, the dose delivered from each separate Co-60 source is identical. Thus, calculation of radiation dose at any point within the coordinates is based on measurements from a single source channel, and then super-

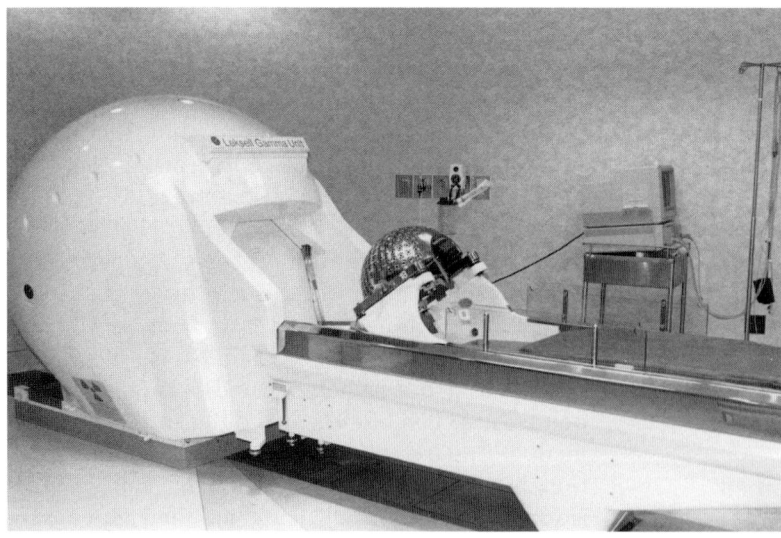

Fig. 6.9. Leksell gamma unit with the 18-mm collimator helmet on the treatment table

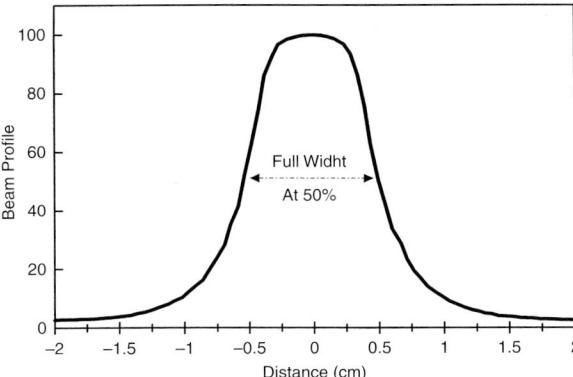

Fig. 6.10. A beam profile for the 8-mm collimator helmet. The measurement was taken along the x-axis in a 16-cm diameter spherical polystyrene phantom with all 201 beams open. The full width at 50% level was about 10.2 cm

imposed from all other active or unplugged sources. The dose calculation at the point of interest for a single beam of a specific collimator requires the patient's skull geometry, the linear attenuation coefficient of Co-60 gamma rays, the transverse radiation dose profile, and the dose rate at the reference point in a tissue-equivalent phantom. For each collimator size, the transverse profile was measured by the manufacturer at a focal distance of 400 mm from the source, with the beam attenuated in a water phantom of 80 mm in depth. The measured data were interpolated and then stored in a table in which each entry is interspaced by a constant difference of the function value other than the independent parameter to achieve maximum accuracy from finite entries.

The Leksell stereotactic head frame system consists of a rectangular base ring with four adjustable posts, two frontal and two occipital, that rigidly attach the head frame to the patient (Fig. 6.11). The system is used for rigid immobilization and target localization as well as treatment (LEKSELL et al. 1987). The head frame is supplied with three sets of plastic indicator plates with fiducial markers for MR imaging (Fig. 6.12), CT scanning, and angiography imaging (AI) localization, respectively. The head frame is locked to the helmet by a pair of trunnions for each treatment shot. The trunnions define the x-coordinates (left to right), while y- (anterior–posterior) and z- (superior–inferior) coordinates can be set on the base ring and attached sliding bars, respectively. Ideally, the stereotactic head frame is placed such that the lesion is as close to the center of the fiducial marker system as possible. Once affixed, the head frame remains in place until the treatment is completed.

Depending on the type of disease to be treated as well as the presence of the surgical metal or device like the pacemaker, different diagnostic imaging techniques including MRI, CT, and AI with orthogonal X-ray films, can be chosen for target localization. A three-dimensional Cartesian coordinate system (x, y, z) is used to specify the target coordinates in stereotactic space. The x-axis (left–right) of the coordinate system lies in the transverse plane, y-axis (anterior–posterior) in the sagittal plane, and z-axis (superior–inferior) in the coronal plane of the patient. The center of the helmet is defined as x=100, y=100, and z=100.

For gamma knife radiosurgery, only a section of the head in interest is normally scanned during image acquisitions. In order to achieve accurate dose calculation, additional information about the skull is needed to take into account the beam attenuation. A special plastic helmet temporarily attached to the head frame is used to measure the distances from the center of the head frame to the surface of the skull for 24 preselected points (Fig. 6.13). These measurements are then entered into the treatment planning system as input data for fitting the parameters of a mathematical model for the surface of the head. The model is used to calculate the distance to the radiation focus from the surface for each beam.

Based on the size, shape, and location of the lesion as seen on CT or MR images, various shots or isocenters are proposed. The radiation dose distribution is calculated within a three-dimensional matrix

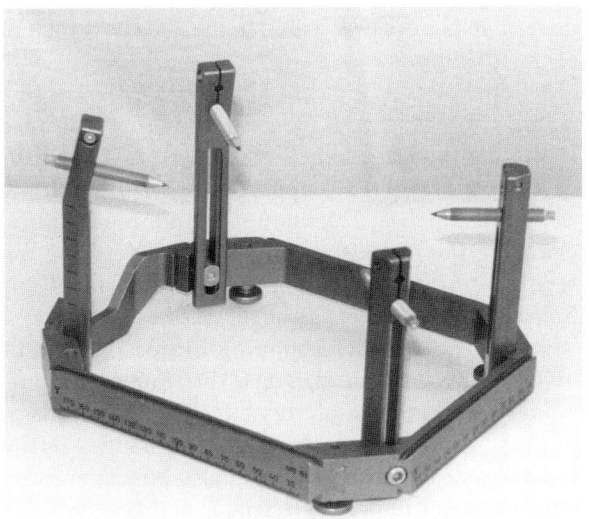

Fig. 6.11. The Leksell stereotactic head frame system

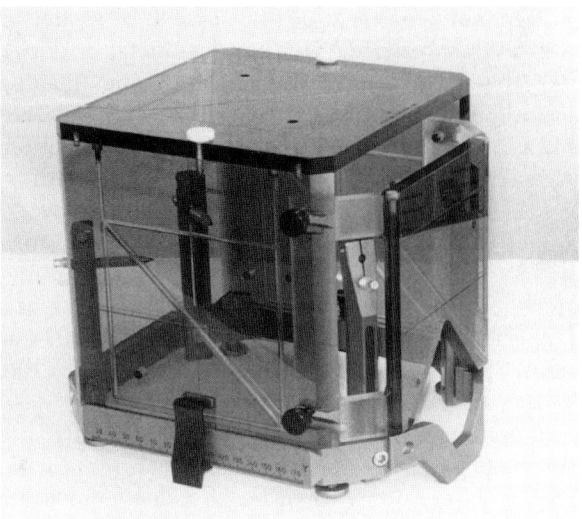

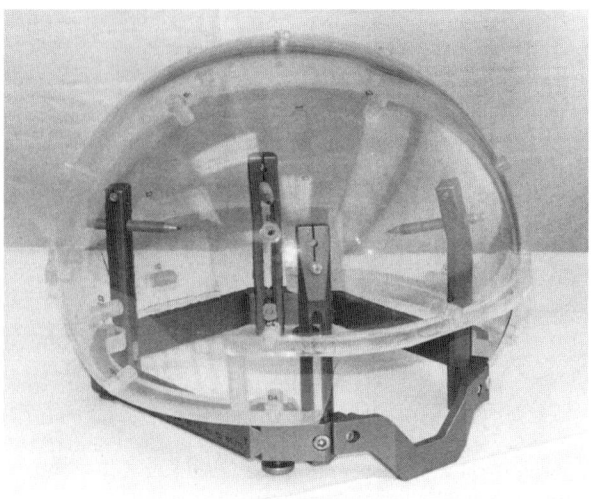

Fig. 6.12. The MR localizer attached to the Leksell head frame

Fig. 6.13. A plastic helmet attached to the Leksell head frame for measurement of the skull geometry

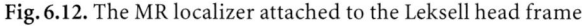

with grid size selected according to the size of lesion. For optimum results and minimum risks, the entire lesion should receive the prescription dose with minimum radiation to the surrounding tissue. This optimization can be achieved by choosing the steepest isodose gradient of the dose distribution to coincide with the periphery of the lesion. For a single isocenter treatment plan, the steepest dose gradient usually falls between the 50 and 80% isodose surfaces. An isodose distribution for the treatment of trigeminal neuralgia with a single isocenter is shown in Fig. 6.14. This treatment with a single 4-mm collimator covered the section of the trigeminal nerve. A dose of 40 Gy was prescribed to the 50% isodose line of the maximum dose.

Often, however, multiple shots with different size collimators are needed to irradiate a lesion, because it is either too large to be covered with a single shot or it is too irregularly shaped. In the case of multiple shots, the isodose distribution can be modified by changing the relative weights which determine the relative duration of the various shots. Individual collimators in the helmet can be replaced by solid plugs, which block the corresponding beams. This technique affects the radiation dose distribution of individual shots, and can be very effective as a means of protecting critical structures. Small changes in the radiation dose distribution can also be achieved by changing the gamma angle, which changes the angle of incidence of the central beam relative to the skull base. This could be useful in the treatment of a pitu-

itary lesion, where the irradiation of the nearby optic chiasm should be avoided. If the lesion is on the periphery of the brain, the treatment position, i.e., prone or supine, can be altered in order to avoid a collision of the head frame or patient's head with the helmet. All these techniques can be used repeatedly for the different shots until the desired optimization is achieved. Finally, the treatment plan is ready to be evaluated by using the dose–volume histogram of the calculation matrix and dose–volume histogram of the target, which provide information about the dose to the whole brain and dose coverage of the target. A typical isodose distribution for treatment of an irregularly shaped pituitary adenoma with eight isocenters is shown in Fig. 6.15. This treatment plan with two 14-mm collimators and two 8-mm collimators was used to deliver a dose of 15 Gy to the 50% isodose volume. Selected beam channels of the 201-channel inner collimator helmet were blocked to reduced radiation exposure to the lens of the eye. Other beam channels were also blocked to shape the irradiation field and reduce the dose to the optic nerves and optic chiasm (Fig. 6.16).

The newly released Leksell GammaPlan (version 5.11 or later) provides an optional Shot Wizard, which features the automatic dose planning in an attempt to help the user to improve a treatment plan or create a treatment plan from scratch. The Shot Wizard consists of two parts, filling the target with shots with given collimators (referred to as fill) and then iteratively adjusting shot positions and their weights

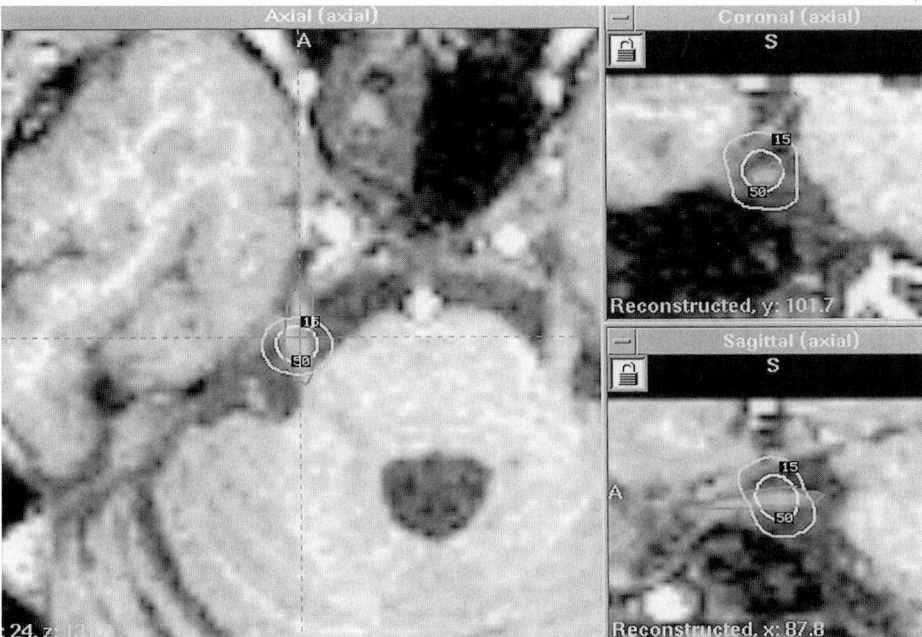

Fig. 6.14. Transverse MR image with 15% and 50% isodose lines for a single 4-mm collimator helmet treatment of a trigeminal neuralgia patient. The coronal and sagittal images reconstructed from the axial images were also shown on the right side of the picture. A section of the right trigeminal nerve was fully covered by the 50% isodose lines relative to the dose maximum of 80 Gy while the 15% lines barely touched the brainstem

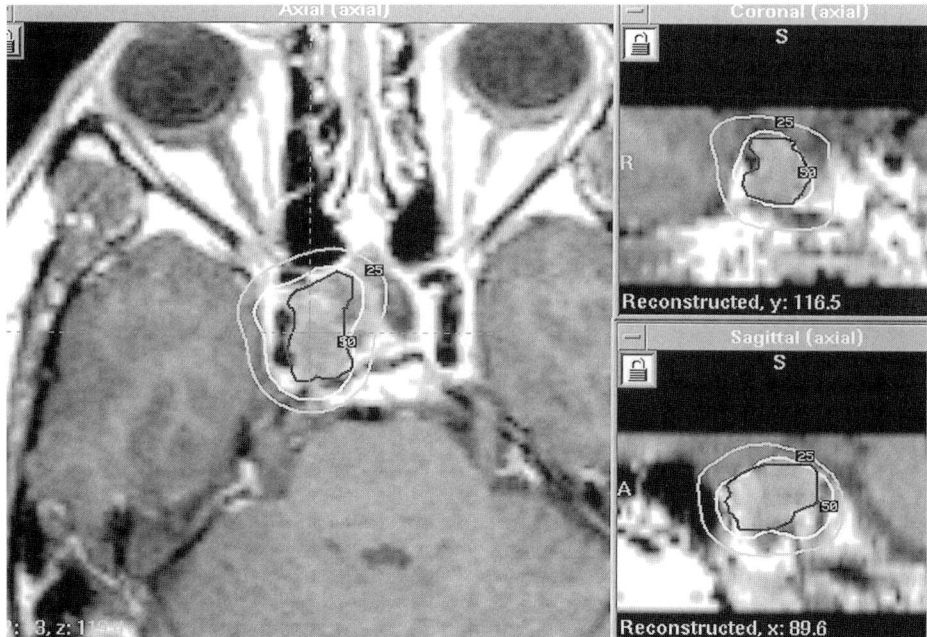

Fig. 6.15. Transverse MR image with superimposed isodose lines of 25% and 50% for treatment of a pituitary adenoma in the right cavernous sinus. The coronal and sagittal images reconstructed from the axial images are also shown on the *right side* of the picture. The irregularly shaped lesion was measured as 2.2 cm^3 in the volume with dimensions of 15.3 mm (x) × 21.2 mm (y) × 15.8 mm (z). The outline of the lesion is indicated by the *darker line* appearing inside the 50% isodose line. The treatment plan was developed with two 14-mm and two 8-mm collimator helmets. The lesion was fully covered with the 50% isodose line (i.e., 15 Gy), relative to the dose maximum of 30 Gy. The maximum dose to the optic chiasms was about 4.5 Gy

by searching for a function minimum (i.e., fine-tune). This is only a suggested new treatment plan, the user still has the responsibility of accepting or discarding it. Personal experience with the Shot Wizard suggests that it is helpful but primitive.

For current models U and B of the gamma unit, each isocenter has to be set up manually. The y-coordinates are set on the adjustable slides of the head frame. The z-coordinates are adjusted by sliding the central part of the slide along its engraved z-coordinate scale. The x-coordinates are set by a pair of trunnions, which also lock the head frame with a patient attached to a collimator helmet. The gamma angle can be read off from a vernier scale on each trunnion.

By shining a small flashlight or laser light through the collimators, one can determine which radiation beams would pass through the lenses of the eyes so that these collimators can be blocked. During the checking process, the patient is advised to close her/his eyes if the laser light is used. This process is repeated for each isocenter.

For gamma radiosurgery, the quality assurance program like that in the linear accelerator-based radiosurgery is extremely important in ensuring a high level of accuracy of patient treatment through optimal performance of the Gamma Unit and patient safety. It includes the procedures required to maintain the accuracy and consistency of dose delivery as well as compliance with the regulatory requirements. The basic programs consist of the daily,

monthly, and annual quality assurance. They mainly reflect two issues:

1. The accuracy of dose delivery
   a) Relative output factors for the helmet
   b) Radiation beam accuracy
   c) Periodical calibration of the radiation measurement instruments
   d) Dose rate for the 18-mm collimator helmet
   e) Timer consistency, linearity, and on–off timer error
   f) Dose profile verifications
   g) Mechanical alignment
2. Radiation safety
   a) Emergency procedures
   b) Radiation monitors, door interlock, emergency-off buttons
   c) Daily visual inspections
   d) Beam-status lights, audiovisual communication system
   e) Radiation leakage test

Detailed references on the gamma knife quality assurance can be found in the literature (Wu et al. 1990, 1992; Berk et al. 1991; Maitz et al. 1995). Two of the issues, the output factor and beam accuracy, will be discussed in greater detail.

In gamma knife radiosurgery, the accuracy of the relative output factor, defined as the ratio of the dose rate for a collimator helmet to that of the 18-mm collimator helmet, directly affects the accuracy of dose delivery to a radiosurgical lesion in patient treatment. This is particularly important for radiosurgical treatment of functional disorders such as Parkinson's disease and trigeminal neuralgia, wherein a single large radiation dose is delivered to the selected target using the 4-mm collimator (LEKSELL 1971b; LINDQUIST et al. 1992; KONDZIOLKA et al. 1996). Elekta's recommended output factors for the 14-, 8-, and 4-mm collimators of the Leksell gamma knife relative to the 18-mm collimator were 0.984, 0.956, and 0.800, respectively. Significant deviations in output factors have been reported from both calculation and measurement, particularly for the 4-mm collimator, ranging from 0.63 to 0.92 (the 7th and 9th International Meetings of the Leksell Gamma Knife Society, 1995 and 1998). Recent data from both calculation and measurement presented at the Leksell Gamma Knife meetings suggest the necessity of an increase of the relative output factor for the 4-mm collimator. New Leksell Gamma Knife and Leksell GammaPlan systems will be delivered with an output factor of 0.87. Elekta recommends all gamma knife customers to consider new results as well as

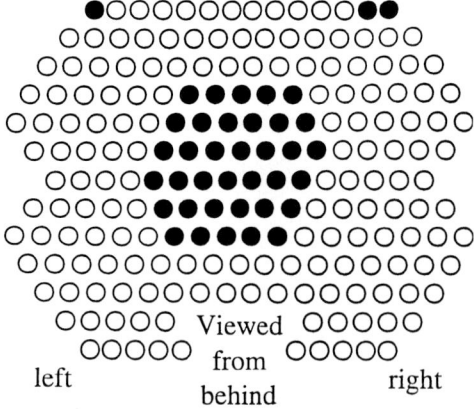

Fig. 6.16. A custom plug pattern to shape the irradiation field and reduce the dose to the optic nerves and optic chiasms for one of the four shots. A total of 39 plugs (*filled circles*) were used. The top two groups (*3 plugs*) were used to protect the lens of the eyes, while the remaining plugs were used to reduce the irradiation of the optic nerves and chiasms

their own measurements to reevaluate their current output factor settings for the gamma knife. The consequence of this change would result in variations of the integral radiation dose, the minimum and maximum dose values, and the dose distribution in terms of the location of the isodose surfaces.

Different radiation dosimetric methods, such as regular film, ion-chamber, diode, thermoluminescent dosimetry (TLD), radiochromic film, and micro-ionization chamber have been developed for measurement of the relative output factors as well as shuttle dose or transit dose at several gamma knife centers. WALTON et al. measured the output factors relative to the 14-mm collimator helmet by using Therados solid-state dosimeters (WALTON et al 1987). They reported output factors of 0.964 and 0.925 for the 8-mm and 4-mm collimator helmets, respectively. These values would be further elevated if normalized to the 18-mm collimator. More recently, WU et al. reported their relative output factor measurements obtained from both the diode and the TLD chips in multiple beam geometry (WU et al. 1990). Their value (0.821) for the 4-mm collimator helmet showed a 3.5% deviation from Elekta's recommended output factors.

At University of Southern California/University Hospital (USCUH), annual output factor measurements for the gamma knife have been carried out by using a high accuracy TLD technique, characterized by the group annealing and sorting (GAS) procedure (YU et al 1999a). For each collimator exposure, one to five LiF TLD $1\times1\times1$-mm^3 cubes were used depending on the collimator size, and the process was repeated until approximately ten TLDs had been exposed for each collimator. Transit radiation dose accumulated during the motion of the treatment couch was measured for each collimator helmet, and the result was subtracted from uncorrected TLD dose measurements. The relative output factors for 5 consecutive years are summarized in Table 6.4. The mean values of the output factors for the 14-, 8-, and 4-mm collimators from last 5 years were 0.985±0.001, 0.948±0.005, and 0.833±0.007, respectively, relative to the 18-mm collimator. These measured relative output factors are virtually identical to the values recommended by Elekta for the 14-mm and 8-mm collimators. The output factor for the 4-mm collimator, however, shows an approximately 4% deviation from Elekta recommend values.

For the acceptance test and annual quality assurance of the Leksell gamma unit, measurement of the beam accuracy, defined as a distance between mechanical and radiological isocenters, poses a chal-

Table 6.4. Relative output factors

Year	Collimator size		
	14 mm	8 mm	4 mm
1994	0.984	0.953	0.824
1995	0.984	0.954	0.836
1996	0.985	0.942	0.842
1997	0.984	0.942	0.838
1998	0.987	0.947	0.826
Average	0.985	0.948	0.833
Elekta	0.984	0.956	0.800

Table 6.5. Measured deviations from the last 6 years

Year	Collimator	
	4 mm	8 mm
1994	0.29 mm	N/A
1995	0.26 mm	0.28 mm
1996	0.22 mm	0.24 mm
1997	0.23 mm	0.18 mm
1998	0.20 mm	0.28 mm
1999	0.29 mm	0.29 mm
Average	0.25 mm	0.25 mm
Elekta	0.29 mm	N/A

N/A, not available

lenge to medical physicists. The specification for the beam accuracy is within 0.5 mm for the 4-mm collimator helmet (Leksell Gamma Unit User's Manual Vol. 2, Elekta, Atlanta, GA). At the University of Southern California gamma knife center, a simple technique was used to analyze the beam accuracy by using a conventional film densitometer with mathematical modeling. A small piece of film was placed inside the film cassette containing a sharp needle. The needle was located such that its tip was exactly positioned at the mechanical isocenter. Before exposure, the film was pierced by the needle. Density profile was accomplished using a densitometer with a spatial resolution of 0.8 mm. The profile was then fitted to a model of the two Gaussian functions, as seen in Fig. 6.17. One is for the radiation field profile, the other for a dip caused by the narrow hole. The difference between the centers of the two Gaussian functions defines the deviation of the beam accuracy from the mechanical center of the unit. The deviations for x, y, and z directions from one of our annual measurements are 0.032 mm, 0.054 mm, and 0.195 mm, respectively. The combined deviation is 0.20 mm, which is well within the specification and in excellent agreement with the results from the manufacture's laser measurement. Beam accuracies for both the 4-mm and 8-mm collimator helmets for 6 consecutive years are summarized in Table 6.5. This technique provides a simple, accurate, and practical tool for measurement of beam accuracy in the acceptance test and annual quality assurance of the Leksell gamma unit.

6.4
Physical Comparison of Stereotactic Techniques

6.4.1
Target Uncertainties

In stereotactic radiosurgery, the accuracy of the target localization is primarily determined by the stereotactic apparatus or rigid head frame and imaging modalities as well as the current knowledge of the neurological abnormality. In that sense it is identical for each of the different radiosurgical techniques. The uncertainty due to the stereotactic apparatus is about 1 mm. The definition of a radiological lesion depends on the resolution of the image (CT or MR) and the relationship of the macroscopic image with the microscopic extent of the disease. The particular uncertainty from the image ranges from 1 mm to 2 mm for different pixel sizes and slice thickness. For gamma knife radiosurgery, the target point is placed at the point of intersection, i.e., the central axes of the radiation sources, or isocenter. Unlike linear accelerators, no parts of the gamma unit move during the treatment. Thus, its theoretical isocenter accuracy is limited only by the machining precision of the collimator helmets. The helmet is machined to within 0.1 mm, while all of the 201 collimators are converged to the isocenter within 0.3 mm (Leksell Gamma Unit User's Manual Vol. 2, Elekta, Atlanta, Ga., USA). On the other hand, the isocenter of the linear accelerators is defined as the intersection of the axes of rotation of the accelerator gantry and the collimator. It is similar for the charged particle beam, except for the stationary port. The accuracy of the isocenter is typically within ±1 mm and can be improved to ±0.5 mm with some minor clinical modifications. FRIEDMAN et al. reported a technique that has achieved a radiation beam accuracy of 0.2 mm by incorporating a mechanical system of precision bearings to control all patient and accelerator movements (FRIEDMAN et al. 1989). Although the isocenter accuracy achievable with linear accelerators may be inferior to that of the gamma unit, it is of the same order as the target localization accuracy possible with modern imaging techniques. The radiosurgery techniques may differ in accuracy of the dose delivery and slightly differ in the dose distribution (PIKE et al. 1987, 1990a,b; PODGORSAK 1989, 1990; GRAHAM et al. 1991, PHILIPS et al. 1994; VERHEY et al. 1998; CARDINALE et al. 1998; SCHWARTZ 1998; YU et al. 1999b); it is unclear whether the differences are clinically significant. The uncertainties in dose delivery for commonly used stereotactic techniques are significantly less than most of the clinical knowledge of the location and extent of the lesion as determined by CT or MRI.

6.4.2
Dosimetric Comparison

In a recent study (YU et al. 1999b), a simulated elongated ellipsoid target, 25 mm in diameter and 35 mm in length, was chosen to examine the dosimetric differences among three commonly used radiosurgery techniques: gamma knife, linear accelerator multiple arcs, and conformally shaped static fields. Single isocenter linear accelerator treatment plans were developed: nine portals for the static shaped field technique, and a seven-arc plan for the multiple arc method. A total of 13 isocenters with three different collimator sizes were used in the gamma knife plan. Such a target is representative of many irregular radiosurgery lesions, since an ellipsoidal enclosing

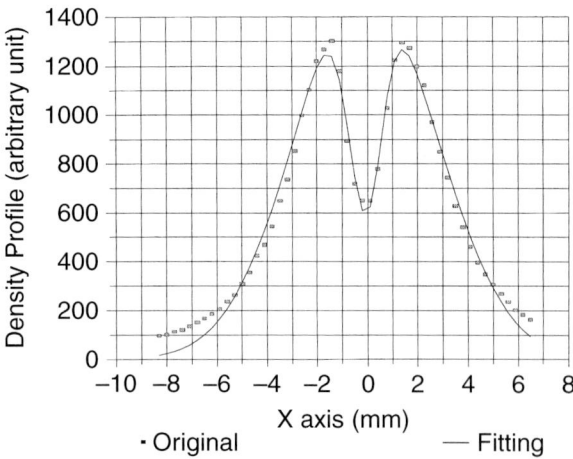

Fig. 6.17. Determination of the beam accuracy for the 4-mm collimator helmet. *Dots* represent the measured data of the density profile. The *solid line* is a fitted curve. It resulted in a deviation of 0.032 mm along the x-axis direction

volume of reasonably close conformation can usually be found for irregularly shaped radiologically defined targets. The alignment of the target was taken to be parallel to the caudo-cephalad axis of the head. Other possible orientations of the target were not considered. It has been shown, however, that it is possible to achieve good conformity with a single isocenter multiple arc radiosurgery treatment plan for a target of this shape for any location and orientation in the head (LUXTON et al. 1994). For all methods, the dose maximum is located within the target, although not at the center. In the transverse plane, high percentile isodose lines for the three radiosurgery techniques are characterized as circular and concentric with the isocenter, but ovoid shaped in the coronal plane. For the gamma knife plan, the low percentile isodose lines are circular in the transverse plane and ovoid in the coronal plane. For the multiple arc technique, peripheral isodose lines are ovoid in the transverse plane and irregular in the coronal plane due to the different projections of multiple arc beams. For static shaped field technique, the peripheral isodose lines are rectangular, as contributed by two pairs of opposed beams in the transverse plane and by lateral-opposed and vertex beams in the coronal plane.

Dose–volume histograms for the elongated ellipsoid target are shown in Fig. 6.18. Dose is normalized to the reference dose or prescribed dose for the individual plans. The target volume (11.5 cm^3) is fully covered by the reference dose in all three stereotactic radiosurgery techniques. Target coverage for the multiple arc and static shaped field techniques are very similar, with the static field plan showing slightly steeper fall-off as the dose increases above 100% of the reference dose. The volume that receives radiation dose above the prescription drops sharply for both linear accelerator techniques. Thus, excellent homogeneity of the dose distribution across the entire target is achieved with these two techniques. On the other hand, in the gamma knife technique there is a greater volume of the target that receives a higher dose, and the fall-off is characterized by a less steep gradient than for the other plans. In this technique, 1.6 cm^3, about 15% of the target volume receives a radiation dose between 170 and 200% of the reference dose as the dose level is increased beyond the prescribed isodose value.

The normal brain cumulative dose–volume histograms (DVH) for the three techniques are compared in Fig. 6.19 after subtracting the target DVHs from the calculation matrix DVHs. Total volume of normal brain tissue covered by the reference dose is 1.7 cm^3 for the gamma knife plan and 2.2 cm^3 for the multiple arc plan as well as 1.8 cm^3 for the shaped field plan. At dose levels from 25% to 100% of the reference dose, the gamma knife plan covers less volume than the multiple arc plan. For example, the gamma knife plan covers 21.4 cm^3 at 50% of the reference dose, compared to 27.3 cm^3 for the multiple

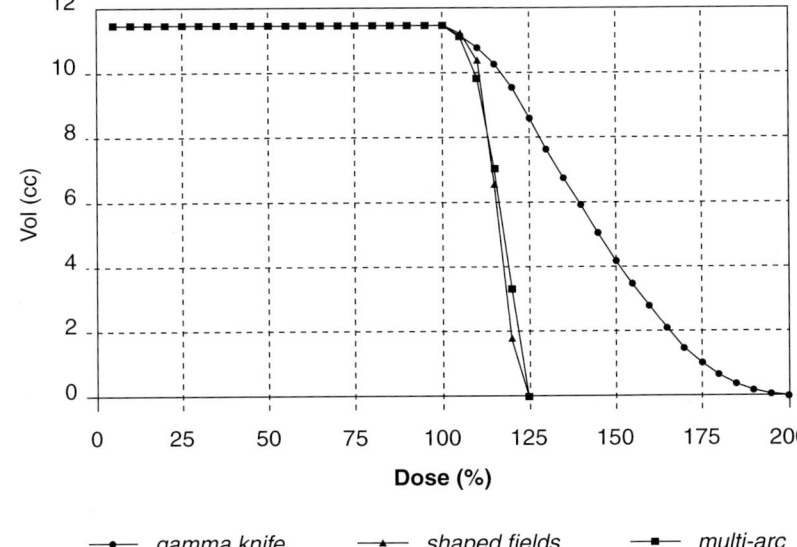

Dose-volume histogram

Fig. 6.18. Dose–volume histograms of the 25×35-mm ellipsoid target calculated for the gamma knife, shaped fields, and multiple arc plans. The filled *ovoids*, *triangles*, and *rectangles* indicate the gamma knife plan, the shaped field plan, and the multiple arcs plan, respectively

Dose-volume histogram

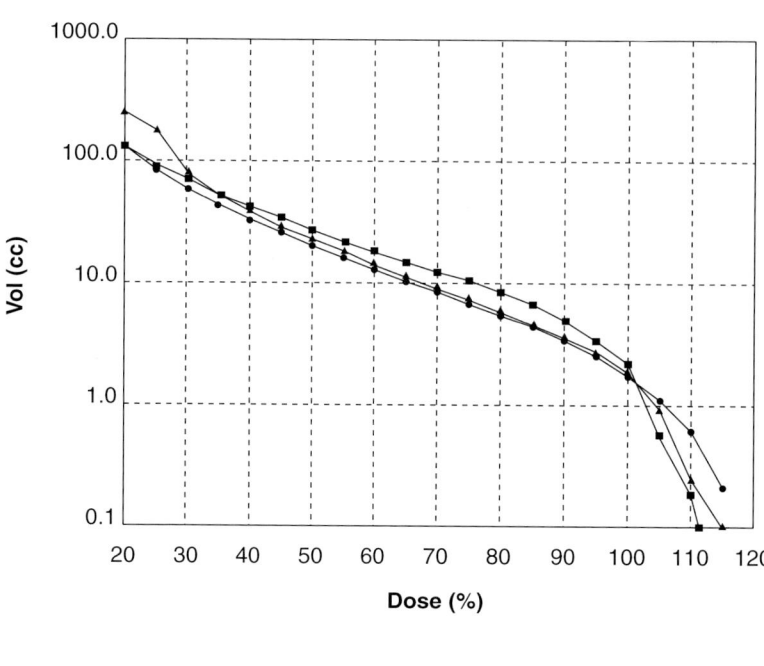

Fig. 6.19. Comparison of normal brain dose–volume histograms in the semilogarithm plot. The horizontal axis is normalized to the respective prescribed dose levels. The filled *ovoids*, *triangles*, and *rectangles* indicate the gamma knife plan, the shaped fields plan, and the multiple arcs plan, respectively

arc plan. The DVH for the multiple arc plan falls more rapidly as the dose is increased above 100% of the reference dose than does the gamma knife plan. For dose levels below 50% of the reference dose, the gamma knife plan covers slightly less volume of normal brain tissue than the shaped field plan. At 50%, the gamma knife plan covers 21.4 cm^3, compared to 22.8 cm^3 for the shaped fixed field plan. At the lower dose levels, the differences are greater. For doses between 50% and 100%, the gamma knife plan and the shaped field plan are virtually identical. As for the multiple arc plan, the shaped field plan treats the target volume with a much faster fall-off at doses greater than 100% of the reference dose than the gamma knife plan. For dose levels below 35% of the reference dose, the multiple arc plan treats less volume of normal brain tissue than the shaped fields plan. For the static shaped field technique, the volume of normal brain receiving radiation doses of 20% of the reference dose is almost twice the volume than with the multiple arc plan or the gamma knife plan. The increase in peripheral dose for the static shaped field plan is caused mainly by opposition of pairs of beams in the transverse plane. Assuming a prescription of 20 Gy defined to the 80% isodose line, 265 cm^3 of normal tissue, instead of 130 cm^3, will receive a dose greater or equal to 4 Gy. Since the morbidity of this dose–volume level is usually acceptable, appro-

priate static shaped fields can be used as a substitute for multiple arc treatment. For dose levels between 35% and 100%, the shaped fields plan covers slightly less volume of normal brain than the multiple arcs plan. At the reference dose, the shaped fields plan treats 1.8 cm^3, slightly lower than the 2.2 cm^3 of the multiple arc plan.

The selected target, a prolate ellipsoid 25 mm in diameter and 35 mm in length, is not ideally matched to the Leksell gamma knife radiosurgery technique. The maximum projection of the target in the transverse plane is 25 mm in this study, whereas the projection of the 50% isodose line from the largest collimator (i.e., the 18-mm collimator) of the gamma knife is about 22 mm in the x-axis (lateral direction), 20 mm in the y-axis (anterior–posterior direction), and 25 mm in the z-axis (superior–inferior direction) in the planes through the isocenter in a 16-cm diameter spherical plastic phantom. Even the largest collimator is too small for this target. Although a smaller number of isocenters could have been used to encompass the target volume, a rather large number of isocenters (13 in total) were actually used in the gamma knife plan to minimize the total non-target volume covered by the 50% isodose surface. Similarly, the multiple isocenter technique could be used for the linear accelerator multiple arc plan. This would presumably result in a dose distribution very similar to that of the gamma knife plan. The multiarc multiple isocenter technique, however, would require considerable complexity in treatment execution, whereas a single isocenter method can in fact provide adequate dose coverage and good neighboring non-target tissue sparing by simply selecting specific arcs, collimator sizes, and nonuniform beam weighting.

Unlike the static shaped field technique, in which the size of the radiation field can be optimized according the two-dimensional projection of the target for each individual field, the circular collimator for conventional multiple arc radiosurgery provides a single degree of freedom in matching the aperture to the projection of the target. In this study, a 40-mm diameter collimator was used for two of seven arcs in the transverse plane in order to achieve the dose coverage in the superior–inferior direction (35 mm plus margins). This resulted in excess coverage in the transverse directions, which may explain the slightly larger volume (2.2 cm^3) of normal brain tissue that would be covered by the prescribed radiation dose in the multiple arc technique as compared to the fixed field technique (1.8 cm^3).

For any shaped target of limited volume, the gamma knife appears to be an appropriate radiosurgery technique, excluding those cases for which the isocenter coordinates would make it impossible to position the patient plus attached head frame inside the collimator helmet. The gamma knife may have the advantage of a higher degree of targeting accuracy than the linear accelerator radiosurgery techniques due to the absence of moving parts during treatment delivery. Special techniques have been used, however, to correct for errors arising from couch rotation in linear accelerator-based radiosurgery (BREZOVICH et al. 1997) and for inaccuracies of gantry rotation (FRIEDMAN et al. 1989), or to minimize the combined effect of both motion-related inaccuracies (LOW et al. 1995). In this study, the gamma knife demonstrated the greatest tissue sparing in the 20–100% dose range relative to the prescribed dose compared with the other techniques considered, although there has been no demonstrated clinical advantage for this degree of reduction in the volume treated with this dose range. The gamma knife is also characterized by simplicity of treatment planning and simplicity of actual treatment. The multiple isocenters introduce a large percent dose inhomogeneity within the target volume while reducing the dose to normal tissue. Thus far, however, there has been no clinical evidence showing adverse consequences of the dose inhomogeneity within the target volume.

In fact, it has been suggested that greater dose inhomogeneity of the type associated with gamma knife treatments might have beneficial consequences (BRENNER et al. 1991; SHAW et al. 1998). On the other hand, for multifraction treatments, dose uniformity within the target could become important (LAX 1993).

For a regular-shaped target, the single isocenter multiple arc technique has certain dosimetric advantages for radiosurgery. It provides better sparing of non-target tissue than the multiple static shaped field at dose levels below 35% of the reference dose and gives a high degree of dose homogeneity within the target. With this technique there is also an inherently high accuracy in the collimation system. For irregular-shaped targets, however, the single isocenter technique with conventional circular aperture may not be capable of minimizing dose to normal tissue as effectively as multiple isocenter techniques. The multiple isocenter technique, which would give a dose distribution similar to that of the multiple isocenter gamma knife plan, is very complex for practical treatment delivery using the multiple arcs for each isocenter. Total treatment time could be substantially increased from each new isocenter setup, particularly if independent quality assurance tests are performed. Furthermore, couch rotation between arcs of each isocenter and possible collimator changes occurring within individual isocenter treatment delivery require entry of staff in the treatment room. The time that is required for this complex treatment delivery could possibly be reduced using the dynamic radiosurgery technique. The ability to choose wider ranges of collimator size does gives the multiple arc technique a distinct advantage over the gamma knife. For example, a 25-mm diameter spherical target could be easily planned and treated with a single isocenter linear accelerator technique, resulting in excellent dose homogeneity, whereas this target would require a gamma knife treatment plan of six to eight isocenters, characterized by dose inhomogeneity within the target.

The static shaped field technique effectively conforms the dose distribution to the shape of the target volume with relative homogeneity within the target volume, similar to that of the proton beam radiosurgery. If dose uniformity within the target is important, the shaped beam techniques with either photons or protons generally have an advantage over other multiple isocenters modalities, particularly in the case of irregular targets. The static shaped photon beam technique is a viable alternative to the other two commonly used photon beam methods. It can easily be used to treat irregular or relatively large targets. It provides a high degree of dose homogeneity within the target as well as better protection of non-target tissue in the 50–100% dose ranges than multiple arc radiosurgery. The multiple-shaped field method, however, treats more normal brain tissue at lower radiation doses, due to the practical limit on the number of beam directions with this technique. On the other hand, new development of intensity modulation with inverse planning capability might be a solution for the limit issue (XING et al. 1998; HARMON et al. 1998; SPIRIDON et al. 1998; BURMAN et al. 1997; LOMAX et al. 1999). Complete systems are now commercially available, such as the Peacock system (Nomos, Sewickley, Pa., USA). The system combines an inverse treatment planning with miniature multileaf modulation collimators to create and deliver the conformal dose distribution (WU et al. 1996). In practice, special precautions in dosimetry should be taken to assure accuracy in dose calculation and measurement when using very small irregularly shaped fields.

Recently, a group from two institutes, headed by VERHEY, reported a collective investigation on comparison of radiosurgery treatment modalities based on physical dose distribution (VERHEY et al. 1998). The study was based on DVH analysis of the treatment plans for the Leksell gamma knife, multiarc linear accelerator, and proton beams radiosurgery. Five clinical cases were selected to represent the typical range of target size, shapes and locations, observed in the practice of stereotactic radiosurgery. The size of the lesions ranged from 1 cm^3 to 26 cm^3. The same stereotactic apparatus and image modality was used for all three techniques. For the gamma knife plans, the number of the isocenter ranged from 1 to 12, with a choice of four different collimator sizes, depending on the size of the lesion. For the proton plans, a single isocenter was used with up to five shaped and fully compensated fields. For the standard linear accelerator plans, up to four isocenters, each with up to six arcs, were used with conventional circular collimators. In addition, complex linear accelerator plans with up to 12 isocenters and 32 arcs were also developed without consideration of any physical limitations, such as number of isocenters and arcs as well as variable arc angles and weightings, in the attempt to achieve more conformal linear accelerator plans. For the five cases, the total of planning and treatment time ranged from 2 to 4 h for the gamma plan, 2 to 5 h for the proton plan, 4 to 7 h for the standard linear accelerator plan, and 4 to 40 h for the complex linear accelerator plan.

They concluded that for a small regular target volume, all three modalities are very much equal in the target coverage and normal tissue sparing, although the proton plan treats slightly more surrounding tissue than the other two modalities. The inferior proton plan for a small target is due to the additional uncertainties of the densities of the tissues. On the other hand, for large irregular targets, both the gamma plan and the complex linear accelerator plan are superior to the standard linear accelerator plan in normal tissue sparing while the proton beam plan has advantages over the other three modalities in that category (SERAGO et al. 1995). For large and irregularly shaped targets, a conformal plan can be generated and implemented relatively easily for the proton beam plan with multiple-shaped and compensated fields, reasonably easily for the gamma plan with multiple isocenters and different collimator sizes, and more laboriously for the standard linear accelerator plan with a limit of a relatively small number of isocenters, and hypothetically for the complex linear accelerator plan. The study on the conformity index, referred to as the ratio of the volume of the prescription isodose surface to the volume of the target, suggested that improved normal tissue sparing could be achieved for the photon beam when using high numbers of isocenters with large diameters. For the peripheral lesion, the standard linear accelerator plan, the complex linear accelerator plan, and the LGU plan are all rather similar to each other in terms of normal tissue sparing; while the proton plan with a single field demonstrates superior advantage in such a situation. In general, the optimal modality for stereotactic radiosurgery depends on target size, shape, and location.

The group mentioned above also reported their comparison study based on complication and control probabilities from the same clinical cases (SMITH et al. 1998). In general, complication probabilities increase with the size of the lesions. Overall, both the complex linear accelerator plans and gamma plans had the lowest complication probability, in contrast to the standard linear accelerator plans. On the other hand, proton plans showed the lowest complication probability for the largest irregularly shaped target and for the very peripheral target, and less advantages for the smaller centrally located volumes, which was consistent with results based on the physical dose distributions (VERHEY et al. 1998).

6.4.3
Conclusion

In general, the optimal treatment modality for stereotactic radiosurgery depends on various factors, such as the target shape, size, and location as well as planning and delivery time. As for the mechanical accuracy concerned, the gamma knife may have an advantage over the linear accelerator. For a target of limited volume and essentially any shape, one can obtain closely conformal dosimetry with the gamma knife. For a regular-shaped target, the single isocenter multiple arc technique gives a more homogeneous dose distribution within the target. Dose distribution for linear accelerator radiosurgery with multiple isocenters and multiple arcs is similar to that of the gamma knife technique with multiple isocenters, except for the relative difficulty of treatment implementation with linear accelerator. The proton beam plan with multiple-shaped and compensated fields can easily generate a conformal dose distribution for large and irregularly shaped targets. Static shaped fields offer an alternative radiosurgery technique, with dosimetry similar to the multiple arc method, applicable to targets of any shape.

References

Adler JR (1994) Image-guided frameless stereotactic Radiosurgery. In Interactive Image-Guided Neurosurgery, Neurosurgical Topics, Vol .6, Maciunas RJ (ed). American Association of Neurological Surgeons.

Adler JR, Cox RS (1996) Preliminary clinical experience with the Cyberkinfe: image-guided stereotactic radiosurgery. In Radiosurgery 1995. Kondziolka D. (ed), Basel, Karger.

Adler JR, Murphy MJ, Chang SD, Hancock SL (1999) Image-guided robotic radiosurgery, Neurosurgery, 44:1299–1307.

Apuzzo MLJ, Chandrasoma PT, Breeze RE, Cohen DM, Luxton G, Mazumder (1988) Applications of image-directed stereotactic surgery in the management of intracranial neoplasms, in Stereotactic Neurosugery Volume 2: Concepts in Neurosurgery, edited by Heilbrun MP, Williams & Wilkins, Baltimore.

Backlund EO (1974) Stereotaxic treatment of craniopharyngiomas. Acta Neurochir [Suppl](Wien) 21:177–183.

Backlund EO (1979) Stereotactic radiosurgery in intracranial tumours and vascular malformations, in Krayenbuhl E (ed): *Advances and Technical Standards in Neurosurgery*, New York, Springer-Verlag, 6:1–37.

Barcia-Salorio JL, Broseta J, Hernandez G, Balester B, Masbout G (1977) Radiosurgical treatment of a carotid-cavernous fistula. Case report, in Szikia G, (ed): *Stereotactic Cerebral Irradiation, INSERM Symposium No. 12.* Amsterdam, Elsevier/North-Holland, pp 251–256.

Barcia-Salorio JL, Hernandez G, Broseta J, Gonzales Darder J, Cuidad J (1982) Radiosurgical treatment of carotid-cavernous fistula. Appi Neurophysiol 45:520–522.

Barendsen GW (1968) Responses of cultured cells, tumors and normal tissues to radiations of different linear energy transfer. Curr Top Radiat Res 4:295–356.

Beatty J, Biggs PJ, Gall Kenneth, Okunieff P, Pardo FS, Harte KJ, Dalterio MJ, Sliski AP (1996) A new miniature x-ray device for interstitial radiosurgery: dosimetry, Med. Phys., 23:53–62.

Berk HW, Agawal SK (1991) Quality assurance of Leksell gamma units, Stereotact Funct Neurosurf 57:106–112.

Betti O, Derechinsky V (1983) Irradiation stereotaxique multifaisceaux. Neurochirurgie 29:295–298.

Betti O, Derechinsky V (1984) Hyperselected encephalic irradiation with a linear accelerator. Acta Neurochir [Suppi] (Wien) 33:385–390.

Betti O, Munari C, Rosier R (1989) Stereotactic radiosurgery with the linear accelerator: Treatment of arteriovenous malformations. Neurosurgery 24:311–321.

Biggs P, Beatty J, Gall K, Harte K, Sliski A (1993) Absolute dosimetry for a new 40 kV x-ray device used for stereotactic radiation therapy. Med. Phys, 20:925 (abstract)

Bourland JD, McCollough KP (1994) Static field conformal stereotactic radiosurgery: Physical techniques. Int J Radiat Oncol Biol Phys 28:471–479.

Bova FJ, Buatti JM, Friedman WA, Mendenhall WM, Yang CC, Liu C (1997) The University of Florida frameless high-precision stereotactic radiosurgery system, Int J Radiat Oncol Biol Phys, 38:875–882.

Brenner DJ, Martel MK, Hall EJ (1991), Fractionated regimens for stereotactic radiotherapy for recurrent tumors in the brain, Int J Radiat Oncol Biol Phys 21:819–824.

Brezovich IA, Pareek PN, Plott WE and Jennelle RLS (1997) Quality assurance system to correct for errors arising from couch rotation in linear accelerator-based stereotactic radiosurgery. Int. J. Radiat. Oncol. Biol. Phys. 38:883–890.

Burman C, Chui CS, Kutcher G, Leibel S, Zelefsky M, LoSasso T, Spirou S, Wu Q, Yang J, Stein J, Mohan R, Fuks Z, Ling CC (1997). Planning, delivery, and quality assurance of intensity-modulated radiotherapy using dynamic multileaf collimator: a strategy for large-scale implementation for the treatment of carcinoma of the prostate. Int J Radiat Oncol Biol Phys. 39:863–73.

Cardinale RM, Benedic SH, Wu Q, Zwicker R, Gaballa HE, Mohan R (1998) A comparison of three stereotactic radiotherapy technique; ARCS vs. noncoplanar fixed fields VS. intensity modulation, Int J Radiat Oncol Biol Phys, 42:431–436.

Caron JL, Souhami L, Podgorsak EB (1992) Dynamic Stereotactic radiosurgery in the palliative treatment of cerebral metastatic tumors. J Neurooncol 12:173–179.

Chen GTY, Singh RP, Castro JR, Lyman JT, Quivey JM (1979) Treatment planning for heavy ion radiotherapy. Int J Radiat Oncol Biol Phys 5:1809–1819.

Chen GTY, Kuchnir FT (1987) Particle therapy 1986, in Kereiakes JG, Elso HR, Born CG (eds): *Radiation Oncology Physics 1986, American Association of Physicists in Medicine, Medical Physics Monograph No. 15.* New York, American Institute of Physics, pp 74–90.

Colombo F, Zanardo A (1984) Clinical application of an original Stereotactic apparatus. Acta Neurochir [Suppi] (Wien) 33:569–573.

Colombo F, Benedetti A, Pozza F, Zanardo A, Avanzo RC, Chierego G, Marchetti C (1985a) Stereotactic radiosurgery utilizing a linear accelerator. Appi Neurophysiol 48:133–145.

Colombo F, Benedetti A, Pozza F, Avanzo RC, Marchetti C, Chierego G, Zanardo A (1985b) External Stereotactic irradiation by linear accelerator. Neurosurgery 16:154–159.

Colombo F, Benedetti A, Pozza F, Avanzo RC, Marchetti C, Dettori P, Bernardi L, Vittore P (1986) Radiosurgery using a 4 MV linear accelerator. Technique and radiobiological implications. Acta Radiol [Suppl] (Stockh) 369:603–607.

Colombo F, Benedetti A, Pozza F, Marchetti C, Chieregi G (1989) Linear accelerator radiosurgery of cerebral arteriovenous malformations. Neurosurgery 24:833–839.

Colombo F, Benedetti A, Pozza F, Marchetti C, Chieregi G, Zanardo A (1990) Linear accelerator radiosurgery of three-dimensional irregular targets. Stereotact Funct Neurosurg 54–55:541–546.

Cosgrove VP, Jahn U, Pfaender M, Bauer S, Budach V, Wurm RE (1999) Commisioning of a micro multi-leaf collimator and planning system for stereotactic radiosurgey, Radiotherapy and Oncology, 50:325–336.

Curtis SB (1977) Calculated LET distributions of heavy ion beams. Int J Radiol Oncol Biol Phys 3:87–91.

Dinsmore M, Harte KJ, Sliski AP, Smith DO, Nomikos PM, Dalterio MJ, Boom AJ, Leonard WF, Oettinger PE, Yanch JC (1996) A new miniature x-ray source for interstitial radiosurgery: device description, Med Phys, 23:45–52.

Fabrikant JI, Lyman JT, Hosobuchi Y (1984) Stereotactic heavy-ion Bragg peak radiosurgery for intra-cranial vascular disorders: Method for treatment of deep arteriovenous malformations. Br J Radiol 57: 479–490.

Fabrikant JI, Lyman JT, Frankel KA (1985) Heavy charge-particle Bragg peak radiosurgery for intracranial vascular disorders. Radiat Res 104[Suppl]:S244-S258.

Fabrikant JI, Frankel KA, Phillips MH, Levy RP (1988) Stereotactic heavy charged-particle Bragg peak radiosurgery for intracranial arteriovenous malformations, in Edwards MSB, Hoffman HJ (eds): Cerebral Vascular Diseases of Childhood and Adolescence. Baltimore, Williams & Wilkins, pp 389–409.

Flickinger JC, Lunsford LD, Wu A, Maitz AH, Kalend AM (1990a) Treatment planning for gamma knife radiosurgery with multiple iso-centers. Int J Radiat Oncol Biol Phys 18:1495–1511.

Flickinger JC, Maitz A, Kalend A, Lunsford LD, Wu A (1990b) Treatment shaping with selected beam blocking using the Leksell gamma unit. Int J Radiat Oncol Biol Phys 19:783–789.

Flickinger JC (1993) Dosimetry and dose-volume relationships in radiosurgery. In: Alexander III E, Loeffler JS, Lunsford LD (ed): Stereotactic Radiosurgery. New York, NY; McGraw-Hill, Inc., pp31–41.

Friedman WA and Bova FJ (1989) The University of Florida radiosurgery system. Surg. Neurol. 32:334–342.

Ginzton EL, Mallory KB, Kaplan HS (1957), The Stanford medical linear accelerator; I. Design and development, Stanford Med. Bull. 15:123–140.

Goetsch SJ, Murphy BD, Schmidt R, Micka J, De Werd L, Chen Y, Shockley S (1999) Physics of rotating gamma systems for stereotactic radiosurgery, Int J Radiat Oncol Biol Phys. 43:689–696.

Goitein M (1983) Compensation for inhomogeneities in charged particle radiotherapy using computed tomography. Int J Radiol Oncol Biol Phys. 4:499–508.

Graham JD, Nahum AE, Brada M (1991) A comparison of techniques for Stereotactic radiotherapy by linear accelerator based on 3-dimensional dose distributions. Radiother Oncol 22:29–35.

Griffin BR, Warcola SH, Mayberg MR, Eenmaa J, Eskridge J, Winn HR (1988) Stereotactic neutron radiosurgery for arteriovenous malformations of the brains. Medical Dosimetry 13:179–182.

Hall EJ (1994) Radiobiology for the Radiologist, Philadelphia, Lippincott, ed 4.

Harmon Jr. JF, Bova F, Meeks S (1998) Inverse radiosurgery treatment planning through deconvolution and constrained optimization, Med. Phys., 25:1850–1857.

Hartmann GH, Schlegel W, Sturm V, Kober B, Pastyr O, Lorenz WJ (1985) Cerebral radiation surgery using moving field irradiation at a linear accelerator facility. Int J Radiat Oncol Biol Phys 11:1185–1192.

Heilbrun M, Roberts T, Apuzzo M, Wells T, Sabshin J (1983) Preliminary experience with Brown-Roberts-Wells (BRW) computerized tomography stereotaxic guidance system. J Neurosurg 59:217–222.

Hosobuchi Y, Fabricant J, Lyman J (1987) Stereotactic heavy-particle irradiation of intracranial arteriovenous malformations. Steinberg 50:248–252.

Houdek PV, Fayos JV, Van Buren JM, Ginsberg MS (1985) Stereotactic radiotherapy technique for small intracranial lesions. Med Phys 12:469–472.

Karzmark CJ, Nunan CS, Tanabe E (1992) Medical Electron Accelerators, New York, McGraw-Hill.

Kjellberg RN, Sweet WH, Preston WM et al (1962) The Bragg peak of a proton beam in intracranial therapy of tumors. Transactions of the American Neurologic Association 87:216–218.

Kjellberg RN, Shintani A, Frantz AG, Kliman B (1968) Proton beam therapy in acromegaly. N Engl J. Med., 278:689–695.

Kjellberg RN (1979) Stereotactic Bragg peak proton radiosurgery results. In Szikia G (ed): Stereotactic Cerebral Irradiation. Boston, Elsevier Press, pp 233–240.

Kjellberg RN, Kliman B (1980) Radiosurgery treatment for pituitary adenoma, in Post KD, Jackson IMD, Reichlin S (eds): The Pituitary Adenoma. New York, Plenum, pp 459–478.

Kjellberg RN, Hanamura T, Davis KR, Lyons SL, Adams RD (1983) Bragg-peak proton-beam therapy for arteriovenous malformations of the brain. N Engi J Med 309:269–274.

Kjellberg RN (1986) Sterotactic Bragg peak proton beam radiosurgery for cerebral arteriovenous malformations. Ann Clin Res 18[Suppl 47]:17–19,.

Kjellberg RN, Abe M (1988) Stereotactic Bragg peak proton beam therapy, in Lunsford LD (ed): Modern Stereotactic Neurosurgery. Boston, Martinus Nijhoff, pp 463–470.

Koehler AM, Schneider RJ, Sisterton JM (1975) Range modulators for protons and heavy ions. Nucl Instr Meth 131:437–440.

Koehler AM, Schneider RJ, Sisterton JM (1977) Flattening of proton dose distributions for large-field radiotherapy. Med Phys. 4:297–301.

Kondziolka D, Lundsford LD, Flickinger JC, Young RF, Vermeulen S, Duma C, Jacques D, Rand R, Regis J, Peragut J, Epstein M, Lindquist C (1996) Stereotactic radiosurgery for trigeminal neuralgia: A multi-institutional study using the gamma unit. J. Neurosurg, 84:940–945.

Laing RW, Bentley RE, Nahum AE, Warrington AP, Brada M (1993) Stereotactic radiotherapy of irregular targets: A comparison between static conformal beams and non-co-planar arcs. Radiother Oncol 28:241–246.

Larsson B, Leksell L, Rexed B, Sourander P, Mair W, Andersson B (1958) The high-energy proton beam as a neurosurgical tool. Nature (Lond) 182:1222–1223.

Larsson B (1961) Pre-therapeutic physical experiments with high energy protons. Br. J. Radiol. 34:143–151.

Larsson B, Liden K, Sarby B (1974) Irradiaton of small structures through the intact skull, Acta Radiologica, Ther. Phyus. Biol. 13:512–534.

Lawrence JH (1957) Proton irradiation of the pituitary. Cancer 10:795–798.

Lawrence JH, Tobias CA, Born JL, Wang CC, Linfoot JH (1962) Heavy-particle irradiation in neoplastic and neurologic disease. J Neuro-surg 19:717–722.

Lawrence JH (1985) Heavy particle irradiation of intracranial lesions. In Wilkins RH, Rengachary SS (eds): Neurosurgery. Philadelphia, Mc Graw-Hill, pp 1113–1135.

Lax I (1993) Target dise versus extra target dose in stereotactic radiosurgery. Acta Oncol. 32–453–457.

Leavitt DD, Gibbs FA, Heilbrun MP, Moeller JH, Takach GA (1991) Dynamic field shaping to optimize radiosurgery. Int J Radiat Oncol Biol Phys 21:1247–1255.

Leksell L (1951) The stereotaxic method and radiosurgery of the brain. Acta Chir Scand 102:316–319.

Leksell L (1968) Cerebral radiosurgery I: Gammathalamotomy in two cases of intractable pain. Acta Chir Scand 134:585–595.

Leksell L (1971a) Stereotaxic radiosurgery in trigeminal neuralgia. Acta Chir Scand 137:311–314.

Leksell L (1971b) A note on the treatment of acoustic tumours. Acta Chir Scand 137:763–765.

Leksell L (1971c) *Stereotaxis and Radiosurgery– an Operative System.* Springfield, Illinois, CC Thomas.

Leksell L (1983) Stereotactic radiosurgery. J Neurol Neurosurg Psychiatry 46:797–803.

Leksell L, Lindquist C, Adler JR, Leksell D, Jernberg B, Steiner L (1987) A new fixation device for the Leksell stereotaxic system. J Neurosurg 66:626–629.

Levy RP, Fabrikant JI, Frankel KA, Phillips MH, Lyman JT (1989) Stereotactic heavy-charged-particle Bragg peak radiosurgery for the treatment of intracranial arteriovenous malformations in childhood and adolescence. Neurosurgery 24:841–852.

Levy RP, Schulte RWM, Slater JD, Miller DW, Slater JM (1999) Stereotactic radiosurgery: the role of charged particles, Acta Oncologica, 38:165–169.

Lindquist C, Steiner L, Hindmarsh T (1992) Gamma Knife thalamotomy for tremor: Report of two cases; in Steiner L (ed): Radiosurgery: Baseline and Trends. New York, Raven Press, pp237–243.

Loeffler JS, Alexander E, Siddon RL, Saunders WM, Coleman CN, Winston KR (1989) Stereotactic radiosurgery for intracranial arteriovenous malformation using a standard linear accelerator. Int J Radiat Oncol Biol Phys 17:673–677.

Lomax AJ, Bortfeld T, Goitein G, Debus J, Dykstra C, Tercier PA, Coucke PA, Mirimanoff RO (1999) A treatment planning inter-comparison of proton and intensity modulated photon radiotherapy. Radiotherapy & Oncology. 51(3):257–71.

Low DA, Li Z and Drzymala RE (1995) Minimization of target positioning error in accelerator-based radiosurgery. Med. Phys. 22:443–448.

Ludewigt BA, Chu WT, Phillips MH, Renner TR (1991) Accelerated helium-ion beams for radiotherapy and Stereotactic radiosurgery. Med Phys 18:36–42.

Lunsford LD, Maitz A, Lindner G (1987) First United States 201 source cobalt-60 gamma unit for radiosurgery. Applied Neurophysiology. 50(1–6):253–6.

Lunsford LD, Flickinger J, Lindner G, Maitz A (1989) Stereotactic radio-surgery of the brain using the first United States 201 cobalt-60 source gamma knife. Neurosurgery 24:151–159.

Lunsford LD, Kondziolka D, Flickinger JC, Bisonette DJ, Jungreis CA, Maitz AH, Horton JA, Coffey RJ (1991) Stereotactic radiosurgery for arteriovenous malformations of the brain. J Neurosurg 75:512–524.

Lunsford LD (1993) Stereotactic radiosurgery at the threshold or at the crossroads, Neurosurgery 21:799–804.

Lutz W, Winston KR, Maleki N (1988) A system for Stereotactic radio-surgery with a linear accelerator. Int J Radiat Oncol Biol Phys, 14:373–381.

Luxton G, Petrovich Z, Jozsel G, Nedzi LA, Apuzzo MLJ (1993) Stereotactic radiosurgery: Principles and comparison of treatment methods, Neurosurgery, 32:241–259.

Luxton G, Jozsef G (1994) Single isocenter treatment planning for homogeneous dose delivery to nonspherical targets in multiarc linear accelerator radiosurgery. Int. J. Radiat. Oncol. Biol. Phys. 31:635–643.

Lyman JT, Howard J (1977) Dosimetry and instrumentation for helium and heavy ions, Int J Radiat Oncol Biol Phys, 3:81–85.

Lyman JT, Fabrikant JI, Frankel KA (1985) Charged-particle Stereotactic radiosurgery. Nucl Instrum Methods Physics Res B l 0/11:110 7–1110.

Lyman JT, Kanstein L, Yeater F, Fabrikant JI, Frankel KA (1986) A helium-ion beam for Stereotactic radiosurgery of central nervous system disorders. Med Phys 13:695–699.

Lyman JT, Phillips MH, Frankel KA, Levy RP, Fabrikant JI (1992) Radiation physics for particle beam radiosurgery, Neurosurgery clinics of North America. 3:1–8.

Maitz AH, Lunsford LD, Wu A, Lindner G, Flickinger JC (1990) Shielding requirements on-site loading and acceptance testing of the Leksell Gamma Knife. Int J Radiat Oncol Biol Phys 18:469–476.

Maitz AH, Wu A, Lunsford LD, Flickinger JC, Kondzioka D, Bloomer WD (1995) Quality assurance for gamma knife stereotactic radiosurgery, 32–1465–1471.

McGinley PH, Butkert EK, Crocker IR, Aiken R (1992) An adjustable collimator for Stereotactic radiosurgery. Phys Med Biol 37:413–417.

Miller CW (1954) An 8 MeV linear accelerator for x-ray therapy, Proc IEE, 101:207–222.

Miller CW (1956) Linear accelerators for x-ray therapy, Eighth International Congress of Radiology, Mexico City.

Nedzi LA, Kooy HM, Alexander E 3d, Svensson GK, Loeffler JS (1993) Dynamic field shaping for stereotactic radiosurgery: a modeling study. International Journal of Radiation Oncology, Biology, Physics. 25(5):859–69.

Ott-Oelschlager S, Schlegel W, Lorenz W (1994) Different collimators in convergent beam irradiation of irregularly shaped intracranial target volumes, Radiotherapy and Oncology, 30:175–179.

Petrovich Z, Luxton G, Formenti SC, Zee CS, Yu C, Jozsef G, Apuzzo MLJ (1997) Stereotactic radiosurgery for benign and malignant diseases of the brain, *Advances in neuro-oncology II*, edited by Walker, K.P.L., Futura Publishing Company, Inc. Armonk, NY, 219–258,.

Phillips MH, Frankel KA, Lyman JT, Fabrikant JI, Levy RP (1990) Comparison of different radiation types and irradiation geometries in Stereotactic radiosurgery. Int J Radiat Oncol Biol Phys 18:211–220.

Phillips MH, Stelzer KJ, Griffin TW, Mayberg MR, Winn HR (1994) Stereotactic radiosurgery: a review and comparison of methods, J. Clinical Oncology, 12:1085–1099.

Pike B, Podgorsak EB, Peters TM, Pla C (1987) Dose distributions in dynamic Stereotactic radiosurgery. Med Phys 14:780–789.

Pike GB, Podgorsak EB, Peters TM, Pla C, Olivier A, Souhami L (1990a) Dose distributions in radiosurgery. Med Phys 17:296–304.

Pike GB, Podgorsak EB, Peters TM, Pla C, Olivier A (1990b) Three-dimensional isodose distributions in radiosurgery. Stereotact Funct Neurosurg 54:519–524.

Podgorsak EB, Olivier A, Pla M, Lefebvre P-Y, Hazel J (1988) Dynamic Stereotactic radiosurgery. Int J Radiat Oncol Biol Phys 14:115–126.

Podgorsak EB, Pike GB, Olivier A, Pla M. Souhami L (1989) Radiosurgery with high energy photon beams: Acomparison among techniques. Int J Radiat Oncol Biol Phys 16:857–865.

Podgorsak EB, Pike GB, Pla M, Olivier A, Souhami L (1990) Radiosurgery with photon beams: Physical aspects and adequacy of linear accelerators. Radiother Oncol 17:349–358.

Podgorsak EB (1992) physics for radiosurgery with linear accelerators, Neurosurgery clinics of North America. 3:9–34.

Saunders WM, Winston KR, Siddon RL, Svensson GH, Kijewski PK, Rice RK, Hansen JL, Barth NH (1988) Radiosurgery for arteriovenous malformations of the brain using a standard linear accelerator: Rationale and technique. Int J Radiat Oncol Biol Phys 15:441–447.

Schell MC, Smith V, Larson DA, Wu A, Flickinger JC (1991) Evaluation of radiosurgery techniques with cumulative dose volume histograms in linear accelerator-based stereotactic external beam irradiation. Int J Radiat Oncol Biol Phys 20:1325–1330.

Schell MC, Kooy H (1994) Stereotactic radiosurgery quality improvement: interdepartmental collaboration, Int J Radiat Oncol Biol Phys. 28:551–552.

Schell MC, Bova FJ, Larson DA, Leavitt DD, Lutz WR Podgorsak EB, Wu A (1995) Stereotactic Radiosurgery, Report of Task Group 42 Radiation Therapy Committee (American Association of Physicists in Medicine), Woodbury, New York.

Schwartz M (1998) Stereotactic radiosurgery: comparing different technologies, CMAJ, 158:625–628

Serago CF, Lewin AA, Houdek PV, Gonzalez-Arias S, Abitbol AA, Marcial-Vega VA, Piscciotti V, Schwade JG (1991) Improved linear accelerator dose distributions for radiosurgery with elliptically shaped fields. Int J Radiat Oncol Biol Phys 21:1321–1325.

Serago CF, Houdek PV, Bauer-Kirpes B, Lewin AA, Abitbol AA, Gonzalez-Arias S, Marcial-Vega VA, Schwade JG (1992) Stereotactic radiosurgery: Dose-volume analysis of linear accelerator techniques. Med Phys 19:181–185.

Serago CF, Thornton AF, Urie MM, Chapman P, Verhey L,

Rosenthal S, Gall KP, Niemierko A (1995) Comparison of proton and x-ray conformal dose distributions for radiosurgery applications, Med. Phys., 22:2111–2116.

Shaw E, Scott C, Souhami L, *et al* (1998) Update of radiation therapy oncology group (RTOG) protocol (9005): Single dose radiosurgical treatment of recurrent brain tumors (abstr.) *Int. J. Radiat. Oncol. Biol. Phys.*; 42(Number 1 supplement):196.

Shiu AS, Kooy HM, Ewron JR, Tung SS, Wong J Antes K, Maor M (1997) Comparsion of miniature multileaf collimation (MMLC) with circular collimation for stereotactic treatment, Int J Radiat Oncol Biol Phys 37:679–688.

Sixel KE, Podgorsak EB (1993) Cylindrical dose distributions in dynamic rotation radiosurgery. Med Phys 20:163–170.

Slater JM, Miller DW, Archambeau JO (1988) Development of a hospital-based proton beam treatment center. Int J Radiat Oncol Biol Phys 14:761–775.

Smith V, Verhey LJ, Serago CF (1998) Comparison of radiosurgery treatment modalities based on complication and control probabiluties, Int J Radiat Oncol Biol Phys, 40:507–513.

Spiridon VS, Chui CS (1998) A gradient inverse planning algorithm with dose-volume constraints, Med Phys. 25:321–333.

Steinberg GK, Fabrikant JI, Marks MP, Levy RP, Frankel KA, Phillips MH, Shuer LM, Silverberg GD (1990) Stereotactic heavy-charged-particle Bragg-peak radiation for intracranial arteriove-nous malformations. N Engi J Med 323:96–101.

Steiner L, Leksell L, Greitz T, Forster DMC, Backlund EO (1972) Stereotaxic radiosurgery for cerebral arteriovenous malformations: Report of a case. Acta Chir Scand 138:459–464.

Steiner L (1984) Treatment of arteriovenous malformations with radiosurgery, in Wilson C, Stein B (eds): *Intracranial Arteriovenous Malformations.* Baltimore, Williams & Wilkins, pp 295–313.

Steiner L, Lindquist C, Steiner M (1988) Radiosurgery with focused gamma-beam irradiation in children, in Edwards MSB, Hoffman HJ (eds): *Cerebral Vascular Diseases of Childhood and Adolescence.* Baltimore, Williams & Wilkins, pp 367–388.

Sterner L, Lindquist C, Sterner M (1992) Radiosurgery. Adv. Tech. Stand. Neurosurg. 19:19–102.

Sturm V, Pastyr O, Schlegel W, Scharfenberg H, Zabel H-J, Netzeband G, Schabbert S, Berberich W (1983) Stereotactic computer tomography with a modified Reichert-Mundinger device as the basis for integrated stereotactic neuroradiological investigations. Acta Neurochir 68:11–17.

Sturm V, Kober B, Hover K-H, Schlegel W, Boesecke R, Pastyr O, Hartmann GH, Schabbert S, Winkel K, Kunze S, Lorenz WJ (1987) Stereotactic percutaneous single dose irradiation of brain metastases with a linear accelerator. Int J Radiat Oncol Biol Phys 13:279–282.

Tobias CA, Lawrence JH, Born JL, McCombs RK, Roberts JE, Anger HO, Low-Beer VA, Huggins CB (1958) Pituitary irradiation with high-energy proton beams: A preliminary report. Cancer Res 18:121–139.

Tobias CA, Lyman JT, Lawrence JH (1971) Some considerations of physical and biological factors in radiotherapy with high-LET radiation including particles, pi mesons, and fast neutrons. In Lawrence JH (ed): Progress in Atomic Medicine: Recent Advances in Nuclear Medicine. New York, Grune & Stratton, Inc.

Tsai J-S, Buck BA, Svensson GK, Alexander E III, Cheng C-W, Mannarino EG, Loeffler JS (1991) Quality assurance in stereotactic radiosurgery using a standard linear accelerator. Int J Radiat Oncol Biol Phys 21:737–748.

Verhey LJ, Smith V, Serago CF (1998) Comparison of radiosurgery treatment modalities based on physical dose distributions, Int J Radiat Oncol Biol Phys, 40:497–505.

Walton L, Bomford CK, Ramsden D (1987) The Sheffield stereotactic radiosurgery unit: Physical characteristics and principles of operation. Br J Radiol 60:897–906.

Weissbluth M, Karzmark CJ, Steele RE (1959) The Stanford medical linear accelerator: II. Installation and physical measurements, Radiology 72:242–253.

Wilson RR (1946) Radiological use of fast protons, Radiology 47:487–491.

Winston KR, Lutz W (1988) Linear accelerator as a neurosurgical tool for stereotactic radiosurgery. Neurosurgery 22:454–463.

Wu A, Lindner G, Maitz AH, Kalend AM, Lunsford LD, Flickinger JC, Bloomer WD (1990) Physics of gamma knife approach on convergent beams in stereotactic radiosurgery. Int J Radiat Oncol Biol Phys 18:941–949.

Wu A (1992), Physics and dosimetry of the gamma knife, Neurosug Clinics of North America, 3:35–50.

Wu A, Johnson M, Chen ASJ, Kalnicki S (1996), Evaluation of dose calculation algorithm of the Peacock system for multileaf intensity modulation collimator, Int J Radiat Oncol Biol Phys, 36:1225–1231.

Xing L, Halmilton RJ, Spelbring D, Pelizzari CA, Chen GTY, Boyer AL (1998) Fast iterative algorithms for three-dimensional inverse treatment planning, Med. Phys., 25:1845–1849.

Yu C, Luxton G (1999a) TLD dose measurement: A simplified accurate technique for the dose range from 0.5 cGy to 1000 cGy, Med. Phys. 26:1010–1016.

Yu C, Luxton G, Jozsef G, Apuzzo MLJ, Petrovich Z (1999b) Dosimetric comparison of three photon radiosurgery techniques for an elongated ellipsoid target. 45:000–000.

7 Imaging of Intracranial and Spinal Neoplasms

Chi Shing Zee, Paul Kim, John L. Go, and Peter Conti

CONTENTS

C. S. Zee, MD
Department of Radiology, Division of Neuroradiology and
PET Imaging, University of Southern California School of
Medicine, 1200 North State Street, Los Angeles, CA 90033,
USA
P. Kim, MD
Department of Radiology, Division of Neuroradiology and
PET Imaging, University of Southern California School of
Medicine, 1200 North State Street, Los Angeles, CA 90033,
USA
J. L. Go, MD
Department of Radiology, Division of Neuroradiology and
PET Imaging, University of Southern California School of
Medicine, 1200 North State Street, Los Angeles, CA 90033,
USA
P. Conti, MD
Department of Radiology, Division of Neuroradiology and
PET Imaging, University of Southern California School of
Medicine, 1200 North State Street, Los Angeles, CA 90033,
USA

7.1
Imaging Techniques for Evaluating Intracranial Neoplasms

Imaging of intracranial and spinal neoplasms is essential to establish diagnosis for treatment planning and to follow the treatment outcome. Current imaging techniques include magnetic resonance imaging (MRI), computed tomography (CT), angiography, myelography, positron emission tomography (PET), proton spectroscopy, and functional imaging. The goals of imaging are to identify the lesion and determine its imaging characteristics (ERNEST et al. 1998), to determine the extent of the lesion and identify the normal structures involved (DEAN et al 1990), and to establish a differential diagnosis and provide the most likely diagnosis (DI CHIRO 1986). In addition, complications related to the tumor, such as hemorrhage, necrosis, impending herniation, trapping of the ventricles, and hydrocephalus, should also be identified. The imaging appearances of intracranial and spinal neoplasms may sometimes provide a reasonable diagnosis in conjunction with clinical information. However, in the majority of cases, a definitive diagnosis that obviates the need for histopathological examination is not possible. Nonetheless, the constellation of imaging findings and clinical history and findings can provide sufficient information in regard to treatment planning, i.e., stereotactic biopsy, surgical biopsy, surgical resection, radiation therapy.

7.1.1
The Role of Contrast Media

Contrast material is commonly used to image and better delineate intracranial and spinal neoplasms. The extent of the lesions or degree of malignancy can be determined, to a certain extent, by the injection of contrast material. However, caution must be exercised in attempting to determine the margin of the glial neoplasm by contrast enhancement. Due to the infiltrative nature of the glial neoplasm, tumor infiltration goes well beyond the area of contrast enhancement. It should be emphasized that contrast enhancement merely reflects the breakdown of the blood–brain barrier and early infiltrative tumor involvement may not cause the barrier to break down. Contrast enhancement can be helpful to determine the degree of malignancy in some cases, but may be misleading in other cases. As a general rule, enhancing intra-axial tumors, such as glioblastoma multiforme, are usually malignant, and non-enhancing intra-axial tumors, such as low-grade gliomas and subependymomas, tend to be low-grade (EARNEST 1988). However, benign tumors, such as pilocytic astrocytoma, enhance intensely following the administration of contrast material, and malignant tumors such as gliomatosis or some of the anaplastic astrocytomas may exhibit no or minimal contrast enhancement. In a study of MR imaging characteristics of tumors, DEAN et al. (1990) concluded that mass effect, cyst formation, and tumor necrosis were almost comparable to histopathological diagnosis for classifying astrocytomas as low-grade, anaplastic, or glioblastoma multiforme.

The goals of imaging are to provide sufficient anatomical and functional information so that the safest approach can be determined for surgery or radiation therapy. The capability of multiplanar imaging, three-dimensional reformation of MRI, makes it the imaging modality of choice. Furthermore, the capability of functional MRI provides critical information for treatment planning. Newer imaging modalities such as magnetoencephalography are evolving, which may also provide functional information in the near future.

Following treatment, imaging plays an important role in determining the result of therapy, identifying residual or recurrent tumor, and complications related to therapy if any.

7.1.2
Interpretation of Imaging Studies

Interpretation of MR imaging involves a challenging task in posttreatment cases – to separate the true extent of the residual or recurrent tumor from postoperative or post radiation changes. In such cases, PET imaging (DI CHIRO 1986; KIM 1992) (Fig. 7.1) or proton MR spectroscopy (GILL 1990; NEGENDANK 1996; HUSTINX 1999; ALGER 1990), which reflect metabolic rather than morphologic features of the tissue, can be employed.

When evaluating computed tomography (CT) or magnetic resonance (MR) imaging for intra-axial neoplasms, the following characteristics of a mass lesion should be assessed: location and extent (ERNEST et al. 1988); mass effect and surrounding edema (DEAN et al. 1990); density on CT or signal intensity on MR (DI CHIRO 1986); and pattern of contrast enhancement (KIM et al. 1992). By carefully assessing these factors, one may arrive at a reasonable differential diagnosis or probable diagnosis. MR is superior to CT in detecting and localizing intrac-

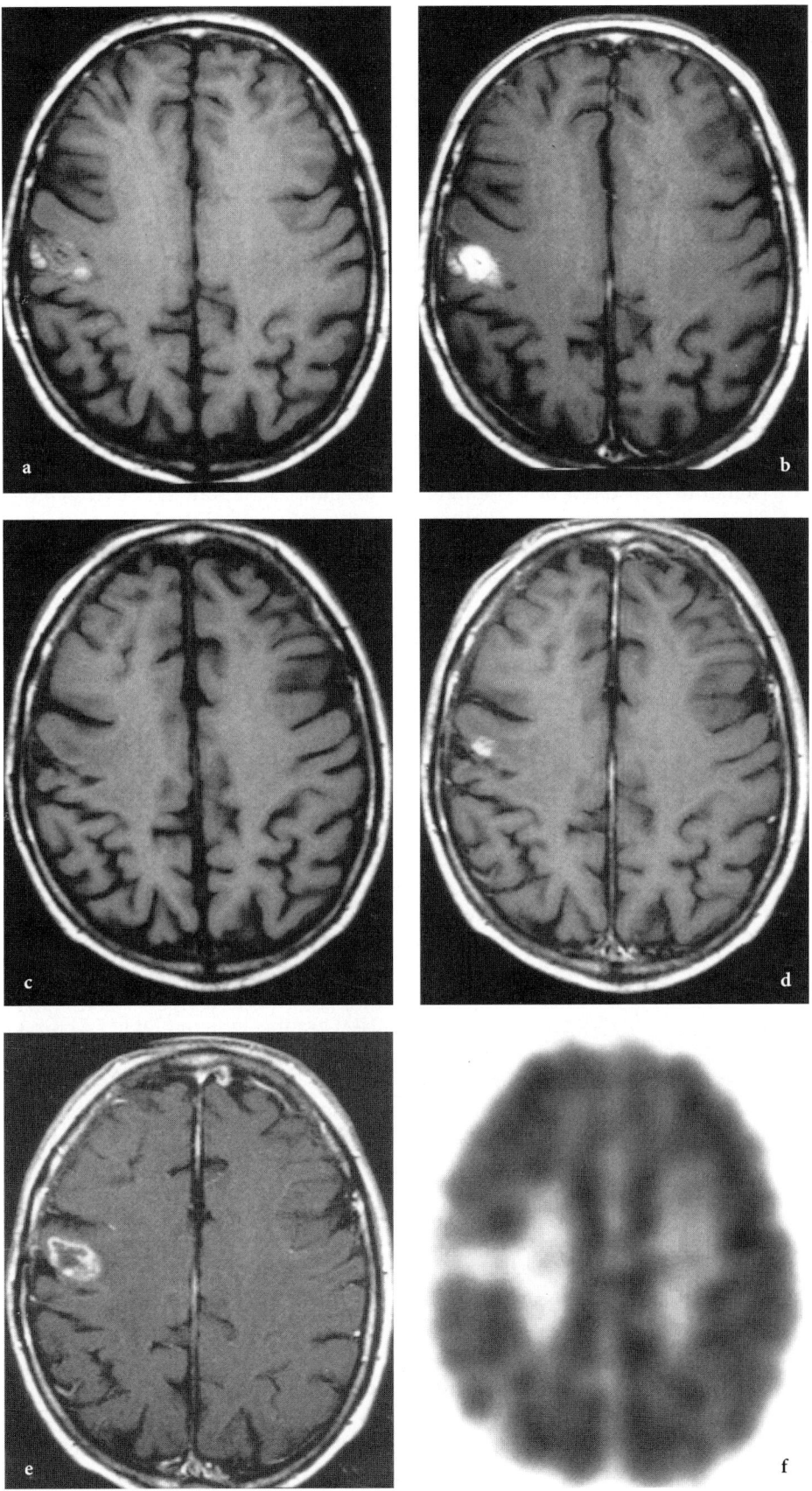

Fig. 7.1a–f. Astrocytoma treated with stereotactic radiosurgery. **a** Initial MR imaging performed in April 1992 showed an area of mixed signal intensity with focal high signal intensity areas on T1-weighted images, and contrast enhancement following the intravenous injection of gadolinium. **b** The findings were consistent with a hemorrhagic neoplasm in the right frontal region. **c** Following stereotactic radiosurgery, multiple/follow-up examinations were performed and progressive reduction in the size of the lesion was seen. A later follow-up examination in June 1994 showed a significant decrease in focal mass effect. **d** A marked decrease in the size of the enhancing lesion, which was consistent with shrinkage of the tumor size. **e** Follow-up examination performed in May 1995 demonstrated increase in the size of the enhancing lesion as well as surrounding edema. A stereotactic biopsy was performed following this study and showed radiation changes without tumor recurrence. **f** PET-FDG image shows an area of hypometabolism corresponding to the area of abnormal signal intensity in the right frontal region seen on MR images. This is consistent with the diagnosis of radiation changes

ranial neoplasms. However, MR is not as highly specific for diagnosing intracranial neoplasms as initially expected. Calcification is important in the differential diagnosis of intracranial neoplasms. CT is superior to MR in the detection of calcification. Non-contrast CT is sometimes required to aid in the differential diagnosis of an intracranial neoplasm (ZEE 1996).

Contrast enhancement of intracranial neoplasms is probably due to multiple factors. In general, tumors have a tendency to provoke the formation of new capillaries. Some of the tumor capillaries in gliomas may be near-normal, while other capillaries in gliomas may be abnormal with fenestrated endothelia [breakdown of the blood–brain barrier (BBB)]. This is probably the basis for explaining why some gliomas enhance and others do not. Metastatic neoplasms contain non-central nervous system (CNS) capillaries (no BBB) that are similar to their tissue of origin. Therefore, metastatic lesions almost always show contrast enhancement, with the exception of very small lesions. Extra-axial neoplasms arise from tissues that contain capillaries without tight junction. This explains why extra-axial neoplasms always exhibit contrast enhancement. The correlation between MR or CT contrast enhancement and hypervascularity on angiography is not good. Hypervascularity is not a prerequisite for contrast enhancement. The explanation of contrast enhancement is presumed to be related to the formation of tumor capillaries lacking blood–brain barrier rather than the destruction of existing blood–brain barrier.

It is important to determine whether an intracranial mass lesion is intra-axial or extra-axial in location. MR permits the separation of an extra-axial mass from the brain surface by demonstrating the presence of cerebrospinal fluid, pial blood vessels, and dura. Normal gray and white matter can be readily identified on MR images, which permits the demonstration of white matter buckling secondary to an extra-axial mass lesion. The multiplanar imaging capability of MR also permits the demonstration of broad-based attachment of the mass lesion to the dura (ZEE 1992). Many extra-axial masses are situated in the posterior fossa, where lesions are often obscured on CT images by beam hardening artifacts due to dense surrounding bone . Contrast-enhanced MR usually demonstrates homogeneous, intense enhancement of the extra-axial mass lesions. The anatomical boundaries of mass lesions are better delineated with contrast-enhanced MR. Sometimes, enhancement of the adjacent dura may be seen with an extra-axial mass lesion, which could represent reactive change in the adjacent dura or infiltration of the neoplasm into the adjacent

dura. This so-called dura tail sign was initially thought to be associated with meningiomas. However, it has been found to be associated with any intracranial mass lesion that has invaded the dura or caused reactive change in the dura (ZEE 1992).

7.2
Supratentorial Intra-Axial Tumors

7.2.1
Incidence and Classification

Brain tumors are uncommon lesions accounting for 1.5% of all malignancies occurring in adults as well as children (Chap. 2 of this volume). The majority of brain tumors in adults are supratentorial in location, whereas approximately half of the brain tumors in children are supratentorial. Supratentorial tumors are more common in neonates and children up to 3 years old, whereas infratentorial tumors are more common in children from 4 to 11 years old.

Approximately one third of the intracranial neoplasms are gliomas, one third are metastatic lesions, and another one third are of other primary origin (including extra-axial neoplasms) (Table 7.1). Gliomas have a slight male predominance of 3:2. Gliomas can be divided into astrocytomas, ependymomas, and oligodendrogliomas. Since the choroid plexus contains modified ependymal cells, choroid plexus neoplasms are considered in the category of gliomas. Three quarters of gliomas are astrocytomas. Astrocytomas are traditionally divided into four grades according to Kernohan's grading system (KERNOHAN and SAYRE 1952) or the WORLD HEALTH ORGANIZATION (WHO) grading system (Table 7.2). Grade 1 and grade 2 astrocytomas are considered low grade and associated with better prognosis. Grade 3 and grade 4 astrocytomas are anaplastic astrocytomas and glioblastoma multiforme, respectively, depending on their histologic features. A total of 25% of astrocytomas are low grade and 75% are high grade (25% anaplastic astrocytoma and 50% glioblastoma multiforme) (BURGER 1985). The majority of high-grade astrocytomas are glioblastoma multiforme.

7.2.2
Juvenile Pilocytic Astrocytoma

Pilocytic astrocytomas in the supratentorial compartment tend to occur in the region of the dien-

Table 7.1. Incidence of brain tumors (100%)

Primary brain tumors 66%		Metastatic tumors 33%
Glial tumors 33%	Nonglial tumors 33%	
Astrocytomas 25%	Meningioma 15%	Lung carcinoma
Oligodendroglioma 4%	PNET 5%	Breast carcinoma
Ependymoma 3%	Schwannoma 4%	Melanoma
Choroid plexus tumors 1%	Pituitary tumor 4%	Renal carcinoma
	Pineal region tumor 2%	Colon carcinoma
Craniopharyngioma 2%		

All percentages are an approximation.

cephalon, including the hypothalamus, visual pathway, optic chiasm, and basal ganglia. The cerebral hemispheres and lateral ventricles are less common locations.

Pilocytic astrocytomas are cystic or multicystic with a mural nodule in 55% and a solid one in 45%. Chiasmatic-hypothalamic pilocytic astrocytomas are usually solid mass lesions (Fig. 7.2) whereas hemispheric pilocytic astrocytomas are more likely to be cystic mass lesions (NAIDICH 1984; LEE 1989) (Fig. 7.3). Chiasmatic-hypothalamic pilocytic astrocytomas are often associated with neurofibromatosis.

Solid masses may or may not show contrast enhancement on CT images. Calcification in a fleck-like pattern may be seen. A cystic mass is seen with an enhancing mural nodule, while the cyst wall typically does not enhance. In CT, cyst fluid is generally of higher density than cerebrospinal fluid owing to its higher protein content.

In MR, solid mass is isointense to hypointense on T1-weighted images and hyperintense on T2-weighted images. Contrast enhancement of the mural nodule of the cystic mass is intense. Occasionally, enhancement of the cyst wall may be seen on MR imaging. Cyst fluid is generally of higher signal intensity than cerebrospinal fluid due to its high protein content.

7.2.3
Low-Grade Astrocytoma

Astrocytomas (all grades) constitute almost 50% of the supratentorial brain tumors in all age groups and 30% of all infratentorial tumors in children.

Low-grade astrocytomas account for about 25% of all cerebral gliomas. Cerebral gliomas constitute approximately 33% of all intracranial neoplasms. Peak incidence for low-grade astrocytomas is between the ages of 20 and 40 years, which is generally 10 years younger than that for glioblastomas. Astrocytomas occur in any part of the cranial hemisphere with the exception of the occipital lobes. Deep structures, such as the corpus callosum and basal ganglia, are frequently involved. Astrocytomas are a group of tumors with heterogeneous histopathological features and variable clinical presentations.

The most common of these tumors in the adult is the diffuse fibrillary astrocytoma. Although these tumors are usually low grade, the incidence of ana-

Table 7.2. Classification of astrocytoma

Tumor	Kernohan	World Health Organization
Pilocytic astrocytoma Subependymal giant cell astrocytoma	Grade 1	Grade I
Low-grade astrocytoma	Grade 1 and 2	Grade II
Anaplastic astrocytoma	Grade 3	Grade III
Glioblastoma multiforme	Grade 4	Grade IV

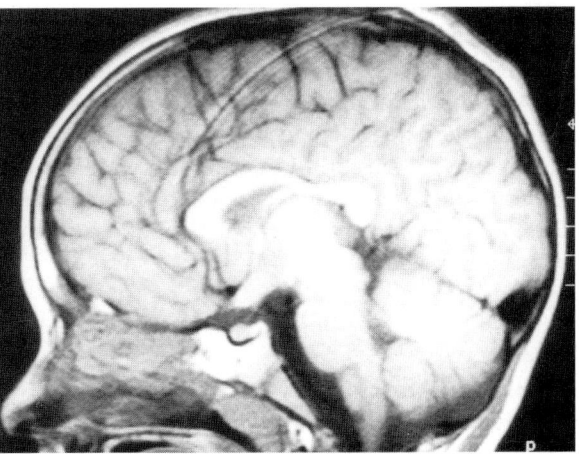

Fig. 7.2. Hypothalamic glioma. Axial T1-weighted image shows enlargement of the hypothalamus and optic chiasm

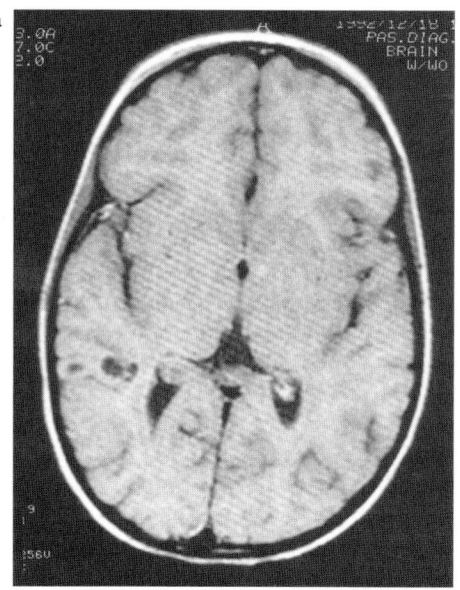
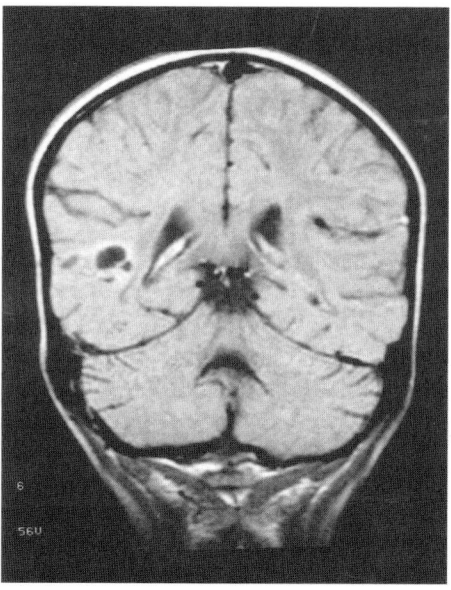

Fig. 7.3a,b. Pilocytic astrocytoma. Axial and coronal post-contrast T1-weighted images show a small multicystic lesion with minimal enhancement in the right temporal lobe

plastic transformation has been shown to be from 10% to 80% (Fig. 7.4). Fibrillary astrocytomas are unencapsulated, infiltrating tumors.

Astrocytomas may show low density or occasionally isodensity on CT images. Peritumoral edema is usually absent to minimal. Tumor calcification is detected in 20% of astrocytomas. In fact, the most common supratentorial tumor with calcification is the astrocytoma, although oligodendrogliomas have the highest frequency of calcification. The pattern of contrast enhancement is quite variable, with 40% of low-grade astrocytomas exhibiting some degree of enhancement.

MR imaging is superior to CT in the evaluation of astrocytomas (Fig. 7.5). Astrocytomas are usually homogeneously hypointense or occasionally isointense on T1-weighted images and slightly hyperintense on T2-weighted images on MR imaging. There is little associated edema or mass effect. Calcification is not seen well on spin echo technique images, but it is seen better on gradient echo technique images.

Contrast-enhanced MR may show a wide variety of enhancing patterns; including no enhancement (Fig. 7.6), inhomogeneous enhancement, or heterogeneous enhancement.

7.2.4
Anaplastic Astrocytomas and Glioblastoma Multiforme

Anaplastic astrocytomas and glioblastoma multiforme constitute 15–20% of all intracranial neo-

plasms. Glioblastoma multiforme makes up 50% of all astrocytomas, whereas anaplastic astrocytoma constitutes 25% of all astrocytomas. Glioblastoma is the most common supratentorial neoplasm in adults. The onset age is higher than that of low-grade astrocytomas. There is a slight male predominance of 3:2.

Glioblastomas tend to spread across the corpus callosum, forming the classic pattern of a butterfly glioma. They have a predilection for white matter of the cerebral hemisphere, especially frontal and temporal lobes. Invasion of the adjacent cortex, leptomeninges, and dura are often seen. Glioblastomas have a median survival of 6 months and anaplastic astrocytomas a median survival of 2 years.

Anaplastic astrocytomas and glioblastomas may be of low density or, more frequently, mixed density on CT images. The margin of the neoplasm is usually not well defined.

Contrast enhancement pattern is variable, including ring-like enhancement, nodular enhancement, heterogeneous enhancement, or occasionally no enhancement.

In MR imaging, they frequently show heterogeneous signal intensity patterns on both T1-weighted and T2-weighted images, and are predominately low-signal intensity mass lesion on T1-weighted images and predominately high-signal intensity on T2-weighted images.

Focal areas of necrosis, hemorrhage, and cystic changes are seen more frequently in glioblastomas.

A contrast enhancement pattern is variable (Fig. 7.7). Contrast enhancement does not reflect actual tumor margin as tumor cells are frequently detected

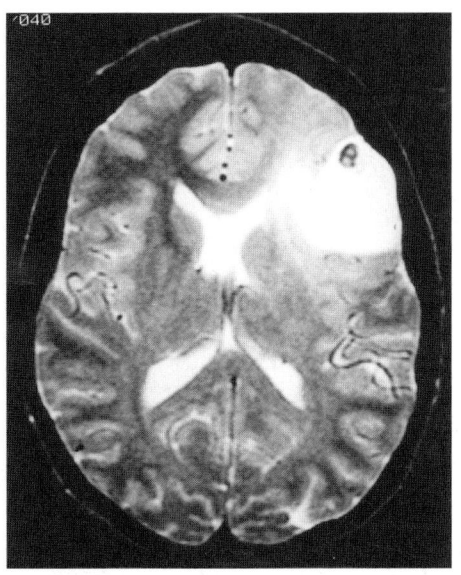

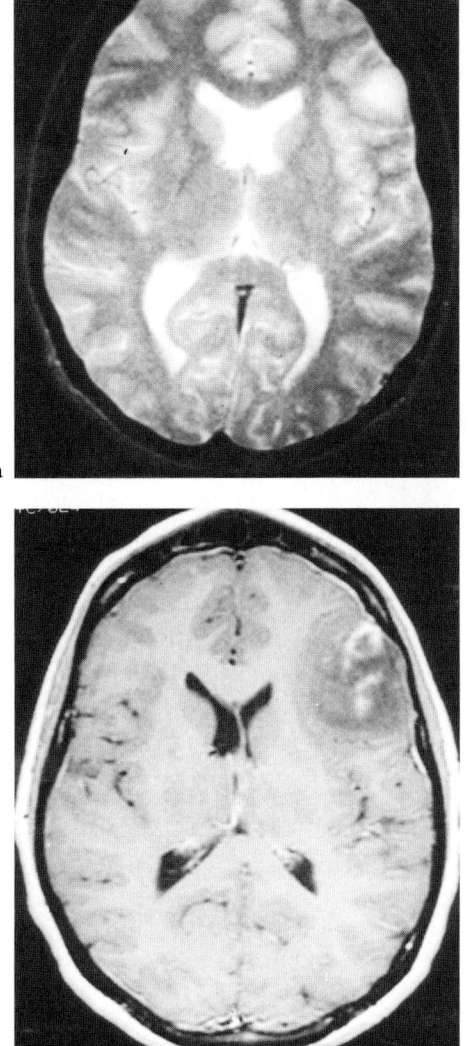

Fig. 7.4a–c. Malignant transformation of low-grade astrocytoma. **a** Axial T2-weighted image shows a small high signal intensity lesion in the left frontal lobe, consistent with a low-grade astrocytoma. This lesion was followed annually by serial CT and MRI for more than 10 years and showed no change in size. **b** A later follow-up MRI T2-weighted image shows a significant increase in the size of the lesion with small calcifications (*dark rings*) seen anteriorly. **c** A later follow-up contrast-enhanced T1-weighted image shows irregular enhancement of the mass. (No contrast enhancement was seen on any previous studies.) This proved to be an anaplastic astrocytoma

beyond the margin of contrast enhancement. YUH et al. (1994) demonstrated that the degree of contrast enhancement is proportional to contrast dose. At higher dose, the contrast enhancement margin may extend beyond the margin of demonstrable T2 signal intensity changes. The enhancement at tumor margins may represent a subtle loss of integrity of the blood–brain barrier due to tumor infiltration.

It is a diagnostic challenge to differentiate recurrent tumor from radiation changes in patients treated with radiation therapy. An absence of increasing mass effect on follow-up imaging studies favors radiation change. However, stereotactic biopsy is often necessary for definitive diagnosis (Fig. 7.8).

7.2.5
Oligodendroglioma

Oligodendrogliomas constitute 5% of all cerebral gliomas and are predominantly seen in young and middle-aged adults. There is a slight male predominance of 3:2. Typically, they involve the cerebral cortex and subcortical white matter in the cerebral hemisphere, especially in the frontal and frontotemporal region. They also occur in the cerebellum and spinal cord and occasionally in the ventricular wall. There is a wide range of grades within the category of oligodendroglioma due to the heterogeneity of histopathology of the tumor.

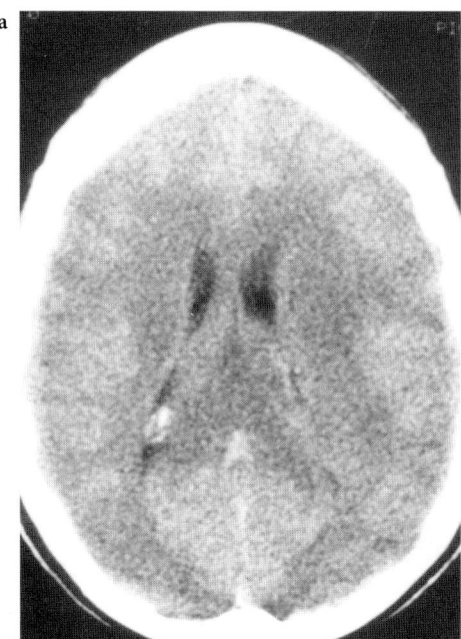

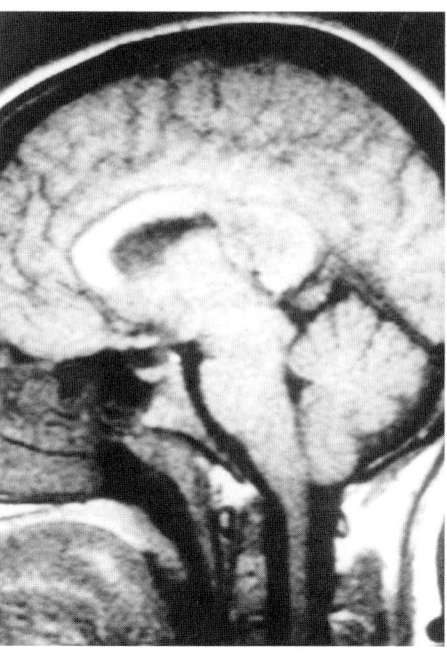

Fig. 7.5a,b. Astrocytoma of the splenium of the corpus callosum. **a** Axial CT shows a subtle low density lesion with an ill-defined margin in the region of the splenium of the corpus callosum. **b** Sagittal T1-weighted image shows enlargement of the splenium of corpus callosum with a low signal intensity mass seen

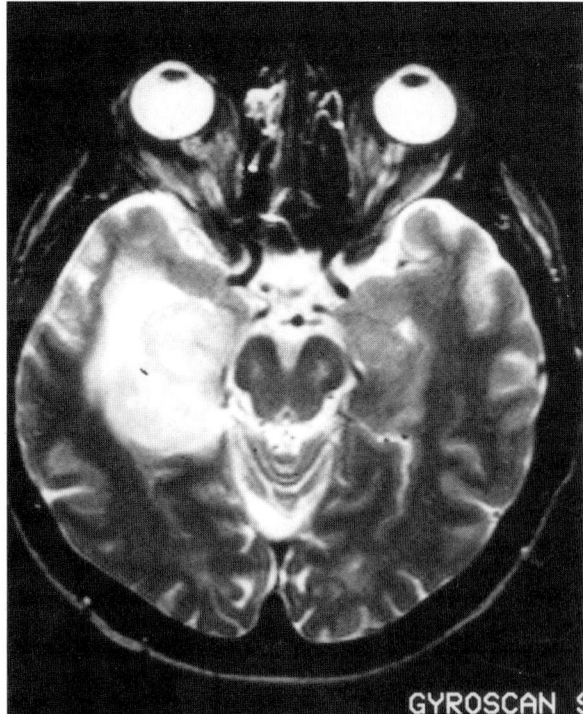

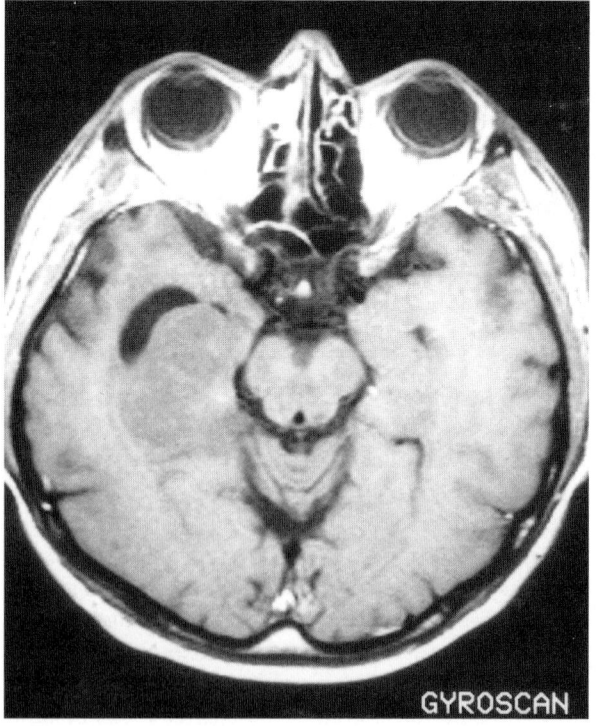

Fig. 7.6a,b. Low-grade astrocytoma. **a** Axial T2-weighted image shows a slightly hyperintense mass lesion with mild surrounding edema in the right temporal lobe. **b** Axial post-contrast T1-weighted image shows no enhancement of the low signal intensity lesion

a 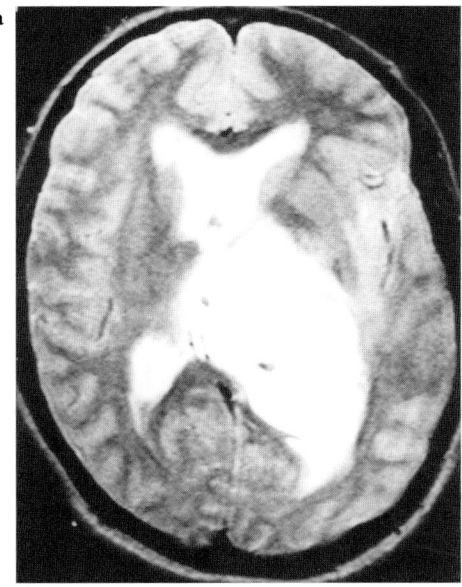 b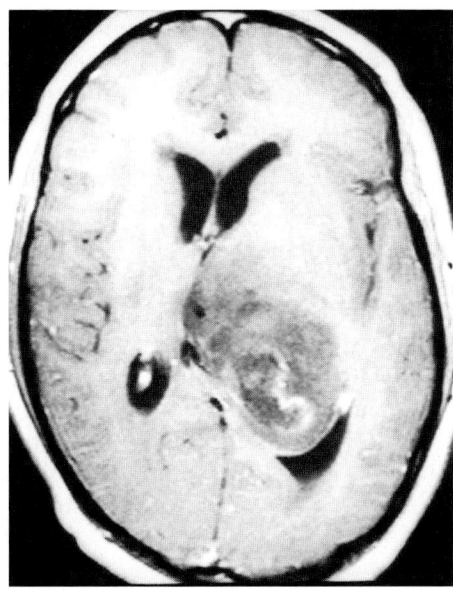

Fig. 7.7a,b. Glioblastoma multiforme. **a** Axial T2-weighted image shows a large high signal intensity mass in the left thalamus with compression of the left lateral ventricle. **b** Axial post-contrast T1-weighted image shows irregular enhancement of the mass

a 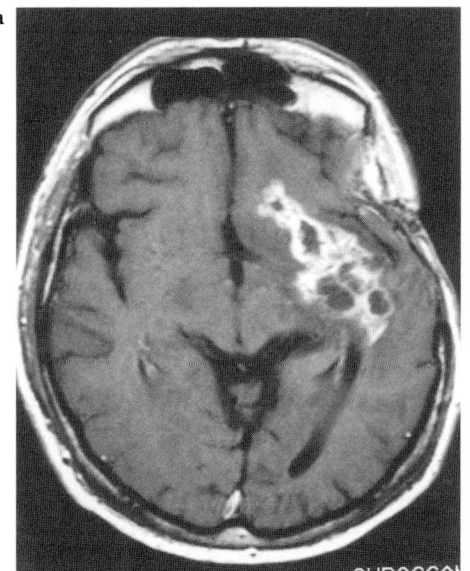 b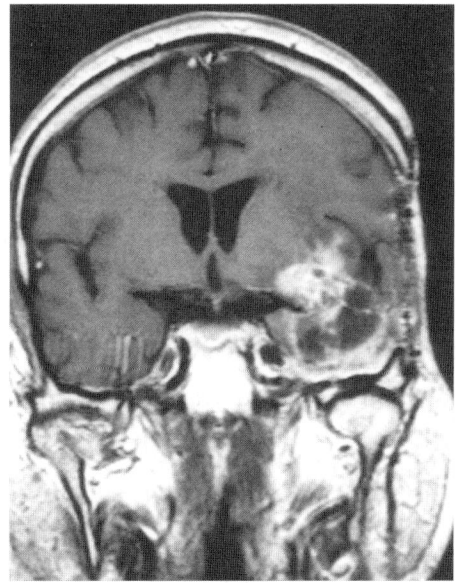

Fig. 7.8a,b. Radiation change. Axial and coronal T1-weighted images show irregular, multicystic contrast enhancement in the left frontotemporal region. This patient had left sided craniotomy for partial tumor resection and radiation therapy. The lesion proved to be radiation change following stereotactic biopsy

Oligodendrogliomas are one of the few intracranial tumors that may be diagnosed on plain roentgenograms of the skull because of the high incidence of popcorn-like calcification (30–40%). Calcification (linear or nodular) is demonstrated on CT images in 50–90% of cases. The usual appearance is that of hypodense to isodense mass with foci of calcification or hemorrhage. About one-half of the tumors will show contrast enhancement while the other half will not enhance. Cystic changes may be seen. Peritumoral edema is mild or absent. Occasionally, erosion of the adjacent bony calvarium may be observed indicating the slow growth of the neoplasm (VONOFAKOS 1979). On MR images, they are heterogeneous in signal intensity, but predominately show isointensity to gray matter on T1-weighted images and hyperintensity on T2-weighted images. Cystic degeneration, hemorrhage, and calcification all contribute to the heterogeneous signal intensity pattern seen on MR imaging. Peritumoral edema is minimal. Following the administration of contrast material, MR imaging is more sensitive in demonstrating tumor enhancement than CT (LEE 1989).

7.2.6
Pleomorphic Xanthoastrocytoma

Pleomorphic xanthoastrocytomas are rare tumors of children and young adults and make up less than 1% of astrocytomas. The temporal lobe is the most common site of tumor origin. Typically, it is a superficially located cystic mass with a mural nodule that abuts the leptomeninges (PAHAPILL 1996).

On CT images, cystic masses are typically present with a mural nodule located superficially, which demonstrates intense contrast enhancement. On MR images, it is usually a well-demarcated cystic mass with a mural nodule, which shows intense contrast enhancement. Occasionally, it can present as solid masses (TONN 1997).

7.2.7
Primitive Neuroectodermal Tumors

Primitive neuroectodermal tumors (PNETs) are common CNS neoplasms in children, consisting of 25% of all intracranial tumors in the pediatric age group. Supratentorial PNETs are rare; 5% of all supratentorial tumors in children are PNETs. The peak incidence is in the first decade of life with a majority presenting before the age of 5 years. Male and female patients are equally affected in the supratentorial compartment. Tumor necrosis and cyst formation is seen in up to 60% of cases, while calcification is seen in up to 70% of cases.

PNET presents as a large, irregular, heterogeneous mass deep in the cerebral white matter. The solid component of the mass is usually hyperdense on CT images. Necrosis, cyst formation, and calcification are frequently seen. Hemorrhage is occasionally observed. Contrast enhancement is seen and may be heterogeneous or ring-like in appearance.

On MR images, the solid component of mass is slightly hypointense on T1-weighted images and slightly to moderately hyperintense on T2-weighted images. Tumor necrosis, hemorrhage, cystic changes, and calcification all contribute to the heterogeneous signal intensity pattern seen on T2-weighted images (DAVIS 1990).

7.2.8
Ependymoma

Ependymomas constitute 2–6% of all gliomas. Only 40% of intracranial ependymomas occur in the su-

pratentorial compartment. The reported incidence of parenchymal origin of the ependymomas varies from 55% to 85%. Parenchymal ependymomas are more commonly seen in the supratentorial compartment. Ependymomas are four to six times more common in children than adults. Infratentorial ependymomas occur more frequently in children, whereas supratentorial ependymomas are evenly distributed among all age groups. In the supratentorial compartment, these tumors have a predilection for frontal and parietal lobes.

On CT images, they are hypodense to isodense to gray matter. Dense, punctate calcification is seen in 50% of cases. Peritumoral edema is seen in about 50% of cases and contrast enhancement is variable from homogeneous to heterogeneous.

On MR images, they are hypointense to isointense on T1-weighted images and hyperintense on T2-weighted images. Heterogeneous signal intensity pattern may be seen due to cystic degeneration, necrosis, calcification, or hemorrhage. The contrast enhancement pattern is variable from homogeneous to patchy heterogeneous (SPOTO 1990) (Fig. 7.9).

7.3
Metastasis

7.3.1
Incidence and Distribution

The brain and its covering may be involved by neoplasms arising in extracranial sites as a result of either direct extension of the primary tumor or more frequently through hematogenous spread. When hematogenous spread is seen, it often occurs at the junction between gray and white matter.

In autopsy series, 20% of patients with systemic cancer have intracranial metastases (see Chap. 21 of this volume). Metastases constitute 15–40% of all intracranial neoplasms and are typically seen at the corticomedullary junction. Uncommon sites for metastasis include the choroid plexus, pineal body, and pituitary gland. Multiple lesions are seen in 50–80% of patients. Metastatic melanoma and breast carcinoma have a higher incidence of multiple lesions than metastatic lung carcinoma and renal cell carcinoma. Supratentorial location is seen in 60–80% of patients with brain metastases.

Subependymal and intraventricular tumor spread occur in lymphoma, melanoma, and occasionally breast carcinoma. Leptomeningeal and du-

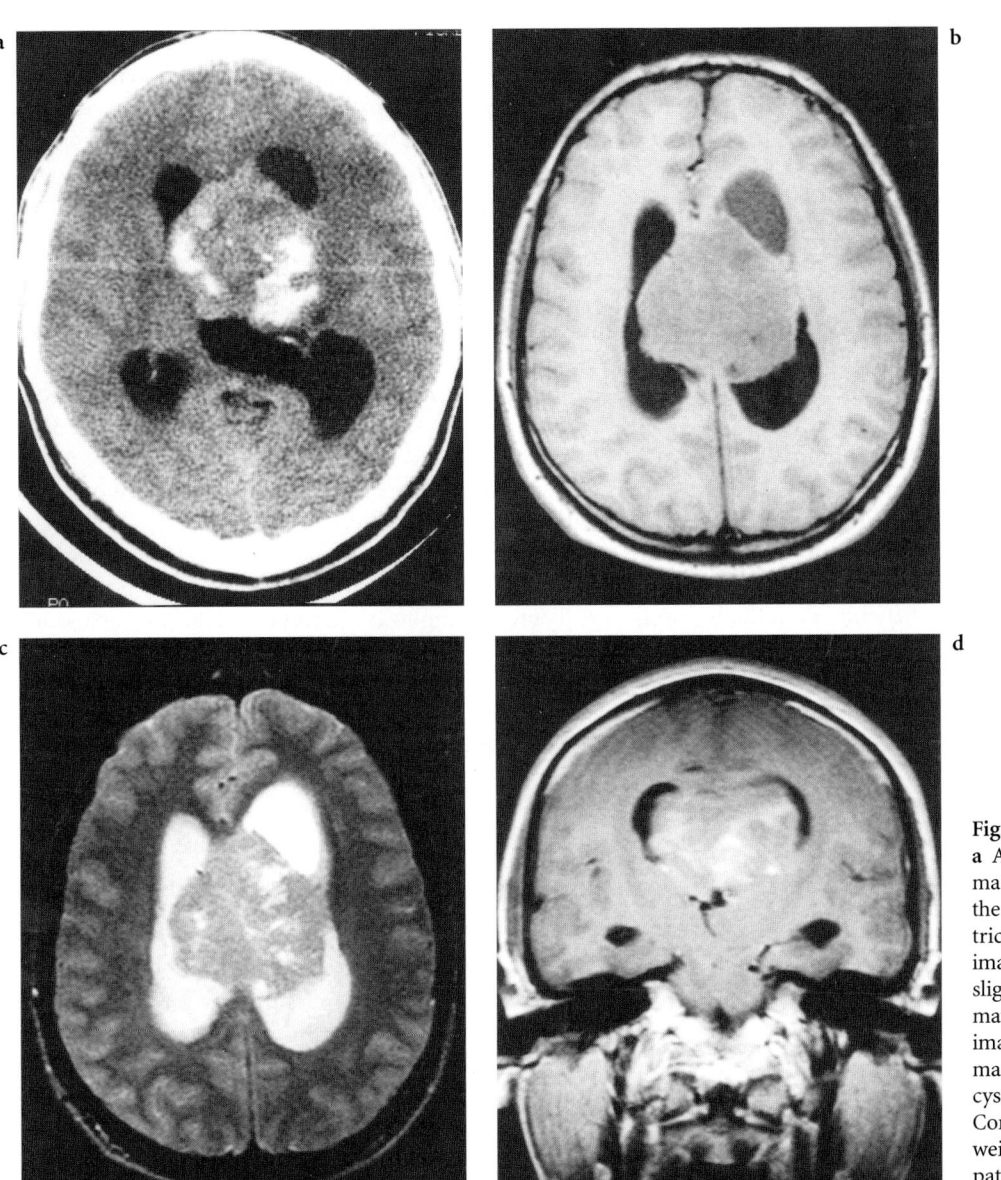

Fig. 7.9a–d. Ependymoma.
a Axial CT shows a large
mass with calcification in
the region of lateral ventricles. b Axial T1-weighted
image shows the mass to be
slightly hypointense to gray
matter. c Axial T2-weighted
image shows an isointense
mass with small areas of
cystic/necrotic changes. d
Coronal post-contrast T1-
weighted image shows
patchy, irregular enhancement of the mass

ral tumor spread may be seen from breast, lung, or
prostate carcinoma.

7.3.2
Imaging Studies

It is recommended to use double-dose (up to 80 g of
organically bound iodine), contrast-enhanced, delayed (up to 45 min) scans for evaluation of metastatic disease with CT imaging. However, contrast-enhanced MR is superior to contrast-enhanced CT for
evaluation of metastatic disease, and CT is only indi-

cated when there is contraindication to MR. Metastatic lesions are of variable density on unenhanced
CT images. Certain lesions show hyperdensity, including melanoma, colon carcinoma, choriocarcinoma, and osteosarcoma. Hemorrhage in metastatic
lesions is seen in 15% of cases and may be seen in
melanoma, choriocarcinoma, bronchogenic carcinoma, and hypernephroma. Calcification is extremely
rare, but may be seen in osteosarcoma and colon
carcinoma. Contrast enhancement is typically seen.
Lesions may show nodular enhancement or thick
ring-like enhancement. Marked vasogenic edema is
commonly seen surrounding the lesion. Occasional-

ly, an enhancing lesion may be seen without significant surrounding edema. CT guided stereotactic biopsy is a useful tool for definitive diagnosis (Fig. 7.10).

Metastases are usually hypointense to isointense (to gray matter) on T1-weighted images and isointense to hyperintense on T2-weighted images. Hemorrhage in metastatic lesions can produce complex signal intensity pattern. Edema presents as peritumoral high-signal areas in the white matter, which may vary from none to marked. Double or triple dose paramagnetic contrast agents (up to 0.3 mmol/kg) have been advocated by some authors (YUH 1992; HAUNSTEIN 1992). Contrast-enhanced MR with magnetization transfer technique is a sensitive way to detect metastatic disease (BOORSTEIN 1994).

Contrast enhancement pattern may be nodular, ring-like, or irregular. Distinction from a primary glioma or abscess may be difficult when the lesion is solitary. Subependymal or intraventricular spread of metastases is best shown on contrast-enhanced MR images. Skull base dural involvement is best shown with gadolinium (Gd)-enhanced, fat-suppressed MR images.

7.4
Lymphoma

Primary lymphoma comprises about 1% of all intracranial tumors. There has been a recent increase in incidence of lymphoma due to an increase in patients with AIDS and immunosuppression (renal transplant, chemotherapy, or other malignancy). Primary CNS lymphoma is more common than secondary involvement by systemic lymphoma (see Chap. 23 of this volume). About 10% of the patients with systemic lymphoma develop CNS involvement on imaging studies, whereas CNS involvement is present in one third of cases at autopsy.

Focal intra-axial lesions are the most common initial presentation of primary CNS lymphoma. The basal ganglia, periventricular white matter, corpus callosum, and septum pellucidum are often involved. Approximately 45% of lesions are multiple and 30% of patients with primary lymphoma develop leptomeningeal disease, which is more common in patients with recurrent disease.

Primary CNS lymphomas are non-Hodgkin's usually of B cell type.

Typical lymphoma (in non-AIDS, non-immunosuppressed patients) exhibits hyperdensity to isodensity to brain parenchyma and uniform enhancement is seen on CT images. In immunosuppressed or AIDS patients, ring-like enhancing lesions with areas of necrosis may be seen. Calcification or hemorrhage is rare.

Typically, on MR images, lymphomas are solid masses that are hypointense to isointense on T1-weighted images and isointense to hyperintense on T2-weighted images. Occasionally, lymphomas could be slightly hypointense on T2-weighted images. Contrast enhancement is intense and uniform in non-AIDS and non-immunosuppressed patients (ROMAN-GOLDSTEIN 1992) (Fig. 7.11). In immunosuppressed or AIDS patients, lymphoma may present as ring-like enhancing lesions or irregular enhancing masses with areas of necrosis (RUIZ 1998). Leptomeningeal seeding is seen better on contrast-enhanced MR than CT.

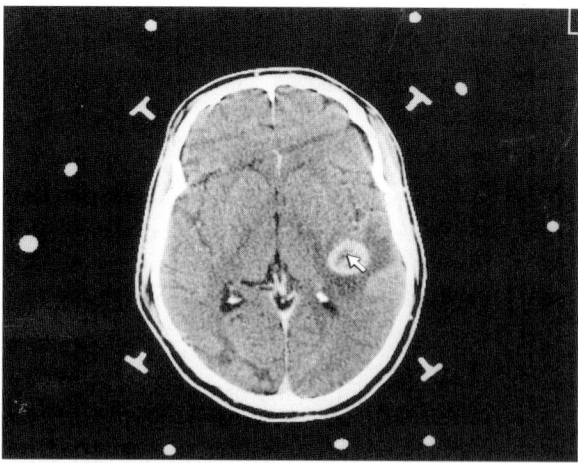

Fig. 7.10. Stereotactic biopsy axial CT performed with stereotactic device attached to the skull. *Arrow* points to the biopsy site within the nodular enhancing mass

7.5
Posterior Fossa Intra-Axial Tumors

7.5.1
Hemangioblastoma

Hemangioblastomas constitute approximately 1–2.5% of all primary CNS neoplasms and 8–12% of all primary posterior fossa neoplasms. They are the most common primary intra-axial posterior fossa neoplasms in adults. Peak age of presentation is be-

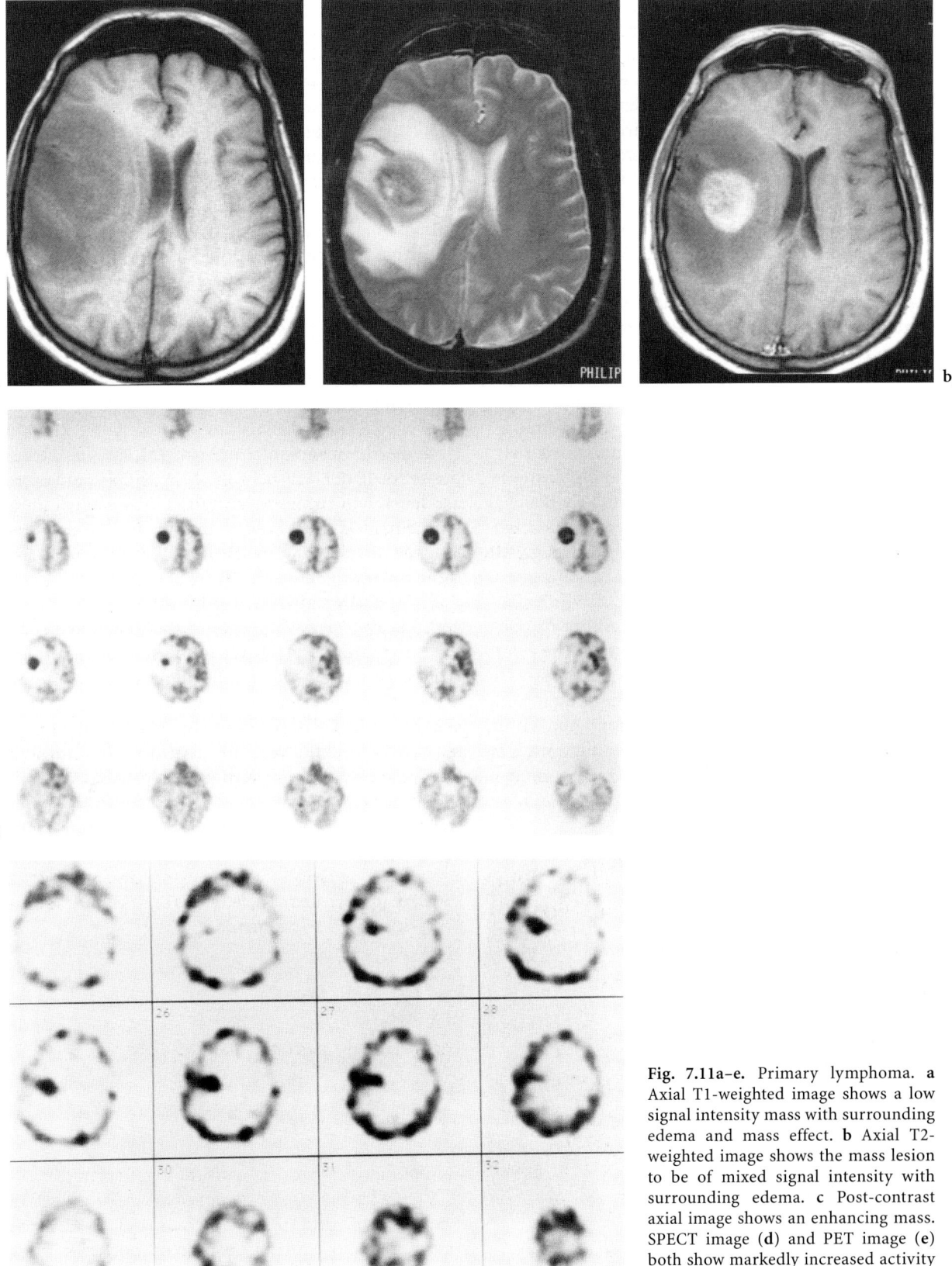

a

b,c

d

e

Fig. 7.11a–e. Primary lymphoma. a Axial T1-weighted image shows a low signal intensity mass with surrounding edema and mass effect. b Axial T2-weighted image shows the mass lesion to be of mixed signal intensity with surrounding edema. c Post-contrast axial image shows an enhancing mass. SPECT image (d) and PET image (e) both show markedly increased activity in the lesion

tween 30 to 40 years. In von Hippel-Lindau syndrome, hemangioblastomas present in younger adults.

They are usually solitary lesions with multiple lesions seen in 10% of von Hippel-Lindau syndrome patients. Multiple lesions are most frequently seen in the cerebellum (>90%), but can be found in the medulla or within the spinal cord. The lesions are typically located at the periphery of the cerebellum with a mural nodule at the pial surface.

Solid hemangioblastomas occur in approximately 40% of cases and the remaining are partially cystic or cystic masses with a mural nodule. About 60% of hemangioblastomas present as a cystic mass with a mural nodule or partially cystic mass and 40% are predominantly solid mass. Cyst fluid may be CSF-like or slightly hyperdense to CSF. The solid component of the mass enhances intensely with contrast material. MR is the most sensitive noninvasive imaging modality for evaluation of hemangioblastoma. Solid lesions presents as a heterogeneously low-signal intensity mass on T1-weighted images and high-signal intensity mass on T2-weighted images. Cystic lesions present as cyst with a pial-based mural nodule that enhances markedly. Linear or curvilinear areas of signal void (vessels) are seen within or adjacent to the solid mass or mural nodule of the cystic mass (Ho 1992) (Fig. 7.12). The cyst fluid has variable signal intensity, depending on the protein content and presence or absence of hemorrhage within it. MR is superior to CT in demonstrating lesions in the cervical cord.

7.5.2
Metastasis

Metastasis is the most common posterior fossa intra-axial tumor in adults, especially in those over the age of 50. Imaging findings of metastatic disease are similar to those of supratentorial lesions.

7.5.3
Primitive Neuroectodermal Tumor (Medulloblastoma)

PNET-MB is the most common posterior fossa neoplasm in children (40%) (ZEE 1993; LUH 1999). Some authors have reported astrocytoma to be the most common posterior fossa neoplasm in children (LEE 1989). PNET-MB constitutes approximately 25% of all pediatric intracranial neoplasms. The peak incidence for PNET-MB is in the first decade, and boys are two to four times more commonly affected than girls. PNET-MB arises from the vermis and may extend to involve the cerebellar hemisphere, brain stem, or fourth ventricle.

PNET-MB originates from poorly differentiated germinative cells of the roof of the fourth ventricle that migrate superolaterally to the external granular layer of the cerebellar hemisphere. PNET-MB may arise anywhere along the path of migration. This concept is useful to explain the fact that medulloblastomas in childhood are usually in the midline along the roof of the fourth ventricle, whereas those

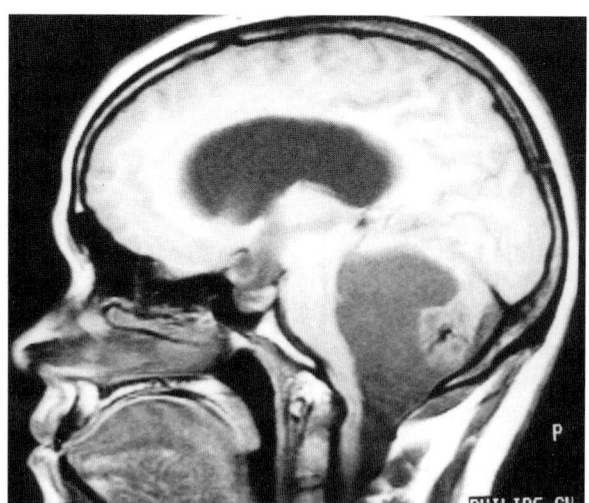
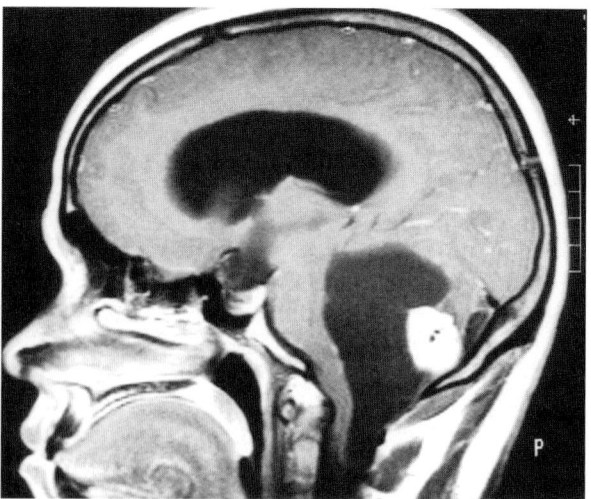

Fig. 7.12a,b. Hemangioblastoma. **a** Sagittal T1-weighted image shows a cystic mass in the posterior fossa with a mural nodule. Curvilinear signal void is seen within the mural nodule, consistent with vessels. **b** Sagittal post-contrast T1-weighted image shows intense enhancement of the mural nodule

in young adults are nearly always located more laterally in the cerebellar hemisphere (KOCI 1993).

PNET-MB generally appears as a uniform high-density lesion on non-contrast CT images. It tends to enhance homogeneously with sharp margins. Atypical features include small cystic or necrotic areas, calcification, hemorrhage, lack of contrast enhancement, eccentric location, and direct supratentorial extension (ZEE 1982).

On MR images, PNET-MB is typically hypointense to isointense to brain parenchyma on T1-weighted images and isointense to hyperintense on T2-weighted images. The pattern of contrast enhancement is similar to CT. However, the greater sensitivity of MR imaging often enables appreciation of a slightly heterogeneous enhancing pattern (MYERS 1992). Occasionally, only minimal contrast enhancement is seen.

Subarachnoid seeding into the intracranial and spinal subarachnoid spaces and ependymal seeding along the ventricular wall occur more commonly with PNET-MB than other pediatric posterior fossa neoplasms.

7.5.4
Astrocytoma

Cerebellar astrocytoma is the second most common posterior fossa tumor in children, being slightly less common than PNET-MB. Approximately 75% of cerebellar astrocytomas are benign juvenile pilocytic astrocytomas, which have a peak incidence in the first decade of life. The remaining 25% are diffuse, infiltrative, fibrillary-type astrocytomas, which have a peak incidence in adolescents and young adults.

7.5.5
Pilocytic Astrocytoma

About 50% of pilocytic astrocytomas are seen in the chiasmatic-hypothalamic region, 30% in the cerebellar vermis and hemisphere. Less common locations for this lesion include the brain stem, basal ganglia, cerebral hemisphere, and in the ventricle. Low-grade fibrillary astrocytomas are more commonly seen in the cerebral hemisphere. Less common locations are the brain stem and cerebellum. High-grade fibrillary astrocytomas are uncommon in the posterior fossa, especially in children.

Cerebellar pilocytic astrocytomas are well-circumscribed masses that are cystic with a small, reddish-tan mural nodule. Brain stem pilocytic astrocytomas are uniform, diffuse infiltrating neoplasm involving the medulla or pons.

Cerebellar astrocytomas are generally large at the time of presentation due to their benign nature and slow growth. Infiltrating fibrillary astrocytomas have a 40% 25-year survival rate. They are unencapsulated tumors that infiltrate diffusely.

Since the majority of cerebellar astrocytomas in children are pilocytic astrocytomas, we will discuss the imaging findings of cerebellar pilocytic astrocytomas only in this section. Imaging findings of low-grade fibrillary astrocytomas are similar to those seen in their supratentorial counterparts.

A common presentation is that of a sharply marginated cystic mass with a mural nodule, which enhances intensely with contrast. Cyst fluid density may be similar to or higher than that of CSF, owing to various degrees of protein content in the fluid. Cystic walls usually do not enhance. Occasionally, tumor involvement of the cyst wall with enhancement may be seen.

On MR images, the tumor presents as a well-demarcated cystic mass with a mural nodule, which enhances intensely with contrast (LEE 1989). Cyst fluid may be of slightly higher signal intensity than CSF due to its high protein content. Cyst walls usually do not enhance and merely represent compressed brain tissue. Occasionally, tumor involvement of the cyst wall with enhancement may be seen. The appearance of cerebellar astrocytomas may resemble that of hemangioblastomas. However, hemangioblastomas are rare in children. The mural nodule of the hemangioblastoma tends to be pial-based and curvilinear areas of signal void vessels are seen within or adjacent to the mural nodule.

7.5.6
Ependymoma

The majority (60%) of intracranial ependymomas are infratentorial in location, particularly in the fourth ventricle. They may also originate in or extend into the cerebropontine angle (CPA) cistern, vallecula, or medulla. Ependymomas have a bimodal age distribution: the larger peak occurs in children and adolescents. The second, much smaller peak occurs in adults (40–50 years). These tumors are four to six times more common in children than in adults. Both sexes are equally affected. Infratentorial ependymomas occur predominantly in children, whereas supratentorial ependymomas are evenly distributed among all age groups.

Ependymomas are gliomas arising from the ependymal cells, usually within the ventricles of the brain or central canal of the spinal cord. Ependymal "rests" in the white matter supratentorially may be the origin of parenchymal ependymomas. Infratentorial ependymomas usually arise from fourth ventricle and its lateral recesses. An especially malignant variant (ependymoblastoma) may grow rapidly within the ventricular system and form a cast of tumor within the ventricular cavity.

Ependymomas are usually slow-growing, firm, often lobulated, well-circumscribed white to grayish avascular masses that arise from ependymal cells lining the walls of ventricles or from ependymal rests in paraventricular white matter. They most commonly arise from the floor of the fourth ventricle and may protrude through foramina into adjacent cisterns (plastic ependymoma). About 50% of ependymomas exhibit calcification. Cyst formation is common but hemorrhage is uncommon (<14%). Larger tumors (over 4–5 cm) more frequently demonstrate cysts, calcification, or hemorrhage.

On CT images, ependymomas appear as hypodense to isodense mass with variable degree of contrast enhancement. Intratumoral cysts are common. Approximately 50% of ependymomas are calcified with the incidence of calcification increased in residual tumors after surgery and/or radiation therapy (Zee 1983).

On MR images, solid components are uniformly (homogeneously) hypo- to isointense to brain, and cystic portions slightly hyperintense to CSF on T1-weighted images. Solid portions of the tumor are hyperintense to brain, and cystic portions isointense to CSF on T2-weighted images. Ependymomas are somewhat lobulated soft tissue masses which may display heterogeneous intratumoral signal due to the presence of necrosis, calcification, tumor vascularity, blood degradation products, and intratumoral cysts. The contrast enhancement pattern is characteristically heterogeneous (Palma 1993; Lizak 1992; Tortori-Donati 1995).

Ependymomas have a distinctive tendency to expand within ventricles and extrude through foramina (e.g., Magendie and Luschka) into surrounding cisterns, the "plastic" configuration.

7.6
Brain Stem Glioma

Brain stem gliomas comprise approximately 10% of all childhood and adolescent brain tumors. They commonly occur before the age of 10 years. There is a male predominance of 2.5:1. The tumors usually arise within the pons and less frequently originate in the midbrain and the medulla.

Most brain stem gliomas (80%) arise from the pons and are fibrillary astrocytomas, which consist of low-grade astrocytomas, anaplastic astrocytomas, and glioblastomas. There is a tendency for low-grade fibrillary astrocytomas to show malignant degeneration. A smaller percentage (20%) of brain stem gliomas arise in the medulla or midbrain and are more likely to be pilocytic astrocytomas.

Approximately 55% of brain stem gliomas are low-grade fibrillary astrocytomas or pilocytic astrocytomas, and 45% of brain stem gliomas are anaplastic astrocytomas or glioblastomas.

On imaging studies, these lesions are hypodense to occasional isodense with enlargement of the brain stem. Contrast enhancement is seen in more than 50% of cases. Exophytic extension of the tumor is frequently seen. MR imaging is superior to CT in evaluating brain stem tumors. Brain stem neoplasms show hypointensity on T1-weighted images and hyperintensity on T2-weighted images (Fig. 7.13).

Pilocytic astrocytomas are usually cystic with enhancing mural nodules (Fig. 7.14). They are more likely to show contrast enhancement than fibrillary astrocytomas (Fischbein 1996; Freeman 1998). There is a tendency for low-grade fibrillary astrocytomas to undergo malignant degeneration with cystic necrosis, hemorrhage, and contrast enhancement.

7.7
Pineal Region Neoplasms

Although pineal region tumors constitute only 0.3–2.7% of all intracranial tumors, they are considered an important clinical entity due to their strategic location. Pineal region neoplasms can be classified into three major groups according to their cell origin: germ cell origin, pineal cell origin, and tumors of other cell origin. Tumors of germ cell origin include germinoma, mature teratoma, malignant teratoma, embryonal cell carcinoma, endodermal sinus tumor, choriocarcinoma, and mixed germ cell tumors. Tumors of pineal cell origin include pineocytoma and pineoblastoma. Tumors of other cell origin include astrocytoma, metastasis, hemangiopericytoma, meningioma, ganglioneuroma, and ganglioglioma. The majority of germ cell tumors are isointense to gray matter on both T1-weighted and T2-weighted images (Zee 1991)

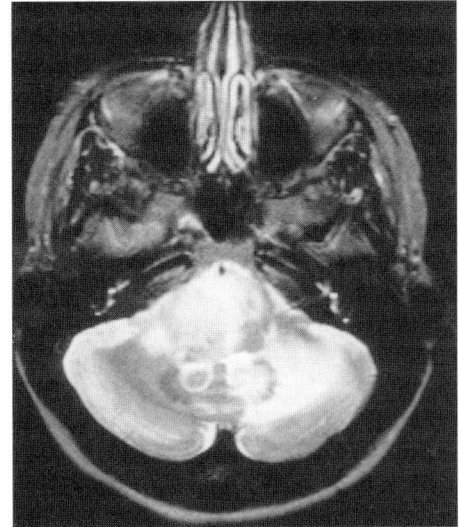

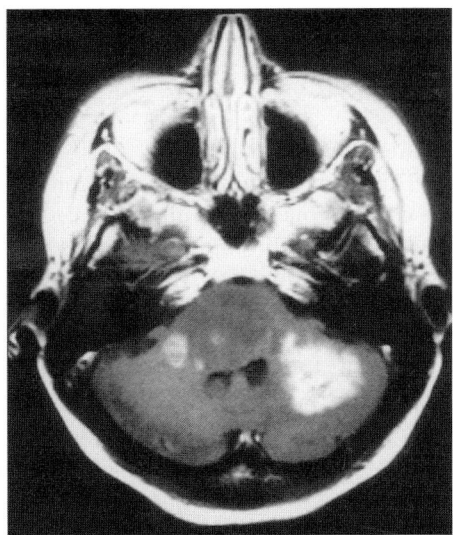

Fig. 7.13a,b. Brain stem glioma and radiation change. **a** Axial T2-weighted image shows abnormal high signal intensity involving the brain stem and left cerebellum. **b** Axial post-contrast T1-weighted image shows an irregular enhancing lesion in the left cerebellum (proven to be radiation change) and small enhancing areas in brain stem and right brachium pontis

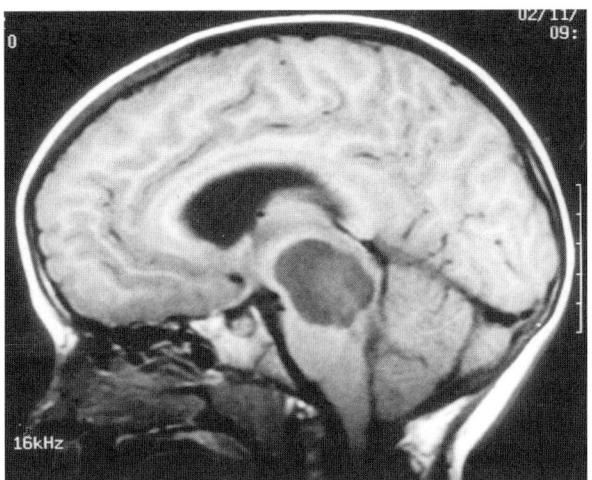

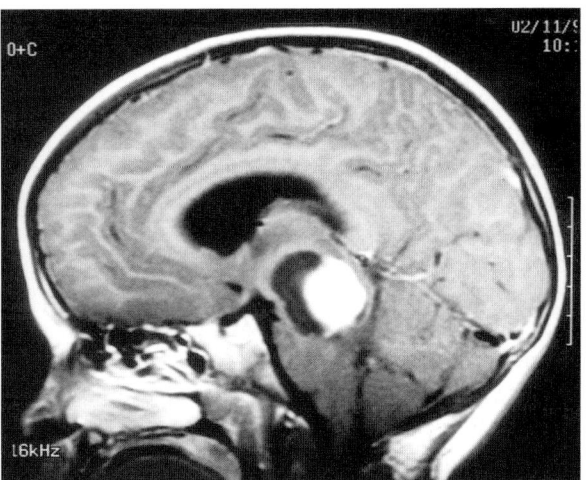

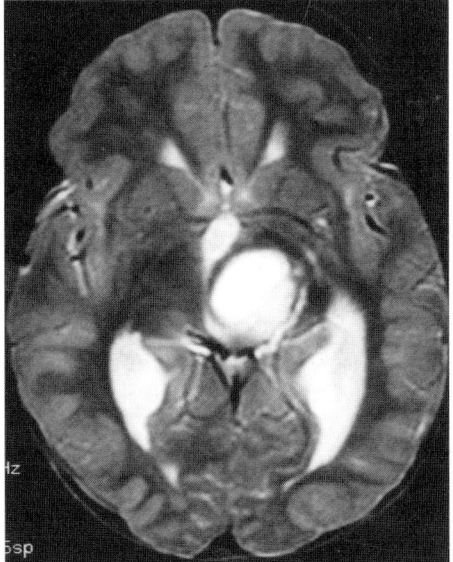

Fig. 7.14a–c. Pilocytic astrocytoma of the brain stem. **a** Sagittal T1-weighted image shows a low signal intensity cystic mass with a low signal mural nodule seen posteriorly. **b** Axial T2-weighted image shows the cystic mass with high signal mural nodule posteriorly. **c** Sagittal T1-weighted image shows intense enhancement of the mural nodule

7.8
Mass Lesions in the Region of the Ventricular System

Approximately 10% of CNS neoplasms are partly or completely intraventricular. The most common lateral ventricular masses are choroid plexus papillomas, meningiomas, followed by ependymomas, subependymomas, subependymal giant cell astrocytomas, and metastases or lymphomas. The most common third ventricular masses are colloid cysts, subependymal giant cell astrocytomas, followed by choroid plexus papillomas, ependymomas, and craniopharyngiomas.

The most common fourth ventricular masses are ependymomas, astrocytomas, choroid plexus papillomas, medulloblastomas, dermoids, epidermoids, subependymomas, and metastases. Cysticercosis cysts, a parasitic disease, can be seen anywhere in the ventricular system.

7.8.1
Ependymoma

Approximately 40% of intracranial ependymomas are supratentorial. Of these, between 66 to 75% are extraventricular mostly near the trigones of the lateral ventricles. Ependymomas adjacent to the lateral ventricle may have an intraventricular component.

About 50% of ependymomas calcify (2/3 infratentorial, 1/3 supratentorial). Cyst formation is commonly seen while hemorrhage is uncommon (<14%). Larger tumors (4–5 cm) more frequently demonstrate cysts, calcification, or hemorrhage.

On CT images they appear as hypodense to isodense masses with variable degree of contrast enhancement. Intratumoral cysts are common. Approximately 50% are calcified (SWARTZ 1982; ZEE 1983). Intraventricular ependymomas may mimic choroid plexus papillomas on CT images. On MR images, solid components of the tumor are uniformly (homogeneously) hypo- to isointense to brain, and cystic portions are slightly hyperintense to CSF on T1-weighted images. On T2-weighted images, solid portions are hyperintense to brain and cystic portions are isointense to CSF. Ependymomas are somewhat lobulated soft tissue masses which may display heterogeneous intratumoral signal due to the presence of necrosis, calcification, tumor vascularity, blood degradation products, and intratumoral cysts. The contrast enhancement pattern is heterogeneous (SPOTO 1990) (Fig. 7.9).

7.8.2
Subependymoma

Subependymomas are relatively rare tumors found primarily in middle-aged and elderly patients. Symptomatic subependymomas, those which cause obstructive hydrocephalus by occluding CSF pathways, present at an average age of 40 years. Asymptomatic subependymomas are usually discovered incidentally at an average age of 60 years.

They arise most frequently from the lower medulla and project into the fourth ventricle. They have also been found in the frontal horns of the lateral ventricles and along the septum pellucidum (~5%) and, less frequently, along the midbody of the lateral ventricles.

Subependymomas are benign, well-circumscribed lobulated tumors which grow by expanding toward ventricles in contrast to gliomas which grow by infiltrating surrounding structures. They also incite less edema, may resemble ependymomas, but are less frequently calcified. Larger tumors (4–5 cm diameter) frequently demonstrate cysts, focal calcification, and hemorrhage.

Subependymomas are typically less heterogeneous, less intense on T2-weighted images and less likely to enhance than ependymomas (SPOTO 1990). Heterogeneity arises primarily from multiple small intratumoral cysts.

7.8.3
Astrocytoma

Intraventricular astrocytomas usually arise from the anterior column of the fornix and may be attached to the ependyma by a pedicle. The frontal horn is the most common intraventricular location. Imaging findings of astrocytomas are similar to those seen in these tumors in other sites of the brain.

7.8.4
Subependymal Giant Cell Astrocytoma

Subependymal giant cell astrocytomas (SGCAs) are found in 10–15% of patients with tuberous sclerosis. They usually occur in patients below 20 years of age. SGCAs occur in the walls of the lateral ventricles after malignant degeneration of hamartoma associated with tuberous sclerosis. The roof of the third ventricle is involved if the tumors grow inferiorly. In such cases, it may obstruct the foramen of Monro.

They are classified as grade I astrocytoma by the WORLD HEALTH ORGANIZATION (WHO).

On CT images, these tumors appear as heterogeneous with mixed hypodense and isodense regions. Calcification and cysts are commonly seen. Inhomogeneous enhancement is seen following the intravenous injection of contrast material.

Cortical tubers are isodense to brain and not seen well on CT images. Subependymal heterotopic nodules are frequently calcified and well demonstrated on CT images.

On MR imaging, they are heterogeneously hypointense on T1-weighted images and heterogeneously hyperintense on T2-weighted images. Contrast enhancement is usually intense but inhomogeneous. Cortical tubers are seen better on MR as areas of high signal intensity on T2-weighted images (JELINEK 1990; TIEN 1991).

7.8.5
Choroid Plexus Papilloma

Choroid plexus papillomas comprise less than 1% of all primary intracranial neoplasms, between 0.5 to 0.6% of intracranial neoplasms in adults and 2–5% of intracranial neoplasms in children. They account for 2–3% of intracranial gliomas. Choroid plexus papillomas are one of the most common brain tumors in children below 2 years of age.

Choroid plexus papillomas occur in locations distributed in rough proportion to the normal distribution of choroid plexus: trigone (atrium) of the lateral ventricle (50%), fourth ventricle (40%), third ventricle, and CPA cisterns (10%). In children, 70% occur in the atria of the lateral ventricles and 10% in the third ventricle. In adults, most occur in the fourth ventricle. Bilateral primary sites are rare (3–4%). Extraventricular primary sites (e.g., in choroid projecting through the foramen of Luschka) are very rare. Seeding along CSF pathways occurs in both benign and malignant tumors, often to the CPA cisterns but also to the suprasellar cistern and pineal region. Choroid plexus papillomas are predominately well-circumscribed, smooth or lobulated masses which may display frond-like margins.

The majority of choroid plexus papillomas are iso- to hyperdense with respect to the brain, but they can be hypodense or mixed in density. Virtually all enhance intensely; most homogeneously, some slightly heterogeneously. On MR imaging, they are isointense to brain on T1-weighted images and iso- to slightly hyperintense to brain on T2-weighted images. Homogeneous contrast enhancement is usually seen. Calci-

fication and hemorrhage are common and may produce signal voids or focal heterogeneities within the tumors. Occasionally a signal void may result from a vascular pedicle (COATES 1989; KEN 1991).

7.8.6
Choroid Plexus Carcinoma

Choroid plexus carcinomas comprise 10–20% of choroid plexus neoplasms. They are malignancies of the pediatric age group with the majority presenting between 2 and 4 years of age (PACKER 1992). The distribution of choroid plexus carcinomas parallels that of papillomas.

Choroid plexus carcinomas cannot be reliably distinguished from choroid plexus papillomas on the basis of imaging characteristics. Both may show local parenchymal invasion and CSF dissemination.

7.9
Sellar and Parasellar Neoplasms

7.9.1
Craniopharyngioma

Craniopharyngiomas comprise 3–5% of all primary intracranial neoplasms, 5–10% of all pediatric intracranial neoplasms, 50% of suprasellar tumors in children, and 15% of supratentorial tumors in children. Craniopharyngiomas have a bimodal age distribution with more than half occurring in children and young adults. A second, smaller peak occurs in the fifth and sixth decade of life. They are the most common neoplasm to calcify in children (70–90% calcify). The incidence of calcification decreases with patient age. Males and females are equally affected. Craniopharyngiomas are both intra- and suprasellar in about 70% of cases, suprasellar only in about 20%, and intrasellar in nearly 10% of cases. Less than 1% arise within an anterior third ventricle.

Craniopharyngiomas are well-circumscribed multilobulated masses, 90% of which have both cystic and solid components. The cystic portions typically have a density approximating CSF but may be hypodense in proportion to cholesterol content or hyperdense in proportion to proteinaceous content. Both enhancement and calcification are more common in pediatric patients. Solid portions, or nodules, enhance in 66% of cases. Calcification is present in 90% of pediatric cases and 50% of adult cases.

On MR imaging, the signal characteristics of the cystic component of craniopharyngiomas are highly variable. Hyperintensity correlates well with high cholesterol or methemoglobin content on T1-weighted images while T2-weighted images are more typically hyperintense (AHMADI 1992). Layering or intermingling of differing cyst components adds to heterogeneity making craniopharyngiomas the most heterogeneous of sellar region masses. Strong but heterogeneous enhancement of the solid component is also seen.

7.9.2
Pituitary Adenoma

The incidence of pituitary microadenomas in autopsy series is approximately 25%. Recent advances in imaging techniques and clinical immunochemistry have improved the diagnosis of pituitary microadenoma and made early diagnosis possible. Non-functioning pituitary macroadenomas usually present with symptoms related to compression of adjacent structures. Functioning pituitary adenomas are usually detected early, before the onset of symptoms related to compression of adjacent structures. Classically, bitemporal hemianopsia is seen with compression of the optic chiasm. Larger tumors may cause obstruction of the foramen of Monro with resultant hydrocephalus. Pituitary macroadenomas are always associated with enlargement of the bony sella turcica.

On CT images, these lesions are isodense to the brain and show contrast enhancement. Calcification is seen in 5% of cases. MR imaging is preferred due to the capability of obtaining sagittal and coronal imaging. On MR images, they are hypointense on T1-weighted images and iso- to hyperintense on T2-weighted images. Contrast enhancement is seen. Cystic and necrotic changes are seen in approximately 15% of cases. MR is superior to CT in the evaluation of cavernous sinus invasion (AHMADI 1985).

7.10
Meningeal Based Neoplasms and Mass Lesions

7.10.1
Meningioma

Meningiomas are the most common non-glial primary neoplasm of the CNS. Meningiomas make up approximately 15% of all operative intracranial tumors (ROSENBAUM 1984). They tend to occur more often in female patients between the ages of 40 and 70 years. The common sites of meningiomas are, in order of decreasing frequency, the following: parasagittal, convexity, sphenoid wing, planum sphenoidale and olfactory groove, parasellar and cavernous sinus, posterior fossa (CPA cistern, foramen magnum), intraventricular, orbital, and pineal region. An association of neurofibromatosis with multiple meningiomas also exists. Multiple meningiomas may also be seen in patients who have received previous radiation therapy or they may be idiopathic in origin.

Classically, benign meningiomas are subdivided into four basic subtypes: fibroblastic, transitional, meningothelial, and angioblastic (Chap. 2). Angioblastic meningiomas consist of angiomatous meningioma, hemangioblastoma, and hemangiopericytoma. Hemangiopericytomas are now considered as a separate entity since they do not arise from meningeal cells (ZEE 1992).

Malignant meningiomas are rare. Invasion of brain parenchyma is generally considered to be evidence of malignancy. However, local invasion of dura, paranasal sinus, regional muscle, or bone may be seen in histologically benign meningiomas.

Grossly, most of the meningiomas are of the globular type, which is a well-demarcated mass with lobulated appearance and attachment to dura. A less common form, meningioma en plaque, has a flattened appearance and follows the contour of the bony calvarium. A rare form, intraosseous meningioma, is seen arising from the diploic space. Bone destruction, bone sclerosis, and hyperostosis are more commonly associated with intraosseous meningiomas. The annual growth rate of meningioma has been reported to range from 0.5% to 21%, with a median growth rate of 3.6%. Meningiomas which occur following radiation treatment of other intracranial neoplasms tend to have a higher growth rate.

The WHO classification subdivides meningiomas into three types: benign (88–94%), atypical (5–7%), and anaplastic or malignant (1–2%). Malignant meningiomas tend to invade the brain. Both benign and malignant forms rarely metastasize extracranially. Between 20–30% of seemingly completely excised meningiomas recur. On CT images, they are a hyperdense or isodense mass lesion with a well-delineated margin. There is usually broad based attachment to the dura.

Meningiomas can be globular or en plaque. En plaque meningiomas may be difficult to detect on CT images. They are more frequently seen at sphenoid ridge convexity and more likely to be associated with hyperostosis (SCHUBEUS 1990). Calcification is seen in 20–50% of cases. Radiologically, the extent of calcification varies markedly. Calcification may be psammomatous (diffuse) or globular (focal) in nature. Hyperostosis is seen in 20% of cases.

The amount of surrounding edema is variable and does not correlate with malignancy, lesion size, or location. Edema is seen in up to 75% of meningiomas. In some cases, there is a large amount of edema associated with meningioma; in other cases there is little or no edema. Uniform contrast enhancement is typically seen in these lesions. Hemorrhage (3%), cystic changes, or necrosis (10%) are uncommon.

A meningioma on MR imaging is isointense(60%) or mildly hypointense (30%) to gray matter on T1-weighted images. On T2-weighted images, the tumors are isointense (50%) or mildly to moderately hyperintense (40%) to gray matter. The remaining 10% of meningiomas have varied signal intensity features. In half of these cases, diffused calcification within the tumor may produce hypointensity on both T1- and T2-weighted images. Cystic meningiomas may exhibit areas of low signal intensity on T1-weighted images and high signal intensity on T2-weighted images. Calcification is less well detected on MR than CT. Gradient echo imaging may improve the detection of tumor calcification. Hemorrhage, cystic changes, and necrotic changes are better demonstrated on MR than CT. Extra-axial location of the mass lesion is better demonstrated on MR. A low signal rim around the tumor margin (CSF cleft, vascular rim, dura) and buckling of the gray–white interface are signs of extra-axial location (ZIMMERMAN 1985).

The tumor can be globular or en plaque. En plaque meningiomas may be hard to detect on non-contrast T1- and T2-weighted images due to their small size, isointensity to brain parenchyma, and lack of surrounding edema. gadolinium enhancement is very useful to demonstrate an en plaque meningioma (Fig. 7.15).

The detection and characterization of meningiomas is markedly enhanced with administration of gadolinium. The majority of meningiomas exhibit intense uniform enhancement. Densely calcified and cystic meningiomas may show inhomogeneous or heterogeneous enhancement. Small tumors that may otherwise be missed are readily shown with gadolinium enhancement, especially those of the en plaque type (ELSTER 1989).

Vasogenic edema within the white matter of the brain is seen around meningiomas in up to 75% of cases. The degree of paratumoral edema in meningiomas has little correlation with tumor size. Some authors have reported increased edema in angioblastic and meningothelial meningiomas as compared with fibroblastic and transitional types.

7.10.2
Meningeal Hemangiopericytoma

Hemangiopericytoma of the meninges is an aggressive, highly vascular neoplasm that is commonly grouped with angioblastic meningiomas. Hemangiopericytoma of the meninges is a distinct entity that arises from the vascular pericytes rather than from meningothelial cells. Imaging features are similar to angioblastic or malignant meningiomas with heterogeneous appearance caused by cystic, necrotic areas and prominent vascular channels (CHIECHI 1996).

7.10.3
Lymphoma

Primary CNS lymphomas were considered to be rare; they constitute about 1% of all intracranial tumors. However, there is a recent increase in incidence due to an increase in patients with AIDS and immunosuppression (renal transplant, chemotherapy, other malignancy). Up to 6% of these patients may have CNS disease.

About 10% of patients with systemic lymphoma develop CNS involvement in clinical series. In autopsy series, secondary CNS involvement by lymphoma may be found in up to 26% of cases. Primary CNS

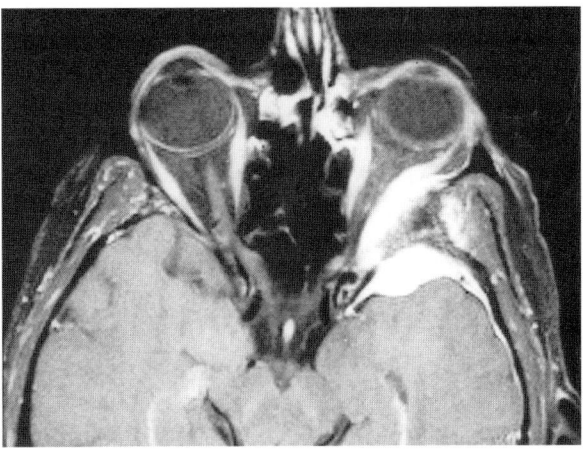

Fig. 7.15. Sphenoid meningioma axial post-contrast T1-weighted, fat-suppressed image shows an enhancing extra-axial mass along the left sphenoid with extension into the left orbit

lymphomas are more common than secondary involvement by systemic lymphoma. All ages are affected. In patients with immunosuppression or AIDS, this happens in the third or fourth decades of life.

A solitary or multicentric location is frequently seen in primary brain lymphoma. Focal intra-axial lesions are the most common initial presentation of primary CNS lymphoma. The basal ganglia, periventricular white matter, corpus callosum, cerebellar vermis, and septum pellucidum are often involved. Approximately 20–40% of lesions are multiple. Of patients with primary lymphoma, 30% develop leptomeningeal disease. Leptomeningeal disease is more common in patients with recurrent disease. Leptomeningeal involvement is also common in secondary CNS lymphoma. Secondary invasion of the brain may occur through the Virchow-Robin spaces producing parenchymal lesions while Secondary invasion of the dura produces dural based mass lesion.

Secondary CNS lymphomas are also of the non-Hodgkin's type. Diffuse varieties of non-Hodgkin' lymphoma affect the CNS more frequently, especially diffuse histiocytic lymphoma. Secondary CNS lymphoma may involve brain parenchyma, leptomeninges, dura, and epidural tissue.

Both primary and secondary lymphoma have similar imaging findings. The typical lymphoma (in non-AIDS, nonimmunosuppressed patients) exhibits hyperdensity to isodensity to brain parenchyma on CT images. Uniform enhancement is seen following the intravenous injection of contrast material. The CT appearance of a dural-based lymphoma may be difficult to differentiate from a meningioma. Leptomeningeal involvement is not well identified with CT.

On MR imaging, lymphomas typically are solid masses that are hypointense to isointense to gray matter on T1-weighted images and isointense to slightly hyperintense on T2-weighted images (ZIMMERMAN 1985). Some cases of lymphoma show hypointensity on T2-weighted images. These signal intensity features make a dural-based lymphoma similar to meningioma. However, lymphoma is often multifocal, and lymphoma may infiltrate the bone to produce an extra-calvarial mass. Furthermore, leptomeningeal and subependymal seeding is often detected on contrast-enhanced MR images.

7.10.4
Metastasis

Common primary sources for dural-based metastases include the breast, prostate, melanoma, and lung in adults and neuroblastoma of the adrenal gland in children. 60% of metastases are seen supratentorially and 40% infratentorially. Metastasis is the most common intra-axial cerebellar tumor in adults. It is the most likely diagnosis for intra-axial cerebellar mass seen in a patient over 50 years of age.

Metastatic disease typically exhibits multiple enhancing lesions in the brain parenchyma at the gray–white junction. Dural-based metastatic lesions are less common and often associated with adjacent bone destruction.

CT has a distinct disadvantage for detecting dural-based metastasis. A thin layer of enhancing tumor along the bony calvarium may be obscured by the high density of the skull. Expanding the window to the proper setting (wide window width) is essential in separating the enhancing neoplasm from dense bony calvarium. Furthermore the majority of metastatic lesions are associated with bone destruction. They are readily detected on bone window images, but could be easily missed on standard soft tissue window images. When intravenous contrast is given to the patient, the enhancing tumor may further masquerade the bone defect. Approximately 10% of patients with leptomeningeal metastasis exhibit hydrocephalus.

MR is superior to CT in demonstrating dural-based metastatic disease (DAVIS 1987). Gd-enhanced MR demonstrated broad-based enhancing lesion along the calvarium (Fig. 7.16). Associated bone destruction can be easily detected. The high signal intensity of normal bone marrow seen on T1-weighted images is reflected by tumor cells, which show low to iso-signal intensity to adjacent muscle on T1-weighted images. On Gd-enhanced T1-weighted images, enhancement of the tumor may show similar signal intensity to fatty marrow. A calvarial metastatic lesion may actually be obscured on Gd-enhanced T1-weighted images. Fat suppression technique is necessary to demonstrate the enhancing lesion. Particularly in the skull base and orbit, Gd-enhanced MR with fat suppression can better demonstrate the enhancing metastatic lesion. The signal intensity pattern of metastatic lesions on T1-weighted and T2-weighted images is variable depending on the primary origin of the neoplasm.

7.10.5
Myeloma (Plasmacytoma)

Primary plasmacytoma of the skull is rare. Secondary involvement of the bony calvarium due to myeloma is more common. The peak incidence is in the sixth and seventh decade of life, similar to metastatic

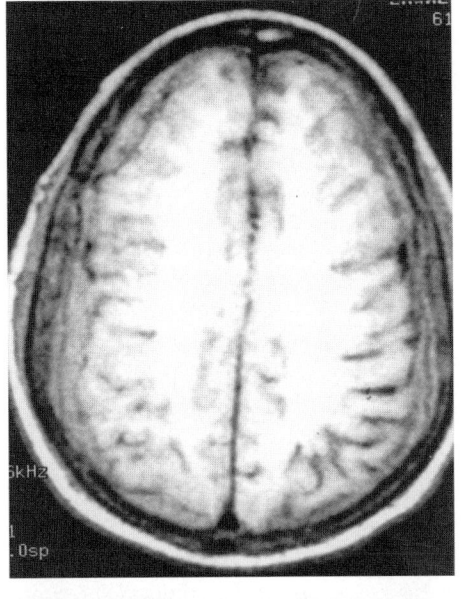

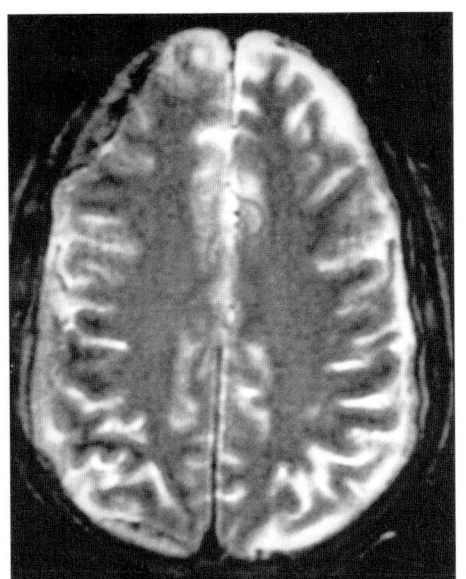

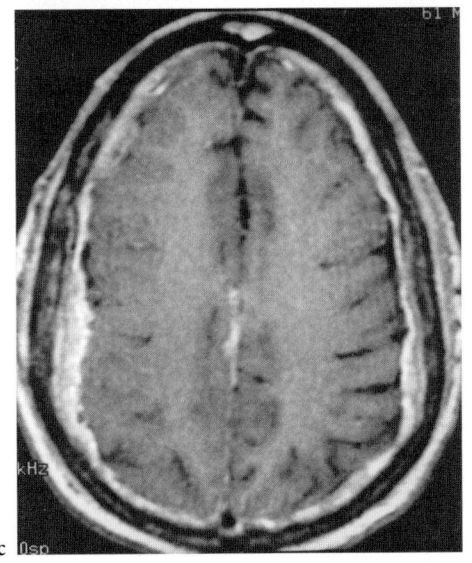

Fig. 7.16a–c. Metastatic prostatic carcinoma to the dura. **a** Axial T1-weighted image shows bilateral extra-axial lesions in both convexity. **b** Axial T2-weighted image shows the lesion is of low to iso-signal intensity. **c** Axial post-contrast T1-weighted image shows enhancement of the bilateral extra-axial lesion

disease. It occurs more frequently in male than female patients. A dural-based mass lesion is usually an extension of a bony lesion. The clivus, skull base, and bony calvarium may be involved.

Radiographs of the skull show multiple lucencies involving the bony calvarium. Destructive lesions may be seen involving the clivus or skull base. CT shows well-defined lucencies in the skull with or without epidural mass. Destructive lesions involving the clivus and skull base with adjacent soft tissue mass may be seen. On MR imaging, plasmacytoma exhibits isointensity to surrounding brain parenchyma on T1-weighted images and hypointensity on T2-weighted images.

The epidural component of the lesion is better seen on MR, especially following intravenous injec-

tion of gadolinium. Mass lesions involving the clivus and skull base are better seen with Gd-enhanced, fat-suppressed images.

7.11
Neoplasms in the Region of Clivus

7.11.1
Chordoma

Rare, slow-growing bone tumors represent 1% of all intracranial neoplasms and 4% of all primary bone tumors. Peak incidence is at the age of 20–40 years.

There is a male predominance with a male:female
ratio of 2:1. Common locations of chordoma include:
sacrococcygeal 50%, clivus 35%, and vertebral body
15%. Clival chordomas tend to occur near spheno-
occipital synchondrosis. CT shows bone destruction
involving the clivus associated with a soft tissue
mass. Calcification is seen in 50% of cases. There is
extension of the soft tissue mass through the dura
posteriorly into the posterior fossa, laterally to the
middle fossa, and anteriorly into the nasopharynx.
Contrast enhancement is seen on post-contrast examinations. On MR imaging, they present as a hypointense mass lesion involving the clivus that replaces
the normal hyperintense fatty marrow on T1-weight-
ed images.

A heterogeneous, hyperintense mass lesion is
seen on T2-weighted images. Heterogeneity may be
secondary to calcification, vascularity, hemorrhage,
or variation in cellular histology. Contrast-enhanced
MR shows intense enhancement. The enhancing
mass may have similar high signal intensity as the
adjacent normal fatty marrows. A fat-suppressed
contrast-enhanced image delineates the mass lesion
as well as the adjacent meningeal involvement and
intracranial extension better. MR is superior to CT
for evaluation of chordomas due to the availability of
sagittal sequence and high tissue contrast resolution
(OOT 1989).

7.11.2
Chondrosarcoma

Approximately 10% of chondrosarcomas occur in
the bones of the face and skull base. They occur
predominantly in patients between 20 and 50 years
of age. The male:female ratio is 2:1.

Chondrosarcomas arise in different locations associated with sutures such as petro-occipital suture.
Other locations include parasellar, retrosellar, cerebellopontine angle, and paranasal sinuses.

Calcification is seen in the chondroid type on CT
images. Bony destruction associated with soft tissue
mass is a frequent finding. Contrast enhancement of
the mass is inhomogeneous, and calcification may
not be detected on MR images.

Chordrosarcoma is hypointense on T1-weighted
images and heterogeneous hyperintense on T2-
weighted images. Gd-enhanced MR may show intense but inhomogeneous enhancement (MYERS
1992) (Fig. 7.17).

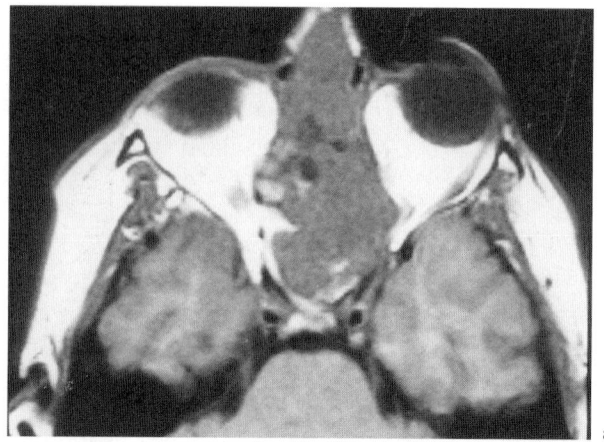

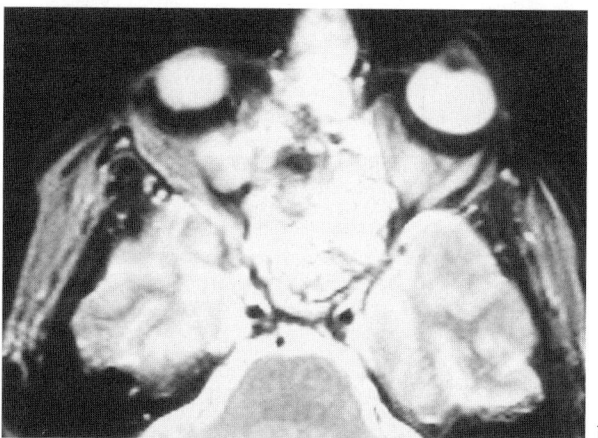

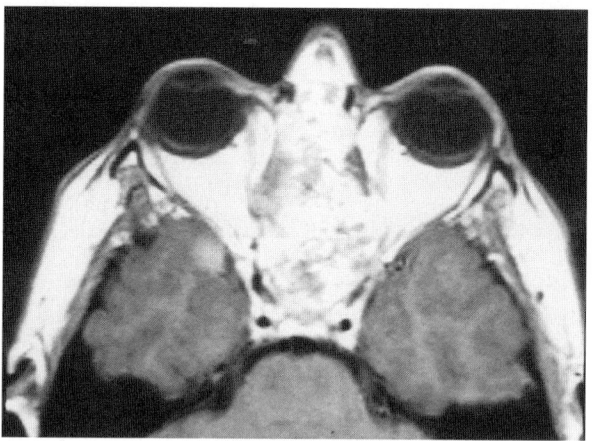

Fig. 7.17a–c. Chondrosarcoma. **a** Axial T1-weighted image
shows a low signal mass in the nasal cavity, ethmoid sinus,
and sphenoid sinus. **b** Axial T2-weighted image shows the
mass to be of predominantly high signal intensity. **c** Axial
post-contrast T1-weighted image shows heterogeneous enhancement of the mass

7.11.3
Metastasis

Primary sites of lesions metastatic to the region of clivus include the breast, prostate, melanoma, and lung. Bone destruction is associated with replacement of normal fatty marrow within the clivus. The T1-weighted sagittal MR image is excellent in demonstration of metastatic disease involving the clivus by exhibiting a low signal intensity mass replacing the high signal fatty marrow. Fat suppression technique in conjunction with Gd-enhancement is superior to CT in detection of intracranial extension of the metastatic disease

7.11.4
Plasmacytoma

Plasmacytoma involving the clivus has radiological findings similar to metastatic disease.

7.11.5
Lymphoma

Lymphoma involving the clivus may present with bone destruction. Lymphoma infiltration of the clivus with replacement of normal fatty marrow may be seen on T1-weighted MR images without discrete bone destruction. Fat suppression technique in conjunction with Gd-enhancement is a good method for demonstrating enhancing infiltrative tumor in the clivus without definite bone destruction.

7.11.6
Nasopharyngeal Carcinoma

Posterior extension of nasopharyngeal carcinoma to involve the clivus and invade the dura with intracranial extension is not uncommon. Frequently, a recurrent nasopharyngeal carcinoma may present with lesions involving the skull base and clivus with intracranial extension, whereas the primary site at the nasopharynx may be normal following previous radiation therapy and chemotherapy. The tumor is isointense to muscle on T1-weighted images and heterogeneously hyperintense on T2-weighted images. Contrast enhancement is inhomogeneous.

7.11.7
Carcinoma of the Sphenoid Sinus

Extension of the carcinoma of the sphenoid sinus to involve the clivus is not common. Neoplasms involving the paranasal sinuses tend to show low to intermediate signal intensity in contrast to the high signal intensity mucosal disease on T2-weighted image. Intense enhancement is seen following the intravenous injection of contrast material.

7.12
Posterior Fossa Extra-Axial Mass Lesions

7.12.1
Vestibular Schwannoma

Vestibular schwannomas are the most common (85%) neoplasm of the cerebellopontine angle. The peak incidence is from 40 to 60 years. Unenhanced CT shows isodense lesion to brain with marked contrast enhancement. Enlargement of the internal auditory canal can be seen on bone window images.

On MR images, vestibular schwannomas show hypointensity on T1-weighted images and marked hyperintensity on T2-weighted images. Gd-enhanced MR shows intense enhancement (Fig. 7.18). The tumor may show cystic or necrotic changes.

7.12.2
Fifth Nerve Schwannoma

Fifth nerve schwannomas occur along the course of the fifth nerve. The tumor may extend from the ambient cistern in the posterior fossa into Meckel's cave and cavernous sinus in the middle fossa. Bone erosion of the petrous apex may be seen. Imaging features are similar to those of eighth nerve schwannomas.

7.12.3
Meningioma

Approximately 10% of meningiomas occur in the posterior fossa and they have similar imaging features as supratentorial meningiomas (Fig. 7.19).

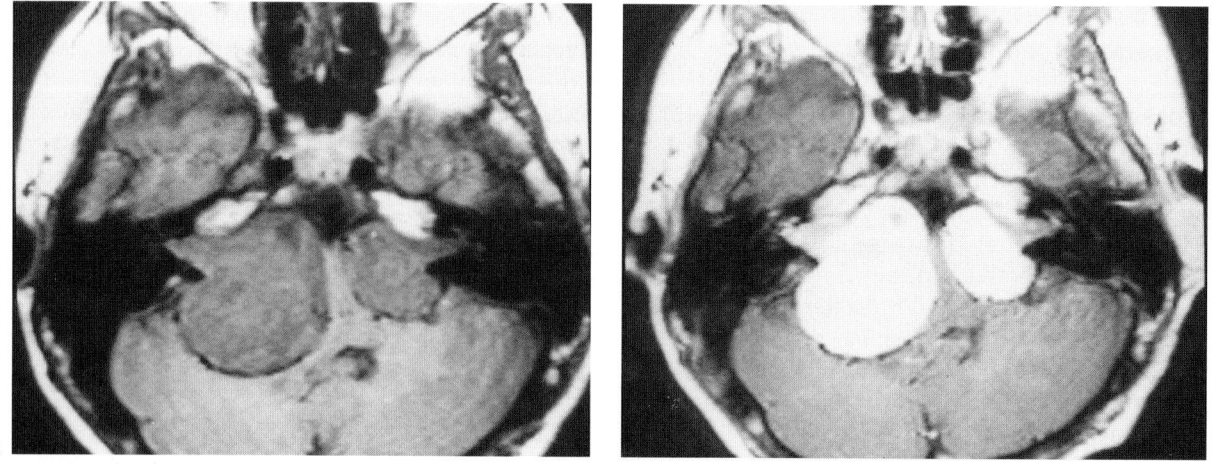

Fig. 7.18a,b. Bilateral vestibular schwannoma. **a** Axial T1-weighted image shows bilateral cerebellopontine angle mass with extension into the internal auditory canals. **b** Axial post-contrast T1-weighted image shows intense enhancement of these masses

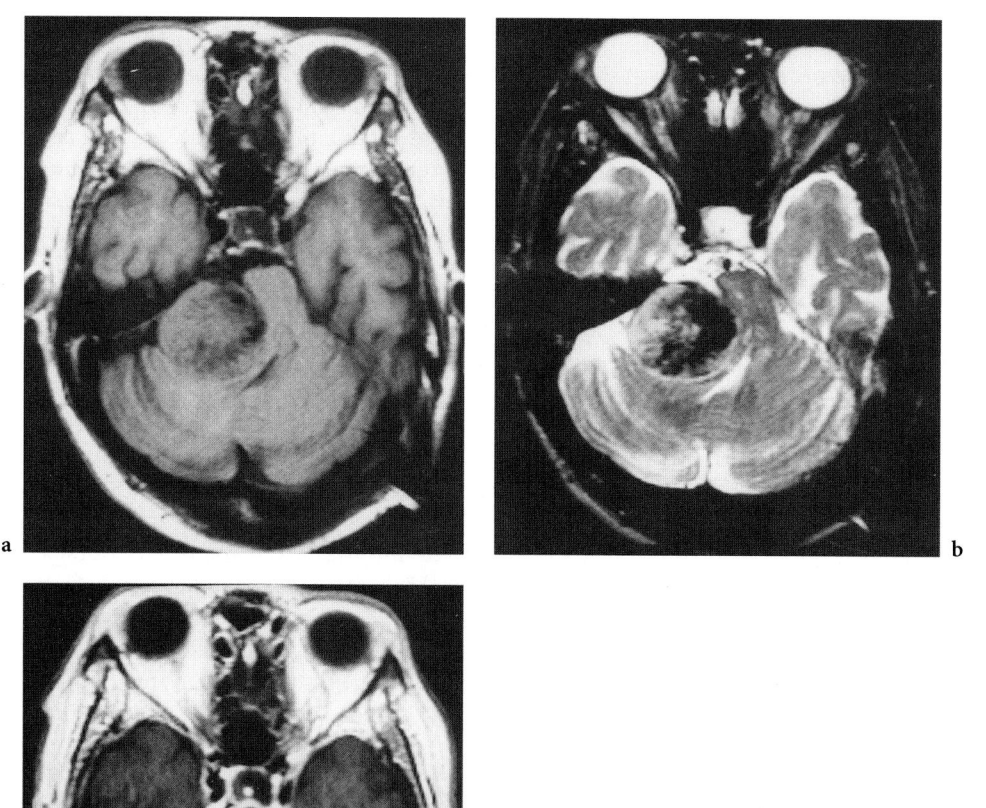

Fig. 7.19a–c. Meningioma. **a** Axial T1-weighted image shows a mixed low and iso-signal mass at the right cerebellopontine angle cistern. **b** Axial T2-weighted image shows the mass to be of predominantly low signal intensity. **c** Axial post-contrast T1-weighted image shows intense contrast enhancement with a focal non-enhancing area due to calcification

7.12.4
Glomus Jugulare Paraganglioma

Glomus jugulare paragangliomas arise in the lateral portion of the jugular foramen. Unenhanced CT shows hyperdense mass and enhanced CT shows intense, homogeneous enhancement. MR shows heterogeneous, mixed intensity lesion with a "salt-and-pepper" appearance on both T1-weighted and T2-weighted images. These small signal voids represent tumor vascularity. Gd-enhanced MR shows intense contrast enhancement (OLSEN 1986).

7.12.5
Metastasis

Metastatic disease can involve the entire skull base. Osteoblastic metastases are usually caused by prostate, breast, colon carcinoma, and Hodgkin's disease. Osteolytic metastases are usually produced by thyroid, renal, and lung carcinoma.

7.13
Imaging Techniques for Tumors of the Spine

The traditional anatomical categorization of spinal tumors into three compartments – extradural (vertebral column and epidural space), intradural extramedullary (within the dura but outside the cord), and intramedullary (within the cord) – is a most useful approach in imaging assessment of spinal lesions. Some lesions, such as nerve sheath tumors, may be found in multiple compartments separately or simultaneously.

MR has become the optimal imaging modality for evaluation of neoplastic disorders of the spine. In particular, the potential of MRI in the evaluation of parenchymal lesions arising from the cord itself was recognized shortly after its inception (HANS et al. 1983; NORMAN et al. 1984). It is superior to myelography and post-myelography computed tomography in the assessment of virtually all tumor categories, including intrathecal subarachnoid metastatic deposits (CARMODY et al. 1989; HEINZ et al. 1995). MRI is also more sensitive than the nuclear scan in detecting primary and metastatic bone lesions of the spine (ALGRA et al. 1991).

Standard MRI protocols change frequently due to the rapid pace of technological development, but routine protocols in the evaluation of neoplastic disease typically include sagittal and axial T1-weighted images with and without intravenous gadolinium-DTPA (Gd-DTPA) contrast, and sagittal and axial T2-weighted images. In the evaluation of bone metastases to the spine, Gd-DTPA contrast is generally unnecessary.

CT and myelography have had limited roles in assessment of spinal tumors since the advent of MRI. Most commonly, they are employed when MRI is contraindicated due to incompatible implant devices or ferromagnetic foreign bodies in potentially precarious anatomic locations. CT may also have a complementary role to MRI in presurgical planning for select cases requiring greater assessment of bone architectural detail. It should be noted, however, that although architectural detail of osseous structures is better visualized with CT, sensitivity to neoplastic involvement of the marrow spaces in the spine is still inferior to MRI (CARMODY et al. 1989).

Unlike MRI, direct acquisition of images of the spine with CT is limited to the axial plane. Sagittal or coronal plane images can then be obtained by reformatting data sets obtained in the axial plane. Routine protocol includes 3-mm cervical and 5-mm thoracic and lumbar slices with soft tissue and bone windowing. Thinner sections may be obtained through an area of interest in the thoracic and lumbar regions. Intravenous contrast has an extremely limited role in CT evaluation of spinal neoplastic disease and may be of limited use only when MRI is contraindicated.

CT of the spine after administration of intrathecal contrast (CT myelography) is typically obtained after conventional plain film myelography. Intrathecal contrast in the subarachnoid space outlines the spinal cord, nerve roots, and filum terminale in detail. Complementary information is obtained from the plain film myelogram which, for instance, affords more detailed visualization of nerve root sleeves.

7.14
Extradural Tumors of the Spine

7.14.1
Benign Extradural Tumors

7.14.1.1
Hemangioma

Hemangiomas are the most common benign tumor of the vertebral column (YOCHUM et al. 1993). They may diffusely replace the vertebral body, but more commonly appear as fairly well-circumscribed geographic lesions. Rarely, they may be primarily extraosseous lesions extending into the epidural space (GOLWYN et al. 1992).

Hemangiomas are typically hyperintense on both T1- and T2-weighted images with a mottled or speckled appearance. Enhancement will be demonstrated if gadolinium is administered, although contrast is not specifically indicated in assessment of these lesions. On MRI images, the main differential diagnostic considerations are bone changes adjacent to degenerative disc disease and metastasis (MODIC 1993). They can usually be readily distinguished from metastatic lesions because, unlike metastatic deposits, hemangiomas will show hyperintense signal on T1-weighted images. However, some hemangiomas with predominantly vascular rather than fatty stroma will show low signal on T1-weighted images and may be difficult to distinguish from metastases (LAREDO et al. 1990). Plain films radiography and CT may be helpful in this instance, showing a striated, "celery stalk" appearance of coarsened, vertically oriented bony trabeculae, which is not a typical feature of metastatic disease. This is identified on CT images as fewer than normal but thickened trabeculae giving rise to a "polka-dot" appearance on axial images (HAUGHTON et al. 1982).

7.14.1.2
Benign Lytic Expansile Tumors

Benign lesions demonstrating similar lytic expansile characteristics include osteoblastoma, aneurysmal bone cyst (ABC), and giant cell tumor (GCT). Because of their similar features, these lesions are usually considered together in radiographic differential diagnosis. Osteoblastoma and aneurysmal bone cysts are benign expansile lytic bone tumors that most commonly involve the posterior arches of the spine, but may involve the vertebral body as well (NEMOTO et al. 1990). Giant cell tumors commonly involve both the anterior and posterior columns, and although typically benign, may behave aggressively with malignant degeneration in 10% of cases (DE SMEDT et al. 1999). With all of these lesions, CT will demonstrate an expansile lytic lesion with a thin sclerotic rim. Osteoblastomas often contain mottled calcifications, while ABCs and GCTs do not. MRI demonstrates predominantly low signal on T1- and high signal on T2-weighted images, with heterogeneous areas of mixed signal due to varying amounts of blood products and, in the case of osteoblastoma, calcifications. ABCs and to a lesser extent GCTs, contain multiloculated cystic

areas containing blood product fluid–fluid levels (AOKI et al. 1991; MUNK et al. 1989). Contrast enhancement is present with gadolinium administration with all of these lesions. Additional differential diagnostic considerations include brown tumors of hyperparathyroidism, malignant tumors such as plasmacytoma, chordoma, or expansile metastases such as thyroid or renal cell carcinoma.

7.14.1.3
Eosinophilic Granuloma

Eosinophilic granuloma (EG) is actually a non-neoplastic lesion primarily affecting children and young adults (POST 1988). This is seen as a geographic lytic lesion without a sclerotic rim in the vertebral body on plain film and CT. It is hyperintense on T2- and variable signal on T1-weighted MR images enhancing strongly with contrast. Near-complete collapse of a vertebral body (vertebra plana) is a common presentation (DE SCHEPPER et al. 1993).

7.14.2
Malignant Extradural Tumors

7.14.2.1
Metastasis

Metastatic tumors are by far the most common extradural malignant neoplasms, most commonly originating in the breast, prostate, and lung carcinoma in adults, and Ewing sarcoma and neuroblastoma in children (BYRNE 1992; KLEIN et al. 1991). Metastases to the spine most frequently involve the vertebral body, but any part of the vertebra may be involved.

Metastases are most commonly lytic lesions with variable degrees of ill-definition of margins and destructiveness on plain radiography and CT appearance. Breast and prostate carcinoma metastases can also be sclerotic (blastic) or mixed lytic–sclerotic. With plain film and CT modalities, myelographic contrast is needed to determine the extent of epidural disease. Nuclear scintigraphy is more sensitive than plain radiographs or CT, but is not specific and may be positive in cases of infection or trauma. MRI is even more sensitive and specific than nuclear bone scanning and also affords evaluation of the extent of epidural tumor and compromise of the spinal canal or neural foramina. Metastatic lesions are typically low signal intensity on T1- and high signal intensity on T2-weighted images.

A common diagnostic problem arises in differentiating pathologic compression fractures due to metastatic disease from acute or subacute benign osteoporotic compression fractures, which show the same general characteristics on MRI. There are only two reliable distinguishing features – extension of abnormal signal into the pedicle and posterior arch, and a significant extraosseous soft tissue component – seen with metastases but typically not with benign disease (BAKER et al. 1990). Involvement of non-compressed vertebral bodies elsewhere also points toward a metastatic process, but ultimately diagnostic overlap cannot be absolutely avoided.

7.14.2.2
Chordoma

Chordomas arise from notochordal remnants within the vertebral body and are most common in the sacrum, followed by the clivus. Only about 15% arise within the vertebral bodies. Vertebral chordomas often involve the adjacent intervertebral disc, and can thus cross disc spaces.

On CT images, some element of bone destruction is always demonstrated. There is a soft tissue mass with frequent calcification and mixed cystic and solid components. On MRI images, chordomas have an inhomogeneous cystic and solid appearance as well, predominantly low signal intensity on T1-weighted images, and, notably as a diagnostic feature, equal or slightly hyperintense signal compared to CSF on proton-density and T2-weighted images. The major radiographic differential diagnosis is giant cell tumor and metastasis (SZE et al. 1988; JEYER et al. 1984).

7.14.2.3
Plasmacytoma and Multiple Myeloma

Plasmacytoma and multiple myeloma are, respectively, the solitary and multicentric forms of the same cellular neoplasm (monoclonal plasma cells), both primarily affecting the elderly. The spine is the most frequent site, and the vertebral body is usually involved before extension into the pedicle. Pathologic fractures and epidural extension are frequent.

Characteristically, bone scans are negative, differentiating these lesions from metastases. Plain X-ray and CT demonstrate a variety of appearances, from diffuse osteopenia due to diffuse marrow infiltration, to sharply circumscribed, "punched out" lesions, to bubbly, lytic expansile lesions (seen with plasmacytoma but typically not with myeloma). On

MRI, signal characteristics are typical for highly cellular lesions with high nucleus:cytoplasm ratios such as lymphoma – intermediate signal intensity on T1- and mildly hyperintense signal on T2-weighted images relative to normal spinal cord signal intensity (LIBSHITZ et al. 1992; RAHMOUNI et al. 1993).

7.14.2.4
Lymphoma

Non-Hodgkin's lymphoma most commonly involves the spine secondarily as metastases, although it can arise in the spine de novo. When arising in the bony skeleton, it more commonly arises in the long bones than in the spine. Hodgkin's disease is much less common and usually occurs in younger patients than non-Hodgkin's lymphoma (PARKER et al. 1980). Pathologic fractures with epidural extension and spinal cord compression can occur and are best delineated by MRI or CT myelography.

Plain film and CT findings of bone involvement show a wide spectrum of appearances, ranging from lytic permeative or moth-eaten patterns to discrete geographic destructive lesions to rare hyperostotic sclerotic lesions, giving rise to the "ivory vertebra" appearance (POST 1988). MRI typically shows intermediate to low signal on T1- and a somewhat heterogeneous mildly hyperintense signal on T2-weighted images. The rare osteosclerotic lesions will show lower signal intensity on all sequences.

7.14.2.5
Sarcomas

Sarcomas include Ewing sarcoma, osteogenic sarcoma, chondrosarcoma, and fibrosarcoma. De novo involvement of the spine in all of these lesions is quite rare.

Ewing sarcoma is the most common of these lesions to involve the spine, but much more commonly as a secondary metastatic process from another site. It is a lesion of older children and young adults and usually involves the vertebral body and epidural space. Plain radiographs and CT are limited in their assessment of marrow space involvement, usually showing only permeative bone changes which can be subtle (GINALDI et al. 1980). CT is able to demonstrate extraosseous soft tissue components as well. MRI more accurately depicts both marrow space and extraosseous disease. Like other highly cellular neoplasms, Ewing sarcoma is typically mildly isointense on T1- and mildly hyperintense on T2-weighted images.

Osteosarcomas, in the rare instances that they arise in the spine, usually occur in previously irradiated bone or in underlying Paget's disease. Plain radiography and CT show a mass with calcified bone tumor matrix formation. MRI appearance varies with the amount of osteoid, bone, calcified matrix, and hemorrhage (OSBORN 1991).

Chondrosarcomas are even less frequent than osteosarcomas in the spine, arising from malignant degeneration of osteochondromas or hereditary multiple exostoses. Plain X-ray and CT show lytic lesions with variable matrix calcification having a characteristic pattern of rings and arcs. They may cross disc spaces to involve contiguous levels. MRI or CT myelography best delineate spinal canal involvement.

Fibrosarcomas are extremely rare and are typically lytic, destructive, somewhat expansile masses without matrix calcification (DORWART et al. 1983).

7.15
Intradural Extramedullary Tumors of the Spine

There are two main categories of intradural extramedullary neoplasms – primary tumors, which include nerve sheath tumors and meningioma, and intradural arachnoid implants or "drop" metastases.

7.15.1
Nerve Sheath Tumors

Nerve sheath tumors are considered under the heading of intradural tumors, which they most commonly are. However, a minority are partially extradural (15%) or completely extradural (27%) in location (GAUTIER-SMITH 1967). In adults, there are two main types of nerve sheath tumors: schwannoma (neurinoma, neurilemoma) and neurofibroma. They are typically benign lesions, but on rare occasions can be malignant de novo or undergo malignant transformation (SORDILLO et al. 1981).

Although schwannomas are typically encapsulated lesions that usually arise eccentrically from the sheath of the parent nerve, while neurofibromas are unencapsulated lesions that envelop, arise within, and expand the parent nerve in fusiform fashion, the two types cannot reliably be distinguished by imaging (OKAZAKI 1983). Schwannomas are generally solitary lesions, while neurofibromas tend to be mul-

tiple and more commonly associated with neurofibromatosis, although both can be isolated lesions.

Plain film findings include posterior scalloping of the vertebral bodies and widening of the neural foramina. On CT images, they are of relatively low attenuation and may appear as the classic "dumbbell" tumor when partially extradural. Myelographic appearance is nonspecific, showing an intradural extramedullary filling defect displacing the cord. Calcification and hemorrhage are rare. On MRI, they are typically lobulated lesions that are isointense to the cord on T1- and markedly hyperintense on T2-weighted images due to the high water content of these lesions, but cystic change, hemorrhage, and necrosis are not uncommon, giving rise to a heterogeneous range of appearances (DEMACHI et al. 1992). They virtually all enhance with contrast administration. There are no reliable features to distinguish benign from malignant forms, but malignant lesions tend to be larger and have more irregular, infiltrative margins (Fig. 7.20). The major differential diagnostic consideration is meningioma (VARMA et al. 1992; LEVINE et al. 1987).

7.15.2
Meningioma

Like nerve sheath tumors, spinal meningiomas can be partially or completely extradural, although much less commonly; they can also be associated with neurofibromatosis syndromes. Plain films are usually unremarkable. The myelographic appearance of

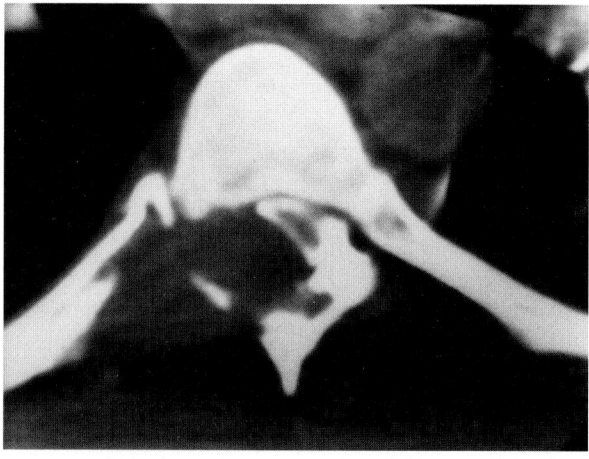

Fig. 7.20. Malignant schwannoma axial post-myelogram CT shows a mass with bone destruction of the right rib and posterior elements. The spinal cord is compressed and displaced anteriorly to the right

meningiomas is nonspecific as is the case with nerve sheath tumors, showing an intradural extramedullary filling defect typically displacing the cord. On CT images without contrast, the occasional presence of calcifications may be a distinguishing feature from schwannomas, which typically do not calcify, and they tend to be of higher attenuation than nerve sheath tumors. MRI is most reliable in distinguishing typical meningiomas from nerve sheath tumors. Unlike schwannomas, meningiomas are isointense to the cord on both T1- and T2-weighted images (Fig. 7.21), and most will show a broad-based dural attachment, sometimes with a "tail" of enhancement along the adjacent dura (the so-called dural tail sign) (MATSUMOTO et al. 1993). As in the brain, there are less common atypical forms of meningioma that may show cystic or necrotic areas, as well as more aggressive or malignant forms that give rise to more variation in imaging appearances.

Hemangiopericytomas are rare aggressive tumors that were previously considered to be an aggressive variant of meningioma, one of the so-called angioblastic forms of meningioma, but they are now considered to be separate entities in the WHO classification of nervous system tumors (RUSSELL et al. 1989; WORLD HEALTH ORGANIZATION 1990). Their imaging characteristics are identical to aggressive angioblastic meningiomas.

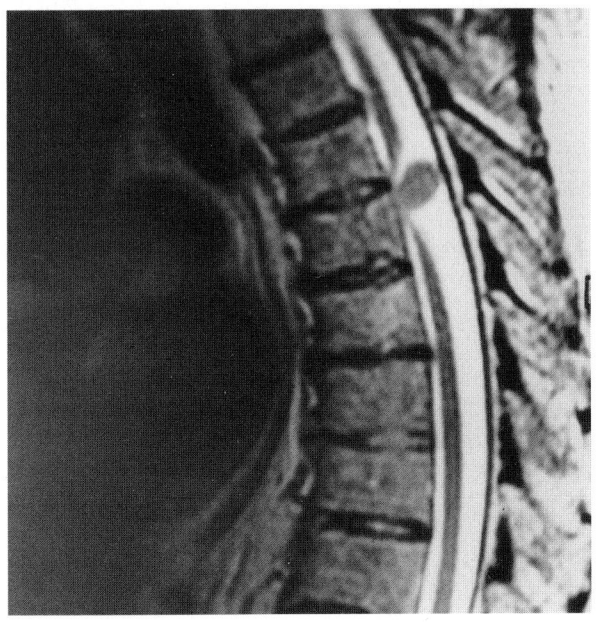

Fig. 7.21. Spinal meningioma sagittal T2-weighted image shows an isointense intradural, extramedullary mass in the thoracic spine

7.15.3
Intradural Implants

The most common tumors to metastasize to the intradural compartment are from the CNS, but systemic tumors outside the CNS may also do so. Overall, the most common leptomeningeal metastatic primary tumor in the pediatric population is the medulloblastoma, with glioblastoma being the next most frequent. Ependymoma, oligodendroglioma, astrocytoma, retinoblastoma, and pineal tumors follow in frequency (BRYAN 1974). Systemic tumors are usually carcinomas from the lung, breast, melanoma, or lymphoma and leukemia, and these frequently involve the dura itself (SCHUKNECHT et al. 1992). Obviously, the need to detect the presence of subarachnoid spread of tumor is of great importance as it generally signifies the need for spinal axis radiation.

Intradural metastases are most common on the pial surface of the cord. There are two main imaging modalities for the detection of subarachnoid metastases – MRI and CT myelography. Overall, MRI is more sensitive than CT myelography if gadolinium contrast is administered (HEINZ et al. 1995). MRI typically shows either enhancing nodules of varying size (usually quite small) or diffuse coating of the cord, nerve roots, or dura. It is particularly in this latter situation of diffuse coating that MRI demonstrates superiority to CT myelography. CT myelography will show either nodular filling defects or areas of irregularity of the thecal sac or nerve roots. CT myelography may occasionally show lesions missed by MRI, usually if the lesions are very localized small nodular lesions or if there is only subtle irregularity of the thecal sac. MRI is superior to CT myelography particularly when there is diffuse coating of the thecal sac and cord (SZE 1996).

It should be noted that direct examination of the CSF is still the most sensitive modality for detection of subarachnoid metastases, despite the sensitivity of MRI. Nevertheless, imaging may be clinically important to optimize spinal axis treatment if there is focal involvement by directing therapy to appropriate areas.

7.16
Intramedullary Tumors

Intramedullary tumors are lesions of the spinal cord, of which gliomas, including ependymoma and astrocytoma, constitute more than 90% of cases. Hemangioblastoma and intramedullary metastases from systemic primaries are very uncommon. Oligodendrogliomas, ganglion cell tumors (ganglioglioma and gangliocytoma), and intramedullary schwannomas have rarely been reported to arise within the spinal cord (ATLAS et al. 1996).

7.16.1
Ependymoma

Ependymomas are overall the most common primary tumor of the spinal cord, although in the pediatric population astrocytomas occur twice as frequently (OSBORN 1991). Because they arise from the ependymal cells or remnants lining the central canal, they tend to be central in location and expand the cord centrifugally.

Plain films are frequently positive, demonstrating widening of the canal with erosion of the pedicles or posterior aspects of the vertebral bodies. CT myelography typically shows bone changes as well as nonspecific widening of the cord, and multisegmental lesions are common (McCORMICK et al. 1990). Unlike ependymomas of the brain, calcification is extremely uncommon in the spine. MRI also delineates these features, but in addition directly demonstrates the tumor, which is typically isointense to the cord on T1- and hyperintense on T2-weighted images. Prominent enhancement is noted with contrast. Mixed, heterogeneous signal will occur if there is cyst formation, hemorrhage, or necrosis, which are common features (NEMOTO et al. 1992). The primary differential diagnosis is astrocytoma, for which there is no reliable feature to differentiate the two, although hemorrhage and sharply circumscribed margins are not as common in astrocytomas. Both frequently show intratumoral cyst formation and extratumoral syrinx formation. Ependymomas are more common in the lower thoracic and lumbar region (Fig. 7.22), while astrocytomas tend to occur in the cervical and thoracic regions. In addition, small tumors of the filum may appear to be intradural extramedullary lesions and can be indistinguishable from schwannomas.

A subtype of ependymoma that arises exclusively in the conus medullaris and filum terminale is the myxopapillary ependymoma. They are slow-growing tumors that can attain a large size, filling and expanding the spinal canal, even expanding into the neural foramina. They typically show a heterogeneous appearance on MRI, reflecting the presence of hemorrhage and cystic degeneration, with an almost plastic, gelatinous configuration within the canal (MOELLEKEN et al. 1992).

7.16.2
Astrocytoma

Most spinal cord astrocytomas are low-grade fibrillary lesions which expand the cord; pilocytic astrocytomas and anaplastic astrocytomas are much less common, and glioblastoma multiforme in the cord is very rare. The cervical cord is the most common location, followed by the thoracic cord (SZE 1996).

Plain films are usually normal, although occasionally, widening of the canal may be seen. CT myelography shows nonspecific enlargement of the cord. MRI demonstrates a lesion that is usually ill-defined and slightly hypointense to the cord on T1-weighted images and hyperintense on T2-weighted images. Contrast enhancement is virtually always present, unlike astrocytomas in the brain which typically enhance significantly only when of higher grade. Intra-

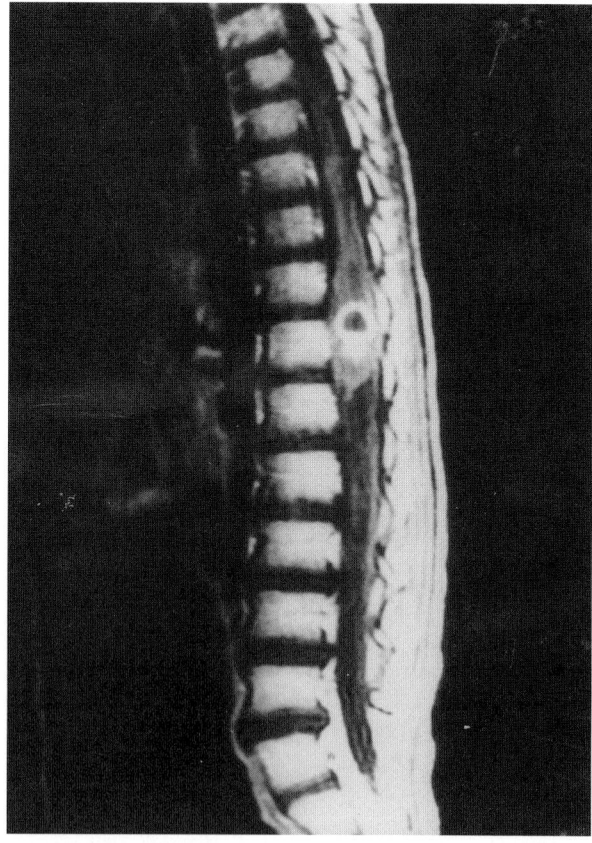

Fig. 7.22. Spinal ependymoma sagittal post-contrast T1-weighted image shows a ring-like enhancing lesion at the conus medullaris with enlargement of the cord

tumoral cyst formation, as well as secondary syrinx formation are common and well-delineated by MRI (GOY et al. 1986). As noted above, the main differential diagnostic consideration is ependymoma.

7.16.3
Hemangioblastoma

Hemangioblastomas are rare, usually solitary tumors of the cord. When multiple, they are usually in association with von Hippel-Lindau disease; in fact, one-third of patients with hemangioblastomas have von Hippel-Lindau disease. Almost all of these lesions arise either in the cervical or thoracic regions, with thoracic lesions slightly more common. They are rare in the lumbar region or conus.

CT myelography typically demonstrates a nonspecific intramedullary mass, but 10–15% have significant extramedullary components and may thus appear as an intradural extramedullary lesion on myelography. The prominent feeding arteries and draining veins associated with their hypervascularity can be seen as serpiginous filling defects on CT and plain film myelography. Angiography demonstrates a highly vascular mass with dense, prolonged tumor stain and enlarged draining veins. On MR imaging, the tumor is solid in less than 50% of cases, with the majority of lesions demonstrating a cyst containing a strongly enhancing nodule. The hypervascularity may be seen as flow voids within the solid portion of the tumor. MRI will also demonstrate flow voids representing the enlarged feeding and draining vessels in the adjacent subarachnoid space (KENDALL et al. 1966; KATTENBERGER et al. 1988). The solid portion of the tumor enhances strongly with contrast administration.

7.16.4
Intramedullary Metastasis

Intramedullary metastasis is an extremely uncommon occurrence, with carcinoma of the lung being the most common systemic neoplasm to metastasize to the spinal cord. The thoracic cord is the most frequent region involved. Plain films are typically normal, unless bone metastases are present. CT and myelography show only nonspecific findings of focal enlargement of the cord. MRI is also not specific, showing a focal cord mass. However, a potentially helpful differentiating feature is that the amount of edema in the adjacent cord is frequently out of proportion to the size of the

tumor. Also, unlike primary tumors, metastatic lesions of the cord rarely have cysts. Virtually all intramedullary metastatic lesions enhance with contrast (JELLINGER et al. 1979; SZE et al. 1988).

7.17
Conclusion

MR imaging is the modality of choice in the evaluation of intracranial and spinal tumors due to its superior soft tissue resolution, multi-planar imaging capability, and flexible data acquisition protocols. It plays a significant role in the diagnosis, in directing stereotactic biopsy and surgical planning, in planning radiation treatment, and in the follow-up evaluation of patients treated with radiation therapy. Despite its superiority to CT, there are times when information obtained from MR imaging is not able to define the true extent of the tumor margin to separate radiation treatment effects from tumor progression. Under these circumstances, functional imaging techniques such as positron emission tomography or MR spectroscopy can be utilized.

References

Ahmadi et al. (1985) Cavernous sinus invasion by pituitary adenomas. AJNR 6:893–898

Ahmadi et al. (1992) Cystic Fluid in craniopharyngioma: MR imaging and quantitative analysis. Radiology 182: 783–785

Alger JR, Frank JA, Bizzi A, et al. (1990) Metabolism of human gliomas: Assessment with H-1 MR spectroscopy and F-18 fluordeoxyglucose PET. Radiology 177:633–631

Algra PR, Bloem JL, Tissing H et al. (1991) Detection of vertebral metastases: comparison between MR imaging and bone scintigraphy. Radiographics 11:219–232

Aoki J, Moriya K, Yamashita K et al. (1991) Giant cell tumors of bone containing large amounts of hemosiderin: MR-pathologic correlation. J Comp Asst Tomogr 15:1024–1027

Atlas SW, Lavi E (1996) Intra-axial brain tumors. In Atlas SW, ed, magnetic Resonance Imaging of the Brain and Spine, 2nd Edition. Philadelphia, Lippincott-Raven Publishers, pp. 315–422

Baker LL, Goodman SB, Perkash I, et al. (1990) Benign versus pathologic compression fractures of vertebral bodies: assessment with conventional spin-echo chemical-shift and STIR MR imaging. Radiology 174:495–502

Boorstein JM, Wong KT, Grossman RI, et al. (1994) Metastatic lesions of the brain: Imaging with magnetization transfer. Radiology 191:799–803

Bryan P (1974) CSF seeding of intracranial tumors: a study of 96 cases. Clin Radiol 25:355–360

Burger PC, Bogel FS, Green SB, et al. ('985) Glioblastomas multiforme and anaplastic astrocytoma: Pathologic criteria and prognostic implications. Cancer 56:1106–1111

Byrne TN (1992) Spinal cord compression from epidural metastases. New England Journal of Medicine 327:614–619

Carmody RF, Yang DJ, Seeley GW, Seeger JF, Unger EC, Johnson JF (1989) Spinal cord compression due to metastatic disease: diagnosis with MR imaging versus myelography. Radiology 173:225–229

Chiechi M, Smirniotopoulos JG, Mena H (1996) Intracranial hemangiopericytomas: MR and CT features. AJNR Am J Neuroradiol 17:1365–1371

Coates TL et al. (1989) Pediatric choroids plexus neoplasms: MR, CT, and pathologic correlation. Radiology 173:81–188

Davis PC et al. (1987) Leptomeningeal metastasis: MR imaging. Radiology 163:449

Davis PC, Wichman RD, Takei Y, et al. (1990) Primary cerebral neuroblastoma: CT and MR findings in 12 cases. AJNR Am J Neuroradiol 11:115–120

De Schepper AMA, Ramon F, Van Marck E (1993) MR imaging of eosinophilic granuloma: report of 11 cases. Skeletal Radiology 22:163–166

Dean BL, Drayer BP, Bird CR, et al. (1990) gliomas: Classificaiton with MR imaging. Radiology 174:411–415

Demachi H, Takashima T, Kadoya M et al (1992) MR imaging of spinal neurinomas with pathological correlation. J Comp Asst Tomogr 14:250–254

Di Chiro G (1986) Positron emission tomography using F-18-fluorodeoxyglucose in brain tumors: A powerful diagnostic and prognostic tool. Invest Radiol 22:360–371

Dorwart RH, LaMasters DL, Watanabe TJ (1983) Tumors. In Newton TH, Potts DG, editors, Computed Tomography of the Spine and Spinal Cord. Clavadel Press, San Anselmo, pp. 115–147

Elster AD et al. (1989) Meningiomas: MR and histopathologic features. Radiology 170:857–862

Ernest F IV et al. (1998) Cerebral astrocytomas: Histopathological correlation of MR and CT contrast enhancement with sterotactic biopsy. Radiology 166:823–827

Fischbein NJ, Prados MD, Wara W, et al. (1996) Radiologic classification of brain stem tumors: Correlation of magnetic resonance imaging appearance with clinical outcome. Pediatr Neurosurg 24:9–23

Freeman CR, Farmer JP (1998) Pediatric brain stem gliomas: A review. Int J Radiat Oncol Biol Phys 40:265–271

Gautier-Smith PC (1967) Clinical aspects of spinal neurofibromatosis. Brain 90:359–393

Gill SS, Thomas DG, Van Bruggen N, et al. (1990) Proton MR spectroscopy of intracranial tumors: In vivo and in vitro studies. J. Comput Assist Tomogr 14:497–504

Ginaldi S, deSantos LA (1980) Computed tomography in the evaluation of small round cell tumors of bone. Rdiology 134:441–446

Golwyn DH, Cardenas CA, Murtagh FR et al. (1992) MRI of a cervical extradural cavernous hemangioma. Neuroradiology 34:68–69

Goy AM, Pinto RS, Raghavenda BN, Epstein FJ, Kricheff II (1986) Intramedullary spinal cord tumors: MR imaging with emphasis on associated cysts. Radiology 161:381–386

Grossman CB, Post JD (1985) The adult spine. In: Gonzalez CF, Grossman CB, Masdeu JM, eds. Head and Spine Imaging. John Wiley & Sons, New York, pp 781–858

Hans JS, Kaufman B, El Yousef SJ, et al. (1983) NMR imaging of the spine. AJNR 4:1151–1159

Haughton VM, Williams AL, eds. (1982) Computed tomography of the Spine. CV Mosby, St. Louis

Haustein J, Laniado M, Niendorf HP, et al. (1992) Administration of gadopentetate dimeglumine in MR imaging of intracranial tumors: Dosage and field strength. AJNR Am J Neuroradiol 13:1199–1206

Heinz R, Wiener D, Friedman H, Tien R (1995) Detection of cerebrospinal fluid metastasis: CT myelography or MR? AJNR 16:1147–1151

Ho VB et al. (1992) Radiologic-pathologic correlation: Hemangioblastoma. AJNR 13:1343–1352

Hustinx R, Alavi A (1999) SPECT and PET Imaging of Brain Tumors. Neuroimaging Clinics of North America, Vol 9, No 4, pp 751–766

Jelinek J, Smirniotopoulos JG, Parisi JE, et al. (1990) Lateral ventricular neoplasms of the brain: Differential diagnosis based on clinical, CT, and MR findings. AJR Am J Roentgenol 155:365–372

Jellinger K, Kothbauer P, Sunder-Plassmann E, Weiss R (1979) Intramedullary spinal cord metastases. Journal of Neurology 22:31–41

Jeyer JE, Lepke RA, Lindfors KKI, et al. (1984) Chordomas: Their CT appearance in cervical, thoracic and lumbar spine. Radiology 15:693–696

Kattenberger DA, Shah CP, Murtagh FR et al (1988) MR imaging of spinal cord hemangioblastoma associated with syringomyelia. J Comp Asst Tomogr 12:495–498

Ken JG et al. (1991) Choriod plexus papillomas of the foramen of Luschka: MR appearance. AJNR 12;1201–1202

Kendall B, Russell J (1966) Hemangioblastomas of the spinal cord. British Journal of Radiology 39:817–823

Kernohan JW, Sayre GP (1952) Atlas of Tumor Pathology. Fascicle 35. Washington, DC, Armed Forces Institute of Pathology

Kim EE, Chung SK, Haynie TP, et al. (1992) Differentiation of residual or recurrent tumors from post-treatment changes with F-18 FDG PET. Radiographics 12:269–279

Klein SL, Sanford RA, Muhlbauer MS (1991) Pediatric spinal epidural metastases. Journal of Neurosurgery 74:70–75

Koci TM et al. (1993) Adult cerebellar medulloblastoma: Imaging features with emphasis on MR. AJNR 14;929–939

Laredo J-D, Assouline E, Gelbert F et al. (1990) Vertebral hemangiomas: fat content as a sign of aggressiveness. Radiology 177:467–472

Lee Y, Van Tassel P, Bruner JM, et al. (1989) juvenile pilocytic astrocytomas: CT and MR characteristics. AJNR Am J Neruoradiol 10:363–370

Lee Y, Van Tassel P (1989) Intracranial oligodendrogliomas: Imaging findings in 35 untreated cases. AJNR Am J Neuroradiol 10:119–127

Levine E, Huntrakoon M, Wetzel LH (1987) Malignant nerve-sheath neoplasms in neurofibromatosis: distinction from benign tumors by using imaging techniques. AJR 149:1059–1064

Libshitz HI, Malthouse SR, Cunningham D et al. (1992) Multiple myeloma: appearance at MR imaging. Radiology 182:833–837

Lizak PF, Woodruff WW (1992) Posterior fossa neoplasms: Multiplanar imaging. Semin Ultrasound, CT, MRI 13:182–206

Luk et al. (1999) Imaging of Brain Tumors in the Pediatric Population. Neuroimaging Clinic of North Am. Vol 9, No 4, pp 691–716

Matsumoto S, Hasu K, Uchino A et al. (1993) MRI of intradural-extramedullary spinal neurinomas and meningiomas. Clinical Imaging 17:46–52

McCormick PC, Torres R, Post KD, Stein BM (1990) Intramedullary ependymoma of the spinal cord. J Neurosurg 62:523–532

Meyers SP et al. (1992) MR imaging features of medulloblastomas. AJR 158:865–895

Meyers SP et al. (1992) Chondrosarcomas fo the skull base: MR imaging features. Radiology 184:103

Modic MT, Steinberg PM, Ross JC, et al. (1988) Degenerative disc disease: Assessment of changes in vertebral body marrow with MR imaging. Radiology 168:177–186

Moelleken SMC, Suger LL, Eckardt JJ, Batzdorf U (1992) Myrxopapillary ependymoma with extensive sacral destruction: CT and MR findings. J Comp Asst Tomogr 16:164–166

Munk PL, Helms CA, Holt RG et al. (1989) MR imaging of aneurysmal bone cysts. AJR 153:99–101

Naidich TP, Zimmerman RA (1984) Primary brain tumors in children. Semin Roentgenol 19:100–114

Negendank WG, Sauter R, Brown TR, et al. (1996) Proton magnetic resonance spectroscopy in patients with glial tumors: A multicenter trial. J Neurosurg 84:449–458

Nemoto O, Moser RP JR, Van Dam BE et al. (1990) Osteoblastoma of the spine: a review of 75 cases. Spine 15:1272–1280

Nemoto Y, Inoue Y, Tashiro T et al. (1992) Intramedullary spinal cord tumors: significance of associated hemorrhage at MR imaging. Radiology 182:793–796

Norman D, Mill C, Brant-Zawadski M, Yeates A, Crooks LE, Kaufman L (1984) Magnetic resonance imaging of the spinal cord and canal: potential and limitations. AJNR 5:9–14

Okazaki H (1983) Fundamentals of Neuropathology. Igaku-Shoin, New York, pp. 208–214

Olsen WI et al. (1986) MR imaging of paragangliomas. AJNR 7:1039

Oot RF et al: (1989) The role of MR and CT in evaluating clival chordomas and chondrosarcomas. AJR 151:567–575

Osborn AG, Post MJD (1991) Handbook of Neuroradiology. Mosby Year-Book, St. Louis, pp. 375–384

Packer RJ et al. (1992) Choroid plexus carcinoma of childhood. Cancer 69:580–585

Pahapill PA, Ramsay DA, Del Maestro RF (1996) Pleomorphic xanthoastrocytoma: Case report and analysis of the literature concerning the efficacy of resection and the significance of necrosis. Neurosurgery 38:822–828

Palma L et al. (1993) Supratentorial ependymomas of the first two decades of life: Long-term followup of 20 cases (including two subependymoma). Neurosurgery 32:169–175

Parker BR, Marglin S, Castllino RA (1980) Skeletal manifestations of leukemia, Hodgkin disease, and non-Hodgkin lymphoma. Semin Roentgenol 15:302–315

Post MJD (1988) Primary spine and cord neoplasms. In: Categorical Course on Spine and Cord Imaging, American Society of Neuroradiology, pp. 58–70

Rahmouni A, Divine M, Mathieu D et al (1993) Detection of multiple myeloma involving the spine: efficiency of fat-suppression and contrast-enhanced MR imaging. AJR 160:1049–1052

Roman-Goldstein SM, Goldman DL, Howieson J, et al. (1992) MR of primary CNS lymphoma in immunologically normal patients. AJNR Am J Neuroradiol 13:1207–1213

Ruiz A, Donovan-Post MJ, Bundschu C, et al. (1998) Primary central nervous system lymphoma in patients with AIDS. Neuroimaging Clin North Am 7:281–296

Russell DS, Rubinstein LJ (1989) Pathology of Tumors of the Nervous System, 5th ed. Williams and Wilkins, Baltimore.

Schubeus P et al. (1990) Intracranial meningiomas: Comparison of plain and contrast-enhanced examinations in CT and MR. Neuroradiology 32:12–18

Schuknecht B, Huber P, Buller B, Nadjmi M (1992) Spinal leptomeningeal neoplastic disease. Eur Neurol 32:11–16

Sordillo PP, Helson L, Hajdu SI, et al. (1981) malignant schwannoma – clinical characteristics, survival and response to therapy. Cancer 10:2503–2509

Spoto GP et al. (1990) Intracranial ependymoma and subependymoma: MR manifestations. AJNR 11:83–91

Swartz JD, Zimmerman RA, Bilaniuk LT (1982) Computed tomography of intracranial ependymomas. Radiology 143:97–101

Sze G (1996) Neoplastic disease of the spine and spinal cord. In Atlas SW, ed, Magnetic Resonance Imaging of the Brain and Spine, 2nd Edition. Philadelphia, Lippincott-Raven Publishers, pp.1339–1385

Sze G, Krol G, Zimmerman RD, Deck MDF (1988) Intramedullary disease of the spine: diagnosis using gadolinium-DTPA enhanced MR imaging. AJNR 9:847–858

Sze G, Uichanco LS III, Brant-Zawadski MN, et al. (1988) Chordomas: MR imaging. Radiology 166:187–191

Tien RD (1991) Intraventricular mass lesions of the brain: CT and MR findings. AJR Am J roentegenol 157:1283–1290

Tonn JC, Paulus W, Warmuth-Metz M, et al. (1997) Pleomorphic xanthoastrocytoma: Report of six cases with special consideration of diagnostic and therapeutic pitfalls. Surg Neurol 47:162–169

Tortori-Donati P, Fondelli MP, Cama A, et al. (1995) Ependymomas of the posterior cranial fossa: CT and MRI findings. Neuroradiology 37:238–243

Varma DGK, Moulopoulos A, Sara AS et al. (1992) MR imaging of extracranial nerve sheath tumors. J Comp Asst Tomgr 16:448–453

Vonofakos d, Marcu H, Hacker H (1979) Oligodendrogliomas: CT patterns with emphasis on features indicating malignancy. J Comput Assist tomogr 3:783–788

World Health Organization (1990) Classification of Brain Tumors. Zurich, WHO.

Yochum TR, Lile RL, Schultz GD et al. (1993) Acquired spinal stenosis secondary to an expanding thoracic vertebral hemangioma. Spine 18:299–305

Yuh WT et al. (1992) Experience with high dose gadolinium MR imaging in the evaluation of brain metastases. AJNR 13:335–345

Yuh WT, Nguyen HD, Tali ET, et al. (1994) Delineation of gliomas with various doses of MR contrast material. AJNR Am J Neuroradiol 15:983–989

Zee CS(1996) Intraaxial and Mass Lesions in the Region of the Ventricular System. Neuroradiology: A Study Guide, pp 153–186, McGraw Hill.

Zee CS et al. (1990) MR imaging of pineal region neoplasms. J CAT 15(1):56–63

Zee CS et al. (1992) Magnetic resonance imaging of meningiomas. Semin Ultrasound CT MRI 13:154–169

Zee CS et al. (1993) Intratentorial Tumors in Children. Neuroimaging Clinics of North America. Vol 3, No 4, pp 705–
  714

Zee CS, Segall H, Apuzzo M, et al. (1991) MR imaging of pineal region neoplasms. J Comput Assist Tomogr 15;56–63

Zee CS, Segall HD, Ahmadi J, et al. (1983) Computed tomography of posterior fossa ependymomas in childhood. Surg
  Neurol 20:221

Zee CS, Segall HD, Miller C, et al.(1982) Less common CT
  features of medulloblastoma. Radiology 144:97–102

Zimmerman RA (1990) Central nervous system lymphoma.
  Radiol Clin North Am 28:697–721

Zimmerman RD et al. (1985) Magnetic resonance imaging of
  meningiomas. AJNR 6:149–157

8 Surgical Management of Pituitary Adenomas

Mark D. Krieger, Arun P. Amar, and Martin H. Weiss

CONTENTS

8.1 Introduction

Pituitary adenomas are benign tumors which originate from any of the multiple cell types of the anterior pituitary gland. These tumors come to clinical attention when they result in signs and symptoms of an endocrinopathy, or when they achieve sufficient size to produce mass effect. Surgical resection is usually curative for these benign lesions. However, ther-

M. D. Krieger, MD
Division of Pediatric Neurosurgery, Children's Hospital of Los Angeles, University of Southern California Keck School of Medicine, 1300 North Vermont, Los Angeles, CA 90027, USA
A. P. Amar, MD
Department of Neurological Surgery, University of Southern California, Los Angeles, CA 90033, USA
M. H. Weiss, MD
Professor and Chairman, Department of Neurological Surgery, University of Southern California School of Medicine, LAC and USC Medical Center, 1200 North State Street, Los Angeles, CA 90033, USA

apeutic conundrums arise when total surgical resection is not feasible.

8.2 General Principles

Pituitary adenomas may present early in their growth if they result in an endocrinopathy. Even small adenomas may cause hormonal abnormalities, resulting in a variety of well-defined clinical syndromes. Currently, these tumors are classified according to their hormone production, which determines the clinical syndrome. The most commonly overproduced hormone is prolactin, which results in the amenorrhea-galactorrhea syndrome, and is frequently discovered during infertility work-up. Growth hormone and corticotrophic hormone are seen with the next highest frequency, resulting in acromegaly or gigantism and Cushing's disease, respectively. Overproduction of thyroid stimulating hormone and gonadotrophic hormone are seen with much lower frequency.

When pituitary tumors grow to a large size, they usually present with mass effect (Fig. 8.1). This pattern is more typical of nonfunctioning pituitary adenomas (null cell adenomas), as functional tumors would be more likely to be detected at an earlier stage due to their associated hormonal abnormalities. However, functioning tumors may go undetected (or the patient may describe a vague complaint of feeling "not quite right," which may have been ignored by his/her primary physician) and present with mass effect. As these tumors grow, they protrude beyond the confines of the sella turcica. The optic chiasm, lying directly above the sella turcica, is particularly susceptible to compression from the enlarging tumor. Compression of the chiasm results in a classic bitemporal hemianopsia. Large tumors may also result in headaches and hypopituitarism from compression of the remaining pituitary gland. Null cell tumors are the most common category of pituitary tumors, presenting later in life than functioning tumors.

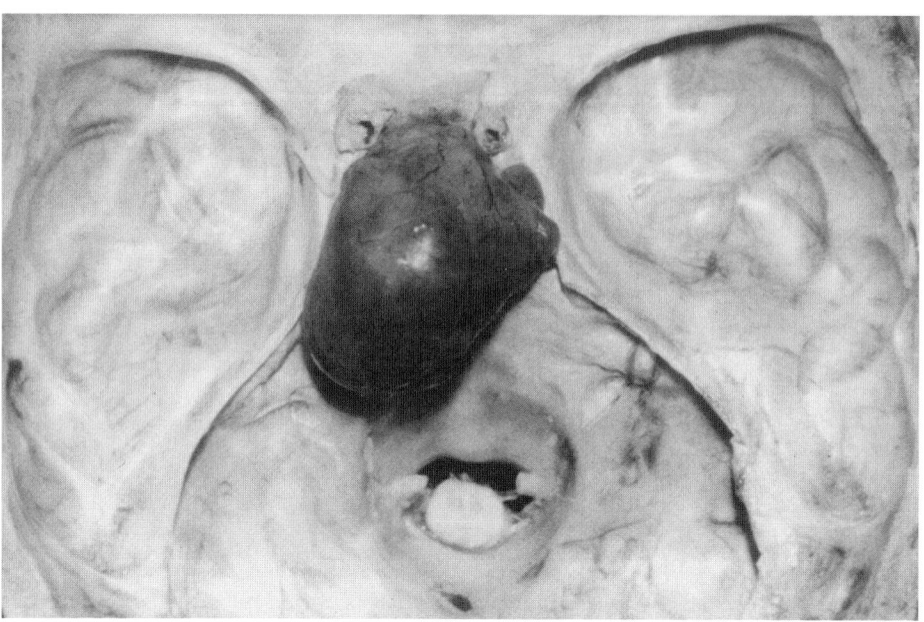

Fig. 8.1. Postmortem examination showing large pituitary tumor with suprasellar extension. Note the proximity of the carotid arteries and remnants of the optic nerves anterior to the tumor

8.2.1
Management

The two major goals for the treatment of all pituitary tumors are: (1) relief of signs and symptoms attributable to mass effect (including visual loss), and (2) correction of associated endocrine abnormalities. It must be kept in mind that even nonsecreting tumors may precipitate hypopituitarism (hormonal undersecretion); thus, a full endocrinologic work-up is always mandated.

Contemporary imaging modalities, such as magnetic resonance imaging (MRI) and computed tomography (CT), combined with the advent of radioimmunoassay techniques to measure minuscule pituitary hormone levels in the blood, have heralded a new era in the detection and management of pituitary adenomas, facilitating the diagnosis, surgical planning, and follow-up care of these patients. Quantification of the hormone levels is particularly important in providing a parameter to determine the response to treatment.

Medical (nonsurgical) therapy is effective only in hypersecreting tumors. Tumors which secrete prolactin or growth hormone are susceptible to this form of management, and medication may be prescribed as a first line treatment. Bromocriptine, a dopamine agonist, suppresses the release of prolactin and results in decreased size of the prolactin-secreting cell population. However, this medication must be taken for life, as the tumor will reachieve its pretherapy size with cessation of the drug. These patients may eventually require surgery if the medication is ineffective or intolerable.

No pharmacologic therapy is available at this point in time for nonfunctioning tumors, or ACTH-, TSH-, or gonadotrope-secreting tumors. The primary mode of treatment for these tumors should therefore be considered surgical, with other options (radiation or observation) reserved for those patients in whom underlying medical conditions preclude surgery.

If the neurosurgeon and the endocrinologist in conjunction agree that an operation is necessary, the usual procedure of choice is a transsphenoidal craniotomy (Fig. 8.2). The transsphenoidal resection of pituitary tumors has a long history of development and refinement since first performed in 1907 by Schloffer, a rhinologist from Innsbruck, Austria. The technique of sphenoid sinus exposure (hence the term "transsphenoidal") was developed by neurosurgeons such as Halstead and Cushing as a more focused approach to this region, with less collateral tissue injury. The technique employs a sublabial incision (under the upper lip) with a submucous dissection of the nasal septum. This technique has greatly increased in popularity over the past 20 years as methods have continued to improve. This may also in part be attributed to the well-recognized inadequacy of other approaches to this region, especially the subfrontal transcranial approach, for removal of the component of the tumor within the

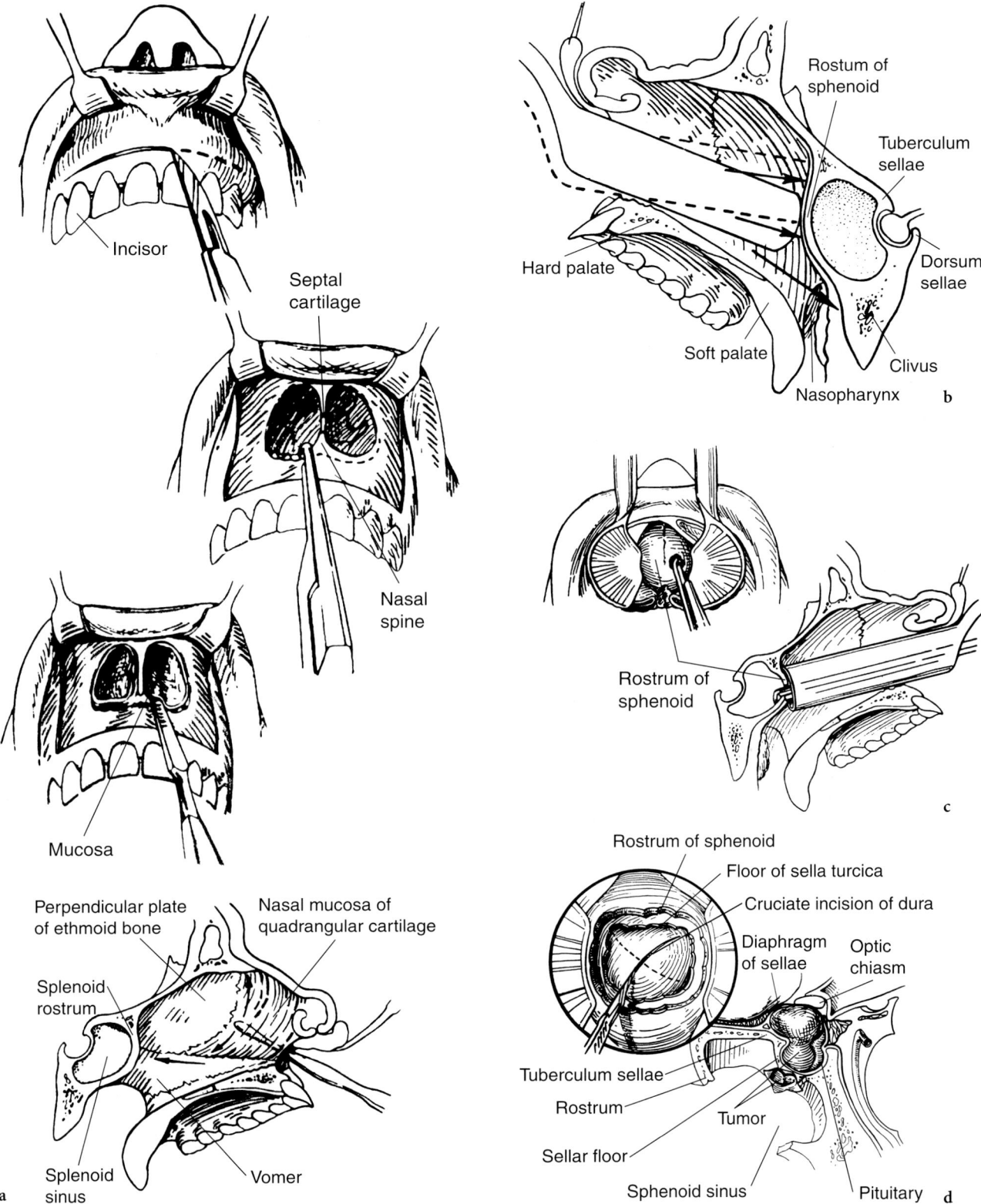

Fig. 8.2a–d. The transsphenoidal craniotomy. **a** Sublabial incision and intranasal mucosal dissection. **b** Advancement of the retractor to the sphenoid and the anatomic relationship of the sella to the sphenoid and nasopharynx. **c** Removal of the rostrum of the sphenoid, allowing access to the sphenoid. **d** Opening of the dura, and the relationship of the tumor to the sphenoid

depths of the sella turcica. The transsphenoidal approach also has proven effectiveness in the treatment of visual disturbances from large adenomas. In addition, there exists clear documentation of the potential for improvement in pituitary function following transsphenoidal tumor resection with careful preservation of normal gland in cases with preexisting hypopituitarism. For smaller hormone-secreting tumors, the efficacy of transsphenoidal surgery in selected patients has been well established, with some reports showing more than 90% tumor control. In series including larger tumors, however, a more realistic 50–80% rate of tumor control is expected with surgery alone. Thus, the efficacy of the transsphenoidal approach in treating small tumors situated deep in the sella and large tumors projecting above the sella establishes this as the approach of choice for the surgical management of most pituitary tumors, regardless of size.

Today, in the hands of an experienced surgeon, mortality of the transsphenoidal operation for pituitary tumors approaches zero. Operative morbidity (adverse outcome) includes transient, or, in some cases, permanent diabetes insipidus (DI), a dysfunction of the posterior lobe of the pituitary gland which results in frequent urination and may require medication to control. The incidence of this ranges from 1.8% permanent DI in one large series to 17% incidence immediately postoperatively with large adenomas, most of which resolved with time. Leakage of cerebrospinal fluid occurs with an incidence of 1–4.4% among different series, depending upon the size of the tumor and the follow-up time, but occurs disproportionately with larger tumors. Other complications are distinctly uncommon. As put forth by all pituitary neurosurgeons, complications amount to a relatively small percentage of the overall surgical experience, emphasizing the relative safety of the procedure. Most patients will leave the hospital after a stay of less than 1 week, with only minimal discomfort.

Although the above procedure is the primary choice for the majority of pituitary tumors, in some instances a transcranial approach may be recommended for a patient harboring a pituitary tumor. Such cases would include tumors with lateral extension out of the sella turcica, or with abnormal courses of the carotid arteries at the base of the skull, which may pose a hazard to the transsphenoidal approach. Both of these circumstances may be anticipated by careful review of the preoperative MRI studies.

8.3
Nonfunctioning Macroadenomas

Transsphenoidal craniotomy is the treatment of choice for typical macroadenomas of the pituitary gland. While the great majority of these lesions present with signs and symptoms of mass effect, usually related to visual compromise, preoperative evaluation must include an assessment of the patient's endocrinologic status. Also requisite are preoperative imaging studies to assess the accessibility and safety of the approach, with MRI predominating as the study of choice. Careful preoperative preparations and the assistance of a well-versed anesthesiologist are critical for the safe use of this technique. In well-trained hands, complications are rare, and can be mitigated with studied technique.

8.3.1
Transsphenoidal Craniotomy
for Macroadenomas: Indications

Pituitary macroadenomas are defined as lesions which are greater than 10 mm in diameter. It must be recognized that, in terms of presentation and treatment, these tumors are distinctly different from microadenomas. Microadenomas commonly come to clinical attention as a result of the signs and symptoms of an endocrinopathy produced by hormonal hypersecretion; they are usually too small to cause significant disruption of surrounding neural structures. Macroadenomas, on the other hand, are usually nonfunctioning: they include null cell tumors, which are the most common type of pituitary adenoma, or they secrete only the alpha subunit, which is not believed to have any endocrinologic effect by itself. This categorization is somewhat self-selecting: since even a small secreting tumor will have a significant endocrinologic effect, most of these tumors come to clinical attention before they achieve the size of a macroadenoma. Exceptional cases do exist, in which a patient (or their physician) ignored longstanding evidence of an endocrinopathy and a functional tumor grew to macroadenoma stature.

Nonfunctional tumors (a better term than "nonsecreting tumors" in light of the discovery of alpha-subunit-secreting tumors, which are nonfunctional but not nonsecreting) typically do not cause signs and symptoms until they grow large enough to compress surrounding intracranial structures. The most common symptoms and signs of this mass effect are headache (believed to be due to impaction on the nociceptively innervated meninges), visual compromise, and hypopituitarism. The visual compromise can be quite variable depending on the fixation of the optic chiasm in relation to the tumor and the concomitant relative compression of the optic nerves versus the chiasm. The classical description is the triad of bitemporal hemianopsia, early loss of central visual acuity, and optic disc pallor (WRAY 1977).

Indications for surgery are largely based on these differences between micro- and macroadenomas. Medical (nonsurgical) therapies are increasingly becoming more useful in the treatment of functional microadenomas. In fact, bromocriptine is now the primary treatment of choice for prolactin-secreting adenomas. Nonfunctioning macroadenomas, however, typically are not amenable to medical management and are thus treated surgically.

One exception to the above delineation concerns the prolactin-secreting adenoma, which, in rare cases, escapes medical intervention and grows to the size of a macroadenoma. These lesions are amenable to medical therapy and should be treated primarily with bromocriptine. While rapid visual loss might elicit concern, it is rapidly reversible in most cases with bromocriptine therapy, and emergency surgery is rarely indicated.

While surgery is the treatment of choice for the typical pituitary macroadenoma, it is simply not an option for the patient whose age or concomitant medical illness increases the risk of general anesthesia and surgery to an unacceptable level. For the elderly patient with only mild, nonprogressive symptoms, a conservative course of careful observation may be undertaken given the benign growth patterns of these tumors. Serial visual field testing, endocrine evaluation, and MRI scans should be obtained to guard against an indolent deterioration.

For the patient with a longer life expectancy, but in whom surgery is still contraindicated, primary radiation therapy should be considered. External beam therapy has received the most attention in the literature to date, although experience is currently being accrued with modalities such as the gamma knife (ARISTZABAL 1977; SHELINE 1974). Local control rates of 50–79% have been described in the major series to date (CHUN 1988; KRAMER 1968; URDANETA 1975). However, radiation also results in a rate of pituitary hormone dysfunction of 40–50% if long-term follow-up is conducted (KJELLBERG 1980). This morbidity makes radiation therapy more acceptable in the patient who already suffers from some de-

gree of hypopituitarism. An additional problem with radiation therapy is that it takes some time for tumor shrinkage to occur (if shrinkage does occur), a serious concern if the patient is losing vision.

With the above exceptions noted, it should be understood that a typical nonfunctioning pituitary macroadenoma requires operative intervention. At this point in time, the transsphenoidal approach is widely recognized as the most appropriate technique for resection of lesions which originate in the sella (BEVIN 1987; CIRIC 1984, 1974; COLLINS 1979; HARDY 1969, 1971; WEISS 1980). Moreover, this approach has been proven to alleviate the visual disturbances caused by the mass effect of these large tumors (CIRIC 1984; WEISS 1980; WILSON 1978). In our initial series of 200 patients who presented with visual loss and received transsphenoidal resections of their tumors, 81% had improvement in their vision, while 16% remained unchanged but did not progress and only 3% had worsening of their symptoms. Transsphenoidal resection has also been shown to improve pituitary function in patients who evidence hypopituitarism from compressive effects of large tumors (ARAFAH 1986; OBER 1988). For the above reasons, there should be little doubt that transsphenoidal resection is the procedure of choice in most cases.

However, this is not to say that there is no role for a transcranial approach. In some cases, an incompetent diaphragma sellae may allow the tumor to grow out laterally into the middle fossa or fossae, without expansion of the sella itself. In these cases, a primary or secondary transcranial procedure may be required. Alternatively, ectatic carotid arteries may obstruct safe access to the full extent of the tumor, prohibiting a transsphenoidal approach. In the majority of these cases, a transcranial approach can be safely conducted, with direct visualization of the tumor and surrounding vascular structures.

8.3.2
Preoperative Evaluation

The three key aspects of preoperative evaluation are the history and neuro-ophthalmologic examination, the radiologic evaluation, and the endocrinologic evaluation. The most straightforward of these is the documentation of the degree and rapidity of visual loss by a detailed ophthalmologic examination which includes visual fields testing. A bitemporal visual field defect can be subtle and might go unnoticed by the patient, necessitating a formal examination in all patients with tumors compressing the optic nerves and/or chiasm.

Radiographic evaluation is important not only in diagnosing the lesion, but also in determining the appropriateness of the transsphenoidal approach and in planning the surgery. In our institution, we have used MRI exclusively since 1982 for its high resolution delineation of intrasellar pathology and vascular anatomy. Coronal, axial, and sagittal sequences are obtained with and without gadolinium (Fig. 8.3). The coronal images are particularly important in that they afford a view of the intracavernous carotid arteries and their spatial relationship to the tumor. Severely ectatic carotid arteries (we have seen cases in which they actually touch each other in the midline!) can block safe access to the tumor via the transsphenoidal approach, and would be considered an absolute contraindication to this approach. The ability of MRI to effectively evaluate the vascular anatomy in this region has obviated the angiogram in most cases.

MRI also provides important information on the anatomy of the sphenoid sinus. The surgeon must note the degree of pneumatization of the sphenoid sinus. While a poorly pneumatized sphenoid (such as that seen in children) does not preclude this approach, it might necessitate the use of an auger or even a drill to gain access to the sella. Additionally, intraoperative imaging might be needed to insure the correct angle of approach. Similarly, the individual variances of the bony anatomy of the sphenoid must be appreciated. Midline and eccentric septa are common in the sphenoid, and can lull the surgeon into thinking the whole sphenoid is opened when in fact the exposure is suboptimal. MRI can also detect

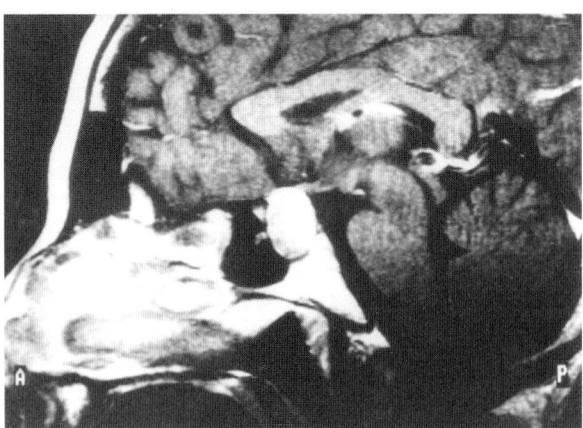

Fig. 8.3. Sagittal MRI showing a large pituitary tumor extending superiorly from the sella, posterior to a large aerated sphenoid sinus

the presence of acute sinusitis, which should result in a delay of the surgery until the inflammation subsides.

There are two key goals in the endocrine evaluation of these patients. The first is to insure that the tumor is truly nonfunctional. The second is to insure that a state of pituitary insufficiency does not exist preoperatively. To accomplish these goals, all patients should have an assay of all adenohypophyseal hormones, with a progression to stimulation studies if any doubt exists as to the presence of an endocrinopathy. The development of the radioimmunoassay over the past two decades has greatly improved the ability to detect such abnormalities.

As was mentioned previously, functioning tumors can grow large enough to be considered macroadenomas. This status would be difficult to miss if the appropriate endocrine work-up is conducted. A more common error, however, is misdiagnosis of a prolactin-secreting adenoma when a large tumor is associated with only mild to moderately elevated serum prolactin levels. In cases where the prolactin level is relatively low given the size of the tumor (for example, a prolactin of less than 200 ng/ml with a tumor greater than 2 cm) a more likely explanation is a "stalk-section effect." In this situation, a large tumor compresses the pituitary stalk, limiting the ability of hypothalamic released dopamine to inhibit prolactin release. The result is mild to moderate hyperprolactinemia, but the tumor will not respond appropriately to bromocriptine therapy.

A more serious diagnostic pitfall would be to miss a clinical or occult state of pituitary insufficiency. This state can be seen with large tumors, which either directly compress the surrounding gland or impair its vascular supply resulting in decreased hormone release. In the perioperative period, the stresses of surgery can precipitate an endocrinologic crisis. For this reason, it is especially important to assess the serum cortisol and thyroxin levels. Occult DI in the preoperative period is also seen, and often can be detected by eliciting a history of urinary frequency and by assessing the electrolyte status of the patient.

8.3.3
Perioperative Preparation

As mentioned above, an occult hormonal deficiency may become manifest in the perioperative period. For this reason, preoperative endocrinologic evaluation is mandatory. If hypothyroidism is detected, thyroid replacement should be initiated. Normalization of thyroid function takes on average 1 week after replacement is begun.

Occult hypocortisolism can be similarly devastating. This problem is somewhat obviated in our institution, as all patients receive preoperative doses of glucocorticoids as a cerebroprotectant. Our standard practice is to administer methylprednisolone at a dosage of 40 mg every 6 h for 24 h preceding the surgery. If neurologic compromise exists or a state of relative hypocortisolism is anticipated, a gradual postoperative taper is used. A serum cortisol level is sent before the patient leaves the hospital, as an assessment of his/her reserve.

8.3.4
Anesthesia Considerations

As with all procedures requiring general anesthesia, an assessment of the patient's general risk factors must be undertaken. It is best to take the time to maximize the patient's medical conditions first; except in the case of rapid visual loss unresponsive to steroids (or bromocriptine, where appropriate) there is rarely a need to rush the patient into surgery.

8.3.5
Transnasal Transsphenoidal Approach

In experienced hands, transsphenoidal craniotomy for macroadenomas can be accomplished with an acceptably low rate of morbidity and mortality. In the large international study reported by ZERVAS (1984), 2677 macroadenomas were treated with a mortality of 0.86%. Major causes of death included hypothalamic injury, infections related to CSF leaks, and vascular injury.

Significant vascular injuries most commonly result from injury to an unrecognized ectatic carotid artery or a carotid artery injury following resection of tumor in the cavernous sinus. Such an injury can cause a fatal hemorrhage, and appropriate steps must be rapidly taken. Surgical cellulose should be placed temporarily against the area of hemorrhage (the arterotomy itself is rarely directly seen). When the hemorrhage is effectively tamponaded, fascia and muscle should be harvested and packed into the cavernous sinus directly against the carotid artery and sella. A postoperative angiogram should be obtained prior to discharge to detect a potential pseudoaneurysm or a carotid-cavernous fistula. Blood pressure

must be maintained to prevent a cerebral infarction, and frequent neurologic exams are mandated.

Another source of morbidity is postoperative DI. Transient postoperative DI is relatively common (17% in Cohen's series) (COHEN 1985), but frequently resolves with time. Permanent DI is less frequent: 1.8% in the 500 cases of LAWS and KERN (1979). To detect this and prevent morbidity, urine volumes and serum sodium levels must be followed in the postoperative period. DDAVP must be used cautiously, as an awake patient will usually readjust his/her electrolytes through intact thirst mechanisms.

8.4
Prolactin-Secreting Pituitary Adenomas

Prolactin (PRL)-secreting adenomas are the most common type of secretory pituitary tumor and are second in frequency only to null cell adenomas in overall incidence (VANCE 1987). In the pediatric population, however, they represent the most frequent type of adenoma overall (MINDERMANN 1995).

Although these tumors are found pathologically at autopsy with equal frequency in men and women, they are clinically significantly more common in women. They are also more common in girls than boys (MINDERMANN 1995). Hyperprolactinemia causes galactorrhea in women and hypogonadism, which are exhibited as anovulatory infertility in the female and impotence in the male (THORNER 1991; EVANS 1984). Presumed abnormalities in pulsatile secretion of growth hormone releasing hormone (GHRH) and gonadotropins precipitate a relative estrogen deficiency (LEYEENDECKER 1980, JACOBS 1976). This hypogonadal state is associated with osteoporosis in women (KLIBANSKI 1986) and both cortical and trabecular osteopenia in men (GREENSPAN 1989). In a personal series of some 392 PRL-secreting pituitary tumors operated on by one of the authors (MHW), 321 (82%) were in female patients (AMAR 1998). The most common presenting symptom in this group was the development of secondary amenorrhea (72%); only about 50% of those with amenorrhea had associated galactorrhea (AMAR 1998). Epidemiologically, approximately 5% of women with primary amenorrhea and 25% of women with secondary amenorrhea (other than those who are pregnant) harbor a PRL-secreting pituitary tumor as the cause of their clinical symptoms. Because of this readily identifiable symptom, these patients generally present relatively early in the course of evolution of the tumors; this is unfortunately not true in the male population. Because the primary symptom of a PRL-secreting tumor in the male is usually a decrease in libido well before true impotence is observed, this problem is frequently ascribed to the aging process or functional causes. About two-thirds of men with hyperprolactinemia due to a PRL-secreting tumor have a low serum testosterone level (HULTING 1985); this condition may be secondary to hyperprolactinemia per se or to mechanical compression of adjacent normal pituitary gland. Thus, males often present at a more advanced age and later in the course of their disease with chiasmal compression and visual compromise. In our series, visual loss ranging in duration from 2 to 24 months was the initial complaint in 60% of males but only 10% of females (AMAR 1989). For the same reasons, large tumors associated with hypothyroidism and adrenal insufficiency are more common in men (HULTING 1985). In the pediatric population, boys tend to have much larger tumors and higher preoperative prolactin levels than girls, and they frequently present with focal neurologic deficit or other signs of significant mass effect (MINDERMANN 1995).

The diagnosis is secured by radiographic evidence of a pituitary lesion with an elevation of serum PRL. High-field thin-section MRI appears to be the most sensitive imaging method for preoperative localization of pituitary adenomas. There exists a rough correlation between the size of the lesion radiographically and pathologically and the serum level of PRL. In addition, local invasion of the tumor into the adjacent venous cavernous sinuses is associated with a marked increase in serum PRL. The diagnosis of pathologic PRL excess should be based on serial blood measurements (ALFORD 1992); PRL levels of more than five times the upper limit of normal are usually associated with a PRL-secreting pituitary tumor (CUNNAH 1991). In the endocrinologic evaluation of patients suspected of harboring a PRL-secreting tumor, it must be appreciated that larger tumors of any endocrine basis may cause a mild to moderate hyperprolactinemia. This is produced by the so-called stalk-section effect, which must be distinguished from a true prolactinoma (LEES 1987). Under such circumstances, it is rare to see PRL levels in excess of 100 ng/ml. Recently, however, we encountered a patient with a preoperative prolactin level above 600 ng/ml, confirmed by serial laboratory testing, that was attributed to stalk-section effect on the basis of immunohistochemical analysis of the tumor, which failed to stain for prolactin (Albuquer-

que). In general, large tumors (>2 cm) associated with PRL levels less than 150 ng/ml (certainly those <100 ng/ml) should be suspected of being nonsecretors when planning management strategies. One would certainly exert caution in expecting such lesions to physically respond to chemical reductions of serum PRL.

A number of reports suggest that neither tumor size nor PRL levels change over a number of years in the majority of women with microprolactinomas (SCHLECHTER 1989; SISAM 1987). In fact, it has been observed that few microprolactinomas progress to macroadenomas (CUNNAH 1991). In one of our series, for instance, only 3 of 27 women harboring microadenomas demonstrated significant tumor growth over a 6-year interval of observation (WEISS 1983). In contrast, macroadenomas, which for reasons described earlier frequently occur in men, may behave in an aggressive manner (ALFORD 1992). They may be associated with invasion of the cavernous sinuses and diffuse invasion of the base of the skull, and they commonly extend to the suprasellar region (LUNDIN 1992). Hemorrhage or cyst formation within the tumor may also occur.

The levels of elevated PRL in a diagnosed pituitary adenoma are of great help in determining subsequent management because the ability to successfully extirpate the tumor is reduced with large or invasive lesions (discussed later).

Bromocriptine is the first-choice drug for therapy of PRL-secreting tumors. The efficacy of bromocriptine (a dopaminergic agonist) in reducing serum PRL, in addition to reducing tumor size and inhibiting further tumor growth, is well established (discussed later). The central considerations related to treating such patients are the ability of the patient to tolerate the medication, the realization that the treatment must continue for the duration of the patient's life, and the implications for fertility.

With PRL-secreting microadenomas, therapeutic options include medical or surgical management. In our series, 225 of 262 patients (86%) undergoing surgery for tumors less than 1 cm had normal (<20 ng/ml) postoperative PRL levels (i.e., chemical cure) (AMAR 1998). Operative mortality was zero, and associated morbidity was low. The experience of other centers corroborates this high rate of surgical success (MASSOUD 1996; LAWS 1996; THOMSON 1994; GIOVANELLI 1996; WEBSTER 1992; WILSON 1984; MOLITCH 1992). Strong consideration should thus be given to surgical intervention in patients harboring smaller tumors without significant hyperprolactinemia.

In cases of larger tumors, however, surgical chemical cures (i.e., serum PRL <20 ng/ml postoperatively) are much less frequent. Those tumors associated with PRL levels greater than 200 ng/ml recur in over 50% of cases following surgery alone (THORNER 1991); the rate of recurrence of hyperprolactinemia following surgery for macroadenomas (with PRL levels >250 ng/ml) exceeds 70% (THORNER 1991; ADAMS 1988). In our personal series, only 63 of 130 (49%) of those patients with tumors greater than 1 cm achieved chemical cure. Although no medical therapy results in cure of a PRL-secreting macroadenoma, only a minority of these patients remain free of their disease following surgery alone. Therefore, bromocriptine should be considered as initial therapy for those patients in whom surgical resection resulting in chemical cure is deemed unlikely (SERRI 1983). On the other hand, some surgeons recommend operative removal in the majority of macroadenomas (WILSON 1984).

At present, it is our practice to place all patients with large or invasive pituitary tumors with endocrinologically documented PRL secretion on a therapeutic trial of bromocriptine initially, and to monitor clinical status and the radiographic appearance of the lesion accordingly. All solid primary PRL-secreting tumors should respond to the medication, both clinically by a reduction in tumor size and by a reduction in PRL level. One exception to this management is larger primary cystic tumors, which are much less likely to respond to pharmacotherapy (WEISS 1983).

The goals of treatment include: (1) reduction of the tumor mass, (2) correction of the hyperprolactinemic state, and (3) preservation of anterior pituitary function (THORNER 1991). The tenet of therapy should be absolute normalization of PRL levels, because a prolonged hyperprolactinemic state may be associated with significant osteoporosis and infertility. Surgical resection of these lesions is indicated in patients who are intolerant to the side effects of the medication, unable to afford the cost of the medication for a prolonged period of time, or in whom sustained tumor reduction is not effected. Furthermore, the Food and Drug Administration (FDA) recommends discontinuing the medication as soon as pregnancy has been established because of concerns about its safety to the mother and fetus (PDR 1997). As discussed below, expansion of the tumor and compression of the optic structures has been reported while off bromocriptine during gestation (PDR 1997). Thus, the desire for fertility constitutes another indication for surgical resection, and in our personal experience, 72 of 96 women (75%) who wanted to achieve pregnancy did so following transsphenoidal surgery (AMAR 1998). Collectively, these reasons necessitate surgery in about 20–25% of patients with microadenomas, while the remaining patients can be successfully treated with bromocriptine alone (MASSOUD 1996; MOLITCH 1992; GRISOLI 1990). Among patients with macroadenomas, however, WILSON and others recommend operative removal in the majority of cases (WILSON 1984).

Subsequent to surgery, if hyperprolactinemia is persistent to some extent, the patient may be able to tolerate markedly reduced doses of bromocriptine to effect long-term control, or one would consider the use of postoperative radiotherapy to bring the residual tumor under control. In our series, all patients who suffered endocrinologic recurrence (relapse of hyperprolactinemia after initial hormonal normalization) or immediate endocrinologic failure (serum prolactin levels >20 ng/ml on the morning after surgery) were able to resume bromocriptine at much lower doses than they had taken preoperatively. All of them tolerated this reduced dose, and although the serum prolactin level was not always restored to normal, no patient has required postoperative radiotherapy (AMAR 1998).

Following radiotherapy for prolactinomas, PRL levels fall slowly over many years, but they rarely reach the normal level (THORNER 1991); thus, these patients may benefit from adjuvant medical therapy with bromocriptine.

Bromocriptine is a dopamine agonist that suppresses PRL production and release by the stimulation of dopamine receptors. This orally active dopamine agonist is a semisynthetic ergot alkaloid that was specifically developed as an inhibitor of PRL secretion. It directly stimulates neuronal and pituitary cell membrane dopamine receptors (CORRODI 1973). A single dose of 2.5 mg results in suppression of serum PRL for up to 14 h (THORNER 1980). The biologic effect, however, may persist for more than 24 h in some patients (VANCE 1987).

At present, bromocriptine is the only dopaminergic analogue that has FDA approval to be used in the clinical treatment of hyperprolactinemia (THORNER 1991). It has proved safe and effective in 15 years of widespread use in the treatment of prolactinomas since its approval in 1978 (VANCE 1987). Initiation of bromocriptine therapy is as described in the previous section for use in GH/PRL-secreting adenomas. Bromocriptine is usually given in a dosage of 2.5 mg three times daily. In some patients with large tumors in whom the tumor size does not decrease or the PRL level is not suppressed by more than 80% of pretreatment levels with the above-mentioned dosage, much larger dosages are required, up to 15–20 mg daily (VANCE 1987; THORNER 1991). However, in certain cases, the dose may be decreased after achievement of adequate suppression (VANCE 1987). Other authors have reported that if reduction in tumor size has not occurred within a 3-month period after starting bromocriptine, it is unlikely that it will occur and medical therapy should be abandoned (THORNER 1991). It has been our observation that patients who do not respond by 6 weeks are unlikely to respond by 3 months, so our current practice is to obtain an MRI scan 6 weeks after initiating medical therapy to document tumor reduction.

In the bromocriptine-treated patient who responds to medication but fails to normalize his/her serum PRL levels and does not achieve restoration of gonadal function, a combined surgical and medical approach should be considered. Following the surgical procedure, hyperprolactinemia is often more responsive to medical therapy, requiring lower doses for control of PRL (THORNER 1991). As mentioned above, reduced doses of bromocriptine have been effective in controlling our patients who were not surgically cured, and adjuvant radiation has not been necessary (AMAR 1998).

Dopamine agonist therapy must be given chronically. In most patients, withdrawal of the drug results in a return of hyperprolactinemia and reexpansion of the tumor (THORNER 1981; ZARATE 1983). Occasionally, patients with a microadenoma or an unidentifiable tumor do not experience a recurrence after discontinuation of therapy (VANCE 1987). In a patient with a microadenoma, bromocriptine can be discontinued every 2 years on a trial basis to determine the need for continued therapy (KLIBANSKI 1991).

Following adequate bromocriptine therapy, PRL levels are usually lowered by over 80% or are normalized (THORNER 1991). The PRL-reducing response to therapy in patients with microadenomas and with macroadenomas is similar, with the exception that in the latter group, the time required for effective lowering of PRL is usually longer (VANCE 1987). In addition, in over 80% of patients, bromocriptine and other dopamine agonists are effective in reversing visual abnormalities and restoring gonadal and anterior pituitary functions (THORNER 1991; CUNNAH 1991). Most female patients begin

menstruation within 6 months of initiating therapy. The restoration of fertility in women with bromocriptine has been well documented (VANCE 1984). However, as stated above, the continuation of bromocriptine during pregnancy is contraindicated, and patients who wish to become pregnant should undergo surgery (PDR 1997).

In addition to reducing PRL secretion, bromocriptine is effective at decreasing tumor size (LANDOLT 1981; WEISS 1983; ZERVAS 1984). Size reduction of the tumor may occur very rapidly, within days of initiation of therapy, and achieve dramatic decompression of the optic chiasm and resolution of headaches and other signs and symptoms of raised intracranial pressure (THORNER 1991). Some tumors are very responsive to bromocriptine and shrink more than 80% within 6 weeks of initiation of therapy (THORNER 1991). Although the vast majority of patients have a satisfactory biochemical and clinical response to medical therapy, there have been isolated case reports of lack of response or progression of disease during bromocriptine therapy (BREIDAHL 1983; CROSIGNANI 1982; MARTIN 1981). Therefore, close monitoring of serum prolactin levels and serial MRI is mandatory. In women, once hyperprolactinemia has been corrected and the menstrual cycle normalized, fertility is usually reestablished and the pregnancy rates are the same as those of normal women in the same age group (GEMZELL 1979; SKRABANEK 1980). Although it is tempting to intuitively suggest that pretreatment with bromocriptine may shrink the tumor and facilitate surgical resection, no study has yet reported higher surgical cure rates after such preoperative treatment with bromocriptine (FAHLBUSCH 1987; HUBBARD 1987). Conversely, as will be discussed later, some surgeons believe that bromocriptine produces adverse effects on the consistency of the adenoma which impede tumor resection (LANDOLT 1981), although this has not been our experience (WEISS 1983).

Pregnant women harboring microprolactinomas rarely develop complications related to tumor expansion, the reported risk being only less than 0.5–1% (VANCE 1987; THORNER 1991). However, in pregnant women with macroprolactinomas, the situation is different; the risk of developing symptoms related to tumor enlargement, such as headache, visual field disturbances, and ophthalmoplegia, is approximately 15%, and that of developing asymptomatic tumor enlargement is 9% (MOLITCH 1985). These complications appear to occur with equal frequency during all trimesters (GEMZELL 1979). Therefore, measures to reduce tumor size such as surgery and radiation are recommended prior to conception in female patients harboring macroadenomas who desire to become pregnant. In the event that the tumor enlarges during pregnancy, bromocriptine has been shown to be safe and effective (CANALES 1981; KONOPKA 1983; VAN ROON 1981). Its administration during pregnancy has not increased the risk of congenital anomalies, spontaneous abortion, or multiple births (TURKALJ 1982, RAYMOND 1985). Motor and psychological development of children born to women treated with bromocriptine during pregnancy were normal (RAYMOND 1985).

If a patient plans to become pregnant while on bromocriptine therapy, a coordinated schedule of follow-up must be observed by the patient, endocrinologist, and neurosurgeon. At present, it is recommended that a woman with a prolactinoma, regardless of tumor size, who wishes to become pregnant while on bromocriptine therapy uses mechanical contraceptive precautions for 3 months. During this period, she should undergo complete endocrine, neuroradiologic, and neuro-ophthalmologic evaluations. After achieving three regular menstrual cycles, she should discontinue the contraceptive precautions. Pregnancy should be suspected when the menses are 2 days overdue, and at that time, the serum beta-human chorionic gonadotropin (hCG) level should be measured; once pregnancy is confirmed, bromocriptine should be discontinued immediately. The woman should then be followed closely for signs and symptoms of tumor expansion. Should visual field abnormalities develop, bromocriptine therapy would be indicated as the clinical situation warrants (VANCE 1987). Following termination of pregnancy, headaches and visual field defects acquired due to tumor expansion resolve as the tumor becomes smaller in all cases.

A rare complication of bromocriptine therapy in patients with large prolactinomas is the development of a cerebrospinal fluid leak during treatment caused by shrinkage of the tumor (KLIBANSKI 1991). In women, galactorrhea may persist even though the PRL level is lowered to the normal range (THORNER 1974). It has been reported that if bromocriptine is given for more than 3 months, the tumor may become fibrous in consistency, which may cause difficulty with surgical resection (LANDOLT 1981), although this has not been our personal experience (WEISS 1983).

Following surgery in a patient harboring a microprolactinoma in whom total resection was thought to be achieved, postoperative measurement of PRL levels are the most sensitive measure of completeness of resection and any recurrence. Because of the short half-life of endogenous PRL, postoperative levels may be checked as early as the morning following surgery. This measurement is repeated at 6 weeks, and it should be performed at routine intervals (every 3 months) in the early postoperative period. Depending on the clinical course, the intervals may be increased accordingly.

We have recently reported the prognostic value of serum prolactin levels obtained immediately following transsphenoidal surgery (AMAR 1998). Our practice is to assess fasting AM prolactin levels on postoperative day (POD) 1 and random serum levels sampled at 6 weeks, 12 weeks, and then every 6 months for a minimum of 5 years. Levels less than 10 ng/ml on POD 1 predict long-term endocrinologic cure, in both patients with microadenomas (100%) as well as those with macroadenomas (93%). In contrast, patients with "normal" levels between 10 and 20 ng/ml on POD 1 remain at risk of endocrinologic recurrence, especially if preoperative tumor size exceeds 10 mm (100% in our series). However, none of our patients with a microadenoma has suffered relapse (AMAR 1998).

In other series, recurrence of hyperprolactinemia after initial hormonal normalization has been reported in 10–50% of patients after transsphenoidal resection, depending on the preoperative size of the tumor and the length of follow-up (MASSOUD 1996; LAWS 1996; THOMSON 1994; WEBSTER 1992; MOLITCH 1992; BUCHFELDER 1991). Differences in surgical technique may also underlie this variation. For instance, based on the hypothesis that delayed recurrences result in situ from residual tumoral cells at the periphery of an adenoma, GRISOLI has proposed performing an "enlarged" rather than selective adenomectomy by removing a layer of normal pituitary gland at the outer edge of the tumor as well as the pituitary capsule in contact with the sellar meninges (GRISOLI 1990). Using this technique in 26 patients with tumors less than 20 mm in diameter, he obtained normal serum prolactin levels in all cases after an average of 16 months. This length of follow-up is short, however, and it remains to be proven whether or not this technique results in a lower incidence of delayed recurrence.

Relapses usually occur within the first few years after surgery, although they have been reported after more than 10 years of follow-up (AMAR 1998, MASSOUD 1996; THOMSON 1994). Often, such recurrences are asymptomatic, but even in patients without overt clinical manifestations, treatment may be indicated in order to prevent osteoporosis (MASSOUD 1996; BUCHFELDER1991). As stated above, reduced levels of bromocriptine are usually well tolerated and often effective in preventing significant enlargement of recurrent tumors (AMAR 1998; MASSOUD 1996).

In most cases, however, imaging of the sella turcica fails to reveal residual or recurrent adenoma, and surgical reexploration is unlikely to achieve chemical cure (AMAR 1998; MASSOUD 1996; LAWS 1996; BUCHFELDER1991). This observation may reflect the fact that, with vigilant protocols for sampling postoperative prolactin levels, most tumor recurrences will be detected early. In our series, for instance, no recurrence was greater than 55 ng/ml (AMAR 1998). Alternatively, this observation may imply that there are other reasons for recurrent hyperprolactinemia besides regrowth of residual tumor remnants, such as a secondary empty sella or a disordered hypothalamic-pituitary axis (MASSOUD 1996; LAWS1996; MAIRA 1989).

The clinical response in impotent men with hyperprolactinemia treated with testosterone is often unsatisfactory until the PRL levels are lowered (EVANS 1984). It is presumed that elevated PRL levels interfere with the peripheral effect of testosterone.

8.5
Growth Hormone-Secreting Pituitary Adenomas

Acromegaly and gigantism are the result of oversecretion of growth hormone (GH) into the somatic circulation. Collectively, they are second in frequency to hyperprolactinemia as pituitary hypersecretory syndromes. They are almost always caused by a somatotroph (i.e., GH-secreting) adenoma of the pituitary gland (more than 99% of cases) as opposed to somatotroph hyperplasia from excess secretion of ectopic GHRH (HO 1991). While the majority of these pituitary tumors exhibit a moderate growth rate, they often present relatively early in their growth due to the detection of a hypersecretory syndrome. In our personal series, over 70% were microadenomas upon presentation (KRIEGER 1997). However, they can present as macroadenomas with extrasellar extension and focal destruction (BAUMANN 1987; FROHMAN 1991; In other series, as many as 85–90% of patients present with macroadenomas

and 10–15% with microadenomas, Ho 1991). Younger patients with acromegaly often harbor larger and more rapidly growing tumors (SERRI 1987). Acromegalic tumors may contain and also secrete prolactin (PRL) or the alpha subunit (common to all the glycoprotein adenohypophyseal hormones) and, rarely, thyrotropin-stimulating hormone (TSH) in addition to GH (BAUMANN 1987). Most patients with large tumors have mixed GH and PRL hypersecretion (WAAS 1990), which results in concomitant hyperprolactinemia in 20–40% of patients (BAUMANN 1987; SERRI 1987). PRL is most often secreted from a tumor containing a mixed population of somatotroph and lactotroph cells (an acidophilic stem cell tumor), but occasionally from a bipotential mammo-somatotroph adenoma (FROHMAN 1991). In patients harboring mammo-somatotroph adenomas, the two hormones, by definition, are present within the same cell, the same secretory granule, or both, and are usually secreted in a similar dynamic pattern (SERRI 1987).

The total amount of GH secreted in a 24-h period is variable among patients harboring GH-secreting tumors and depends on cell activity, but it roughly correlates with the size of the tumor (RANDALL 1991). GH oversecretion results in elevated plasma insulin-like growth factor (IGF)-1 levels (BAUMANN 1987) that are fairly stable and reflect the integrated pulsatile 24-h secretion of GH. As GH levels increase, IGF-1 rises linearly until GH reaches about 20 ng/ml, after which the IGF-1 level plateaus. As a corollary, to achieve any measure of successful treatment, GH must decrease to a level below 20 fg/l for IGF-1 levels to drop or clinical improvement to occur (HO 1991). However, there is a poor correlation between plasma GH levels and clinical manifestations of acromegaly, presumably because of variable responsiveness of peripheral tissues to GH excess (BAUMANN 1987).

The clinical manifestations of excess secretion of GH depend on the age of the patient. If the excess secretion occurs in childhood or adolescence, before the epiphyses of long bones have fused, the result is gigantism; individuals with such a condition may attain great height if the disease progresses unchecked [often greater than 7 ft (2.13 m)]. After fusion of the epiphyses, excess GH results in the syndrome of acromegaly in adults, with soft tissue and bony enlargement in characteristic locations. Clinical manifestations of these soft tissue changes include coarsening of facial features, laryngeal enlargement, goiter, thick heel pads, acanthosis nigricans, cardiomegaly, and hepatomegaly. Bony changes are extensive, producing facial prognathism, enlargement of the mandible with increased spacing between the teeth, and bony enlargements of hands and feet. Soft tissue and bony changes may produce compressive neuropathies and arthropathies (Fig. 8.4). Metabolic manifestations include associated hypertension, diabetes mellitus and goiter, and commonly hyperhidrosis. Deficiencies in adrenocorticotropic hormone (ACTH) and TSH are found in less than 10–20% of patients. Hypogonadism occurs in 30–40% of patients, but it may be attributable to associated hyperprolactinemia (BAUMANN 1987), and may result in osteoporosis. Acromegaly affects men and women with approximate equal frequency.

The diagnosis is made by assessing GH secretion. A basal fasting GH level greater than 10 ng/ml is present in 90% of acromegalics. However, because GH is secreted in several peaks throughout the day, a single fasting level may fail to demonstrate an elevated level in some patients. Therefore, the suspected diagnosis can be confirmed by the glucose suppression test. In the acromegalic, an oral administration of 100 g of glucose fails to suppress the serum GH level to less than 5 ng/ml at 60 min. The measurement of serum IGF-1 levels are elevated in acromegalics, and prove to be a more reliable measure of the disease and its response to treatment. Radiographic imaging (MRI, CT, or both) demonstrates the presence of a pituitary adenoma in more than 90% of patients with endocrinologically documented acromegaly. At present, high-field thin-section MRI scans appear to be the most sensitive imaging method for preoperative localization of pituitary ade-

nomas. On unenhanced images, focal glandular hypodensity identified on coronal images is the most sensitive predictor of adenoma location. Radiographic evaluation should consist of coronal, sagittal, and axial MRI, with large tumors usually having similar signal intensity to that of brain on T1-weighted images. The normal pituitary gland, infundibulum, and cavernous sinuses enhance immediately after administration of gadolinium-DTPA, allowing contrast between the enhancing normal glandular tissue and the low-intensity adenomas. At present, a T1-weighted image following the infusion of gadolinium-DTPA is the method of choice for the delineation of intrasellar pathology. Shortly after administration, the normal vascular pituitary increases in signal intensity, and a pituitary tumor is visible but remains less intense, being slower to perfuse with the contrast agent.

Excess secretion of GH should be considered a malignant endocrinopathy, which may result in life-threatening medical complications, and thus should be treated aggressively once diagnosed. Left untreated, the mortality is double that of healthy age-matched controls, from complications including hypertension, cardiac disease, diabetes, pulmonary infections, and associated malignancies (NABARRO 1987; BENGTSSON 1988; MELMED 1990; WRIGHT 1970). The goals of therapy in management of a GH-secreting pituitary adenoma include: (1) resolution of tumor mass effect, (2) restoration of normal GH physiology [absolute normalization of GH and somatomedin-C (IGF-1) levels], and (3) replacement of any associated hormone deficiencies.

To date, there are no generally accepted criteria for assessment of cure of acromegaly (ARAFAH 1987; BARKAN 1992; GIANNELLA-NETO 1988; MELMED 1990). Various biochemical tests have been proposed in the postoperative period, including basal GH level, mean GH levels, GH response to the oral glucose tolerance test, GH response to thyrotropin-releasing hormone, and IGF-1 (or somatomedin C) levels. Each of these tests has been found limited in determining cure. Many authors now believe that criteria for successful therapy (chemical cure) include 24-h integrated GH concentration of less than or equal to 2.5 ng/ml, together with normalization of the circulating IGF-1 level (FROHMAN 1991; Ho 1990).

In our institution, we use normalization of the IGF-1 level as the ultimate determinant of successful therapy (chemical cure). We have found that in 99% of cases, an early postoperative growth hormone level of 2 ng/ml or less correlates with long-term nor-

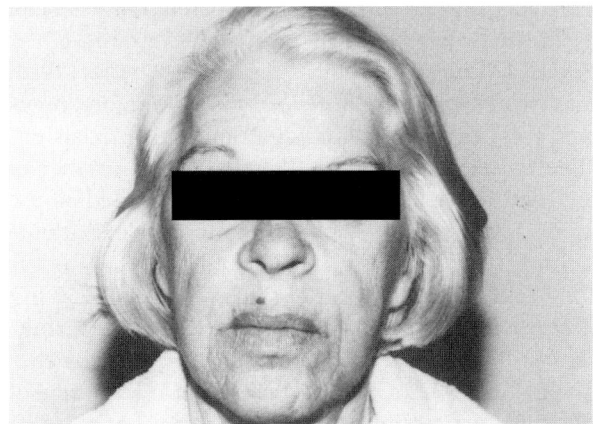

Fig. 8.4. The typical facies of an acromegalic patient. Note the coarsening of the facial features and prognathism

malization of the IGF-1 level and thus long-term disease remission. However, higher levels of GH rarely indicate long-term chemical cure (KRIEGER 1997).

In the patient harboring a GH-secreting microadenoma, surgical resection should be considered as the optimal first choice of management if he/she is medically stable to undergo a surgical procedure. Transsphenoidal microsurgical adenomectomy is currently the most accepted and efficient first-line therapy for the GH-secreting tumors of acromegaly (ARAFAH 1980; ARON 1995; BASKIN 1982; BUCHFELDER 1991; DAVIS 1993; FAHLBUSCH 1992; GRISOLI 1990; HARDY 1979; LAWS 1985; MELMED 1990; ROSS 1988; SERRI 1985; TINDALL 1993; TUCHER 1980). Some authors indicate that transnasal dissection in the acromegalic patient with associated soft tissue and bony changes may present an added challenge for the surgeon. However, in our personal experience, this has never been a limiting factor in the use of the transsphenoidal approach. Such tumors may be cured by chemical criteria in the majority of cases. A large combined analysis of 1360 acromegalics by ROSS and WILSON documented an overall postoperative cure rate of 60.4% (ROSS 1988). Microadenomas have an even higher rate of cure, exceeding 76–84% in recent large surgical series (ARAFAH 1980; BUCHFELDER 1991; DAVIS 1993; FAHLBUSCH 1992; LEAVENS 1977; MELMED 1990; TINDALL 1993; TUCKER 1980). In our personal series, 78% of patients with microadenomas undergoing transsphenoidal resection achieved normal long-term IGF-1 levels, and were considered cured. This rate was determined using very stringent criteria for cure: a postoperative growth hormone level less than or equal to 2 ng/ml, a normal 5-year IGF-1, and clinical evidence of disease remission at 5 years (KRIEGER 1997). Postoperative persistent elevation of GH or IGF-1 levels would be an indication for pharmacotherapy or radiation therapy (discussed later).

The patient harboring a GH-secreting macroadenoma poses a more difficult management dilemma. Certainly, the likelihood of cure is low in cases of large tumors with frank cavernous sinus invasion; in our series, only 31% of all patients with a macroadenoma achieved chemical cure by surgery alone(KRIEGER 1997). Pharmacotherapy or radiotherapy should thus be considered as integral components in the overall management plan. In these cases, initial pharmacotherapy may be indicated; however, surgical resection may be helpful in decreasing the tumor load to effect an absolute normalization of IGF-1 levels by pharmacotherapy.

Pharmacotherapy should be considered in: (1) patients in whom surgery is contraindicated; (2) patients whose GH and IGF-1 levels are still elevated after surgery, as an alternative for radiotherapy at this stage; and (3) patients with elevated GH and IGF-1 levels after surgery and radiation therapy (Ho 1991). Medical therapy may be administered in conjunction with radiation therapy to provide interim GH suppression while awaiting the beneficial effects of the radiation.

Native somatostatin is believed to control GH secretion by suppression of GH release from the pituitary gland and GHRH from the hypothalamus (MASUDA 1989). At present, there is only one FDA-approved analogue appropriate for clinical use – octreotide (Sandostatin, Sandoz, East Hanover, N.J., USA; previously designated SMS 201–995) (BAUER 1982). Octreotide contains the active sequence of somatostatin, and it appears to similarly control GH secretion by suppression of GH release from the pituitary gland and by suppression of GHRH from the hypothalamus (MASUDA 1989). In comparison to the native hormone, it has enhanced binding affinity to the somatostatin receptor and a prolonged half-life of 110 min after subcutaneous injection of a 50–100-µg dose, providing an overall duration of effect of 6–8 h (BARNARD 1986). A single injection of octreotide produces a decrease in GH levels within 30–60 min, with maximum suppression of GH levels occurring in 2–4 h (LAMBERTS 1988). Analogues are under investigation that have greater biologic potency than octreotide and are more specific for the pituitary gland (FROHMAN 1991).

The usual initial dosage is 100 µg subcutaneously every 8 h, and this dosage should be increased until adequate suppression is achieved. In acromegalics treated with octreotide, a close correlation has been found between the mean 24-h GH levels and IGF-1 levels before and during therapy (OPPIZZI 1986; LAMBERTS 1987a,b; BARKAN 1988). Therefore, regular IGF-1 measurements on an outpatient basis enable optimization of the daily dose and number of octreotide injections needed for each individual patient (LAMBERTS 1987a,b,). The majority of patients achieve control with 300–600 µg/day (LAMBERTS 1988). In a recent national survey, doses of 750 µg/day resulted in increased frequency of tumor shrinkage without adding any biochemical or clinical benefit (EZZAT 1992). Over a 6-month period, the size of the pituitary tumor was reduced in 34% of patients receiving this latter dose versus 17% of patients receiving 300 µg/day. At present, the maximum recommended dose is 1500 fg/day (FROHMAN 1991). As many as 50% of patients can be maintained on a twice-daily regimen (CHRISTENSEN 1987), but some patients may achieve better control by receiving the same daily dose every 6 h instead (FROHMAN 1991). In this regard, continuous subcutaneous pump infusion of 100–600 µg/day has been shown to provide superior and more stable suppression of mean 24-h GH levels (CHRISTENSEN 1987).

Of acromegalic patients, 75–90% experience some biochemical, clinical, and metabolic improvement with octreotide therapy. Clinical improvement may be heralded by the disappearance or the amelioration of excessive sweating, headaches, paresthesia, soft-tissue swelling, joint pain, and improvement of nerve entrapment symptoms, together with a general sense of well-being (FROHMAN 1991; EZZAT 1992). Immediate and prolonged relief of headaches is experienced in some patients with acromegaly, generally in those with evidence of suprasellar tumor extension (WILLIAMS 1987). Visual field improvement has been noted, in many cases without demonstrable change in tumor size (discussed later) (FROHMAN 1991). In some patients, dose- and time-related symptoms indicative of drug dependency occur (POPOVIC 1987), which may be mediated by the binding of octreotide to the opioid receptor (FROHMAN 1991).

Effective decreases of GH and IGF-1 levels occur in 30–53% and in 40–68% of patients, respectively, according to various studies (FROHMAN 1991; BARNARD 1986; LAMBERTS 1988; EZZAT 1992; SANDLER 1987; McKNIGHT 1991) In most patients, IGF-1 levels fall within 1 week of the start of treatment and tend to normalize in 37–81% of patients with continued therapy (EZZAT 1992; PAGE 1990; LAMBERTS 1985; BARKAN 1988; HARRIS 1988). GH and IGF-1 levels have been shown to continue to decrease with long-term treatment of 1.5–2 years when compared with levels at 6–12 months (LAMBERTS 1988). Long-term responsiveness can be predicted by the acute GH-suppression effect of a single test injection of 50 µg of octreotide. The mean hourly GH level from 2 to 6 h after drug injection exhibits a high degree of correlation with the 24-h integrated GH level after long-term (1–2 years) therapy (LAMBERTS 1989). The plasma IGF-1 and GH level response 2 h after drug injection or anytime during subcutaneous infusion are also useful predictors of efficacy (FROHMAN 1991). Plasma PRL levels in patients with mixed GH/PRL-containing tumors have been shown to be suppressed by octreotide in about one-half of cases

(LAMBERTS 1988). Elevated concentrations of the alpha subunit, which can be found in about 35% of acromegalic patients (WHITE 1986), respond to octreotide in a similar fashion to the changes in GH level (LAMBERTS 1988).

Preoperative treatment with octreotide causes the tumor to become soft in consistency and to exhibit a grayish red color at surgery (SPINAS 1987). Several neurosurgical groups have concluded that pretreatment with octreotide to soften the adenoma has facilitated surgical resection (SPINAS 1987; LANDOLT 1985). Long-term octreotide therapy produces a slight decrease in pituitary tumor size in about 20–50% of acromegalic patients (LAMBERTS 1987; BARKAN 1988; EZZAT 1992; JACKSON 1986). Complete tumor shrinkage has been reported in isolated cases (SADOUL 1992). Tumor size may increase soon after the drug is stopped (CHAREST 1989), but in occasional patients, a period off the drug may subsequently permit comparable control to be achieved at a lower dose. This phenomenon is possibly explained by a reversal of somatostatin receptor downregulation (FROHMAN 1991).

Although the drug is generally well tolerated, several side effects have been reported. Within the first few days of administration, a transient decrease in gastrointestinal motility and slowed absorption occur in most patients. The patient may experience transient abdominal pains and bloating. Steatorrhea, presumably due to a reduction in pancreatic exocrine secretion (PAGE 1990), occurs less frequently but may persist with long-term therapy. Treatment with pancreatic enzymes, if necessary, is usually effective (HO 1991). Nutritional deficiency has not been reported. Toxic hepatitis has occurred very infrequently. Inhibition of insulin secretion can lead to hyperglycemia, although the concomitant improvement in glucose tolerance as a consequence of a decrease in GH secretion is generally sufficient to prevent this. Although somatostatin inhibits TSH secretion, hypothyroidism has not been reported during long-term octreotide therapy (LAMBERTS 1985, 1987; BARKAN 1988). The side effect of greatest concern is cholelithiasis due to suppression of cholecystokinin secretion and a resulting decrease in bile flow. The incidence of gallstone formation in patients on long-term octreotide therapy is 40–50% (HO 1990; WASS 1989); thus, all patients should be screened regularly for the development of gallstones during treatment (PAGE 1990). No allergic problems related to octreotide have been reported, although antibodies to octreotide have been detected in one patient (Wass 1990). Tachyphylaxis and desensitization have not been observed during long-term treatment (Lamberts 1988). Although the injections are often painful, the pain may be minimized by slow injection of the drug.

With the advent of a pharmacotherapeutic agent effective in a large percentage of these tumors, it is hoped that the need for radiation therapy in these patients will diminish. At our institution, radiation therapy is considered only for those patients in whom chemical cure through surgery has not been achieved and in whom medical therapy is contraindicated, not tolerated, or demonstrated to be ineffective.

Radiotherapy has been advocated for the management of pituitary tumors since 1907 (Gramegna 1909). Radiotherapy per se, however, should not be considered a completely benign therapy or an equivalent alternative to microsurgical resection (Chun 1988). Adverse effects from radiation in this region may range from mild to severe. It carries a significant risk of worsening of preexisting hypopituitarism, with an overt 10–15% frequency of panhypopituitarism (Noell 1980); may increase the rate of atherogenesis in the major vessels in the field; and may cause visual impairment (Chun 1988). These complications increase as a function of total treatment dose (Aristzabal 1977). The visual impairment may result from one of several mechanisms, including empty sella syndrome, treatment failure, and direct radiation damage to optic pathways. This latter complication is seen with significant frequency with daily fractionation greater than 220 cGy (Aristzabal 1977). Other minor complications from radiation therapy include epilation, scalp swelling, and otitis (Baglan 1981).

Should radiotherapy be indicated in an acromegalic patient, a dose of 4000 cGy by external beam is considered optimal by most radiotherapists (Aristzabal 1977; Sheline 1974). In a reported series of 12 patients treated with radiotherapy alone, Chun and colleagues (Chun 1988) described a 50% recurrence rate, with a 75% incidence of local control following salvage treatment. Other authors report a local control rate of 50–79%, with an adequate salvage in cases of recurrence (Kramer 1968; Urdaneta 1975). The rationale for the use of postoperative radiation therapy is to reduce the incidence of recurrence, with several studies suggesting improved tumor control with the combination of surgery plus radiotherapy (Chun 1988; Noell 1980; Bloom 1973; Ciric 1984). This is especially true in large and invasive lesions, which exhibit an increased rate of recurrence. This treatment, however,

by no means ensures recurrence-free survival, but the time to recurrence may be prolonged. Valtonen and Myllymaki (Valtonen 1986) have reported a surprisingly high 36% recurrence rate in patients with so-called total removal following transfrontal craniotomy and postoperative radiation therapy, with recurrences having occurred up to 18 years following therapy. Thus, published recurrence rates may be misleading in series with short follow-up times.

The development of focal radiotherapy techniques (i.e., stereotactic radiosurgery) offers a potentially improved method in delivering accurate lethal dosages of radiation to the tumor while limiting toxicity to the surrounding visual and neural structures. Clinical trials are currently under way.

As noted earlier, the majority of patients with microadenomas achieve postoperative amelioration of their endocrinopathy. Overall, 78% of patients with microadenomas and 64% of all patients (microadenomas and macroadenomas) in our personal series achieved normal postoperative IGF-1 levels (Krieger 1997).

Although the surgical experience with microadenomas has been satisfying, cure with restoration of intact pituitary function is rarely achieved with large macroadenomas (Alford 1992). In our series, only 31% of patients who harbored macroadenomas achieved a chemical cure from surgery alone (Krieger 1997). Even when normal GH levels are achieved postoperatively, normal pulsatile secretion of GH and glucose suppression are often not restored (Frohman 1991). Clinically, the physical manifestations of acromegaly are rarely reversed; however, there appears to be little progression of the clinical manifestations of disease when GH levels are below 5 ng/ml.

All acromegalic patients, regardless of initial tumor size, must be followed assiduously for recurrence of their endocrinopathy after surgery. This vigilance is mandated by the increased morbidity and mortality associated with persistent disease. Physical examination for progression of acromegaly and for the development of hypopituitarism is indicated. Whereas GH levels less than 5 ng/ml are not usually associated with persistent clinical disease, levels greater than 2 ng/ml indicate a risk for recrudescent disease and must be monitored closely. After an initial postoperative IGF-1 level obtained at 6 weeks, follow-up measurements of GH or IGF-1 should be performed every 6 months (Baumann 1987). If octreotide is administered after irradiation, it is withdrawn for 2 weeks every 1–2 years, and GH and IGF-1 levels are measured. If they are normal, the drug should be discontinued (Ho 1991).

8.6
ACTH-Secreting Pituitary Adenomas

Cushing's syndrome is the name given to systemic hypercortisolemia. It is accompanied by protean symptoms, including fatigue, emotional lability, and muscle pain and weakness. The physical examination is notable for truncal obesity, abdominal striae, easy bruisability, and moon facies (Fig. 8.5). However, hypercortisolemia is also a malignant endocrinopathy, associated with hypertension, diabetes mellitus, osteoporosis, obesity, and immune compromise. There are many systemic etiologies for Cushing's syndrome. However, in most adult cases, hypercortisolemia is caused by an ACTH-producing pituitary adenoma. These cases are described by the term "Cushing's disease."

The diagnosis of Cushing's disease, and its differentiation from Cushing's syndrome, can be difficult. These typically small tumors often evade detection on MRI. Hypercortisolemia is demonstrated by measurement of plasma- and urinary-free cortisol levels. Differentiation between pituitary, adrenal, and metastatic sources of hypercortisolemia can be done by studying the dexamethasone suppressed levels of cortisol, as well as by measuring plasma ACTH levels. In some cases, corticotropin-releasing hormone (CRH) measurements or the CRH stimulation test can add additional information. When the diagnosis is still uncertain, petrosal sinus ACTH sampling with CRH stimulation can be helpful. Petrosal sinus sampling will also aid in the localization of the tumor within the pituitary gland when the imaging studies are nondiagnostic.

The treatment of choice for Cushing's disease is surgical resection of the adenoma. This is accomplished in most cases by transsphenoidal adenomectomy. However, in some cases, the adenoma itself cannot be localized on preoperative imaging studies or intraoperatively. In these cases, partial hypophysectomy can be performed, guided by results from petrosal sinus sampling.

Surgical resection can fail in cases of invasive adenomas. In this situation, radiation therapy may be indicated. Surgery also is relatively ineffective in cases of hypercortisolemia caused by a diffuse proliferation of ACTH-producing cells in the pituitary gland.

Medical therapy does exist to treat the symptoms of hypercortisolemia. Ketoconazole, for example, inhibits adrenal steroidogenesis. It can be titrated to result in normal serum cortisol levels. Perhaps more effective, however, is its use for complete adrenal suppression, with subsequent administration of exogenous steroids.

8.7
Glycoprotein-Secreting Pituitary Adenomas

TSH, luteinizing hormone (LH), and follicle-stimulating hormone (FSH) constitute the glycoprotein hormones. Each is composed of two subunits: an alpha subunit, which is common to all three, and a beta subunit which is specific for each hormone. Adenomas of each type exist, although these are rare. More commonly seen are the so-called alpha subunit

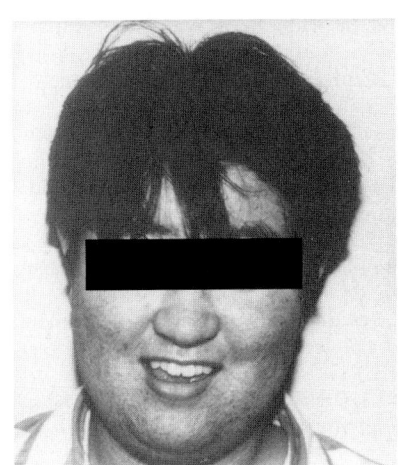
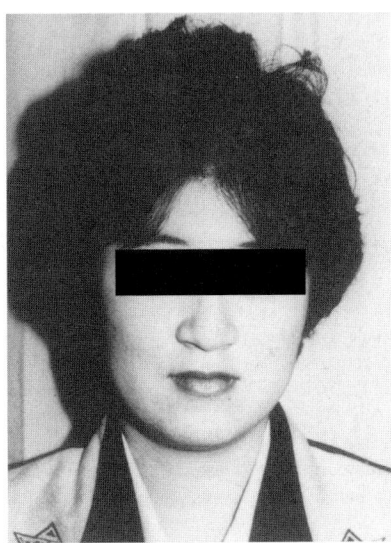

Fig. 8.5. The typical facial changes of a patient with Cushing's disease. Note the moon facies, skin changes, and plethora

adenomas, which secrete only the alpha subunit.

Rare TSH-secreting tumors can present as hyperthyroidism, and need to be distinguished from Grave's disease. The other three types of adenomas (secreting FSH, LH, or alpha subunit) do not usually result in clinically evident endocrinopathies. These tumors typically come to clinical attention when they grow large enough to cause compressive or mass effect symptoms.

Treatment of these lesions can be difficult. Because they typically do not present until they have grown to macroadenoma size, surgery has a relatively lower rate of cure. Radiation therapy can be used to control tumor growth, albeit with concomitant side effects. In most cases, palliation can be achieved with multimodal therapy.

8.8
Conclusions

Pituitary tumors result in a wide variety of clinical syndromes. Their management is often predicated on the type of tumor at hand. In many cases, excellent results can be achieved by employing a rational course of diagnosis and treatment. Vigilance in the post-therapy period is requisite to insure long-term success.

References

Adams CBT: (1988) The management of pituitary tumours and post-operative visual deterioration. Acta Neurochir (Wien) 94:103–116

Albuquerque FC, Hinton DR, Weiss MH: Elevation of serum prolactin due to stalk section effect. J Neurosurg. In press

Alford FP, Arnott R: (1992) Medical management of pituitary tumors. Med J Austr 157:57–60

Amar AP, Chen JCT, Couldwell WT, Weiss MH: (1998) Predictive value of immediate serum prolactin levels following transsphenoidal surgery. J Neurosurg 88:392A–393 A (abstract)

Arafah B: (1986) Reversible hypopituitarism in patients with large nonfunctioning pituitary adenomas. J Clin Endocrinol Metab 62:1173

Arafah BH, Brodkey JS, Kaufman B, Velasco M, Manni A, Pearson OH. (1980) Transsphenoidal Microsurgery in the Treatment of Acromegaly and Gigantism. J Clin Endocrinol Metab 50:578

Arafah BM, Rosenzweig JL, Fenstermaker R, Salazar R, McBride CE, Selman W. (1987) Value of growth hormone dynamics and somatomedin C (insulin-like growth factor I) levels in predicting the long-term benefit after transsphenoidal surgery for acromegaly. J Lab Clin Med 109: 346–354

Aristzabal S, Caldwell WL, Avila J: (1977) The relationship of time–dose fractionation factors to complications in the treatment of pituitary tumors by irradiation. Int J Radiat Oncol Biol Phys 2:667–673

Aron DC, Tyrrell JB, Wilson CB. (1995) Pituitary Tumors. Current Concepts in Diagnosis and Management. West J Med 162: 340–352

Baglan R, Marks J: (1981) Soft–tissue reactions following irradiation of primary brain and pituitary tumors. Int J Radiat Oncol Biol Phys 7:455–459

Barkan A, Lloyd RV, Chandler WF, et al: (1988) Treatment of acromegaly with SMS 201–995 (sandostatin): Clinical, biochemical and morphologic study, in Lamberts SWJ (ed): Sandostatin in the treatment of acromegaly. New York, Springer, pp 103–108

Barkan AL, Kelch RP, Hopwood NJ, Beitins IZ: (1988) Treatment of acromegaly with the long-acting somatostatin analog SMS 201–995, J Clin Endocrinol Metab 66:16–23

Barkan AL: (1992) Acromegaly. Trends Endocrinol Metab 3: 205–210

Barnard LB, Grantham WG, Lamberton P, et al: (1986) Treatment of resistant acromegaly with a long-acting somatostatin analogue (SMS 201–995). Ann Intern Med 105:856–861

Baskin DS, Boggan JE, Wilson CB: (1982) Transsphenoidal microsurgical removal of growth hormone-secreting pituitary adenomas. A review of 137 cases. J Neurosurg 56: 634–641

Bauer W, Briner U, Doepfner W, et al: (1982) SMS 201–995: A very potent selective octapeptide analogue of somatostatin with prolonged action. Life Sci 31:1133–1140

Baumann G: (1987) Acromegaly. Endocrinol Metab Clin North Am 16:685–702

Bengtsson, BA, Eden S, Ernest I, Oden A, Sjogren B: (1988) Epidemiology and long term survival in acromegaly. Acta Med Scandinav 223: 327–335

Bevin JS, Adams CBT, Burke CW et al: (1987) Factors in the outcome of transsphenoidal surgery for prolactinoma and non-functioning pituitary tumor, including pre-operative bromocriptine therapy. Clin Endocrinol 26:541

Bloom HTG: (1973) Radiotherapy of pituitary tumors, in Jenkins JS (ed): Pituitary Tumors. Butterworth, London, pp 165–197

Breidahl HD, Topliss DJ, Pike JW: (1983) Failure of bromocriptine to maintain reduction in size of a macroprolactinoma. Br Med J 287:451–452

Buchfelder M, Brockmeier S, Fahlbusch R, Honegger J, Pichl J, Manzl M. (1991) Recurrence following Transsphenoidal Surgery for Acromegaly. Horm Res 35: 113–118

Buchfelder M, Fahlbusch R, Schott W, Honegger J: (1991) Long-term follow-up results in hormonally active pituitary adenomas after primary successful transsphenoidal surgery. Acta Neurochir Suppl 53:72–76

Canales ES, Garcia IC, Ruiz JE, et al: (1981) Bromocriptine as prophylactic therapy in prolactinoma during pregnancy. Fertil Steril 36:524–526

Charest L, Comtois R, Beaureguard H, Serri O: (1989) Growth hormone rebound after cessation of SMS 201–995 treatment in acromegaly. Can J Neurol Sci 16:442–445

Christensen SE, Weeke J, Orskov H, et al: (1987) Continuous subcutaneous pump infusion of somatostatin analogue

SMS 201–995 versus subcutaneous injection schedule in acromegalic patients. Clin Endocrinol 27:297–306

Chun M, Masko GB, Hetelekidis S: (1988) Radiotherapy in the treatment of pituitary adenomas. Int J Radiat Oncol Biol Phys 15:305–309

Ciric I, Mikhael M, Stafford T, et al: (1984) Transsphenoidal microsurgery of pituitary macroadenomas with long-term follow-up results. J Neurosurg 59:395–401

Ciric IS, Tarkington J: (1974) Transsphenoidal microsurgery. Surg Neurol; 2:207

Cohen AR, Cooper PR, Kupersmith MJ et al: (1985) Visual recovery after transsphenoidal removal of pituitary adenomas. Neurosurg 17:446

Collins WF: (1979) Pituitary tumor management: an overview. P. 179. In Tindall GT, Collins WF (eds): Clinical Management of Pituitary Disorders. Raven Press, New York

Corrodi H, Fuxe K, Hokfelt T, et al: (1973) Effect of ergot drugs on central cathecolamine neurons: Evidence for stimulation of central dopamine neurons . Pharm Pharmacol 25:409

Crosignani PG, Mattei A, Ferrari C, et al: (1982) Enlargement of a prolactin-secreting pituitary macroadenoma during bromocriptine. Br J Obstet Gynecol 89:169–170

Cunnah D, Besser M: (1991) Management of prolactinomas. Clin Endocrinol 34:231–235

Davis DH, Laws ER, Ilstrup DM, Speed JK, Caruso M, Shaw EG, Abboud CF, Scheithauer BW, Rood LM, Schleck C. (1993) Results of surgical treatment for growth hormone-secreting pituitary adenomas. J Neurosurg 79: 70–75

Evans WS, Thorner MO: (1984) Mechanisms for hypogonadism in hyperprolactinemia. Semin Reprod Endocrinol 2:9–22

Ezzat S, Snyder PJ, Young WF, et al: (1992) Octreotide treatment of acromegaly. A randomized, multicenter study. Ann Intern Med 117:711–718

Fahlbusch R, Buchfelder M, Schrell U: (1987) Short-term preoperative treatment of macroprolactinomas by dopamine agonists. J Neurosurg 67:807–815

Fahlbusch R, Honegger J, Buchfelder M. (1992) Surgical Management of Acromegaly. Endocrin and Met Clinics North America 21: 669–692.

Frohman LA: (1991) Therapeutic options in acromegaly. J Clin Endocrinol Metab 72:1175–1181

Gemzell C, Wang CF: (1979) Outcome of pregnancy in women with pituitary adenoma. Fertil Steril 31:363–372

George SR, Kovacs K, Asa SL, et al: (1987) Effect of SMS 201–995, a long-acting somatostatin analogue, on the secretion and morphology of a pituitary growth hormone cell adenoma. Clin Endocrinol (Oxf) 26:395–405

Giannella-Neto D, Wajchenberg BL, Mendonca BB, Almeida SF, Macchione M, Spencer EM. (1988) Criteria for the cure of acromegaly: comparison between basal growth hormone and somatomedin C plasma concentrations in active and non-active acromegalic patients. J Endocrinol Invest 11:57

Giovanelli M, Losa M, Mortini P, Acerno S, Giugni: (1996) Surgical results in microadenomas. Acta Neurochir Suppl 65:11–12

Gramegna A: (1909) Un cas d'acromegalie traitJ par la radiotherapie. Rev Neurol 17:15

Greenspan SL, Oppenheim DO, Klibaski A: (1989) Importance of gonadal steroids to bone mass in men with hyperprolactinemic hypogonadism. Ann Intern Med 110:526–531

Grisoli F, Brue T, Graziani N, et al: (1990) Enlarged adenomectomy for enclosed prolactinomas: A preliminary study of 26 cases. Acta Neurochir (Wien) 103:92–98

Hardy J, Somma M: (1979) Acromegaly: surgical treatment by transsphenoidal microsurgical removal of the pituitary adenoma, in Tindall GT, Collins WF (eds): Clinical Management of Pituitary Disorders. New York: Raven Press, pp209–217

Hardy J: (1971) Transsphenoidal hypophysectomy. J Neurosurg 34:582

Hardy J: (1969) Transsphenoidal microsurgery of the normal and pathological pituitary. Clin Neurosurg 16: 185.

Harris AG, Prestele H, Herold K, et al: (1988) Long-term efficacy of sandostatin (SMS 201–995, octreotide) in 178 acromegalic patients: Results from the International Multicenter Acromegaly Study Group, in Lamberts SWJ (ed): Sandostatin in the Treatment of Acromegaly. New York, Springer, pp 117–125

Ho KY, Weissberger AJ, Marbach P, Lazarus L. (1990) Therapeutic efficacy of the somatostatin analog SMS 201–995 (octreotide) in acromegaly. Ann Intern Med 112:173–181

Ho PJ, Barkan AL: Acromegaly, in Bardin CW (ed): (1991) Current Therapy in Endocrinology and Metabolism, 4th ed. Philadelphia, B.C. Decker Inc, pp 38–43

Hubbard JL, Scheithauer BW, Abboud CF, Laws ER Jr: (1987) Prolactin-secreting adenomas: The preoperative response to bromocriptine treatment and surgical outcome. J Neurosurg 67:816–821

Hulting AL, Muhr C, Lundberg PO, Werner S: (1985) Prolactinoma in men: Clinical characteristics and the effect of bromocriptine treatment. Acta Med Scand 217:101–109

Jackson I, Barnard LB, Lamberton P: (1986) Role of long-acting somatostatin analogue (SMS 201–995) in the treatment of acromegaly. Am J Med 81(Suppl 6-):94–100

Jacobs HS, Franks S, Murray MAF, et al: (1976) Clinical and endocrine features of hyperprolactinemic amenorrhea. Clin Endocrinol (Oxf) 5:439–454

Kjellberg RN, Kliman B, Swisher BJ. (1980) Radiosurgery for pituitary adenoma with Bragg peak proton beam. In Derome PJ, Jedynak CP, Peillon F, eds. Pituitary adenomas, biology, physiopathology and treatment: Second European Workshop La Pitie-Salpetriere, Paris. Paris: Asclepios Publishing 209–217

Klibanski A, Greenspan SL: (1986) Increase in bone mass after treatment of hyperprolactinemic amenorrhea. N Engl J Med 315:542–546

Klibanski A, Zervas NT: (1991) Diagnosis and management of hormone-secreting pituitary adenomas. N Engl J Med 324:822–831

Konopka P, Raymond JP, Merceron RE, et al: (1983) Continuous administration of bromocriptine in the prevention of neurological complications in pregnant women with prolactinomas. Am J Obstet Gynecol 146:935–938

Kramer S: (1968) The value of radiation therapy for pituitary and parapituitary tumors. Can Med Assoc J 99:1120–1127

Krieger MD, Couldwell WTC, Weiss MH: (1987) Assessment of Surgical Cure of Acromegaly. J Neurosurg 86:351 A

Lamberts SWJ, del Pozo E: (1988) Somatostatin analog treatment of acromegaly: New aspects. Hormone Res 29:115–117

Lamberts SWJ, Uitterlinden P, del Pozo E: (1987a) SMS 201–995 induces a continuous decline in circulating growth hormone and somatomedin-C levels during therapy of acromegalic patients for over two years. J Clin Endodrinol Metab 65:703–710

Lamberts SWJ, Uitterlinden P, Verleun T: (1987b) Relationship between growth hormone and somatomedin-C levels in untreated acromegaly, after surgery and radiotherapy and during medical therapy with Sandostatin (SMS 201–995). Eur J Clin Invest 17:354–359

Lamberts SWJ, Uitterlinden P, Verschoor L, et al: (1985) Long-term treatment of acromegaly with the somatostatin analogue SMS 201–995. N Engl J Med 313:1576–1580

Lamberts SWJ, Van Koetsveld P, Hofland L: (1989) A close correlation between the inhibitory effects of insulin-like growth factor-1 and SMS 201–995 on growth hormone release by acromegalic pituitary tumours in vitro and in vivo. Clin Endocrinol (Oxf) 31:401–410

Lamberts SWJ: (1988) The role of somatostatin in the regulation of anterior pituitary hormone secretion and the use of its analogs in the treatment of human pituitary tumors. Endocr Rev 9:417–436

Landolt AM, Osterwalder V, Jantzer R, Stuckmann G: (1985) Pre-operative treatment of acromegaly with SMS 201–995: Surgical and pathological observations. Neuro Endocrinol Lett 7:94

Landolt AM. (1981) Surgical treatment of pituitary prolactinomas: Postoperative prolactin and fertility in seventy patients. Fertil Steril 35:620–625

Laws ER, Fode NC, Redmond MJ. (1985) Transsphenoidal surgery following unsuccessful prior therapy. J Neurosurg 63: 823–829

Laws ER, Kern EB: (1979) Complications of transsphenoidal surgery. p. 435. In Tindall GT, Collins WF (eds.): Clinical Management of Pituitary Disorders. Raven Press, New York

Laws ER. (1996) Comment on paper by Massoud et al. Surg Neurol 45:344–345

Leavens ME, Samaan NA, Jesse RH, Byers RM. (1977) Clinical and endocrinological evaluation of 16 acromegalic patients treated by transsphenoidal surgery. J Neurosurg 47: 853–860,

Lees PD, Pickard JD: (1987) Hyperprolactinemia, intrasellar pituitary tissue pressure, and the pituitary stalk compression syndrome. J Neurosurg 767:192–196

Leyeendecker G, Struve T, Plotz EJ: (1980) Induction of ovulation in chronic intermittent (pulsatile) administration of LH–RH in women with hypothalamic and hyperprolactinemic amenorrhea. Arch Gynecol 229:177–190

Lundin P, Nyman R, Burman P, et al: (1992) MRI of pituitary macroadenomas with reference to hormonal activity. Neuroradiology 34:43–51

Maira G, Anile C, DeMarinis L, Barbarino A: (1989) Prolactin-secreting adenomas: Surgical results and long-term follow-up. Neurosurgery 24:736–743

Martin NA, Hales M, Wilson CB: (1981) Cerebellar metastasis from a prolactinoma during treatment with bromocriptine. J Neurosurg 55:615–619

Massoud F, Serri O, Hardy J, Somma M, Beauregard H: (1996) Transsphenoidal adenomectomy for microprolactinomas: 10 to 20 years of follow-up. Surg Neurol 45:341–346

Masuda A, Shibasaki T, Kim YS, et al. (1989) The somatostatin analog octreotide inhibits the secretion of growth hormone (GH)-release hormone, thyrotropin and GH in man. J Clin Endocrinol Metab 69:906–1000

Mcknight JA, McCance DR, Sheridan B, et al. (1991) Long-term dose–response study of somatostatin analogue (SMS 201–995, octreotide) in resistant acromegaly. Clin Endocrinol 34:119–125

Melmed S. (1990) Acromegaly. NEJM 322:966–977

Molitch ME: (1992) Pathologic Hyperprolactinemia. Endocrinol Metab Clin North Am 21:877–901

Molitch ME: (1985) Pregnancy and hyperprolactinemic woman. N Engl J Med 312:1364–1370

Moyse E, Le Dafniet M, Epelbaum J, et al: (1985) Somatostatin receptors in human growth hormone and prolactin-secreting pituitary adenomas. J Clin Endocrinol Metab 61:98–103

Nabarro JDN. (1987) Acromegaly. Clin Endorinol 26:481–512

Noell KT (1980) Prolactin and other hormone producing pituitary tumors: Radiation therapy. Clin Obstet Gynecol 23:441–452

Ober K, Kelly D: (1988) Return of gonadal function with resection of nonfunctioning pituitary adenoma. Neurosurg 22:386

Oppizzi G, Petroncini MM, Dallabonzana D, et al: (1986) Relationship between somatomedin-C and growth hormone levels in acromegaly: Basal and dynamic evaluation. J Clin Endocrinol Metab 63:1348–1353

Page MD, Millward ME, Hourihan M, et al: (1990) Long-term treatment of acromegaly with octreotide (Sandostatin). Horm Res 33(Suppl 1):20–31

Physicians' desk reference, ed. 51. Medical Economics Company, 1997, pp 2411–2413

Popovic V, Paunovic VR, Micic D, et al: (1987) The analgesic effect and development of dependency to somatostatin analogue (octreotide) in headache associated with acromegaly. Horm Metab Res 20:250–251

Randall RV: (1991) Acromegaly and gigantism, in DeGroot LJ (ed): Endocrinology, 2nd ed. Philadelphia, W.B. Saunders Copp 330–350

Raymond JP, Goldstein E, Konopka P, et al: (1985) Follow-up of children born of bromocriptine-treated mothers. Horm Res 22:239–246

Reubi JC, Landolt AM: (1989) The growth hormone responses to octreotide in acromegaly correlate with adenoma somatostatin receptor status. J Clin Endocrinol Metab 68:844–850

Ross DA, Wilson CB. (1988) Results of transsphenoidal microsurgery for growth hormone-secreting pituitary adenoma in a series of 214 patients. J Neurosurg 68: 854–867

Sadoul J-L, Thyss A, Freychet P: (1992) Invasive mixed growth hormone/prolactin secreting pituitary tumour: Complete shrinking by octreotide and bromocriptine and lack of tumour growth relapse 20 months after octreotide withdrawal. Acta Endocrinol 126:179–183

Sandler LM, Burrin JM, Williams G, et al: (1987) Effective long-term treatment of acromegaly with a long-acting somatostatin analog (SMS 201–995). Clin Endocrinol (Oxf) 26:85–95

Schlechte J, Dolan K, Sherman B, et al: (1989) The natural history of untreated hyperprolactinemia: A prospective analysis. J Clin Endocrinol Metab 68:412–418

Serri O, Rasio E, Beauregard H, et al: (1983) Recurrence of hyperprolactinemia after selective transsphenoidal adenomectomy in women with prolactinoma. N Engl J Med 309:280–283

Serri O, Robert F, Comtois R, et al: (1987) Distinctive features of prolactin secretion in acromegalic patients with hyperprolactinaemia. Clin Endocrinol 27:429–436

Serri O, Somma M, Comtoid R, et al: (1985) Acromegaly: biochemical assessment of cure after long term follow-up of transsphenoidal selective adenomectomy. J Clin Endocrinol Metab 61: 1185–1189

Sheline GF: (1974) Treatment of non-functioning chromophobe adenomas of the pituitary. Am J Roentgenol 120:553–561

Sisam DA, Sheehan JP, Sheeler LR: (1987) The natural history of untreated microprolactinomas. Fertil Steril 48:67–71

Skrabanek P, McDonald D, Meager D, et al: (1980) Clinical course and outcome of thirty-five pregnancies in infertile hyperprolactinemic women. Fertil Steril 33:391–395

Spinas GA, Zaph J, Landolt AM, et al: (1987) Pre-operative treatment of 5 acromegalics with a somatostatin analogue: Endocrine and clinical observations. Acta Endocrinol (Copenh) 114:249–256

Thomson JA, Davies DL, McLaren EH, Teasdale GM: (1994) Ten year follow up of microprolactinoma treated by transsphenoidal surgery. Br Med J 309:1409–1410

Thorner MO, McNeilly AS, Hagen C, et al: (1974) Long-term treatment of galactorrhea and hypogonadism with bromocriptine. Br Med J 2:419–422

Thorner MO, Perryman RL, Rogol AD, et al: (1981) Rapid changes of prolactinoma volume after withdrawal and reinstitution of bromocriptine. J Clin Endocrinol Metab 53:480–483

Thorner MO: Prolactinoma, in Bardin CW (ed): (1991) Current Therapy in Endocrinology and Metabolism, 4th ed. Philadelphia, B.C. Decker Inc, pp 35–38

Tindall GT, Oyesiku NM, Watts NB, Clark RV, Christy JH, Adams DA. (1993) Transsphenoidal adenomectomy for growth hormone-secreting pituitary adenomas in acromegaly: outcome analysis and determinants of failure. J Neurosurg 78: 205–215

Tucker HS, Grubb SR, Wigand JP, Watlington CO, Blackard WG, Becker DP. (1980) The Treatment of Acromegaly by Transsphenoidal Surgery. Arch Intern Med 140: 795–802.

Turkalj I, Braun P, Krupp P: (1982) Surveillance of bromocriptine in pregnancy. JAMA 247:1589–1591

Urdaneta N, Chessin H, Fisher JJ: (1975) Pituitary adenomas and craniopharyngiomas. Analysis of 99 cases treated with radiation therapy. Int J Radiat Oncol Biol Phys 1:895–902

Valtonen S, Myllymaki K: (1986) Outcome of patients after transcranial operation for pituitary adenoma. Ann Clin Res 18(Suppl 47):43–45

Van Roon E, Van der Vijver JCM, Gerretsen G, et al: (1981) Rapid regression of a suprasellar extending prolactinoma after bromocriptine treatment during pregnancy. Fertil Steril 36:173–177

Vance ML, Evans WS, Thorner MO: (1984) Drugs five years later: Bromocriptine. Ann Intern Med 100:78–91

Vance ML, Thorner MO: (1987) Prolactinomas. Endocrinol Metab Clin 16:731–753

Wass JAH, Anderson JV, Besser GM, Dowling RH: (1989) Gall stones and treatment with octreotide for acromegaly. Br Med J 299:1162–1163

Wass JAH: (1990) Octreotide treatment of acromegaly. Horm Res 33(Suppl 1):1–6

Wass JAM, Thorner MO, Morris DV, et al: (1977) Long-term treatment of acromegaly with bromocriptine. Br Med J 1:875–878

Webster J, Page MD, Bevan JS, Richards SH, Douglas-Jones AG, Scanlon MF: (1992) Low recurrence rate after partial hypophysectomy for prolactinoma: The predictive value of dynamic prolactin function tests. Clin Endocrin 36:35–44

Weiss MH, Teal J, Gott P, et al: (1983) Natural history of microprolactinomas: Six year follow-up. Neurosurgery 12:180–182

Weiss MH, Wycoff RR, Yadley R, et al: (1983) Bromocriptine treatment of prolactin-secreting tumors: Surgical implications. Neurosurgery 12:640–642, 1983

Weiss MH: (1980) In Horvath K, Kaufman F, Kovacs E, Wiess MH (eds.): Pituitary Diseases. CRC Press, Bocan Raton, FL, p 180

White MC, Newland P, Daniels M, et al: (1986) Growth hormone secreting pituitary adenomas are heterogeneous in cell culture and commomly secrete glycoprotein hormone alpha-subunit. Clin Endocrinol (Oxf) 25:173–179

Williams G, Ball J, Lawson R, et al: (1987) Analgesic effect of somatostatin analogue (octreotide) in headache associated with pituitary tumors. Br Med J 295:247–248

Wilson CB, Dempsey LC: (1978) Transsphenoidal microsurgical removal of 250 pituitary adenomas. J Neurosurg; 48:13.

Wilson CB: (1984) A decade of pituitary microsurgery. J Neurosurg 61:814–833

Wray SH: (1977) Neuro-opthalmologic manifestations of pituitary and parasellar lesions. Clin Neurosurg; 24:86

Wright AD, Hill DM, Lowry C, Fraser TR: (1970) Mortality in acromegaly. Q J Med 39: 1–16

Zarate A, Canales ES, Cano C, Pilonieta CJ: (1983) Follow-up of patients with prolactinomas after discontinuation of long-term therapy with bromocriptine. Acta Endocrinol (Copenh) 104:139–142

Zervas NT: (1984) Surgical results for pituitary adenomas: Results of an international survey, in Black PMcL, Zervas NT, Ridgeway EC (eds): Secretory tumors of the pituitary gland. New York, NY, Raven Press, pp 377–385

9 Radiotherapy for Pituitary Adenomas

Anca-Ligia Grosu, Martin Kocher, Jürgen Voges,
Rolf-Peter Müller, and Michael Molls

9.1
Introduction

Pituitary adenomas represent about 12% of all intracranial tumors. The clinical classification into

A.-L. Grosu MD; M. Molls MD, PhD
Department of Radiotherapy, Klinikum Rechts der Isar,
Technische Universität Munich, Ismaninger Strasse 22, 81675
Munich, Germany
M. Kocher MD; R.-P. Müller MD
Department of Radiotherapy, Universität zu Köln, Joseph
Stelzmann Strasse 9, 50924 Cologne, Germany
J. Voges, MD
Department of Stereotactic and Functional Neurosurgery, Universität zu Köln, Josef Stelzmann Str. 9, 50931 Cologne, Germany

hormone-secreting and nonsecreting tumors, defined on the basis of serum level, is widely used. Surgery, radiotherapy, and medication are the three key elements of the treatment strategy.

The treatment of choice for adenomas with mass effect is transsphenoidal microsurgery, followed, in cases of partial resection or recurrence, by radiotherapy. In patients with hormone-secreting adenomas, with the exception of prolactinomas, transsphenoidal microsurgery is the first treatment step. The persistence or recurrence of a high hormonal level is an indication for radiotherapy. Irradiation needs months or even years to exert its effect, and during this time a medical treatment is indicated. In most cases of prolactinoma, a medical therapy with dopamine agonists reduces the tumor mass and the prolactin level within a few hours but after cessation of this treatment recurrences occur. Radiotherapy is indicated after incomplete surgical resection and/or persistence of high prolactin levels.

Radiotherapy is a well-established treatment for pituitary adenomas. The aim of the treatment is to control the tumor cell proliferation and, in endocrine tumors, to reduce the hypersecretion. These goals should be achieved with minimal injury to the surrounding normal tissue. The use of radiotherapy in the treatment of pituitary adenomas was first described in 1909 for a patient with acromegaly (Gramegna et al. 1909). Although there are no randomized studies comparing the role of radiotherapy with surgery or medical management, the clinical experience accumulated over a century, as well as many retrospective studies, clearly demonstrates the importance of this therapy in the management of pituitary adenomas. However, many problems concerning optimal patient selection and radiation treatment remain unsolved.

The goal of radiation treatment planning should be conformal coverage of the tumor with maximal sparing of the surrounding normal tissue. A total dose of 45 Gy in 1.8-Gy fractions, 5+/week, is generally recommended. A high rate of tumor control with a very low rate of side-effects is achieved by this procedure. Radiosurgery may be indicated in individual cases. The main advantage seems to be a reduction of the hormonal level within a shorter time. The role of radiotherapy will be discussed in relation to other therapeutic options, namely surgery and medical management.

9.2
Anatomical, Physiological, and Pathological Considerations

The difficulty in treating pituitary tumors lies firstly in the location and secondly in the complex function of this endocrine gland. The pituitary (hypophysis) is located in the sella turcica, in the body of the sphenoid bone, and is separated from the brain by the diaphragma sellae, an extension of the dura mater. The cavernous sinus, lateral to the sella, contains the internal carotid arteries and cranial nerves III, IV, V, and VI. The optic chiasm is situated anterior to the pituitary stalk. The hypothalamus extends anteriorly to the optic chiasm and posteriorly to include the mamillary bodies. Lateral to the cavernous sinus are the temporal lobes with the hippocampus.

The posterior lobe of the pituitary, the neurohypophysis, is an extension of the hypothalamus and releases antidiuretic hormone (vasopressin) and the milk let-down factor (oxytocin) into the bloodstream. Tumors intrinsic to the neurohypophysis are unknown. The anterior and intermediate lobe, the adenohypophysis, is a pharyngeal derivative (Rathke's pouch). It releases trophic hormones, under hypothalamic control, which regulate the major endocrine axes. There are seven known hypothalamic hormones: corticotropin-releasing hormone (CRH), thyrotropin-releasing hormone (TRH), growth hormone-releasing hormone (GH-RH), growth hormone release-inhibiting hormone (GH-RIH) or somatostatin, follicle-stimulating hormone-releasing hormone (FSH-RH), luteinizing hormone-releasing hormone (LH-RH), and prolactin-inhibiting hormone (PIH). These seven hormones control the production of six anterior pituitary hormones: adrenocorticotropic hormone (ACTH), thyroid-stimulating hormone (TSH), growth hormone (GH), follicle-stimulating hormone (FSH), luteinizing hormone (LH), and prolactin. The adenohypophysis is prone to the formation of benign and malignant tumors.

The modern pathological classification of pituitary adenomas is based on electron microscopy and immunocytochemistry. Distinction is drawn between growth hormone cell, prolactin cell, mixed growth hormone–prolactin cell, acidophilic stem cell, corticotropic cell, gonadotropic cell, and undifferentiated cell adenomas (Kovacs et al. 1977).

9.3
Epidemiology

Pituitary tumors have been reported to account for at least 12% of all intracranial tumors (Kernohan and Sayre 1956). The prevalence is 200 cases per 1 million population and the incidence is 15 new cases yearly per 1 million. (Ambrosi et al. 1991). Clinically asymptomatic adenomas are found in 1.5%–27% of autopsies (Burrow et al. 1981; Muhr et al. 1981; Abd El-Hamid et al. 1988; Kontogeorgos et al. 1991; Camaris et al. 1995; Auer et al. 1996). The development of high-resolution computed tomography (CT) and magnetic resonance imagining (MRI) has led to an increase in incidentally diagnosed pituitary tumors, called incidentalomas (Molitch and Russel 1990; Feldkamp et al. 1999). In an MRI study, Hall et al. (1994) found about 10% of the normal adult population to have abnormalities comparable with the diagnosis of asymptomatic pituitary adenoma.

9.4
Pathogenesis

The etiology of pituitary adenomas is unknown. Analysing the pathogenesis of pituitary adenomas, Molitch et al. (1987) concluded that perhaps 80%–90% of GH-, PRL- and ACTH-secreting tumors have a pituitary origin. The remaining cases could be a result of underlying hypothalamic dysregulation. Herman et al. (1990) support the hypothesis that genetic mutation(s) in the hypophysis may play the essential role in the pathogenesis of pituitary adenomas but do not exclude a facilitative role of the hypothalamus, perhaps by inducing clonal expansion of a genomically altered cell.

9.5
Clinical Manifestations

The clinical symptoms are caused by the local tumor growth with pressure effect or by the malfunction of the pituitary. The most common findings are visual field changes, initially characterized by bitemporal hemianopsia. Headaches and ocular palsies due to tumor invasion of the cavernous sinus may occur. The neuroendocrine dysfunction is a consequence of the hormone hypersecretion, of the tumor compression, or of both. As already mentioned, the clinical classification into secreting and nonsecreting tumors, defined on the basis of the serum hormone level and the presence of the clinical syndrome of hypersecretion, is widely used (LANDOLT 1975). The clinical abnormalities in patients with pituitary tumors are summarized in Table 9.1.

9.6
Treatment

9.6.1
Surgery

The goals of surgery are: (1) to remove the tumor mass, (2) to decompress quickly the chiasm and the optic nerves and, therefore, to improve the vision acuity, (3) to normalize the hormonal status in endocrine adenomas, if possible with preservation of the remaining normal pituitary tissue, (4) to achieve a histological diagnosis, which may influence the therapeutic decision. Using transsphenoidal microsurgery, which replaced frontal surgery, these goals can be achieved with a reduced risk of side-effects. Relevant details regarding surgical therapy can be found in Chap. 8.

Summarizing the data in the literature, CHANSON (1998) found 99 recurrences (26%) among a total of 377 patients treated with surgery of a nonsecreting pituitary adenoma, in comparison with 45 recurrences (11%) among 426 patients treated with combined surgery and postoperative fractionated radiotherapy (EBERSHOLD et al. 1986; JAFFRAIN-REA et al. 1993; HAYES et al. 1971; SHELINE et al. 1981; CIRIC et al. 1983; CHUN et al. 1988; VLAHOVITCH et al. 1988; GITTOES et al. 1998). However, several surgical studies have demonstrated that transsphenoidal microsurgery can be very effective and safe in the initial treatment of pituitary adenomas and that postoperative radiotherapy is not required: COMTOIS et al. (1991) summarized the results in 126 patients with nonsecreting pituitary adenomas treated with transsphenoidal microsurgery alone and found a 21% recurrence rate at 6.4 years. LAWS and THAPAR (1995) reported that 10 years after transsphenoidal microsurgery the recurrence rate was about 8% for acromegaly, 12% for Cushing's disease, 17% for nonsecreting adenomas, and 24% for prolactinomas. Finally, LILLEHEI et al. (1998) found a 6% recurrence rate 5.5 years after radical resection of nonsecreting tumors.

The result of surgery, based on the surgeon's report and on the MRI and hormone investigations, is important in the choice between postoperative radiotherapy and a wait-and-see strategy. However, the follow-up of patients with secreting adenomas has shown that in the majority of cases the operation is imperfect. Several studies have documented a high correlation between the grade of tumor invasiveness

Table 9.1. Clinical manifestations of pituitary tumors

Disease and hormonal dysfunction	Clinical manifestations
Hyperprolactinemia Prolactin hypersecretion	Amenorrhea, oligomenorrhea, infertility in females Impotence in males Galactorrhea Hypopituitarism, enlarged sella
Acromegaly Growth hormone hypersecretion	Gigantism in children and acromegaly in adults Hyperhidrosis, heat intolerance, fatigue, weight gain, paresthesias, arthralgias, headache, enlargement of sella, visual impairment, glucose intolerance, hypogonadism, hypoadrenalism, hypothyroidism
Cushing's disease, ACTH hypersecretion	Adrenal hyperplasia and hypercortisolism, obesity, hypertension, glucose intolerance, hirsutism, easy bruising, striae, osteoporosis, psychological changes, hypogonadism, rarely hypopituitarism
Hormone-inactive pituitary tumor, hormonal dysfunction due to tumor compression	Gonadotropin deficiency leading to secondary hypogonadism, hypothyroidism, hypoadrenalism, headache, visual disturbance, panhypopituitarism, enlarged sella

Modified from GRIGSBY 1998

in the neighboring structures (cavernous sinus, dorsum sellae, clivus, sphenoid sinus) and the risk of recurrence after transsphenoidal microsurgery (FAHLBUSCH et al. 1992). However, CIRIC et al. (1983) found that invasive tumors recurred in 15% of cases and noninvasive tumors in 12%. The risk of side-effects after transsphenoidal microsurgery has been decreased by the use of modern operative techniques (COMTOIS et al. 1991): mortality, 0.4%–1.6%; cerebral fluid lake, 2%–4.8%; meningitis, 2%; cranial nerve palsy, 1.6%; permanent diabetes insipidus, 5.6%, etc.

9.6.2
Radiotherapy

The classical indications for radiotherapy are: (1) incompletely excised or recurrent tumors, (2) medically inoperable patients or patients who refuse surgery, and (3) secretory tumors uncontrolled by surgery or medical management.

9.6.2.1
Techniques of Radiotherapy

The location of the hypophysis between important anatomical and functional structures and the clinical treatment results showing that grave side-effects can occur (although their incidence is very low) indicate the need to develop an optimal irradiation technique. The goal should be conformal coverage of the tumor with maximal sparing of the surrounding normal tissue. Various treatment techniques and their advantages and disadvantages will be discussed.

9.6.2.1.1
STANDARD COPLANAR AND
NONCOPLANAR IRRADIATION TECHNIQUES

Conventional radiation techniques are used in many departments. However, the tendency is to replace these techniques with three-dimensional (3-D) conformal radiotherapy. The most widely used irradiation techniques are summarized in Table 9.2. A linear accelerator with 6-, 10-, or 18-MV radiation beams, rather than a cobalt-60 therapy apparatus, is used to deliver the radiation. The patient's head is fixed using a thermoplastic relocatable mask. The treatment volume encompasses the macroscopic tumor region and the area of supposed microscopic invasion, and includes a 10- to 20-mm margin for possible uncertainties with respect to tumor borders and for variations in the day-to-day setup. The portals are in general no more than 4+4 cm to 6+6 cm in size. Wedge filters are used to obtain a homogeneous dose distribution.

SOHN et al. (1995) compared these techniques using a 3-D irradiation planning system. The goal was to identify the optimal technique for minimizing the dose of irradiation in the surrounding normal tissue. The evaluation was done by comparing dose-volume histograms for the eye and for the frontal and temporal lobe and analyzing the isodose distribution for different anatomical areas. The authors found that a radiation technique using four noncoplanar arcs delivered less dose to the frontal and temporal lobes

Table 9.2. Principal radiation treatment techniques used for pituitary adenoma

Technique	Field arrangement	Arc start angle	Arc stop angle	Wedge	Characteristics of dose distribution
Two-field	Two laterals	–	–	–	High percentage of the prescribed dose to the temporal lobe
Three-field	Two laterals	–	–	–	Improved dose distribution throughout the temporal lobe, approx. 20 Gy to 30% of the frontal lobe
	One vertex	–	–	15°	
110° bilateral arc	Arc 1	250°	360°	30°	Superior to the two- and three-field techniques in sparing the temporal lobe, approx. 10 Gy to 62% of the frontal lobe
	Arc 2	360°	110°	30°	
330° arc	Arc 1	195°	165°	–	
Four arc noncoplanar, 90° span; table angle 45° between each arc	Arc 1 (table angle=68°)	30°	120°	–	More effectively limited dose delivery to the temporal and frontal lobes than with the rotational arc technique
	Arc 2 (table angle=23°)	40°	130°	–	
	Arc 3 (table angle=292°)	240°	330°	–	
	Arc 4 (table angle=337°)	230°	320°	–	

Modified from SOHN et al. (1995)

than the other techniques; however, it delivered more dose to the eyes. They concluded that each technique has advantages and disadvantages and that the radiation technique should be chosen on an individual basis.

9.6.2.1.2
3-D Radiation Treatment Planning

In the era of CT and MRI, 3-D radiation treatment planning has replaced the conventional techniques.

The gross tumor volume, the planning tumor volume, and the critical structures (chiasm, optic nerves, hypothalamus, brainstem, temporal lobe with hippocampus, and eyes with lens) are defined on the basis of fusion imaging CT-MRI. For all these anatomical structures, dose-volume histograms are calculated.

9.6.2.1.3
Stereotactic Radiosurgery and
Stereotactic Fractionated Radiotherapy

Stereotactic radiosurgery (SRS) is a very precise technique for the delivery of focused radiation beams to small targets, with maximal sparing of the normal brain tissue. Three methods are available: heavy charged particle beams (proton, helium, neon, etc.) emitted from a cyclotron, gamma irradiation beams produced from a fixed array of cobalt-60 sources (gamma knife), and high-energy photon irradiation delivered from an adapted linear accelerator (LINAC) (see Chaps. 5, 6 and 19 for the relevant data). The treatment can be administered in a single fraction (radiosurgery: SRS) or multiple fractions (stereotactic fractionated radiotherapy: SFR). Using SRS the intent is to produce cell death within a well-defined target volume. The intense radiobiological effects of a high irradiation dose may produce important side-effects on the surrounding normal tissue. SFR combines the precision of target location and dose application of SRS with the radiobiological advantage of fractionation for the normal tissue (Fig. 9.1).

Facilities for heavy charged particle irradiation are available only in a limited number of centers. Use of a gamma knife and adapted LINAC to deliver the SRS and SFR is more widespread and in the past two decades extensive clinical experience has been accumulated.

The most important steps in the performance of stereotactic irradiation are: (a) fixing the patient's

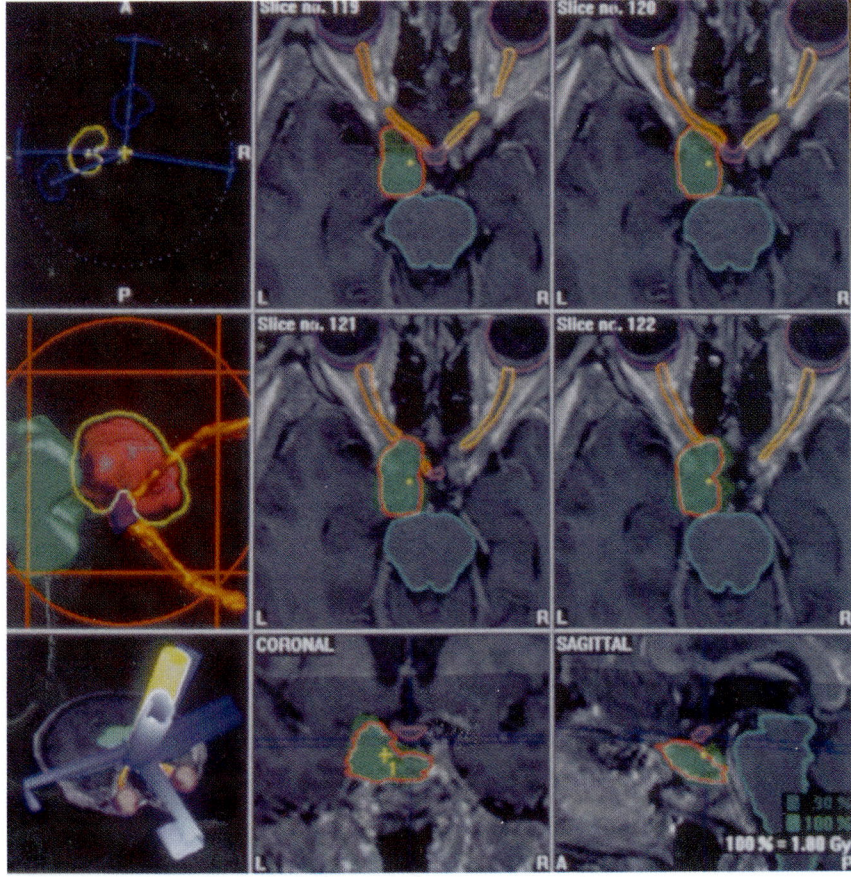

Fig. 9.1. Stereotactic fractionated radiotherapy treatment of a patient with pituitary adenoma, using static fields (Department of Radiation Oncology, Technische Universität, Munich, Germany; BrainLab System). The tumor margins are marked in pink. The green area represents the 100% isodose distribution. The optical nerve (orange), chiasm (violet), brain stem (green) and hypothalamus are not incorporated in high isodose area, although they are located closely to the tumor. On the left the conformal shaped irradiation fields are shown.

head using a stereotactic frame; (b) performing a CT and/or MRI scan that includes the whole head and the stereotactic system, attached to the frame; (c) defining the target volume and the critical structures using CT-MRI fusion images; (d) planning treatment using 3-D dose distribution reconstructions; (e) positioning the patient for irradiation using the 3-D stereotactic coordinate system; and (f) performing the irradiation as a single or fractionated treatment.

9.6.2.1.4
Implantation of Radioactive Sources
(Yttrium-90 and Gold-198)
Fraser et al. (1973) used this technique in 200 patients with pituitary adenomas and achieved a remission rate of 60% in patients with Cushing's disease and normal GH levels in 20% of patients with acromegaly. The disadvantage is the unclear dose distribution and the high rate of side-effects (50%).

9.6.3
Treatment Results

9.6.3.1
Local Control

Pituitary adenomas are benign tumors characterized by slow proliferation, so long-term follow-up is essential for the evaluation of treatment results. Tumor is considered to have been "locally controlled" when there is reduction or stabilization of the tumor mass as demonstrated by radiographic studies, and, in the case of secreting adenomas, when there is normalization of hormonal levels. The rationale for radiotherapy for benign tumors and the concept of cure after therapy are subjects of controversy in the literature. Herman et al. (1990) and Jacoby et al. (1990) postulated that pituitary adenomas are slowly proliferating clonal tumors and that late recurrences may be explained as a growth delay effect of radiation. Discussing this aspect, Brada et al. (1993) concluded that, considering the median age of the population with pituitary adenomas of 47 years, tumor control in 94% of patients at 10 years and 88% at 20 years is a real and worthwhile endpoint.

Reported progression-free survival (PFS) at 10 years after surgery and postoperative radiotherapy ranges between 77% (Hughes et al. 1993) and 95% (Brada et al. 1993; McCord et al. 1997). PFS 10 years after radiotherapy alone ranges between 60% (Hughes et al. 1993) and 100% (Halberg and Sheline 1987; McCollough et al. 1991). Zaugg et

al. (1995) reported 100% PFS 10 years after radiotherapy alone in patients with postoperative recurrences. The greatest number of recurrences occur between 4 and 8 years after treatment. At 30 years after surgery and radiotherapy, Grigsby et al. (1989) recorded a PFS of 44% in comparison to 73.5% after radiotherapy alone. The authors concluded that extended follow-up is necessary before pituitary adenomas can be considered "cured." Breen et al. (1998) found a tumor control rate of 64.7% at 30 years after radiotherapy (± surgery) (Table 9.3).

Various prognostic factors have been analyzed: age, gender, race, performance status, histology, tumor extension, hormonal and visual status, radiotherapy fields, radiotherapy dose, surgical approach, and the use of CT and MRI in the treatment planning (Table 9.4). In the majority of studies, age, gender, race, and performance status have been found not to be significant predictors of outcome. However, Tsang et al. (1994) found, in a multivariate analysis of tumor control, that young age was predictive of a worse outcome. They found a higher risk of recurrence in patients younger than 20 years and older than 60 years. However, this finding should be interpreted very cautiously in the younger group because of the small number of patients (three patients, with one failure). The reason for the higher recurrence rate in older patients is, as in the case of other tumors, unclear (in the aforementioned study there were 32 patients older than 60 years, with seven failures). Grabenbauer et al. (1996) also found a higher rate of failure in patients older than 60 years (univariate analysis), but age above 60 years was not statistically significant on multivariate analysis. In a multivariate analysis, McCord et al. (1997) observed that young age was predictive of worse control (median age of patients 48 years, range 17–89 years).

Surprisingly, in many studies no significant relation has been found between tumor extension or invasiveness in the dura and neighboring structures and the rate of recurrence after radiotherapy, illustrating the special biological behavior of pituitary adenomas. Grigsby et al. (1989), found a disease-free survival at 10 years of 77.8% for patients without extrasellar extension compared with 91.3% for patients with extension of disease beyond the sella. Similar treatment results have been reported by other investigators, including Tran et al. (1991), Hughes et al. (1993), Brada et al. (1993), Tsang et al. (1994), and McCord et al. (1997).

The presence of visual field deterioration at diagnosis was a significant prognostic factor in 70 patients treated between 1954 and 1982 with radio-

Table 9.3. Treatment outcomes in patients with pituitary adenoma

Reference	Patients	Follow-up	Treatment	RT dose	Tumor control/progression free survival
Chun et al. 1988	126	1970–1985 Med. 6.5 yr	S: 60 P S+RT: 54 P RT: 12 P	40–55 Gy 1.8–2 Gy/day	S: 85% (TC) S+RT: 93% (TC) RT: 50% (TC)
Grigsby et al. 1989	210	1954–1982 Med. 13 yr	S+RT: 121 P RT: 70 P S(failure)RT: 19 P	S+RT: mean 44.9 Gy RT: mean 39.8 Gy	S+RT: 92.8%, 10 yr (PFS) 71.2%, 20 yr (PFS) 44.0%, 30 yr (PFS) RT: 80.5%, 10 yr (PFS)
				73.5%, 20 yr (PFS)	73.5%, 30 yr (PFS)
Tran et al. 1991	95	1967–1985 Mean 7 yr	S+RT: 70 P RT: 25 P	44–55 Gy Mean 49 Gy 1.8–2.5 Gy/day	NFA: 83% (TC) GH: 60% (TC) PL: 44% (TC) NS: 3/5 (TC) CS: 3/3 (TC)
Salinger et al. 1992	68	1961–1986 RT: 39 P	S+RT: 29 P Med. 50 Gy	45.7–56 Gy 94%, 10 yr (PFS) 1–2 Gy/day Med. 2 Gy	S+RT: 100%, 5 yr (PFS) RT: 86%, 5 and 10 yr (PFS)
Hughes et al. 1993 Boost (79 P)	268	1962–1986 RT: 108 P	S+RT: 160 P 20–25 fractions	45–50 Gy RT: 60%, 10 yr (PFS) 60–100 Gy	S+RT: 77%, 10 yr (PFS)
Brada et al. 1993	411	1962–1986 Med. 10.5 yr	S+RT: 348 P RT: 73 P Max. 1.8 Gy/day	40–60 Gy Med. 45 Gy	S+RT: 95%, 10 yr (PFS) RT: 91%, 10 yr (PFS)
Tsang et al. 1994[a]	160	1972–1986 8.3 yr	S+RT: 128 P S(failure)RT: 29 P	40–50 Gy Med. 45 Gy 1.9–2 Gy/day	S+RT: 91%–10 yr (TC) S(failure)RT: 78%, 10 yr (TC)
Zaugg et al. 1995	89	1973–1992 Mean 8.1 yr	S+RT: 66 P S(failure)RT: 23 P	40–45 Gy 1.8–2.25 Gy/day	S+RT: 90.3%, 10 yr (PFS) S(failure)RT: 100%, 10 yr(PFS)
Zierhut et al. 1995	138	1972–1991 6.5 yr	S+RT: 99 P S(failure)RT: 23 P RT: 16 P	40–60 Gy Mean 45.5 Gy 2 Gy/day	94.9% (TC)
Grabenbauer et al. 1996[a]	50	1983–1990 Med. 4–5 yr	S+RT	46–63 Gy Med. 48 Gy 1.9–2.1 Gy	94% (TC)
Rush et al. 1997	70	1973–1985 Med. 8 yr	S+RT	43.2–50.4 Gy Med. 45 Gy 1.8 Gy/day	97.1% (TC)
McCord et al. 1997	141	1965–1993 Med. 9.2 yr	S+RT: 98 P Failure: S+RT: 10 P RT: 23 P Failure: RT: 10 P	42–55 Gy Med. 47.2 Gy 1.4–2 Gy/day Med. 1.8 Gy/day	S+RT: 95%, 10 yr (TC) RT: 90%, 10 yr (TC)
Breen et al. 1998[a]	120	1960–1991 Med. 9 yr	S+RT: 91 P RT: 29 P	37.6–65.6 Gy Med. 46.7 Gy 1.5–2.5 Gy/day Med. 1.95 Gy/day	87.5%, 10 yr (TC) 77.6%, 20 yr (TC) 64.7%, 30 yr (TC)

S, surgery; RT, radiotherapy; TC, tumor control; PFS, progression-free survival

[a] Endocrine inactive tumors

therapy alone (Grigsby et al. 1988). Zaugg et al. (1995) reported similar treatment results in 89 patients with macroinvasive adenomas treated between 1973 and 1992 with combined surgery and radiotherapy or with radiotherapy alone. The visual symptoms are certain indirect signs of tumor extension,

Table 9.4. Important prognostic factors in the treatment of patients with pituitary adenoma

Study	Age	Gender	Performance status	Tumor histology	Tumor extent	Hormonal status	Visual status	RT field	RT dose	Surgical	CT/MRI approach
GRIGSBY et al. 1989											
S+RT	NS	NS	–	–	NS	NS	NS	NS	S	NS	–
RT	NS	NS	–	–	NS	NS	S	NS	NS	–	–
FLICKINGER et al. 1989	NS	NS	NS	–	–	–	–	S	NS	–	NS
TRAN et al. 1991	NS	NS	–	–	NS	PL(–)	–	–	–	NS	–
HUGHES et al. 1993											
S+RT	NS	NS	NS	–	NS	PL (–), NSA (+)	NS	NS	S	S	–
RT	NS	NS	NS	–	NS	PL (–), NSA (+)	NS	S	NS	–	–
BRADA et al. 1993[a]	NS	NS	NS	NS	NS	NSA (+)	NS	–	–	NS	–
TSANG et al. 1994[a]	S	NS	–	–	NS	–	–	S	NS	–	–
ZAUGG et al. 1995	–	–	–	S	S°	PL (–), GH(–)	S	–	–	–	–
ZIERHUT et al. 1995	–	–	–	–	–	–	–	–	S	–	–
GRABENBAUER et al. 1996[a]	NS	–	–	–	–	–	–	–	NS	–	–
McCORD et al. 1997	S	NS	–	–	NS	PL (–), ACTH (–)	NS	–	NS	NS	–
BREEN et al. 1998[a]	NS	NS	–	S	–	–	NS	NS	NS	–	NS

S, Significant; NS, not significant; PL, prolactinoma; NSA, nonsecreting adenoma; GH, growth hormone; ACTH, adrenocortico-tropic hormone; (–), negative prognostic factor; (+), positive prognostic factor; RT, radiotherapy; S+RT, surgery plus radiotherapy
[a] Endocrine inactive adenoma

important especially for the CT and MRI era. Like tumor extension, visual field deterioration has been shown in many studies not to have a statistically significant impact on the prognosis (Table 9.4).

The classical histology (chromophobe, eosinophil, basophil, and mixed adenomas) was found not to be a significant prognostic factor in the study by BRADA et al. (1993). BREEN et al. (1998) found tumor progression after radiotherapy significantly more often in patients with oncocytoma than in patients with nononcocytic adenoma. PEGOLO et al. (1995) showed that routine histology is not useful in defining the aggressive tumors. Modern histological investigation seems to be more important in the selection of pituitary adenomas with a high risk of recurrence. Various immunohistochemical staining techniques have been developed in an attempt to define new markers for tumor proliferation: PCNA, Ki-67, MIB-1, nm-23, p53, and p 27. Discussing the correlation of these factors with tumor behavior, PLOWMAN (1999) suggests that the next step could be to select the predictors of aggressive adenomas that most closely correlate with recurrence and to in-

tegrate them in the selection criteria for postoperative radiotherapy.

Analyses of dose-response data have revealed an increased tumor control rate in patients treated with radiation doses from 30 Gy to 54 Gy. GRIGSBY et al. (1989) reported a tumor control rate of 94.1% in patients receiving 50–54 Gy, 85% for radiation doses of 40–49.99 Gy, 75% for 30–39.99 Gy and 28.6% for doses lower than 30 Gy. In that study the only prognostic variable identified by univariate analysis was radiation dose. The authors recommended radiation doses of 50.4 Gy in 1.8-Gy fractions for microscopic or small residual tumors and 54 Gy, also at 1.8 Gy per fraction, for gross tumors. SHELINE and WARA (1975) also demonstrated a dose-response relationship in the radiation treatment of pituitary nonsecreting adenomas and acromegaly: 55.6% failures at 30 Gy, 11.1% at 30–40 Gy and 5.9% at doses higher than 40 Gy. ZIERHUT et al. (1995) found a statistically significant dose-response relationship in favor of radiation doses of 45 Gy or higher: 10.9% of patients treated with doses lower than 45 Gy suffered a tumor recurrence whereas failure was diagnosed in only 1.2% of patients receiving doses higher than 45 Gy. They recommended a dose of 45–48 Gy with the use of conventionally fractionated radiotherapy (1.8 Gy). It is important to mention that dose escalation up to 70 Gy in the study by HUGHES et al. (1993) did not yield a better tumor control rate: only 40% of patients receiving 60 Gy or more had PFS at 10 years, compared with 78% of patients treated with a lower dose.

Many studies have used generally uniform treatment: 45–50 Gy, at 1.8–2 Gy/day (BRADA 1993; TSANG 1994; GRABENBAUER 1996; McCORD 1997). FLICKINGER et al. (1989) used radiation doses from 35.72 Gy to 62.32 Gy. No improvement in tumor control could be observed at higher total radiation doses. The authors concluded that, although the dose-response curve for nonfunctional pituitary adenomas is probably not completely flat from 38 Gy to 50 Gy, treatment with doses higher than 47.5 Gy (in 25 fractions) is not indicated; any improvement in tumor control would be too small to justify the increased risk of side-effects. BREEN et al. (1998) reported new data from the University of Pittsburgh: analyzing 120 patients with nonsecreting pituitary adenomas they found slightly less tumor control at doses greater than 47 Gy (possibly expressing a dose escalation in bigger tumors). On the other hand they found that oncocytic tumors seem to be a subpopulation with poorer tumor control at this dose. The authors postulated that future molecular genetic studies may be able to separate tumor subpopulations with different radiation dose-response relationships. For now they recommend doses from 40 Gy to 45 Gy in 20–25 fractions.

Several studies have found a significantly lower incidence of tumor control in lesions treated with larger radiation fields (FLICKINGER et al. 1989; HUGHES et al. 1993; TSANG et al. 1994). The explanation could be that larger field sizes correspond to larger tumors. However, many studies have shown no significant correlation between tumor volume and control rates obtained after irradiation (Table 9.4), and also no correlation between field size and tumor control (GRIGSBY et al. 1989; HUGHES et al. 1993; BREEN et al. 1998).

The role of the surgical approach in tumor control after postoperative irradiation has been analyzed in many studies. GRIGSBY et al. (1989) compared the transfrontal with the transsphenoidal approach and found no correlation between the surgical approach and the disease control rate. Similar data were reported by TRAN et al. (1991), BRADA et al. (1993), and McCORD et al. (1997). Comparing the tumor control after irradiation in patients with complete surgery, incomplete surgery, or biopsy only, BRADA et al. (1993) found no statistically significant difference in the treatment outcome. In the study of McCORD et al. (1997) there was no difference in tumor control between patients operated on with gross total versus subtotal resection. Actually, the rate of tumor control after surgery was generally comparable to the rate of tumor control after primary radiotherapy or after radiotherapy for surgical failure (Table 9.4). Considering these findings, TSANG et al. (1994) recommended that in favorable cases in which small tumors have been totally removed, a postoperative course of radiotherapy should be given only when surgical failure occurs. In the study of HUGHES et al. (1993) the extent of surgical excision was the only significant prognostic factor identified in a multivariate analysis. However, CORNETT et al. (1996) found a higher tumor control rate after surgery and postoperative radiation in comparison with radiation alone and suggested that immediate radiotherapy may be superior to radiation for surgical or medical failures.

9.6.3.2
Survival

The disease-specific survival rate after radiotherapy or surgery and radiotherapy following surgery in patients with pituitary adenomas is high. In the study of GRIGSBY et al. (1989), 5 (4%) of 121 patients died due to progression of disease after surgery plus radiotherapy and 3 (4%) of 70 patients died due to tumor growth after radiotherapy alone. BRADA et al. (1993) reported a study of 411 patients of whom four (1%) died of progressive disease after treatment. TSANG et al. (1994) reported a study of 160 patients with six (%) patients dying of tumor progression while BREEN et al. (1998) reported two (2%) deaths among 120 treated patients. However, although the risk of death directly attributable to tumor growth is very low, BRADA et al. (1993) showed that the overall survival probability in the group of patients with pituitary adenomas was 77% at 10 years and 58% at 20 years posttreatment. These survival rates were dissimilar to those seen in a matched group of the normal population. During the follow-up, 109 of the 411 patients treated died, a significantly higher number than the expected figure of 62 patients calculated on the basis of age-, time period-, and sex-specific mortality rates in England and Wales. The relative risk of 1.76 ($P<0.001$) was interpreted as an indicator of the adverse effect of the disease and possibly of the treatment on survival rate. The explanation for this finding could be the presence of endocrine syndromes (acromegaly) but, considering that excess mortality was also observed in nonsecreting adenomas, the authors postulate that hypopituitarism may also play an important role in increasing the mortality in these patients.

9.7
Clinical Entities

9.7.1
Prolactinoma

Hyperprolactinemia is defined as a plasma level of prolactin higher than 20 ng/ml. Microadenomas (tumors <1 cm) are associated with levels of less than 250 ng/ml, whereas macroadenomas (tumors >1 cm) cause serum levels to exceed 250 ng/ml (BAMBERG et al. 1996). For microprolactinomas the treatment of choice is the dopaminergic agonists (BAMBERG et al. 1996). Quinagolide or cabergoline seem to be more effective and better tolerated than bromocriptine (VILAR and BURKE 1994; COLAO et al. 1997). Transsphenoidal surgery is reserved for those with unresponsive adenomas. Analyzing the data of the literature, MOLITCH (1995) reported on 1224 patients with microadenomas treated with transsphenoidal resection. Permanent normalization of the prolactin level was observed in 71.2% of the patients. At UCSF 93% of patients treated with transsphenoidal surgery for microprolactinomas showed tumor control (HALBERG and SHELINE 1987). HARDY et al. (1978) reported a disease-free survival of 90%. Late regrowth of microadenomas was also observed: RODMAN et al. (1984) found 17% late relapses, whereas SERRI et al. (1983) reported a 50% recurrence rate. Consideration of radiotherapy is generally not necessary in this group of patients (BAMBERG et al. 1996).

In patients with macroprolactinomas, dopaminergic agonists are initially recommended. Reduction of tumor mass with a decompression effect can be achieved within a few hours. A decrease in tumor volume can be observed in about 77% of patients and a lower prolactin level is obtained in 73%–95% of patients (MOLITCH 1995; COLAO et al. 1997). In more than a half of patients treated, bromocriptine is not well tolerated. In these cases other dopaminergic agonists like quinagolide or cabergoline can be used. The disadvantage of the dopaminergic agonists

alone is that they do not lead to a permanent reduction in tumor volume and prolactin levels. After cessation of administration, recurrences occur, and this obliges the patient to accept lifelong drug use, with all its potential side-effects (CHANSON 1998). Surgical resection, indicated to reduce compression (especially in tumors that do not respond to dopaminergic agonists) and to lower the prolactin level, is less successful than in microadenomas. Summarizing the data from the literature, MOLITCH (1995) found a control rate after surgery of 31.8% in 1256 patients with macroadenomas. RODMAN et al. (1984) found a rate of late relapse of 20% whereas the recurrence rate reported by SERRI et al. (1983) was 80%. The data of HARDY et al. (1984) indicate that tumor control probably correlates well with tumor size and hormone levels before the treatment.

Radiotherapy is indicated after incomplete surgical resection and/or persistence of high prolactin levels. The reported results of radiotherapy vary widely. GRIGSBY et al. (1988) reported 82.3% disease-free survival 10 years after radiotherapy alone. In other studies, the rate of tumor control after radiotherapy alone or surgery plus radiotherapy has been significantly lower, ranging between 15% and 30% (SHELINE 1979; GROSSMAN and BESSER 1985; HUGHES et al. 1993; ZIERHUT et al. 1995). The treatment response occurs over several months or years following administration of radiotherapy. CLARKE et al. (1993) reported a response rate (complete plus partial response) of 86%, with a median time to response of 6.6 months. TRAN et al. (1991) reported a normalization of hormonal levels in 41% of patients after surgery and radiotherapy and in 56% of those receiving radiotherapy alone (the latter group, however, comprised only a small number of patients). The time to measured response varied from 1.2 to 6 years, with a mean time of 3 years. Until a normal prolactin level is achieved, dopaminergic agonists are indicated. The control rate seems to be inversely related to the prolactin level. In the study of TRAN et al. (1991) on tumors with a prolactin level lower than 200 ng/ml, the control rate was 75%. On the other hand, for those with prolactin levels higher than 200 ng/ml it was only 20%. Several authors have suggested that elevation of the prolactin level after surgery or radiotherapy does not necessarily imply the recurrence or persistence of the tumor. This elevation may be due to disturbance of normal delivery of prolactin-inhibiting factor (PIF) to the adenohypophysis as a consequence of impairment of the pituitary stalk by tumor and/or treatment (KLEINBERG 1977).

9.7.2
Acromegaly

The treatment of choice for patients with acromegaly is transsphenoidal resection. Using the strict new criteria of remission for microadenomas (MELMED 1995; FROHMAN 1996), which include a growth hormone (GH) level of £2.5 ng/ml and a normal insulin-like growth factor I (IGF-I) level, tumor control was found to range between 61% (Sheaves et al. 1996) and 88% (FREDA et al. 1998). The reported remission rate for macroadenomas was 26% (SHEAVES et al. 1996) and 60% (ROELFSEMA et al. 1985).

In patients with an incomplete resection and persistence of high GH serum levels, radiotherapy is indicated to reduce both mass effect and hormone level. However, the endpoint of therapy has been variably defined in the surgery and radiotherapy literature, so that many authors have considered a fasting GH level of less than 5 ng/ml or 10 ng/ml as remission (HALBERG and SHELINE 1987; CLARKE et al. 1993). Generally, progression-free survival at 10 years after radiotherapy ranges between 64% (HUGHES et al. 1993) and 80%–100% (ZAUGG et al. 1995). The results of radiotherapy are a function of the initial GH level and of time. SHELINE and WARA (1975) were the first to document this fact, observing that all 17 patients with GH levels <50 ng/ml achieved a normal GH serum level at 3 years, in comparison with only five of seven patients who had an initial GH serum level of 50 ng/ml or more. These observations have been confirmed in many other studies (BLOOM and KRAMER 1984; WASS et al. 1986). ZAUGG et al. (1995) reported 10-year progression-free survival with GH levels lower than 2 ng/ml in 80% of patients having initial GH levels higher than 100 ng/ml and in 100% of patients with initial GH levels lower than 100 ng/ml (P=0.03). The most important disadvantage of radiotherapy is the long time needed to normalize the hormonal level. The rate of GH decrease is about 10%–30% per year, so that several years may be required to normalize the hormonal status (EASTMAN et al. 1979). In this time an adapted medical therapy is required.

The dopamine agonists reduce the GH concentration in less than 10% (JAFFE et al. 1992). The somatostatin analogs (octreotide LP and lanreotide LP) have to be administered until a complete response to radiotherapy is achieved. The tumor control rate ranges between 18% (EZZAT et al. 1992) and 76% (GIUSTI et al. 1996) for GH normalization to <2.5 ng/ml.

9.7.3
Cushing's Disease

The first patient with Cushing's disease treated successfully with irradiation was reported in 1932 by Cushing himself. ACTH-secreting tumors are generally microadenomas. Transsphenoidal surgery is the first treatment option, leading to an immediate decrease in circulating hormone and a high rate of tumor control that ranges in the reports of the past decade between 75% (TAHIR et al. 1992) and 92% (RAM et al. 1994). In an evaluation of 668 surgical patients, BOCHICCHIO et al. (1995) found a tumor control rate of 76% (501 of 668 patients) with a recurrence rate of 12.7% (65 of 501 patients) after a mean time of 46 months. If resection fails to correct the hypercortisolism, radiotherapy is indicated. The tumor control after radiotherapy ranges between 50% (SHELINE 1979) and 100% at 10 years (GRIGSBY et al. 1988). As in the case of other hormone-secreting adenomas, the results are dependent on the criteria used to define the tumor control. The time to remission after treatment is generally nearly 1 year, but in some cases it may be as long as 3 years (HOWLETT et al. 1989; ESTRADA et al. 1997). Anticortisol therapy (mitotane) is indicated until the late effect of irradiation has been achieved.

Previously, bilateral adrenalectomy was the therapy of choice for patients with Cushing's disease. Unfortunately, 10%–30% of these patients developed enlarging pituitary adenomas with increased skin pigmentation after this procedure (Nelson's syndrome). This seems to have occurred independently of previous pituitary irradiation (MOORE et al. 1976; HALBERG and SHELINE 1987). In such cases tumor resection was performed, followed by irradiation in patients with incomplete resection and an elevated ACTH serum level. Tumor control was reported in about 50% of patients (NELSON et al. 1965; MOORE et al. 1976).

9.7.4
Thyrotropin-Secreting Pituitary Adenomas

Thyrotropin (THS)-secreting adenomas are rare. Usually they are macroadenomas with autonomous TSH secretion. The therapy consists in transsphenoidal resection followed, in the case of tumor persistence, by radiotherapy. Somatostatin analogs are indicated while waiting for the delayed effects of radiotherapy.

9.7.5
Adenomas with Mass Effects

About 30% of pituitary tumors are nonsecreting adenomas. These tumors often show invasion into the cavernous sinus, hypothalamus, or bone and are not completely resectable. The results of resection with and without radiotherapy are discussed in Chap. 8. The rate of tumor control after radiotherapy is very high, ranging at 10 years between 87.5% (BREEN et al. 1998) and 97% (BRADA et al. 1993) (Table 9.3). Since radiotherapy given at the time of tumor recurrence leads to progression-free survival rates comparable to those achieved following primary radiotherapy, TSANG et al. (1994) suggested that these patients be observed postoperatively for signs of recurrence: once a recurrence has been diagnosed, patients should be offered salvage irradiation. By contrast, BRADA et al. (1993), also on the basis of the excellent tumor control data and a low incidence of treatment toxicity, recommended a limited surgical decompression (e.g., transsphenoidal resection) followed by conventional fractionated external beam radiotherapy.

9.7.6
Incidentalomas

In the era of contemporary imaging with CT and MRI, a new clinical entity has been described, namely the pituitary adenoma discovered incidentally on a radiological examination performed for an unrelated reason. Such a tumor has been designated an "incidentaloma" (MOLITCH and RUSSEL 1990; HALL et al. 1994). FELDKAMP et al. (1999) reported a series of 67 patients with incidentalomas of the pituitary gland followed prospectively over a mean period of 2.7 years. Of these 67 patients, 63% had micro-adenomas and 37% macroadenomas. On ophthalmological and endocrinological examinations, visual field defects were present in 4.5% of patients, partial deficiency of anterior pituitary function in 15%, and prolactinomas in 12%. An increase in tumor size during the period of observation was noted in 3% of microadenomas and 26% of macroadenomas. A wait-and-see strategy was recommended in all patients with incidentalomas without clinical symptoms, with periodic imaging studies and careful clinical observation.

9.8
Complications of Fractionated External Beam Radiotherapy

Acute complications of external beam radiotherapy include minor, localized swelling of the scalp, reversible focal epilation, and, in some cases, otitis. There is a low incidence of late complications but, if they appear, they may have major clinical implications. Late side-effects include hypopituitarism, injury to the visual apparatus, brain necrosis, neurocognitive deficit, and carcinogenesis, of which the risk is very low.

9.8.1
Hormonal Dysfunction

Radiation-induced hypopituitarism is the most frequent late complication of conventional fractionated radiotherapy in patients with pituitary adenoma and can occur many years after the treatment. Pituitary hormone deficiency has been reported following irradiation for nasopharyngeal carcinoma (SAMAAN et al. 1979; LAM et al. 1991) or primary brain tumors (HARROP et al. 1976; DUFFNER et al. 1985), as well as in children after prophylactic cranial irradiation for acute lymphoblastic leukemia or total body irradiation.

The pathogenesis of the radiation-induced damage is not completely understood. Analyzing the hormonal status in children and adults with brain tumors who underwent radiotherapy CONSTINE et al. (1993) showed that the hypothalamus is more sensitive than the anterior pituitary. SAMAAN et al. (1979) evaluated late effects occurring from 3 to 20 years after irradiation in patients with extracranial tumors (nasopharyngeal carcinoma) who had been treated with 30–85 Gy (92% of doses being at least 45 Gy). In 54 (83%) of the 65 patients treated, a hypothalamic-pituitary impairment was diagnosed and in 25 (38%) patients primary hypopituitarism was found. A further argument supporting the hypothalamus as the first target for radiation injury is the lower combined incidence of corticotropin and TSH deficiency after yttrium-90 brachytherapy in the pituitary gland in patients with adenomas. JADRESIC et al (1987) reported that 14 years after yttrium-90 treatment, 39% of patients had combined corticotropin–TSH deficiency (JADRESIC et al. 1987), whereas the figure was 90% 10 years after conventional radiotherapy in which the hypothalamus was completely included in the irradiation field (LITTLEY et al. 1989). Actually, the hormonal suppression seen in patients with radiation-induced injury generally corresponds to the characteristic hormonal findings in patients with pathologically documented hypothalamic disease (SHALET et al. 1993). It remains unclear whether vascular or direct neuronal changes following radiotherapy are primarily responsible for the hypothalamic injury. Additionally, it is unknown why there is such a low incidence of diabetes insipidus in these patients. However, recognition of the hypothalamus as the most important site of radiation injury may have an important influence on the radiation treatment planning. Using conformal radiotherapy techniques such as stereotactic radiotherapy, the hypothalamus can to a large extent be excluded from receiving therapeutic doses of radiotherapy. Another implication of these findings is the importance of a specifically and physiologically designed hormonal therapy (O'HALLERAN and SHALET 1996).

LITTLEY et al. (1989) demonstrated that radiation-induced hypopituitarism is dependent on the radiation dose. The first affected hormone is GH; the gonadotropin and corticotropin axes are the next in radiation sensitivity, while the least sensitive hormone is TSH. The explanation for this hierarchy in the radiation response is another open question. In a review of all types of pituitary adenomas, SNYDER et al. (1986) reported the incidence of adrenal, thyroid, and gonadal hormone deficiency to be 13%, 13%, and 0% respectively after surgery alone, 55%, 15%, and 50% respectively after radiotherapy alone, and 67%, 55%, and 67% respectively following combined surgery and radiotherapy. HUGHES et al. (1993) reported an incidence of hypopituitarism of 34% after radiotherapy alone and 74% after surgery plus radiotherapy. In the analysis of FEEK et al. (1984), 47% of patients were hypogonadal 10 years after radiotherapy alone, 30% were hypoadrenal, and 16% were hypothyroid. The incidence was 70%, 54%, and 38% respectively after surgery plus radiotherapy. These results show that the risk of hypopituitarism is lower after surgery or radiotherapy alone and higher after the use of combined treatment.

In patients with hypopituitarism an increased incidence of cerebrovascular mortality has been noted, probably due to an inadequate substitution of pituitary hormones, especially GH (FLICKINGER et al. 1989; ROSEN and BENGTSSON 1990; BÜLOW et al. 1997). These findings are arguments for long-term endocrinological follow-up and for the importance of an adequate substitution treatment (see Sect. 9.6.3.2).

9.8.2
Visual Injury

The optic nerve and optic chiasm are included in the radiation field in most patients treated with external beam radiotherapy for pituitary adenoma. Reports of visual impairment are generally very rare (Table 9.5). The total radiation doses and daily radiation fractions shown in Table 9.5 represent radiotherapy in patients with serious visual injury and therefore do not necessarily represent dose schedules used in the treatment of all patients. In cases where no specific radiation dose was associated with visual complications, the treatment prescribed for the entire group of patients has been cited. HARRIS and LEVEN (1976) diagnosed optic nerve or chiasm radiation neuropathy in five (9%) of the 55 patients treated. All patients with this radiation injury received 2.5-Gy daily fractions. No patient who received less than 2.5 Gy per day showed visual loss. In this report the delivered dose per fraction was more important in the development of optic nerve or chiasm injury than was the total radiation dose given. Similar findings were also demonstrated in the studies of ARISTIZABAL et al. (1977) and PARSON et al. (1994). However, total doses not greater than 45 Gy sharply decrease the risk of complications and assure a high tumor control rate (HALBERG and SHELINE 1987; McCORD et al. 1997; BREEN et al. 1998). Higher doses may primarily increase the risk of side-effects without a corresponding increase in the tumor control rate. Using daily dose fractions lower than 1.8 Gy to a total dose ranging from 40 to 60 Gy, with a median dose of 45 Gy, BRADA et al. (1993) found that only 2 (0.5%) of 411 patients had late and otherwise unexplained visual deterioration, in neither case leading to blindness. In a considerable number of studies of patients treated with radiotherapy for pituitary adenoma no damage to the optic pathway has been reported (JONES 1991; TRAN et al. 1991; TSANG et al. 1994; MOVSAS et al. 1995; RUSH et al. 1997). Acromegaly, Cushing's disease, hypertension, preexisting vascular disease, age, and tumor compression of the chiasm of long duration are important factors predisposing to chiasm or optic nerve atrophy after radiotherapy (KRAMER 1973; ARISTIZABAL et al. 1977; ATKINSON et al. 1979; PARSON et al. 1994).

9.8.3
Carcinogenesis

The risk of carcinogenesis after radiotherapy of pituitary adenomas is the subject of controversy discussed

Table 9.5. Chiasm or optic nerve injuries in the reported radiotherapy series

Author	Total dose (Gy)	Daily fraction (Gy)	Patients, injury
HARRIS and LEVENE 1976	45	2.5	3/55 P: blindness right eye, 6 mo; blindness both eyes, 9 mo; tunnel vision, 2 yr
	50	2.5	1/55 P: bitemporal hemianopsia, 3 yr
	70	2.5	1/55 P: (craniopharyngioma?) virtual blindness, 2 yr
ARISTIZABAL et al. 1977	50	Lower than 2	0/7P
	50	2–2.2	1/99 P: optic nerve atrophy, 13 mo
			1/99 P: progressive blindness, 10 mo
	50	Higher than 2.2	2/16 P: progressive blindness, 14 mo, 15 mo
SHELINE 1979	45–50	2.25	1/181 P: optic injury
CHUN et al. 1988	40–55	1.8–2	3/126 P: decrease in visual acuity
GRIGSBY et al. 1988/89	46.8	0.5–2, med. 1.6	1/70 P: optic neuritis
RT alone	18.8		1/70 P: visual deterioration during RT
S+RT	50.4	1.1–2, med. 1.8	1/121 P: unilateral optic nerve atrophy 6 yr
	18		1/121 P: visual deterioration during RT
JONES 1991	45	1.8	0/332 P: no damage to optic pathways
TRAN et al. 1991	44–55	1.8–2.5	0/95 P: no damage to optic pathways
HUGHES et al. 1993	50	2.5	1/268 P: optic atrophy
BRADA et al. 1993	40–60 Med. 45	Max. 1.8	2/411 P: visual deterioration, none became blind
FISHER et al. 1993	50	2	2/134 P: visual deterioration, optic atrophy
TSANG et al. 1994	40–50 Med. 45	1.9–2 Gy	0/160 P: no damage to optic pathways
ZAUGG et al. 1995	40	2	3/89 P: intermittent visual deterioration, 6 yr; right temporal loss of visual field, 15 yr; deterioration of visual field, 1.5 yr
	44	2	1/89 P: deterioration of acuity 9.5 yr
ZIERHUT et al. 1995	46	2	1/138 P: completely lost vision left eye 4 yr
	52	2	1/138 P: worsening of already existing impaired vision 3 yr
MOVSAS et al. 1995	45–59.4 Med. 50	1.8–2	0/21 P: no damage to optic pathways
GRABENBAUER et al. 1996	63	2.1	1/50 P: optic neuropathy 6 yr
	58.75	1.9–2.25	1/50 P: optic neuropathy 1.5 yr
RUSH et al. 1997	43.2–50.4	1.8	0/70 P: no damage to optic pathways
McCORD et al. 1997	42–55	1.4–2	4/141 P: visual loss
BREEN et al. 1998	50	1.67	2/120 P: unilateral visual loss 7 mo, 12 mo

P, Patients

in the literature. Evaluating the reported results in the literature for a period of 10 years (1988–1998), we found a total of 17 (0.85%) secondary tumors in 2000 patients irradiated for pituitary adenomas (Table 9.6). The age of patients at the time of radiotherapy ranged from 26 to 67 years. The time from treatment to the diagnosis of a second tumor ranged from 6 to 28 years (Table 9.6). Of these 17 patients with secondary tumors, 13 had malignant tumors (0.65%) and four had meningiomas (0.2%). Therefore, in the clinical decision-making process, the minimal risk of developing a secondary tumor has to be balanced against the well-established advantages of the treatment. In a group of 1946 patients treated with radiotherapy (Table 9.3), one case of radionecrosis (0.05%) was described, located in the temporal lobe and diagnosed 5 years after radiotherapy with 54 Gy, 2 Gy/day, 5+/week (GRABENBAUER et al. 1996).

9.8.4
Neuropsychological Abnormalities

Diagnosis of neuropsychological abnormalities due to external beam radiotherapy is difficult as such cases have uncommonly been reported in the literature. A study evaluating neuropsychological problems in 65 patients with pituitary tumors revealed impairment of memory and executive function independent from the effects of radiotherapy or surgery. The outcome of this study lent support to the hy-

Table 9.6. Reported second malignant lesions in patients treated for pituitary adenoma

Author	Patients	Second brain tumor
CHUN et al. 1988	126	0
GRIGSBY et al. 1989	210	0
TRAN et al. 1991	95	0
JONES 1991	332	1 glioma, 1 neuroectodermal tumor, 2 myelogenous leukemia
SALINGER et al. 1992	68	0
HUGHES et al. 1993	268	0
BRADA et al. 1992	411	2 gliomas, 2 meningiomas, 1 meningeal sarcoma
TSANG et al. 1993	367	4 gliomas
BLISS et al. 1994	193	1 lymphoma (?), 1 meningioma
ZAUGG et al. 1995	89	0
ZIERHUT et al. 1995	138	0
GRABENBAUER et al. 1996	50	0
RUSH and COOPER 1997	70	0
McCORD et al. 1997	141	0
BREEN et al. 1998	120	1 glioblastoma, 1 meningioma
Total	2000	17 secondary tumors (0.85%)

pothesis that pituitary and hypothalamic hormones have an active role in the modulation of memory and behavioral pathways (GRATTAN-SMITH et al. 1992). However, there are few reported data in the literature showing neuropsychological changes after radiotherapy for pituitary adenoma. PEACE et al. (1997) observed fewer symptoms of depression in patients treated with surgery than in those treated with radiotherapy. ZAUGG et al. (1995) reported that of 89 patients treated with radiotherapy alone or surgery followed by radiotherapy, four (4.5%) developed lapse of memory, sleeplessness, and reduced physical efficiency but the authors mentioned that these symptoms could also have been related to increasing patient age. Neurocognitive sequelae after surgery and radiotherapy were also reported by McCORD et al. (1997). Although data on the neuropsychological effects of radiotherapy for pituitary adenomas are insufficient and unclear, the limbic system, responsible for highly differentiated cognitive and emotional functions, is located in the vicinity of the hypophysis and late morphological and physiological changes are possible. This region has to be defined as a risk area and has to be considered in the irradiation treatment planning.

In summary: acute complications of radiotherapy for pituitary adenoma are uncommon and of no major clinical significance. Hypopituitarism is the most frequent late complication of pituitary irradiation and regular endocrinological follow-up is indicated over a long period following radiotherapy. Visual injury, brain necrosis, neurocognitive deficits, and carcinogenesis are extremely rare complications in contemporary radiotherapy. Stereotactic radiosurgery can potentially further reduce the incidence of these complications by sparing critical anatomical structures in the vicinity of the volume of interest. Future studies have to aim to establish better criteria of patient selection for radiotherapy and improved definition of the role of modern treatment techniques such as radiosurgery and stereotactic fractionated radiotherapy.

9.9 Reirradiation

A number of cases of reirradiation have been reported in the literature. SCHOENTHALER et al. (1992) described follow-up of 15 patients treated with a second course of radiotherapy 2–17 years (median 9 years) after the first treatment. The median initial dose was 48.84 Gy and the median dose given during the salvage radiotherapy was 42 Gy. Tumor control was achieved in 12 of these patients. One patient developed a recurrence and two patients had pituitary carcinomas. Two patients developed temporal lobe injuries, with no visual complications recorded. FLICKINGER et al. (1989) analyzed the clinical results of ten patients, including six with pituitary adenomas, reirradiated for treatment failure (first dose 36–53.65 Gy and second dose 35–49.6 Gy, interval 0.6–16.5 years). All six patients with pituitary adenomas remained free of disease progression 0.2–9.7 years after the second course of irradiation. One patient developed optic neuropathy. In the treatment of external beam radiotherapy failures, radiosurgery can also be used, on condition that the volume of the recurrent tumor can be well defined and that it does not include critical structures such as the chiasm.

9.10 Radiosurgery

Proton and heavy ion beams have been used mainly for primary therapy of secreting adenomas. KJELLBERG et al. (1984) treated more than 250 patients with both GH- and ACTH -secreting tumors using a single-fraction proton beam therapy. With the limitations resulting from an incomplete follow-up, it seems that 50% of the treated patients with acromegaly and 80% of those with ACTH hypersecretion reached normal hormone levels within 5 years (KJELLBERG et al. 1984; KLIMANN et al. 1984). The same results were achieved by LEVY et al. (1991, 1996) using hypofractionated helium ion beam therapy. Neurotoxic side-effects affected only a few of the patients and were mainly restricted to the nerves passing through the cavernous sinus and the temporal lobe. However, in conjunction with both techniques, hypopituitarism requiring hormone replacement was observed in up to 50% of the patients. Given the above-mentioned limitations of the conventional imaging techniques, it was likely not possible to selectively irradiate the adenoma and spare the normal hypophyseal tissue.

Gamma-knife radiosurgery was initially also used without CT- or MRI-based treatment planning (DEGERBLAD et al. 1986), with doses of 35–50 Gy defined to the 50% isodose surface. Hormonal normalization rates were as high as with heavy particle beam radiosurgery, but hypopituitarism was also frequent (incidence of up to 55%). Later, treatment planning was based on MRI and doses were reduced to 10–35 Gy at the tumor periphery (20–70 Gy maximum dose) (THOREN et al. 1991; WITT et al. 1996). Due to the high efficacy of surgical therapy, only patients with persistent or recurrent hypersecretion following one or more surgical procedures were selected for radiosurgery at that time. With the aid of

the high spatial resolution of CT and MR images, highly conformed dose distribution in relation to target volumes can be generated by the use of multiple isocenters. The results of this refined treatment technique are promising. At median follow-up times of 2–3 years, 50%–70% of patients have been found to achieve normal hormone levels, with minor neurotoxicity and only a 0%–15% rate of hypopituitarism. Encouraged by these results, some Asian centers have again started to treat patients primarily with radiosurgery. At a median follow-up of about 2 years, 40%–100% of the patients so treated have achieved hormonal normalization (LIM et al. 1998; PAN et al. 1998). Reported treatment toxicity is very low in these series.

The treatment results obtained with a linear accelerator-based radiosurgery are more preliminary. Unfortunately, most of the centers using LINAC radiosurgery have treated patients with pituitary adenomas by a simple technique with only one isocenter and a limited number of arcs. While treatment effects in terms of hormonal normalization seem to be comparable to the gamma knife series, significant neurotoxicity (visual deterioration, temporal lobe necrosis) has been observed (ROCHER et al. 1995; MITSUMORI et al. 1998; YOON et al. 1998). As a consequence, the Boston group recommended the use of fractionated stereotactic radiotherapy instead of single-dose radiosurgery (MITSUMORI et al. 1998).

Our group started to treat patients with single-dose LINAC radiosurgery in 1990 (University of Cologne, Germany). Emphasis was put on sophisticated treatment planning, using two to five isocenters each irradiated with seven to ten arcs in order to cover the irregular target volumes as optimally as possible. So far, 79 patients with recurrent pituitary adenomas have been treated with 12–20 Gy referred to the 65%–80% isodose surface. Neurotoxicity (temporal lobe necrosis) has been observed in two of the patients treated (VOGES et al. 1996a). Following adoption of the guidelines resulting from a risk analysis for radionecrosis (VOGES et al. 1996b) and integration of MRI into the treatment planning procedure, no further severe side-effects related to damage to the temporal lobe or optic system have been observed in the group of subsequently treated patients. Including all patients, pituitary insufficiency occurred in 12%, temporary blood-brain barrier disruption of the temporal lobe in 3%, and visual field disturbances in 2%. An analysis of a total of 55 patients with a follow-up period of more than 1 year revealed a hormonal normalization rate of 44% (acromegaly) to 50% (Cushing's disease) (VOGES, unpublished data).

From these results it can be concluded that only patients with small, well-demarcated adenomas benefit from treatment with single-dose radiosurgery. The distance between the adenoma and the optic pathways should be more than 3(–5) mm in order to keep the dose to the optic nerves below a threshold dose of 8 Gy. Sophisticated treatment planning according to the above-mentioned guidelines is needed to avoid unnecessary irradiation of the temporal lobes. Thus, these patients will probably achieve normal hormonal levels much faster than those treated with conventionally fractionated irradiation (LANDOLT et al. 1998).

9.11
Conclusion

Clinical data accumulated over a century have shown that fractionated external beam radiotherapy is followed by control of tumor growth in a high percentage of patients for a very long period. In hormone-secreting tumors, radiotherapy can decrease or normalize the hormonal level, but the decrease can be protracted, requiring months or years. During this time patients depend on medical therapy. Late side-effects are rare. Future studies have to better define both diagnosis and therapy criteria:

1. Immunohistochemical assays are required to describe the pathological profile of tumors and to define selection criteria for radiotherapy.
2. The hormonal response after radiotherapy must be quantified over a time axis in clinical studies using strictly defined endocrinological criteria.
3. The role of SRS, especially in the normalization of the hormonal level, needs to be analyzed after a long follow-up.
4. The anatomical areas at risk, such as the optic chiasm, optic tract, optic nerves, infundibulum, and hypothalamus, have to be exactly defined by the use of MRI and CT. Modern 3-D radiation techniques, especially SRS and SFR, spare these critical structures better than does the traditional procedure of external beam radiotherapy. Ophthalmological and endocrinological investigations and neuropsychological tests have to be correlated with dose distributions and dose volume histograms in these anatomical areas.

References

Abd el-Hamid MW, Joplin GF, Lewis PD (1988) Incidentally found small pituitary adenomas may have no effect on fertility. Acta Endocrinologica 117:361–364

Abd el-Hamid MW, Joplin GF, Lewis PD (1988) Incidentally found small pituitary adenomas may have no effect on fertility. Acta Endocrinologica 117:361–364

Ambrosi B, Faglia G (1991) Epidemiology of pituitary tumors. In: Faglia G, Beck-Peccoz P, Ambrosi B, Travaglini P, Spada A (eds) Pituitary adenomas: new trends in basic and clinical research. Excerpta Medica, Amsterdam, pp 159–169

Aristizabal S, Caldwell WL, Avila J (1977) The relationship of time dose fractionation factors to complications in the treatment of pituitary tumors by irradiation. Int J Radiat Oncol Biol Phys 2:667–673

Atkinson AB, Aller IV, Gordon DS, et al. (1979) Progressive visual failure in acromegaly following external pituitary irradiation. Clinical Endocrinology 10: 469–479

Auer RN, Alakija P, Sutherland GR (1996) Asymptomatic large pituitary adenomas discovered at autopsy. Surgical Neurology 46:28–31

Bamberg M, Hess CF, Kortmann RD (1996) Zentralnervensystem–Hypophysenadenome. In: Scherer E, Sack H (eds) Strahlentherapie. Radiologische Onkologie. Springer, Berlin, pp780–784

Bliss P, Kerr GR, Gregor A (1994) Incidence of second brain tumours after pituitary irradiation in Edinburgh 1962–1990. Clinical Oncology 6:361–363

Bloom B, Kramer S (1984) Conventional radiation therapy in the management of acromegaly. In: Black P, et al. (eds) Secretory tumors of the pituitary gland (Progress in Endocrine Research and Therapy, Vol. 1. Raven Press, New York pp179–190

Bochicchio D, Losa M, Buchfelder M (1995) Factors influencing the immediate and late outcome of Cushing's disease by transsphenoidal surgery: a retrospective study by the European Cushing's Disease Survey Group. J Clin Endocrinol Metab 80:3114–3120

Brada M, Ford D, Ashley S (1992) Risk of second brain tumour after conservative surgery and radiotherapy for pituitary adenoma. British Medical Journal 304:1343–1346

Brada M, Rajan B, Traish D, et al. (1993) The long-term efficacy of conservative surgery and radiotherapy in the control of pituitary adenomas. Clinical Endocrinology 38:571–578

Breen P, Flickinger JC, Kondziolka D, et al. (1998) Radiotherapy for nonfunctional pituitary adenoma: analysis of long-term tumor control. J Neurosurg 89:933–938

Bülow B, Hagmar L, Mikoczy Z, et al. (1997) Increased cerebrovascular mortality in patients with hypopituitarism. Clinical Endocrinology 46:75–81

Burrow G, Worzman G, Rewcastle NB, et al. (1981) Micro-adenomas of the pituitary and abnormal sellar tomo-grams in an unselected autopsy series. N Engl J Med 304:156–158

Camaris C, Balleine R, Little D (1995) Microadenomas of the human pituitary. Pathology 27:8–11

Chonson P (1998) Traitment des adenomes hypophysaires. Presse Med 27:2077–2087

Chun M, Masko GB, Hetelekidis S (1988) Radiotherapy in the treatment of pituitary adenomas. Int J Radiat Oncol Biol Phys 15:305–309

Ciric I, Mikhael M, Stafford T, et al. (1983) Transsphenoidal microsurgery of pituitary macroadenomas with long term follow-up results. J Neurosurg 59:395–401

Clarke SD, Woo SY, Butler EB (1993) Treatment of Secretory Pituitary Adenoma with Radiation Therapy. Radiology 188:759–763

Colao A, Di Sarno A, Landi ML (1997) Long-term and low-dose treatment with cabergoline induces macroprolactinoma shrinkage. J Clin Endocrinol Metab 82:3574–3579

Comtoi R, Beauregard H, Somma M (1991) The Clinical and Endocrine Outcome to Trans-Sphenoidal Microsurgery of Nonsecreting Pituitary Adenomas. Cancer 68:860–866

Constine LS, Woolf PD, Cann D, et al. (1993) Hypo-thalamic.pituitary dysfunction after radiation for brain tumors. N Engl J Med 328:87–94

Cornett MS, Paris KJ, Spanos WJ (1996) Radiation Therapy for Pituitary Adenomas. A Retrospective Study of the University of Louisville Experience. Am J Clin Oncol 19:292–295

Degerblad M, Rahn T, Bergstrand G, et al. (1986) Long-term results of stereotactic radiosurgery to the pituitary gland in Cushing's disease. Acta Endocrinol Copenhagen 112:310–314

Duffner PK, Cohen ME, Voorhess ML, et al. (1985) Long-Term Effects of Cranial Irradiation on Endocrine Function in Children with Brain Tumors. A Prospective Study. Cancer 56:2189–2193

Eastman RC, Gorden P, Roth J (1979) Conventional supervolt-age irradiation is an effective treatment for acromegaly. J Clin Endocrinol Metab 48:931–940

Ebersold MJ, Quast LM, Laws Jr ER, et al. (1998) Long-term results in transsphenoidal removal of nonfunctioning pituitary adenomas. J Neurosurg 64:713–719

Estrada J, Boronat M, Mielgo M, et al. (1997) The long-term outcome of pituitary irradiation after unsuccessful transsphenoidal surgery in Cushing's disease. N Engl J Med 336:172–177

Ezzat S, Snyder PJ, Young WF, et al. (1992) Octreotide treatment of acromegaly. A randomized, multicenter study. Ann Intern Med 117:711–718

Feek CM, McLelland J, Seth J, et al (1984) How effective is external pituitary irradiation for growth hormone-secreting pituitary tumors? Clin Endocrinol 20:401–408

Feldkamp J, Santen R, Harms E, et al. (1999) Incidentally discovered pituitary lesions: high frequency of macroadenomas and hormone-secreting adenomas – results of a prospective study. Clin Endocrinol 51:109–113

Fisher BJ, Gaspar LE, Noone B (1993) Radiation Therapy of Pituitary Adenoma: Delayed Sequelae. Radiology 187:843–846

Flickinger JC, Deutsch M, Lunsford LD (1989) Repeat megavoltage irradiation of pituitary and suprasellar tumors. Int J Radiat Oncol Biol Phys 17:171–175

Flickinger JC, Nelson BP, Taylor FH, et al. (1989) Incidence of cerebral infarction after radiotherapy for pituitary adenoma. Cancer 63:2404–2408

Flickinger JC, Nelson PB, Martinez AJ, et al. (1989) Radio-therapy of Nonfunctional Adenomas of the Pituitary Gland. Cancer 63:2409–2414

Fraser R, Doyle F, Joplin GF, et al (1973) The assessment of endocrine effect and the effectiveness of ablative pituitary treatment by Y90 and Au 198 implantation. In: Kohler PO, Ross GT (eds) Pituitary Tumors. New York, Elsevier, pp 35–47

Freda PU, Wardlaw SL, Post KD (1998) Long-term endocrinological follow-up evaluation in115 patients who underwent transsphenoidal surgery for acromegaly. J Neurosurg 89:353–358

Frohman LA (1996) Acromegaly: what constitutes optimal therapy? (editorial) J Clin Endocrionol Metab 81:443–445

Gisti M, Gussoni G, Cuttica CM, et al. (1996) Effectiveness and tolerability of slow release lanreotide treatment in active acromegaly: six-month report on an Italian multicentric study. Italian Multicenter Slow Release Lanreotide Study Group. J Clin Endocrinol Metab 81:2089–2097

Gittoes NJL, Bates AS, Tse W (1998) Radiotherapy for non-functioning pituitary tumors. Clin Endocrinol 48:331–337

Grabenbauer GG, Fietkau R, Buchfelder M, et al. (1996) Non-Functioning Adenomas: Results and Late Effects after Resection and External Radiotherapy. Strahlentherapie und Onkologie 172:193–197

Grattan-Smith PJ, Morris JGL, Shores EA, et al. (1992) Neuropsychological abnormalities in patients with pituitary tumors. Acta Neurol Scand 86:626–631

Grigsby PW (1998) Pituitary. In: Perez CA, Brady LW (eds) Principles and Practice of Radiation Oncology.Third Edition. Lippincott-Raven, Philadelphia pp829–848

Grigsby PW, Stokes S, Marks JE, et al. (1988) Prognostic factors and results of radiotherapy alone in the management of pituitary adenomas. Int J Radiat Oncol Biol Phys 15:1103–1110

Grigsby PW, Simpson JR, Emami BN, et al. (1989) Prognostic factors and results of surgery and postoperative irradiation in the management of pituitary adenomas. Int J Radiat Oncol Biol Phys 16:1411–1417

Grigsby PW, Simpson JR, Fineberg B (1989) Late regrowth of pituitary adenomas after irradiation and/or surgery. Cancer 63:1308–1312

Griming A (1909) Un cas d'acromegalie trait'par la radio-therapie. Rev. Neurol. 17:15

Grossman A, Besser GM (1985) Prolactinomas (regular review). Br Med J 290:182–184

Halberg FE, Sheline GE (1987) Radiotherapy of pituitary tumors. Endocrinology and Metabolism Clinics 16:667–683

Hall WA, Luciano MG, Doppman JL, et al. (1994) Pituitary magnetic resonance imaging in normal human volunteers: Occult adenomas in the general population. Annals of Internal Medicine 120:817–820

Hardy J, Beauregard H, Robert F (1978) Prolactin-secreting pituitary adenomas: Transsphenoidal microsurgical treatment. In: Robyn C, Harter M (eds) Progress in Prolactin Physiology and Pathology. Elsevier/North Holland, New York, p 361

Harris JR, Levene MB (1986) Visual complications following irradiation for pituitary adenomas and craniopharyngiomas. Radiology 120:167–171.

Harrop JS, Davies TJ, Capra LG, et al. (1976) Hypothalamic-pituitary function following successful treatment of intracranial tumours. Clin Endocrinol 5:313–321

Hayes TP, Davis RA, Raventos A (1971) The treatment of pituitary chromophobe adenomas. Radiology 98:149–153

Herman V, Fagin J, Gonsky R, et al. (1990) Clonal origin of pituitary adenomas. J Clin Endocrinol Metab 71:1427–1433

Howlett TA, Plowman PN, Wass JA, et al. (1989) Megavoltage pituitary irradiation in the management of Cushing's disease and Nelson's syndrome: long-term follow-up. Clin Endocrinol (Oxf) 31:309–323

Hughes MN, Llamas KJ, Yelland ME, et al. (1993) Pituitary adenomas: long-term results for radiotherapy alone and post-operative radiotherapy. Int J Radiat Oncol Biol Phys 27:1035–1043

Jacoby L, Hedley-Whyte T, Pulaski K, et al. (1990) Clonal origin of pituitary adenomas. Journal of Neurosurgery 73:731–735

Jadresic A, Jimenez LE, Joplin GF (1987) Long-term effect of 90-Y pituitary implantation in acromegaly. Acta Endocrinol (Copenh) 115:301–306

Jaffe CA, Barkan AL (1992) Treatment of acromegaly with dopamine agonists. Endocrinolog Metab Clin North Am 21:713–735

Jaffrain-Rea ML, Derome P, Bataini JP, et al. (1998) Influence of radiotherapy on long-term relapse in clinically non-secreting pituitary adenomas. A retrospective study (1970–1988). Eur J Med 2:398–403

Jones A (1991) Radiation oncogenesis in relation to the treatment of pituitary tumors. Clinical Endocrinology 35:379–397

Kernohan JW, Sayre GP (1956) Tumors of the pituitary gland and infundibulum. Section X, fascicle 26, Washington DC, Armed Forces Institute of Pathology.

Kjellberg RN, Kliman B, Swisher B, et al. (1984) Proton beam therapy of Cushing's disease and Nelson's syndrome. In: P McL Black (ed). Secretory tumors of pituitary gland. Raven Press, New York, pp 295–307

Kleinberg DL, Noel GL, Frantz AG (1977) Galactorrhea: A study of 235 cases including 48 with pituitary tumors. N Engl J Med 28:589–600

Kliman B, Kjellberg RN, Swisher B, et al. (1984) Proton beam therapy of acromegaly: A 20 year experience. In: P McL Black (ed). Secretory tumors of pituitary gland. Raven Press, New York, pp 191–211

Kontogeorgos G, Kovacs K, Horvath E, et al. (1991) Multiple adenoma of the human pituitary. A retrospective autopsy study with clinical implications. Journal of Neurosurgery 74:243–247

Kovacs K, Horvath E, Ezrin C (1977) Pituitary adenomas. In: Sommers SC (ed) Pathology Annual. Norwalk CT Appleton-Century-Crofts

Kramer S (1973) Indications for, and results of, treatment of pituitary tumors by external radiation. In: Kohler PO, Ross GT (eds) Diagnosis and Treatment of Pituitary Tumors. Excerpta Medica, New York p 217

Lam KSL, Tse VKC, Wang C, et al. (1991) Effects of cranial irradiation on hypothalamic-pituitary function – a 5-year longitudinal study in patients with nasopharyngeal carcinoma. Q J Med 78:165–176

Landolt AM (1975) Ultrastructure of human sella tumors: Correlation of clinical findings and morphology. Acta Neurochir 22:1

Landolt AM, Haller D, Lomax N, et al. (1998) Stereotactic radiosurgery for recurrent surgically treated acromegaly: comparison with fractionated radiotherapy. J Neurosurg 88:1002–1008

Laws ER, Thapar K (1995) Surgical management of pituitary adenomas. In: Fagin J (ed) Pituitary tumours. Bailliere's Clinical Endocrinology and Metabolism. Bailliere Tindall, London, pp 391–406

Lillehei KO, Kirschman DL, Kleinschmidt-Demasters BK, et al. (1998) Reassessment of the role of radiation therapy in the treatment of endocrine inactive pituitary macroadenomas. Neurosurgery 43:432–439

Lim YJ, Leem W, Kim TS, et al. (1998) Four years' experience in the treatment of pituitary adenomas with gamma knife radiosurgery. Stereotact Funct Neurosurg 70 (suppl. 1): 95–109

Littley MD, Shalet SM, Beardwell CG, et al. (1989) Hypopituitarism following external radiotherapy for pituitary tumours in adults. Q J Med 70:145–160

Littley MD, Shalet SM, Beardwell CG, et al. (1989) Radiation induced hypopituitarism is dose-dependent. Clin Endocrinol 31:363–373

Littley MD, Shalet SM, Morgenstern GR, et al. (1991) Endocrine and reproductive dysfunction following fractionated total body irradiation in adults. Q J Med 78:265–274

McCollough WM, Marcus RB, Rhoton AL, et al. (1991) Long-term follow-up of radiotherapy for pituitary adenoma: the absence of late recurrence after 45 Gy (1991). Int J Radiat Oncol Biol Phys 21:607–614

McCord MW, Buatti JM, Fennell EM, et al. (1997) Radiotherapy for pituitary adenoma: long-term outcome and sequelae (1997) Int J Radiat Oncol Biol Phys 39:437–444

Melmed S, Ho K, Klibanski A, et al. (1995) Clinical Review 75: Recent advances in pathogenesis, diagnosis, and management of acromegaly. J Clin Endocrinol Metab 80:3395–3402

Mitsumori M, Shrieve DC, Alexander III E, et al. (1998) Initial clinical results of linac-based stereotactic radiosurgery and stereotactic radiotherapy for pituitary adenomas. Int J Radiat Oncol Biol Phys 42:573–580

Molitch ME (1987) Pathogenesis of Pituitary Tumors. Endocrinol Metab Clin 16: 503–527

Molitch ME (1995) Prolactinoma. In: Melmed S (ed) The pituitary. Blackwell Science, Boston pp 443–477

Molitch ME, Russel EJ (1990) The pituitary "incidentaloma". Annals of Internal Medicine112:925–931

Moore TJ, Dluhy RG, Williams GH, et al. (1976) Nelson's syndrome: Frequency, prognosis and effect of prior pituitary irradiation. Ann Intern Med 85:731–734

Movsas B, Movsas TZ, Steinberg SM, et al. (1995) Long-term visual changes following pituitary irradiation. Int J Radiat Oncol Biol Phys 33:599–605

Muhr C, Bergstrom K, Grimelius L, et al. (1981) A parallel study of the roentgen anatomy of the sella turcica and the histopathology of the pituitary gland in 205 autopsy specimens. Neuroradiology 21:55–65

Nelson DH, Meakin JW, Thorn GW (1965) ACTH-producing pituitary tumors following adrenalectomy for Cushing's syndrome. Proc R Soc Med 52:560–569

O'Halleran DJ, Shalet SM (1996) Radiotherapy for pituitary adenomas: an endocrinologist's perspective. Clinical Oncology 8:79–84

Pan L, Zhang N, Wang E, et al. (1998) Pituitary adenomas: The effect of gamma knife radiosurgery on tumor growth and endocrinopathies. Stereotact Funct Neurosurg 70 (suppl. 1):119–126

Parsons JT, Bova FJ, Fitzgerald CR, et al. (1994) Radiation optic neuropathy after megavoltage external-beam irradiation: analysis of time-dose factors. Int J Radiat Oncol Biol Phys 30:755–763

Peace KA, Orme SM, Sebastian JP, et al. (1997) The effect of treatment variables on mood and social adjustment in adult patients with pituitary disease. Clinical Endocrinology 46:445–450

Pegolo G, Buckwalter JG, Weiss MH, et al. (1995) Pituitary adenomas. Correlation of the cytological appearance with biological behaviour. Acta Cytologica 39:8890–8892

Plowman PN (1999) Pituitary adenoma radiotherapy – when, who and how? Clinical Endocrinology 51:265–271

Plowman PN, Grossman A (1990) Radiotherapy in the treatment of pituitary tumors. Int J Radiat Oncol Biol Phys 19:229–230

Ram Z, Nieman LK, Cutler GB Jr, et al. (1994) Early repeat surgery for persistent Cushing's disease. J Neurosurg 80:37–45

Rocher FP, Sentenac I, Berger C (1995) Stereotactic radiosurgery: The Lyon experience. Acta Neurochir [Wien] suppl 63:109–114

Rodman EF, Molitch ME, Kalmon DP, et al. (1984) Long-term follow-up of transsphenoidal selective adenomectomy of prolactinoma. JAMA 252:921–924

Roelfsema F, van Dulken H, Frohlich M (1985) Long-term results of transsphenoidal pituitary microsurgery in 60 acromegalic patients. Clin Endocrinol (Oxf) 23:555–565

Rush S, Cooper PR (1997) Symptom resolution, tumor control, and side effects following postoperative radiotherapy for pituitary macroadenomas. Int J Radiat Oncol Biol Phys 37:1031–1034

Rush SC, Newall J (1989) Pituitary adenoma: the efficacy of radiotherapy as the sole treatment. Int J Radiat Oncol Biol Phys17:165–169

Salinger DJ, Brady LW, Miyamoto CT (1992) Radiation Therapy in the Treatment of Pituitary Adenomas. Am J Clin Oncol 15(6):467–473

Samaan NA, Vieto R, Schultz PN (1982) Hypothalamic, pituitary and thyroid dysfunction after radiotherapy to head and neck. Int J Radiat Oncol Biol Phys 8:1857–1867

Schoenthaler R, Albright NW, Wara WM, et al. (1992) Reirradiation of pituitary adenoma. Int J Radiat Oncol Biol Phys 24:307–314

Serri O, Rasio E, Beauregard H, et al. (1983) Recurrence of hyperprolactinemia after selective transsphenoidal adenomectomy in women with prolactinoma. N Engl J Med 309:280–283

Shalet SM (1993) Radiation and pituitary dysfunction. N Engl J Med 328:131–133

Sheaves R, Jenkins P, Blackburn P, et al. (1996) Outcome of transsphenoidal surgery for acromegaly using strict criteria for surgical cure. Clin Endocrinol (Oxford) 45:291–298

Sheline GE (1979) The role of conventional radiation therapy in the treatment of functional pituitary tumors. In: Linfoot JA (ed) Recent advances in the diagnosis and treatment of pituitary tumors. Raven, New York, pp 289–313

Sheline GE (1981) Pituitary tumors: radiation therapy. In: Beardwell C, Robertson GL (eds) Clinical Endocrinilogy 1. The pituitary. Butterworths, London, pp 106–139

Sheline GE, Wara WM (1975) Radiation therapy of acromegaly and nonsecretory chromophobe adenomas of the pituitary. In: Seydel HG (ed): Tumors of the Central Nervous System. NewYork, Wiley, pp119–131

Snyder PJ, Fowble BF, Schatz NJ, et al. (1986) Hypopituitarism following radiation therapy of pituitary adenomas. Am J Med 81:457–462

Sohn JW, Dalzell JG, Suh JH, et al. (1995) Dose-volume histogram analysis of techniques for irradiating pituitary adenomas. Int J Radiat Oncol Biol Phys 32:831–837

Tahir AH, Sheeler LR (1992) Recurrent Cushing's disease after transsphenoidal surgery. Arch Intern Med 152:977–981

Thoren M, Rahn T, Guo WY, et al. (1991) Stereotactic radiosurgery with the cobalt-60 gamma unit in the treatment of growth hormone-producing pituitary tumors. Neurosurg 29:663–668

Tran LM, Bluont L, Horton D, et al. (1991) Radiation Therapy of Pituitary Tumors: Results in 95 Cases. Am J Clin Oncol 14:25–29

Tsang RW, Brierley JD, Panzarella T, et al. (1994) Radiation Therapy for Pituitary Adenoma: Treatment Outcome and Prognostic Factors. Int J Radiat Oncol Biol Phys 30:557–565

Vilar L, Burke CW (1994) Quinagolide efficacy and tolerability in hyperprolactinaemic patients who are resistant to or intolerant of bromocriptine. Clin Endocrinol (Oxf) 41:821–826

Vlahovitch B, Reynaud C, Rhiati J, et al. (1988) Treatment and recurrence in 135 pituitary adenomas. Acta Neurochir 42:120–123

Voges J, Sturm V, Deuss U, et al. (1996) LINAC-radiosurgery (LINAC-RS) in pituitary adenomas: Preliminary results. Acta Neurochir suppl 65:41–43

Voges J, Treuer H, Sturm V, et al. (1996) Risk analysis of linaer accelerator radiosurgery. Int J Rad Oncol Biol Phys 36:1055–1063

Wass JAH, Laws ER Jr, Randall RV, et al. (1986) The treatment of acromegaly. Clin Endocrinol Metab 15:683–707

Witt TC, Kondziolka D, Flickinger JC, et al. (1996) Stereotactic radiosurgery for pituitary tumors. Radiosurgery 1:55–65

Yoon SC, Suh TS, Jang HS (1998) Clinical results of 24 pituitary macroadenomas with linac-based stereotactic radiosurgery. Int J Radiat Oncol Biol Phys 41:849–853

Zaugg M, Adaman O, Pescia R, et al. (1995) External irradiation of macroinvasive pituitary adenomas with telecobalt: a retrospective study with long-term follow-up in patients irradiated with doses mostly of between 40–45 Gy (1995). Int J Radiat Oncol Biol Phys 32:671–680

Zierhut D, Flentje M, Adolph J, et al. (1995) External Radiotherapy of Pituitary Adenomas. Int J Radiat Oncol Biol Phys 33:307–314

10 Craniopharyngiomas: Surgical Management

LARRY T. KHOO, JEREMY FLAGEL, MARK LIKER, and MICHAEL L. LEVY

CONTENTS

10.1 Introduction

Craniopharyngiomas are an unusual group of epithelial tumors thought to be derived from the embryonic remnants of an incompletely involuted hypophyseal-pharyngeal duct (ERDHEIM 1904). The name of the tumor was first introduced by Cushing in 1932, and has been considered by many to be a misnomer as Rathke's pouch is actually an evagination of the primitive stomodeum and not the pharynx proper. They are encountered primarily in the sellar and parasellar regions but can be found anywhere along the developmental path of Rathke's pouch (PODOSHIN et al. 1970). They occur with a peak incidence between 5 to 15 years of age but can present at any age (SUNG et al. 1981). Visual loss and impairment, headache, apathy, depression, incontinence, hypersomnia, cognitive deficits, memory loss, sexual dysfunction, and growth failure are typical symptoms. Hydrocephalus and endocrine disorders are often present at the time of diagnosis (CARMEL 1982). Due to the slow growth rate of these tumors, they are often quite large before becoming symptomatic. They typically originate within the sellar and suprasellar regions but can frequently extend to the cavernous sinus, interpeduncular fossa, hypothalamic, and third ventricular regions at the time of diagnosis. Their size and central location thereby makes achieving adequate surgical exposure generally problematic (HAKUBA et al. 1986; MATSON and CRIGLER 1969; SWEET 1988). Dissection of the tumor is further complicated by the its propensity to cause an intense gliosis and dense arachnoid adhesions to the surrounding brain parenchyma and neurovascular structures (KEMPE 1968). More than 60% of incompletely resected lesions will demonstrate tumor progression within 3 years of surgery (SUNG et al. 1981). Although recent advances in the past decade have demonstrated an encouraging role for adjuvant radiation in cases of subtotal tumor resection, total removal still offers the best chance of cure for the patient.

L. T. KHOO, MD
Clinical Instructor, Department of Neurosurgery, University of Southern California Keck School of Medicine, 1200 North State Street, Suite 5046, Los Angeles, CA 90033-0804, USA
J. FLAGEL, BS
Medical Student, University of Southern California Keck School of Medicine, 1200 North State Street, Suite 5046, Los Angeles, CA 90033-0804, USA
M. LIKER, MD
Clinical Instructor, Department of Neurosurgery, University of Southern California Keck School of Medicine, 1200 North State Street, Suite 5046, Los Angeles, CA 90033-0804, USA
M. L. LEVY, MD
Assistant Professor, Division of Pediatric Neurosurgery, Children's Hospital of Los Angeles, University of Southern California Keck School of Medicine, 1300 North Vermont, Suite 906, Los Angeles, CA 90027, USA

10.2 Epidemiology

Craniopharyngiomas are the most common intracranial tumors of nonglial origin in the pediatric population (HOFFMAN et al. 1992). They constitute between 1.2–4% of all brain tumors and 6–9% of pediatric tumors (SANFORD and MUHLBAUR 1991). There are 0.5 to 2 new cases per million population occurring each year. Approximately 54% of all sellar chiasmatic region tumors in childhood are craniopharyngiomas (EINHAUS and SANFORD 1999). From an autopsy series of 3000 consecutive intracranial tumors, craniopharyngiomas represented 1.3% of the lesions and 13% of all sellar and suprasellar tumors for all ages (ZÜLCH 1986). Although craniopharyngiomas account for a greater percentage of intracranial tumors during childhood, over one-half of the total cases are actually found in adults (ADAMSON et al. 1990). Indeed, craniopharyngiomas are overall less common in the pediatric population than in adults and should no longer be mistaken for a "childhood" lesion.

Craniopharyngiomas can occur at any age; however, the primary incidence peak for craniopharyngiomas is between 5 and 14 years of age. A second peak occurs in the fourth to sixth decades of life. CHOUX et al. (1991) reviewed over 30 series containing more than 3200 cases and noted that 60% of patients were over 16 years old and 40% were under this age. Cases have been reported at the extremes of life with unusually large tumors in the newborn and even in utero (HURST et al. 1988; SNYDER et al. 1986). Rare cases have also been documented in patients over the age of 70 (van EFFENTERRE et al. 1991). The gender distribution is essentially equal with a slight male predominance of 55% for all ages (BARKOVICH 1995).

Overall, no clear genetic or inherited predisposition has been firmly established for craniopharyngiomas. However, anecdotal cases of siblings with tumors and familial clusters have been reported (VARGUS et al. 1981; THOMSETT et al. 1980; WALD et al. 1982). Although no well-defined risk factors or premorbid conditions exist for these tumors, numerous reports of associated pathologies exist. These include concurrent astrocytomas, meningiomas, prolactinomas, angiomas, pinealomas, germinomas, congenital malformations, precocious puberty, polydactyly, and low-lying ears (CHOUX et al. 1991; WAKAI et al. 1984; DRAZIN et al. 1980).

10.3
Pathogenesis

Craniopharyngiomas usually occur in the prechiasmatic suprasellar, retrochiasmatic suprasellar, or sellar regions; however, other rare locations have been reported. These include the nasopharynx, ventricle, posterior fossa, pineal gland, or within the chiasm (EINHAUS and SANFORD 1999). Using roentgenograms and surgical findings, ROUGERIE and FARDEAU (1962) originally categorized these tumors by location into intrasellar (11%), intra- and suprasellar with anterior (51%) or posterior involvement (36%), and giant or atypical lesions (2%). With the advent of MRI and other modern imaging techniques, craniopharyngiomas have been classified into four major anatomic types: intrasellar, infundibulum-tuberan, intraventricular, and dumbbell-shaped tumors (RAYBAUD et al. 1991). From a surgical perspective, the degree of vertical and anteroposterior extension is important for operative planning and exposure. As such, numerous classification schemata have also been developed to quantify the anatomic extent of craniopharyngiomas (YASARGIL et al. 1990).

The tumors are benign and have no malignant cells (SWEET 1994). Craniopharyngiomas can vary greatly in size and shape and are usually solid and cystic, although they can be entirely cystic or completely solid. Pediatric series have revealed a predominance of cystic (40%) and mixed lesions (50%), whereas adult lesions are typically solid in nature (HETELEKIDIS et al. 1993). On rare occasions, completely solid craniopharyngiomas occur with only microscopic cyst formation. Small lesions are sometimes diagnosed due to pituitary dysfunction and can be mistaken for pituitary adenomas. Conversely, other lesions may remain silent and achieve tremendous proportions before presenting with hydrocephalus and compressive symptoms.

On surgical and gross examination, craniopharyngiomas are typically smooth, multilobulated lesions with a capsule of variable appearance. The capsule can be thin and translucent in some areas and thick and grayish in others. This capsule often serves as a good demarcation from surrounding brain tissue, although finger-like extensions of tumor into the surrounding brain parenchyma with attendant gliosis is extremely common. On cut-section, the tumors are variegated with pale, granular solid areas punctuated by multiple spongiomatous, cystic regions (RUSSEL and RUBINSTEIN 1989). The cysts contain a lipid-rich oily secretion that has been likened to machinery oil. This secretion is composed mostly of desquamated squamous epithelial cells rich in membrane lipids, especially cholesterol and triglycerides. The fluid also contains keratin from the cytoskeleton. Cholesterol crystals in the fluid can often be seen grossly and can be confirmed by microscopic examination under polarized light. Gritty areas are often encountered with calcifications seen on histology. Childhood lesions almost invariably contain such calcium deposits and occur in approximately half of adult lesions (MILLER 1994). For craniopharyngiomas, calcifications should be considered a secondary by-product of tumor degeneration and not a sign of hamartomatous change. Indeed, return of calcifications after complete resection correlates well with tumor recurrence (PANG 1993). On rare occasions, lamellar bone and actual teeth formation can be found within the lesion. Careful differentiation of craniopharyngiomas from calcifying odontogenic cysts and teratomas is needed for such cases (ALVAREZ-GARIJO et al. 1981). Figure 10.1A demonstrates a sagittal section of a specimen with a massive lesion filling the third ventricle. Gritty nodules are seen in the anterior and inferior portion of the lesion representing calcifications. The dark cystic fluid is not present as it has drained away during preparation and fixation of the specimen.

10.3.1
Histopathology

The craniopharyngioma is a cystic epithelial neoplasm. Its histopathology can be classified into three types according to the microscopic pattern of the epithelium: adamantinomatous, squamous papillary, and mixed.

The classic adamantinomatous craniopharyngioma is the main histologic type seen in children. It also occurs in adults, though less frequently. This epithelium resembles that of tumors of tooth-forming tissues (adamantinomas) which are seen in the oropharynx (SEEMAYER et al. 1992). The epithelium creates a varied histologic pattern with the formation of sheets, lobules, anastomosing trabeculae, cloverleaves, and cysts.

Adamantinomatous craniopharyngiomas display three principal epithelial layers. These include a palisading basal layer of small cells demonstrating high

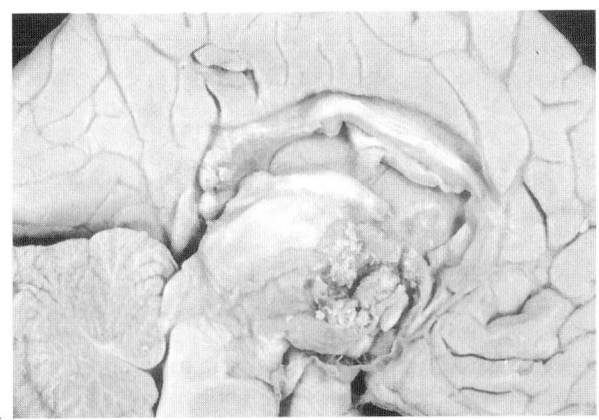
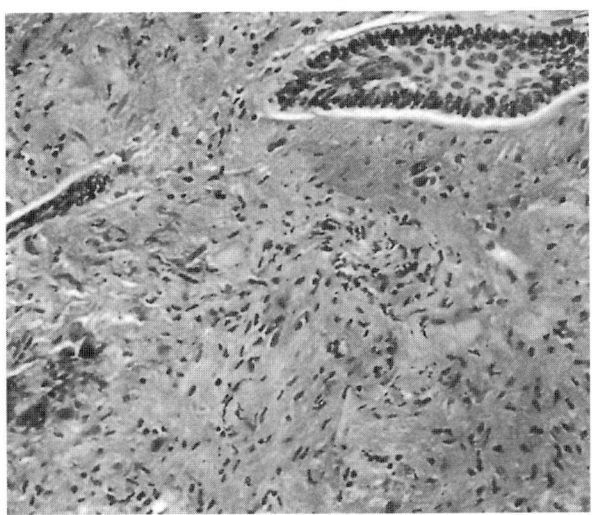
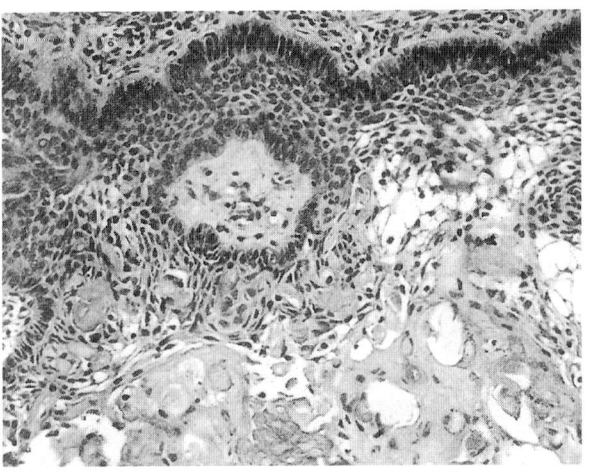

Fig. 10.1. A Sagittal cross-section through a gross specimen of a large craniopharyngioma filling the third ventricle of a patient's cerebrum. The optic apparatus and hypothalamus are severely deformed. Gritty calcifications are evident within the tumor parenchyma. **B** A medium-power view of the typical histologic findings in craniopharyngioma. A complex epithelial pattern of growth is seen at the tumor margin which is bordered by gliotic brain. Keratin formation and calcifications are also seen. Wet keratin and fluid filled cystic areas are evident as well. The epithelium demonstrates an area of palisading with transition to a looser pattern. **C** A view demonstrating a finger-like pseudopod pushing into the adjacent brain parenchyma, creating the appearance of invasion. These irregular contours of the tumor are often cut tangentially to give a false impression of islands of tumor. Also note the surrounding intense gliosis around the finger of tumor that is sometimes mistaken for astrocytoma

mitotic activity; an intermediate layer of variable thickness above the basal layer composed of a loose collection of stellate cells; and a top layer where the cells are abruptly enlarged, flattened, and keratinized to flat, plate-like squamous cells. The epithelial structures also contain nodules of keratin, often described as "wet keratin" because its appearance is entirely unlike the flaky keratin of epidermoid cysts. These wet keratin nodules are a hallmark of the adamantinomatous subtype. An example of these classic histologic findings is provided in Fig. 10.1B. Dystrophic calcification often occurs due to the accumulation of calcium salts in the keratin-rich surface cells of the top histologic layer. In rare instances, this leads to actual metaplastic bone formation, in which there may be bone marrow development. Additional histologic features include fibrosis, chronic inflammation, and cholesterol clefts (EINHAUS and SANFORD 1999).

The squamous papillary type is the predominant pattern seen in adults and is rarely found is children (ADAMSON et al. 1990). The epithelium in these tumors is solid and compact with no loose stellate zone. It is arranged around fibrovascular cores and sometimes forms pseudopapillae. The epithelium has been said to resemble the metaplastic changes one may see in respiratory epithelia in various pathological states. Unlike adamantinomatous tumors, squamous papillary tumors rarely undergo calcification, they do not form keratin nodules or desquamate large stacks of dying squamous cells into their lumens. The cyst contents in these tumors are less oily and dark than in adamantinomatous craniopharyngiomas. Grossly, these tumors tend to be more solid than cystic and are frequently found in the third ventricle (EINHAUS and SANFORD 1999).

Occasionally, mixed tumors are found that contain separate foci with histologic features of both adamantinomatous and squamous papillary types. Because of the presence of these mixed tumors, it has been suggested that craniopharyngiomas represent single spectrum tumors with a wide sprawl of characteristics. These characteristics range from the purely adamantinomatous type through a mixed variety to the squamous papillary type.

Although histologically benign, craniopharyngiomas can invade in a fingerlike fashion into adjacent brain tissue. The most frequent site of invasion is the hypothalamus. This invasion complicates attempts at total resection and it is not uncommon to find small tumor foci in the brain tissue adjacent to resected tumor specimens (MILLER 1994). Brain invasion is most commonly associated with the child-

hood adamantinomatous variety, but on rare occasions has been associated with the squamous papillary type as well (ADAMSON et al. 1990). Whether or not these remaining foci are responsible for recurrences is debated. Some assert that recurrent craniopharyngiomas are more likely with multiple remaining foci, but others maintain that their presence is not predictive (WEINER et al. 1994).

Another pathological feature of craniopharyngiomas is the frequent formation of a dense, fibrillary gliosis in the immediately adjacent brain. This gliosis is especially frequent when the tumor is in contact with or invading the hypothalamus (SWEET 1994). Invasions of the epithelial material from the neoplasm into the gliotic material constitutes the invasive behavior of craniopharyngiomas. Small islands of cells erroneously thought to be carcinomatous invasion can be found in many specimens where this reactive gliosis has pinched off small masses of tumor cells (SANFORD and MUHLBAUR 1991). An example of such pseudopod-like extension of tumor with intense surrounding gliosis is shown in Fig. 10.1C. The combination of brain invasion and gliosis may complicate surgical removal, or the glial reaction may create a cleavage plane that aids in tumor removal (WEINER et al. 1994).

10.3.2
Tumor Biology

The traditional belief concerning the origin of craniopharyngiomas takes into account their location, their relationship to tumors of tooth-forming cells, and the known embryologic contribution of Rathke's pouch to the formation of the adenohypophysis. Craniopharyngiomas can be formed anywhere along the path of development of Rathke's pouch. It has long been believed that these tumors evolve from rests or remnants of the pharyngeal epithelium left over during embryogenesis, and later transformed into neoplastic cells (ERDHEIM 1904; PODOSHIN 1970).

Squamous papillary tumors, on the other hand, do not resemble tumors of tooth-forming epithelium and arise almost exclusively in adults. Rathke's pouch remnants are not usually a stratified squamous epithelium, thus it is difficult to ascribe the same etiological hypothesis to these tumors as adamantinomatous tumors (MILLER 1994). Another hypothesis for the embryogenesis of craniopharyngiomas is that they are derived from residual metaplastic squamous epithelium found in the adenohypophysis and anterior infundibulum.

It is convenient and tempting to attribute adamantinomatous tumors to Rathke's pouch remnants, and squamous papillary tumors to metaplastic foci. However, two separate etiologies would not account for the mixed histology tumors. Based on available data, it is probably best to consider the different histologic patterns of craniopharyngiomas as part of a spectrum of differentiation within a single metaplastic category. These lesions are believed to be a part of a continuum of ectodermally derived cystic epithelial lesions with the same origin as Rathke's cleft cysts, epithelial cysts, epidermoid cysts, and dermoid cysts and are all found within and around the sella (HARRISON et al. 1994).

The dark cystic fluid produced by craniopharyngiomas has been extensively studied. The pattern of mucus found is very similar to that of the oropharynx. The epithelial cells of the tumor contain zymogen granules with secretory activity seen within the microcysts. Thus, the cystic fluid is not purely the result of degenerative changes as previously postulated (SZEIFERT et al. 1991). Additionally, insulin-like growth factor (IGF)-II has also been demonstrated in the cyst fluid by means of gel analysis. From fetal rat studies, the most intense IGF-II expression in the CNS was found within Rathke's pouch (ZUMKELLER et al. 1991). These findings together add further support to the postulated origin of craniopharyngiomas from Rathke's pouch.

Whereas a great deal of information has been published on the structural characteristics of craniopharyngiomas, far less data on their genetic and biological potential is available. One of the major reasons for this is that craniopharyngioma cells are extremely difficult to maintain in tissue culture. The first reported successful culture line was that of COBB and WRIGHT (1959) who were only able to achieve a single epithelial layer from implanted cells. Two decades later, LISZCZAK et al. (1978) were able to develop a more aggressive culture line with more microvilli, irregular nuclei, and cytoplasmic basophilia. Since then, little to no data on the genetic make-up of craniopharyngiomas has been published. VAGNER-CAPODANO et al. (1992) did demonstrate a loss of chromosome Y and aneuploidy in three cases, but these findings are rare and inconsistent for the majority of tumors. Cytogenic analysis of craniopharyngiomas is needed for a more thorough understanding of their biological potential.

SHIBUYA et al. (1993) examined the proliferative potential of craniopharyngiomas via an assay with monoclonal Ki-67, anti-DNA polymerase alpha, and bromodeoxyuridine antibody labeling. From a small study of seven tumors, six had low proliferation indices whereas the remaining tumor had a very high number of labeled cells. This finding underscores the observation that these tumors have a highly variable clinical behavior and regrowth rate. As a whole, craniopharyngiomas are thought of as slow-growing, histologically benign lesions (RUSSELL and RUBINSTEIN 1989). Whereas recurrence of these tumors at the primary or at contiguous sites is extremely common even after complete surgical resection, primary seeding or distal metastases are virtually unheard of (ZÜLCH 1986). Rare cases of malignant degeneration and very aggressive behavior have been reported, but it is generally agreed that these tumors do not undergo malignant degeneration (LISZCZAK et al. 1978). The one such reported case of malignant change occurred after the patient had been irradiated (NELSON 1988).

10.4
Clinical Presentation

Craniopharyngiomas are slow-growing extra-axial tumors that can often reach a large size before producing symptoms. These symptoms are caused by compression on adjacent neural structures. The development of symptoms can be protracted and can range from 1 to 2 years. They frequently become large enough to obstruct cerebrospinal fluid (CSF) pathways, resulting in hydrocephalus and increased intracranial pressure (ICP) (CARMEL 1990). Overall, three major clinical syndromes are observed: (1) ICP and hydrocephalus, (2) endocrine dysfunction, and (3) visual deficits from compression of the optic apparatus. At presentation, common complaints are headache, nausea, vomiting, and visual disturbance. Headache is the most frequent presenting complaint, and is reported in 55–86% of patients. Obstructive hydrocephalus is found in about 30–40% of cases at presentation. Visual disturbance is observed in 37–68% of patients at presentation, and papilledema is observed in approximately 40% (MATSON and CRIGLER 1969). Children are often inattentive to visual loss and will tolerate a significant amount without complaint. Of the 20–30% of children who do complain of visual dysfunction, a great number will have complete loss in one eye at diagnosis (PANG 1993). Conversely, almost 80% of adults will complain of visual loss with typically smaller deficits on presentation. On formal visual testing and examination, bitemporal hemianopia, unilateral temporal hemianopia, and unilateral and bilateral decrease of visual acuity may be documented. Severe cases may show optic atrophy or near total blindness with see-saw nystagmus. Other cranial nerve abnormalities are rarely present at diagnosis (GRAHAM et al. 1992). Cognitive dysfunction, neuropsychological problems, mentation deficits, memory loss, incontinence, frontal disinhibition, apathy, and Korsakoff's syndrome are more common from large bilateral masses of the frontal basilar region (KAHN and CROSBY 1972). Seizures are very rare but have been reported from lesions extending to the sylvian fissure and after cases of cyst rupture and aseptic meningitis.

Endocrine dysfunction is also commonly evident at presentation and can be documented in 66–90% of new pediatric patients (CARMEL 1982). Only a minority of patients, however, reach medical attention specifically for an endocrine related complaint. Short stature, hypothyroidism, or diabetes insipidus (DI) remain the three most common endocrine abnormalities found at initial presentation. The classic description of a craniopharyngioma pediatric patient is that of a child who is short, obese, dull, half-blind, and has a progressively deteriorating school performance (PANG 1993). Short stature (height less than the third percentile) is present in 23–45%, although growth hormone (GH) deficiency has been reported in up to 75% (THOMSETT et al. 1980). DI, characterized by symptoms such as excessive thirst, frequent urination, and decreased urine-specific gravity, is present in 7.5–24% of cases. Hypothyroidism is present in 12–25% and is commonly characterized by weight gain, lethargy, fatigue, and poor intellectual performance in patients with craniopharyngioma (SANFORD and MUHLBAUR 1991). Luteinizing hormone (LH) and follicle-stimulating hormone (FSH) deficiency has been reported in 40%, adrenocorticotropic hormone (ACTH) in 25%, and thyroid-stimulating hormone (TSH) in 25% has also been reported. Hypogonadism is also quite common and can be manifest in several ways. For children, delayed sexual development or precocious pseudopuberty can result. In adults, amenorrhea in women and a loss of libido in men is typically found. In addition, prolactin may be elevated in 20% of children at presentation (SKLAR 1994). Other less common presenting features include obesity in 11–18%, diplopia in 8–11%, and mentation disturbance in 5–15% of children (EINHAUS and SANFORD 1999). Integrity of the hypothalamic-pituitary axis is essential for normal psychological and social development as well. Even moderately sized lesions of these areas have been related to behavioral dysfunction especially in children (PALM et al. 1992).

Spontaneous ruptures of craniopharyngioma cysts have been reported. This rare phenomenon can produce headache, fever, and nuchal rigidity secondary to a chemical meningitis. The CSF of these patients occasionally contains cholesterol crystals, which can aid in diagnosis (OKAMOTO et al. 1985). Rare cases of spontaneous intracranial hemorrhage and tumor drainage through the nose have also been reported (KUBOTA et al. 1980; MAIER 1985). Craniopharyngiomas can also be rarely discovered incidentally by skull X-ray and head CT after trauma or migraines. Enlargement or erosion of the dorsum and tuberculum sellae is typically seen along with tumor calcification within or superior to the sella (BARKOVICH 1995).

The clusters of symptoms produced by craniopharyngiomas are closely related to their location. There are three predominant locations: prechiasmatic suprasellar, retrochiasmatic suprasellar, and sellar. Tumors located in the prechiasmatic suprasellar region usually grow anteriorly between the optic nerves. Their growth pushes the chiasm posteriorly. This growth may elevate the A1 segments of the anterior cerebral arteries, but they rarely encroach upon the third ventricle, thus obstructive hydrocephalus is uncommon. Children with prechiasmatic tumors tend to show decreased visual acuity, field cuts, and optic atrophy. Tumors located in the retrochiasmatic suprasellar region displace the chiasm anteriorly against the tuberculum sellae. They may also fill the third ventricle and can travel inferiorly along the clivus and into the posterior fossa. The symptoms of this growth pattern most frequently include obstructive hydrocephalus and sequelae due to increased ICP (SWEET 1988; SUNG et al. 1981). Extension into the third ventricle also brings the tumors within reach of the hypothalamus, including the supraoptic and paraventricular nuclei. Further retrochiasmatic extension may involve the thalamus; with potential damage to important endocrine control and memory system (MILLER 1994). Sellar craniopharyngiomas are frequently small and expand the sella turcica. They may invade the pituitary gland, but usually do not compress the overlying optic nerves or chiasm or displace the anterior cerebral arteries. Thus, patients typically present with headaches and endocrine disturbance. Craniopharyngiomas can also exhibit both anterior and posterior growth, resulting in a combination of the symptoms described for prechiasmatic and retrochiasmatic tumors (LEVY et al. 1997).

10.5
Diagnostic Evaluation

10.5.1
Imaging

Whereas clinical diagnosis and the neurological exam formed the mainstay of lesion localization in the past, modern neuroimaging now provides rapid anatomic information with precise accuracy. Computed tomographic scanning (CT) and magnetic resonance imaging (MRI) are now the standard for visualizing craniopharyngiomas and their regional anatomy. Plain radiographs are used with decreasing frequency, but can still be helpful as an initial modality. Changes of the bony skull base are frequently observed in patients with craniopharyngioma. Two-thirds of adults and almost half of children will demonstrate such osseous changes (BANNA 1973; BANNA et al. 1973). Lesions with marked suprasellar extension may be associated with an eroded dorsum sellae and anterior clinoids. Nearly 50% will possess an enlarged sella at the time of diagnosis (NAIDICH et al. 1976). Calcifications can also be seen on skull X-ray in about 40% of adults and 80% of children with craniopharyngiomas (SUNG et al. 1981). An example of these calcifications as well as erosion and thinning of the sella is provided in Fig. 10.2.

Whereas cerebral angiograms had widely been used in the past for intracranial tumors, they are now rarely used to delineate craniopharyngiomas. For newly diagnosed lesions, the small vessels typically supplying the tumor are very difficult to identify on routine angiography. Large caliber feeding vessels are rarely observed (CARMEL 1990). For recurrent cases, examination of the cerebral vessels may be quite important as postoperative fusiform dilations of major vessels have been reported (SUTTON et al. 1991). The recent improvements in MR angiography, however, have decreased the need for invasive studies even in these cases (SAMII and BINI 1991). Also of historical interest are the use of ventriculography and pneumoencephalography, which were widely used in the past to localize craniopharyngiomas and other neoplasms.

With the advent of CT scanning and the use of intravenous contrast enhancement, the extent and margins of craniopharyngiomas became much easier to define preoperatively. Areas of cystic change, solid tumor, and intratumoral calcifications are readily identified with CT scanning. However, some lesions which demonstrate dense, homogeneous contrast-enhancement on CT may actually contain cysts or microcysts on equivalent MRI sequences (CARMEL 1996). The cyst fluid content is typically hypodense to the CSF, but may have areas of hyperintensity due to calcifications in the tumor walls. Thin section CT images (1.5 mm thickness) are particularly helpful to define the extent of the tumor's skull base involvement, bony changes, and intratumoral calcifications.

Improvements in MRI quality over the last decade have made it the first choice in precisely defining the three-dimensional architecture of a craniopharyngioma. The ability to view the lesion in multiple axial, sagittal, and coronal planes makes MRI particularly helpful for preoperative planning. MRI is superior to CT in identifying the soft-tissue involvement around the tumor and also the location of nearby vital neurological structures (i.e., optic chiasm, pituitary stalk and gland, hypothalamus, third ventricle). Additionally, MRI demonstrates cystic spread of the tumor into bone and pneumatized skull base areas better than CT. The exact MRI appearance of a craniopharyngioma is highly variable and is correlated with the amount of cholesterol, hemorrhage, keratin, and calcifications contained within (RAYBAUD et al. 1991). Table 10.1 demonstrates the typical constellation of MRI characteristics. Cystic portions of the tumor often demonstrate a high, uniform T1-weighted signal for both isodense and hypodense lesions as defined by CT

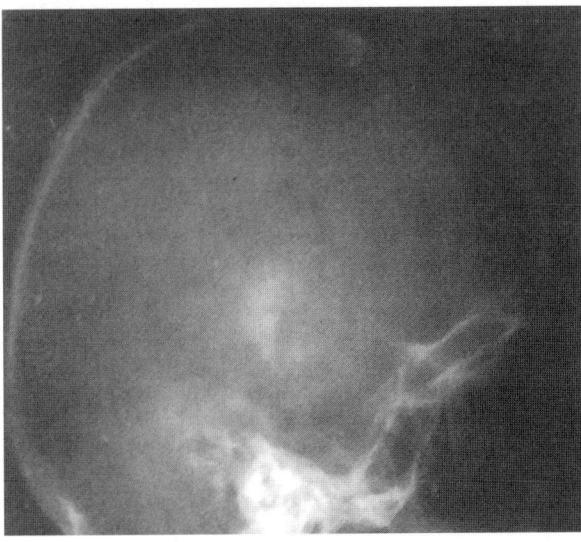

Fig. 10.2. A plain lateral skull radiograph demonstrates the intense calcifications often seen in large suprasellar craniopharyngiomas. Also of note are the changes seen in the sella and frontal skull base

Table 10.1. Craniopharyngioma MRI characteristics

Tumor class	T1	T2	Contents
Cystic	–	+	Cholesterol
	+	+	Hemorrhage
	–	–	Keratin
Solid	–	+	Typical
	+	+	Hemorrhage or cholesterol
	+	–	Cholesterol

(HUK et al. 1990). Calcification produces characteristic low signal on MRI. Injection of gadolinium (Gd-DTPA) intravenous contrast produces a marked, homogeneous increase in signal intensity for solid portions of the tumor. This is particularly helpful in differentiating craniopharyngiomas from other cystic suprasellar lesions (HUA et al. 1992). For adequate preoperative planning, most surgeons view CT and MRI as complimentary procedures and ideally obtain both before attempting a resection (Figs. 10.3, 10.4).

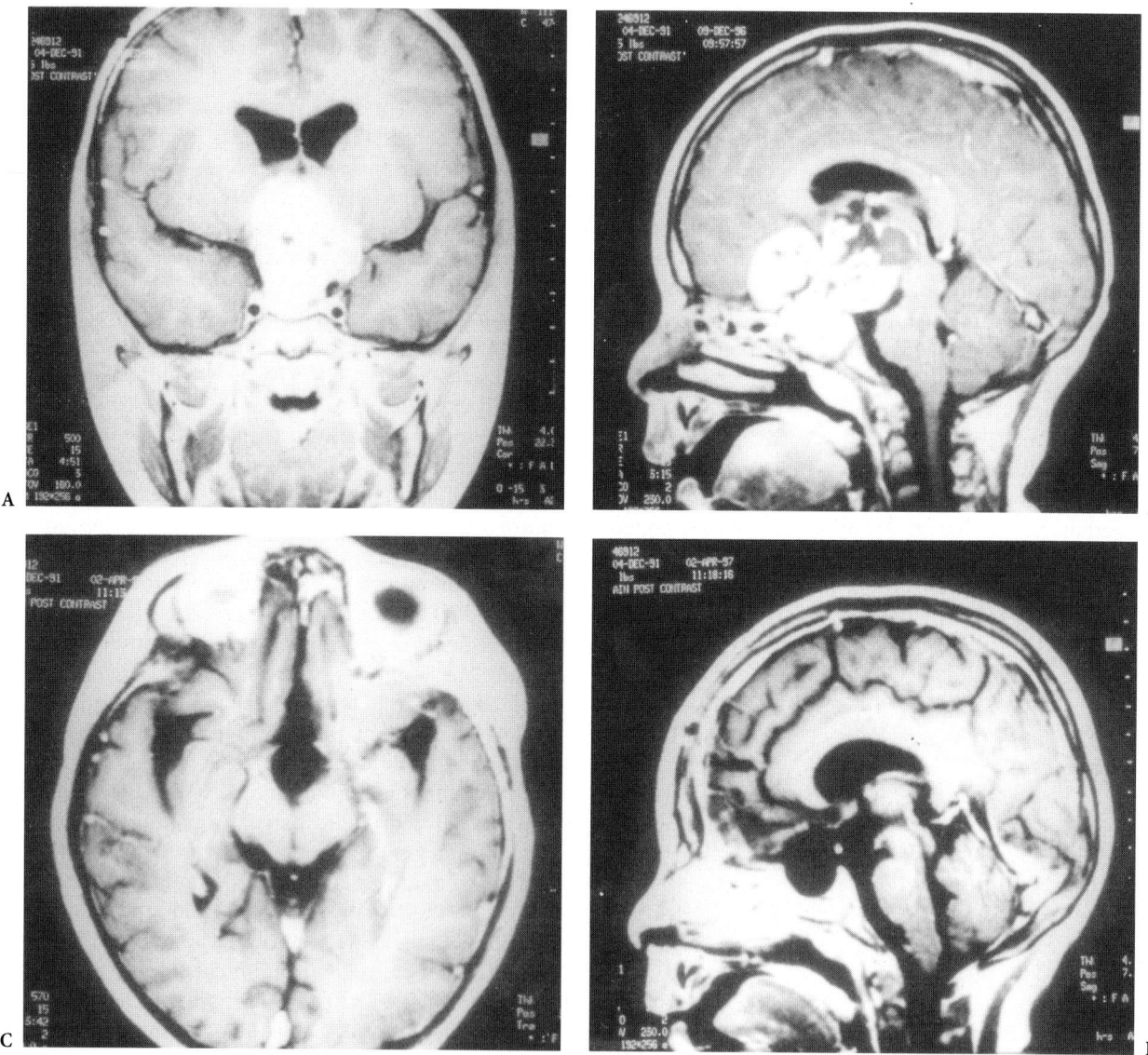

Fig. 10.3A–D. A 5-year-old boy presented with a 1-year history of headache, progressive visual loss, and difficulty with ambulation. These MR images document the presence of a large heterogeneous lesion with extension into the interpeduncular fossa and third ventricle. The patient was operated on via a FOZT approach with total resection achieved as based on the postoperative images. **A,B** Preoperative gadolinium T1-weighted coronal and sagittal images. **C,D** Postoperative gadolinium T1-weighted axial and sagittal images

Neonatal and intrauterine ultrasounds have also been responsible for detecting several large craniopharyngiomas during the perinatal period. Calcifications are frequently visible in the tumor which can sometimes occupy up to 70% of the intracranial volume (HELMKE et al. 1984; SNYDER et al. 1986; HURST et al. 1988). The cranial perimetry for such cases was usually enlarged beyond 40 cm. Intraoperative use of ultrasound has also become increasingly popular to refine the extent of the resection and also to localize cystic aspects of the tumor.

10.5.2
Clinical Tests

As craniopharyngiomas often have profound effects on neuroendocrine and homeostatic mechanisms, they can cause significant physiological and biochemical alterations in patients with such lesions. Identification of these derangements is crucial to ensure complete treatment of the entire patient and not just of the tumor. Timely laboratory-based identification of physiological problems will allow for

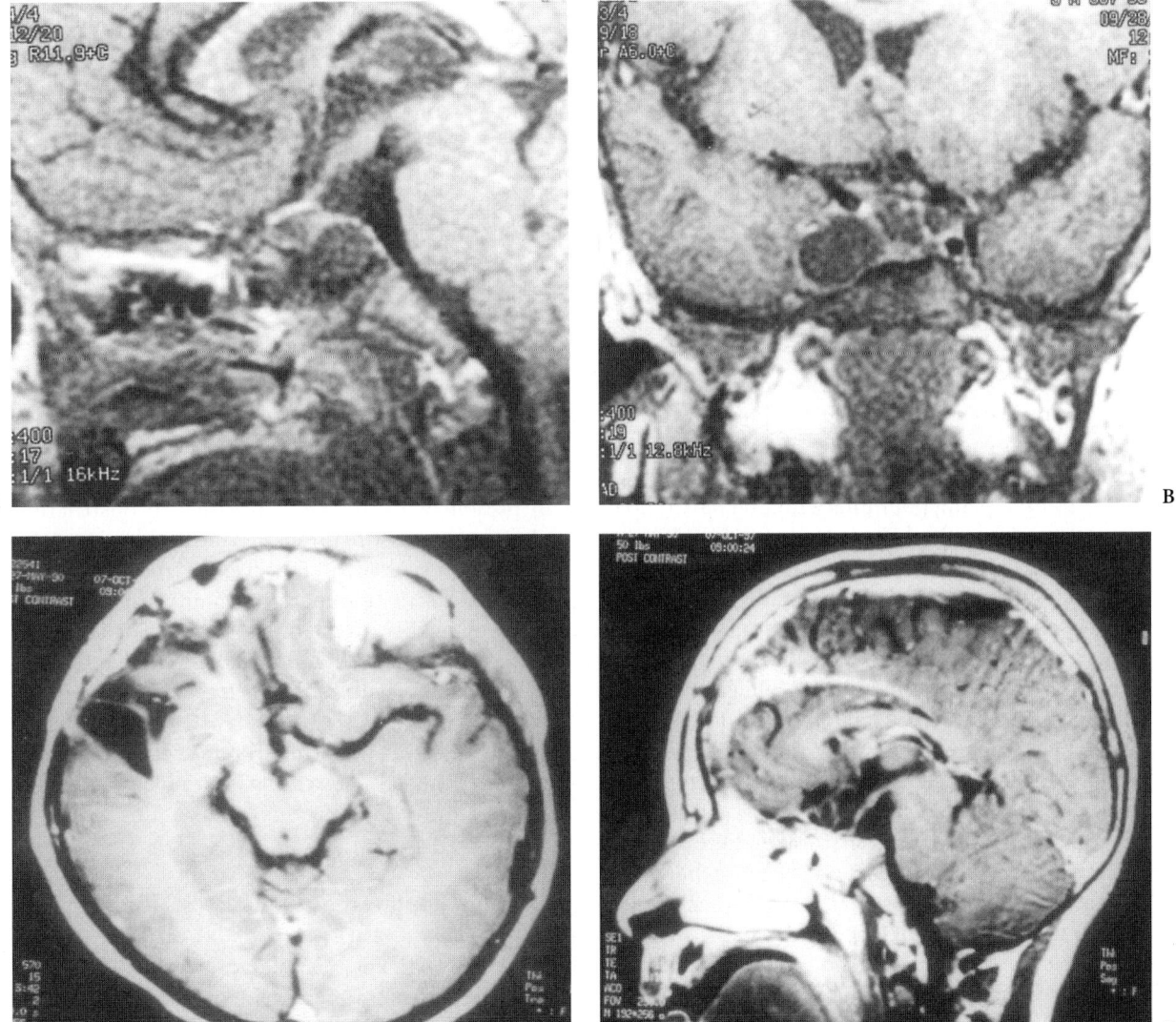

Fig. 10.4A–D. The case of a 41/2-year-old boy who was referred to the Children's Hospital of Los Angeles for a history of incompletely resected craniopharyngioma in the suprasellar and right cavernous sinus region. The patient was taken to the OR where the FOZT approach provided an excellent exposure of the tumor, sellar, third ventricle and cavernous sinus regions. A generous but subtotal resection was achieved. **A,B** Preoperative gadolinium T1-weighted sagittal and coronal images **C,D** Postoperative gadolinium T1-weighted axial and sagittal images

adequate correction prior to surgery thereby also minimizing the operative morbidity and mortality.

Craniopharyngiomas typically cause a compressive dysfunction of the hypothalamic-pituitary complex. This essential neuroendocrine system regulates the important secretion of somatropin, thyrotropin, corticotropin, gonadotropin, vasopressin, prolactin, and other peptides and neurotransmitters (ERZIN and WEISS 1990). Even small tumors within the anatomic confines of this system can cause significant derangements. Generally, these resultant dysfunctions can be grouped into several syndromes including those of endocrine deficits, thirst disturbances, and problems of osmolarity and water balance (STREETEN et al. 1987). The most common laboratory findings are DI and hypogonadism. Some of these endocrine findings have already been discussed (see Sect. 10.3).

Through the use of simple blood sampling and biochemical analysis, the majority of these endocrine alterations can be identified. Thorough preoperative evaluation of the neuroendocrine axis as well as assessment of the patient's blood chemistries, CBC, and volume status are mandatory to prevent potentially devastating problems. Importantly, hypoadrenalism, hypothyroidism, and DI must be identified and corrected prior to surgery as they can cause fatal perioperative complications. Such laboratory testing may not be immediately helpful for cases where radical resection is planned as the patient is generally expected to have panhypopituitarism afterwards; however, this information is very useful in planning replacement therapy for less invasive procedures (i.e., intracystic therapy or stereotactic radiosurgery) and also for long-term management. Treatment with glucocorticoid, thyroid, and other hormone replacements can take some time during which temporary CSF diversion may be needed for cases with critically elevated ICP. The exact tests used for each patient can be individualized based on the acuity of the presentation as well as on the clinical suspicion. A battery of screening tests can be used first with additional tests ordered if needed. It is important to realize that only a few patients will have clear clinical findings suggestive of endocrine insufficiency whereas the majority will have derangements on blood analysis. Table 10.2 summarizes the typical biochemical panel used to assess the integrity of the hypothalamic-pituitary axis.

In addition to biochemical evaluation of the endocrine and physiological derangements associated with craniopharyngiomas, preoperative evaluation of the patients functional and behavioral status is also prudent. As discussed previously, integrity of the hypothalamic axis plays a direct role in cognition and

behavior. Furthermore, large tumors involving the frontal, temporal, or parietal lobes can also cause further emotional and psychological dysfunction. As such it is wise to establish the patient's baseline functional status prior to surgery. This is particularly important for patients who may undergo subsequent radiation. Multiple batteries of neuropsychological tests are available for both adult and pediatric patients. These include the Wechsler Intelligence Scale for Adults and Children (WISC), Wechsler Memory Scale and its modified pediatric form, verbal and nonverbal selection recall tests, complex figure duplication, and a variety of other frontal lobe function subtests (CAVAZZUTI et al. 1983). Unfortunately, few adequate tests exist for children under the age of 6 years. Finally, a thorough assessment of the patient's visual ability should be completed by a qualified neuro-ophthalmologist. Subtle deficits and field-cuts are generally present and can be frequently missed by simple bedside testing. This is especially true for children whose vision is particularly difficult to evaluate using only standard techniques.

10.6
Preoperative Management

A large proportion of craniopharyngioma patients will present with increased ICP due to obstruction and with a host of neuroendocrine and homeostatic derangements. As such, clinical experience has shown that a significant amount of morbidity and mortality is present in this preoperative period. For such patients, management should thus begin well before actual treatment with either surgery, radiation, or intracystic therapy (TOMITA 1988). Only after the hydrocephalus and endocrine dysfunction is corrected should definitive treatment be undertaken.

10.6.1
Hormonal Replacement

Once a thorough endocrinological work-up has been completed, hormonal replacement should begin immediately to correct any identified deficiencies. As discussed earlier, such deficiencies are present in 50% of children and up to 80% of adult patients. Appropriate thyroid replacement can take several days to 2 weeks with oral L-thyroxine (T4) and should thus be initiated as early as possible for hypothyroid patients. Untreated hypothyroidism carries with it significant

Table 10.2. Endocrinological evaluation tests

Axis	Screening tests	Additional tests
LH-FSH	Serum testosterone, estrogen	LH, RH
ACTH	Serum ACTH, fasting cortisol Urinary cortisol level	Hypoglycemic cortisol test Insulin induced hypoglycemia
ADH	Chem 20 panel, urine and blood Osmolarities, 8-h Water deprivation test	24-h water deprivation test Tagged red cell, CVP catheter
Growth	Weight, size, bone age, growth chart Somatomedin-C	Bone biopsy Stimulation tests
PRL	Serum and fasting prolactin level	TRH stimulation
TSH	Serum free and total T3 and T4 Thyroglobulin, TIBG	TRH stimulation

surgical risks and should be avoided. In cases of extremis when immediate surgical decompression or CSF diversion is needed, intravenous T4 infusion can be given cautiously with careful monitoring for arrhythmias and myocardial enzymes. Patients who are very young often require dosages that are disproportionately large compared to body size. Appropriate expert endocrinological consultation should always be sought to help manage hormonal therapy dosing. For euthyroid patients, L-thyroxine replacement can be initiated on an elective basis 1–2 weeks after surgery using the free-T4 level as a guide.

Even more importantly, corticosteroid replacement is mandatory for all but the smallest craniopharyngiomas and should be initiated early on for most patients. For example, thyroid replacement should never be started until cortisone replacement has begun as acute adrenocortical insufficiency can be precipitated by an increased metabolic rate from correction of hypothyroidism (INGBAR 1987). Additionally, larger doses to cover the stress of any procedures or concurrent medical problems should be given. This is especially true for the physiological stress produced during the induction of general anesthesia. For lesions associated with significant peritumoral or white matter edema, high dose dexamethasone can also be used to treat both brain swelling and cortisone deficiency at the same time. Prior to surgery, adequate stress doses are typically three times that of average daily cortisol production. For most patients over 1 year old, the mean physiological requirement is 13–15 mg/m^2 per day. This dose can be given as an intravenous infusion of Solu-Cortef the night before surgery or as intramuscular injections of cortisone acetate for children. During surgery, it is prudent to continue coverage with either a continuous intravenous drip or intermittent infusion of glucocorticoids.

As the patient's fluid and electrolyte balance are of crucial concern to the surgeon, correction of dehydration and DI is also mandatory prior to surgery. Accurate assessment of the patient's water balance and appropriate treatment with intravenous or intranasal doses of antidiuretic hormone (desmopressin or arginine vasopressin) should be completed during this time. Patients who have borderline function of this hormonal axis will often be made worse after surgery. Careful monitoring of the electrolytes and fluid balance is thus critical during the perioperative period. Furthermore, careful attention is needed so as not to over correct DI and cause fluid overload and iatrogenic SIADH (syndrome of inappropriate antidiuretic hormone).

10.6.2
Control of Hydrocephalus

Up to 60% of children and a significant percentage of adults with craniopharyngiomas will present with increased ICP and obstructive hydrocephalus (EINHAUS and SANFORD 1999). For patients who are not in crisis, it is generally preferable to postpone CSF diversion until the time of surgery. This will help to reduce the attendant morbidity and mortality of temporary external CSF drainage. During the operation, a ventriculostomy or similar form of external ventricular drain can be placed. This will allow for perioperative drainage of the CSF as well as for intraoperative brain relaxation. For the majority of cases, the hydrocephalus typically resolves after the obstructing tumor is resected or significantly debulked (PANG 1993).

The ventriculostomy is usually set at a physiological level of 10–12 cm above the auditory meatus for 3–5 days after surgery. This period of drainage allows for resolution of perioperative edema, hemorrhage, and surgical debris which can occlude the CSF circulation. As the CSF absorptive capacity and flow improves, the drainage parameter is gradually increased to see if there is any increase in the ICP or if the patient develops any neurological changes. It is generally prudent to obtain a non-contrast CT scan during this period to assess the ventricles. If the patient remains asymptomatic and the CT reveals no evidence of worsening ventriculomegaly, a trial of clamping off the drain for 24–48 h can be undertaken after which the drain can be removed.

For patients who present in extremis due to a critically elevated ICP, untreated preoperative hydrocephalus has been statistically correlated with a negative effect on postoperative outcome and mean survival (WEN et al. 1992). Some authors have routinely shunted such patients preoperatively with success (CARMEL 1990). On the other hand, we believe that it is preferable to place a temporary external ventricular drain rather than to shunt the patient prior to resection. Based on our experience with craniopharyngiomas, there are several reasons for this practice. First, the risk of shunt infection is significantly increased from the usually prolonged exposure time of the hardware and CSF during a radical tumor resection operation. Secondly, the incidence of shunt obstruction and malfunction is also increased by the blood and debris that inevitably enters the CSF after surgical resection of a tumor. Lastly, many of these patients who present in hydrocephalic crisis will have return of normal CSF circulation after a successful surgery. Based on these observations, we generally reserve ventriculoperitoneal shunting for only those patients who fail weaning from a ventricular drain 5–7 days after surgery. Serial exchanges or replacements of the ventriculostomy are sometimes needed to reduce the risk of infection for periods of prolonged external CSF diversion.

10.7
Surgical Treatment

10.7.1
Surgical Anatomy and Planning

Craniopharyngiomas possess certain characteristics that make their surgical extirpation particularly challenging. Their central location and large size often make complete resection through any one surgical corridor extremely difficult. The tumors are usually intimately involved with several areas of the skull base that in and of themselves often require specialized approaches. These include the peri-third ventricular and interlaminar regions, the interpeduncular fossa, clivus and the cavernous sinus region. Our experience as well as that of others has been that such widespread tumor extension can sometimes necessitate a staged operative procedure (CARMEL 1996).

Historically, a diverse number of operative approaches have been used in the management of these lesions including the subfrontal, bifrontal, pterional, translamina terminalis, transsphenoidal, transcallosal, and transcortical approaches (EINHAUS 1999; FUJITSU 1992; KEMPE 1968; MATSON and CRIGLER 1969; SWEET 1988; SYMON and SPRICH 1985). Whereas each particular technique has both its strengths and weaknesses, the surgeon must choose the approach that provides the optimal exposure which maximizes the chances for total resection. The subfrontal or frontobasal approach and the pterional approach have been most commonly employed for resection of craniopharyngiomas. As exposure of each is limited to a certain degree, we have employed a modified version of the fronto-orbitozygomatic (FOZT) approach in many of our patients with larger lesions with great success (LEVY et al. 1997).

Ultimately, the choice of surgical access is dictated by the individual characteristics of the tumor and its affect on the regional neurovascular structures. Preoperative high-resolution imaging is essential in visualizing the sagittal relationships of craniopharyngiomas to the optic nerve and the anterior portion of the circle of Willis. It is also important to appreciate the inferior extent of the tumor and erosion of the sella turcica, the relationship of the tumor to the third ventricle, any cavernous sinus involvement, and the degree of obstruction of CSF pathways. By clearly defining the three-dimensional boundaries of the tumor and its relationship to entrapped and adjacent structures, an appropriate corridor of surgical access can be chosen to maximize the chances of gross total or near-total resection. The specific operative corridor chosen will ultimately depend on the anatomy of each individual tumor as noted on these preoperative MR and CT images.

Craniopharyngiomas commonly derive the bulk of their blood supply from the anterior circulation (FUJITSU and KUWABARA 1985; MATSON and CRIGLER 1969). As mentioned, particular care must also be taken to preserve the arterial anastomotic ring surrounding the median eminence. Typically, the blood supply is derived primarily from small arterial feeders of the anterior circulation. Direct branches from the internal carotid, posterior-communicating arteries, and cavernous sinuses were also seen. Occasionally, lesions involving the third ventricle will parasitize blood from the posterior cerebral and basilar arteries, though this is rare. Although tumor feeders are seen in this region, the perforators from the circle of Willis also concurrently supply the undersurface of the chiasm and optic tracts. Adequate visualization along the length of the major vessel surfaces is thus crucial to prevent unnecessary blood loss and to avoid ischemic injury to adjacent structures. Accidental division of small feeders can lead to visual loss and hypothalamic injury (CARMEL et al. 1982). Skeletonization of the major circle of Willis vessels with removal of as much tumor tissue as possible is a crucial part of achieving a gross total resection. Unfortunately, tumor tissue is often so adherent to vessel walls that safe removal may be impossible.

The choice of surgical exposure used is also dependent on the position of the tumor in relation to the optic chiasm which must be preserved. To this end, PANG (1993) categorized craniopharyngiomas into one of four broad categories. One third of tumors are retrochiasmatic and displace the optic apparatus superior and anterior towards the tuberculum sellae. These patients are often mistaken for having a prefixed chiasm when, in actuality, it has been pushed forward by the mass. A subfrontal approach to large retrochiasmatic lesions is often greatly hampered by the limited space around the pseudoprefixed chiasm. The second third of craniopharyngiomas are subchiasmatic and push the chiasm directly upward while moving the pituitary stalk posteriorly. The optic nerves are thus placed on stretch in such cases. Another 20–30% of tumors are prechiasmatic and displace the chiasm inferior and posterior. The final 10–15% of tumors primarily expand within the sella itself and thus cause pituitary dysfunction earlier on in the clinical course (OLIVECRONA 1967). Some of these are amenable to a transsphenoidal route of excision, but total resection of the superior portions of the tumor may be limited by its often dense adherence to structures above.

The first two types, the retrochiasmatic and subchiasmatic, are usually solid in nature and thus have a hard, firm consistency. As such, these tumors typically invaginate and push the floor of the third ventricle upwards toward the foramen of Monro. The hypothalamic structures usually maintain their normal ana-

tomic relationships and accommodate by moving laterally. True intraventricular extension of craniopharyngiomas is very uncommon and probably arises from dislocated tuberal ectoblastic cells as opposed to direct tumor invasion (VAN DEN BERGH 1970). For the majority of cases, the tumor remains outside of the third ventricle no matter how thinned the floor is and despite the MRI finding of the tumor appearing to be within the third ventricle. Transventricular approaches for such cases are associated with a high incidence of hypothalamic dysfunction as the floor is often hard to identify and inadvertently sectioned (PANG 1993). The incidence of purely compressive hypothalamic dysfunction is actually surprisingly rare in pediatric cases (CAVAZZUTI et al. 1983; THOMSETT et al. 1980).

Prechiasmatic lesions are more frequently cystic and tend to burrow underneath and eventually expand within the frontal lobes. As a result, these tumors can often reach enormous proportions with the soft cystic portions reaching out with pseudopod-like extensions to the sylvian fissure, the dorsum sellae, and the prepontine cistern. Such lesions frequently become extensively multilobulated with a high occurrence of psychomotor seizures and cranial neuropathies due to their many areas of compression and cortical irritation.

The intense glial reaction that usually accompanies these lesions further complicates operative dissection (LANDOLT 1972). These tumors are tenaciously adherent to the major arteries, nerves, and perforators located at the skull base (SYMON and SPRICH 1985). As craniopharyngiomas are thought to be noninvasive tumors, some authors have advocated dissection along this "glial envelope" (HAKUBA et al. 1986; MATSON and CRIGLER 1969). When possible, one should attempt to remain within this subarachnoid plane as delineated by the cisternal arachnoid membrane, but this is often broadly fused to the tumoral arachnoid membrane. The dense calcifications and multiple cysts that are encountered frequently contribute to an already piecemeal delivery of the lesion.

Despite these many obstacles hampering the tumor dissection, one should strive for the removal of all tumor that can be safely resected. Careful inspection of all neural and vascular structures entrapped within and adjacent to the tumor must be attempted. This often requires additional skeletonization and mobilization of vessels and nerves. When needed, further bony drilling both intra- and extradurally is helpful as well. As long as such aggressive exposure and dissection does not compromise the underlying tissue, an attempt should be made to remove any tumor tissue that is encountered. The arteries of the circle of Willis, hypothalamus, and pituitary stalk are the most common sites of residual tumors and recurrence (SUNG et al. 1981; CARMEL 1996; SYMON and SPRICH 1985).

To better visualize these problematic regions, we feel that an extended subfrontal exposure is afforded by the FOZT approach by drilling the sphenoid and removing the orbital roof down to the superior orbital fissure. This allows for direct visualization of the median eminence, its anastomotic vascular ring, and the pituitary stalk in many cases. Using its unique portal vein striations to differentiate it from surrounding suprasellar structures, the pituitary stalk can often be located as it penetrates the diaphragma sellae (SAMII and TATAGIBA 1997). Identification of the stalk is basic to its preservation. The good visualization of the FOZT approach in this region thereby helps to insure its integrity. The benefit of this approach over a subfrontal one is that the surgeon has direct visualization of the tumor in relationship to the inferior aspect of the optic chiasm. Tumor dissection can thus be completed sharply with the preservation of all inferior perforating vessels to the chiasm while minimizing the chance of causing ischemic compromise to the optic apparatus.

Numerous other approaches have also been utilized in the resection of craniopharyngiomas. These include the subfrontal (PANG 1993), trans-lamina terminalis, transsphenoidal (LAWS 1980; PATTERSON and DANYLEVICH 1980), pterional (YASARGIL et al. 1990), subtemporal (HAKUBA et al. 1985), fronto-orbitozygomatic (LEVY et al. 1997), transcallosal (APUZZO et al. 1982), transcortical (BUSCH 1944; YASARGIL et al. 1990), transfacial (FUJITSU et al. 1992), and transpetrosal approaches. A detailed discussion of all the operative exposures and surgical techniques needed for safe resection of craniopharyngiomas is beyond the scope of this text. Rather, we will briefly present some of the more commonly used surgical techniques – the subfrontal, trans-lamina terminalis, transsphenoidal, and the pterional approach. An expanded discussion of the FOZT approach is then provided to elucidate its relative merits. Table 10.3 summarizes some of the merits and disadvantages of several of these approaches. Figure 10.5 graphically illustrates the different trajectories afforded by some of these different approaches. *Arrow 1* represents the standard pterional trajectory. *Arrow 2* follows the path taken by a subtemporal or temporopolar approach. *Arrow 3* illustrates the trajectory of the fronto-orbitozygomatic technique. Lastly, *arrow 4* demonstrates the midline approach of the subfrontal craniotomy.

Table 10.3. Comparison of surgical approaches

Orbitozygomatic

Pros: Short approach to the sella
Direct visualization of parasellar/retrosellar region
Exposes clivus and anterior brain stem
Three fossa exposure
Cons: Unilateral exposure
Large bony removal
Limited intraventricular exposure

Interhemispheric/transcallosal

Pros: Good exposure to lateral and third ventricles
Good visualization of vascular tissue and choroid
Cons: Landmarks difficult to identify
Forniceal and anterior callosal damage

Transsphenoidal

Pros: Excellent cosmesis
Minimal encroachment on neurovascular tissue
Shorter convalescent period
Excellent sellar exposure
Cons: Poor exposure of chiasmal, suprachiasmatic, tuberculum, clival, or supra-cavernous sinus extension
Limited field of view
Blind curettage of tumor in lateral gutters, cavernous sinus
Difficult hemostasis

Subfrontal/transbasal

Pros: Wide lateral, clival, and sella region exposure
Direct visualization of ipsilateral carotid arteries, chiasm, and optic nerves
Anterior third ventricular approach via lamina terminalis
Intra- and extradural exposure
Cons: Bifrontal incision increases operative time and morbidity
Hypothalamic damage via trans-lamina terminalis approach

10.7.2
Surgical Approaches

10.7.2.1
Subfrontal Approach

The subfrontal approach has been the most commonly utilized surgical approach in the resection of craniopharyngiomas (CHOUX et al. 1991; SWEET 1994). Many premier neurosurgeons who have dealt with these difficult lesions preferentially employ it to resect tumors of the midline sellar region (PANG 1993; SAMII and TATAGIBA 1997). It is advantageous as it allows for direct exposure of the frontal skull base in

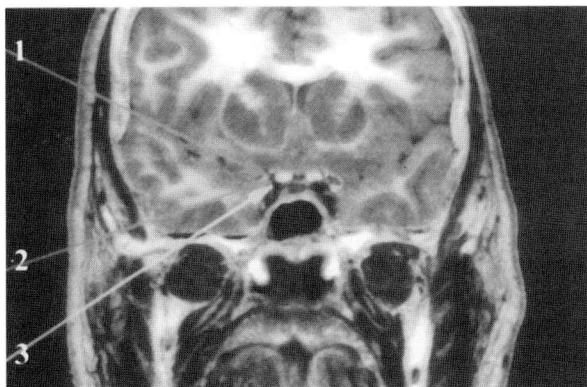

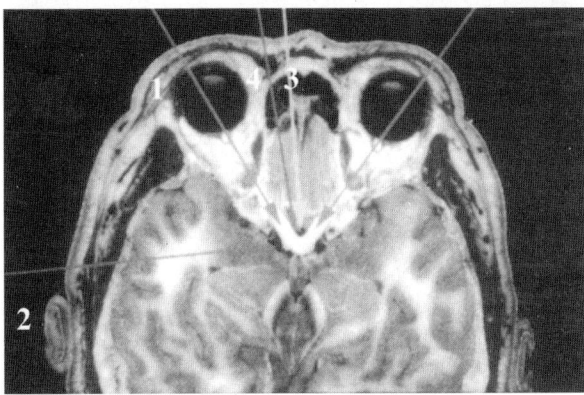

Fig. 10.5. Demonstration of the differences in surgical trajectory of the various surgical approaches as seen in the coronal (**A**) and axial (**B**) plane. The *numbered arrows* represent the various trajectories: *1*, pterional approach; *2*, subtemporal and temporopolar approach; *3*, fronto-orbitozygomatic approach; *4*, subfrontal or frontobasal approach

the midline. As craniopharyngiomas are generally midline lesions that push neurovascular structures from the midline (*arrow 4*, Fig. 10.5B), the subfrontal approach allows for a good view of both the tumor and the displaced regional anatomy. Additionally, the lamina terminalis of the third ventricle can be opened from a safe anterior corridor to achieve an intraventricular view.

The patient is usually positioned supine with the head placed neutrally or sometimes turned slightly away from the more involved side. Whereas a bicoronal scalp flap is fashioned behind the hairline for better cosmesis, usually only a unilateral bone flap is required. Use of only such unilateral frontal lobe retraction typically provides more than adequate exposure and can help prevent debilitating bifrontal lobe contusion and injury. For truly midline lesions, a right-sided craniotomy and frontal lobe elevation is performed as it is technically easier for a right-handed surgeon. Tumors which are more eccentric

should be approached from the ipsilateral side. After elevating an appropriate pericranial and scalp flap, an osteoplastic right frontal craniotomy is fashioned such that the medial edge of the bone flap crosses the midline by 1–1.5 cm to allow for control of the anterior portion of the superior sagittal sinus (SSS). The anterior, inferior limit of the flap lies immediately on the orbital roof itself (Fig. 10.6A). For additional exposure, a section of the orbital roof can actually also be included in the bone flap. Bony removal can be further extended along the roof back to the sphenoid ridge to allow for a more pterional-like trajectory if desired (Fig. 10.6B). Numerous variations of the basic subfrontal approach are possible and should be individualized to the needs of each case.

After exposure of the dura and careful removal of the bone flap from over the sinus, the SSS is usually doubly ligated and sectioned. The anterior falx is then detached sharply from the crista galli. In the case of larger lesions, it is sometimes necessary to divide the ipsilateral olfactory tract as well. Although many patients are anosmic at presentation, bilateral division of the olfactory nerves should be avoided if possible. Malleable retractors are then placed to gently elevate the frontal lobe off the skull base. Drainage of CSF via an external ventriculostomy combined with diuresis can facilitate brain relaxation and minimize traction injury. The subfrontal retraction is then gradually deepened along with the retractors. In order, the ipsilateral optic nerve, chiasm, and carotid artery will then come into view. Sharp dissection and opening of the carotid and prechiasmal cisterns along a horizontal plane extending from the temporal lobe to the contralateral carotid cistern will allow for further CSF drainage and brain relaxation.

At this point, the tumor is typically visible behind a veil of dense, thickened arachnoid that is adherent between the ipsilateral optic nerve and carotid artery. In essence, the tumor thus lies behind this neurovascular lattice comprised of the internal carotid artery, basilar artery, anterior cerebral arteries, temporal lobe, optic nerve, optic chiasm, and sylvian fissure and vessels. Tumor extraction is thus accomplished by a piecemeal delivery of small pieces through the various portals or spaces of the lattice. These portals include the space between the optic nerves (interoptic space), the area between the optic nerve and carotid (carotico-optic space), and the region between the carotid and the lateral sylvian fissure (caroticosylvian space) (Fig. 10.6C). As most craniopharyngiomas are soft, they should be internally debulked through a combination of sharp curettage and aspiration with attention to meticu-

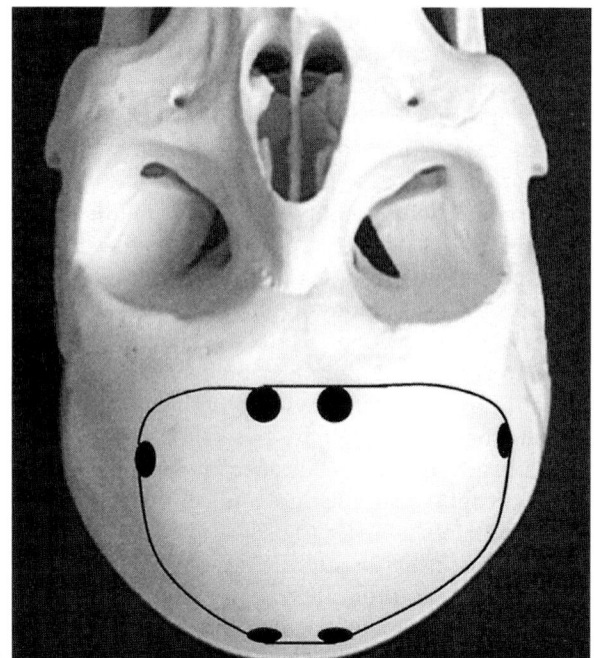

A

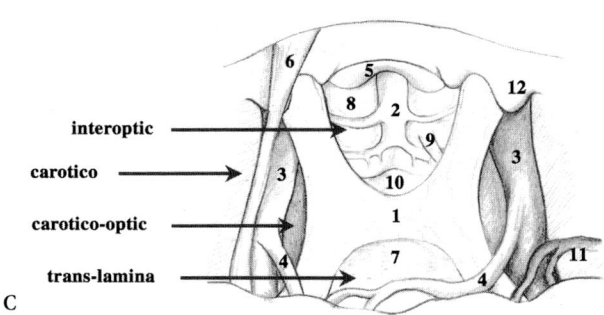

interoptic →

carotico →

carotico-optic →

trans-lamina →

C

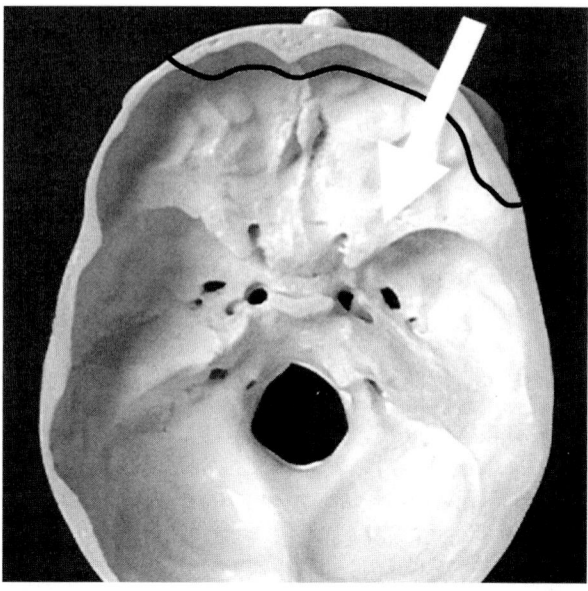

B

Fig. 10.6A–C. These diagrams demonstrate the craniotomy flap, trajectory, and overall exposure afforded by the subfrontal approach. **A** A right-sided unilateral frontal craniotomy is diagrammed. Note the placement of burr holes around the sagittal sinus for hemostatic control. **B** The extent of bony removal from the orbital rim and frontal bone is outlined. The overall trajectory is demonstrated for a pterional modification of the subfrontal approach. **C** Illustration of the anatomic view seen during a subfrontal approach. *Arrows* point out the various surgical windows through which tumor resection is achieved. The following structures are labeled: *1*, optic chiasm; *2*, basilar artery; *3*, internal carotid; *4*, anterior cerebral artery; *5*, dorsum sellae; *6*, olfactory nerve; *7*, lamina terminalis; *8*, brain stem; *9*, third cranial nerve; *10*, hypothalamus; *11*, sylvian vein; *12*, clinoid

lous hemostasis at every step. As the lesion is collapsed, the small morsels of tumor are then brought out through these named anatomic windows.

Some authors have recommended stereotyped sequences of maneuvers to ensure safe resection of a tumor. An example of this includes: (1) interoptic debulking, (2) separation of the tumor capsule from the optic structures, (3) lateral dissection of the tumor edges, (4) removing the upper pole of the tumor from the hypothalamus and the floor of the third ventricle, (5) dissection of the posterior aspect of the lesion from the basilar tip and membrane of Liliequist, and finally, (6) extirpation of the remaining tumor from the sella and dorsum (PANG 1993). As long as meticulous attention is paid to preserving vital structures, avoiding injury to feeding vessels, and dissecting as much tumor as is possible, any combination of these steps would be appropriate.

After fixing the retractors, the resection is generally begun by aspirating the cystic portions of the tumor. If adequate brain relaxation via CSF drainage from the adjacent cisterns or from external ventricular drainage has not been accomplished, it should be initiated at this time to allow for better exposure. By first decompressing the portion of tumor between the optic nerves, the chiasm eventually will fall away from the tuberculum thereby enlarging the window of the interoptic space. With gentle traction placed on the capsule as it pulls away from the chiasm and nerves, an arachnoid plane is often revealed underneath these structures. This plane should be utilized to safely peel off the tumor from the optic apparatus. Whereas the arterial feeders to the capsule from the anterior cerebral and anterior communicating arteries need to be divided, one must be very careful not to divide the vessels which go on to feed the inferior aspect of the chiasm and optic nerves. After interruption of this anterior blood supply to the tumor, the only remaining vascular supply to the tumor at this point is usually small vessels arising laterally from the posterior communicating arteries and inferiorly from the meningohypophyseal arteries.

Thus, lateral dissection on either side of the tumor serves to divide the blood supply from the posterior communicating arteries and to detach the lesion from the medial temporal lobe and carotid artery. On the right side, this resection is best accomplished through the carotico-optic space. With gentle medial retraction of the tumor capsule, feeders are placed on stretch and can be cauterized and divided. On the other hand, thalamotuberal perforators that normally supply the basal ganglia are left loose and can be thus spared. For tumors with more lateral extension, the caroticosylvian space may also have to be utilized to completely free the tumor from its lateral attachments. On the left side, the lateral dissection can often be easily accomplished by working through the already enlarged interoptic space and by rotating the patient slightly to the left away from the surgeon.

After thus debulking the lateral aspects of the lesion, the superior pole of the tumor can now be pulled down from its attachments to the hypothalamus through the interoptic space. Although often compressed and thinned, the tumor and the floor of third ventricle are still usually separated from the tumor by a layer of arachnoid. Unfortunately, this layer is usually fused to the capsule near the region of the hypothalamus and infundibular stalk. Interestingly, this portion of the tumor is often best delivered by a firm grasping and pulling motion rather than by sharp, sweeping dissection. The technique involves the alternating use of micro-forceps to gradually pull the baggy tumor mass out of this deep hole. By pulling the tumor forcibly out of this region, some authors believe that the tumor pseudopods are avulsed intact from the gliotic underlying brain rather than being amputated and left behind. This may also help to reduce the incidence of recurrence (PANG 1993). After extirpating the tumor in this fashion, a distorted pituitary stalk can sometimes be identified by its pathognomonic striated, long, portal vessels (CARMEL 1979). In such cases, it can be carefully preserved. The stalk is, however, often encased within the tumor mass and must be sacrificed.

The posterior aspect of the tumor can be rolled forward into the interoptic space as well. There are usually no feeding vessels to the tumor from the posterior circulation. The thick, double-layered membrane of Liliequist usually serves to prevent tumor attachment to the brain stem and basilar artery. Thus the majority of tumors can be pulled forward and removed by sectioning the arachnoid adhesions. The small remaining inferior portion of the tumor can usually be lifted up at this point from the diaphragma or the dura overlying the sella. The lower portion of the capsule rarely fuses with these structures. The few remaining meningohypophyseal branches to the tumor can be coagulated and sectioned.

10.7.2.2
Trans-Lamina Terminalis Approach

For patients with a lesion that is retrochiasmatic or for those rarer cases that truly have a prefixed optic chiasm, resection of extensive craniopharyngiomas through the interoptic and carotico-optic spaces is severely limited by the small space afforded. An additional working space can be obtained by opening the lamina terminalis and obtaining additional access to the dome of such retrochiasmatic tumors. In this regard, the trans-lamina terminalis approach can be viewed as an extension or modification of the standard subfrontal technique described above. CHOUX and his group (1991) reported on the use of this technique in the majority of 54 consecutive cases of adult craniopharyngioma with excellent results.

The lamina terminalis typically delimits the anterior and inferior portion of the third ventricle. In cases with a normal third ventricular floor, opening of the lamina does not directly expose the dome of the tumor which is further separated by the floor. For very large tumors with long-standing compression, the tuberal portion of the hypothalamus bounded by the mamillary bodies and chiasm can be stretched quite thin by the dome of the tumor. The lamina and tuberal portion of the hypothalamus can sometimes form what appears to be a single, translucent membrane in such cases. This membrane typically is stretched between the splayed-out optic tracts (Fig. 10.6C). In either case, the tumor dome can either be directly removed by opening the floor of the third ventricle or by pulling the lesion downward and then delivering it through either a subchiasmatic or lateral (carotico-optic or caroticosylvian) portal (MATSON and CRIGLER 1969). As the basal hypothalamic nuclei have generally been slowly displaced laterally by the tumor, section of the lamina terminalis is not associated with a high incidence of hypothalamic deficiency.

10.7.2.3
Transsphenoidal Approach

Although completely intrasellar lesions are less common and comprise less than 15% of craniopharyngiomas, a fair number of tumors will at least have some component of tumor within the sella. When the preoperative images show wide expansion of the sella with accompanying clinoid erosion, the lower aspect of the tumor capsule is generally densely adherent to the sellar dura and cavernous sinus walls at that point. The surgeon must thus be prepared to pursue alternate means of removing this sellar component as it will not be accessible through a standard subfrontal corridor (HONEGGER et al. 1992; HARDY and VEZINA 1976).

For lesions which are still intrasellar or suprasellar but subdiaphragmatic, a primary transsphenoidal resection via either a nasoseptal or sublabial route can be used with great success. The enlarged, ballooned pituitary fossa often seen in such cases is very helpful as it provides even more surgical exposure than one normally encounters while operating on pituitary adenomas. We would direct the reader to the reports of other authors much more experienced with this approach for a more detailed explanation of the approach (LAWS 1980; THAPAR and LAWS 1997). However, certain technical points merit consideration. During the dural opening, great caution must be exercised to not inadvertently enter the cavernous sinuses as the regional anatomy can be greatly deformed by the tumor. Furthermore, the pituitary gland is often pushed downward and forward by the mass such that transection of the anterior lobe is needed to gain access to the tumor. When debulking the tumor capsule, every attempt should be made to dissect it free from the dura. The superior portion of the capsule, however, is frequently densely fused with the overlying diaphragma sella. For such cases, extra care to identify the pituitary stalk is mandatory before blindly curetting the superior portion of the tumor. More often than not, the infundibulum and stalk should be able to be preserved. When lesions contain ample calcifications, complete extirpation is often impossible and will also require a staged transcranial procedure. The recent use of endoscopic assistance has added a further new dimension to the transsphenoidal approach as well (HALVES and SORENSEN 1982)

For lesions that have both intrasellar and suprasellar supradiaphragmatic components, direct access to the sella can be obtained via a subfrontal transsphe-

noidal approach as described by PATTERSON and DANYLEVICH (1980). This technique begins with a standard subfrontal exposure. After this, a high-speed drill is used to break through the tuberculum sellae into the sphenoid sinus. The mucosa is then swept away to reveal the anterior sellar wall which is then removed. This approach is particularly helpful during subfrontal exposures of patients with sellar extensions and prefixed or pseudoprefixed chiasms. During exposure, the circular and cavernous sinuses may bleed profusely but can usually be controlled by simple venous tamponade. This technique may also be combined with the trans-lamina terminalis procedure as detailed previously to gain even further exposure.

Whether approached from above or below, the sella and the sphenoid sinus, if violated, should be packed with fat and fascia lata to prevent brain herniation and postoperative CSF leak. For cases where the sphenoid mucosa and arachnoid have both been violated, it is often prudent to perform some form of lumbar drainage to help prevent prolonged CSF drainage through the operative site.

10.7.2.4
Pterional Approach

There has been increasing use of the laterally based pterional or frontotemporal to resect even large craniopharyngiomas. Some authors use this approach preferentially to resect these tumors often in conjunction with a combined or staged transsphenoidal or transcallosal approach (YASARGIL et al. 1990; DEROME 1991). The approach is based on a curvilinear scalp incision beginning at the root of the zygoma slightly anterior to the tragus which then proceeds superiorly and slightly anteriorly to end past midline slightly in front of the hairline. Osseous exposure is afforded by an oval-shaped bone flapped based on the pterion to include the basal aspects of the parietal, frontal, and temporal bones. This approach provides a trajectory essentially based on the sphenoid wing. Such a surgical corridor provides much greater lateral exposure of craniopharyngiomas but sacrifices some of the anterior basal exposure afforded by a subfrontal approach. This corridor of access is illustrated by *arrow 1* in Fig. 10.5A,B. Modifications of the pterional approach to include zygoma removal and inclusion of portions of the orbit and frontal floor provide even greater flexibility to the approach. As a standard pterional approach is well known to most neurosurgeons, we will not go into great depth regarding its technical aspects. For a detailed discussion, we would refer readers to YASARGIL (1984) for an excellent description of the technique which he helped to pioneer.

Like the subfrontal approach, tumor resection through a pterional approach is accomplished by a piecemeal delivery of the tumor through several anatomic windows or portals formed by the regional neurovascular anatomy. These include the parachiasmal, prechiasmatic, carotico-optic, and carotidoentorial triangles. Further corridors include the triangle superior to the carotid bifurcation and through the opening of the ipsilateral lamina terminalis. We have utilized a modification of this approach (fronto-orbitozygomatic) to resect larger lesions at one sitting thus obviating the need for staged or combined procedures in many cases.

10.7.2.5
Fronto-Orbito Zygomatic Approach

The fronto-orbito zygomatic (FOZT) technique takes its roots from Yasargil's standard pterional craniotomy and the temporopolar approach of Dolenc (1987) and Sano (1980). We have used the FOZT approach for lesions in and around the basilar bifurcation, above the dorsum sellae, posteriorly pointing apex lesions, and lesions adjacent to the posterior clinoid process. The overall trajectory of the FOZT craniotomy is demonstrated by arrow 3 in Fig. 10.5. The principle advantages of the FOZT approach are the preservation of anterior temporal venous draining veins, decreased brain retraction, and a wider operative corridor that allows for movement of the microscope through an arc of nearly 90 . The key anatomic features of this approach include removal of the extradural sphenoid wing and anterior clinoid process, skeletonization-decompression of the optic canal superior orbital fissure and foramen rotundum, extradural retraction of the temporal tip, transcavernous mobilization of the carotid and oculomotor nerve, and transcavernous removal of the posterior clinoid if needed.

The initial preparation, positioning, and skin incision is similar to that used for a routine pterional approach. The skin incision extends inferiorly over the root of the zygoma. A more basal-to-vertex trajectory is usually required for the exposure of tumors that extend above the dorsum sella. Removal of the zygoma in combination with removal of the orbital rim adds significantly to the exposure. This is an important consideration when we approach large

tumors that extend into the suprasellar, interpeduncular, and clival regions. To allow for orbital retraction, the orbital rim is removed with the bone flap as a single unit.

Zygoma removal is initiated with a cut made parallel to the long axis of the zygoma at its junction with the temporal bone. The second cut, perpendicular to the first, is made along the orbital zygomatic process near the lateral orbital rim. Two views of the overall FOZT bone flap are provided in Fig. 10.7A,B. This maneuver allows for inferior retraction of the temporalis muscle, enabling the operating microscope to be radically deviated to gain a more lateral-to-medial and inferior-to-superior trajectory.

Once the craniotomy flap is removed, dural elevation is initiated from the anterolateral middle fossa to expose the foramen rotundum and superior orbital fissure, and continued medially to expose the floor of the anterior cranial fossa. The lateral limit of dural elevation is the foramen ovale and the medial limit the anterior superior ethmoidal artery. The sphenoid ridge is shaved along with any irregularities of the orbital roof and anterior middle fossa floor using the high-speed drill with cutting and diamond burrs and copious irrigation. Continued meticulous drilling of the lateral dural wall of the superior orbital fissure allows for increased mobility of the superior orbital fissure. The foramen rotundum is then unroofed using the high-speed drill beginning laterally and medially and finally over the nerve exposing the second trigeminal branch. The optic canal is additionally unroofed extradurally to achieve modest mobility of the optic nerve which is often fixed by the tumor.

The anterior clinoid process is removed by initially drilling and debulking the center of the process. This leaves a thin shell of bone which is progressively chipped away and then removed. One should be aware of the potential for a pneumatized anterior clinoid and in such cases the chance for a postoperative CSF fistula. The optic strut is additionally flattened and removed. When the extradural bone removal is completed, the dura propria of the temporal tip is elevated from the inner cavernous membrane. The middle fossa dura is stripped away allowing extradural mobilization of the temporal tip. Further separation of the middle fossa dura from the true cavernous membrane will minimize temporal lobe retraction. Initially, the meningo-orbital vessels are divided at the apex of the superior orbital fissure and a cleavage plane formed originating at the junction of the temporal dura and the periorbital fascia.

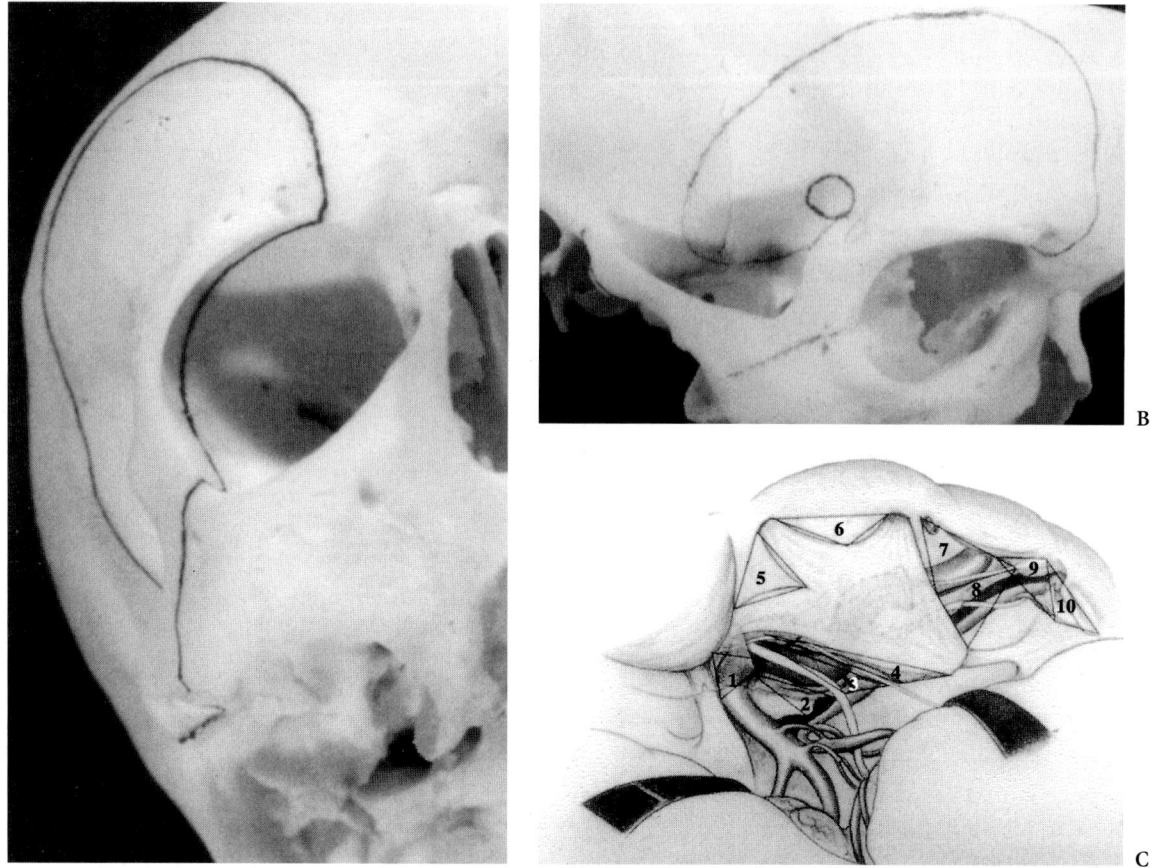

Fig. 10.7A–C. These diagrams demonstrate the craniotomy flap and overall exposure afforded by the fronto-orbitozygomatic approach. **A** Anterior view of craniotomy flap. **B** Lateral view showing extent of zygoma resection and orbital rim removal. **C** A view of the typical anatomic exposure provided by the FOZT approach. The trigeminal nerve can be seen clearly with several branches of the internal carotid artery in view. Further, the lateral wall of the cavernous sinus has been removed

The dura is then sharply elevated from the true cavernous membrane extending from the superior orbital fissure along the second trigeminal branch and continuing posteriorly to the foramen ovale. The true cavernous membrane is composed of thin connective tissue contiguous with the nerve sheaths of the third, fourth, and fifth cranial nerves and surrounds the venous plexus of the cavernous sinus. The limits of dural reflection of the true cavernous membrane are the third trigeminal branch posteriorly and the tentorial edge medially. Finally, the medial tentorial incisura is incised and separated from the inner cavernous membrane near the third cranial nerve. A picture of the lateral-to-midline view afforded by the FOZT approach is seen in Fig. 10.7C.

The removal of the anterior clinoid process with skeletonization of the optic canal, superior orbital fissure and foramen rotundum allows for the safe manipulation of the optic nerve, carotid artery, superior orbital fissure contents, and the second branch of the trigeminal nerve without compromise from overlying bony surfaces. Additional mobility of the third nerve is often helpful in gaining access to portions of tumor located in and around the cavernous sinus and interpeduncular fossa. Opening the porus oculomotorius will allow for extra length of the third nerve to further improve retractability and potentiate safe tumor removal from the third nerve and prevent injury. The dura is opened over the sylvian fissure extending to the optic nerve sheath dura and then medially along the frontal base for 2–3 cm forming an L shape. Perneczky's ring is opened and the carotid artery freed of its dural attachment laterally. If required, retractors are placed extradurally allowing for posterolateral retraction of the temporal lobe and posteromedial retraction of the frontal lobe. The temporal tip veins are thus protected and preserved with the anterior temporal dura. The anterior 2–3 cm of the sylvian fissure is sharply opened allowing for increased exposure of the superior aspect of the clival region.

At this point, the tumor is commonly encountered and found to be densely adherent to the brain, cranial nerves, and vascular structures. The tumor is exposed by opening the cisternal arachnoid along the edge of the now drilled-away sphenoid ridge, over the optic nerves, and over the tumor bulk. An attempt is made to distinguish the multiple layers of arachnoid and to differentiate the cisternal from the tumor arachnoidal plane and thus avoid unnecessary parenchymal injury. Accordingly, care is taken not to anneal arachnoid to the tumor capsule as this would obliterate the subarachnoid plane of dissection. With larger craniopharyngiomas, however, the arachnoidal layers are often fused over a significant portion of the tumor surface.

Continued slow, cautious sharp dissection allows for visualization of the internal carotid and proximal A1 and M1 segments. The triangle between the oculomotor and trochlear nerves (superior triangle of the cavernous sinus) can also be opened sharply if required. Tumor involvement in, around, and through this triangle is frequently seen. The oculomotor nerve is then exposed from its origin at the midbrain to its dural entrance into the superior orbital fissure. At this point in the approach, the oculomotor nerve and trochlear nerves can be mobilized as needed to maximize exposure of the tumor. The third nerve can be gently retracted laterally only after first covering it with a soft cottonoid. The internal carotid artery can now also be mobilized medially or laterally as it has been freed from its dural attachment anteriorly. Whenever possible, an attempt is made to aspirate any cystic regions as this often provides additional room for dissection.

Sharp microdissection of the arachnoid as described will now allow for additional retraction in order to widen the corridors to the sella, posterior clinoid, and membrane of Liliequist. When enough of the tumor surface is exposed, the tumor is debulked internally. Calcifications are sometimes encountered that need to be crushed before they can be delivered through the small windows of access. Small arterial feeders are cautiously coagulated and divided.

Larger lesions that extend farther superiorly in the suprasellar region involve the basilar region and interpeduncular fossa or extend into the third ventricle, require additional surgical exposure. To gain increased visualization of the interpeduncular fossa region, the arachnoid membrane is sharply opened lateral to the internal carotid artery. To complete the exposure, the posterior clinoid can be removed intradurally with a high-speed drill. This increases the exposure of the basilar artery below the sella. Removal of the posterior clinoid process expands the working space for management of giant lesions as well as providing for temporary occlusion of the mid-portion of the basilar artery if warranted. The superior and posterior aspects of tumors in this region and those that extended into the third ventricle usually do not have a major arterial supply. Dense arachnoid adhesions are often encountered where the tumor is adjacent to the basilar and posterior cerebral arteries.

After resection of the tumor mass, a careful inspection of the sellar and parasellar structures is made to insure that no resectable portions of tumor tissue remain. At the conclusion of the procedure, the dura is closed in a watertight fashion, utilizing pericranium and fibrin glue. The pericranium is preserved during opening for this purpose. The en bloc free bone flap and zygomatic arch are then reattached with the use of titanium mini-plates. For cosmetic purposes, the anterior and superior portions of the bone flap are preferentially aligned.

Two representative cases demonstrating the utility of the FOZT approach are provided. The first case demonstrates a large complex, multilobulated lesion that was eccentric to the right side. This 5-year-old boy was originally admitted to the Children's Hospital of Los Angeles for a 1-year history of headache, progressive visual loss, and difficulty with ambulation. Due to the lesion's large size and wide extension both superiorly and posteriorly, the decision to attempt resection through a FOZT approach was made. The other option was to perform a combined subfrontal and pterional procedure. A FOZT approach was accomplished with excellent tumor resection and no evidence of residual tumor on the follow-up images (Fig. 10.3). Except for worsening of the patient's pre-existing DI and a transient third nerve palsy, the postoperative course was unremarkable.

The second case was a 4/12-year-old boy who was referred to the Children's Hospital of Los Angeles for a history of incompletely resected craniopharyngioma in the suprasellar and right cavernous sinus region. He had originally presented with hydrocephalus and had been operated on via a right pterional approach. Early postoperative MRI revealed residual tumor adjacent to the circle of Willis and around the right cavernous sinus region. The patient was taken to the OR where the FOZT approach provided an excellent exposure of the tumor, sellar, third ventricle and cavernous sinus regions. Posterior mobilization of the temporal tip with gentle traction and sparing of the bridging veins provided improved visualization of the third ventricular region without increased risk of venous infarct as had occurred during the first operation. A generous but subtotal resection was achieved (Fig. 10.4). No intraoperative surgical complications were encountered.

10.7.2.6
Combined or Staged Surgical Approaches

Due to the often tremendous proportions of craniopharyngiomas at the time of presentation, it is necessary to perform combined or staged procedures to achieve a good, complete resection. This is especially true for tumors that have a complex, multilobulated morphology with far lateral, inferior, or superior extensions. As no single approach will be able to address all sides of these difficult lesions, several authors have utilized various combinations of procedures to both maximize the extent of surgical resection and to preserve as much of the native anatomy as possible (Koos and MILLER 1971; CARMEL 1996). Fig. 10.8 demonstrates the frequency with which we have used the various surgical approaches for craniopharyngioma patients at our institution over the recent years (L. T. Khoo et al., unpublished data). Of note is the large proportion of cases requiring staged or combined approaches (40%).

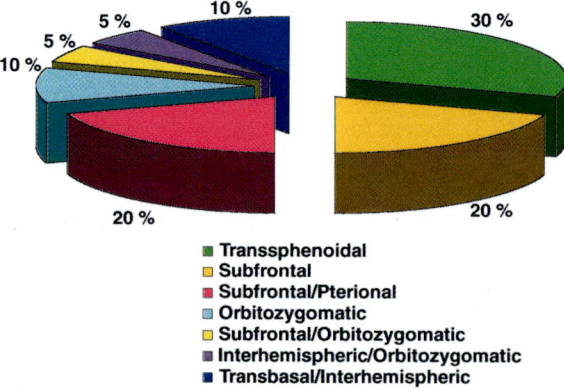

Fig. 10.8. Frequency of approaches used for craniopharyngioma

10.8
Surgical Results

10.8.1
Postoperative Complications

Although most series agree that gross total or complete resection of craniopharyngiomas affords the best chance for long-term cure and prevention of recurrence, radical resection also carries with it a higher chance of neurological injury and deterioration. Indeed, the tenacious and adherent nature of craniopharyngiomas often makes complete resection impossible without sacrifice or injury to the adjacent neurovascular structures. As such, a compromise must always be reached between these two goals of resection and preservation of the local anatomy. Unavoidably, craniopharyngioma resection carries with it an significant amount of attendant morbidity.

Of the iatrogenic neurological deficits associated with surgery, visual loss or deterioration is by far the most common (PANG 1993). This can be due to either direct injury to the optic apparatus or, more commonly, to ischemic injury from damage to vital nutrient vessels supplying the nerves, tract, and chiasm. The preoperative visual status is the most important prognostic variable in predicting the outcome of the patient. Those with limited vision or near-blindness are unlikely to regain meaningful function, whereas those with partial deficits may experience significant improvement after resection. Patients with less than 1-year history of visual dysfunction have a three-times better chance of improvement after surgery than those with more than 1 year of disability (ARTERO et al. 1984). Similarly, postoperative deficits lasting more than a few days are unlikely to recover much as well.

After visual loss, injury to the pituitary stalk and gland accounts for the bulk of postoperative complications after craniopharyngioma resection. Such injury can range from mild, transient deficits to profound, long-term panhypopituitarism. Due to almost unavoidable manipulation of the stalk, a postoperative period of DI is extremely common. This is the most common endocrinological complication after tumor resection (SAMII and TATAGIBA 1997). Classically, a triphasic pattern or course is encountered. Heavy diuresis and fluid loss typically begins within 24 h after surgery due to acute interruption of normal ADH transport from the infundibulum. As wallerian degeneration of the hypophyseal tract and pitressin-neurophysin-containing axons then takes place, agonal release of ADH occurs from stored vesicles to cause paradoxical water retention after 48–96 h (SHUCART and JACKSON 1976). Extremely cautious management of the patient during this critical window is needed to avoid fluid overload and uncontrollable brain swelling from water intoxication. Use of shorter acting agents such intravenous DDAVP (desmopressin) is prudent during this period. The final phase of the triad sets in several days later when the remaining ADH is depleted and the permanent diuretic state ensures. Interestingly, 10–15% of patients with permanent DI from presumed stalk sectioning will experience a partial return of endogenous ADH production within 3 years. Although unclear, some have postulated that new neurovascular ADH-containing centers are formed in the supraoptic and paraventricular nuclei (ANTUNES et al. 1979).

Hypoadrenalism from decreased ACTH production is well documented for most patients with large craniopharyngiomas preoperatively. These patients typically receive hormonal replacement prior to surgery as well as larger stress doses of glucocorticoids during the perioperative period. The primary danger in such patients occurs when the steroids are gradually tapered off after surgery. It must be assumed that the majority of postoperative patients are even more hypoadrenal after surgery due to both operative manipulation and iatrogenic adrenal suppression from exogenous steroids. As such, endocrinological consultation is needed to accurately assess the patients' endogenous cortisone production before prematurely tapering the patients off their perioperative regimen (HOFFMAN et al. 1977). Some authors have also advocated the use of cortisone acetate or similar preparations as glucocorticoids have little mineralocorticoid effect (CARMEL 1996).

Partial dysfunction of other endocrine axes also occurs after sectioning of the pituitary stalk. As such, a complete endocrine work-up should be repeated for all patients after recovering from the acute phase of surgery. Laboratory data should then be compared to that of the preoperative work-up and appropriate changes made to the hormonal replacement regimen. Some degree of hypothyroidism is very common after surgery and is seen in 60–80% of patients with stalk injury (PANG 1993). FSH and LH deficiencies that occur after surgery are usually permanent and will require replacement to ensure normal growth and sexual maturation of the patient. As the arcuate nucleus and the sexual hormone system are highly complex and sensitive, recovery after stalk injury has not been observed to date. For males,

simple testosterone replacement is usually enough to maintain libido, although sperm production will often still be abnormal. For females, ovulation must be maintained through a complex and expensive procedure involving multiple stimulating hormones and gonadotropins (GLASS 1978). Replacement of testosterone and estrogen must be postponed, however, in young children as they can accelerate premature closure of the epiphyseal plates in long bones thereby arresting growth. This must be weighed against the psychological and social stigmata that will result from delaying sexual maturity. Children after stalk sectioning will require growth hormone replacement as well, but such therapy is typically postponed for 6–9 months after surgery (AYRAL et al. 1980). This is done because a sizable number of these children will continue to grow despite a lack of growth hormone. Numerous hypotheses have been formulated to explain this phenomenon. These include a hyperinsulinemic state, hypersecretion of prolactin owing to reduced prolactin-inhibiting factor secretion, and elevated levels of insulin-like growth factors (IGF) (COSTIN 1976; PANG 1993).

In the past, rare cases of operative death occurred from a clinical syndrome of hyperpyrexia, loss of thirst sensation, dyssomnia. This was attributed to direct injury to the thirst, thermoregulation, and circadian centers of the anterior hypothalamus (CARMEL 1996). With improvements in microneurosurgical techniques, this grave complication has been encountered with far less frequency. Hypothalamic syndromes are still encountered, however, but in more minor forms. Some degree of central hyperphagia and weight gain from injury to hypothalamic satiety centers is quite common 1–6 months after surgery. Such food-seeking behavior often requires strict behavioral modification, psychological counseling, and external support (PANG 1990). Abulia minor can also occur after trans-lamina terminalis resection via either subfrontal or pterional approaches. This unusual syndrome is characterized by a flattening of the affect, apathy, a reduction of spontaneous action and behavior, and psychomotor retardation (UNGERSTEDT 1971). Although not well established, abulia minor is thought to result from injury to the mesolimbic pathways projecting from the rostral midbrain to the medial septal nuclei, nucleus accumbens, cingulate gyrus, and other limbic structures (LEKSELL et al. 1967). Overall, neuropsychological disorders have been reported in anywhere from 30 to 60% of patients after surgery (CHOUX et al. 1991). Although patients can compensate for many of these problems over time, the long-term effect of these changes can continue to impact their quality of life for many years (FISCHER et al. 1990).

10.8.2
Outcome

The overall survival rate of craniopharyngiomas after satisfactory resection, as a group, has been estimated at approximately 90% at 10 years (CHOUX et al. 1991). As these tumors are not malignant at a cellular level, managing them is more an issue of local control and recurrence prevention than it is a problem of survival. The major long-term impact of craniopharyngiomas is due to the secondary effects of tumor growth and iatrogenic complications of surgery and radiation. As such, endocrine dysfunction, functional disability, and cognitive decline contribute the lion's share of the morbidity and mortality associated with these troublesome lesions.

The global risks and mortality associated with surgery have also varied widely among published series. For most contemporary reports, an estimated 1–2% mortality has been reported in the perioperative period (HOFFMAN et al. 1992; SHAPIRO et al. 1979; YASARGIL et al. 1990). Similarly, a 5–10% incidence of serious postoperative morbidity is generally quoted (CARMEL 1982; SWEET 1976). Some series have reported radical resection and minimal residual tumor volume with zero surgical mortality and little morbidity (HOFF and PATTERSON 1972; HOFFMAN et al. 1977; SWEET 1980). Much of these data are, however, difficult to interpret as many patients in these series had multiple operations for either residual tumor or recurrence.

The majority of neurosurgeons agree that total resection should be the starting goal for all craniopharyngiomas. The many obstacles which serve to limit surgical success make such a goal only achievable in 30–90% of cases (KATZ 1975; SHAPIRO et al. 1979; SYMON and SPRICH 1985). One of the problems complicating the outcome analysis of craniopharyngioma patients is how to decide what a "total" resection actually is. Whereas the majority of series base this decision on the judgment of the operative surgeon, the phenomenon of a "false-cure" is well documented. As there are many blind corners and numerous pseudopod extensions of the typical operative case, small pieces of residual tumor are frequently left behind in cases where the surgeon feels that a "complete" resection has been accomplished. Indeed,

almost every large series of craniopharyngiomas has reported a sizable number of early local recurrences after supposed total tumor removal. In a multi-series review of 92 total removals, AMACHER (1980) found over 17 cases of early recurrence at the surgical site. Although the use of endoscopes, operating microscopes, and even small micromirrors to look around such blind spots has helped to reduce this phenomenon, such overestimation on the surgeon's part continues to be problematic (CARMEL 1996, 1979). Thus, we advocate an early high-quality MRI gadolinium-enhanced image of the tumor bed within 24–48 h after surgery to gain a more accurate assessment of the degree of surgical resection.

When one speaks of long-term craniopharyngioma outcomes, it is usually in terms of local recurrence rates. The majority of recurrences after surgical resection of these lesions occur within 3–5 years after surgery (CARMEL 1996; SAMII and TATAGIBA 1997). In a long-term analysis by KATZ (1975) of many cases, he found a 25% recurrence rate anywhere from 4 to 19 years after total surgical resections. Since then, other authors have reported similar findings of 10–30% recurrence rates after complete extirpation (CARMEL 1982; HOFFMAN et al. 1977; SHAPIRO et al. 1979; SWEET 1976; YASARGIL et al. 1990). The survival for such patients has been estimated to be around 80–90% at 10 years (PANG 1990). When only a subtotal or incomplete excision has been achieved, the recurrence rate rises precipitously. CHOUX in his review of their institutions' experience found a 28% overall recurrence rate with a 19% rate in completely resected lesions and a 57% incidence of recurrence for subtotal resections (1991). Overall, adults (20%) had a lower recurrence rate than children (20%). From a review of several large series, a combined recurrence rate of 75% is estimated for patients having subtotal resection without adjuvant irradiation (CARMEL 1996; HOFFMAN et al. 1977; CABEZUDO et al. 1981; LICHTER et al. 1977). The 10-year survival for such patients was equally poor at around 25%. For patients with recurrence, most surgeons have advocated an attempt at re-resection. Such reoperations have a significantly decreased chance of affecting complete removal due to scarring and deformation of the normal anatomy. Additionally, they are associated with a higher incidence of morbidity and postoperative neuroendocrine and behavioral dysfunction.

With the addition of postoperative radiation for cases with subtotal resection, several centers have reported significantly improved survivals of up to 75 and 80% (TIBERIN et al.1958; SHAPIRO et al. 1979; MANAKA et al. 1985). Some long-term follow-up studies comparing combined modality treatment with subtotal surgery and radiation versus subtotal resection only have consistently demonstrated better survival rates for the first group (REGINE and KRAMER 1992). Because of this excellent 10-year survival rate with such a combined management, some surgeons have intentionally adopted a protocol of intentional subtotal resection followed by radiotherapy to decrease the incidence of postoperative neurological deficits and surgical complications (FISCHER et al. 1990). However, not all series utilizing such a combined modality have had such optimistic results. SUNG et al. (1981) in his analysis of 108 cases found only a 52% survival of subtotally resected adults at 10 years follow-up. The survival of children with partial resections was even worse at 31%. Although the desire to minimize postoperative morbidity from neurological and endocrine injury is understandable, we still attempt a complete surgical resection whenever possible at our institution. Many neurosurgeons, including ourselves, express deep concerns over the harmful effects of irradiating children and young adults (AMACHER 1980). Conventional external beam therapy has been associated with its own unique set of problems as well. Visual failure, hypopituitarism, organic brain syndromes, dementia, sensorimotor deficits, learning disabilities from frontal lobe changes, de novo malignant mesenchymal tumors, vasculopathy, and radiation necrosis have been seen with irradiation of craniopharyngiomas (KRAMER et al. 1968; SWEET 1980; BACKLUND 1980; MARTIN et al. 1977; HARRIS and LEVINE 1976; NISHIZAWA et al. 1991; CARMEL 1990). Furthermore, some long-term studies have demonstrated that irradiation after subtotal resection does not affect or delay tumor recurrence (HOFF et al. 1972). For these reasons, we continue to advocate gross or complete resection for tumors whenever it is safe to do so. For cases where total extirpation of the tumor is deemed too risky as it is adherent to vital structures or for patients who are too old or frail to undergo radical resection, subtotal resection combined with radiation is a completely reasonable alternative. Recent advances in stereotactic radiosurgery and continuing experience with intracavitary brachytherapy for cystic tumors have brought a new dimension to nonsurgical management of craniopharyngiomas. A detailed discussion of radiation therapy and other treatment modalities for craniopharyngiomas follows in Chap. 11 of this volume.

References

Adamson TE, Wiestler OD, Kleijues P, et al. (1990) Correlation of clinical and pathological features in surgically treated craniopharyngiomas. J Neurosurg 73:12–17

Alvarez-Garijo JA, Froufe A, Taboada D, Vila M (1981) Successful surgical treatment of an odontogenic ossified craniopharyngioma. Case report. J Neurosurg 55:832–835

Amacher AL (1980) Craniopharyngioma: the controversy regarding radiotherapy. Childs Brain 6:57–64

Antunes JL, Carmel PW, Zimmerman EA, Ferin M. Regeneration of the magnocellular system of the rhesus monkey following hypothalamic lesions. Ann Neurol 5:462–469

Apuzzo MLJ, Chikovani OK, Gott PS, et al. (1982) Transcallosal, interforniceal approaches for lesions affecting the third ventricle: surgical considerations and consequences. Neurosurgery 10:547–554

Artero JMC, Crespo SN. Status of vision following surgical treatment of craniopharyngiomas. Acta Neurochir (Wien) 73:165–177

Ayral D, Talot L, David M, Lecornu M, Francois R (1980) Etude de la croissance paradoxale de certains enfants apres chirurgie hypothalamo-hypophysaire en depit de l'absence d'hormone de croissance. Pediatrie 35:389–401

Backlund EO. (1980) Stereotactic treatment of craniopharyngiomas – 15 years experience. Presented at the 32nd Annual Meeting of the Scandinavian Neurosurgical Society; September 5, 1980; Linkoping, Sweden. Abstract

Banna M (1973) Craniopharyngioma in adults. Surg Neurol 1:202–204

Banna M, Hoare RD, Stanley P, Till K (1973) Craniopharyngioma in Children. J Pediatr 83:781–785

Barkovich AJ (1995) Craniopharyngiomas. Brain tumors of childhood. In Barkovich AJ, ed. Pediatric Neuroimaging, 2 ed. New York: Raven; pp. 381–386

Busch E (1944) New approach for the removal of tumors of third ventricle. Acta Pyschiatr 19:57–60

Cabezudo JM, Vaguero J, Areitia E, et al (1981) Craniopharyngiomas: a clinical approach to treatment. J Neurosurg 55:371–375

Carmel PW, Antunes JL, Ferrin M. (1979) Collection of blood from the pituitary stalk and portal veins in monkeys, and from the pituitary sinusoidal system of monkey and man. J Neurosurg 50:75–80

Carmel PW, Antunes JL, Change CH (1982) Craniopharyngiomas in children. Neurosurgery 11: 382–389

Carmel PW (1990) Brain tumors of disordered embryogenesis. In: Youmans JR (ed) Neurological Surgery, 3rd edn, vol.5., WB Saunders, Philadelphia, pp.3223–3249

Carmel PW (1996) Craniopharyngiomas. In Wilkins RR and Rengachary SA, eds.: Neurosurgery, 2nd edn, vol.1. New York, McGraw-Hill, pp. 905–916

Cavazzuti V, Fischer EG, welch H, Belli JA, Winston JR (1983) Neurological and psychological sequelae following different treatment of craniopharyngioma for children. J Neurosurg 59:409–417

Choux M (1991) Craniopharyngioma surgery: techniques, complications, and alternatives. Presented at the 59th Annual Meeting of the American Association of Neurological Surgeons. New Orleans, April 23

Choux M, Lena G, Genitori L (1991) Le craniopharyngiome de l'enfant. Neurochirurgie (Paris) 37 (suppl 1):12–165

Cobb JP, Wright JC (1959) Studies of craniopharyngioma in tissue culture. I. Growth characteristics and alterations produced following exposure to two radiometric agents. J Neuropath Exp Neurol 18:563–568

Costin G, Hogut MD, Philips LS, Daughaday WH. Craniopharyngioma: the rate of insulin in promoting postoperative growth. J Clin Endocrinol Metab 42:370–379

Derome P (1991) Opinions. In: Choux M, Lena G, Genitori L (eds) Le craniopharyngiome de l'enfant. Neurochirurgie (Paris) 37:167

Drazin MB, Sterlin MW, Johanson AJ (1980) Silver-Russel syndrome and craniopharyngioma. J Pediatr 96: 887–889

Einhaus SL, Sanford RA (1999) Craniopharyngiomas. In Albright L, Pollack I, Adelson D, eds. Principles and Practice of Pediatric neurosurgery. New York: Theime Medical Publishers, Inc.; pp.545–562

Erdheim J (1904) Ueber Hypophysengangsgeshwulste un Hirncholesteatome. Sitzungsber. Akad. Wiss (Wien), 113: 537–726

Fischer EG, Welch K, Shillito J, et al (1990) Craniopharyngiomas in children. Long-term effects of conservative surgical procedures combined with radiation therapy. J Neurosurg 73:534–540

Fujitsu K, Kuwabara T (1985) Zygomatic approach for lesions in the interpeduncular cistern. J Neurosurg 62:340–343

Fujitsu K, Saijo M, Aoki F, et al (1992) Cranio-nasal median splitting for radical resection of craniopharyngiomas. Neurol Res 14:345–351

Glass RH. Infertility. In: Yen SSC, Jaffe RB (eds). (1978) Reproductive endocrinology: Physiology, pathophysiology and clinical management. WB Saunders, Philadelphia,pp.398–417

Graham PH, Gattamaneni HR, Birch JM (1992) Paediatric craniopharyngiomas: A regional Review. Br J Neurosurg. 6:187–194

Hakuba A, Nishimura S, Inoue Y (1985) Transpetrosal-transtentorial approach and its application in the therapy of retrochiasmatic craniopharyngiomas. Surg Neurology 24:405–415

Hakuba A, Liu S, Nishimura S (1986) The orbitozygomatic infratemporal approach: A new surgical technique. Surg Neurol 26: 271–276

Halves E, Sorensen (1982) Indications for the trans-sphenoidal approach to craniopharyngioma operations in youth and childhood. In: Voth D, Gutjahr P, Langmaid C (eds) Tumors of the central nervous system in infancy and childhood. Springer, Berlin, pp.270–275

Hardy J, Vezina JL (1976) Transsphenoidal neurosurgery of intracranial neoplasm. Adv Neurol 15:261–274

Harris JR, Levine MB (1976) Visual complications following irradiation for pituitary adenomas and craniopharyngiomas. Radiology 120:167–171

Harrison MJ, Morgello S, Post KD (1994) Epithelial cystic lesions of the sellar and parasellar region: a continuum of ectodermal derivatives. J Neurosurg 80:1018–1025

HelmkeK, Hausdorf G, Moehrs D, Laas R (1984) CCT and sonographic findings in congenital craniopharyngioma. Neuroradiology 26: 523–526

Hetelekidis S, Barnes PD, Tao ML, et al (1993) 20-Year experience in childhood craniopharyngioma. Int J Rad Onc Biol Phys 27:189–195

Hoff JT, Patterson RH (1972) Craniopharyngiomas in children and adults. J Neuosurg 36:299–302.

Hoffman HJ, Hendrick EB, Humphreys RP, et al. (1977) Management of craniopharyngioma in children. J Neurosurg 47:218–227

Hoffman HJ, DeSilva M, Humphreys RP, et al. (1992) Aggressive surgical management of craniopharyngiomas in children. J Neurosurg 76:47–52

Honnegger J, Buchfelder M, Fahlbusch R, et al. (1992) Transsphenoidal microneursurgery for craniopharyngioma. Surg Neurology 37:189–196

Hua F, Asato R, Miki Y, et al. (1992) Differentiation of suprasellar nonneoplastic cysts from cystic neoplasms by Gd-DPTA MRI. J Comp Assist Tomo 16:744–749

Huk WJ, Gademann G, Friedmann G (1990) MRI of central nervous system diseases. Springer, Berlin, pp.268–270

Hurst RW, McLlhenny J, Park TS, Thomas WO (1988) Neonatal craniopharyngioma. CT and ultrasonographic features. J Comp Assis Tomo 12:858–861

Ingbar Sh (1987) Diseases of the thyroid. In: Braundwald E, Isselbacher KJ, Petersdorf RG, et al (eds) Harrison's Principles of internal medicine, 11th edn, vol 2. McGraw-Hill, New York, pp.1732–1752

Kahn EA, Crosby EC (1972) Korsakoff's syndrome associated with surgical lesions involving the mamillary bodies. Neurology 22:117–125

Katz EL (1975) Late results of radical excision of craniopharyngiomas in children. J Neurosurg 42:86–90

Kempe LG (1968) Operative Neurosurgery. Vol.1. New York, Springer-Verlag, pp.90–93

Koos WT, Miller MH (1971) Intracranial tumors of infants and children. Stuttgart, Thieme.

Kramer S, Southard M, Mansfield CM (1968) Radiotherapy in the management of craniopharyngiomas:further experiences and late results. Am J Roentgenol 103:44–52

Kubota T, Fuji H, Ikeda K, et al. (1980) A case of intraventricular craniopharyngioma with subarachnoid hemorrhage. No Shinkei Geka 8:495–501

Landolt AM (1972) Die Ultrastruktur des Kranio-pharyngeoms. Schweiz Arch Neurol Neurochir Psychiatr 111:313–329

Laws ER Jr (1980) Transsphenoidal microsurgery in the management of craniopharyngioma. J Neurosurg 52:661–666

Leksell L, Backlund EO, Johansson L (1967) Treatment of craniopharyngiomas. Acta Chir Scand 133:345–350

Levy ML, Khoo LT, Day JD, et al. (1997) Optimization of the operative corridor for the resection of craniopharyngiomas in children: the combined frontoorbitozygomatic temporopolar approach. Neurosurg Focus 3(6): Article 5

Lichter AS, Wara WM, Sheline GE, et al. (1977) The treatment of craniopharyngiomas. Int J Radiat Oncol Biol Phys 2:675–683

Liszczak T, Richardson EP Jr, Phillips JP, et al. (1978) Morphological, biochemical, ultrastructural, tissue culture and clinical observations of typical and aggressive craniopharyngiomas. Acta Neuropathologica (Berlin) 43:191–203

Maier HC (1985) Craniopharyngioma with erosion and drainage into the nasopharynx. An autobiographical case report. J Neurosurg 62:132–134

Manaka S, Teramoto A, Takakura K (1985) The efficacy of radiotherapy for craniopharyngiomas. J Neurosurg 62:648–656

Martin AM, Johnston JS, Henry JM, Stoffel TJ, Di Chiro G. (1977) Delayed radiation necrosis of brain. J Neurosurg 47:336–345

Matson DD and Crigler JF (1969) Management of craniopharyngiomas in childhood. J Neurosurg 30: 377–390

Miller DC (1994) Pathology of craniopharyngiomas: clinical import of pathological findings. Pediatr Neurosurg. 21(suppl 1):11–17

Naidich TP, Pinto RS, Kushner MJ, et al. (1976) Evaluation of sellar and parasellar masses by computed tomography. Radiology 120:91–99

Nishizawa S, Ryu H, Yokoyama T, et al. (1991) Post-irradiation vasculopathy of intracranial major arteries in children. Report of two cases. Neurol Med Chir (Tokyo) 31:336–41

Okamoto H, Harada K, Uozumi T, Goishi J (1985) Spontaneous rupture of a craniopharyngioma cyst. Surg Neurol 24:507–510

Olivercrona H (1967) The surgical treatment of intracranial tumors. In: Olivercrona H, Tonnis W (eds) Handbuch der Neurochirurgie. Springer-Verlag, Heidelberg, pp.1–301

Palm L, Nordin V, Elmqvist D, et al.(1992) Sleep and wakefulness after treatment for craniopharyngioma in childhood; influence on the quality and maturation of sleep. Neuropediatrics 23:39–45

Pang D (1990) Cranipharyngiomas. In: Deutsch M (ed) Management of Childhood Brain Tumors. Kluwer Publishers: Norwell, Mass; pp.285–307

Pang D (1993) Surgical management of craniopharyngioma. In: Sekhar LN, Janecka IP (eds) Surgery of cranial base tumors. Raven Press, New York., pp.787–807

Patterson RH, Danylevich A. (1980) Surgical removal of craniopharyngiomas by a transcranial approach through the lamina terminalis and sphenoid sinus. Neurosurgery 7:111–117

Podoshin L, Rolan L, Altman MM, et al. (1970) Pharyngeal craniopharyngioma. J Larynogol.Otol. 84: 93–99

Raybaud C, Rabehanta P, Girard N (1991) Aspects radiologiques des cranipharyngiomes. In: Choux M, Lena G, Genitori L (eds) Le craniopharyngiome de l'enfant. Neurochirurgie (Paris(37 (suppl 1):44–58

Regine WF, Kramer S (1992) Pediatric craniopharyngiomas: long-term results of combined treatment with surgery and radiation. Int J Radiat Oncol Biol Phys 24:611–617

Rougerie J, Fardeau M (1962) Les cranio-pharyngeomes. Masson, Paris, pp.1–217

Russell DS, Rubinestein LJ (1989) In: Bigner DD, McLendon R, Bruner JM (eds.), Pathology of tumors of the nervous system, 6th edn. Williams & Wilkins, Baltimore, pp.695–704

Sanford RA, Muhlbaur MS (1991) Craniopharyngioma in children. Neuro Clin 9(2):453–465

Samii M, Tatagiba M (1997) Craniopharyngioma. In: Kaye AH, Laws ER (eds) Brain Tumors- An Encyclopedic Approach. Churchill Livingstone, Edinburgh, pp.873–894

Samii M, Bini W (1991) Surgical management of craniopharyngiomas. Zentralblatt fur Neurochirurgie 52:17–23

Seemayer TA, Blundell JS, Wiglesworth FW (1972) Pituitary craniopharyngioma with tooth formation. Cancer 29:423–430

Shapiro K, Till K, Grant DN. (1979) Craniopharyngiomas in childhood: a rational approach to treatment. J Neurosurg 50:617–623

Shibuya M, Ito S, Miwa T, et al. (1993) Proliferative potential of brain tumors. Analyses with Ki-67 and anti-DNA polymerase alpha monoclonal antibodies, bromodeoxyuridine labeling, and nucleolar organizer region counts. Cancer 71:199–206

Shucart WA, Jackson I (1976) Management of diabetes insipidus in neurosurgical patients. J Neurosurg 44:65–70

Sklar CA. (1994) Craniopharyngioma:endocrine abnormalities at presentation. Pediatr Neurosurg 21 (suppl 1):18–20

Snyder JR, Lustig-Gillman I, Milio L, et al. (1986) Antenatal ultrasound diagnosis of an intracranial neoplasm (craniopharyngioma). J Clin Ultrasound 14:304–306

Streeten DHP, Moses AM, Miller M (1987) Disorders of the neurohypophysis. In: Braunwald E, Isselbacher KJ, Petersdorf RG, et al (eds) Harrison's Principles of Internal Medicine, 11th edn, vol 2. McGraw-Hill, New York, pp.1722–1732

Sung DI, Chang CH, Harisiadis L, et al. (1981) Treatment results of craniopharyngioma. Cancer 47: 847–852

Sweet WH (1976) Radical surgical treatment of craniopharyngioma. Clin Neurosurg 23:52–79

Sweet WH (1980) Recurrent craniopharyngiomas: therapeutic alternatives. Clin Neurosurg 27:206–229

Sweet WH (1988) Craniopharyngiomas (with a note on Rathke's cleft cysts). In Schmidek HH, ed. Operative Neurosurgical Techniques. Orlando, Grune & Stratton.

Sweet WH (1994) History of surgery for craniopharyngiomas. Pediatr Neurosurg 21(suppl 1):23–28

Symon L, Sprich W (1985) Radical excision of craniopharyngioma. Results in 20 patients. J Neurosurg 62:174–181

Szeifert GT, Julow J, Szabolcs M, et al. (1991) Secretory component of cystic craniopharyngiomas: A mucino-histochemical and electron-microscopic study. Surg Neurology 36:286–293.

Thapar K, Laws ER (1997) Pituitary Tumors. In: Brain Tumors. An Encyclopedic Approach. Churchill Livingstone, Edinburgh, pp.759–776

Thomsett MJ, Conte FA, Kaplan SL, et al. (1980) Endocrine and neurological outcome in childhood craniopharyngiomas. Review of effect of treatment in 42 patients. J Pediatr 97:728–735

Tiberin P, Goldberg GM, Schwartz A (1958) Craniopharyngiomas in the aged. Neurology 8:31–54

Tomita T (1988) Management of craniopharyngiomas in children. Pediatric Neuro 14:204–211

Ungerstedt U (1971) Stereotaxic mapping of the dopamine pathways in the rat brain. Acta Physiol Scand 367(suppl): 1–48

Vagner-Capodano AM, Gentet JC, Gambarelli D, et al. (1992) Cytogenetic studiies in 45 pediatric brain tumors. Ped Hem Onc 9(3):225–235

Van den Bergh R (1970) The transventricular approach in craniopharyngioma of the third ventricle: neurosurgical and neuropathological aspects. Neurochirurgie 16:51–65

Van Efferente R, van Efferente G, Cabanis EA, et al. (1991) Tumeurs suprasellaires chez les sujets ages de plus de 70 ans. Interet d'une craniectomie fronto-temporale limitee. Resultats visuels. A propos de 5 cas. Neurochirurgie 37:330–337

Vargas JR, Pino JA, Murad TM (1981) Craniopharyngiomas in two siblings. JAMA 16:1807–1808.

Wakai S, Arai T, Nagai M (1984) Congenital brain tumor. Surg Neurol 21:597–609

Wald SL, Liwnicz BH, Truman TA, Khobadad G (1982) Familial primary nervous system neoplasms in three generations. Neurosurgery 11:12–15

Weiner HL, Wisoff JH, Rosenberg ME, et al. (1994) Craniopharyngiomas: a clinicopathological analysis of factors predictive of recurrence and functional outcome. Neurosurg 35(6):1001–1011

Wen DY, Seljeskog EL, Haines SJ (1992) Microsurgical management of craniopharyngioma. Br J Neurosurg 6:467–474

Yasargil MG (1984) Microneurosurgery. Volume 1. Microsurgical Anatomy of the Basal Cisterns and Vessels of the Brain, Diagnostic Studies, General Operative Techniques and Pathological Considerations of the Intracranial Aneurysms. Stuttgart: Georg Thieme, pp.215–233

Yasargil MG, Curcic MC, Kis M, et al (1990) Total removal of craniopharyngiomas. Approaches and long-term-results in 144 patients. J Neurosurg 73:3–1

Zülch KJ (1986) Brain tumors. Their biology and pathology, 3rd edn. Springer, New York, pp.426–433

Zumkeller W, Saaf M, Rahn T, Hall K (1991) Demonstration of insulin-like growth factors I, II and heterogeneous insulin-like growth factor binding proteins in the cyst fluid of patients with craniopharyngiomas. Neuroendocrinology 54:196–201

11 Radiation Therapy for Craniopharyngioma

Michael Selch

CONTENTS

11.1
Introduction

The craniopharyngioma is a histologically benign parasellar tumor that can occur at any age. There is no known etiology for craniopharyngioma although tumor growth during the course of successive pregnancies has been reported (AYDIN et al. 1999). The tumor generally follows a protracted course, but patients with rapid evolution have been described (BARTLET 1971; SCOTT et al. 1995; ARGINTEANU et al. 1997). The clinical presentation is dominated by endocrine and visual disturbances. Complete removal is often difficult due to proximity of the lesion to critical central nervous system structures. The role of radiation therapy for this unusual tumor remains controversial. This chapter will discuss the results of external beam irradiation, stereotactic radiosurgery, and radioisotope instillation for craniopharyngioma.

M. SELCH, MD
Professor of Radiation Oncology, University of California Los Angeles, 200 Medical Plaza, Suite B265, Los Angeles, CA 90095, USA

11.2
Embryology

The embryologic derivation of craniopharyngioma has been the subject of much investigation. In embryonic development, the anterior lobe of the pituitary gland is formed by union of the infundibular pouch of the central nervous system with the stomodeal pouch (INGRAHAM and SCOTT 1946). The stomodeal pouch is a diverticulum of the embryonic buccal cavity and has been eponymously termed "Rathke's pouch". The stomodeal pouch is composed of squamous epithelium of ectodermal origin. As the anlage of the anterior hypophysis, persistent squamous cell rests of the involuted Rathke's pouch can be found at necropsy in the absence of craniopharyngioma (INGRAHAM and SCOTT 1946). These squamous cell rests are typically located on the anterior surface of the adenohypophysis and the infundibulum. The neoplastic cells of craniopharyngioma are, in turn, derived from proliferation of vestigial remnants of Rathke's pouch within the sella or above the diaphragma sella (GHATAK et al. 1971).

The complex embryogenesis of craniopharyngioma has resulted in a number of synonyms for this tumor. The following are among the more frequently encountered terms in the literature: suprasellar cyst, interpeduncular cyst, craniobuccal cyst, suprasellar epithelioma, Rathke's pouch tumor, hypophyseal duct tumor, craniopharyngeal duct tumor, and pituitary adamantinoma. The term craniostomodeal cyst reflects more accurately the embryogenesis of craniopharyngioma since the tumor is derived from embryonic buccal epithelium rather than pharyngeal epithelium (INGRAHAM and SCOTT 1946).

11.3
Histology

The craniopharyngioma is composed of anastomosing trabeculae of epithelial cells associated with an epithelial lined cyst (GHATAK et al. 1971; PETITO et al. 1976). The epithelial cells resemble closely the squamous components of skin (GHATAK et al. 1971). The neoplastic cells are embedded in a loose, fibrous connective tissue stroma and are arranged in one of two distinctive patterns (PETITO et al. 1976; GIANSPERO et al. 1984; ADAMSON et al. 1990; CROTTY et al. 1995). The most common appearance is the adamantinomatous variant. In this form, tumor tissue recapitulates the fetal tooth bud and resembles the adamantinoma/ameloblastoma arising in the jaw of adults. The tumor is composed of solid nests of uniform epithelial cells surrounded by a single layer of palisading cells, a loose stellate reticulum, and discrete keratin nodules (KAHN et al. 1973; GHATAK et al. 1971; CROTTY et al. 1995). This variant is virtually always cystic and calcified. It can occur in adults or children. A less common variant is termed papillary squamous (ADAMSON et al. 1990; WEINER et al. 1994; CROTTY et al. 1995). The tumor is composed of non-palisading, mature stratified squamous epithelium without keratin nodules. This variant occurs almost exclusively in adults and rarely calcifies. Cyst formation occurs in approximately one-half of papillary squamous variants (CROTTY et al. 1995). A small biopsy of this variant could be mistaken for a Rathke's cyst. Transitional forms demonstrating features of both variants have been reported (PETITO et al. 1976; WEINER et al. 1994; CROTTY et al. 1995). WEINER and associates have described the histologic appearance of 56 craniopharyngiomas (WEINER et al. 1994). Among adults, 66% demonstrated adamantinomatous features, 28% were papillary squamous, and 6% were mixed. Among the pediatric patients, 96% were adamantinomatous and 4% were mixed. Calcification was noted in 95% of the adamantinomatous or mixed tumors compared to one of eight papillary squamous lesions.

Carcinomatous features are rarely reported at diagnosis of craniopharyngioma. One or more mitotic figures have been reported in 7% of adamantinomatous tumors compared to 25% of papillary squamous lesions (WEINER et al. 1994). The presence of mitotic figures alone is not sufficient for designating a craniopharyngioma malignant. Malignant histology appears restricted to the adamantinomatous variant (INGRAHAM and SCOTT 1946). Malignant degeneration has been reported 8 years following radiation therapy for a benign craniopharyngioma (NELSON et al. 1988). The recurrent tumor displayed the usual constellation of findings observed in frankly malignant neoplasms: nuclear pleomorphism, atypical nuclei, mitoses, and necrosis. The malignant region of the recurrent tumor blended with areas of typical benign craniopharyngioma.

The cyst wall of craniopharyngioma is composed of epithelial cells varying from a single layer to stratified squamous (KOBAYASHI et al. 1981). A variable amount of cyst stroma correlates directly with the size of the cyst. The cyst is filled with an oily liquid composed of desquamated, liquefied epithelial cells and cholesterol crystals. Rupture of the cyst results in aseptic ventriculitis or meningitis.

11.4
Microscopic Anatomy

The microstructure of craniopharyngioma is of importance to radiation oncologists. The tumor is typically circumscribed; however, nests or islands of isolated epithelial cells can be identified in surrounding connective tissue. The phenomenon of finger-like projections of epithelial cells was recognized as early as 1939 and gives the impression of invasive tumor (SWEET 1976; STENO 1985; NELSON et al. 1988). The nests of tumor cells, nevertheless, retain the benign histologic features of the parent tumor. These neoplastic extensions are more common with the adamantinomatous than the papillary squamous variant (PETITO et al. 1976; ADAMSON et al. 1990). Brain invasion has been noted in 37% of adamantinomatous tumors compared to 13% of papillary squamous lesions (WEINER et al. 1994). The solid portion of tumor is more likely to display tumor islands than is the cystic component. Accurate quantification of the extent of tumor projections has not been performed but appears limited to a few millimeters at most (BARTLET 1971; KOBAYASHI et al. 1981; HOFFMAN et al. 1977).

Neoplastic cell extensions of craniopharyngioma evoke a variable gliotic reaction (GHATAK et al. 1971; SWEET 1976; BRUCE et al. 1981; STENO 1985). Reactive glial tissue is composed of fibrillary astrocytes and Rosenthal fibers (GHATAK et al. 1971). Glial reactive tissue is more typical of rapidly progressive than indolent craniopharyngioma and more typical of the solid portion of tumor than the cystic component (BARTLET 1971). Gliotic reactive tissue was noted in 65% of adamantinomatous tumor compared to 50% of papillary squamous lesions (WEINER et al. 1994). Gliosis can extend from several hundred microns to several millimeters and directly adhere to surrounding tissue (GHATAK et al. 1971). In a series of 75 craniopharyngiomas, dense adhesions of tumor to the hypothalamus were noted in 14, major vessels in 12, and to both structures in 3 (DE VILE et al. 1996). Several authors have stated that craniopharyngiomas lack a true capsule and there is no obvious cleavage plane between the reactive gliosis and the surrounding brain tissue (BRUCE et al. 1981; YASARGIL et al. 1990). Others argue just as strongly that reactive gliosis is easily dissected from normal brain tissue and represents a surgical margin of safety (SWEET 1976; HOFFMAN et al. 1977; WEINER et al. 1994). No difference has been found in the rate of gross total resection between adamantinomatous and papillary variants despite their varying incidences of apparent brain invasion (WEINER et al. 1994).

11.5
Clinical Presentation

Craniopharyngioma can arise in children or adults. In combined series of patients, median age varies from 19 to 37 years of age (MANAKA et al. 1985; BASKIN and WILSON 1986; RAJAN et al. 1993; FAHLBUSCH et al. 1999) There are two reported age peaks for this tumor. The earlier occurs in the first two decades of life and the later between the fifth and sixth decades (SUNG et al. 1981; FAHLBUSCH et al. 1999). Median age in strictly pediatric series varies from 7 to 9 years, compared to 48 years for adult patients (HOFFMAN et al. 1992; HETELEKIDIS et al. 1993; WEINER et al. 1994; KHAFAGA et al. 1998). A case occurring at 82 years of age has been reported (LEDERMAN et al. 1987).

The embryogenesis of craniopharyngioma determines the location of tumor. Purely infradiaphragmatic/intrasellar tumors are rare. In a combined experience with 92 children, tumor was confined to the sella in four cases (THOMSETT et al. 1980; HOFFMAN et al. 1992). More commonly, the tumor is partially or entirely suprasellar (YASARGIL et al. 1990). Supradiaphragmatic craniopharyngioma can extend in either a prechiasmatic direction and protrude between the optic nerves or in a retrochiasmatic direction, filling the third ventricle. Despite suprasellar growth, extension of craniopharyngioma through the optic foramen is unusual. These two types of extension occur with equal frequency (HOFFMAN et al. 1992).

Craniopharyngioma is frequently cystic. In a series of 245 cases from the Air Force Institute of Pathology (AFIP), exclusively or predominantly cystic tumors occurred in 70% (PETITO et al. 1976). Predominantly solid or mixed cystic-solid tumors each occurred in 15% of cases. In a series of 148 patients from the University of Erlangen, 10% of tumors were entirely solid and 28% predominantly solid, while the remainder were exclusively or predominantly cystic (FAHLBUSCH et al. 1999). In several smaller series, purely solid tumors were noted in 2–24% of patients (WEN et al. 1989; MARK et al. 1995; HABRAND et al. 1999). A cystic component is particularly common in pediatric patients. Cyst formation was noted in 34 of 36 children evaluated with CT scan (HETELEKIDIS et al. 1993).

Radiographic calcification of the solid tumor component occurs in approximately 80% of pediatric patients and 30–40% of adults (THOMSETT et al. 1980; CARMEL et al. 1982; HOOGENHOUT et al. 1984; WEN et al. 1989; HETELEKIDIS et al. 1993; FAHLBUSCH et al. 1999). If histologic examination is included, reported rates of calcification for children and adults are 90% and 50%, respectively (LEDDY and MARSHALL 1951; SUNG et al. 1981; HETELEKIDIS et al. 1993). Calcification is usually particulate but may be extensive and, occasionally, bone-like.

Tumor size is variable. Although typically a median of 3–4 cm, craniopharyngiomas ranging from 1 to 11 cm have been reported (WEISS et al. 1989). Uncontrolled tumor can extend into the cerebral hemispheres, brain stem, hypothalamus, and caudate (GROVER and RORKE 1968). Tumors 3 cm or larger have been reported in 91% of children compared to 60% of adults (WEN et al. 1989). Tumor volume was recorded in a series of 51 patients by DE VILE et al. (1996). Tumors less than 50 cm^3 occurred in 57% of the group, 50–100 cm^3 in 14%, and larger than 100 cm^3 in 29% (DE VILE et al. 1996).

The signs and symptoms of craniopharyngioma are related to tumor location and pattern of extension. In a 25-year experience with pediatric lesions, HABRAND et al. (1999) noted endocrinopathy in 78%, visual disturbance in 62%, and other neurologic alteration in 73%. Endocrine disorders in this experience included growth retardation (49%), panhypopituitarism (22%), diabetes insipidus (22%), obesity (8%), and precocious puberty (3%). Visual disturbances included abnormal fields (30%), oculomotor palsy (16%), amblyopia (11%), and unilateral blindness (5%). Neurologic alterations included hydrocephalus (62%), psychiatric disorder (8%), other cranial neuropathy (8%), motor dysfunction (5%), and seizure(3%). Endocrinopathy has been reported in15–80% of children and 13–76% of adults (SUNG et al. 1981; CARMEL et al. 1982; HOOGENHOUT et al. 1984; WEISS et al. 1989; WEINER et al. 1994). Visual disturbance occurs in 35–95% of children compared with 60–88% of adults (SUNG et al. 1981; CARMEL et al. 1982; HOOGENHOUT et al. 1984; WEISS et al. 1989; WEINER et al. 1994). The majority of patients present with multiple signs and symptoms. Patients are symptomatic for 4–14 months prior to diagnosis (HOFF and PATTERSON 1972; THOMPSON et al. 1978; THOMSETT et al. 1980; SUNG et al. 1981; CARMEL et al. 1982). Duration of symptoms is longer in adults than children.

11.6
History of Radiation Therapy

The role of radiotherapy for craniopharyngioma has been debated for decades. Many investigators initially concluded that the tumor was refractory to irradiation (Leddy and Marshall 1951). Early experiences were compromised by inferior imaging technology and low-energy photon beam equipment. The unavoidable outcome was delivery of inadequate dose and failure to encompass the tumor within treatment portals. Lack of appreciation of the slow radiation response of benign tumors also contributed to therapeutic nihilism. Although the craniopharyngioma could be assumed to be radioresistant based upon histologic appearance, some authors demonstrated reduction in cyst fluid reaccumulation and prevention of solid tumor progression (Carpenter et al. 1937; Ingraham and Scott 1946; Kerr 1948; Leddy and Marshall 1951). These observations indicated radiotherapy was not entirely fruitless for craniopharyngioma. Carpenter and coworkers, in fact, concluded as early as 1937 that the results of cyst aspiration plus radiation therapy were superior to attempted total removal (Carpenter et al. 1937). Prior treatment planning and dose delivery limitations are now no more relevant to the role of radiotherapy for craniopharyngioma than the historic risks of postoperative edema and hypopituitarism are to the role of modern neurosurgery.

Simon Kramer and associates at Thomas Jefferson University were the first to publish the systematic use of high dose, continuous course, megavoltage therapy in conjunction with minimal surgery for craniopharyngioma (KRAMER et al. 1961). Their initial patients received either paired 180 arcs with a 90 separation or a 360 rotation field. Air contrast studies were used to design circular fields. Pediatric patients received 5500 cGy and adults 7000 cGy using cobalt-60 beam. In the authors' first report, all six children and two of four adults were free of progression after a minimum of 6 years follow-up. One adult required aspiration of an enlarging cyst and was considered a treatment failure. One other adult died of an unrelated cause, free of progressive tumor. An update of this series with 8 more years of follow-up revealed all children still free of progressive tumor (KRAMER et al. 1968). Two further adults had died of unrelated illnesses with no evidence of recurrent craniopharyngioma. In their update, KRAMER et al. (1968) added the results of 16 additional patients. This second group received a single 220 coronal arc. The authors stressed that the center of arc rotation for this approach must be placed eccentrically ("past pointing") to ensure tumor dose homogeneity. Four of six children were free of recurrence. Two relapsed within 3 years of treatment, apparently with progressive solid component. Seven of ten adults were free of relapse 1.5–11 years after irradiation. Two died of unrelated causes and were free of identifiable tumor at autopsy. Histopathologic complete response of craniopharyngioma to radiotherapy has since been confirmed by other authors (WEISS and RASKIND 1969; ONOYAMA et al. 1977; AMACHER 1980). One adult relapsed but it is unclear whether there was cyst enlargement or growth of the solid component.

The Thomas Jefferson University group recently published the results for all 19 children irradiated at this center (REGINE and KRAMER 1992). After a median follow-up of 21 years, 13 patients remain free of recurrent tumor. Five patients (26%) relapsed 2.2–17.5 years after radiotherapy. Four of these succumbed to recurrent tumor and another died of an in-field malignant glioma. Several factors were found to influence survival or recurrence. Twelve children were irradiated immediately after their initial surgery; 10- and 20-year survival rates in this group were 82% and 80%, respectively. The remaining children were treated for recurrent tumor a median of 16 months after initial surgery; 10- and 20-year survival rates in this group were 60% and 25%, respectively. Despite this survival difference, the local relapse rates following immediate and delayed radiotherapy were 25% and 29%, respectively. Three of 6 recurred after receiving 5400 cGy or less compared to 2 (15%) of 13 receiving higher doses. One (14%) of 7 treated in the CT era relapsed compared to 4 (33%) of 12 irradiated in an earlier era.

11.7
Radiation Therapy

The experience of KRAMER and coworkers documented the beneficial role of modern radiotherapy for craniopharyngioma. (KRAMER et al. 1968). Subsequent reports from multiple centers serve to confirm these pioneering efforts. Table 11.1 enumerates the long-term relapse-free survival rates for patients irradiated after a variety of incomplete surgical interventions (CABEZUDO et al. 1981; CARMEL et al. 1982; FLICKINGER et al. 1990; RAJAN et al. 1993; HETELEKIDIS et al. 1993; MARK et al. 1995; KHAFAGA et al. 1998; HABRAND et al. 1999). Five-year relapse-free rates vary from 78% to 96%. Ten-year rates vary from 41% to 95%. RAJAN et al. (1993) reported 79% 20-year relapse-free survival in a series of 173 pa-

tients, the largest available radiotherapy experience. The results in series with uniform use of CT are, in general, superior to those with sporadic use of CT or those from the pre-CT era. Table 11.2 displays results from series utilizing crude local relapse as a therapeutic end point (ONOYAMA et al. 1977; THOMPSON et al. 1978; SHAPIRO et al. 1979; THOMSETT et al. 1980; SUNG et al. 1981; CALVO et al. 1983; DANOFF et al. 1983; BASKIN and WILSON 1986; WEN et al. 1989; WEISS et al. 1989; FISCHER et al. 1990; HOFFMAN et al. 1992; HOOGENHOUT et al. 1984). Only the series of WEISS et al. (1989) utilized routine CT scanning. The overall local failure in this group of 323 patients was 18%. In an earlier literature review, local relapse was recorded in 42 of 138 (30%) patients (AMACHER 1980). Finally, Table 11.3 lists overall survival rates following radiation therapy for craniopharyngioma

Table 11.1. Progression-free survival rates following radiotherapy for craniopharyngioma

Series	Patients	Age	Progression-free period(%)		
			5-year	10-year	20-year
SUNG et al. 1981	32	A, P	78 (P)	78 (P)	–
	–	–	82 (A)	41 (A)	–
CABEZUDO et al. 1981	22	A, P	–	94	–
CARMEL et al. 1982	14	P	78	78	–
FLICKINGER et al. 1990	21	A, P	95	95	–
RAJAN et al. 1993	173	A, P	–	83	79
HETELEKIDIS et al. 1993	37	P	–	86	–
KHAFAGA et al. 1990	19	P	–	62	–
MARK et al. 1995	25	A, P	96	–	–
HABRAND et al. 1990	32	P	78	56	–

A, adult; P, pediatric.

Table 11.2. Local recurrence following radiotherapy for craniopharyngioma

Series	Patients	Age	Follow-up	Recurrence
THOMPSON et al. 1978	11	A, P	5 years median	3
CALVO et al. 1983	18	A, P	2–12 years	0
DANOFF et al. 1983	19	P	8 years median	3
HOOGENHOUT et al. 1984	13	A, P	2–22 years	3
SHAPIRO et al. 1979	29	P	–	11
WEN et al. 1989	27	A, P	1–28 years	7
HOFFMAN et al. 1977	18	A, P	2–14 years	5
WEISS and RASKIND 1969	13	P	5 years median	1
FISCHER et al. 1990	27	A, P	10 years minimum	1
BASKIN and WILSON 1986	67	A, P	–	6
ONOYAMA et al. 1977	32	A, P	–	7
THOMSETT et al. 1980	17	A, P	6–192 months	3
SUNG et al. 1981	32	P	–	8
	323	–	–	58 (18%)

A, adult; P, pediatric.

Table 11.3. Survival rates following radiotherapy for craniopharyngioma

Series	Patients	Age	Survival rates (%) 5-year	10-year	20-year
RICHMOND et al. 1980	12 (STR)	A, P	100	88	–
	8 (Bx)	A, P	88	57	–
MANAKA et al. 1985	34	A, P	91	81	–
CARMEL et al. 1982	14	P	90	80	–
ONOYAMA et al. 1977	32	A, P	69	60	–
FLICKINGER et al. 1990	21	A, P	89	89	–
RAJAN et al. 1993	173	A, P	–	77	66
MARK et al. 1995	25	A, P	96	96	–
HABRAND et al. 1999	32	P	91	65	–

A, adult; P, pediatric; STR, subtotal resection; Bx; biopsy.

(ONOYAMA et al. 1977; RICHMOND et al. 1980; CARMEL et al. 1982; MANAKA et al. 1985; FLICKINGER et al. 1990; RAJAN et al. 1993; MARK et al. 1995; HABRAND et al. 1999). SHAPIRO et al. (1979) cautioned that "overall survival is inadequate as an index of therapeutic efficacy" since recurrent craniopharyngioma may be amenable to salvage therapy and compatible with prolonged survival. Reported 5-year survival rates vary form 69% to 100% and 10-year survival rates range from 57% to 96%. In the large series of RAJAN et al. (1997), 22 (13%) patients died of recurrent craniopharyngioma while 24 (14%) succumbed to unrelated causes.

11.7.1
Prognostic Factors

A number of factors have been analyzed for their potential impact on outcome following radiation therapy for craniopharyngioma. Small patient numbers and the lack of stratified clinical trials hamper analysis of putative prognostic factors. Survival of pediatric or young adult patients is superior to that of more elderly patients according to some authors (ONOYAMA et al. 1977; DANOFF et al. 1983; WEN et al. 1989) but not others (RICHMOND et al. 1980; MANAKA et al. 1985). RAJAN et al. (1993), using multivariate analysis, found overall survival significantly better for patients less than 40 years of age. This same group, however, reported no independent impact of age on relapse-free survival. WEN and co-workers demonstrated a significant influence of timing of radiotherapy (WEN et al. 1989). The local control rate for patients irradiated after initial surgery was 90%. If radiotherapy was administered after first or second relapse, control rates were 69% and 33%, respectively. ONOYAMA et al. (1977) reported superior overall survival for patients irradiated after first operation compared to treatment after reoperation. The survival difference between these groups was lost after 7 years of follow-up. Many other investigators report no influence of radiotherapy timing on relapse-free survival (THOMPSON et al. 1978; WEISS et al. 1989). Patients undergoing aspiration prior to radiotherapy had superior survival compared to those undergoing partial resection in a series of 19 patients (DANOFF et al. 1983). Several groups, on the other hand, report superior outcome in patients partially resected compared to those merely aspirated prior to irradiation (SHAPIRO et al. 1979; HOFFMAN et al. 1992). The majority of reports, including the multivariate analysis of RAJAN et al. (1993), document no prognostic influence of extent of incomplete surgery when radiotherapy is employed (MANAKA et al. 1985; FLICKINGER et al. 1990). Predominantly cystic lesions demonstrate superior survival or relapse-free survival in some reports (SHAPIRO et al. 1979; DANOFF et al. 1983). Other series document no significant impact of tumor morphology on outcome (RICHMOND et al. 1980; WEN et al. 1989; MANAKA et al. 1985). In primary surgical series, a higher relapse rate has been demonstrated for the adamantinomatous variant (KAHN et al. 1973; ADAMSON et al. 1990). Histologic subtype of craniopharyngioma does not influence prognosis in series utilizing radiotherapy (MANAKA et al. 1985; CROTTY et al. 1995). Female gender has been associated with improved survival in one report (ONOYAMA et al. 1977). There is no influence of gender in all other series analyzing this factor (WEN et al. 1989; MANAKA et al. 1985; RAJAN et al. 1993; HABRAND et al. 1999). Tumor calcification, sellar enlargement, increased intracranial pressure, and diabetes insipidus are not prognostic in radiotherapy series (WEN et al. 1989; MANAKA et al. 1985; RAJAN et al. 1993).

11.7.2
Radiation Therapy Technique

A variety of radiotherapy techniques have been utilized for craniopharyngioma. Portal arrangement, traditionally coplanar, includes opposed lateral fields, multiple static fields and arc rotations. There is no impact of portal arrangement on local control rate (WEN et al. 1989). Field size is related to tumor dimension and has varied from 4+4 to 11+12 cm in the literature. Several groups found no relation between field size and local relapse (FLICKINGER et al. 1990; HABRAND et al. 1999). There is no impact, furthermore, of tumor size in series employing routine postoperative radiotherapy (MANAKA et al. 1985). HETELEKIDIS and associates reported a significantly higher local failure rate for tumors larger than 4 cm compared to smaller tumors (HETELEKIDIS et al. 1993). Not all patients in that series, however, received radiotherapy. Few institutions discuss the margin of normal tissue included within the radiotherapy volume. A margin of 2 cm around the tumor volume is typically employed in the CT era (MARK et al. 1995; HABRAND et al. 1999). Regardless of field size or normal tissue margins, relapse outside the field of treatment is extraordinarily uncommon for craniopharyngioma. Relapse in the epidural space 20 years after surgery and radiotherapy has been reported (MALIK et al. 1992). The rarity of failure outside the radiotherapy field implies that a margin of several centimeters provides adequate irradiation of microscopic tumor extensions, eliminating the risk of marginal recurrence. The minimum effective margin has not been determined. Insufficient treatment volume may permit growth of microscopic tumor nests. Marginal recurrence due to inadequate tumor delineation in the pre-CT era has been reported (HOOGENHOUT et al. 1984). SUNG and coworkers reported two relapses in the third ventricle but do not comment on use of CT (SUNG et al. 1981). HETELEKIDIS and associates reported a frontal lobe relapse in a patient with attempted total resection (HETELEKIDIS et al. 1993). Cyst expansion, furthermore, is possible during radiotherapy (vide infra). Provision of an inadequate margin may result in underdosage of part of an enlarging cyst.

The use of modern neuroimaging studies is essential for accurate planning of radiotherapy fields. Although all relapses were in-field in the experience of HABRAND et al. (1999), the authors demonstrated a significant impact of CT scanning on outcome. The 10-year event-free survival of patients treated in the CT era was 54% compared to 20% for those from an earlier era. The development of "conformal" techniques now permits definition of tumor and normal anatomy in three dimensions using slice-by-slice CT image data. One millimeter axial slices throughout the target volume are recommended (HABRAND et al. 1999). Using this technique, the high-dose region can be better conformed to the tumor volume, thus reducing unnecessary normal tissue irradiation. An increased number of beams, including non-coplanar fields, may be possible using three-dimensional conformal radiotherapy treatment planning (PURDY 1999).

Investigators at Columbia Presbyterian Hospital reported an apparent dose–response relationship for craniopharyngioma (SUNG et al. 1981). Local relapse occurred in 47% of patients receiving less than 5000 cGy. The rate of recurrence following 5500–5750 cGy and 6000 cGy or greater was 16% and 20%, respectively. Relapse in the highest dose group was outside of the radiotherapy field. HABRAND and colleagues reported a 10-year event-free survival rate of 65% for those receiving at least 5500 cGy compared to 45% following lower doses (HABRAND et al. 1999). Other authors, however, demonstrate no impact of dose over the range of 5000–7000 cGy on outcome (ONOYAMA et al. 1977; WEN et al. 1989; FLICKINGER et al. 1990; HETELEKIDIS et al. 1993). The minimum effective dose for craniopharyngioma has not been determined. Several authors report local relapse if less than 4000 cGy is utilized (CABEZUDO et al. 1981; HOFF and PATTERSON 1972). Given the available data, a total dose of 5000–5500 cGy is reasonable for either pediatric or adult craniopharyngioma.

The impact of beam quality is uncertain. RAJAN and associates reported a significantly better survival and a trend toward superior relapse-free survival for patients irradiated with 6 MV photons compared to 2 MV photons (RAJAN et al. 1993). The authors pointed out that the use of higher energy photons corresponded with the more frequent utilization of modern neuroimaging for diagnosis and treatment of craniopharyngioma.

11.7.3
Treatment Failure

The interval from completion of radiotherapy to documented relapse varies from several months to as long as 15 years (HETELEKIDIS et al. 1993). The typical median time to progression is 12–24 months (RAJAN et al. 1993; THOMSETT et al. 1980). Many investigators, however, fail to define the criteria for radiotherapy relapse. Others require imaging evidence of enlargement of the solid or cystic component of tumor. CABEZUDO et al. (1981) defined failure of therapy as any recurrence of symptoms. It must be stressed that symptomatic deterioration or cyst enlargement following radiation therapy does not necessarily represent true tumor relapse. RAJAN and coworkers reported an acute deterioration, manifested as worsening symptoms, in 26 of 188 (14%) irradiated patients (RAJAN et al. 1997). Two patients deteriorated prior to instituting radiation therapy, 17 deteriorated during treatment, and 7 within 2 months of completing irradiation. Symptomatic deterioration was associated with cyst enlargement in 16 and hydrocephalus in 6 patients. Eighteen patients underwent surgical intervention including aspiration and/or shunting. All 18 recovered and their long-term survival was equivalent to irradiated patients without acute deterioration. Six (75%) of the eight patients that did not undergo surgical intervention died within 3 months of deterioration. The authors found no patient, tumor, or treatment factors that were predictive of acute deterioration. BASKIN et al. (1986) described three patients recurring within 8 months of radiotherapy but provided no further details (BASKIN and WILSON 1986). Despite being categorized by the authors as treatment failures, these patients were successfully managed by repeated aspirations through an Ommaya reservoir "until radiotherapy took effect". Finally, CONSTINE and associates reported two patients with cyst enlargement within 5 months of radiotherapy (CONSTINE et al. 1989). There was progressive cyst shrinkage thereafter without surgical intervention.

These findings indicate that cyst expansion, particularly if the onset is during or shortly after radiotherapy, does not necessarily represent failure of treatment. Cyst expansion is a manifestation of the inherently slow response of benign cells to ionizing irradiation. Cyst fluid accumulation may continue despite the damage done by radiation therapy to the reproductive capacity of craniopharyngioma cells.

11.8
Morbidity of Conventional Radiation Therapy

Serious long-term morbidity due to radiation therapy is unusual following treatment for craniopharyngioma. Several groups report no new visual or endocrine dysfunction with follow-up periods ranging from 2 to 12 years (THOMPSON et al. 1978; RICHMOND et al. 1980; CALVO et al. 1983; HOOGENHOUT et al. 1984). DANOFF and colleagues reported two patients with new endocrinopathy but these were ascribed to the effects of local recurrence or hydrocephalus (DANOFF et al. 1983). Serious morbidity following radiotherapy is largely a function of dose. Blindness has been reported only following doses in excess of 6100 cGy or following treatment with phosphorus-32 for cyst enlargement after external irradiation (FLICKINGER et al. 1990; MARK et al. 1995). The Thomas Jefferson University group reported nine children with endocrinopathy after irradiation (REGINE and KRAMER 1992). Endocrine dysfunction occurred in 4 of 5 (80%) patients receiving more than 6100 cGy compared to 5 of 14 (36%) children treated with lower doses. Investigators at the University of Pittsburgh reported a significantly higher rate of any serious complication (endocrine plus visual deficit) among patients receiving more than 6000 cGy compared to lower doses (FLICKINGER et al. 1990).

Several groups have attempted to compare functional outcome of patients undergoing surgery alone with those undergoing minimal surgery and radiotherapy. CAVAZUTTI and colleagues, in particular, analyzed multiple end points in a series of 17 radically resected patients and 18 undergoing minimal surgical intervention followed by radiotherapy (CAVAZUTTI et al. 1983). Visual performance and sorting test scores were significantly worse in the radically resected group. Profound dyslexia occurred only among the radically resected group. The authors also demonstrated a greater incidence of visual deficits and oculomotor palsies among the resected patients. Anosmia occurred in 12 (71%) resected patients compared to none of the irradiated patients. Measures of IQ, word fluency, manual dexterity, and memory were equivalent between the groups. Other series document the favorable outcome of irradiated patients. Several authors have reported that irradiated children demonstrate no significant difference in school performance or incidence of psychosocial problems compared to those patients managed with surgery alone (HOOGENHOUT et al. 1984; FISCHER et al. 1990). THOMSETT and coworkers reported a good neurologic performance score in 70% of irradiated patients compared to 57% following radical resection (THOMSETT et al. 1980). The reported incidence of new diabetes insipidus following radiation therapy varies from 22% to 38% compared to 70% to 100% following attempted total resection (HETELEKIDIS et al. 1993; RICHMOND et al. 1980; CALVO et al. 1983).

Malignant brain tumors arising within the fields of radiotherapy have been reported in seven patients with craniopharyngioma (Sogg et al. 1978; Maat-Schieman et al. 1985; Liwnicz et al. 1985; Fischer et al. 1990; Regine and Kramer 1992; Hetelekidis et al. 1993; Habrand et al. 1999). The latency from irradiation to diagnosis of a second brain tumor varies from 8 to 25 years. Radiotherapy dose for the primary treatment of craniopharyngioma has varied from 5760 to 6000 cGy. Brada et al. (1992) reviewed experiences with 334 pituitary tumors receiving 4500 cGy. Treatment of this tumor represents a useful model for the induction of second brain tumors following therapy for craniopharyngiomas. After a minimum follow-up of 6 years, five in-field neoplasms were documented. The relative risk of a brain tumor compared to the non-irradiated population was 9.4. The actuarial 10- and 20-year risks of a radiation-associated neoplasm were 1.3% and 1.9%. Although the absolute risk of an induced brain tumor is low, the potential for this complication should be kept in mind when recommending conventional irradiation for children with craniopharyngioma.

Radiation necrosis within the treatment volume has been reported on several occasions (Kramer et al. 1968; Martins et al. 1977; Flickinger et al. 1990; Habrand et al. 1999). Although Habrand and associates reported a case following 5500 cGy, all other cases in the literature followed doses in excess of 6880 cGy. Other unusual late effects of radiotherapy for craniopharyngioma include moya-moya syndrome, neurovascular insufficiency, and deafness (Regine and Kramer et al. 1992; Hetelekidis et al. 1993; Hoogenhout et al. 1993).

11.9
Integration of Resection and Radiotherapy

There is no role for radiation therapy following gross total removal of craniopharyngioma confirmed by modern imaging studies (see Chap. 10 of this volume). Several authors report 5-year relapse-free survival rates of 87% to 89% following gross total resection confirmed by CT scan (De Vile et al. 1996; Fahlbusch et al. 1999). Ten-year relapse-free rates vary from 79% to 81% in these same reports. Patients thought to have complete tumor removal by intraoperative assessment consistently demonstrate residual tumor or presence of calcification upon postoperative imaging (Carmel et al. 1982; Weiss et al.

1989; Hetelekidis et al. 1993; De Vile et al. 1996; Fahlbusch et al. 1999). Even a scant amount of residual calcification has been associated with eventual tumor regrowth. Weiss and colleagues reported 18 patients thought to have undergone gross total resection (Weiss et al. 1989). There were two (14%) recurrences among the 14 patients who had no evidence of residual tumor on postoperative CT scan. Four (29%) patients had evidence of persistent tumor on CT scan and tumor recurred in all of these. Conventional radiographs are insufficiently sensitive for evaluation of degree of resection. In the pre-CT era, relapse was distressingly frequent following apparent gross total removal. Amacher reviewed the literature prior to 1980 and reported relapse following unconfirmed total resection in 17 (19%) of 92 patients (Amacher 1980). Subsequently, Sung and associates reported 5- and 10-year progression-free survival rates of 77% and 47%, respectively, for pediatric patients undergoing unconfirmed total resection (Sung et al. 1981). Relapse-free rates for adult patients at similar postoperative intervals were 37% and 16%. Overall relapse rates of 23–50% are reported from other centers relying upon intraoperative impression of surgical completeness or sporadic CT scanning (Richmond et al. 1980; Carmel et al. 1982; Calvo et al. 1983; Wen et al. 1989; Mark et al. 1995). Significant factors limiting resection include: tumor size, hydrocephalus, tumor extension to the third ventricle, and extensive calcification (De Vile et al. 1996; Fahlbusch et al. 1999). Patients with these factors should be strongly considered for adjunctive radiotherapy if they have undergone unconfirmed "total resection".

Partial resection is associated with high relapse rates. In Amacher's review, 83 out of 111 patients recurred following partial resection (Amacher 1980). Sung et al. (1981) reported 5- and 10-year progression-free survival rates of 14% and 7% for partially resected pediatric patients. Progression-free rates for adults were 10% at each period. Multiple authors have since documented relapse rates of 47–100% following incomplete resection alone for craniopharyngioma (Shapiro et al. 1979; Thomset et al. 1980; Carmel et al. 1982; Calvo et al. 1983; Manaka et al. 1985; Wen et al. 1989; Hoffman et al. 1992; Khafaga et al. 1998). The mean time to relapse following partial surgery varies from 12 to 30 months, considerably shorter than after unconfirmed gross total removal. Weiss et al. (1989) demonstrated a significantly better relapse-free survival for patients treated with radiotherapy after partial resection compared with those patients managed with surgery alone who had evidence of postoperative residual disease, including those with apparent total removal but positive postoperative CT scan. There was no difference in outcome following subtotal removal plus radiotherapy compared to CT-confirmed total resection.

11.10
Stereotactic Radiosurgery and Radiotherapy

Stereotactic radiosurgery (SRS) involves delivery of a large dose of ionizing irradiation in a single fraction to an intracranial target (see Chaps. 6 and 19 of this volume). The technique depends upon precise target definition using the principles of stereotaxis. SRS can be delivered by a multisource cobalt-60 unit (gamma knife) or modified linear accelerator. Linear accelerator SRS requires precise isocentric rotation of the treatment couch and the source gantry. Dose deposition by any SRS approach is characterized by a steep gradient, thus protecting normal tissue. A full discussion of the technique and technology of SRS is beyond the scope of this chapter. The reader is referred to several reviews of the concepts and results of SRS (LOEFFLER and ALEXANDER 1990; FLICKINGER et al. 1994).

Investigators at the Karolinska Institute were the first to report the use of the gamma knife for craniopharyngioma. The solid portion of the tumor was irradiated, in the belief that this component was the substrate for cyst fluid production (BACKLUND 1973). Early gamma knife collimators were rectangular and of limited aperture. As a result, craniopharyngiomas less than 2 cm in diameter were selected for treatment and frequently multiple isocenters were required to irradiate the target. The first patient received an isocenter dose of 2000 cGy and recurred within 4 months. Histopathologic analysis revealed extensive central tumor disruption but also a thin rim of surviving peripheral cells corresponding to the fall-off dose of 100–200 cGy. Later patients received an isocenter dose of 5000 cGy to ensure a minimum peripheral dose of at least 300 cGy (BACKLUND 1974, 1979).

Japanese investigators reported results of SRS for 10 patients in a more recent gamma knife series (KOBAYASHI et al. 1994). These patients received a mean of six isocenters with a dose defined to the 50% isodose line encompassing the solid portion of the lesion. The mean maximum and minimum doses

were 2760 and 1430 cGy, respectively. After mean follow-up of 14 months, seven (70%) tumors responded and three (30%) were stable but demonstrated loss of central contrast enhancement on MRI scan. Tumor reduction was noted over 15 months. Loss of enhancement on MRI, thought to represent tumor necrosis, had an onset 9 months following SRS. One patient experienced visual deterioration and one had worsening of hypopituitarism after SRS. Both patients, however, received SRS for recurrent tumors after prior therapy, including 6000 cGy conventional radiotherapy in one patient.

The major limitation of SRS for craniopharyngioma is proximity of the tumor to the optic chiasm. The radiation tolerance of the central nervous system is a strong function not only of total dose but also of dose per fraction. The tolerance of the chiasm to SRS is estimated to be 800 cGy (TISCHLER et al. 1994). Given this single fraction tolerance, craniopharyngiomas suitable for SRS are those not closer than 3–5 mm to the chiasm.

Several authors state that the tolerance of the chiasm to fractionated radiotherapy is 5000 cGy if dose per fraction is no more than 200 cGy (HARRIS and LEVENE 1976; PARSONS et al. 1983). The fractionated dose tolerated by the chiasm is within the range reported effective for craniopharyngiomas. Fractionated stereotactic radiotherapy (SRT) is a recent innovation that utilizes the steep dose gradient characteristic of SRS and exploits the biologic advantages of dose fractionation. Development of SRT has been aided by the introduction of noninvasive, relocatable stereotactic head frames for targeting and immobilization (GILL et al. 1991; KOOY et al. 1994). These frames are applicable to pediatric patients.

Investigators at the Harvard Joint Center for Radiation Therapy published the only SRT experience for craniopharyngioma (TARBELL et al. 1994, 1995). The authors irradiated 21 patients, 13 (62%) with tumor recurrent after prior surgery. SRT was delivered with circular collimators at least 27.5 mm in diameter using multiple non-coplanar arcs directed about a single isocenter. The authors encompassed the target within the 90–95% isodose contour, but do not comment on the margin of normal tissue included within the treatment volume or if both solid and cystic components were irradiated. Time–dose considerations were similar to conventional radiotherapeutic techniques: 5040–5400 cGy in 28–30 fractions of 180 cGy each. All patients were free of progression after a 15-month median follow-up. Given the relapse interval following conventional radiotherapy cited above, these results must be considered preliminary. One patient experienced acute headache and visual deterioration during SRT. Cyst enlargement was documented and the patient finished SRT without further incident after aspiration. Two other patients demonstrated cyst enlargement within 8 months of SRT. Cysts decreased in both patients without specific intervention. These data, once again, indicate that cyst enlargement after radiotherapy does not indicate inevitable treatment failure.

A further refinement of SRT involves shaping the spherical dose distribution produced by circular collimators through the use of a minimultileaf collimator (Novalis). This innovation (BrainLab, Heimstetten, Germany) permits tailoring of the SRT dose to spherical tumors. Beam-shaping results in less normal tissue irradiated than does use of a single large circular collimator. This technique also results in superior target dose homogeneity compared to the use of multiple isocenters. At the University of California, Los Angeles, virtually all patients with craniopharyngioma receive SRT with shaped fields unless they are unable to tolerate frame relocation. Treatment planning utilizes CT–MR image fusion. The target volume includes the solid and cystic components. The treatment volume includes the target plus a margin of 5–10 mm of apparently normal tissue (Fig. 11.1). The aim of treatment planning is to encompass the treatment volume within the 90% isodose contour. The treatment volume receives 4500–5040 cGy using 180 cGy fractions. The total dose and/or fraction size is altered if the chiasm receives more than 200 cGy per day or a total dose of more than 5000 cGy.

11.11
Radioisotope Instillation

Intracystic brachytherapy using a beta-emitting colloidal radioisotope is a third method for treating craniopharyngioma. Radioisotope instillation delivers a high dose of irradiation to the cyst wall resulting in destruction of the epithelial lining and reduction in fluid formation. Intracystic brachytherapy is not an effective method for treatment of the solid component of tumor given the short range of the beta particle. As a result, radioisotope therapy is advocated for predominantly cystic craniopharyngiomas. Radioisotopes in common use are yttrium-90 in Europe and phosphorus-32 in the United States (Pollock et al. 1995). These isotopes are pure beta

emitters. Yttrium-90 has a 2.7-day half-life, a maximum particle energy of 2.27 MeV, and a half-value layer in tissue of 1.1 mm. Phosphorus-32 has a 14.2-day half-life, a maximum energy of 1.71 MeV, and a tissue half-value depth of 0.8 mm. Other isotopes that have been used include gold-198 and rhenium-186. Both of these isotopes, however, emit a gamma ray photon. Commercial rhenium-186, in addition, converts to a water soluble compound that may distribute systemically. Since introduction of radioisotope instillation by Leksell in 1952, most investigators deliver a minimum of 15,000 cGy to the cyst wall (Leksell et al. 1967). The activity required to administer this dose depends directly upon the volume of the cyst. Methods to calculate this volume began with air contrast radiography but now rely on the radioisotope dilution approach or CT/MR. Studies demonstrate that these methods are comparable (Strauss et al. 1982). Puncture of the cyst for instillation is performed with stereotactic guidance. Multicystic tumors must have separate volume calculations and individual instillation punctures unless intercystic communications are demonstrated. MR scan is ideal for detecting these communications. Backlund (1994) and coworkers cautioned that altering the cyst volume during instillation of the isotope could render dosimetry calculations inaccurate (Backlund 1972a,b). Isotope leakage following instillation can be detected by scintigraphy. Leakage rates following instillation of yttrium-90 vary from 10% to 20% (Van den Berge et al. 1992; Voges et al. 1997). Negligible leakage occurs after phosphorus-32 therapy (Lunsford et al. 1995). Yttrium-90 activity measured in the cerebrospinal fluid varies from 0.005% to 0.025% of the total instilled activity (Van den Berge et al. 1992). No activity within the bloodstream is detected following instillation of yttrium-90 or phosphorus-32. Huk and Mahlstedt (1983) described an indwelling radioisotope delivery system to eliminate any risk of leakage.

Intracystic radioisotope instillation is successful in arresting cyst progression. The majority of cysts respond to brachytherapy, but the extent of response is debated. Voges et al. (1997) reported response in 55 (83%) of 66 cysts treated with yttrium-90. Response was complete in 32 and partial in 23 cases. Pollock et al. (1995) reported response in 28 (87%) of 32 cysts treated with phosphorus-32. Complete response occurred in only three (11%) patients and there was no significant impact of dose over the range of 20,000–30,000 cGy on response rate. There is no difference in response rate if brachytherapy is administered as primary therapy compared to deliv-

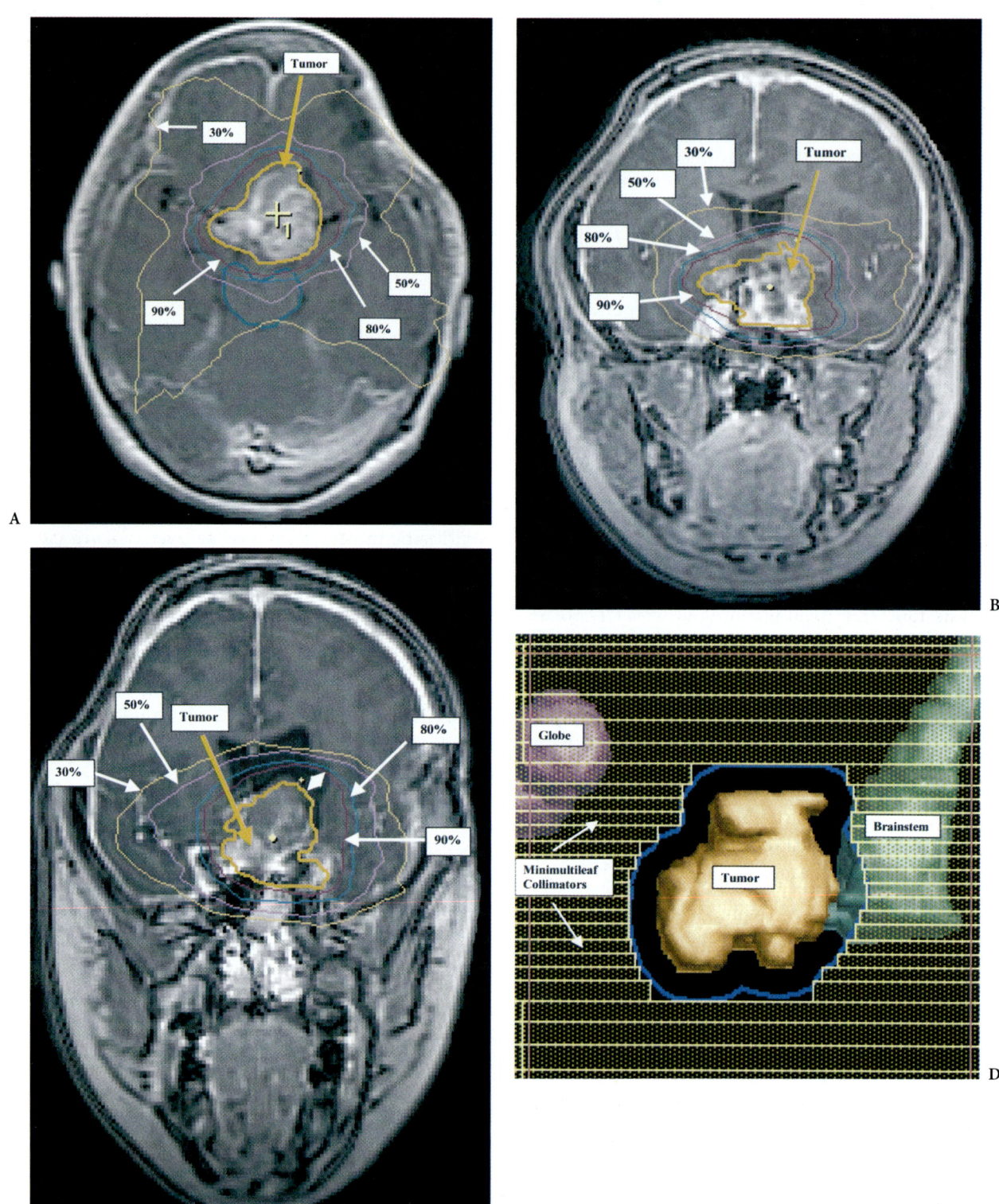

Fig. 11.1. A Axial MR displaying craniopharyngioma in an 8-year-old boy. The patient was treated with nine individually shaped, static, non-coplanar beams and a single isocenter. The patient received a total of 4500 cGy using 180 cGy fractions prescribed to the 90% isodose line. The maximum tumor dose was 5000 cGy. The 95% isodose line included the optic chiasm and this structure received 4750 cGy. **B** Coronal MR of the same patient. **C** Coronal MR displaying isodose lines and margin around the cystic component of tumor (*double arrowhead*). **D** Beam's-eye-view of one of nine shaped radiosurgery beams produced by the Novalis system

ery after documented relapse. Complete histologic response of cysts to brachytherapy has been documented (SZEIFERT et al. 1990). No adhesions can be demonstrated between the irradiated cyst and surrounding tissue (BACKLUND 1994). Approximately 10–20% of cysts are stable following brachytherapy. Cyst progression rates following radioisotope instillation vary from 0 to 10%. Patients with cyst progression after instillation may have prolonged progression-free survival after a single aspiration (POLLOCK et al. 1995). The beneficial effects of brachytherapy on cyst dynamics are delayed. Cyst reduction occurs several months after treatment and response continues for as long as 2 years (STRAUSS et al. 1992; POLLOCK et al. 1995). Cyst aspiration for control of symptoms present prior to instillation may also be necessary due to the delay in radiotherapy effects (POLLOCK et al. 1995). Aspiration following brachytherapy, particularly with yttrium-90, is safe for medical personnel since 95% of the planned dose is delivered within the first five isotope half-lives. Aspiration is rarely required if the cyst volume is less than 10 cm^3 (POLLOCK et al. 1995). Formation of new cysts following successful brachytherapy has been reported (VOGES et al. 1997; POLLOCK et al. 1995). Many authors, furthermore, note progression of the solid component of craniopharyngioma following radioisotope therapy for mixed tumors (VAN DEN BERGE et al. 1992; POLLOCK et al. 1995). Survival following intracystic brachytherapy is related to tumor size and morphology. Mean and long-term survival are better for patients with monocystic tumors compared to those with multicystic or mixed cystic-solid lesions (VOGES et al. 1997). Tumors larger than 30 cm^3 or multicystic tumors are associated with a higher mortality rate (VAN DEN BERGE et al. 1992).

Radioisotope therapy is not free of morbidity. VAN DEN BERGE et al. (1992) evaluated 64 eyes following yttrium-90 therapy. A decline in visual acuity was noted in 37 eyes, 14 of which were rated serious. A restriction of visual fields occurred in 33 eyes, 29 of which were rated serious. Visual deterioration occurred despite frequent cyst reduction. The authors stated that solid tumor growth and new cyst formation could explain some of the visual decline following brachytherapy. Visual decline has been reported in 11 (37%) of 30 patients treated with phosphorus-32 (POLLOCK et al. 1995). Two of these patients were thought to have optic neuropathy. Visual deterioration in the remainder could be ascribed to solid tumor growth, new cyst formation, or cyst progression. VOGES et al. (1997) reported new diabetes insipidus in three patients receiving yttrium-90. Two of these,

however, had received prior treatment with this isotope. Endocrine and visual morbidity following radioisotope instillation appears related to cyst wall doses in excess of 50,000 cGy (POLLACK et al. 1988).

11.12 Conclusions

Craniopharyngioma can serve as a model for the combined modality therapy for central nervous system tumors. Following cyst decompression, conventional external beam radiation therapy represents effective adjunctive treatment for patients with craniopharyngioma. A total dose of 5000–5500 cGy delivered to the cystic and solid components of tumor results in tumor control and quality of life equivalent to radical surgical extirpation. Development of image-based treatment planning systems should permit irradiation of craniopharyngioma with reduced normal tissue exposure. In centers with expertise in stereotaxis, fractionated stereotactic radiotherapy and radioisotope instillation represent useful therapy for managing craniopharyngioma.

References

Adamson TE, Wiestler OD, Kleihues P, et al. (1990) Correlation of clinical and pathologic features in surgically treated craniopharyngioma. J Neurosurg 73: 12–17

Amacher AL (1980) Craniopharyngioma: The controversy regarding radiotherapy. Child's Brain 6: 57–64

Argineteanu MS, Hague K, Zimmerman R, et al. (1997) Craniopharyngioma arising de novo in middle age. J Neurosurg 86: 1048–1056

Aydin Y, Can M, Gulkilik A, et al. (1999) Rapid enlargement and recurrence of a preexisting intrasellar craniopharyngioma during the course of two pregnancies. J Neurosurg 91: 322–324

Backlund EO (1972a) Studies on craniopharyngiomas I. Treatment: past and present. Acta Chir Scand 138: 743–747

Backlund EO (1972b) Studies on craniopharyngiomas II. Treatment by stereotaxis and radiosurgery. Acta Chir Scand 138: 749–759

Backlund EO (1973) Studies on craniopharyngiomas IV. Stereotaxic treatment with radiosurgery. Acta Chir Scand 139: 344–351

Backlund EO (1974) Stereotaxic treatment of craniopharyngiomas. Acta Neurochir (Suppl) 21: 177–183

Backlund EO (1979) Solid craniopharyngiomas treated by stereotactic radiosurgery In: Szikla G (ed) Stereotactic cerebral irradiation. INSERM symposium no. 12, Elsevier, North Holland Biomedical Press, pp 271–281

Backlund EO (1994) Treatment of craniopharyngioma: the multimodality approach Pediatr Neurosurg 21: 82–89

Baskin DS, Wilson CB (1986) Surgical management of craniopharyngiomas. J Neurosurg 65: 22–27

Bartlet JR (1971) Craniopharyngiomas: an analysis of some aspects of symptomatology, radiology and histology. Brain 94: 725–732

Brada M, Ford D, Ashley S, et al. (1992) Risk of second brain tumor after conservative surgery and radiotherapy for pituitary adenoma. British Med J 204: 1343–1346

Bruce DA, Schut L, Rorke LB (1981) Craniopharyngioma in a capsule? Concepts in Ped Neurosurgery 1: 29–35

Cabezudo JM, Vaquero J, Areitio E, et al. (1981) Craniopharyngiomas: a critical approach to treatment. J Neurosurg 55: 371–375

Calvo FA, Hornedo J, Arellano A, et al. (1983) Radiation therapy for craniopharyngiomas. Int J Radiat Oncol Biol Phys 9: 493–496

Carmel PW, Antunes J, Chang CH (1982) Craniopharyngiomas in children. Neurosurgery 11: 382–389

Carpenter RC, Chamberlain GC, Frazier CH (1937) The treatment of hypophyseal stalk tumors by evacuation and irradiation. Am J Roentgenol 38: 162–177

Cavazutti V, Fischer EG, Welch K, et al. (1983) Neurological and psychological sequelae following different treatments of craniopharyngioma in children. J Neurosurg 59: 409–417

Constine LS, Randall SH, Rubin P, et al. (1989) Craniopharyngiomas: fluctuation in cyst size following surgery and radiation therapy. Neurosurgery 24: 53–59

Crotty TB, Scheithauer BW, Young WF, et al. (1995) Papillary craniopharyngioma: a clinicopathological study of 48 cases . J Neurosurg 83: 206–214

Danoff BF, Cowchock FS, Kramer S (1983) Childhood craniopharyngioma: survival, local control, endocrine and neurologic function following radiotherapy. Int J Radiat Oncol Biol Phys 9: 171–175

De Vile CJ, Grant DB, Kendall BE, et al. (1996) Management of childhood craniopharyngioma: can the morbidity of radical surgery be predicted? J Neurosurg 85: 73–81

Fahlbusch R, Honegger J, Paulus W, et al. (1999) Surgical treatment of craniopharyngiomas: experience with 168 patients. J Neurosurg 90: 237–250

Fischer EG, Welch K, Shillito J, et al. (1990) Craniopharyngiomas in children. Long term effects of conservative surgical procedures combined with radiation therapy. J Neurosurg 73: 534–540

Flickinger JC, Lunsford LD, Singer J, et al. (1990) Megavoltage external beam irradiation of craniopharyngiomas: analysis of tumor control and morbidity. Int J Radiat Oncol Biol Phys 19: 117–122

Flickinger JC, Loeffler JS, Larson DA (1994) Stereotactic radiosurgery for intracranial malignancies. Oncology 8: 81–98

Ghatak NR, Hirano A, Zimmerman HM (1971) Ultrastructure of a craniopharyngioma. Cancer 27: 1465–1475

Gianspero F, Burger PC, Osborne, et al. (1984) Suprasellar papillary squamous epithelioma ("papillary craniopharyngioma"). Am J Surg Pathol 8: 57–64

Gill SS, Thomas DGT, Warrington AP, et al. (1991) Relocatable frame for stereotactic external beam radiotherapy. Int J Radiat Oncol Biol Phys 20: 599–603

Grover WD, Rorke LB (1968) Invasive craniopharyngioma. J Neurol Neurosurg Psychiat 31: 580–582

Habrand JL, Ganry O, Couanet D, et al. (1999) The role of radiation therapy in the management of craniopharyngioma: a 25-year experience and review of the literature. Int J Radiat Oncol Biol Phys 44: 255–263

Harris JR, Levene MB (1976) Visual complications following irradiation for pituitary adenomas and craniopharyngiomas. Radiology 120: 167–171

Hetelekidis S, Barnes PD, Tao ML, et al. (1993) 20-year experience in childhood craniopharyngioma. Int J Radiat Oncol Biol Phys 27: 189–195

Hoff JT, Patterson RH (1972) Craniopharyngiomas in children and adults. J Neurosurg 36: 299–302

Hoffman HJ, Hendrick EB, Humphreys RP, et al. (1977) Management of craniopharyngioma in children. J Neurosurg 47: 218–227

Hoffman HJ, De Silva M, Humphreys RP, et al. (1992) Aggressive surgical management of craniopharyngiomas in children. J Neurosurg 76: 47–52

Hoogenhout J, Otten BJ, Kazem I, et al. (1984) Surgery and radiation therapy in the management of craniopharyngiomas. Int J Radiat Oncol Biol Phys 10: 2293–2297

Huk WJ, Mahlstedt J (1983) Intracystic radiotherapy (^{90}Y) of craniopharyngiomas: CT-guided stereotaxic implantation of indwelling drainage system. Am J Neuroradiol 4: 803–806

Ingraham FD, Scott HW (1946) Craniopharyngiomas in children. J Pediatr 29: 95–116

Kahn EA, Gosch HH, Seeger JF, et al. (1973) Forty-five years experience with the craniopharyngioma. Surg Neurol 1: 5–12

Kerr HD (1948) Irradiation of pituitary tumors. Am J Roentgenol 60: 348–355

Khafaga Y, Jenkin D, kanaan I, et al. (1998) Craniopharyngioma in children. Int J Radiat Oncol Biol Phys 42: 601–606

Kobayashi T, Kageyama N, Yoshida J, et al. (1981) Pathological and clinical basis of the indications for treatment of craniopharyngiomas. Neurol Med Chir (Tokyo) 21: 39–47

Kobayashi T, Tanaka T, Kida Y (1994) Stereotactic gamma radiosurgery of craniopharyngiomas. Pediatr Neurosurg 21 :69–74

Kramer S, McKissock W, Concannon JP (1961) Craniopharyngioma: treatment by combined surgery and radiation therapy. J Neurosurg 18: 217–226

Kramer S, Southard M, Mansfield CM (1968) Radiotherapy in the management of craniopharyngiomas. Am J Roentgenol 103: 44–52

Lederman GS, Recht A, Loeffler JS, et al. (1987) Craniopharyngioma in an elderly patient. Cancer: 1077–1080

Leddy ET, Marshall TM (1951) Roentgen therapy of pituitary adamantinomas. Radiology 56:384–393

Leksell L, Backlund EO, Johansson L (1967) Treatment of craniopharyngiomas. Acta Chir Scand 133: 345–350

Liwnicz BH, Berger TS, Liwnicz RG, et al. (1985) Radiation-associated gliomas: a report of four cases and an analysis of postradiation tumors of the central nervous system. Neurosurgery 17: 436–445

Loeffler JS, Alexander E (1990) The role of stereotactic radiosurgery in the management of intracranial tumors. Oncology 4: 21–37

Lunsford LD, Pollock BE, Kondziolka DS, et al. (1994) Stereotactic options in the management of craniopharyngioma. Pediatr Neurosurg 21: 90–97

Maat-Schieman MLC, Bots GTAM, Thomeer RTWM, et al. (1985) Malignant astrocytoma following radiotherapy for craniopharyngioma. Brit J Radiology 58: 480–482

Malik JM, Cosgove GR, VandenBerg SR (1992) Remote recurrence of craniopharyngioma in the epidural space. J Neurosurg 77: 804–807

Manaka S, Teramoto A, Takakura K (1985) The efficacy of radiotherapy for craniopharyngioma. J Neurosurg 62: 648–656

Mark RJ, Lutge WR, Shimizu KT, et al. (1995) Craniopharyngioma: treatment in the CT and MR imaging era. Radiology 197: 195–198

Martins AN, Johnston JS, Henry JM, et al. (1977) Delayed radiation necrosis of the brain. J Neurosurg 47: 336–345

Nelson GA, Bastian FO, Schlitt M, et al. (1988) Malignant transformation in craniopharyngioma. Neurosurgery 22: 427–429

Onoyama Y, Ono K, Yabamuto E, et al. (1977) Radiation therapy of craniopharyngioma. Radiology 125: 799–803

Parsons JT, Fitzgerald CR, Hood IC, et al. (1983) The effects of irradiation on the eye and optic nerve. Int J Radiat Oncol Biol Phys 9: 609–622

Petito CK, DeGirolami U, Earle KM (1976) Craniopharyngioma: a clinical and pathological review. Cancer 37: 1944–1952

Pollack IF, Lunsford LD, Slamovits TL, et al. (1988) Stereotaxic intracavitary irradiation for cystic craniopharyngiomas. J Neurosurg 68: 227–233

<referePollock BE, Lunsford LD, Kondziolka D, et al. (1995) Phosphorus-32 intracavitary irradiation of cystic craniopharyngiomas: current technique and long-term results. Int J Radiat Oncol Biol Phys 33: 437–446

Purdy JA (1999) 3-D treatment planning and intensity-modulated radiation therapy. Oncology 13: 155–168

Rajan B, Ashley S, Gorman CC, et al. (1993) Craniopharyngioma – long-term results following limited surgery and radiotherapy. Radiother Oncology 26: 1–10

Rajan B, Ashley S, Thomas DGT, et al. (1997) Craniopharyngioma: improving outcome by early recognition and treatment of acute complications. Int J Radiat Oncol Biol Phys 37: 517–521

Regine WF, Kramer S (1992) Pediatric craniopharyngiomas: long term results of combined treatment with surgery and radiation complications. Int J Radiat Oncol Biol Phys 24: 611–617

Richmond IL, Wara WM, Wilson CB (1980) Role of radiation therapy in the management of craniopharyngiomas in children. Neurosurgery 6: 513–517

Shapiro K, Till K, Grant DN (1979) Craniopharyngiomas in childhood. J Neurosurg 50: 617–623

Sogg RL, Donaldson SS, Yorke CH (1978) Malignant astrocytoma following radiotherapy of a craniopharyngioma. Case report. J Neurosurg 48: 622–627

Strauss L, Sturm V, Georgi P, et al. (1982) Radioisotope therapy of cystic craniopharyngiomas. Int J Radiat Oncol Biol Phys 8: 1581–1585

Steno J (1985) Microsurgical topography of craniopharyngioma. Acta Neurochir 35: 94–100

Sung DI, Chang CH, Harisiadis L, et al. (1981) Treatment results of craniopharyngioma. Cancer 47: 847–852

Sweet WH (1976) Radical surgical treatment of craniopharyngioma. Clin Neurosurg 23: 52–79

Szeifert GT, Julow F, Balint K, et al. (1990) Pathological changes in cystic craniopharyngiomas following intracavital ^{90}yttrium treatment. Acta Neurochir 102: 14–18

Tarbell NJ, Barnes P, Scott RM, et al. (1994) Advances in radiation therapy for craniopharyngiomas. Pediatr Neurosurg 21: 101–107

Tarbell NJ, Scott RM, Goumnerova LC, et al. (1995) Craniopharyngioma: preliminary results of stereotactic radiation therapy. In: Kondiolzka D (ed) Radiosurgery, Karger, Basel, pp 75–82

Tischler RB, Loeffler JS, Lunsford LD, et al. (1994) Tolerance of the cranial nerves of the cavernous sinus to radiosurgery. Int J Radiat Oncol Biol Phys 27: 215–221

Thompson IL, Griffin TW, Parker RG, et al. (1978) Craniopharyngioma: the role of radiation therapy. Int J Radiat Oncol Biol Phys 4: 1059–1063

Thomsett MJ, Conte FA, Kaplan SL (1980) Endocrine and neurologic outcome in childhood craniopharyngiomas: review of effect of treatment in 42 patients. J Pediatr 97: 728–735

Van Den Berge JH, Blaauw G, Breeman WAP, et al. (1992) Intracavitary brachytherapy of cystic craniopharyngiomas. J Neurosurg 77: 545–550

Voges J, Sturm V, Lehrke R, et al. (1997) Cystic craniopharyngioma: long-term results after intracavitary irradiation with stereotactically applied colloidal b-emitting radioactive sources. Neurosurgery 40: 263–270

Wen BC, Hussey DH, Staples J, et al. (1989) A comparison of the roles of surgery and radiation therapy in the management of craniopharyngiomas. Int J Radiat Oncol Biol Phys 16: 17–24

Weiner HL, Wisoff JH, Rosenberg ME, et al. (1994) Craniopharyngiomas: a clinicopathological analysis of factors predictive of recurrence and functional outcome. Neurosurgery 35: 1001–1011

Weiss SR, Raskind R (1969) Non-neoplastic intrasellar cysts. Int Surgery 51: 282–288

Weiss M, Sutton L, Marcial V (1989) The role of radiation therapy in the management of childhood craniopharyngioma. Int J Radiat Oncol Biol Phys 17: 1313–1321

Yasargil MG, Curcic M, Kis M, et al. (1990) Total removal of craniopharyngiomas. Approaches and long-term results in 144 patients. J Neurosurg 73: 3–11

12 Management of Vestibular Schwannomas

Sanjay Ghosh and Steven Giannotta

CONTENTS

12.1
Introduction

The modern management of vestibular schwannomas represents a triumph of surgery and medicine. What was once a fatal disease with an almost equally fatal treatment is now curable with relatively little morbidity or mortality.

S. Ghosh, MD
Department of Neurological Surgery, University of Southern California School of Medicine, 1200 North State Street, Room 5046, Los Angeles, CA 90033, USA
S. Giannotta, MD
Department of Neurological Surgery, University of Southern California School of Medicine, 1200 North State Street, Room 5046, Los Angeles, CA 90033, USA

12.1.1
Historical Background

The earliest recorded attempt to remove an acoustic neuroma was by Charles McBurney in 1891. After removing the occipital skull with a mallet and chisel, he was unable to remove any tumor. Unfortunately, this initial effort proved fatal for the patient. Later that decade, a British surgeon named Charles Ballance successfully removed a vestibular schwannoma by a lateral suboccipital route (Stone 1999). Dr. Ballance performed the surgery in a staged manner with the craniotomy on one day and the tumor resection at a later date. He used blunt finger dissection to free the tumor from the pons and cranial nerves. Reportedly, the patient lived 18 years after the surgery, albeit with persistent facial and trigeminal nerve palsies (Stone 1999). The lateral suboccipital craniotomy that Charles Ballance employed became the standard approach for the early pioneers of vestibular schwannoma surgery.

The early attempts at surgical treatment of vestibular schwannomas carried substantial mortality, up to 78% by 1913 (Jackler 1994). Harvey Cushing, one of the great pioneers of neurosurgery, was successful in reducing the mortality rate to 20% by 1917 (Cushing 1921). Dr. Cushing emphasized the need to be gentle with the structures of the central nervous system and associated cranial nerves, arteries, and veins. In addition, he obtained meticulous hemostasis with the use of bone wax, silver clips, and electrocautery. Walter Dandy, a pupil of Dr. Cushing, further advanced the field by advocating complete tumor removal by gently stripping the capsule of the tumor away from the pons and cerebellum. Cushing, in contrast, chose to leave a small cap of tumor behind to avoid injury to the brain stem, arteries, and cranial nerves. The technical contributions of both surgeons were instrumental in reducing the mortality rate to 10% by 1931 (Jackler 1994). Despite this reduction in mortality, these pioneering surgeons were unable to remove tumors without critically injuring the facial nerve. The incidence of facial nerve palsy after removal of an acoustic neuroma was on the order of 60% by 1960. William House introduced the surgical techniques that were necessary to completely remove acoustic neuromas while preserving the pons, facial nerve, and anterior inferior cerebellar artery (HOUSE 1964).

12.1.2
Contemporary Surgery

Dr. House employed the middle fossa approach to the internal auditory canal, and he refined translabyrinthine craniotomy in the early 1960s (HOUSE 1964). The middle fossa approach provided exposure of the internal auditory canal, which was difficult to access by the more popular suboccipital approach. Translabyrinthine craniotomy (translab) provided more direct access to the cerebellopontine angle than suboccipital craniotomy, with less injurious cerebellar retraction than the suboccipital route. Dr. House was able to successfully utilize these approaches by employing the operating microscope and the high-speed drill in these surgeries. The operating microscope allowed for precise dissection of the tumor away from the facial nerve, brain stem, cerebellum, and cerebellar arteries. The high-speed drill enabled the surgeon to precisely remove the bony coverings of the auditory canal and cerebellopontine angle without injuring the adjacent neurovascular structures. These were impossible to achieve with the older techniques utilizing a mallet and chisel. These early attempts at translabyrinthine craniotomy were met with considerable resistance. Cushing felt that, "there is no possible route more dangerous or difficult" (HOUSE and HOUSE 1964). By utilizing microscope magnification and a high-speed drill, Dr. House was able to overcome such hurdles and remove small tumors with very little risk of facial nerve injury and very low mortality for the time (HOUSE and HITSELBERGER 1964). In 1964, Dr. House reported 5% mortality amongst all of his surgical patients, and partial or complete preservation of facial nerve function in all 41 patients who had translabyrinthine surgery for acoustic neuroma removal (HOUSE and HITSELBERGER 1964).

Neurosurgeons later adopted the operating microscope and high-speed drill for suboccipital craniotomy as well. Large tumors were eventually resected by the suboccipital route with little injury to adjacent neurovascular structures and low mortality.

DI TULLIO et al. (1978) reported 91% success in complete tumor removal with only 12% facial nerve palsy and 3.7% mortality. More recent series report even better outcomes with 99% incidence of complete tumor removal and less than 1% mortality with the suboccipital, retrosigmoid approach (EBERSOLD 1992; GORMLEY 1997).

12.1.3
Stereotactic Radiosurgery

A major revolution in the management of vestibular schwannomas occurred with the development of the gamma knife stereotactic radiosurgical unit. In 1968, a pioneering neurosurgeon named Lars Leksell designed the first stereotactic unit to deliver gamma radiation to treat arteriovenous malformations and tumors of the brain (LEKSELL 1983). Stereotactic radiosurgery allows the neurosurgeon to treat intracranial lesions without the attendant risks of craniotomy including cerebellar contusion, cerebrospinal fluid (CSF) leak, and meningitis. The major disadvantage of this treatment modality is that radiosurgery fails to eradicate the tumor; rather, it only ceases the tumor growth.

In the early 1980s, NOREN et al. (1983), presented some of the earliest cases of vestibular schwannomas treated with stereotactic radiosurgery. The authors initially reported reduction of the tumor size among 30% of their patients and arrest of growth among 60%. These data were viewed with considerable skepticism at the time, since radiosurgeries did not result in tumor removal, only in the control of tumor growth. To confirm that the treatment truly controls tumor growth, 10–20 years of follow-up is necessary. These long-term follow-up data are now beginning to emerge. As a result, stereotactic radiosurgery now has an important role in the management of vestibular schwannomas (LEKSELL 1983; LINSKEY et al. 1990; LUNSFORD et al. 1990, 1992; FLICKINGER et al. 1991, 1993, 1996, 1998; LUNSFORD and LINSKEY 1992; KONDZIOLKA and LUNSFORD 1993; KONDZIOLKA et al. 1998; FLICKINGER 1999).

As we enter a new millennium, the neurosurgeon and neurotologist have four important tools to treat vestibular schwannomas. A judicious combination of the suboccipital craniotomy, translabyrinthine craniotomy, middle fossa approach, and stereotactic radiosurgery represents the complete armamentarium in the modern management of vestibular schwannomas.

12.2
Cerebellopontine Angle

12.2.1
Surgical Anatomy

Acoustic neuromas are actually schwannomas that arise from one of the cranial nerves within the cerebellopontine (CP) angle. The CP angle is a space that lies ventral and lateral to the pons and upper medulla. The CP angle is bound by the cerebellum posteriorly and medially, and the petrous portion of the temporal bone laterally. The CSF-filled space between the pons and the petrous portion of the temporal bone is referred to as the superior CP angle cistern. This CSF-filled space is bound by the ambient cistern superiorly and the inferior CP angle cistern inferiorly.

Several critical neural and vascular structures are in very close opposition in the CP angle. Superiorly, the trigeminal nerve (CN V) exits from the ventrolateral pons and traverses the CP cistern towards the cavernous sinus and middle fossa. Inferior to the fifth cranial nerve, the facial nerve and vestibulocochlear nerves emanate from the ventromedial pons and cross the CP cistern towards the porus acusticus of the internal auditory canal. The facial nerve originates from the lower pons at the lateral end of the cleft between the pons and medulla called the pontomedullary sulcus (RHOTON and TEDESCHI 1992). Just 1–2 mm lateral and posterior to the facial nerve along the pontomedullary sulcus, the vestibulocochlear nerve originates from the pons. This is the greatest distance between the facial and vestibulocochlear nerves as they travel to the internal auditory canal. Just 2–3 mm inferior to the facial nerve, lie the rootlets of the glossopharyngeal (CN IX), vagal (CN X), and accessory nerves (CN XI) all emanating from the ventrolateral medulla. Management of acoustic neuromas is a challenge by any treatment modality due to the close proximity of these vital cranial nerves within the CP angle. Injury to these nerves results in many of the complications associated with both open surgery and radiosurgery such as facial numbness, corneal anesthesia, gait imbalance, vertigo, dysphagia, dysarthria, hoarseness, and aspiration.

The facial nerve, the nervus intermedius, the cochlear nerve, and the superior and inferior vestibular nerves enter the porus acusticus of the internal auditory canal. The relative position of the nerves shifts as they travel towards the lateral portion of the canal. Laterally, the nerves are separated by a horizontal crest of bone called the transverse or falciform crest. The facial and superior vestibular nerves are superior to the crest, and the cochlear and inferior vestibular nerves are inferior to the crest. The vestibular nerves are both located posteriorly to the facial and cochlear nerves at this lateral part of the canal. Consequently, tumors within the canal tend to push the facial and cochlear nerves anteriorly. Because the relationship of the nerves shifts within the internal auditory canal, it is impossible to preferentially treat tumors within the canal with radiosurgery. It must be assumed that any intracanalicular tumor that is treated with radiosurgery results in full radiation exposure for the cochlear and facial nerves as well.

The anterior inferior cerebellar artery (AICA) is the principal vascular structure of the CP angle. This vessel originates from the basilar artery along the ventral brain stem and encircles the inferior pons along the pontomedullary sulcus. With respect to the facial and vestibulocochlear nerves, the artery may course above, below, or between them. Tumors most commonly displace the AICA inferiorly; however, they may displace the vessel anteriorly or superiorly depending upon the previous relationship of the vessel (RHOTON and TEDESCHI 1992). The AICA provides the internal auditory artery to the facial and cochlear nerves, the subarcuate artery of the porus acusticus, and recurrent perforating arteries which supply the brain stem. Occlusion of the AICA may result in a lateral pontine infarction. This would potentially result in ipsilateral ataxia, facial numbness, ptosis, miosis, facial anhydrosis, facial weakness, deafness, and gaze palsy. The lateral pontine syndrome could also result in contralateral loss of pain and temperature sensation over the body, as well as nystagmus, nausea, and vomiting. Clearly, preservation of the AICA is critical in the management of acoustic neuromas.

12.2.2
Tumor Origin

The term acoustic neuroma is actually a misnomer. These are in fact tumors of Schwann cell origin. Over 95% of the time, the schwannoma arises from the superior vestibular nerve, inferior vestibular nerve, or both (SLATTERY et al. 1997). Less than 3% of the time, the schwannoma actually arises from the cochlear nerve, facial nerve, or the nervus intermedius.

Consequently, the more appropriate name for this tumor is vestibular schwannoma. This more accurately reflects the pathology of the tumor. In this chapter, both terminologies are used interchangeably.

The precise origin of the schwannoma has important clinical implications. Tumors that arise from the vestibular nerves may be treated while preserving cochlear and facial nerve function. This is not the case for tumors originating from the facial nerve. In such a situation, the nerve must be sectioned to remove the tumor, and a cable interposition nerve graft must be used to reapproximate the free ends of the facial nerve (Slattery et al. 1997).

The close proximity of so many vital neural and vascular structures within the CP angle makes the treatment of acoustic neuromas a formidable challenge. The measurement of treatment outcome cannot be based on tumor extirpation alone. Facial nerve function and hearing preservation are critical factors in evaluating treatment outcome and efficacy.

12.3
Facial Nerve Grading System

Dr. John House developed a simple yet elegant system to grade facial nerve function (Table 12.1.) (HOUSE 1983). The facial nerve function is scored on a scale of I–VI. A score of I is normal facial nerve function. A score of II is mild dysfunction where the patient has normal facial symmetry at rest, but has mild asymmetry with maximal effort. A score of III is moderate dysfunction with some asymmetry at rest and significant asymmetry with maximal contraction of the facial musculature. A score of IV is

Table 12.1. House facial nerve grading system (from HOUSE 1983)

Grade I	Normal facial nerve function
Grade II	Mild dysfunction; normal symmetry at rest, asymmetry with maximal contraction of facial musculature
Grade III	Moderate dysfunction; asymmetry at rest; able to close eye completely
Grade IV	Moderately severe dysfunction; asymmetry at rest; unable to completely close eye
Grade V	Severe dysfunction; trace facial muscle activity; unable to close eye
Grade VI	Total paralysis

moderately severe dysfunction with impaired ability to completely close the eye. Inability to completely close the eye is a potential source of morbidity as the patients cannot protect their cornea from foreign objects nor can they lubricate the cornea and sclera. These patients must have an eye shield and perform meticulous eye care in order to avoid corneal abrasions or conjunctivitis. This problem is compounded if the patient has corneal anesthesia from trigeminal nerve dysfunction. A House grade V is severe facial nerve dysfunction with incomplete eye closure and only a twitch of facial motion with maximal effort. Grade VI is total paralysis of the face.

In most clinical studies of vestibular schwannoma treatment, excellent facial nerve function is considered a House grade I or II. Acceptable or good facial nerve function is considered grade III in most series, and grade III or IV in some series. Poor facial nerve function is grade V or VI in all series. A comparison of facial nerve function after treatment is critical when evaluating different treatment modalities.

12.4
Audiology

At one time, any attempt to treat vestibular schwannomas resulted in complete loss of ipsilateral hearing. Refinements in surgical technique and diagnostic imaging have made hearing preservation a realistic goal (Gardner et al. 1983; Shelton et al. 1989a,b, 1990; Shelton and House 1990; Shelton 1992; Samii et al. 1991; Samii and Matthies 1997).

The two measurements of hearing function that are pertinent to acoustic neuroma treatment are pure tone audiometry (PTA) and speech discrimination score. PTA is a measure of a patient's ability to hear different frequencies of sound. At each frequency from 125 to 8000 Hz, the decibel level at which the patient can first detect sound is recorded. Normal hearing has been established and each patient's score is relative to normal hearing. A patient that hears a frequency at the mean threshold for the population would receive a score of 0 dB for that frequency. A patient that can only first hear a frequency when it is 30 dB greater than that detected by the average population has a score of 30 dB for that frequency. A higher score in PTA signifies a more significant hearing loss.

Speech discrimination score (SDS) is a measurement of patients' ability to understand speech when it is delivered above their normal threshold of sound reception. The SDS is reflected as a percentage of words that were recognized from 1 to 100. A lower SDS signifies a more significant hearing loss.

GARDNER and ROBERTSON (1988) developed a classification of hearing that is often used to evaluate hearing ability after the treatment of acoustic neuromas (Table 12.2.). Patients are scored on a scale from I to V. Class I patients have a PTA of 0–30 dB and an SDS of 70–100%. Class II, III, and IV patients have progressively poorer hearing ability as measured by PTA and SDS. Class V represents no hearing whatsoever.

Patients in class I have normal or excellent hearing. Patients in class II have good or functional hearing while those in class III have poor hearing. Patients in classes IV and V are functionally and completely deaf, respectively.

Table 12.2. Gardner and Robertson hearing classification (from GARDNER and ROBERTSON 1988)

Class	Pure tone audiometry	Speech discrimination
Class I	0–30 dB	70–100%
Class II	31–50 dB	50–69%
Class III	51–90 dB	5–49%
Class IV	Over 91 dB	1–4%
Class V	No hearing	0%

12.5
Surgical Options

12.5.1
Suboccipital Craniotomy

The anatomic boundaries of the suboccipital craniotomy are the tentorium cerebelli and transverse sinus superiorly, the sigmoid sinus anteriorly, and the foramen magnum inferiorly. This surgical approach provides access to the cerebellar hemisphere and the lateral brain stem from the upper pons to medulla.

12.5.1.1
Technique

Suboccipital craniotomy is performed with the patient in either the supine or sitting position. The exposure starts with a curvilinear incision starting above the pinna of the ear, extending 3 cm behind the ear, and inferiorly just below the mastoid process.

The skin and subcutaneous tissue are dissected and mobilized anteriorly to the external auditory canal. The muscular fascia is incised in a figure seven with the horizontal limb just above the transverse sinus and the vertical limb paralleling the skin incision. This muscular and fascial layer is reflected anteriorly to just before the external auditory canal and inferiorly to the digastric groove of the mastoid process. Next, craniotomy is performed, and the occipital skull is removed from the transverse sinus superiorly to the sigmoid sinus anteriorly, and the posterior lip of the foramen magnum inferiorly. It is important to bring the anterior margin of the craniotomy to the sigmoid sinus. This allows for maximal exposure of the CP angle, while minimizing injurious retraction of the cerebellum. Some surgeons refer to this as the retrosigmoid modification of the suboccipital approach.

Next, the dura is opened up to the boundaries of the sigmoid and transverse sinuses, thus exposing the cerebellar hemisphere. The arachnoid over the cisterna magna is carefully incised to allow drainage of CSF. This allows the cerebellum to relax, and facilitates medial retraction of the cerebellar hemisphere. The trigeminal (V), facial (VII), vestibular (VIII), cochlear (VIII), glossopharyngeal (IX), vagus (X), and accessory (XI) nerves are all visualized with minor adjustments in retraction (RHOTON and TEDESCHI 1992). The AICA is observed to emanate from the basilar artery and travel in proximity to the facial and vestibulocochlear nerves. With large tumors, the surgeon may encounter the superior cerebellar artery near the trigeminal nerve superiorly, and the posterior inferior cerebellar artery (PICA) crossing cranial nerves X and XI inferiorly. Often, vestibular schwannomas displace the facial and cochlear nerves anteriorly (RHOTON and TEDESCHI 1992; TEDESCHI and RHOTON 1994). If the tumor extends into the internal auditory canal, the surgeon may drill the posterior lip of the internal auditory canal to expose the medial portion of the canal.

12.5.1.2
Decision Making

Suboccipital craniotomy has some distinct advantages in the management of acoustic neuromas. First, it allows for resection of the tumor while preserving hearing in that ear. Acoustic neuromas most commonly arise from either the superior or inferior vestibular nerves. The cochlear nerve and its blood supply are often in intimate association with the tumor.

This makes hearing preservation in the management of acoustic neuromas a challenge by any treatment modality. In one report, surgeons were able to preserve useful hearing in 41% of their patients treated with suboccipital craniotomy (UMEZU and AIBA 1994; UMEZU et al. 1996). TATAGIBA et al. (1992) observed a similar trend with hearing preservation in 49% of their patients managed by the suboccipital approach. SAMII and MATTHIES (1997) were able to preserve the integrity of the cochlear nerve in 682 (68%) of 1000 cases. They observed good cochlear nerve function and hearing preservation in 39.5% of all 1000 cases (SAMII and MATTHIES 1997). In a small series of patients, HAINES and LEVINE (1993) observed a rate of 80% hearing preservation among their patients with acoustic neuromas less than 10 mm in size. The principal determinant in the preservation of hearing among these patients is tumor size. As would be expected, tumors greater than 3 cm in diameter require substantial dissection. The extra manipulation that is necessary with large tumors is more likely to lead to disruption of the inner ear labyrinth or retraction and ischemia of the cochlear nerve. Both of these will result in hearing loss (TATAGIBA et al. 1992). Early detection and treatment are critical to the preservation of hearing in acoustic neuromas.

EBERSOLD et al. (1992) accomplished gross total tumor removal in 97% of their 256 cases. After surgery, they reported excellent or good facial nerve function (House-Brackman grades I, II, and III) among 79% of their patients, and poor or absent function (House-Brackman grades IV, V, and VI) among the remaining 21%. As is the case with hearing preservation, tumor size is a significant determinant in the preservation of facial nerve function. GORMLEY et al. (1997) observed excellent facial nerve function among 96% of their patients with small tumors (<2.0 cm), among 74% of patients with medium tumors (2.0–3.9 cm), and 38% of those with large tumors (>4.0 cm). This group achieved gross total resection among 99% of their 150 patients managed by retrosigmoid craniotomy. Furthermore, they observed no recurrence among these patients with a mean of 70 months follow-up (GORMLEY et al. 1997). Both series of surgical cases had 1% mortality, with deaths due to pulmonary embolism and myocardial infarction. There were no deaths resulting from the procedure itself in either series. The most frequent complication of retrosigmoid craniotomy is CSF leak. GORMLEY et al. (1997) observed a CSF leak among 15% of their patients (26 of 179). Most of the patients had resolution of their CSF leaks with temporary diversion of the CSF using a lumbar drain. Some patients required another surgery to repair the fistula. EBERSOLD et al. (1992) observed an 11% incidence of CSF leakage in their series. In contrast to GORMLEY et al. (1997), this group elected to treat CFS leakages with early surgery. They felt that the most common cause of fluid leakage was the entry of CSF into the mastoid air cells, which in turn tracked into the middle ear and eustachian tube (EBERSOLD et al. 1992). Upon reoperation, these clinicians further exposed the mastoid air cells and filled the middle ear canal with autologous fat. Other, much less frequent complications include aseptic meningitis, hydrocephalus, wound infection, lower cranial nerve palsy, and ataxia. The suboccipital, retrosigmoid craniotomy provides the neurosurgeon with an effective means to resect acoustic neuromas while occasionally preserving hearing, and frequently preserving facial nerve function depending on the tumor size. With this approach, neurosurgeons and neurotologists are able to treat these tumors with very little morbidity and mortality.

At the University of Southern California (USC), the retrosigmoid approach is used almost exclusively as a hearing preservation strategy. In 40 cases employed in patients with preoperative serviceable hearing, 33% had a Gardener Robinson score of I with 25% experiencing scores of II or III; 42% had poor or no hearing. All had total removal of their tumors without permanent facial weakness.

12.5.1.3
Case Report

Figure 12.1a demonstrates the intraoperative view through a retrosigmoid craniotomy of a 2-cm tumor in a 39-year-old female who presented with subtle hearing loss and tingling of the face. Her audiogram demonstrated only a 7-dB speech reception threshold (SRT) and 92% speech discrimination. Figure 12.1b shows complete microscopic removal of the lesion with the facial and cochlear nerve preserved but splayed apart. A follow-up audiogram 3 months postoperatively showed a 22-dB SRT and 96% discrimination.

12.5.2
Translabyrinthine Craniotomy

Translabyrinthine (translab) craniotomy is the most effective means to treat acoustic neuromas in pa-

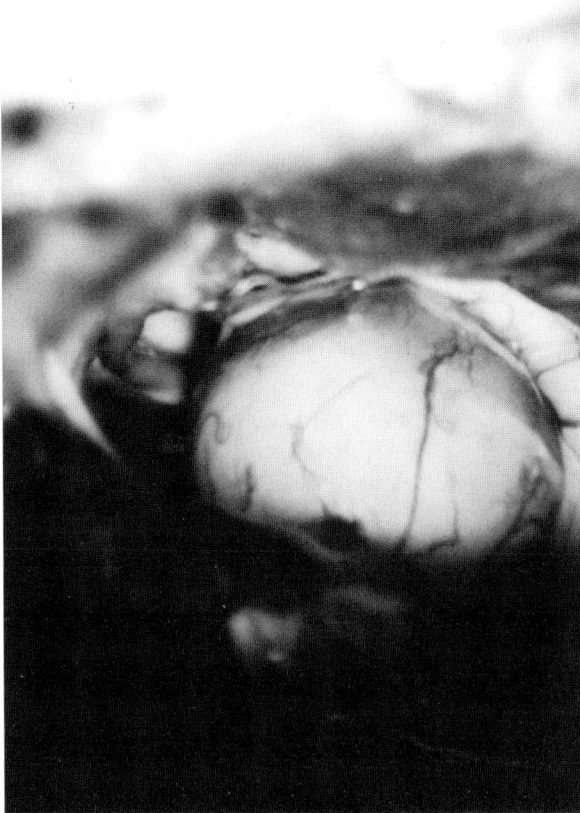
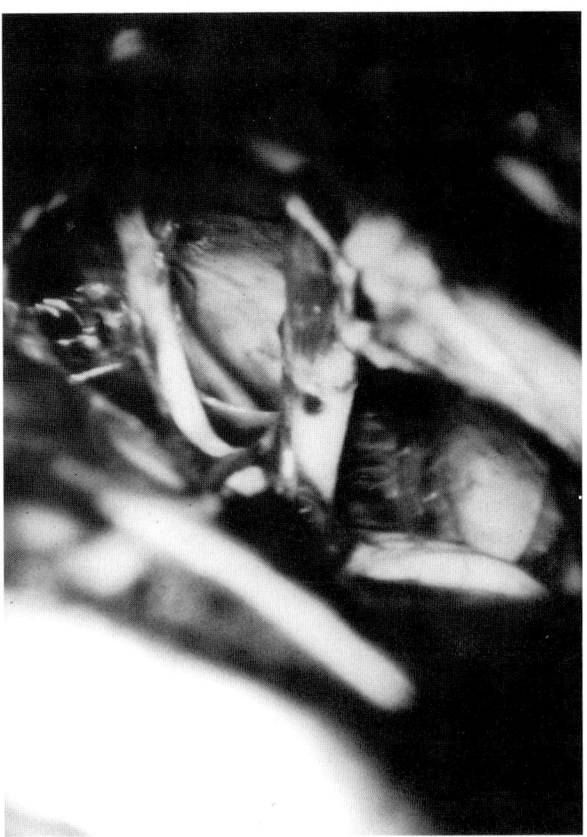

a   b

Fig. 12.1. a An intraoperative view of a vestibular schwannoma that was exposed through a suboccipital craniotomy. The anterior inferior cerebellar artery is displaced inferiorly by the tumor. **b** An intraoperative view after microsurgical resection of the tumor. The cochlear and facial nerves are splayed apart from the tumor

tients who have already lost hearing from the tumor. This approach is advantageous over retrosigmoid craniotomy in that it provides a shorter absolute distance to the CP angle and provides direct access to the entire internal auditory canal (HOUSE 1964). Furthermore, the translabyrinthine approach requires no cerebellar retraction. (BRACKMANN and GREEN 1992). The translabyrinthine approach also provides excellent exposure of the facial nerve from its pontine origin to the stylomastoid foramen. Consequently, it is much easier to perform a primary repair of the facial nerve with the translabyrinthine approach compared to the suboccipital approach (BRACKMANN and GREEN 1992). One significant disadvantage of the translabyrinthine approach is that it is not possible to preserve hearing in the ipsilateral ear. Therefore, it is not the appropriate approach for patients with serviceable hearing preoperatively. Another limitation of the translabyrinthine technique is that it provides little exposure to the foramen mag-

num and lower cranial nerves. Consequently, tumors that extend inferiorly towards the foramen magnum are more easily treated with retrosigmoid craniotomy (TEDESCHI and RHOTON 1994).

12.5.2.1
Technique

Translabyrinthine craniotomy starts with a skin incision and fascial dissection similar to that of the retrosigmoid approach. After the mastoid process is exposed, the surgeon must drill through the cortical bone of the mastoid process, temporal bone, and occipital bone. The sigmoid sinus marks the posterior limit of bone dissection. The middle fossa dura and petrosal sinus demarcate the superior limit. The external auditory canal lies along the anterior boundary, and the digastric ridge and jugular bulb lie inferiorly (TEDESCHI and RHOTON 1994; GIANNOTTA 1992). Next, the surgeon exposes the mastoid antrum followed by the structures of the inner ear; specifically, the horizontal semicircular canal followed by the posterior and superior semicircular canals. The semicircular canals provide the necessary landmarks to identify and expose the facial nerve within the temporal bone. Removal of the semicircular canal and vestibule results in exposure of the internal auditory canal. The horizontal or tympanic section of the facial nerve also provides an important landmark in the identification of the internal auditory canal. The facial nerve is exposed to the stylomastoid foramen. The dura is then opened with incisions parallel to the superior petrosal and sigmoid sinuses, and parallel to the course of the internal auditory canal. This provides exposure of the trigeminal, facial, vestibular, and cochlear nerves. In addition, the anterior inferior cerebellar, superior cerebellar, and basilar arteries are visualized. Depending on the position of the jugular bulb, it may be impossible to visualize the hypoglossal and vagal nerves as they enter the jugular foramen; but they are easily identified adjacent to the choroid plexus emerging from the foramen of Lushka (TEDESCHI and RHOTON 1994).

12.5.2.2
Decision Making

Translabyrinthine craniotomy allows the neurotologist and neurosurgeon to safely and effectively remove acoustic neuromas with little morbidity and mortality. In Dr. House's original article on the translabyrinthine approach, all 41 patients had preservation of facial nerve function after tumor removal (HOUSE and HITSELBERGER 1964). KING and MORRISON (1980) reported on their experience with the translabyrinthine approach. These surgeons achieved gross total resection of tumor in all 150 patients treated, with a 2% incidence of mortality (KING and MORRISON 1980). They achieved preservation of facial nerve function in 100% of the small tumors (<1 cm), 80% of medium tumors (1–2.5 cm), and 20% of large tumors (>2.5 cm). The most frequent complication was CSF rhinorrhea in 14% of cases and CSF wound leak in 7% of all cases. These authors reported no cases of recurrence with a mean of 4 years of follow-up; however, this was before the availability of magnetic resonance imaging. More recently, HARDY et al. (1989) reported on their experience with 100 translabyrinthine operations with gross total resection in 97% of cases. These clinicians reported 3 (3%) perioperative deaths, from a brain

stem infarction in one patient, a CP angle hematoma in another patient, and a pulmonary embolus in a third. All of these patients had a tumor that was larger than 3.5 cm in diameter. The most common complication was CSF leak, which occurred 13% of the time, most of which required another surgery.

The initial tumor size has a very important impact on the ultimate treatment outcome. Almost 90% of all patients with tumors that were less than 2.5 cm in size had excellent functional outcomes and were able to return to their previous employment. In contrast, only 60% of all patients with tumors greater than 4.5 cm were able to return to their previous vocation (HARDY et al. 1989). Facial nerve function is also dependant on the initial size of the tumor. HARDY et al. (1989) found that patients with small tumors had excellent facial nerve function (House grade I or II) in 94% of all cases after translabyrinthine resection.

ARRIAGA et al. (1994) observed a similar trend in the management of small tumors. They observed excellent postoperative facial nerve function 91% of the time after translabyrinthine removal of acoustic neuromas less than 1.5 cm in size. The incidence of facial nerve injury is significantly higher in the management of larger tumors.

LANMAN et al. (1999) presented a series of 190 patients with large acoustic neuromas (>3 cm) that were managed with the translabyrinthine approach. These surgeons achieved gross total resection of tumor in 96% of all cases, with anatomic preservation of the facial nerve in 94% of their patients. The patients experienced excellent facial nerve function (House grade I or II) 1 year after surgery in 53% of all cases, and acceptable facial nerve function (House grade I–IV) in 81% of all cases. The facial nerve outcome was directly related to tumor size.

Translabyrinthine craniotomy is a safe and effective means to treat acoustic neuromas where hearing preservation is not the goal. Experienced neurosurgeons and neurotologists are able to completely resect small tumors over 97% of the time, with complete preservation of facial nerve function 91% of the time in some series (ARRIAGA et al. 1994). The modern series report little to no mortality from this approach, even when dealing with larger tumors (LANMAN et al. 1999).

At USC, the translabyrinthine approach is relied upon heavily as a strategy for all large tumors and those where it is unlikely that functional hearing will result. In the senior author's series of 294 patients, 96% resulted in a microscopic total removal. Facial nerve function at 1 year was excellent (grade I or II) in 90% of patients.

12.5.2.3
Case Report

Figure 12.2 illustrates a patient who was managed with a translabyrinthine craniotomy. This patient had a 4-cm tumor arising from the left superior vestibular nerve. The tumor was causing significant mass effect upon the pons, and was compressing the fourth ventricle. The patient had no serviceable hearing in the left ear; therefore, a translabyrinthine craniotomy was performed to resect the tumor. In this case, the translabyrinthine approach provided access to the lateral portion of the internal auditory canal, and averted retraction on the cerebellum.

12.5.3
Middle Fossa Approach

The middle fossa approach is the most effective surgical treatment for small schwannomas that extend into the lateral portion of the internal auditory canal. Dr. William House initially used the middle fossa approach to remove bone from the internal auditory canal to relieve pressure on the cochlear nerve. He performed this with the intention of improving hearing (HOUSE and HOUSE 1964). As a result of these efforts, he recognized the utility of the middle fossa approach to gain access to the entire internal audi-

tory canal. He found that he could develop an excellent view of the superior and inferior vestibular nerves, cochlear nerve, facial nerve, and nervus intermedius all the way to the lateral most portion of the internal auditory canal. Such lateral exposure was very difficult to achieve through the suboccipital route. The most significant limitation of the middle fossa approach is that it provides very little exposure to the rest of the posterior fossa. Consequently, tumors that extend more than 1.5 cm from the porus acusticus cannot be managed by the middle fossa route.

Dr. House was the first to successfully remove vestibular schwannomas using the middle fossa approach (HOUSE and HOUSE 1964). Subsequent technical modifications have made it an excellent treatment modality for the removal of small tumors while preserving both facial nerve function and hearing (SAMII et al. 1991; BRACKMANN 1992; HAINES and LEVINE 1993; ARRIAGA et al. 1994; BRACKMANN et al. 1994; SLATTERY and BRACKMANN 1995; SLATTERY et al. 1997).

12.5.3.1
Technique

The middle fossa approach is performed with the patient in supine position and the head turned away from the side of the tumor. An incision is made no more than 5 mm anterior to the tragus of the ear to avoid the frontal branch of the facial nerve. The incision is extended in a curvilinear manner past the

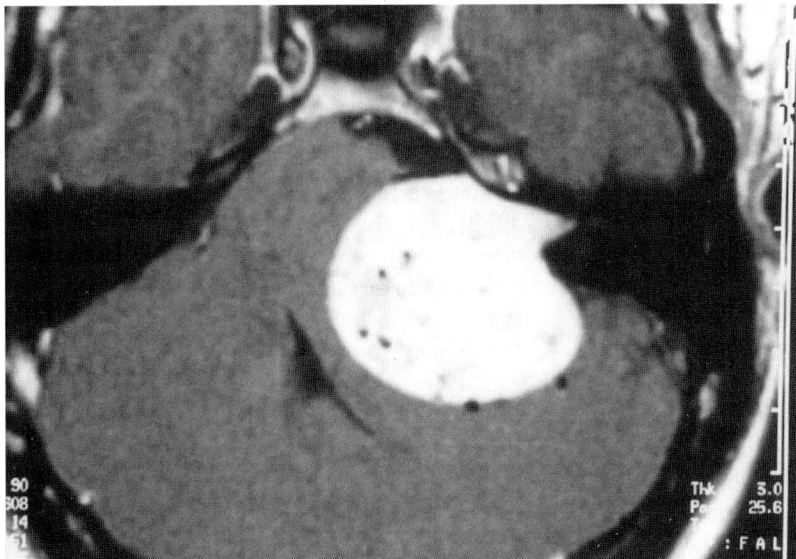

Fig. 12.2. An axial T1-weighted image of the brain with contrast reveals a 4-cm tumor that is compressing the pons and extending laterally into the internal auditory canal

superior temporal line. The subcutaneous fat and galea are incised, and the superficial temporal artery branches are cauterized if necessary. The temporalis muscle and fascia are incised. The muscle is reflected off the squamous portion of the temporal bone and retracted anteriorly and inferiorly. The root of the zygoma approximates the floor of the middle fossa, and this is used to guide the lower margin of the craniotomy. The craniotomy is extended approximately 3 cm anterior to the external auditory canal and 2 cm posterior to the canal. The upper margin of the bone flap is the superior temporal line.

Next, the dura is dissected from the middle fossa floor until the arcuate eminence, the greater superficial petrosal nerve, and the middle meningeal artery at the foramen spinosum are identified. The dura and temporal lobe are then gently retracted superiorly. The point where the greater superficial petrosal nerve exits, the temporal bone is identified and removed using a coarse diamond burr. This reveals the geniculate ganglion of the facial nerve. From this point, the bone overlying the labyrinthine portion of the facial nerve is removed, thus following the nerve medially to the internal auditory canal. The roof of the internal auditory canal is thinned to eggshell thickness all the way to the porus acusticus. The bone around the porus acusticus is then removed almost circumferentially to an arc of 270° (BRACKMANN et al. 1994). Laterally, near the vertical crest that separates the superior vestibular nerve from the facial, an arc of only 90° of bone is removed due to the proximity of the cochlea anteriorly and the semicircular canal posteriorly. Violation of either of these inner ear structures will result in hearing loss. The bone is then gently removed from the porus acusticus medially to the vertical crest laterally (Bill's Bar). The dura is then opened parallel to the long axis of the internal auditory canal, directly over the superior vestibular nerve, which is posterior to the facial nerve at the vertical crest. Under high magnification, the superior vestibular nerve is cut, and the tumor is gently dissected free from the facial nerve. Great care must be taken to preserve the internal auditory artery, which lies within the canal. Sacrifice or spasm of this artery may lead to cochlear injury and hearing loss (BRACKMANN et al. 1994). The tumor is removed in a medial to lateral direction to prevent traction on the nerve as it enters the modiolus (BRACKMANN et al. 1994). At the end of surgery, BRACKMAN et al. (1994) recommend irrigation of the internal auditory canal with the calcium channel antagonist papaverine to relieve spasm of the arterial supply of the inner ear and preserve hearing.

12.5.3.2
Decision Making

The middle fossa approach to acoustic neuroma resection is a technically demanding yet effective means to remove small tumors while preserving hearing and facial nerve function. In a small series of patients, preservation of hearing in six of seven patients managed with the middle fossa approach for small tumors limited to the internal auditory canal was reported (HAINES and LEVINE 1993). BRACKMANN et al. (1994) reported 71% hearing preservation among their 24 patients managed with the middle fossa craniotomy. Later, the same group presented their data on 151 patients managed with the middle fossa approach and observed 68% incidence of preservation of hearing. The tumors in these series ranged from 0.5 to 2.5 cm in diameter with a mean of 1.2 cm (SLATTERY et al. 1997).

Facial nerve preservation is usually excellent. ARRIAGA et al. (1994) reported 96% incidence of excellent facial nerve function among their 48 patients treated with the middle fossa approach. SLATTERY et al. (1997), maintained anatomic integrity of the facial nerve in 150 of 151 cases. The only case that required sectioning of the facial nerve was when the schwannoma arose from the facial nerve itself. These authors observed excellent facial nerve function amongst 95% of their patients.

Other reported complications from middle fossa approach include CSF leakage amongst 7% of cases, and meningitis in 2% of all cases. No deaths have been reported in recent series of the middle fossa approach (SLATTERY et al. 1997). It is important to note, however, that these outstanding results are achieved at centers of excellence for acoustic neuroma surgery. Given the technical demands of this procedure, it is unlikely that surgeons with less experience than that of the aforementioned authors are likely to achieve such excellent outcomes. With this important point in mind, the middle fossa craniotomy is still a definitive means to completely remove small acoustic neuromas from the internal auditory canal while preserving hearing in a majority of cases, and conserving facial nerve function over 95% of the time.

At USC, the middle fossa approach is employed for exclusively intracanalicular lesions with functional hearing, especially those tumors impacted laterally in the internal canal. In 33 cases, hearing preservation in the grade I–II range totaled 52%. Total removal was obtained in all and there was no prolonged facial nerve morbidity.

12.5.3.3
Case Report

Figure 12.3 depicts a patient with a small schwannoma of the vestibular nerve that is located primarily within the internal auditory canal. Because this patient had functional hearing in that ear, a translabyrinthine craniotomy would not have been the appropriate approach. The lateral portion of the tumor would have been very difficult to access by the suboccipital approach without compromising the inner ear (HABERKAMP et al. 1998). The middle fossa approach was used in this patient to completely dissect the tumor free from the facial and cochlear nerves while preserving both facial nerve function and hearing. Some neurosurgeons would advocate stereotactic radiosurgery for this lesion; however, that will be further addressed in the next section.

12.6
Stereotactic Radiosurgery

Lars Leksell was instrumental in the development of the first stereotactic Gamma Unit in 1968 (LEKSELL 1983). The radioactive source that he used was cobalt 60. With this Gamma Unit, it was possible to make very sharply circumscribed, disc-shaped lesions. Initially, this was used for functional neurosurgery to make precise lesions in the basal ganglion and thalamus. Subsequently, the Gamma Unit was used to treat deep-seated tumors and vascular malformations in the brain and along the skull base. Dr. Leksell felt that the Gamma Unit was well suited for such lesions because this radiosurgical technique obvi-

ated the need for technical ability and surgical skill (LEKSELL 1983). It requires significant training and technical competence to safely obtain surgical access to lesions within the ventricles, basal ganglion, posterior fossa, or skull base. As a result, treatment outcome is affected by the skill of the surgeon when it comes to complex, deep-seated lesions such as craniopharyngiomas, arteriovenous malformations, and acoustic neuromas. Dr. Leksell felt that the gamma knife eliminated the need for such technical competence on the part of the neurosurgeon (LEKSELL 1983). At USC we feel it is imperative that the treating neurosurgeon is familiar with both the open surgical and the stereotactic radiosurgical approaches to acoustic neuromas.

12.6.1
Technique

Radiosurgery starts with the stereotactic frame placement. At USC we perform this with an anesthesiologist in attendance. Prior to frame placement, the patient receives a combination of intravenous Versed, alfentanyl, Zofran, and propofol. The frame is aligned on the patient's head to bring the lesion as close to the center of the frame as possible. A solution of Marcaine with epinephrine is injected in the subperiosteal space along the sites of pin placement. Four pins are used to secure the frame to the outer table of the skull. This use of monitored sedation and local anesthetic allows for frame placement without any perceived pain on the part of the patient.

The patient receives gadolinium contrast intravenously, followed by a magnetic resonance image of the brain. The axial images are downloaded to a

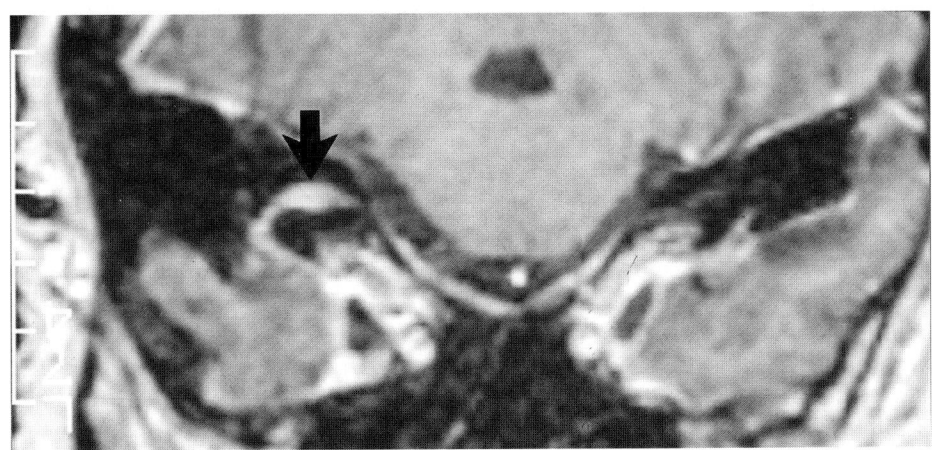

Fig. 12.3. An axial T1-weighted image of the brain with contrast reveals a small vestibular schwannoma in the right internal auditory canal (*arrow*). The tumor has a small extension into the cerebellopontine angle cistern

workstation where treatment is planned using the Leksell Gamma Plan software. In treating acoustic neuromas, we often utilize the 8-mm collimator. The small collimator helps to keep the 50% isodose line as close to the contour of the tumor as possible. Due to the small volume obtained with the use of the 8-mm collimator, several separate isocenters (shots) are required to achieve tumor coverage. However, it is possible to minimize radiation dose to the pons, anterior inferior cerebellar artery, and nearby cranial nerves by using small collimators with multiple shots. The prescribed dose is generally 14 Gy to the 50% isodose line, with 28 Gy maximum dose. The maximum dose delivered to the pons is limited to 5 Gy.

After treatment, the frame is removed. Bleeding from the pin sites is most often controlled with gentle pressure. Occasionally, the scalp must be closed with a suture to control bleeding from branches of the occipital, superficial temporal, or supraorbital arteries. The pin sites are then dressed with antibiotic ointment and local dressings, and the patient is monitored in the recovery room. The patients are discharged home later that day.

12.6.2
Decision Making

Stereotactic radiosurgery is an effective means to treat acoustic neuromas that are less than 2.5 cm in size in patients who are elderly, medically unsuitable for general anesthesia, or refusing open surgery. In Dr. Leksell's early series, he presented seven patients treated with the gamma knife with 5–12 years of follow-up (LEKSELL 1983). He observed control of tumor growth in five of the seven patients treated. One of the patients had a recurrence 12 years after the initial treatment. Dr. Leksell ascribed this recurrence to an insufficient amount of radiation delivered to that region of the tumor. It is clear from these early data that stereotactic radiosurgery can slow tumor growth; however, these patients require a very long period of follow-up to confirm that the tumor has been functionally eradicated.

NOREN et al. (1983) described the radiation dosages that were initially used to treat acoustic neuromas in Sweden. These clinicians used a 14-mm collimator in most cases and a central target dose of 50–125 Gy. The maximum dose to the tumor periphery in this series of 14 patients was 17–49 Gy. The authors reported control of tumor growth in 78% of their patients at 4 years, and an increase in tumor size

among the remaining 12% of patients. Based on their clinical data and experimental evidence, they stated that a minimal dose of 20 Gy to the periphery of the tumor is necessary to control acoustic neuroma growth. With such a high dose of radiation, they observed a high complication rate. They had an 80% incidence of hearing loss among patients with hearing preoperatively. Transient facial nerve palsy was noted in 28% and permanent facial sensory loss in 7% of patients. One elderly patient died from pneumonia 6 months after treatment. It is possible that this was related to the effects of radiation (NOREN et al. 1983). This yields a mortality rate of 7% for this small series.

LINSKEY et al. (1990), reported the first American series using the gamma knife for acoustic neuromas. In order to minimize complications of radiation, these neurosurgeons used the minimal effective dose as described by NOREN et al. (1983), 20 Gy to the 50% isodose line in most cases (LINSKEY et al. 1990). The tumor size ranged from 8 to 33 mm in this small series of 26 patients. With a mean follow-up of 8 months after treatment, these clinicians observed a modest decrease in tumor size among 58% of patients, and no change in tumor size among 42% of patients. A dose of 20 Gy resulted in unacceptable cochlear nerve dysfunction. Only three of seven patients with serviceable hearing prior to treatment maintained their hearing after treatment. A hearing preservation rate of 43% is lower than that obtained by other treatment modalities. The patients also experienced 31% incidence of new onset or aggravated facial nerve palsy and 27% new onset trigeminal nerve dysfunction. Other complications included gait imbalance, vertigo, headache, and nausea and vomiting. Average time of onset of these cranial nerve symptoms ranged from 3 to 6 months after gamma knife treatment.

In order to decrease the incidence of cranial neuropathy after gamma knife, several investigators have tried to decrease the prescription dose of radiation delivered to the tumor. MILLER et al. (1999) initially used 20 Gy to the 50% isodose line for tumors with diameters less than 2 cm, 18 Gy for tumors 2.1–3 cm in diameter, and 16 Gy for tumors 3.1–4 cm in diameter. In the latter group of patients, they decreased the prescription doses to 16, 14, and 12 Gy for each respective tumor size. These clinicians found that the greatest risk factor in the development of facial neuropathy was a tumor margin dose of 18 Gy or greater. They observed a 38% incidence of lasting facial neuropathy among the patients treated with the increased dose protocol, and only 8% complication rate with the decreased dose. In this series, useful hearing preservation was achieved in 39% of cases at 2 years follow-up. There were no cases of mortality in this series of 82 patients. The authors did not observe any progression in tumor size; however, their short follow-up time does not allow for any meaningful conclusions about tumor control with the decreased radiation dose. One of the major limitations to the existing literature that addresses radiosurgery for acoustic neuromas is a relatively short follow-up. Up to 70% of all untreated acoustic neuromas will show no growth over a period of 3.5 years (WIET et al. 1995; DEEN et al. 1996; FUCCI et al. 1999). Consequently, it is not possible to draw significant conclusions about the long-term efficacy of stereotactic radiosurgery unless the follow-up is much greater than 4 years.

Effective stereotactic radiosurgery must strike a balance between the complications of too high a radiation dose and the inefficacy of too low a dose. The optimal dose to obtain long-term control of acoustic neuroma growth while minimizing radiation effects remains to be determined. In their original articles, both LEKSELL (1983) and NOREN et al. (1983) felt that 20 Gy was the minimal dose necessary to permanently inhibit acoustic neuroma growth. Leksell described a patient with neurofibromatosis who developed tumor recurrence 12 years after the initial treatment. He ascribed this failure in treatment to an insufficient radiation dose; however, in these early studies, they used up to 45 Gy to the tumor periphery (NOREN et al. 1983). Such doses are significantly higher than those used in modern series. If it is possible to develop recurrence at 12 years with such a high dose of radiation, it is logical to assume that it is even more likely to develop delayed recurrences with the lower doses that are in use today.

KONDZIOLKA et al. (1998) presented one of the largest series of long-term outcome after stereotactic radiosurgery. These neurosurgeons evaluated 162 patients from 5 to 10 years after gamma knife treatment of acoustic neuromas. The tumors ranged in size from 8 to 39 mm with a mean of 22 mm. The patients were treated with three different dose regimens. Early in the series, the patients received 18–20 Gy to the 50% isodose line. The dose was decreased to 16 Gy 2 years into the study. The dose was further decreased to 14 Gy 5 years into the study in order to help decrease the incidence of cranial nerve injury (OGUNRINDE et al. 1995; NIRANJAN et al. 1999). These authors observed a decrease in lesion size amongst 62% of tumors, no change in size amongst 33% of tumors, and an increase in size in 9% of cases.

It is important to note that the follow-up was 10 years for patients with the high dose regimen. The follow-up was only 5 years for patients who received 14–16 Gy. According to the early pioneers of the gamma knife, Leksell and Noren, 5 years is an insufficient amount of time to determine whether tumor growth is indeed arrested on a permanent basis (LEKSELL 1983; NOREN et al. 1983).

In the series of KONDZIOLKA et al. (1998), their patients experienced a 16% incidence of permanent complications. Over 53% of patients with useful hearing before radiosurgery lost useful hearing after radiosurgery. In addition, 21% of patients experienced a marked decrease in facial nerve function after stereotactic radiosurgery. Other complications included balance difficulty, facial spasm, tinnitus, hydrocephalus, and facial numbness.

The early data on stereotactic radiosurgery demonstrate that acoustic neuroma growth can be controlled for 10 years or more using 20 Gy to the tumor margin. At this point, there are no long-term follow-up data to prove whether 14 Gy provides the same control of tumor growth that is achieved with 20 Gy. For this reason, at USC, we recommend stereotactic radiosurgery among patients who are more than 60 years of age with tumors less than 2.5 cm in size. In the elderly population, we treat tumors that have demonstrated growth on serial magnetic resonance imaging. We also recommend radiosurgery for patients with small tumors who cannot tolerate general anesthesia. Some patients are unwilling to accept the small risk of mortality associated with open surgery, and we counsel them that stereotactic radiosurgery is effective in the early control of tumor growth, but it is of unproven benefit in permanently controlling tumor growth. We will perform stereotactic radiosurgery in this circumstance, if the patients opt for this over microsurgery.

Figure 12.4 demonstrates a patient who was treated with stereotactic radiosurgery at USC. This is a vestibular schwannoma in a 75-year-old man with a history of tinnitus and unilateral sensorineural hearing loss. The planning was performed to keep the 50% isodose line as close to the margin of the tumor as possible, so as to minimize the radiation dose delivered to the pons. One treatment with the 14-mm collimator and five treatments with the 8-mm collimator were used to deliver 12 Gy to the 50% isodose line. The total target volume was 2.4 cm^3, and the total volume within the 50% isodose line was 3.6 cm^3. The maximum dose of radiation delivered to the pons was 6 Gy. A similar clinical problem is demonstrated in Fig. 12.5a,b.

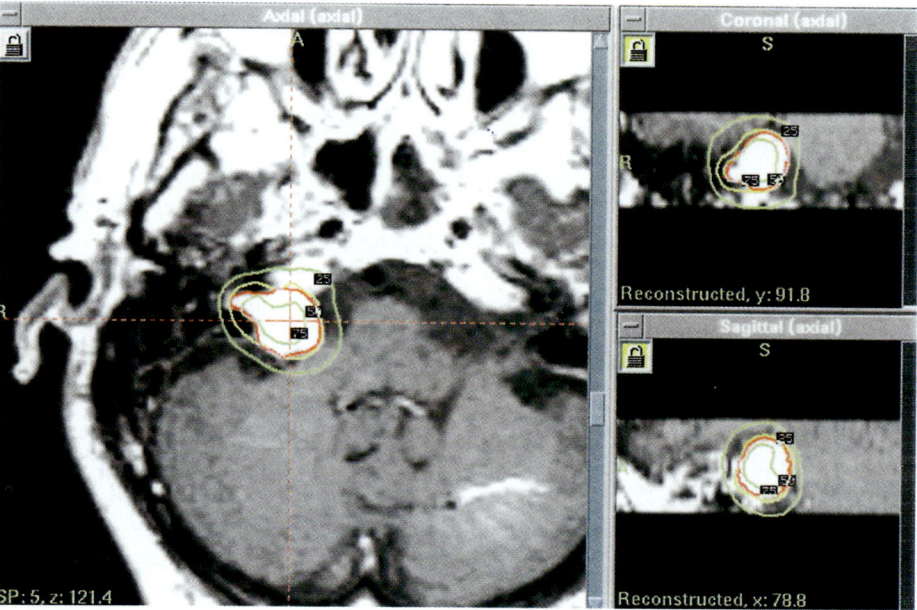

Fig. 12.4. T1-weighted MRI of the brain with contrast demonstrates an acoustic neuroma in a 75-year-old man. The tumor has a small extension into the internal auditory canal on the left. The treatment planning was performed to have the 50% isodose line conform as close to the tumor volume as possible. This is important to minimize the radiation dose delivered to the pons or other cranial nerves

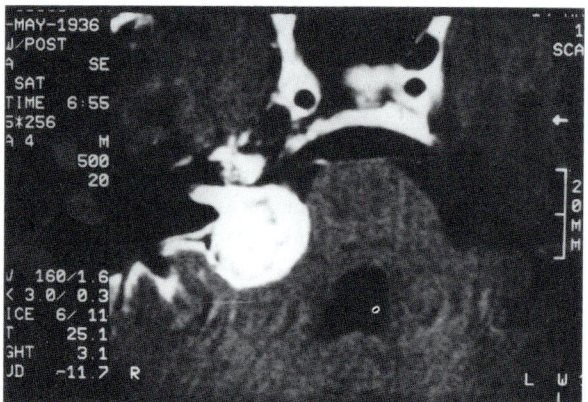

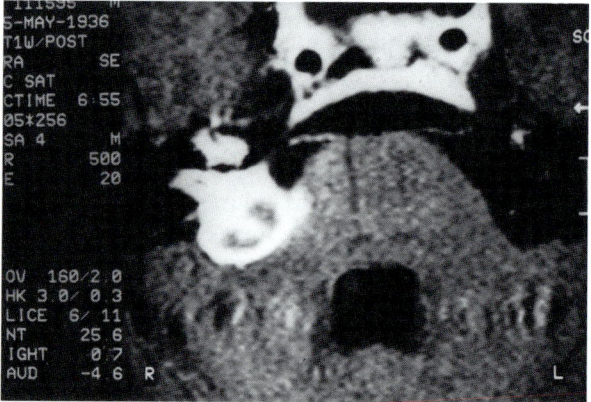

Fig. 12.5. a An axial magnetic resonance image with contrast shows a 2-cm schwannoma that is extending into the internal auditory canal on the right. This patient could not undergo microsurgery due to a bleeding diathesis. He was treated with stereotactic radiosurgery. **b** An axial MRI after radiosurgery reveals a loss of contrast enhancement within the center of the tumor, and a slight decrease in the size of the tumor

12.6.3
Stereotactic Radiosurgery After Microsurgery

In certain circumstances, it is not possible to achieve gross total tumor resection. CUSHING (1921), in his original papers, was emphatic that it was necessary to leave a capsule of tumor behind to prevent injury of the pons and cranial nerves. In the modern era, gross total resection is achieved up to 98% of the time (SAMII and MATTHIES 1997). In certain circumstances, the tumor is firmly adherent to the pons or other cranial nerves. It is occasionally necessary to leave a capsule of tumor behind to preserve these

vital structures. SAMII and MATHIES (1997) found it necessary to deliberately perform subtotal tumor resection in 21 (2.1%) of 1000 cases. In 10 (1%) cases, the goal of surgery was only to decompress the brain stem in elderly, debilitated patients. In 11 (1.1%) cases, they left a small cap of tumor with the intent of preserving hearing in the only hearing ear. When it is not possible to completely resect the tumor, we have found adjunctive stereotactic radiosurgery useful in controlling tumor growth.

The use of stereotactic radiosurgery after microsurgery was analyzed in a number of studies by POL-LOCK et al. (1998a,b,c). Most of their patients had a recurrence after deliberate subtotal surgical resection. Of their 79 patients, 33% had had prior gross total resections with recurrence. These clinicians reported control of tumor growth in 94% of patients with a mean follow-up of 43 months. This study demonstrates the efficacy of stereotactic radiosurgery in controlling tumor growth over short periods of time; however, the study has important limitations. Early in their study, the patients were treated with 18–20 Gy to the tumor margin. Later in the study, the dosage was decreased to 12 or 14 Gy. This decrease in radiation dose significantly improved facial nerve function. With treatment greater than or equal to 18 Gy, Pollock et al. observed a 57% incidence of deterioration of facial nerve function. With 15–17 Gy, they observed a 22% facial nerve injury rate, and with 12–14 Gy a 14% facial nerve injury rate. It remains to be seen whether 12–14 Gy will have a lasting impact on tumor growth; however, radiosurgery seems to be a useful adjunct when complete tumor resection is not possible.

Another situation where stereotactic radiosurgery is a potential option is during recurrence after a previously complete microsurgical resection. Samii and Matthies (1997) observed tumor recurrence in 6 (0.7%) of 880 patients who had a prior gross total resection with suboccipital craniotomy. These clinicians managed their recurrences with a second operation. Shelton (1995) observed a recurrence rate of 0.3% after complete removal of unilateral acoustic neuromas by the translabyrinthine approach. In this series, the time to recurrence was on the order of 10–12 years after initial resection, and recurrences were managed with surgical resection. At USC, we recommend a second surgery in the rare event of a recurrence after prior gross total resection, unless the patient meets the criteria previously set forth for gamma knife. If the patient can no longer tolerate general anesthesia, is of advanced age, or refuses another surgery, we will consider treating the tumor with stereotactic radiosurgery.

The series of images in Fig. 12.6 exemplifies a patient that was managed with a combination of microsurgery and stereotactic radiosurgery. Figure 12.6a,b shows axial images without and with contrast of a large acoustic neuroma. The tumor is compressing the pons and obstructing the flow of CSF within the fourth ventricle. Figure 12.6c shows the extent of the tumor from the tentorial incisura to the foramen magnum in the coronal plane. Figure 12.6d highlights the same tumor in the sagittal plane. This reveals significant compression of the pons. The patient was managed with a suboccipital craniotomy, and a mi-

crosurgical resection was performed. Part of the tumor was found to be firmly adherent to the pons, medulla, facial nerve, and lower cranial nerves. It was elected to leave a capsule of tumor in the interest of preserving these critical structures. Figure 12.6e,f shows postoperative axial images without and with contrast. These images show that the mass effect on the pons is relieved, and the patency of the fourth ventricle is restored. Figure 12.6g demonstrates the residual lesion along the medulla and lower cranial nerves. This was treated with 14 Gy defined to the 50% isodose line. The plan was obtained to limit the radiation dosage to the pons and medulla to 4 Gy. Please note a good conformance of the 50% isodose line to the size and shape of the treated lesion.

12.6.4
Microsurgery After Stereotactic Radiosurgery

As acoustic tumors continue to grow, they can exert mass effect upon other cranial nerves and the brain stem. Such mass effect can ultimately result in noncommunicating hydrocephalus, cranial nerve palsies, and even quadriparesis or coma. Currently, the only way to reliably relieve such mass effect is with microsurgery. With stereotactic radiosurgery, it is impossible at the present time to have such a significant impact on the mass effect of the tumor. For that reason, tumors greater than 2.5 cm in size must be managed surgically.

In certain circumstances, radiosurgery has proven ineffective, thus necessitating microsurgery after radiosurgery. Pendl et al. (1996) presented six cases of acoustic neuromas with macrocystic components. In all six cases, the cystic component increased significantly in size. In half of the cases, urgent microsurgery had to be performed to relieve the mass effect of the expanding cysts (Pendl et al. 1996). It appears that tumors with cystic components carry a risk of acutely expanding after radiosurgery.

The use of microsurgery after failed radiosurgery was analyzed by Pollock et al. (1998a,b). These clinicians evaluated 452 patients at a mean of 41 months follow-up. The authors found it necessary to perform microsurgery on 2.9% of all patients. The neurosurgeons reported increased surgical difficulty compared to their experience with untreated tumors in 8 of 13 cases. The increased difficulty was related to tumor fibrosis in one case, loss of the peritumoral arachnoid plane in four patients, and scarring in three patients. The treatment outcome for this group of patients was significantly worse than for patients

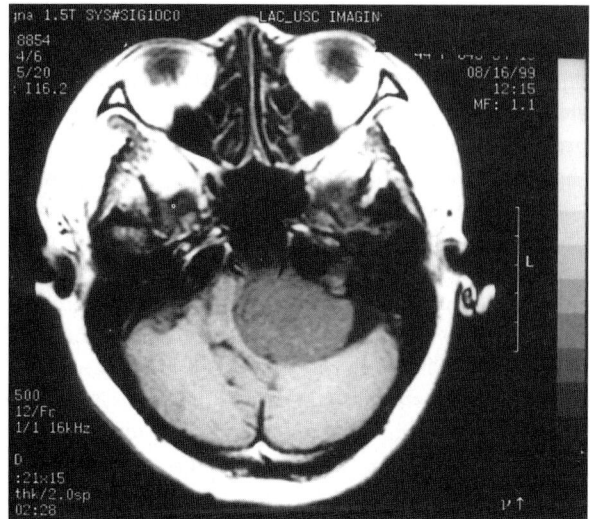

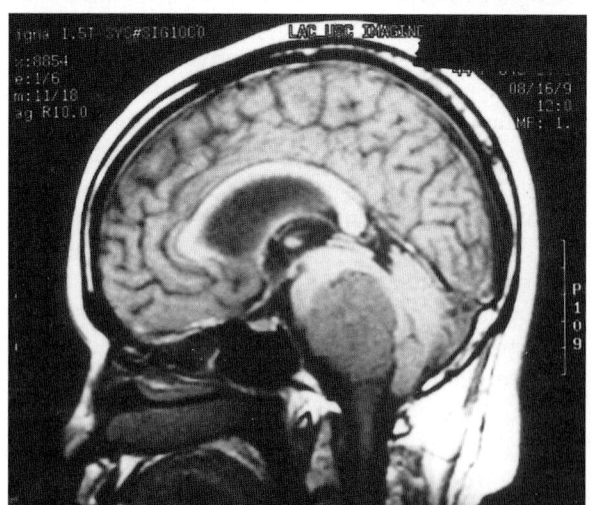

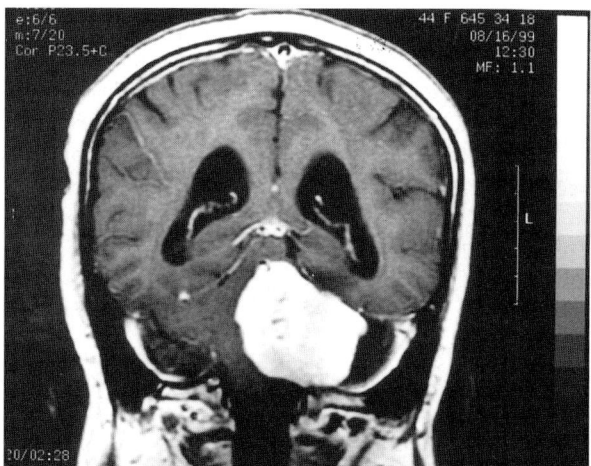

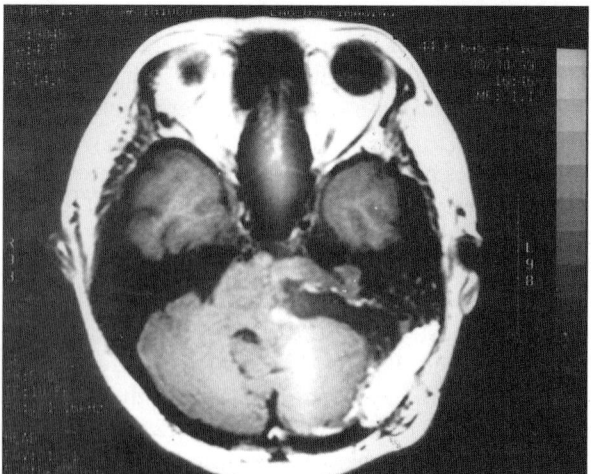

Fig. 12.6. a Axial, T1-weighted MRI of the brain without contrast reveals a large tumor of the cerebellopontine angle that is slightly hypointense to the pons and cerebellum. It is causing severe compression of the pons and cerebellum. The mass is occluding the fourth ventricle, and impairing cerebrospinal fluid dynamics. **b** An axial T1-weighted image of the brain reveals significant contrast enhancement of the tumor with extension into the internal auditory canal laterally. **c** A coronal T1-weighted image of the brain with contrast reveals the magnitude of the tumor. The tumor extends from the tentorium superiorly to just above the foramen magnum inferiorly. The ventricles are dilated due to hydrocephalus. **d** A sagittal T1-weighted image of the brain without contrast further illustrates the deformation of the pons and brain stem from this very large vestibular schwannoma. **e** Axial T1-weighted image of the brain without contrast reveals a small residual cap of tumor along the pons and facial nerve. The deformation of the pons has been relieved. The fourth ventricle is now patent, thus reestablishing CSF flow. **f** Axial T1-weighted image of the brain with contrast further delineates the small residual tumor. **g** This T1-weighted MRI of the brain with contrast is the gamma knife treatment plan for this patient. The residual tumor was treated with 14 Gy to the 50% isodose line

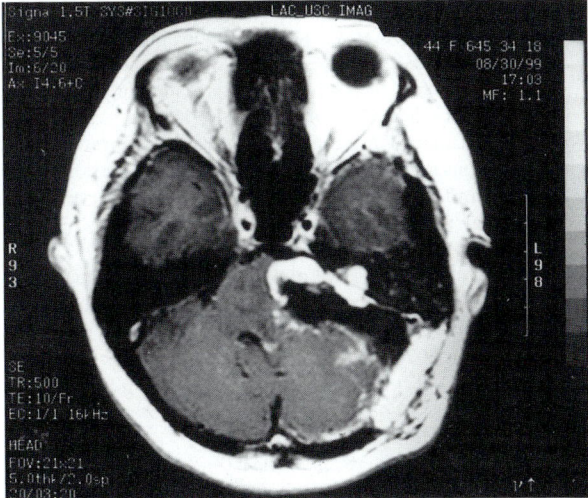

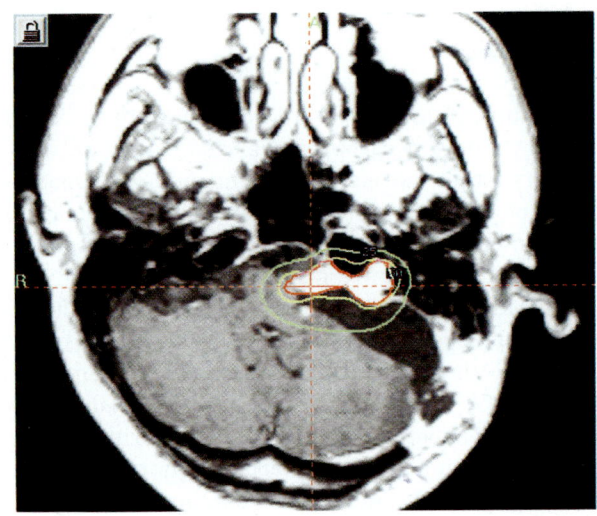

who had not had prior radiosurgery. There was a significant decrease in facial nerve function (House grades IV–VI) after microsurgery in 70% of the patients with normal facial nerve function (House grade I or II) prior to delayed microsurgery.

SLATTERY and BRACKMAN (1995) observed a similar difficulty with microsurgery after prior radiosurgery. These surgeons presented five patients who required microsurgery for tumor progression despite radiosurgery. The surgeons reported significant scarring of the tumor to the facial nerve in all cases. They ascribed the poor outcome of facial nerve function after surgery to this scarring and loss of normal anatomic planes. It is likely that radiosurgery adversely affects the microvasculature of the cranial nerves. Consequently, the trigeminal, facial, and cochlear nerves are less able to withstand surgical manipulation after previous radiosurgery. As long-term data on the patients who are treated with lower radiation doses emerge, it is likely that neurosurgeons and neurotologists will be faced with this surgical dilemma even more frequently.

12.7
Conservative Management and Natural History

In certain circumstances, small acoustic neuromas may be managed conservatively. WIET et al. (1995) followed 53 patients with small acoustic neuromas ranging from 0.2 to 3 cm in size. They observed an average tumor growth rate of 1.6 mm a year. More importantly, 60% of the patients had no demonstrable tumor growth at an average of 2.1 years of follow-up. FUCCI et al. (1999) observed similar findings amongst elderly patients with small tumors. They followed 119 patients with a mean age of 65 years. The range of follow-up was 5 months to 8 years with a mean of 2.5 years. During this period, only 30% of the tumors demonstrated any growth, 66% showed no growth, and 4% showed regression of tumor size without treatment.

DEEN et al. (1996) also demonstrated the indolent nature of some acoustic tumors. These clinicians analyzed 68 patients who were managed conservatively. In this study, the 68 patients did not receive treatment due to advanced age, patient preference, minimal symptoms, poor medical condition, asymptomatic tumor, or tumor in the only hearing ear. With a mean follow-up of 3.4 years, 71% of the patients showed no tumor growth. The patients that went on to require treatment had a tumor growth rate of 3 mm a year. The patients that had tumor growth, but still did not need treatment, had a tumor growth rate of only 0.36 mm a year. These data suggest that acoustic tumors may manifest a full spectrum of biological activity, from complete indolence to more persistent growth. Those tumors that manifest symptoms or rapid growth should be treated. Those tumors that do not show progression on serial imaging may be managed conservatively.

12.8
Conclusion

The suboccipital craniotomy, translabyrinthine craniotomy, middle fossa approach, and stereotactic radiosurgery are all vital elements in the modern management of vestibular schwannomas. At the present, we recommend microsurgical removal of these tumors whenever possible. We instrument the suboccipital approach for all tumors in patients with functional hearing preoperatively, and for very large tumors that extend to the foramen magnum or to the tentorial margin. We use the translabyrinthine craniotomy when the patient has lost functional hearing. When the tumor is limited to the internal auditory canal and hearing preservation is the goal, we employ the middle fossa approach. We utilize the gamma knife for tumors less than 2.5 cm in patients over 60 years of age, those who cannot tolerate general anesthesia, or those who refuse open surgery. We also use stereotactic radiosurgery as an adjunct when the tumor cannot be safely removed by microsurgical means.

References

Arriaga MA, Luxford WM, et al. (1994) Facial nerve unction following middle fossa and translabyrinthine acoustic tumor surgery: a comparison. Am J Otol 15(5):620–624

Brackmann DE (1992) Middle fossa approach for acoustic tumor removal. Clin Neurosurg 38: 603–618.

Brackmann DE and Green JD (1992) Translabyrinthine approach for acoustic tumor removal. Otolaryngol Clin North Am 25(2): 311–329

Brackmann DE, House JR.3rd, et al. (1994) Technical modifications to the middle fossa craniotomy approach in removal of acoustic neuromas." Am J Otol 15(5): 614–9.

Cushing H (1921) Further Concerning the Acoustic Neuromas. Laryngoscope 31(4): 209–228

Deen HG, Ebersold MJ, et al. (1996) Conservative management of acoustic neuroma: an outcome study. Neurosurgery 39(2): 260–4; discussion 264–266

DiTullio MV,Jr., Malkasian D, et al. (1978) A critical comparison of neurosurgical and otolaryngological approaches to acoustic neuromas. J Neurosurg 48(1): 1–12.

Ebersold MJ, Harner SG, et al. (1992) Current results of the retrosigmoid approach to acoustic neurinoma [see comments]. J Neurosurg 76(6): 901–909

Flickinger JC (1999) Observation versus early stereotactic radiotherapy of acoustic neuroma: what are you waiting for? [editorial; comment]. Int J Radiat Oncol Biol Phys 44(3): 481–482

Flickinger JC, Kondziolka D, et al. (1998) Clinical applications of stereotactic radiosurgery. Cancer Treat Res 93: 283–297

Flickinger JC, Kondziolka D, et al. (1996) Evolution in technique for vestibular schwannoma radiosurgery and effect on outcome. Int J Radiat Oncol Biol Phys 36(2): 275–280

Flickinger JC, Lunsford LD, et al. (1991) Radiosurgery of acoustic neurinomas. Cancer 67(2): 345–353

Flickinger JC, Lunsford LD, et al. (1993) Gamma knife radiosurgery for acoustic tumors: multivariate analysis of four year results. Radiother Oncol 27(2): 91–98

Fucci MJ, Buchman CA, et al. (1999). Acoustic tumor growth: implications for treatment choices. Am J Otol 20(4): 495–499.

Gardner G and Robertson JH (1988) Hearing preservation in unilateral acoustic neuroma surgery. Ann Otol Rhinol Laryngol 97(1): 55–66

Gardner G, Robertson JH, et al. (1983) 105 patients operated upon for cerebellopontine angle tumors – experience using combined approach and CO2 laser." Laryngoscope 93(8): 1049–1055.

Giannotta SL (1992) Translabyrinthine approach for removal of medium and large tumors of the cerebellopontine angle. Clin Neurosurg 38: 589–602

Gormley WB, Sekhar LN, et al. (1997) Acoustic neuromas: results of current surgical management [see comments]. Neurosurgery 41(1): 50–8; discussion 58–60

Haberkamp TJ, Meyer GA, et al. (1998). Surgical exposure of the fundus of the internal auditory canal: anatomic limits of the middle fossa versus the retrosigmoid transcanal approach. Laryngoscope 108(8 Pt 1): 1190–1194

Haines SJ and Levine SC (1993) Intracanalicular acoustic neuroma: early surgery for preservation of hearing. J Neurosurg 79(4): 515–520

Hardy DG, Macfarlane R, et al. (1989) Surgery for acoustic neurinoma. An analysis of 100 translabyrinthine operations [see comments]. J Neurosurg 71(6): 799–804

House HP and House WF (1964) Historical Review and Problem of Acoustic Neuroma. Archives of Otolaryngology 80: 601–605

House JW (1983) Facial nerve grading systems. Laryngoscope 93(8): 1056–1069

House WF (1964) Evolution of Transtemporal Bone Removal of Acoustic Tumors. Archives of Otolaryngology 80: 731–742

House WF and Hitselberger WE (1964) Morbidity and Mortality of Acoustic Neuromas. Archives of Otolaryngology 80: 752–756

Jackler RK (1994) Acoustic Neuroma. Neurotology. 1: 729–785

King TT and Morrison AW (1980) Translabyrinthine and transtentorial removal of acoustic nerve tumors. Results in 150 cases. J Neurosurg 52(2): 210–216

Kondziolka D and Lunsford LD (1993) Preservation of hearing in acoustic neurinoma surgery [letter; comment]. J Neurosurg 78(1): 154–156

Kondziolka D, Lunsford LD, et al. (1998) Long-term outcomes after radiosurgery for acoustic neuromas [see comments]. N Engl J Med 339(20): 1426–1433

Lanman TH, Brackmann DE, et al. (1999) Report of 190 consecutive cases of large acoustic tumors (vestibular schwannoma) removed via the translabyrinthine approach. J Neurosurg 90(4): 617–623

Leksell L. (1983) Stereotactic radiosurgery. J Neurol Neurosurg Psychiatry 46(9): 797–803

Linskey ME, Lunsford LD, et al. (1990) Radiosurgery for acoustic neurinomas: early experience. Neurosurgery 26(5): 736–44; discussion 744–745

Lunsford LD, Kamerer DB, et al. (1990) Stereotactic radiosurgery for acoustic neuromas. Arch Otolaryngol Head Neck Surg 116(8): 907–909

Lunsford LD, Kondziolka D, et al. (1992) Radiosurgery as an alternative to microsurgery of acoustic tumors. Clin Neurosurg 38: 619–634

Lunsford LD and LINSKEY ME (1992) Stereotactic radiosurgery in the treatment of patients with acoustic tumors. Otolaryngol Clin North Am 25(2): 471–491

Miller RC, Foote RL, et al. (1999) Decrease in cranial nerve complications after radiosurgery for acoustic neuromas: a prospective study of dose and volume. Int J Radiat Oncol Biol Phys 43(2): 305–311

Niranjan A, Lunsford LD, et al. (1999) Dose reduction improves hearing preservation rates after intracanalicular acoustic tumor radiosurgery. Neurosurgery 45(4): 753–62; discussion 762–765

Noren G, Arndt J, et al. (1983) Stereotactic radiosurgery in cases of acoustic neurinoma: further experiences. Neurosurgery 13(1): 12–22

Ogunrinde OK, Lunsford DL, et al. (1995) Cranial nerve preservation after stereotactic radiosurgery of intracanalicular acoustic tumors. Stereotact Funct Neurosurg 64(Suppl 1): 87–97

Pendl G, Ganz JC, et al. (1996) Acoustic neurinomas with macrocysts treated with Gamma Knife radiosurgery. Stereotact Funct Neurosurg 66(Suppl 1): 103–111

Pollock BE, Lunsford LD, et al. (1998a) Vestibular schwannoma management. Part I. Failed microsurgery and the role of delayed stereotactic radiosurgery. J Neurosurg 89(6): 944–948

Pollock BE, Lunsford LD, et al. (1998b) Vestibular schwannoma management. Part II. Failed radiosurgery and the role of delayed microsurgery. J Neurosurg 89(6): 949–955

Pollock BE, Lunsford LD, et al. (1998c) Vestibular schwannoma management in the next century: a radiosurgical perspective. Neurosurgery 43(3): 475–481; discussion 481–483

Rhoton AL, Jr. and Tedeschi H (1992) Microsurgical anatomy of acoustic neuroma. Otolaryngol Clin North Am 25(2): 257–294

Samii M and Matthies C (1997) Management of 1000 vestibular schwannomas (acoustic neuromas): hearing function in 1000 tumor resections. Neurosurgery 40(2): 248–260; discussion 260–262

Samii M, Matthies C, et al. (1991) Intracanalicular acoustic neurinomas. Neurosurgery 29(2): 189–198; discussion 198–199

Shelton C (1992) Hearing preservation in acoustic tumor surgery. Otolaryngol Clin North Am 25(3): 609–621

Shelton C (1995) Unilateral acoustic tumors: how often do they recur after translabyrinthine removal? Laryngoscope 105(9 Pt 1): 958–966

Shelton C, Brackmann DE, et al. (1989a) Acoustic tumor surgery. Prognostic factors in hearing conversation. Arch Otolaryngol Head Neck Surg 115(10): 1213–1216

Shelton C, Brackmann DE, et al. (1989b) Middle fossa acoustic tumor surgery: results in 106 cases. Laryngoscope 99(4): 405–408

Shelton C, Hitselberger WE, et al. (1990) Hearing preservation after acoustic tumor removal: long-term results. Laryngoscope 100(2 Pt 1): 115–119

Shelton C and House WF (1990) Hearing improvement after acoustic tumor removal. Otolaryngol Head Neck Surg 103(6): 963–965

Slattery WH,3rd, and Brackmann DE (1995) Results of surgery following stereotactic irradiation for acoustic neuromas. Am J Otol 16(3): 315–319; discussion 319–321

Slattery WH,3rd, Brackmann DE, et al. (1997). Middle fossa approach for hearing preservation with acoustic neuromas [published erratum appears in Am J Otol 1997 Nov;18(6):796]. Am J Otol 18(5): 596–601.

Stone JL (1999). Sir Charles Ballance: pioneer British neurological surgeon. Neurosurgery 44(3):610–631; discussion 631–632

Tatagiba M, Samii M, et al. (1992) The significance for postoperative hearing of preserving the labyrinth in acoustic neurinoma surgery. J Neurosurg 77(5): 677–684

Tedeschi, H. and A. L. Rhoton, Jr. (1994) Lateral approaches to the petroclival region. Surg Neurol 41(3): 180–216

Umezu H and Aiba T (1994) Preservation of hearing after surgery for acoustic schwannomas: correlation between cochlear nerve function and operative findings. J Neurosurg 80(5): 844–848

Umezu H, Aiba T, et al. (1996) Early and late postoperative hearing preservation in patients with acoustic neuromas. Neurosurgery 39(2): 267–71; discussion 271–272

Wiet RJ, Zappia JJ, et al. (1995) Conservative management of patients with small acoustic tumors. Laryngoscope 105(8 Pt 1): 795–800

13 Surgical Therapy and Problems in the Treatment of Meningiomas

Bernard George

CONTENTS

13.1
Introduction

Meningiomas are generally benign tumors of the central nervous system that are usually described as highly curable lesions. Some meningiomas, however, may present at sites that make surgical treatment difficult. Moreover, even those meningiomas appearing benign on histological examination may be clinically aggressive. Multiple clinical and histological parameters are helpful in defining optimal management and the correct level of treatment. These parameters may relate to the following:

1. Biological behavior of the tumor
2. Location of the tumor
3. Gross appearance of the tumor on an imaging study
4. Presence of tumor extension to neighboring structures
5. Patient's general and neurological status
6. The presence or absence of previous treatment(s)

Some of the above parameters guide the neurosurgeon in selection of the most appropriate treatment modality for a given patient. The most frequently used management options in patients with meningiomas are: surgery, radiotherapy, chemotherapy or follow-up only without a specific treatment. If surgical treatment is selected, a detailed decision on the use of the most appropriate surgical technique is needed in order to optimize the extent of tumor resection and to make it compatible with the best possible quality of life of the treated patient.

13.2
Biological Behavior

Meningiomas originate from cells of the arachnoid capsule and are most frequently benign tumors characterized by a slow rate of growth. Progressive tumor growth may produce compression of the neighboring structures with their subsequent displacement, and sometimes encasement without actual invasion. Therefore, a plane of cleavage may be found between the meningioma capsule and nerve sheaths, blood vessels or the brain (spinal cord) surface. This cleavage plane is initially represented by the arachnoid membranes, which may remain intact for a very long period of time. Therefore, a fundamental principle of meningioma resection is opening of the plane between the tumor surface and the arachnoid. Subsequently, dissection is carried out as much as possible away from the arachnoid membrane. In fact, as long as the surgeon follows this principle, the important functional elements are kept on the other side of the arachnoid and there is a very low risk of complications. Even in the case of the tumor embedding nerves or blood vessels, the arachnoid membrane surrounding them is, at least initially, intact. This usually permits preservation of these important structures.

Following what is usually a long period of time, tumor growth produces a transgression of the arachnoid membrane and the pia mater, eventually exposing the cortical surface. This leads to several difficulties regarding the surgical resection. The first is the recruitment of feeding blood vessels from arterial branches supplying the brain or nerve sheaths or

B. George, M.D.
Professor and Chief of Service, Department of Neurosurgery, Hôpital Lariboisière-Paris-France, Service de Neurochirurgie, Hôpital Lariboisière, 2 rue Ambroise Paré, 75010 Paris, France

blood vessels (SINDOU and ALAYWAN 1998). These vessels cannot be surgically controlled as easily as vessels primarily supplying the tumor. For cranial meningiomas, the primary blood supply comes from branches of the external carotid artery, which may be embolized or surgically occluded with very minimal risk to the patient. When the arachnoid membrane is transgressed, the arterial blood supply also comes from branches of the internal carotid artery, which makes dissection even more difficult. The second problem relates to a loss of an open plane between the surrounding structures and the tumor surface. Obviously, the separation and preservation of these structures may become questionable. The third problem is a development of peritumoral edema, which is generally much more significant in case of arachnoid and pia mater involvement (Fig. 13.1). The severity of the peritumoral edema may be linked to other factors such as tumor size, the degree of brain compression, or venous occlusion. However, an involvement and transgression of the meningeal covering of the brain leads to increased permeability of the blood–brain barrier. Clearly, the presence of edema in the brain surrounding meningiomas makes their dissection much more difficult. Several recent studies have emphasized the relation between brain invasion and the presence of peritumoral edema, and between edema, vascular supply, magnetic resonance imaging (MRI) appearance and tumor resectability (Go et al. 1988; HINO et al. 1990; ILDAN et al. 1999; KAWASE et al. 1985; MANTLE et al. 1999; SALPIETRO et al. 1994). In one study, it was found that the probability of brain invasion increases by 20% for every centimeter of peritumoral edema (MANTLE et al. 1999). Moreover, 100% of patients with malignant meningiomas have well-expressed peritumoral edema. ILDAN et al. (1999) found a significant correlation between the T2 MRI signal of meningiomas and the brain–tumor interface, which the authors graded into the three following groups:

1. Smooth
2. Intermediate
3. Invasive

Another study demonstrated a linear relation between peritumoral edema and the presence of tumor in the cortical surface (Go et al. 1988). SINDOU and ALAYWAN (1998) showed that vascular tumoral supply by cortical arteries is associated with edema and invasion of the cortical surface. In fact, all of the above factors are linked. Tumor presence in superficial layers of the cortex, the presence of arterial blood supply to the tumor from cortical arteries and development of edema result in:

1. Greater difficulty in safely finding the plane of separation between brain and tumor surface
2. The need for more surgical manipulations of the brain

As a consequence, the rate of total resection decreases, severe post-operative edema is more likely to occur and post-operative morbidity increases.

In more aggressive meningiomas there is invasion of the surrounding structures. True invasion of intradural structures such as brain, nerves or blood vessels does not exist in benign forms of meningioma. However, infiltration of extradural elements is not uncommon and may involve adjacent muscles, bone, nerve sheaths and blood vessels (CAHAN et al. 1948; INOUE et al. 1984; LEONETTI et al. 1993; Fig. 13.2). Obviously, invasion of the arterial wall never occurs at primary presentation, but is only observed in the intradural space in patients who have undergone previous surgery or radiotherapy. It is also commonly observed in those with extradural tumor extension (Fig. 13.3). The common finding in such cases is a lack of the subarachnoid membrane, which has disappeared after previous treatments and does

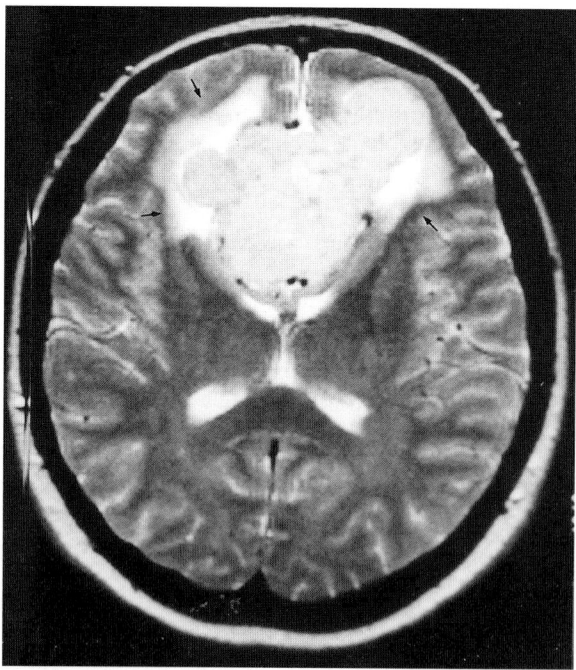

Fig. 13.1. Olfactory groove meningioma with bilateral extension. T2 MRI axial view. Notice the edema (*white hypersignal*) surrounding the tumor and the vessels (*black signal void*) stretched over the tumor margins

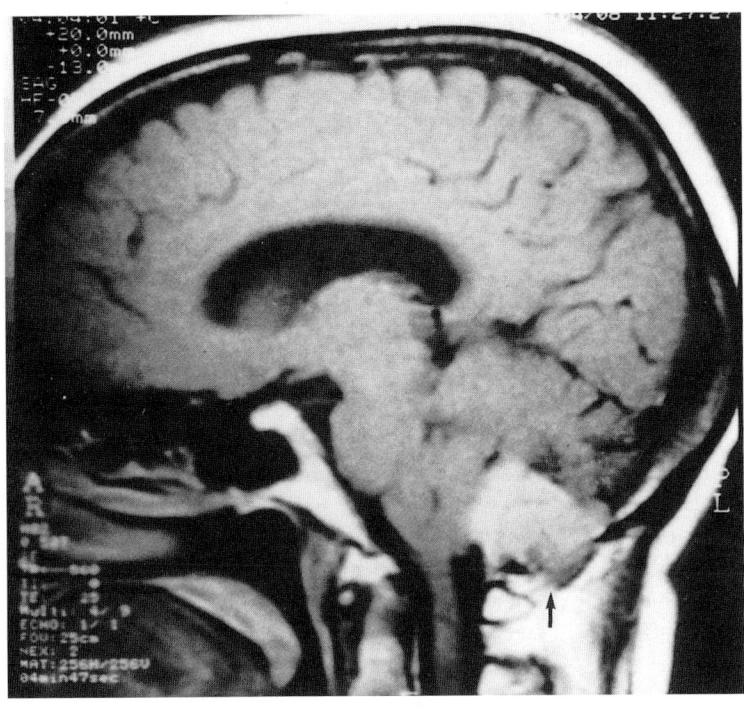

Fig. 13.2. Meningioma of the cerebellar convexity with bone and muscular extension. MRI sagittal view

not exist in the extradural space. At this point, the cavernous sinus should be considered as the extradural space. Tumor invasion of the internal carotid artery wall and oculomotor nerve sheaths has clearly been demonstrated in this meningioma location (Huvos et al. 1973; Kotapka et al. 1994; Shaffrey et al. 1999).

A particularly aggressive biological behavior may be clearly explained in some cases by the histological features of the tumor. Many different histological classifications have been proposed for meningiomas since 1922 (Oberling 1922). Hemangiopericytoma was once considered a subtype of meningioma but was removed from this tumor classification. Hemangiopericytomas are most commonly invasive tumors with disruption of meningeal membranes, the presence of arterial cortical feeders, and peritumoral edema. They often invade the dura, bone and subcutaneous tissues. About 25% of patients present with metastasis (Goellner et al. 1978). In fact, the currently used classification (Kleihues et al. 1993) follows the World Health Organization (WHO) definition of meningioma, which includes only tumors derived from meningothelial

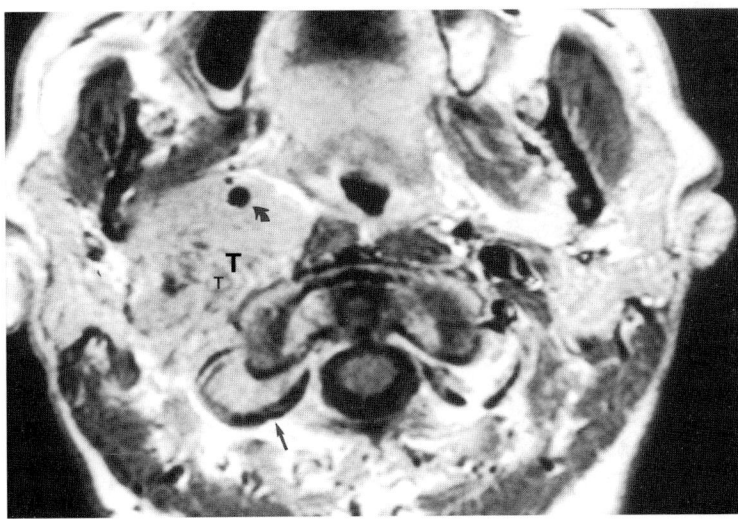

Fig. 13.3. Extracranial meningioma (*T*) embedding the vertebral artery (*arrow*) at the C1 level and the carotid artery (*curved arrow*)

cells and excludes those developed from connective elements of the meninges. In the WHO classification, three grades are distinguished according to histological criteria such as number of mitosis, cell density, nuclear/cytoplasmic ratio, presence of necrosis and modification of tissue architecture. Therefore, following the WHO classification, some types of meningiomas are clearly benign (grade I), among which meningothelial, fibromatous, and transitional meningiomas are the most common. Some other types of meningioma, which are obviously malignant (grade III), include: meningiosarcomas, anaplastic and papillary forms (CAHAN et al. 1948; INOUE et al. 1984; PASQUIER et al. 1986; THOMAS and BERRY 1981). The intermediate forms are considered as having the potential for aggressiveness, but this is not always demonstrated (grade II). Radiation-induced meningioma is another category that includes tumors with aggressive biological behavior, as reflected by their multiple sites of presentation, malignancy and high incidence of recurrence (CAHAN et al. 1948; HARRISON and SUNDARESAN 1991; KUMAR et al. 1987; MANN et al. 1953; MODAN et al. 1974; RUBINSTEIN et al. 1984; SOFFER et al. 1989). However, there are some exceptions especially among presumably benign types of tumors which may nonetheless rapidly recur with locally invasive features (Fig. 13.4), or even with metastasis (CLAVERE et al. 1990; MILLER et al. 1985; NOTTERMAN et al. 1987).

Moreover among „true" benign meningiomas, the rate of growth is highly variable. Therefore, deciding at surgery to leave part of a tumor that is located near an important structure in order to avoid the risks of post-operative sequellae may be:

1. A good decision in case of a slow-growing tumor, since it lets the patient enjoy a normal life for a long period of time.
2. A poor decision because, in the case of a fast-growing benign meningioma, it does not give the patient an optimal chance of a cure through a radical resection, while the function of a tumor-involved structure will be impaired shortly after surgery.

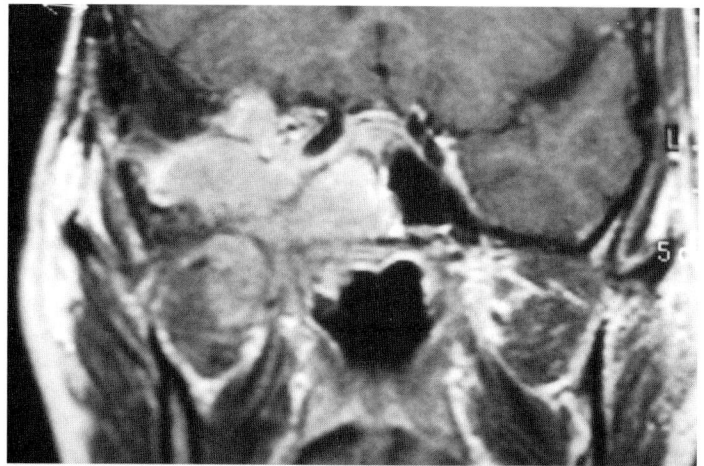

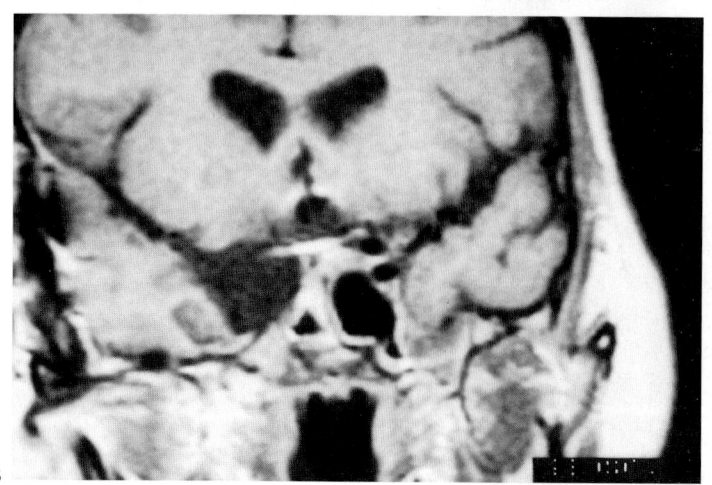

Fig. 13.4A,B. Early recurrence (12 months) of a histologically benign clinoid meningioma with cavernous sinus; sphenoid sinus and infratemporal extension. **A** Pre-operative MRI coronal view. **B** Post-operative MRI coronal view after exenteration of the cavernous sinus

Currently there is a lack of data on the natural evolution of the individual types of meningioma, such as regarding tumor growth rate and local invasiveness. There are a number of other important parameters, such as mitotic index (MIB1), antigen Ki67 and bromodeoxymidin (BrDU) incorporation. However, at this point in time these cannot be considered as sufficiently reliable predictors of tumor behavior (MATSUNO et al. 1996; McCORMICK et al. 1993; IDE et al. 1996; OHTA et al. 1994; PLATE et al. 1990; SHIBUYA et al. 1992), although they do provide information on the phases of tumor cell division. The specimens are all obtained at surgery and therefore give information a posteriori. Moreover even with qualitative assessments, the results of recently published studies still present conflicting information. Therefore, before making a decision on the appropriateness and extent of surgery (more or less radical resection), it may be useful to propose a short-term period of observation with the use of frequent MRI. This policy is especially warranted in older patients (>70 years) or in any patient in poor general condition in whom there is a higher risk of complications either due to general anesthesia or post-operatively. In some cases, surgery clearly needs to be carried out, for example, with large meningiomas with severe brain compression and meningiomas with clear signs of aggressiveness, such as the presence of extradural invasion or extensive peritumoral edema. Meningiomas in the close vicinity of the optic nerve also need to be removed without delay. In such cases, waiting for demonstration of local tumor progression is likely to lead to a much more surgically risky situation because of tumor extension into the optic canal or the cavernous sinus. In the vast majority of other cases, a 1- or 2-year follow-up may provide very useful information, allowing better definition of tumor behavior and thus the appropriate therapeutic decision. A follow-up period may help to avoid unnecessary surgery or provide a more solid basis for proposing a surgical resection.

Meningiomas occurring in children present different problems and may more frequently require surgical resection. Meningiomas in patients under 15 years of age are rare (CHOUX et al. 1991). They represent only 1%–2% of all intracranial tumors of infancy and childhood (DRAKE et al. 1985; MERTENS et al. 1974) and only 1%–2% of all meningiomas (DRAKE et al. 1985; MERTENS et al. 1974). They are often multiple and are found in association with neurofibromatosis. They are also more likely to be

malignant. Some reports also mention the presence of a more frequent extradural extension and underline the generally more aggressive tumor behavior (CHOUX et al. 1991; CROUSE and BERG 1972; MATSON 1969; MERTENS et al. 1974).

13.3
Tumor Location

The location of meningiomas markedly influences the ease and the extent of surgical resection (CHAN et al. 1984; JAASKELAINEN et al. 1991; KALLIO et al. 1992; MIRIMANOFF et al. 1985; SUTHERLAND and SIMA 1991; THOMAS and BERRY 1981; Table 13.1). In the convexity, where meningiomas most frequently occur, surgical access is straightforward and removal of the base of implantation may be performed with a wide margin. However, even in tumors arising in the convexity, the rate of recurrence is not as low as their quality of resection should suggest. According to a study reported by SIMPSON (1957), the extent of resection should correlate with the rate of recurrence. He recommended the use of the following grading system: grade I, the dura at the site of tumoral attachment is resected and recurrence should be uncommon; grade II, dura is left in place but coagulated; grade III, a piece of meningioma is left attached to the dura; grade IV, a partial resection is achieved. In meningiomas arising in the convexity, Simpson grade I resection can be performed in most cases, the noticeable exception

Table 13.1 Location of meningiomas

	Benign SUTHERLAND CANTORE (1991)		CANTORE and SIMA (1991)	(1991)
SUTHERLAND and SIMA (1991)				
	$N=169$	$N=625$	$N=14$	$N=65$
Supratentorial				
Convexity	35%	23%	50%	–
Parasagittal	23%	32.5%	30%	33%
Sphenoid ridge	18%	20%	20%	28%
Tuberculum sellae	4%	6.5%	–	6%
Olfactory groove	3.5%	6.7%	–	10%
Tentorial	4%	4.8%	–	9%
Orbital	2.4%	2%	–	3%
Infratentorial	9%	4%	–	12%

being tumors close to the venous sinus (Fig. 13.5), such as parasagittal meningiomas (BEKS et al. 1988; BONNAL AND BROTCHI 1978; KONDZIOLKA et al. 1998). In an important study on 657 single meningiomas of benign type, 165 patients (25%) had tumors arising in the convexity (JAASKELAINEN et al. 1991). Of these 165 patients, 159 (96%) had a Simpson grade I resection and eight (5%) recurrences were observed, while six had a grade II resection with one (17%) recurrence being noted. Conversely, there were 136 parasagittal meningiomas with nine (9%) recurrences following grade I resection (N=105) and five (16%) after grade II resection (N=31). The overall results showed a 5.4% incidence of recurrence in convexity meningiomas as compared to a 10% incidence of recurrence in parasagittal meningiomas. The recurrence rate was 21% in olfactory groove meningiomas and 16% in sphenoid ridge meningiomas. In skull base meningiomas, the rate of recurrence has been reported to be up to 30% of patients. In Jaaskelainen's study, the recurrence rate in the total series of 657 patients was estimated by life-table analysis to be 19% at 20 years (JAASKELAINEN et al. 1991). The observed median time to recurrence was 7.5 years. Three factors correlated strongly and independently with the incidence of recurrence: coagulation or removal of the dura,

tumor attachment to bone and tumor consistency (soft vs hard). Tumor location was analyzed separately as it would have divided the series into groups that were too small to allow for meaningful analysis. At 20 years post-treatment, the estimated recurrence rate was 18%, 21%, 29% and 36%, respectively for convexity, parasagittal, sphenoid ridge and olfactory groove meningiomas. In a multivariate analysis with the three factors mentioned above, the observed recurrence rate at 20 years was 11% with none of the factors present, 15%–24% with one factor present and 32%–56% with two factors present. This study excluded atypical and anaplastic forms of meningioma and thus showed the importance of the quality of resection, especially resection of the adjacent dura. However, it must be stressed again that the rate of recurrence after grade I resection is at least 5% for convexity meningiomas and an average of 15% for the overall series. This means that the location of the tumor and its biological behavior are important factors predicting tumor recurrence following surgical resection.

Some additional parameters are also known to influence the incidence of tumor recurrence. The presence of bone involvement has been a matter of debate for a long time. In some cases, it corresponds to a simple hyperostosis in relation to bone hypervascularization, while in others, it represents real tumoral extension into the bone, which requires extensive bone resection (ARANA et al. 1996; AZAR-KIA et al. 1974; DEROME and GUIOT 1978; MAROON et al. 1994; PIEPER et al. 1999; POMPILI et al. 1981; Fig. 13.6). Therefore, radical tumor removal should not only include resection of the dural attachment but also removal of the bone adjacent to the tumoral insertion. Another important factor is the dura surrounding the true zone of tumor attachment (TOKUMARO et al. 1990; WILMS et al. 1989). On MRI scanning, it is often seen as a contrast enhancement of the dura mater widely exceeding the dural attachment (Figs. 13.7, 13.8). As for the bone, the question is our ability to differentiate the presence of reactive hypervascularization vs true bone involvement by meningioma. If it corresponds to a tumoral extension into the bone, resection should include the involved bone. Histological studies of surgical specimens have shown that both explanations may be correct (BOROVICH AND DORON 1986; SCHÖRNER et al. 1990). In some studies, nests of meningioma cells have been found at a relatively remote distance (up to 2 cm) from the gross tumor (BOROVICH AND DORON 1986).

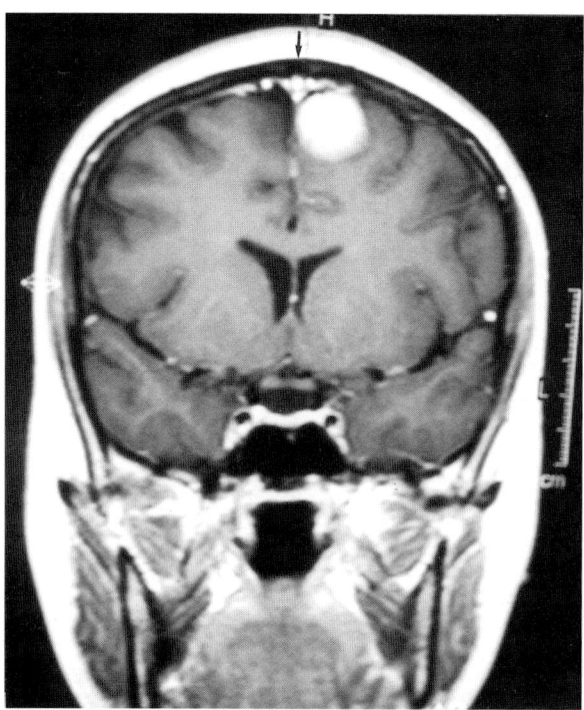

Fig. 13.5. Parasagittal meningioma attached on the lateral wall of the superior sagittal sinus. MRI coronal view

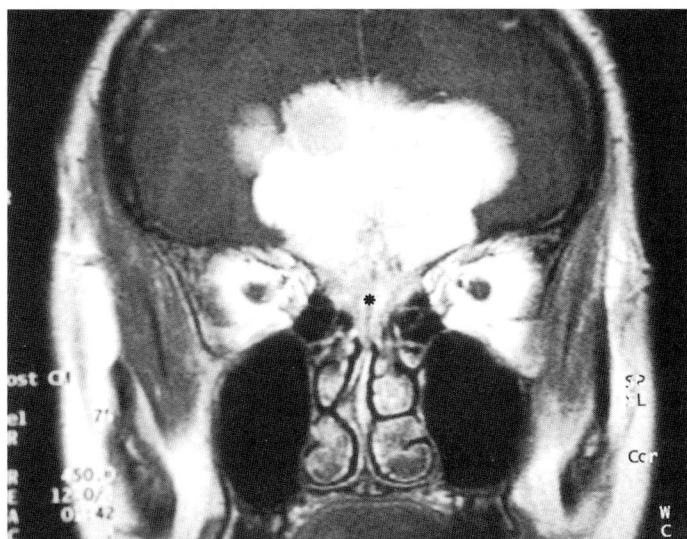

Fig. 13.6. Olfactory groove meningioma. T1 MRI coronal view. Notice the ethmoidal extension (*)

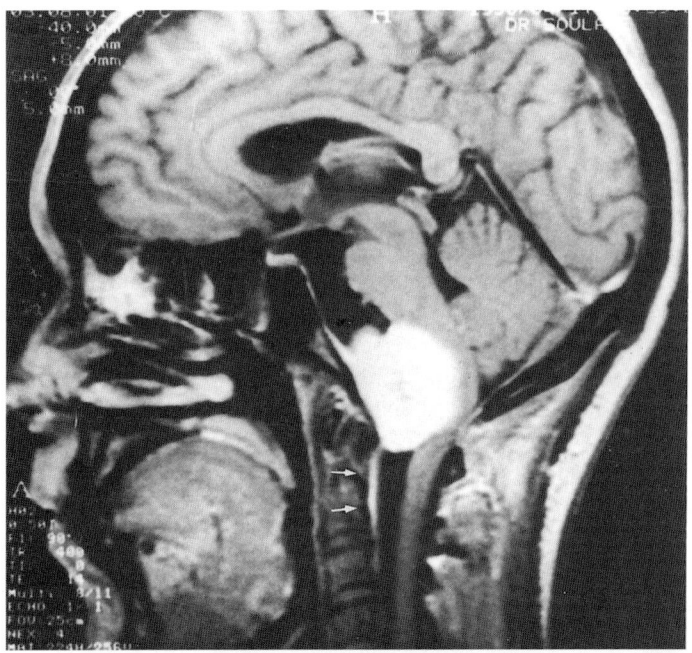

Fig. 13.7. Contrast enhancement of the dura above and below the attachment of a foramen magnum meningioma. MRI sagittal view

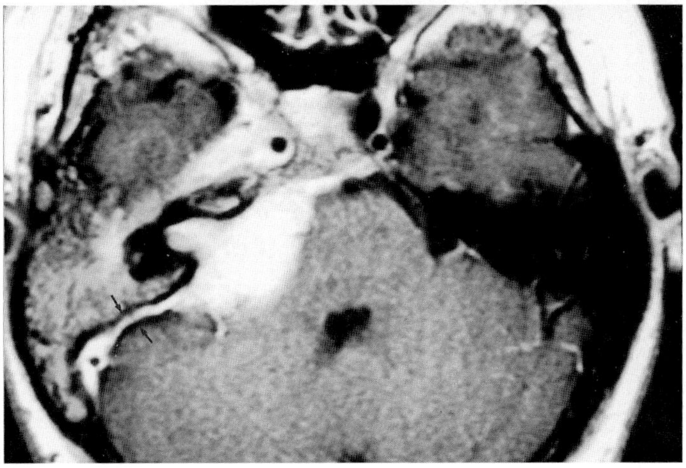

Fig. 13.8. En plaque meningioma of the petrous bone. Notice the contrast enhancement of the surrounding dura (compared with the opposite side)

In practice, surgical margins of 2 cm, which include extensive resection of the adjacent dura and bone, can be obtained in convexity meningiomas. For meningiomas arising in the other sites such margins are either impossible to obtain or the risk of complications is too high (Fig. 13.9). In surgical management of parasagittal meningiomas, the involvement of the venous sinus may be of major importance. In case of limited involvement of one wall, a resection and reconstruction with a graft taken from the falx or the pericranium is advisable (BONNAL AND BROTCHI 1991). More extensive involvement of the venous sinus needs a revascularization, which is associated with an unacceptable morbidity and mortality (BEDERSON et al. 1995; HAKUBA et al. 1979; SINDOU and HALLACQ 1966; STEIGER et al. 1989). A better choice is to let a small tumor remnant remain unresected, as tumor progression eventually will occlude the venous sinus. This „natural" occlusion is well-tolerated since it occurs slowly and progressively giving sufficient time for collateral vascular pathways to develop. A reoperation several years later will then resect the sinus without the need for revascularization (BONNAL AND BROTCHI 1978; BONNAL AND BROTCHI 1991; HARTMANN and KLUG 1975). However, it cannot be a wide resection that significantly extends beyond the gross tumor, as it would include a patent part of the sinus and functioning collateral cortical veins (CZERNICKI et al. 1991; GIOMBINI et al. 1984). In this situation, some authors have recently proposed a radiosurgical treatment of the tumor remnant involving the sinus, which can be performed electively following the first surgery (KONDZIOLKA et al. 1998). A similar problem is observed at the skull base with the

cranial nerves. Except for the facial nerve, which can be grafted with an acceptable success rate, other cranial nerves have to be preserved or deliberately sacrificed. The sacrifice at surgery of a fully functional nerve is not commonly acceptable. Therefore, in most cases, the surgeon has to choose between:

1. Leaving a part of the tumor adjacent to a nerve, removal of which is estimated as too risky for the preservation of nerve function
2. An attempt at resection, with a high probability of a transient nerve palsy and the hazard of a permanent deficit

The best example of this problem is cavernous sinus meningioma involving the oculomotor nerve. To the above comments, it must be added that, for the oculomotor nerves, a partial or even a subtotal recovery has a limited value for the patient since it results in the same problem of diplopia regardless of the degree of severity of the nerve palsy.

A special problem is presented by meningiomas of the optic nerve sheath. It is technically possible to resect these meningiomas but the resection leads without exception to complete blindness due to severance of all the tiny vascular branches supplying the nerve.

Over the past 10 years, major improvements have been made in surgical techniques combining microsurgery, computer-assisted surgery and various tools such as laser, ultrasonic aspirators and endoscopy. Currently, it is possible to drill the bone of any part of the skull base, to enter the cavernous sinus and to safely reach any part of the clivus. In spite of these surgical advances, radical resection of skull base

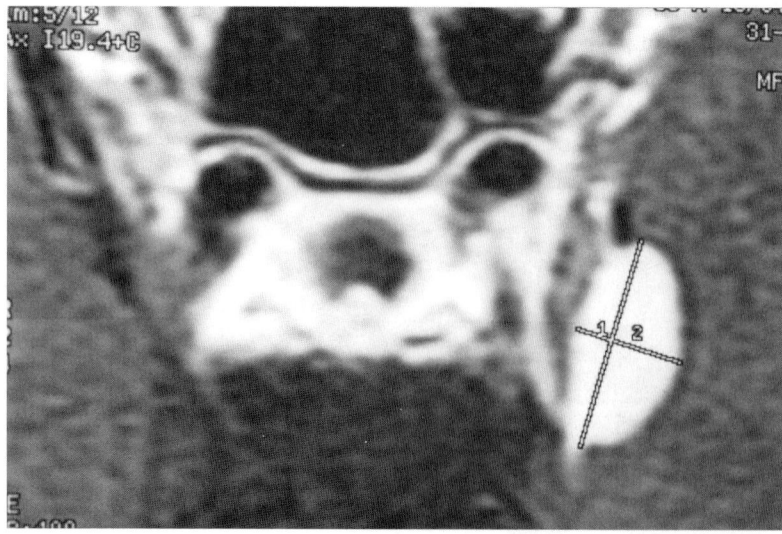

Fig. 13.9. Small meningioma attached to the lateral wall of the cavernous sinus. MRI axial view

Table 13.2 Suprasellar meningiomas

	N	Total removal	Mortality	Recurrence	Improved vision	Worsened vision
AL MEFTY et al. (1991)	35	91%	9%	8.7%	25%	3%
CONFORTI et al. (1991)	68	80%	16%	8.7%	59%	13%
GÖKALP et al. (1993)	88	67%	18%	4.5%	54%	19%
RUBIN et al. (1994)	67	85%	9%	7%	56%	9%
PUCHNER et al. (1998)	50	84%	2%	8%	67%	25%

meningiomas with wide resection of bone and dura is impossible to achieve. As an example, in Table 13.2, the rate of total tumor removal and the incidences of recurrence and improvement of vision are given for suprasellar meningiomas (PUCHNER et al. 1998). In the best-reported series, total tumor removal was achieved in 91% of patients but with vision improvement in only 25% and about a 9% incidence of tumor recurrence. The only case in which the term „radical resection" can be used is when exenteration of one area is performed. Obviously exenteration requires sacrificing the nerves and blood vessels passing through the resected area. Exenteration of the cavernous sinus including the internal carotid artery and all the nerves has been performed in ten cases (Fig. 13.4). In all ten patients, the relevant nerve function was already impaired, a high rate of tumor growth was documented or an early recurrence had been demonstrated.

13.4
En Plaque and Extradural Meningiomas

En plaque meningiomas are particular forms of the tumor, different from the most common type which is a globulous with a small zone of attachment. En plaque meningiomas present as a wide area of meningeal thickening with generally limited intradural extension (Fig. 13.8). They generally widely involve the adjacent bone. En plaque meningiomas may be observed at any sites but most frequently occur on the sphenoid ridge, where they may also present with an intraorbital extension (Fig. 13.10). Their radical removal needs a much more extensive dura and bone resection than the more common forms of meningioma. Consequently, after surgical resection the orbital walls have to be reconstructed. As in many cases of skull base meningiomas, the bone resection may open air cells of sphenoid or ethmoid sinus. In such cases, careful repair of the

dura is mandatory to avoid cerebrospinal fluid leak.

Another type of meningioma is a primary extradural lesion. It is similar to an intradural meningioma in that the tumor extends extradurally. This type of meningioma is known for its propensity to exhibit invasive features such as invasion of adjacent bone and soft tissues including muscles, nerves and sheaths of blood vessels (LEONETTI et al. 1993; PIEPER and AL MEFTY 1999; SUTHERLAND and SIMA 1991). Fortunately, these tumors are very uncommon. I consider these forms of meningiomas as locally malignant tumors and propose an aggressive plan of therapy combining surgery and radiotherapy.

13.5
Management of Recurrent Meningiomas

Recurrent meningiomas raise the problem of the interface between tumor and brain or other structures. The arachnoid has been opened by previous surgery and a surgical scar has developed; therefore, separation of the functional structures from the meningioma surface is much more difficult. Dissection is still more difficult in patients with previously irradiated meningiomas. Patients with recurrent meningiomas have a high incidence of significant peritumoral edema.

13.6
Adjuvant Therapy

Based on the above discussion, it is clear that the truly benign nature of meningioma is questionable even in the relatively common and simple-looking forms such as globular convexity meningiomas. Therefore, adjuvant treatment needs to be considered in some patients. This, of course, is not necessary in cases of previously untreated meningiomas in which Simpson

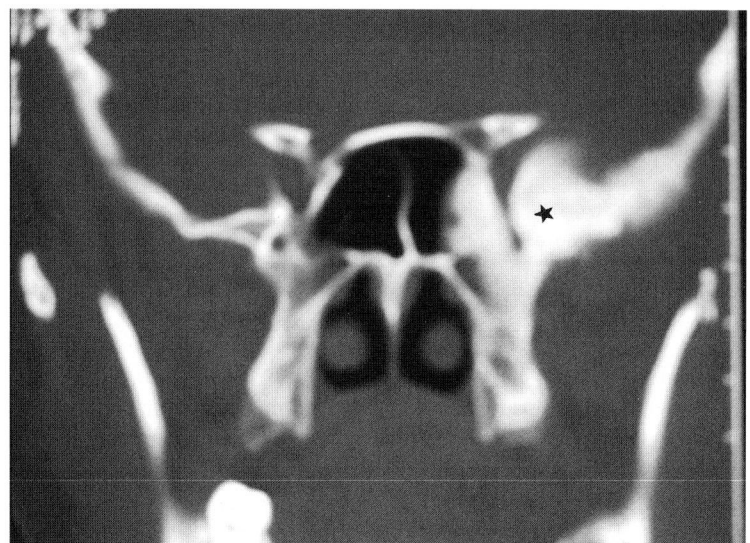

A

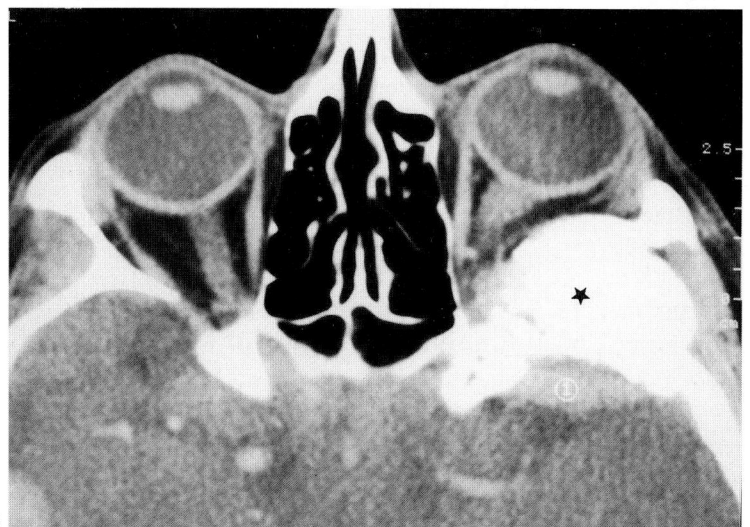

B

Fig. 13.10A,B. Spheno-orbital meningioma. **A** CT coronal view with bone window. Tumoral bone involvement of the temporal fossa (greater sphenoidal wing) up to the sphenoidal fissure, root of the pterygoid process and lateral wall of the sphenoid sinus. **B** CT axial view with soft tissue window. Thickening of the bone compressing the orbit content (*black star*). Notice the meningeal plaque (*1*)

grade I or II resection has been performed, except for those tumors with histologically identifiable malignant features. These malignant forms require post-operative radiotherapy occasionally in association with chemotherapy (hydroxyurea). In practice, adjuvant radiotherapy has very rarely been proposed in patients with benign meningiomas following the first resection attempt, even if the resection is incomplete. In fact, there is generally not enough data available on the natural history of such tumors to be able to anticipate a rapid recurrence. However, in some cases, a treatment strategy may be devised that includes deliberate partial surgical resection followed by radiosurgery focused on the tumor remnant (KONDZIOLKA et al. 1991, 1998). The main indication for such an approach is cavernous sinus meningioma in patients

with normal oculomotor nerve function. The purpose of this surgery is to obtain a histological diagnosis and to remove the meningioma – as long as the oculomotor nerves are not placed at risk. Another goal of surgery is to increase the margin between the meningioma and the optic chiasm and/or nerve so that these important structures are not exposed to the therapeutic dose of radiation delivered during radiosurgery. This generally means removal of the part of the tumor that is located outside the cavernous sinus and, to a limited extent, inside the sinus.

Conversely in patients with recurrent tumors, radiotherapy has certainly to be questioned when the delay before regrowth is relatively short (less than 2 years). In those patients where early recurrence is suspected, a planned early course of postoperative radiotherapy should be carried out shortly after reoperation and preferentially by a method which can irradiate the whole area of dural involvement. The area at risk for recurrence often corresponds to a surface too wide for radiosurgery and therefore, requires the use of involved fields conventional radiotherapy.

13.8
Conclusion

Although meningiomas are considered to be benign tumors, their management raises many technical problems for the surgeon. Surgery remains the best method of treatment for these lesions but the belief that most meningiomas can be cured with surgery is not realistic. Even in patients presenting with the most common and simple benign tumors, recurrence is not rare. Therefore, careful follow-up is mandatory to be able to detect tumor recurrence as early as possible and to apply appropriate treatment in a timely fashion. Our policy is to perform a post-operative MRI at 2 months which is used as a reference examination, and then to follow with studies at 1, 3, 6 and 10 years.

One or several reliable indices providing data on the biological behavior of meningiomas is lacking. This kind of information would allow surgeons and clinicians to adjust the aggressiveness of treatment (surgery and radiotherapy) according to the aggressiveness of each type of meningioma.

References

al Mefty O, Ayoubi S (1991) Clinoidal meningiomas. Acta Neurochir Suppl (Wien) 53: 92–97

Arana E, Diaz C, Latorre FF, et al. (1996) Primary intraosseous meningiomas. Acta Radiologica 37: 937–942

Azar-Kia B, Sarwar M, Marc JA, et al. (1974) Intraosseous meningioma. Neuroradiol 6: 246

Bederson JB, Eisenberg MB (1995) Resection and replacement of the superior sagittal sinus for treatment of a parasagittal meningioma: technical case report. Neurosurgery 37: 1015–1018

Beks JF, de Windt HL (1988) The recurrence of supratentorial meningiomas after surgery. Acta Neurochir (Wien) 95: 3–5

Bonnal J, Brotchi J (1978) Surgery of the superior sagittal sinus in parasagittal meningiomas. J Neurosurg 48: 935–945

Bonnal J, Brotchi J (1991) Reconstruction of the superior sagittal sinus in parasagittal meningiomas. In: Schmidek (ed) Meningiomas and their surgical treatment. Saunders WB, Philadelphia, PA, pp 221–229

Borovich B, Doron Y (1986) Recurrence of intracranial meningiomas: the role played by regional multicentricity. J Neurosurg 64: 58–63

Cahan WG, Woodard HQ, Higinbotham NL (1948) Sarcomas arising in irradiated bone, report of eleven cases. Cancer 1: 3–29

Cantore G, Delfini R, Domenicucci M (1991) Recurrence of intracranial meningioma. In: Schmidek (ed) Meningiomas and their surgical treatment. Saunders WB, Philadelphia, PA, pp 526–534

Chan RC, Thompson GB (1984) Morbidity, mortality, and quality of life following surgery for intracranial meningiomas: a retrospective study in 257 cases. J Neurosurg 60: 52–60

Choux M, Lena GL, Genitori L, et al. (1991) Meningiomas in children. In: Schmidek (ed) Meningiomas and their surgical treatment. Saunders WB, Philadelphia, PA, pp 93–102

Clavere P, Roullet B, Loubert R, et al. (1990) Métastases osseuses et pulmonaires díun méningiome bénin et récidivant. La Presse Médicale 19: 1304

Conforti P, Moraci A, Albanese V, et al. (1991) Microsurgical management of suprasellar and intaventricular meningiomas. Neurochirurgia (Stuttg) 34: 85–89

Crouse SK, Berg BO (1972) Intracranial meningiomas in childhood and adolescence. Neurology (Minneap.) 22: 135

Czernicki Z, Grochowski W, Uchman G, et al. (1991) Occlusion of the superior sagittal sinus caused by meningioma, intracranial volume-pressure relations and brain edema. Neurol Neurochir Pol 25: 580–586

Derome PJ, Guiot G (1978) Bone problems in meningiomas invading the base of the skull. Clin Neurosurg 25: 435–451

Drake JM, Hendrick EB, Becker LE, et al. (1985) Intracranial meningiomas in children. Pediatr Neurosci 12: 134–139

Giombini S, Solero CL, Lasio G, et al. (1984) Immediate and late outcome of operations for parasagittal and falx men ingiomas: report of 342 cases. Surg Neurol 21: 427–435

Go KG, Wilmink JT, Molenaar WM (1988) Peritumoral brain edema associated with meningiomas. Neurosurgery 23: 175–179

Goellner JR, Laws ER Jr, Soule EH, et al. (1978) Hemangiopericytoma of the meninges. Mayo Clinic Experience. Am J Clin Pathol 70: 375–380

Gökalp, et al. (1993) This reference will follow from author.

Hakuba A, Huh CW, Tsujikawa S, et al. (1979) Total removal of a parasagittal meningioma of the posterior third of the sagittal sinus and its repair by autogenous vein graft. Case report. J Neurosurg 51: 379–382

Harrison MJ, Sundaresan N (1991) Radiation-induced meningiomas. In: (ed) Schmidek Meningiomas and their surgical treatment. Saunders WB, Philadelphia, PA, pp 34–41

Hartmann K, Klug W (1975) Proceedings: recurrence and possible surgical procedures in meningiomas of the middle and posterior parts of the superior sagittal sinus. Acta Neurochir (Wien) 31: 283

Hino A, Imahori Y, Tenjin H, et al.(1990) Metabolic and hemodynamic aspects of peritumoral low-density areas in human brain tumor. Neurosurgery 26: 615–621

Huvos AG, Leming RH, Moore OS (1973) Clinicopathologic study of the resected carotid artery. Am J Surg 126: 570–574

Ide M, Jimbo M, Yamamoto M, et al. (1996) MIB-1 staining index and peritumoral brain edema on meningiomas. Cancer 78: 133–143

Ildan F, Tuna M, Iskender GoÁer A, et al. (1999) Correlation of the relationships of brain-tumor interfaces, magnetic resonance imaging, and angiographic findings to predict cleavage of meningiomas. J Neurosurg 91: 384–390

Inoue H, Tamura M, Koizumi H, et al. (1984) Clinical pathology of malignant meningiomas. Acta Neurochir(Wien) 73: 179–191

Jaaskelainen J, Haltia M, Kallio M, et al. (1991) Recurrence of histologically benign intracranial meningioma after seemingly complete removal. In: Schmidek (ed) Meningiomas and their surgical treatment. Saunders WB, Philadelphia, PA, pp 517–525

Kallio M, Sankila R, Hakulinen T, et al. (1992) Factors affecting operative and excess long-term mortality in 935 patients with intracranial meningioma. Neurosurgery 31: 2–12

Kawase T, Ohira T, Murakami H, et al. (1985) Influence of peritumoral edema on rCBF and on cerebral function: analysis by xenon-enhanced CT and EEG topography; In: Inaba Y, Klatzo I, Spatz M (eds) Brain Edema. Springer-Verlag, Berlin, pp 484–489

Kleihues P, Burger PC, Scheithauer BW (1993) The new WHO classification of brain tumors. Brain Pathol 3: 255–268

Kondziolka D, Lunsford LD, Coffey RJ, et al. (1991) Stereotactic radiosurgery of meningiomas. J Neurosurg 74: 552–559

Kondziolka D, Flickinger JC, Perez B (1998) Gamma Knife Meningioma Study Group: Judicious resection and/or radiosurgery for parasagittal meningiomas: outcomes from a multicenter review. Neurosurgery 4: 405–414

Kotapka MJ, Kalia KK, Martinez J, et al. (1994) Infiltration of the carotid artery by cavernous sinus meningioma. J Neurosurg 81: 252–255

Kumar PP, Good RR, Skultety FM, et al. (1987) Radiation-induced neoplasms of the brain. Cancer 59: 1274–1282

Leonetti JP, Al-Mefty OA, Eisenbeis JF, et al. (1993) Orbitocranial exposure in the management of infratemporal fossa tumors. Otolaryngol Head Neck Surg 109: 769–772

Mann J, Yates PC, Ainslie JP (1953) Unusual case of double primary orbital tumour. Br J Ophtalmo 37: 758–762

Mantle R E, Boleslaw L, Delgado MR, et al. (1999) Predicting the probability of meningioma recurrence based on the quantity of peritumoral brain edema on computerized tomography scanning. J Neurosurg 91: 375–383

Maroon JC, Kennerdell JS, Vidovich DV,et al. (1994) Recurrent spheno-orbital meningioma.J Neurosurg 80: 202–208

Matson DD (1969) Neurosurgery of infancy and childhood. In: Charles C. Thomas (ed) Springfield, IL, pp 607–608

Matsuno A, Nagashima T, Matuvra R, et al. (1996) Correlation between MIB-1 staining index and the immunoreactivity of P53 protein in recurrent and non recurrent meningiomas. Am J Clin Pathol 106: 776–781

McCormick D, Chong H, Hobbs C (1993) Detection of the Ki-67 antigen in fixed and was-embedded sections with the monoclonal antibody MIB-1. Histopathol 22: 355–360

Merten DF, Gooding CA, Newton TH, et al. (1974) Meningiomas of childhood and adolescence. J Pediatr 84: 696–700

Miller DC, Ojemann RG, Proppe KH, et al. (1985) Benign metastazing meningioma. J Neurosurg 62: 763–766

Mirimanoff RO, Doseretz DE, Linggood RM, et al. (1985) Meningioma: analysis of recurrence and progression following neurosurgical resection. J Neurosurg 62:18–24

Modan B, Baidatz D, Mart H, et al. (1974) Radiation-induced head and neck tumours. Lancet 7852: 277–279

Notterman J, Depierreux M, Raftopoulos C, et al. (1987) Les métastases de méningiomes. Neurochirurgie 33: 184–189

Oberling C (1922) Les tumeurs des méninges. Bull Fr Cancer 11: 365

Ohta M, Iwaki T, Kitamoto T, et al. (1994) MIB-1 staining index and scoring of histologic features in meningioma. Cancer 74: 3176–3189

Pasquier B, Gasnier F, Pasquier D, et al. (1986) Papillary meningioma: clinicopathologic study of seven cases and review of literature. Cancer 58: 299–305

Pieper DR, al Mefty O (1999) Management of intracranial meningiomas secondarily involving the infratemporal fossa: radiographic characteristics, pattern of tumor invasion, and surgical implications. Neurosurgery 45: 231–238

Pieper DR, al Mefty O, Hanada Y, et al. (1999) Hyperostosis associated with meningioma of the cranial base: secondary changes or tumor invasion. Neurosurgery 44: 742–747

Plate KH, Ruschoff J, Behnke J, et al. (1990) Proliferative potential of human brain tumours as assessed by nucleolar organizer regions (Ag NORs) and Ki-67 immunoreactivity. Acta Neurochir (Wien) 104: 103–109

Pompili A, Derome PJ, Visot A, et al. (1982) Hyperostosing meningiomas of the sphenoid ridge-clinical features, surgical therapy, and long-term observations: review of 49 cases. Surg Neurol 17: 411–416

Puchner MJA, Fischer-Lampsatis RCM, Herrmann HD, et al. (1998) Suprasellar meningiomas. Neurological and visual outcome at long term follow-up in a homogeneous series of patients treated microsurgically. Acta Neurochir (Wien) 140: 1231–1238

Rubin G, Ben David U, Gornish M, et al. (1994) Meningiomas of the anterior cranial fossa floor. Review of 67 cases. Acta Neurochir (Wien) 129: 26–30

Rubinstein AB, Shalit MN, Cohen ML, et al. (1984) Radiation-induced cerebral meningioma: a recognized entity. J Neurosurg 61: 966–971

Salpietro FM, Alafaci C, Lucerna S, et al. (1994) Peritumoral edema in meningiomas: microsurgical observations of different brain tumor interfaces related to computed tomography. Neurosurgery 35: 638–642

Schörner W, Schubeus P, Henkes H, et al. (1990) "Meningeal sign": a characteristic finding of meningiomas on contrast-enhanced MR images. Neuroradiology 32: 90–93

Shaffrey ME, Dolenc VV, Lanzino G, et al. (1999) Invasion of the internal carotid artery by cavernous sinus meningiomas. Surg Neurol 52: 167–171

Shibuya M, HoshinoT, Ito S, et al. (1992) Meningiomas: clinical implications of a high proliferative potential determined by Bromodeoxyuridine labeling. Neurosurg 30: 494–498

Simpson D (1957) The recurrence of intracranial meningiomas after surgical treatment. J Neurol Neurosurg Psychiatry 20: 22–39

Sindou MP, Alaywan M (1989) Most intracranial meningiomas are not cleavable tumors: anatomic-surgical evidence and angiographic predictability. Neurosurgery 42: 476–480

Sindou M, Hallacq P (1966) Microsurgery of the venous system in meningiomas invading the major dural sinuses. In: Hakuba A (ed) Surgery of the intracranial venous system. Springer-Verlag, Tokyo pp 226–236

Soffer D, Gomori JM, Siegal T, et al. (1989) Intracranial meningiomas after high dose irradiation. Cancer 63: 1514–1519

Steiger HJ, Reulen HJ, Huber P, et al. (1989) Radical resection of superior sagittal sinus meningioma with venous interposition graft and reimplantation of the rolandic veins. Acta Neurochir (Wien) 100: 108–111

Sutherland GR, Sima AAF (1991) Incidence and Clinopathologic features of meningioma. In: Schmidek (ed) Meningiomas and their surgical treatment. Saunders WB, Philadelphia, PA, pp 10–21

Thomas HG, Dolman CL, Berry K (1981) Malignant meningioma: Clinical and pathological features. J Neurosurg 55: 929–934

Tokumaru A, Ouchi T, Eguchi T, et al. (1990) Prominent meningeal enhancement adjacent to meningioma on Gd-DTPA enhanced MR images: histopathologic correlation. Radiology 175: 431–433

Villani R, Gori G (1974) Long-term clinical results of the surgical treatment for meningiomas of infancy and adolescence. In: Bushe KA, et al. (ed) Progress in Pediatric Neurosurgery, Hippocrates-Verlag, Stuttgart, pp 26–54

Wakai S, Ochiai C, Takakura K, et al. (1980) Meningiomas in childhood. Nervous System in Children (Jap) 5: 1

Wilms G, Lammens M, Marchal G, et al. (1989) Thickening of dura surrounding meningiomas: MR features. J Comput Assist Tomogr 13: 763–768

14 Radiotherapy for Meningioma

Zbigniew Petrovich, Gabor Jozsef, Chi-Shing Zee, and Cheng Yu

CONTENTS

14.1
Introduction

14.1.1
Incidence

Meningioma is a relatively common primary intracranial tumor arising from the meninges. This tumor represents approximately 20% of all intracranial neoplasms (Prados et al. 1998; Mahaley et al. 1989; Walker et al. 1985; Laws and Thapar 1993). It is of interest to note that this incidence was nearly twice as high in the state of Minnesota (Walker et al. 1985). The reason for this higher incidence of meningioma in this state was not immediately apparent. Peak incidence of meningioma is 55 years of age, although this tumor has been reported at any age, including its uncommon incidence in children. Meningioma occurs primarily in women, with a reported female to male ratio of 2–3:1 (Prados et al. 1998;

Z. Petrovich, MD; G. Jozsef, PhD; C.-S. Zee, MD; C. Yu, PhD
Department of Radiation Oncology University of Southern California School of Medicine, 1441 Eastlake Avenue, Los Angeles, CA 90033, USA

Laws and Thapar 1993). Over the past 20 years a substantial body of evidence has been accumulating about the hormonal influence on tumor growth, with particular reference to increased tumor growth rate during pregnancy (Lesch et al. 1987; Schrell and Fahlbusch 1991). It is also to be noted that this tumor is more common in those with breast cancer (Rubinstein et al. 1989), and there is good evidence for the presence of progesterone and estrogen receptors in meningioma cells (Lesch et al. 1987; Schrell and Fahlbusch 1991; Rubinstein et al. 1989).

14.1.2
Prognostic Factors

Over 90% of patients with meningioma present with tumors of benign histology, with the remaining 10% of patients presenting with malignant, anaplastic and atypical meningioma. See Chap. 2 for relevant details on the pathology of these tumors. From the clinical point of view the histological categories of relevance include malignant meningioma, aggressive tumors, and benign meningioma (Hoffmann et al. 1995). The natural history of benign meningioma is that of a slow progressive local expansion and a low incidence of recurrence following surgery (Stafford et al. 1998). On the other hand, malignant meningioma is a widely infiltrating and rapidly growing tumor, which is known to have multifocal potential. Surgical resection is usually followed by tumor recurrence rapidly leading to death. Anaplastic meningioma displays an intermediate behavior. Occasionally, meningioma may present metastasis usually to the lung.

The primary treatment in the management of meningioma is surgery, with radiotherapy having an important role as a postoperative therapy or as primary therapy in highly selected patients (see Chap. 13). In the case of complete tumor resection there is a very low probability of recurrence. On the other hand, incomplete tumor removal or malignant histology may result in >50% incidence of tumor recurrence (Miramanoff et al. 1985; Jaaskelainen 1986;

QUEST 1978; HOFFMAN et al. 1995). The extent of tumor resection is an important factor predicting treatment outcome and can help to define the need for adjuvant radiotherapy. A useful grading system based on this extent of surgical resection was proposed in the late 1950s (SIMPSON 1957). Table 14.1 presents this useful grading system in detail. It is apparent that patients with benign histology (grade I) or grade II resection need no further therapy. Patients with grade III resection have relative indications for postoperative radiotherapy while those with grade IV and V tumors have strong indications for the adjuvant treatment. Other important factors favorably affecting patient prognosis include: age<60 years, benign histology, Karnofsky performance status (KPS) >70 and intact neurological status of the patient (Table 14.2) (MAHALEY et al. 1989). Excellent long-term survival rates have been routinely obtained in patients treated with surgery, and again there has been a good correlation between extent of surgery and survival. The 5-year actuarial survival in the National Survey of Pattern of Care for Brain Tumors was: biopsy only 63%, subtotal resection 78%, and total resection 96% (MAHALEY et al. 1989). Similarly, the 5-year survival rates for patients with <70 on the KPS scale was 80.5% while it was 95% for those >70 on the KPS scale (MAHALEY et al. 1989).

Table 14.1. Classification by extent of resection in patients with meningiomas (from SIMPSON 1957)

Grade	Extent of resection
I	Gross total tumor resection, dural attachment, and abnormal bone
II	Gross total tumor resection, coagulation of dural attachment
III	Gross total tumor resection without resection or coagulation of dural attachment or, alternatively, of its extradural extensions
IV	Partial tumor resection
V	Simple decompression (biopsy)

Table 14.2. Important prognostic parameters in patients with intracranial meningioma (modified from MAHALEY et al. 1989)

Parameter	Favorable	Unfavorable
Patient age (yrs)	<60	>70
Neurological status	Normal	Impaired
Seizures	Present	Absent
Extent of resection	Complete	Incomplete
Increased intracranial pressure	Absent	Present
Atypical histological features	Absent	Present

14.2 External Beam Radiotherapy

In the 1950s and 1960s the indications for radiotherapy in the management of patients with meningioma were not well defined. This treatment was used as definitive therapy in patients who were poor risk for surgery, and frequently in the postoperative period in those with incomplete resection or with malignant histology. In recent years consensus has emerged on a more systematic approach to the use of radiotherapy in meningioma. Ultimately, close working interaction between a neurosurgeon and radiation oncologist is necessary to find the optimal treatment for a given patient.

An important early study on the indications for radiotherapy in patients with meningioma was published by the University of California San Francisco (UCSF) (SHELINE 1977). A total of 176 meningioma patients were treated during a 20-year period, including 84 (48%) who in the opinion of an attending surgeon had complete resection. During the period of observation there has been no tumor recurrence in this latter group of patients with complete resection. In the remaining 92 patients who had an incomplete resection, 34 (37%) received postoperative irradiation and 10 (29%) had tumor recurrence as opposed to 43 (74%) of the 58 who received no postoperative irradiation. Local recurrence in surgery-alone patients who had an incomplete resection was most frequently recorded within 5 years of resection, while some patients in this group showed local recurrence >10 years following surgery. A subsequent UCSF study of 140 patients (benign, $n=117$ and malignant, $n=23$) treated with contemporary radiotherapy consisting of 54 Gy demonstrated the overall 5-year actuarial survival for patients with benign and malignant histology to be 85% and 58%, respectively ($P=0.02$) (GOLDSMITH et al. 1994). The 5-year progression-free survival was 89% and 48%, respectively ($P=0.001$). The 10-year overall and progression-free survival was 77%. Important prognostic factors significantly improving disease-free survival in patients with benign tumors were younger patient age and treatment after 1980, but not the tumor size. There were no predictive prognostic values in patients with malignant meningioma. The authors concluded that patients with incomplete resection who are treated with contemporary postoperative radiotherapy have a similar outcome to those patients who have had complete tumor resection. Other investigators (BLOOM 1982; SOLAN and KRAMER 1985) reported similar data. In the series of

37 patients treated in the Royal Marsden Hospital with radiotherapy alone, the 5- and 10-year disease-free survival was 73% and 60%, respectively, and this was similar to the outcome in 65 patients receiving postoperative irradiation following incomplete resection (BLOOM 1982). A more recently published experience with 186 meningioma patients also treated at Royal Marsden Hospital demonstrated even better treatment results obtained with radiotherapy in terms of overall and disease-free survival (GLAHOLM et al. 1990).

In the Thomas Jefferson University series of 32 patients treated with postoperative radiotherapy, 17 (68%) out of 25 benign histology patients were long-term disease-free survivors, whereas only two of seven (29%) with malignant meningioma were alive (SOLAN and KRAMER 1985). An interesting study of 91 meningioma patients treated with radiotherapy was reported from Bordeaux, France (MAIRE et al. 1995). The indications for radiotherapy in this study included: (1) incomplete resection, $n=29$; (2) post-surgical tumor recurrence, $n=14$; (3) complete resection in those with angioblastic, aggressive benign, and anaplastic tumors, $n=8$; (4) poor surgical risk patients and those with unresectable lesions, $n=44$. Contemporary radiotherapy techniques were used for the treatment of these patients, who received a median dose of 52 Gy. Median follow-up was 40 months. The 5- and 10-year actuarial survival rates were 71% and 40%, respectively. The most significant influence on survival but not on the incidence of tumor recurrence was the age of patients at the time of treatment. It is of interest to note that of the 60 symptomatic study patients who had neurological deficit, 43 (72%) showed neurological improvement. This improvement included recovered cranial nerve palsies. A new report on the management of meningioma patients was recently published from Bordeaux, France, supporting the outcomes of the former study (VENDRELY et al. 1999).

Two reports from the University of Gainesville, Florida, presented treatment outcomes in 132 and 262 patients, respectively (TAYLOR et al. 1988; CONDRA et al. 1997). The median follow-up in the second report was 8.2 years. Treatment groups included: (1) surgery alone, $n=229$ (74%); (2) postoperative irradiation, $n=21$ (8%); (3) radiotherapy alone, $n=7$ (4%); and (4) radiosurgery alone, $n=5$ (2%). Local tumor control at 15 years was 76% in patients with total excision, 76% in those with incomplete resection followed by postoperative irradiation, and 30% in those who had incomplete resection without adjuvant radiotherapy ($P=0.0001$). This study concluded that outcome is similar following total surgical excision or subtotal excision followed by external beam radiotherapy. Incomplete surgical excision without adjuvant irradiation is not a recommended treatment. Others (FORBES and GOLDBERG 1984; MIRALBELL et al. 1992) have presented similar findings.

Virtually all published reports have demonstrated poor treatment outcomes in patients with malignant meningioma (SOLAN and KRAMER 1985; GOLDSMITH et al. 1994; GLAHOLM et al. 1990; HOFFMANN et al. 1995; CONDRA et al. 1997; HAIE-MEDER et al. 1995). Patients with malignant meningioma tend to have wide infiltration of adjacent tissue, show early recurrence following even "complete" surgical excision, and suffer recurrence following adequate contemporary radiotherapy. The recommended radiation dose for these patients is approximately 60 Gy, or 10% higher than the commonly used radiation dose for benign meningioma. Anaplastic or atypical histological patterns have a better prognosis than malignant meningioma but a much worse prognosis than benign meningioma.

Two recent reports addressed the issues relevant to the management of patients with malignant meningioma. The first report was on 38 patients treated with 48 resections (total resection, $n=28$; subtotal resection, $n=20$) at Baylor College of Medicine in Houston, Texas (DZIUK et al. 1998). Of these 48 resections, 25 were performed as a part of the initial treatment and 23 were used to treat recurrent disease. In these 48 resections the histological diagnosis was anaplastic meningioma in 32 (67%) (in 13 patients who originally had benign meningioma, malignant transformation was noted at the time of second resection), hemangiopericytoma in 11 (23%), papillary meningioma in three (6%), and meningiosarcoma in two (4%). A total of 19 patients received postoperative irradiation consisting of a median dose of 54 Gy. No indications for radiotherapy were provided in the report. Additionally, five (13%) of the 38 patients were excluded from analysis, including two who were lost to follow-up and three who had perioperative mortality, and median follow-up was not provided (range 3–144 months). The 5-year actuarial disease-free survival (DFS) was 39% in patients with complete resection whereas none of the patients with incomplete resection survived 5 years ($P=0.001$). Adjuvant irradiation in those with complete resection nearly doubled their 5-year DFS (NS). Postoperative radiotherapy as a planned part of the initial treatment increased the 5-year DFS from 15% to 80% ($P=0.002$). In the management of recurrent lesions, radiotherapy increased the 2-year actuarial DFS from 50% to 89%. Multivariate analysis showed extent of resection, postoperative irradiation, and recurrent disease to be independent prognostic factors.

The second report was from Thomas Jefferson University presenting treatment outcome in nine atypical and eight malignant meningioma patients (COKE et al. 1998). Complete resection was performed in 12 patients, and incomplete resection in four (extent of resection was unknown in one patient). Postoperative irradiation with a mean dose of 61 Gy was given to 15 (88%) study patients. The overall 5- and 10-year actuarial survival was 87% and 58%, respectively, and for those with atypical meningioma it was likewise 87% and 58%, respectively. In patients with malignant meningioma, 5- and 10-year actuarial survival was 60% and 60%, respectively. It is of interest to analyze causes of failure in these patients. Of the five patients who died, three received <54 Gy, which led to local recurrence. Local recurrence was documented in 11 patients (65%) after surgery and in three (18%) after radiotherapy. Apparently, aggressive treatment in this group of patients resulted in relatively good survival rates. There was no difference in treatment outcomes between patients with atypical or malignant meningioma.

An important study was published by Princess Margaret Hospital in Toronto, Canada (MILOSEVIC et al. 1996). This study was based on treatment outcomes in 59 patients, including 42 (71%) with malignant meningioma and 17 (29%) with atypical meningioma. The 5-year actuarial overall and disease-specific survival was 28% and 34%, respectively. In multivariate analysis, age <58 years, treatment after 1975, and a radiation dose >50 Gy were independent prognostic factors associated with higher DFS. This study again validated the need for a well-planned course of postoperative radiotherapy with higher radiation doses (60 Gy). Similarly, stereotactically guided conformal or intensity-modulated radiotherapy is an important treatment in patients with meningioma in order to optimize radiation dose delivery and lower its toxicity (ALHEIT et al. 1999; GRANT 1998). Other recent reports on patients with malignant meningioma have demonstrated similar treatment results to the above-presented studies (SHIMIZU et al. 1995; DEVRIES et al. 1999).

In an important study to identify factors predicting tumor response to radiotherapy, PCNA index was evaluated (COLVETT et al. 1997). PCNA is a DNA polymerase found at the highest levels in the most radioresistant part of the generation cycle (S-phase). Meningioma patients with a high PCNA index were noted to be least likely responders to radiotherapy

($P<0.001$). This PCNA index may help in the formulation of appropriate treatment strategies in the management of patients with meningioma.

14.2.1
Skull Base Tumors

Meningioma presenting at the skull base creates a special problem since complete surgical excision is very difficult (MAYBERG and SYMON 1986; FRIEDLANDER et al. 1999). Excellent treatment results, with a low incidence of treatment toxicity, have been reported with the use of well-planned external beam radiotherapy (FRIEDLANDER et al. 1999; NUTTING et al. 1999; MAGUIRE et al. 1999; KINJO et al. 1997; PEELE et al. 1996). In a study on 28 patients treated with fractionated external beam radiotherapy for cavernous sinus meningioma (subtotal resection, $n=22$, and unresectable, $n=6$), the 8-year overall and disease-free survival was 96% and 81%, respectively. The median radiation dose was 53.1 Gy. This study provides a treatment alternative to the use of stereotactic radiosurgery, which is the most frequently used form of radiotherapy in the management of patients with cavernous sinus tumors. This question has also been evaluated in a study from the United Kingdom (SIBTAIN and PLAOMAN 1999).

14.2.2
Optic Pathway Meningioma

Patients with optic pathway meningioma represent a small but very important group of tumors. Meningioma in adults occurs primarily between the ages of 30 and 60, with slow tumor growth rate being most frequently reported (CAPO and KUPERSMITH 1991). The same tumor is clinically much more aggressive in children. The symptom of greatest importance in these tumors is a progressive loss of vision. Treatment of choice has to date been surgical excision, which frequently cannot be total and results in visual complications. Conformal radiation therapy, consisting of about 54 Gy, in patients with progressive loss of vision is a good alternative to surgical treatment. It can also be successfully used in patients who have had an incomplete tumor resection. Conformal radiotherapy allows for a sharp reduction of brain tissue irradiated to therapeutic doses, thus reducing the incidence of late radiation toxicity (ENG et al. 1992; CAPO and KUPERSMITH 1991; LEE et al. 1996). In spite of these new developments in contemporary radiotherapy, the issue of routine use of radiotherapy in patients with optic pathway meningioma remains controversial.

14.3
Charged Particle Radiotherapy

Charged particle radiotherapy is an interesting treatment modality in skull base tumors, including meningioma. A report was published from University of California Lawrence Berkeley Laboratory in Berkeley, California on the treatment of 29 patients with meningioma, including 26 skull base and three spinal meningiomas (KAPLAN et al. 1993). All patients were treated with helium ion beam using a mean radiation dose of 60 Gy equivalent (range 53–80.4 GyE). The 10-year rates of local control and survival were 84%, and 80%, respectively. The incidence of complications was low with 60 GyE. Local failures occurred only in massive, recurrent tumors. The authors concluded that helium ion beam is an effective therapy in patients with unresectable skull base meningiomas. Similar conclusions were reported with the use of charged particle beams for other skull base tumors in addition to meningioma (CASTRO et al. 1994). Excellent treatment results were obtained at Harvard University treating meningioma patients with 160-MV proton beam (MIRALBELL et al. 1992). The main problem preventing greater utilization of charged particle beams in the management of patients with meningiomas is the very high cost of constructing and operating such facilities.

14.4
Brachytherapy

The use of brachytherapy in the management of patients with meningioma has been infrequently reported in the literature. In a report from University of Nebraska Medical Center in Omaha, Nebraska, 13 patients with intracranial meningioma were treated with high-activity iodine-125 permanent implants (KUMAR et al. 1993). The total radiation dose was 100–500 Gy delivered at a rate of 5–25 cGy per hour. Patients selected for brachytherapy included those with postsurgical recurrence or with unresectable lesions. This treatment program was well tolerated without evidence of late toxicity. Of the 13 study patients, nine (69%) had complete response and four (31%) had >50% tumor volume resolution. Similar good results

with the use of iodine-125 brachytherapy were reported in elderly parasellar-clival meningioma patients treated at University of Helsinki, Helsinki, Finland. In view of these good treatment results and the low incidence of treatment toxicity, it is surprising that so few medical centers are interested in the use of this procedure in the management of patients with meningioma.

14.5
Stereotactic Radiosurgery

Stereotactic radiosurgery (SRS) has emerged as an important and minimally invasive treatment modality in the management of selected patients with malignant, benign, and vascular lesions in addition to its usefulness in functional disorders. See Chaps. 5 and 6 for principles of the physics of SRS, and Chaps. 19–21 for clinical applications of frameless stereotaxy and conventional SRS. Dosimetric parameters and radiation dose distribution are similar for linear accelerator-based, proton beam-based, and gamma knife SRS. Of these three treatment modes, the fastest growing is gamma knife SRS. Worldwide data on the frequency of gamma knife use are now available by courtesy of the Leksell Gamma Knife Society. The most recent report published by this society was in June 1999. Based on reports from more than 100 gamma knife facilities, 103,000 patients had received such treatment for various indications up to June 1999. Of these 103,000 patients, 42,242 had been treated for benign lesions, including 14,212 with a diagnosis of meningioma (Table 14.3). The indica-

Table 14.3. Benign tumors treated with gamma knife SRS worldwide up to June 1999 (courtesy of Leksell Gamma Knife Society, Necross, Georgia)

Tumor	No.	% Benign lesions	% All lesions
Meningioma	14,212	33.6	12.8
Acoustic neuroma	11,201	26.5	10.1
Pituitary adenoma	10,651	25.2	9.4
Pineal	1,481	3.5	1.3
Craniopharyngioma	1,404	3.3	1.3
Trigeminal Neuroma	698	1.5	0.6
Chordoma	650	1.5	0.6
Schwannoma	619	1.5	0.5
Hemangioblastoma	617	1.5	0.5
Other benign lesions	709	1.7	0.6
Total	42,242	100	37.1

tions for SRS and the frequency of applications of this treatment are expanding rapidly in the United States and in the rest of the world. The use of SRS in patients with meningioma has also been increasing, as evidenced by the fact that nearly 34% of all patients treated with SRS for benign lesions are being treated for meningioma (Table 14.3). The reasons for this increase in the use of SRS for this disease include the 6%–19% incidence of tumor recurrence, morbidity of 23%–27%, and mortality of 5%–16% reported in contemporary surgical series in patients treated for meningioma (CHANG et al. 1998). In contrast, published reports on the use of SRS demonstrate 94% mean incidence of tumor stabilization or regression, morbidity of <3%, and a mean mortality of 0.7% (CHANG et al. 1998). Additionally, there is well-documented radiobiological support for the use of SRS in patients with meningioma (HALL and BRENNER 1993). See Chap. 4 for relevant details on radiobiology.

Linear accelerator-based SRS was used in the treatment of 55 patients with skull base meningioma at Stanford University Medical Center (CHANG and ADLER 1997). Mean tumor volume was 7.33 cm^3 (range 0.45–27.65 cm^3) and mean follow-up was 48.4 months (range 17–81 months). Radiation treatment parameters were: mean dose to the tumor periphery of 18.3 Gy (range 12–25 Gy), and mean isocenters 2.2 (range 1–5). Of the 55 patients treated, 38 (69%) had tumor stabilization, 16 (29%) had tumor regression, and only one (2%) showed tumor progression. The 2-year actuarial tumor control was 98%. The study patients tolerated this treatment program very well, and only temporary cranial nerve dysfunction was noted, with no significant or clinically important late toxicity. Similar excellent treatment outcomes with linear accelerator-based SRS have been reported by other investigators (HAKIM et al. 1998; VALENTINO et al. 1993).

SRS with 180-MeV proton beam was used in the treatment of 19 patients with unresectable skull base meningiomas in Uppsala, Sweden (GUDJONSSON et al. 1999). A total dose of 24 Gy was given in four 6-Gy consecutive daily fractions. Minimum follow-up was 3 years. None of the treated patients showed tumor progression during the period of observation. Of the 19 patients treated, two (10%) developed peritumoral edema, which responded well to corticosteroid therapy.

A multicenter study was reported on the treatment with gamma knife SRS of 203 patients with benign parasagittal meningiomas (KONDZIOLKA et al. 1998). The median follow-up was 3.5 years. Mean tumor volume was 10 cm^3. A total of 66 (33%) patients

were treated with primary SRS and their 5-year actuarial tumor control was 93%. No clinical failure was reported among patients (n=41) with tumor volume <7.5 cm^3 who never had surgery. Tumor control rate in patients who had had prior surgery was 60%, with an incidence of local control in the SRS-treated volume of 85%. Most of the other failures were due to tumor growth elsewhere in the brain. There was a 16% incidence of temporary peritumoral edema occurring within 2 years of SRS and its incidence was tumor volume dependent. Multivariate analysis identified the following factors as adversely affecting the tumor control rate: increasing tumor volume (P=0.002) and previous neurological deficit. Based on this study the authors recommended the use of SRS alone in patients with tumors <3 cm in diameter and patent sagittal sinus. Patients with tumors >3 cm in size and/or progressive neurological deficit should have open surgery first, to be followed by SRS to a much-reduced residual tumor volume. In another study using gamma knife SRS, 99 consecutive patients treated at Pittsburgh University Medical Center received a mean dose to the tumor periphery of 16 Gy (KONDZIOLKA et al. 1999a). The clinical control rate was 93%. It is of interest that between 5 and 10 years after SRS, 96% of patients who were surveyed expressed their satisfaction with the treatment outcome. A similar treatment outcome was reported by these authors in another study (KONDZIOLKA et al. 1999b) and in patients with petroclival meningioma (SUBACH et al. 1998).

SRS is the optimal treatment modality in the management of patients with meningioma involving the cavernous sinus (KONDZIOLKA et al. 1999b; KURITA et al. 1997). See Chap. 19 for treatment results in these patients obtained at USC (unpublished data).

An interesting report addressing treatment toxicity in 88 patients with skull base meningiomas and treated with gamma knife was published by the group from Mayo Clinic, Rochester, Minnesota (MORITA et al. 1999). Prior treatment consisting of surgery was received by 49 (56%) patients, while four (4%) patients received prior fractionated external beam radiotherapy. All patients who received prior therapy had good evidence of tumor progression. The most common signs and symptoms at presentation were cranial nerve dysfunction such as: trigeminal in 24 (27%), abducent in 24 (27%), visual changes in 20 (23%), oculomotor palsy in 19 (21%), trochlear nerve palsy in 9 (10%). Other signs and symptoms were present in 50 (57%). Many of these 88 patients had more than one sign or symptom present. Of the 88 patients treated, 66 (75%) had tumors in the cavernous sinus and petroclival region. The median dose to the periphery of tumors was 16 Gy. The 5-year progression-free survival was 95%, with only two (2.3%) patients demonstrating tumor progression following SRS treatment. At the time of last evaluation, 60 (68%) lesions were smaller and 26 (29.5%) remained unchanged. Clinical improvement in cranial nerve dysfunction occurred in 15 patients. Of the nine patients with new trigeminal nerve dysfunction, all received a radiation dose of 19 Gy or more. Based on their data, the authors recommended the use of gamma knife SRS for patients with skull base meningiomas. The knowledge on radiation dose limitations to the normal structures such the optic apparatus or other cranial nerves is expected to minimize the probability of clinically significant neurological dysfunction.

14.6
The USC Experience

14.6.1
Gamma Knife Stereotactic Radiosurgery

Between 1994 and 1999, a total of 107 patients received gamma knife SRS at USC School of Medicine (Petrovich et al., unpublished data). Of these patients, 80 were females and 27 males, and their median age was 60 years (range 16–91 years). Of the 107 study patients, 48 (45%) had undergone a prior open surgical procedure, while a majority (55%) of patients were treated de novo. The reason for SRS treatment was either poor risk for a craniotomy or a tumor in a relatively inaccessible location for open surgery. Nearly 60% of patients had asymptomatic tumors. The most common (31%) tumor location was the cavernous sinus, followed by frontal and temporal regions with an incidence of 14% and 9%, respectively (Table 14.4). It is of interest to note that a total of 15 tumors were adjacent to the pons or brainstem or were present in the cerebellopontine angle, with substantial encroachment on these critical structures. Histological confirmation of meningioma was available in all patients who had prior craniotomy, while in those without prior surgery the diagnosis was based on imaging studies (MRI). Median follow-up was 30 months.

Details on the SRS treatment techniques used in the management of these patients are presented elsewhere in this volume (Chaps. 6, 19, and 21). Basically, all patients were treated on an outpatient basis un-der conscious systemic sedation with local anesthesia used for the stereotactic frame placement. There was a neuroanesthesiologist in attendance. Nearly 98% of the treated patients were discharged from the hospital within 1 h of completion of stereotactic treatment. In a few elderly patients who had coexisting medical problems, it was elected to keep them in hospital overnight. In the 107 study patients, a total of 117 SRS treatments were given to manage 128 lesions. The median tumor volume was 4.7 cm^3, with a range from 0.2 to 29.9 cm^3 (Table 14.5). The usual prescribed radiation dose to the lesion periphery was 16 Gy defined to the 50% isodose line (Table 14.5). A median of five isocenters (range 1–12) was used in the treatment of these patients.

Representative examples of recently treated patients are shown in Figs. 14.1 and 14.2. Figure 14.1 concerns a 37-year-old male patient who in the past had undergone subtotal resection of a skull base meningioma. The residual tumor was adjacent to the left optic nerve. The patient received a dose of 15 Gy defined to the 50% isodose line using seven isocenters in order to optimize SRS treatment (Fig. 14.1). Figure 14.2 shows MR images of a 52-year-old female patient who had undergone two extensive surgical resections

Table 14.4. Distribution of gamma knife-treated meningiomas at USC by tumor site

Site	No.	%
Cavernous sinus	40	31
Frontal	18	14
Temporal	12	9
Infratentorial	9	7
Parietal	8	6
Occipital	7	5
Pons	5	4
Cerebellopontine angle	5	4
Brainstem	5	4
Clivus	4	3
Other	15	12
Total	128	100

Table 14.5. Important treatment parameters in 128 lesions treated at USC

	Prescribed Dose (Gy)	Dose max. (Gy)	Tumor volume (cm^3)	Treated volume (cm^3)	No. of iso-centers
Maximum	24	44	29.9	47.5	12
Minimum	9	18	0.2	0.6	1
Mean	15.7	30.6	5.7	9.1	5
Median	16.0	32	4.7	71	5

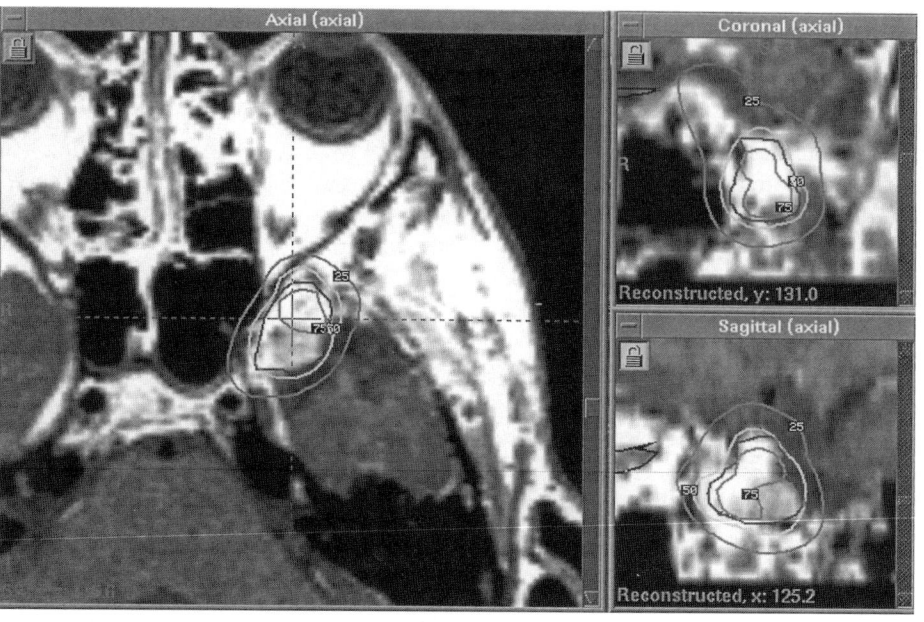

Fig. 14.1. Axial, coronal, and sagittal postcontrast MR images demonstrating a well-enhancing mass adjacent to the left optic nerve in a 37-year-old male. Tumor dimensions were: $x=14.4$ mm, $y=18.1$ mm, $z=27.5$ mm, and tumor volume was 2.9 cm^3. A total of 100% of the tumor volume was treated, with a total treated volume of 4.9 cm^3 receiving the prescribed dose of 15 Gy. The dose was defined to the 50% isodose line and seven isocenters were used to treat this lesion

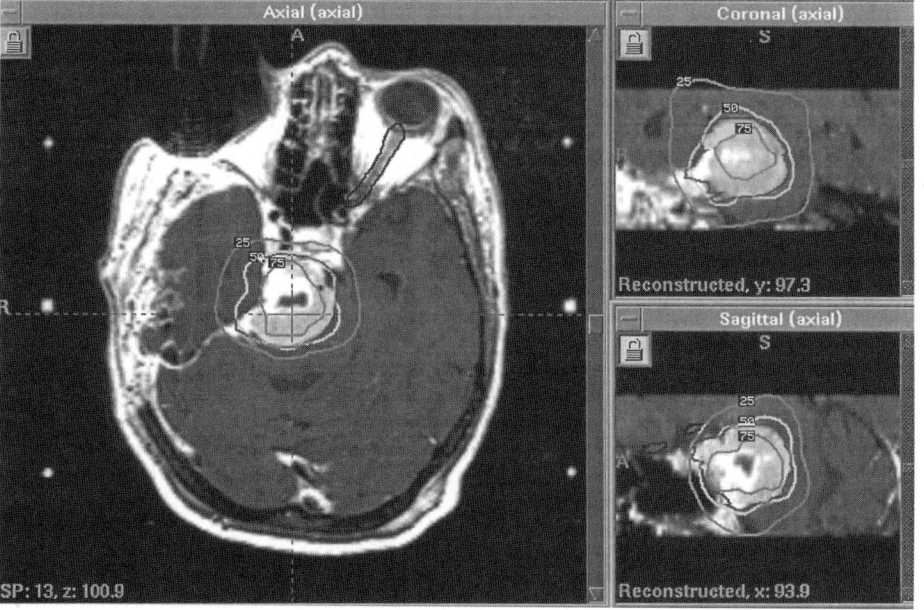

Fig. 14.2. Axial, coronal, and sagittal MR postcontrast images showed a large, well-enhancing lesion involving the cavernous sinus and clivus in a 52-year-old female. This lesion was histologically confirmed as meningioma. The lesion dimensions were: $x=43$ mm, $y=44$ mm, and $z=34.9$ mm. Tumor volume was 20 cm^3 and the tumor treated volume was 19 cm^3 with a total 25 cm^3 of tissue receiving the prescribed dose. A total of 12 isocenters were used to treat this patient to a dose of 15 Gy defined to the 50% isodose line

for a skull base meningioma. This patient presented with a recurrent lesion involving the right cavernous sinus and the clivus. The patient received a total dose of 15 Gy defined to the 50% isodose line, to this large (25 cm^3) tumor, using 12 isocenters. Both of these patients had an excellent treatment tolerance and showed no evidence of tumor progression during the period of follow-up.

SRS was very well tolerated in this group of 107 patients. Mild fatigue of short duration was noted in about 40% of patients. Nausea lasting for up to 2 days

was recorded in four (4%) patients of whom two had experienced a few hours of vomiting, which was well controlled with oral antiemetic medications. Of the 40 patients with cavernous sinus meningiomas, 38 (95%) had no tumor progression or a slight decrease in tumor dimensions. Treatment failure was noted in two (5%) patients, who had progressive tumor growth leading to death. The first patient had a malignant meningioma and the second a very large anaplastic meningioma. Transient IVth nerve palsy appearing several months following SRS and lasting for up to 6 months was recorded in two patients. One patient, who presented with an extensive bilateral meningioma involving the cavernous sinus and bilateral internal carotid artery narrowing 6 months following SRS, experienced signs and symptoms of an impending stroke and required surgery to bypass the occluded vessel. This patient did well following this surgical procedure. It is not clear whether the internal carotid artery occlusion could be attributed to gamma knife SRS. Of the remaining 67 (63%) patients, three (4%) developed imaging evidence of moderate-degree peritumoral edema, which was associated with signs and symptoms resulting from the presence of this focal edema. Two of these patients responded well to corticosteroid therapy while one required resection of a necrotic focus. Surgical treatment resulted in a rapid improvement in signs and symptoms in the latter patient.

14.6.2
External Beam Radiotherapy

During the same 5-year period as above, 78 patients with a diagnosis of meningioma were treated with conformal external beam radiotherapy. Patients referred for this treatment typically had:

1. Larger lesions, which precluded the application of gamma knife SRS
2. Extensive residual involvement following skull base surgery
3. Extensive sagittal sinus involvement following subtotal tumor resection
4. A lesion involving a critical structure such as the chiasm, contraindicating the use of SRS

Of the study patients, 60 (77%) were females and 18 (23%) were males; their median age was 58 years.

Of the 78 patients, five (6%) had malignant meningioma, two (3%) had anaplastic meningioma, and three (4%) were classified as having "aggressive tumors." Radiotherapy was given using a 3-D conformal approach. The patient's head and neck was immobilized and computerized tomography was obtained with fiducial markers. The resulting images were reconstructed in 3-D and a treatment plan was devised. In patients with benign meningioma a <1-cm margin of normal tissue was used, while in those with malignant meningioma 2-cm margins were used. Radiation dose was 54 Gy for benign histology and 60 Gy for those with malignant meningioma. The dose was usually defined to the 95% isodose line. This treatment program was very well tolerated by our patients, with

acute toxicity being of no clinical significance. All five patients with malignant meningioma failed the treatment and died within 2 years of radiotherapy. An overwhelming (95%) majority of the remaining patients showed no tumor regression or a slight decrease in tumor dimensions. Of the four patients who failed radiotherapy, two developed multiple progressive tumors, one had pulmonary metastases, and the fourth had progressive tumor growth leading to death. Typical examples of meningioma patients treated with external beam radiotherapy are shown below.

Patient 1 is a middle-aged male who had had two prior surgical resections and presented with suprasellar meningioma involving the right optic nerve and located less than 2 mm from the chiasm (Figs. 14.3, 14.4). Based on the above findings, the patient was felt not to be a candidate for gamma knife SRS. External beam conformal radiotherapy was given to a total dose of 54 Gy, in daily fractions of 1.8 Gy. Figures 14.5 and 14.6 show the treatment plan for this patient. Patient 2 is a 32-year-old female with an extensive meningioma of the floor of the posterior fossa. A partial tumor resection was performed. The residual tumor was encroaching on a wide area extending superiorly from the pons to the upper part of the C2 spinal cord level (Figs. 14.7–14.9). External beam radiotherapy was felt to be the only viable treatment option. Treatment setup and radiation dose distribution are shown in Figs. 14.10 and 14.11.

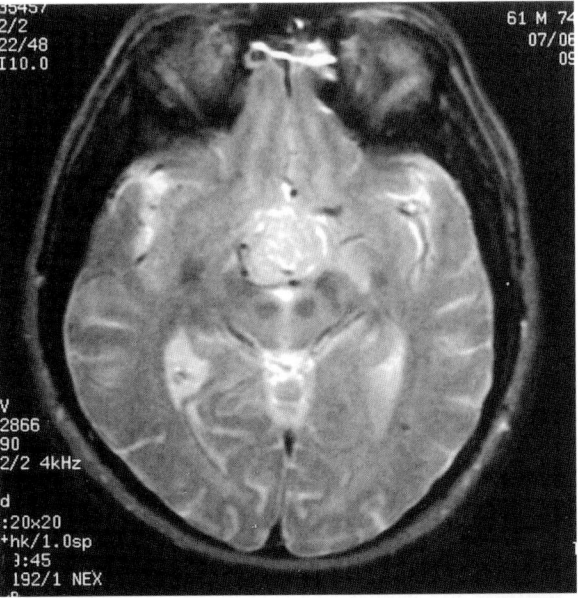

Fig. 14.3. Axial T2-weighted MR image showed a slightly hyperintense mass lesion in the suprasellar region in this middle-aged male

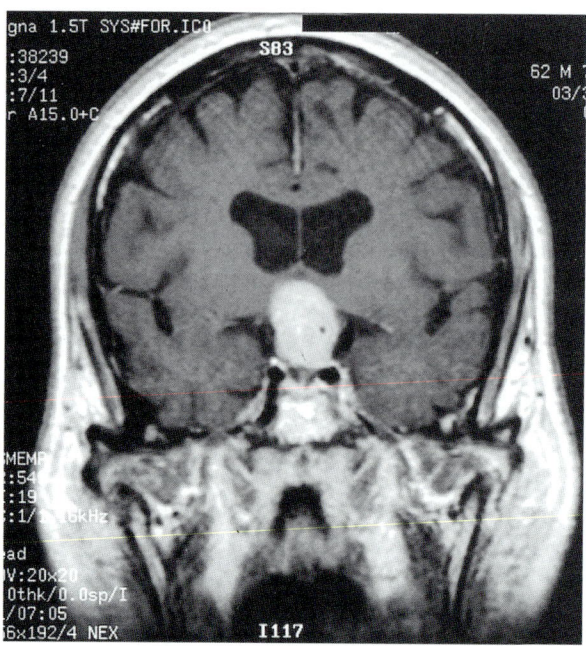

Fig. 14.4. Coronal post-contrast T1-weighted MR image showing an intensely enhancing mass in the suprasellar region (same patient as in Fig. 3)

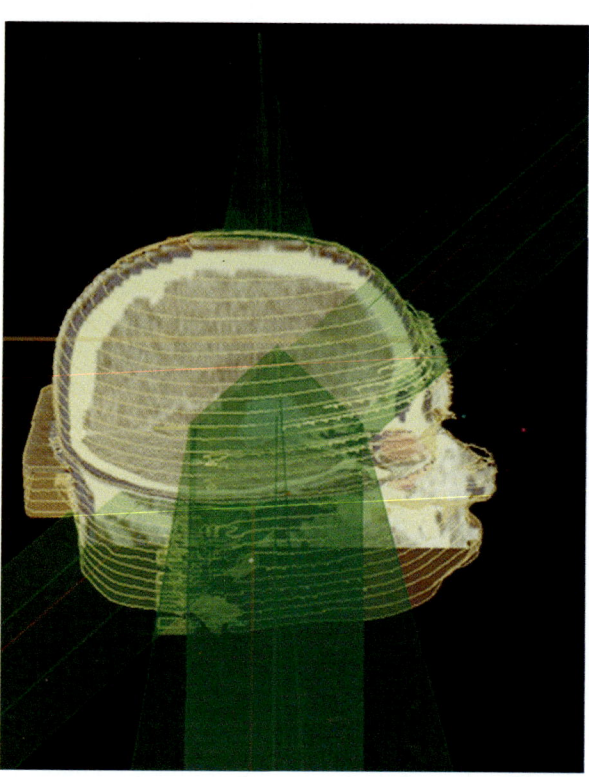

Fig. 14.5. Three-field setup for the management of the suprasellar meningioma shown in Figs. 14.3 and 14.4. The plane of the central rays is an oblique plane, rotated 40° towards the top of the head from the transverse plane. Two lateral and cephalocaudal/anteroposterior oblique fields are used. The collimators of the lateral fields are rotated to match the edges of the oblique fields. A similar setup with smaller field sizes is frequently used for the management of pituitary adenomas

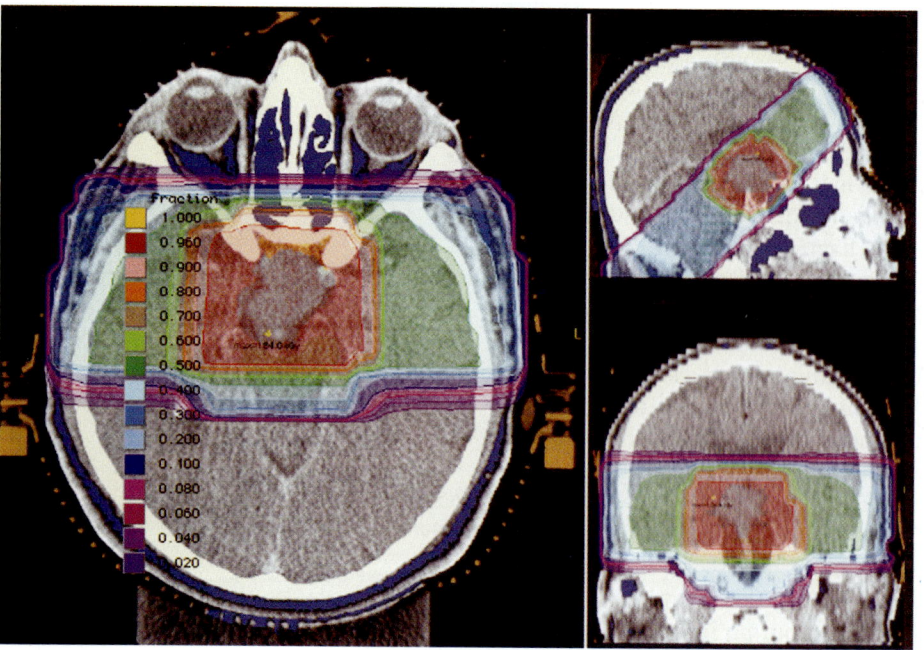

Fig. 14.6. Demonstration of dose distribution of the three-field setup shown in Fig. 14.5. This patient was treated to a total dose of 54 Gy, given in 1.8-Gy daily fractions. The dose is defined to the 95% isodose surface, relative to the global dose maximum. Radiation dose distribution is shown in axial, sagittal, and coronal planes

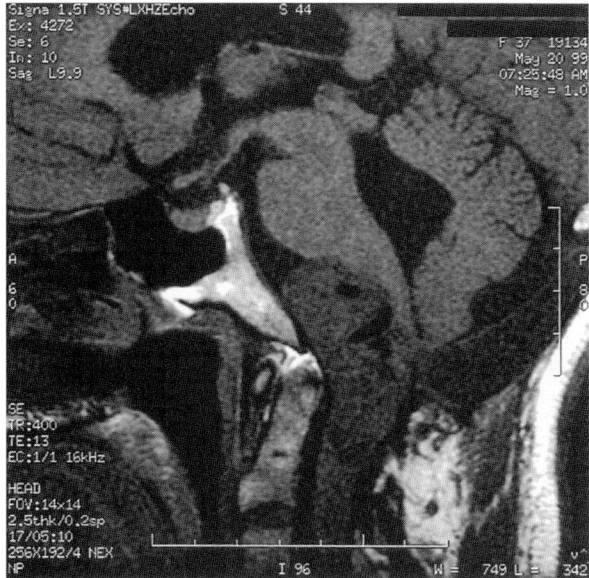

Fig. 14.7. Sagittal, T1-weighted MR image showing an extra-axial mass with anterior compression of the brainstem and upper cervical cord in a 32-year-old female. The mass is slightly hypointense compared with the brain parenchyma

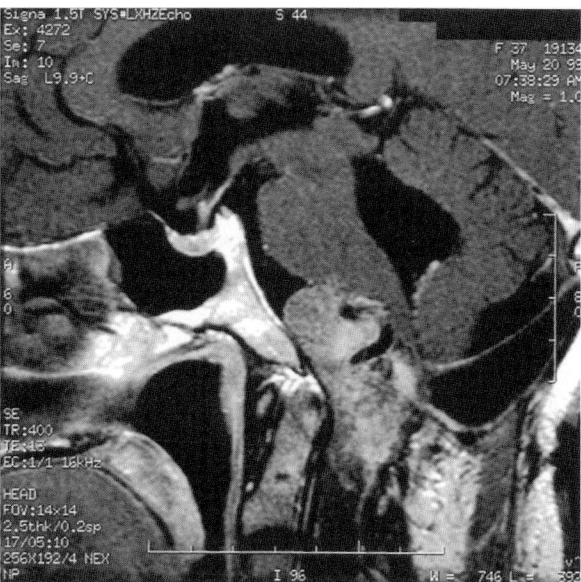

Fig. 14.8. Sagittal, post-contrast T1-weighted MR image showing good enhancement of the mass illustrated in Fig. 14.7. This mass is seen encasing the left vertebral artery (curvilinear signal void)

14.7
Conclusion

Based on the published data (ALHEIT et al. 1999; BARBARO et al. 1987; CARELLA et al. 1982; CONDRA et

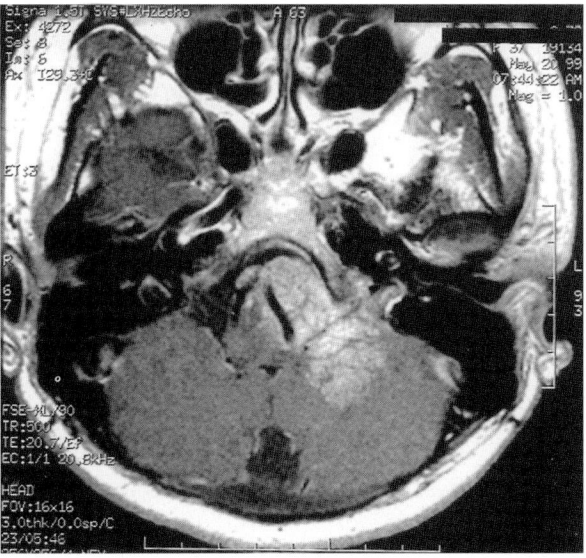

Fig. 14.9. Same patient as in Figs. 14.7 and 14.8. Axial, post-contrast T1-weighted MR image showing an enhancing mass anterior and to the left side of the medulla, involving the left perimedullary and cerebellopontine angle cistern. The medulla is compressed and displaced to the right side

al. 1997; GLAHOLM et al. 1990; KONDZIOLKA et al. 1998; KONDZIOLKA et al. 1999b; MORITA et al. 1999) and the experience at our institution, we would make the following recommendations:

1. All patients with meningioma of malignant or anaplastic histology should undergo external beam radiotherapy irrespective of Simpson's grade.
2. External beam radiotherapy should be used in nearly all patients with aggressive tumors (atypical histology).
3. External beam radiotherapy should also be employed in patients with benign histology and Simpson's grade IV or V.
4. Those with grade III resection should also be considered for postoperative irradiation.
5. Patients who are poor surgical risk should be considered for definitive irradiation, either conformal external beam radiotherapy or SRS.
6. Patients with optic nerve sheath meningiomas should be considered for definitive conformal external beam radiotherapy.
7. Tumors >35 mm in greatest dimension and those in close proximity (<5 mm) to the chiasm or optic nerves should be considered for conformal external beam radiotherapy.
8. The above recommendation also applies to tumors encroaching on the midbrain or a similar critical structure.

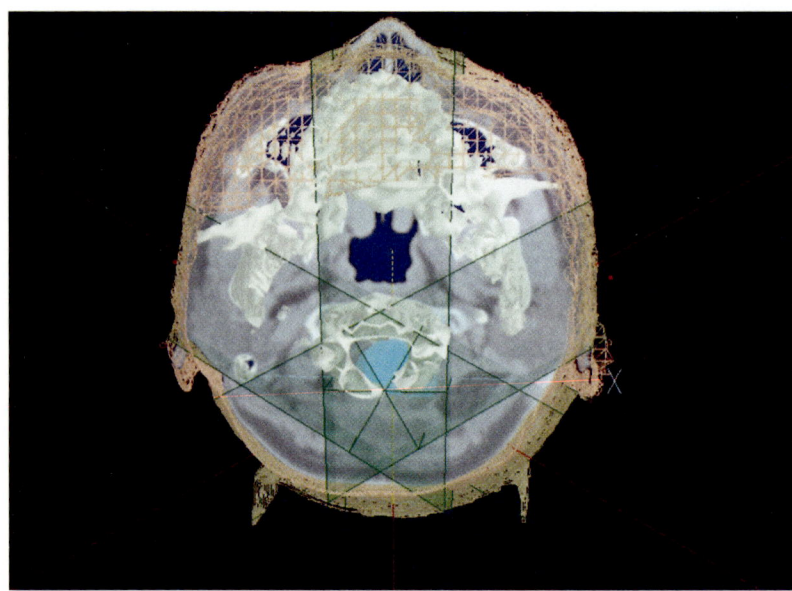

Fig. 14.10. A three-field setup for the treatment of the lesion described in Figs. 14.7–14.9. The plane of the central rays is the transverse plane through the center of the treated lesion. One posterior and two lateral oblique fields are employed. The oblique fields are +120° apart from the posterior field

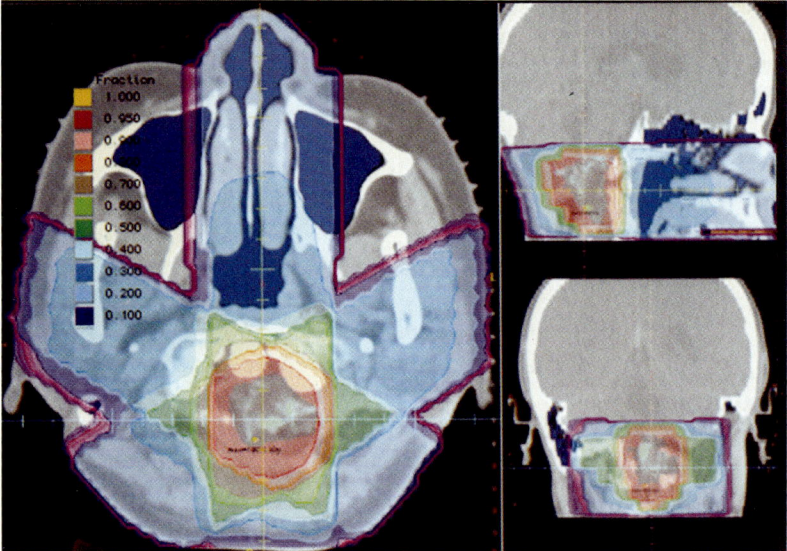

Fig. 14.11. Radiation dose distribution of the three-field setup demonstrated in Fig. 14.10. A total dose of 54 Gy was planned to be given at 1.8 Gy daily. The dose was defined to the 95% isodose line, relative to the global dose maximum. Radiation dose distribution is shown in axial, coronal, and sagittal planes through the center of the lesion

9. Lesions <35 mm and >5 mm from the chiasm or optic nerves should be considered for stereotactic radiosurgery.

10. Smaller (<35 mm) symptomatic or asymptomatic lesions anywhere within the cranial cavity should be considered for stereotactic radiosurgery.

11. The incidence of treatment toxicity of clinical importance in patients with meningioma who have been properly selected for contemporary external beam radiotherapy or SRS is expected to be very low.

12. Both external beam radiotherapy and SRS produce excellent treatment results (>90% incidence of local tumor control) in properly selected patients with intracranial meningioma.

References

Alheit H, Saran FH, Warrington AP, et al. (1999) Stereotactically guided conformal radiotherapy for meningiomas. Radiotherapy & Oncology 50(2):145–150

Barbaro NM, Gutin PH, Wilson CB, Sheline GE, Boldrey EB, Wara WM (1987) Radiation therapy in the treatment of partially resected meningiomas. Neurosurgery 20(4):525–528

Bloom HJG (1982) Intracranial tumors: Response and resistance to therapeutic endeavors, 1970–1980. Int J Radiat Oncol Biol Phys 8:1083–1113

Carella RJ, Ransohoff J, Newall J (1982) Role of radiation therapy in the management of meningioma. Neurosurgery 10(3):332–339

Castro JR, Linstadt DE, Bahary JP (1994) Experience in charge particle irradiation of tumors of the skull base: 1977–1992. Int J Radiat Oncol Biol Phys 29:647–655

Chang SD, Adler JR Jr. (1997) Treatment of cranial base meningiomas with linear accelerator radiosurgery. Neurosurgery 41(5):1019–1025; discussion 1025–1027

Chang SD, Adler JR, Hancock SL (1998) Clinical uses of radiosurgery. Oncology 12: 1181–1191

Coke CC, Corn BW, Werner-Wasik M, Xie Y, Curran WJ Jr. (1998) Atypical and malignant meningiomas: an outcome report of seventeen cases. Journal of Neuro-Oncology 39(1):65–70

Colvett KT, Hsu DW, Su M, Lingood RM, Pardo FS (1997) High PCNA index meningiomas resistant to radiation. Intl J of Radiat Oncol Biol Phys 38(3):463–468

Condra KS, Buatti JM, Mendenhall WM, et al. (1997) Benign meningiomas: primary treatment selection affects survival. Int J of Radiat Oncol Biol Phys 39(2):427–436

DeVries A, Munzenrider JE, Hedley-Whyte T, Hug EB (1999) The role of radiotherapy in the treatment of malignant meningiomas. Strahlentherapie und Onkologie 175(2):62–67

Dziuk TW, Woo S, Butler EB, et al. (1998) Malignant meningioma: an indication for initial aggressive surgery and adjuvant radiotherapy. Journal of Neuro-Oncology 37(2):177–188

Eng TY, Albright NW, Kuwahara G, et al. (1992) Precision radiation therapy for optic nerve sheath meningiomas. Intl J of Radiat Oncol Biol Phys 22(5):1093–1098

Forbes AR, Goldberg ID (1984) Radiation therapy in the treatment of meningioma: the Joint Center for Radiation Therapy experience 1970 to 1982. Journal of Clinical Oncology 2(10):1139–1143

Friedlander RM, Okemann RG, Thornton AF (1999) Management of meningiomas of the cavernous sinus: conservative surgery and adjuvant therapy. Clinical Neurosurgery 45:279–282

Glaholm J, Bloom HJ, Crow JH (1990) The role of radiotherapy in the management of intracranial meningiomas: the Royal Marsden Hospital experience with 186 patients. Intl J of Radiat Oncol Biol Phys 18(4):755–761

Goldsmith BJ, Wara WM, Wilson CB, Larson DA (1994) Postoperative irradiation for subtotally resected meningiomas. A retrospective analysis of 140 patients treated from 1967 to 1990. Journal of Neurosurgery 80(2):195–201

Grant W 3rd, Cain RB (1998) Intensity modulated conformal therapy for intracranial lesions. Medical Dosimetry 23(3):237–241

Gudjonsson O, Blomquist E, Nyberg G, et al. (1999) Stereotactic irradiation of skull base meningiomas with high energy protons. Acta Neurochirurgica 141(9):933–940

Haie-Meder C, Brunel P, Cioloca C, et al. (1995) Role of radiotherapy in the treatment of meningioma. Beulletin du Cancer Radiotherapie 82(1):35–9

Hakim R, Alexander E 3rd, Loeffler JS, et al. (1998) Results of linear accelerator-based radiosurgery for intracranial meningiomas. Neurosurgery 42(3):446–453; discussion 453–454

Hall EJ, Brenner DJ (1993) The radiobiology of radiosurgery: Rationale for different treatment regimes for AVM's and malignancies. Int J Radiat Oncol Biol Phys 25:381–385

Hoffman W, Muhleisen H, Hess CF (1995) Atypical and anaplastic meningiomas –does the new WHO-classification of brain tumours affect the indication for postoperative irradiation? Acta Neurochirurgica 135(3–4):171–178

Jaaskelainen J (1986) Seemingly complete removal of histologically benign intracranial meningioma: late recurrence rate and facts predicting recurrence in 657 patients. Surg Neurol 26:461–469

Kaplan ID, Castro JR, Phillips TL (1994) Helium charged particle radiotherapy for meningioma: experience at UCLBL. University of California Lawrence Berkeley Laboratory. Intl J of Radiat Oncol Biol Phys 28(1):257–261

Kinjo T, Mukawa J, Koga H, Shingaki T (1997) An extensive cranial base meningioma extending bilaterally into Meckel's case report. Neurosurgery 40(3):615–617; discussion 617–619

Kondziolka D, Flickinger JC, Perez B (1998) Judicious resection and/or radiosurgery for parasagittal meningiomas: outcomes from a multicenter review. Gamma knife Meningiomas Study Group. Neurosurgery 43(3):405–13; discussion 413–414

Kondziolka D, Levy EI, Niranjan A, et al. (1999a) Long-term outcomes after meningiomas radiosurgery: physician and patient perspectives. Journal of Neurosurgery 91(1):44–50

Kondziolka D, Niranjan A, Lunsford LD, Flickinger JC (1999b) Stereotactic radiosurgery for Meningiomas. Neurosurgery Clinics of North America 10(2):317–325

Kumar PP, Patil AA, Leibrock LG, et al. (1993) Continuous low dose rate brachytherapy with high activity iodine-125 seeds in the management of meningiomas. Intl J of Radiat Oncol Biol Phys 25(2):325–328

Kurita H, Sasaki T, Kawamoto S, et al. (1997) Role of radiosurgery in the management of cavernous sinus meningiomas. Acta Neurologica Scandinavica 96(5):297–304

Laws ER, Thapar K (1993) Brain tumors. Ca Cancer J Clin 43: 263–271

Lee AG, Woo SY, Miller NR, et al. (1996) Improvement in visual function in an eye with a presumed optic nerve sheath meningioma after treatment with three-dimensional conformal radiation therapy. Journal of Neuro-Ophthalmology 16(4):247–251

Lesch KP, Schott W, Engl HG, et al. (1987) Gonadal steroid receptors in meningiomas. J Neurol 234:328–333

Maguire PD, Clough R, Friedman AH, Halperin EC (1999) Fractionated external-beam radiation therapy for meningiomas of the cavernous sinus. Intl J of Radiat Oncol Biol Phys 44(1):75–79

Mahaley MS, Mettlin C, Natarajan N, et al. (1989) National survey of pattern of care for brain-tumor patients. J Neurosurg 71:826–836

Maire JP, Caudry M, Guerin J, et al. (1995) Fractionated radiation therapy in the treatment of intracranial meningiomas: local control, functional efficacy, and tolerance in 91 patients. Intl J of Radiat Oncol Biol Phys 33(2):315–321

Mayberg MR, Symon L (1986) Meningioma of the clivus and apical petrous bone. J Neurosurg 65:160–167

Milosevic MF, Frost PJ, Laperriere NJ, Wong CS, Simpson WJ (1996) Radiotherapy for atypical or malignant intracranial meningioma. Intl J Radiat Oncol Biol Phys 34(4):817–822

Miralbell R, Linggood RM, de la Monte S, et al. (1992) The role of radiotherapy in the treatment of subtotally resected benign meningiomas. Journal of Neuro-Oncology 13(2):157–164

Miramanoff RO, Dosoretz DE, Linggood RM et al. (1985) Meningioma: analysis of recurrence and progression and progression following neurosurgical resection. J Neurosurg 62:18–24

Morita A, Coffey RJ, Foote RL, et al. (1999) Risk of injury to cranial nerves after gamma knife radiosurgery for skull base meningiomas: Experience in 88 patients. J Neurosurg 90:42–49

Nutting C, Brada M, Brazil L, et al. (1999) Radiotherapy in the treatment of benign meningioma of the skull base. Journal of Neurosurgery 90(5):823–827

Peele KA, Kennerdell JS, Maroon JC, et al. (1996) The role of postoperative irradiation in the management of sphenoid wing meningiomas. A preliminary report. Ophthalmology 103(11):1761–1766

Quest DO (1978) Meningiomas: An update. Neurosurg 3:219–225

Prados MD, Berger MS, Wilson CB (1998) Primary central nervous system tumors: Advances in knowledge and treatment. Ca Cancer J Clin 48:331–360

Rubinstein AB, Schein M, Reichenthal E (1989) The association of carcinoma of the breast with meningioma.. Surg Gynecol Obstet 169:334–336

Schrell UMH, Fahlbusch R (1991) Hormonal manipulation of cerebral meningiomas. In. Al-Meftey O, Ed., Meningiomas, New York, Raven Press, pp 273–283

Sheline GE (1977) Radiation therapy of brain tumors. Cancer 39: 873–881

Shimizu T, Iijima M, Tanaka Y (1995) Radiotherapy for intracranial meningioma: special reference to malignant and high risk benign meningioma. Nippon Igaku Hoshasen Gakkai Zasshi – Nippon Acta Radiologica 55(15):1047–1052

Sibtain A, Plaowman PN (1999) Stereotactic radiosurgery. VII. Radiosurgery versus conventionally-fractionated radiotherapy in the treatment of cavernous sinus meningiomas. British Journal of Neurosurgery 13(2):158–166

Simpson D (1957) The recurrence of intracranial meningiomas after surgical treatment. J Neurol Neurosurg Psych 20: 22–39

Solan MJ, Kramer S (1985) The role of radiation therapy in the management of intracranial meningiomas. Intl J of Radiat Oncol Biol Phys 11(4):675–677

Stafford SL, Perry A, Suman VJ, et al. (1998) Primarily resected meningiomas: outcome and prognostic factors in 581 Mayo Clinic patients, 1978 through 1988. Mayo Clinic Proceedings 73(10):936–942

Subach BR, Lunsford LD, Kondziolka D, Maitz AH, Flickinger JC (1998) Management of petroclival meningiomas by stereotactic radiosurgery. Neurosurgery 42(3): 437–443; discussion 443–445

Taylor BW Jr., Marcus RB Jr., Friedman WA, Ballinger WE Jr., Million RR (1988) The meningioma controversy: postoperative radiation therapy. Intl J of Radiat Oncol Biol Phys 15(2): 299–304

Valentino V, Schinaia G, Raimondi AJ (1993) The results of radiosurgical management of 72 middle fossa meningiomas. Acta Neurochir (Wien) 122:60–70

Vendrely V, Maire JP, Carrouzet V, et al. (1999) Fractionated radiotherapy of intracranial meningiomas: 15 years' experience at the Bordeaux University Hospital Center. Cancer Radiotherapie 3(4):311–317

Vuorinen V, Heikkonen J, Brander A, et al. (1996) Interstitial radiotherapy of 25 parasellar/clival meningiomas and 19 meningiomas in the elderly. Analysis of short-term tolerance and responses. Acta Neurochirurgica 138(5):495–508

Walker AE, Robins M, Weinfeld FD (1985) Epidemiology of brain tumors: The National Survey of Intracranial Neoplasms. Neurol 35:219–226

Winkler C, Dornfeld S, Schwart R, Friedrich S, Baumann M (1998) The results of radiotherapy in meningiomas with a high risk of recurrence. A retrospective analysis. Strahlentherapie und Onkologie 174(12):624–628

15 Management of Low-Grade Gliomas: A Surgical Perspective

LARRY T. KHOO and MICHAEL L. J. APUZZO

CONTENTS

L. T. KHOO, MD
Clinical Instructor, Department of Neurosurgery, University of Southern California School of Medicine, 1200 North State Street, Suite 5046, Los Angeles, California 90033, USA
M. L.J. APUZZO, MD
Edwin M. Todd and Trent H. Well Jr. Professor, Department of Neurosurgery and Radiation, Oncology, Biology and Physics, University of Southern California School of Medicine, 1200 North State Street, Suite 5046, Los Angeles, California 90033, USA

15.1 Introduction

Low-grade gliomas pose a daunting challenge to all clinicians involved in their management. Far from a single clinicopathological entity, this group of tumors is characterized by numerous histologic subtypes each possessing their own unique biological characteristics and behavior. Subdivisions of these neoplasms include low-grade astrocytomas (LGAs), pilocytic astrocytomas, oligodendrogliomas, gangligliomas, dysembryonic neuroepithelial tumors, pleomorphic xanthoastrocytomas, and subependymal giant cell astrocytomas. As each subgroup is overall clinically distinct, this chapter will focus primarily on the most common type of low-grade glioma – the astrocytomas. We will also further restrict our review to grade I and grade II astrocytomas, as defined by the Kernohan classifications, or grade II tumors, as categorized by Daumas-Duport. Although some of the observations and recommendations suggested by this chapter may also apply to other types of low-grade gliomas, the lack of consistent literature on these rarer entities makes them even more difficult to analyze. By limiting our discussion to this group of gliomas, we hope to eliminate much of this confounding information and thereby gain a clearer picture of these particular tumors' behavior. For a broader discussion of these other types of gliomas as well as LGAs, we would direct readers to our two earlier monographs, *Benign Cerebral Gliomas* (vols. I, II), on the subject (APUZZO 1995).

Within the supposedly discrete group of LGAs, there is also a striking amount of additional clinical heterogeneity observed. Whereas some patients with LGAs may survive for an extended period of time, other patients with lesions of the same histologic grade may have a more rapid clinical course with early progression and demise. Interpretation of the available literature on low-grade gliomas has thus been particularly problematic. Our aim in this chapter is thus to review in detail the available information on LGAs and to distill some broad management principles from it.

15.2
Epidemiology

In the adult population, tumors of neuroglial cells comprise nearly 50% of all primary central nervous system tumors. For children, this proportion rises to almost 80%. Of these, diffuse or low-grade astrocytomas account for approximately 25%–35% of these neoplasms. Taken as a whole, well-differentiated astrocytomas thereby comprise 10%–15% percent of all brain tumors in adults and 25%–30% percent in children (Russell and Rubenstein 1989). From the available international population data, the annual incidence rate of gliomas has been estimated at 5.4 cases per 100,000. The calculated incidence rate for LGAs would thereby be 25%–35% percent of this or 1.35–1.89 new cases per 100,000 persons per year (Radhakrishnan et al. 1993).

Unlike their more malignant counterparts, diffuse astrocytomas occur much earlier in life with a predilection for middle age. The peak incidence of these lesions falls between 35 and 45 years of age with a second minor peak in early adolescence (Helseth et al.1989; Laws et al. 1984). This childhood peak is also characterized by a predilection for pilocytic and cerebellar type lesions (Leibel et al. 1975). As far as is known, this distribution is consistent across different national and racial subgroups. Although no sexual predilection is associated with low-grade gliomas, males typically constitute between 55 and 65% of the cases (Guthrie and Laws 1990).

15.3
Pathology and Biology

Like all tumors, gliomas likely arise from either the oncogenetic transformation of pluripotent tissue or from the dedifferentiation of mature cells. Although the cell of origin of LGAs continues to elude identification, exciting insights into the mechanisms of malignancy have begun to unfold. Rather than simply being academic trivia, an up-to-date understanding of the pathobiology behind these lesions assists clinicians by providing valuable prognostic information and optimizing therapy for each individual patient. Thus it behooves the internist, surgeon, and oncologist to be well-versed in such seemingly esoteric details.

15.3.1
Surgical Pathology

Astrocytic tumors, as a group, usually originate within the white matter of the cerebrum and then grow in a centrifugal fashion. The anatomic predilection of LGAs is thus directly proportional to the relative white matter content of each of the brain's hemispheres. Approximately 40%–50% occur in the frontal lobes, 25%–30% in the parietal lobes, 25%–30% in the temporal lobe white matter (Vertosick et al. 1991; Zulch 1986). Although comprising less than 11% of all LGAs, tumors of the deep white and gray matter (i.e., thalamus) are generally associated with a dismal prognosis. Such patients often deteriorate due to the local spread of the tumor in a vital area rather than as a result of dedifferentiation or malignant transformation (Krouwer et al. 1995; Mccormack et al. 1992).

Astrocytomas comprise a spectrum of histologic features that range from the normal and benign to the bizarre and malignant. Traditionally, LGAs have been subdivided into fibrillary, protoplasmic, gemistocytic, and giant cell subtypes by order of frequency. The gemistocytic type is associated with the highest incidence of degeneration and, as a result, a much poorer overall prognosis (Krouwer et al. 1991). Gemistocytic lesions are characterized by fiber-rich cytoplasm with brightly eosinophilic bodies resembling Rosenthal fibers. Due to the aggressive nature of these gemistocytes and the frequent coexistence of early anaplastic features, many pathologists equate their presence with the diagnosis of a grade III astrocytoma (Burger et al. 1991; Schieffer et al. 1987).

Protoplasmic astrocytomas typically involve the cortical gray matter and have been associated with a decreased tendency toward malignant transformation. Protoplasmic lesions characteristically expand the cortical surface and appear as a superficial soft-grayish prominence. Examination of the cut specimen usually reveals a soft, gelatinous homogenate with poorly defined borders, cysts, and involvement of the subjacent white matter. Conversely, the more common fibrillary type is found in white matter lesions and is usually more dense and firmer to palpation (Fig. 15.1). As such, lower grade fibrillary lesions may be more difficult to smear than softer protoplasmic or higher grade tumors. Due to its whitish-yellow coloration and tumor cell infiltration, fibrillary tumors may be even harder to distinguish from the surrounding white matter. Similarly, the adjacent

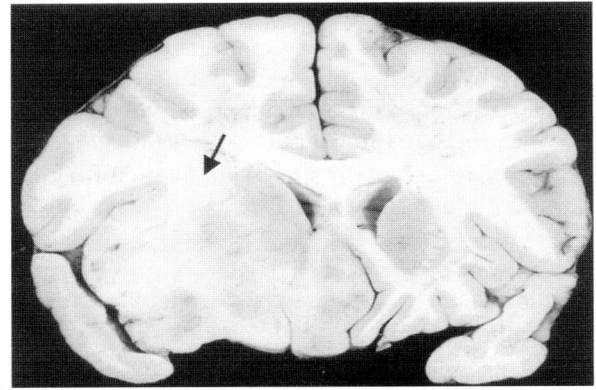

Fig. 15.1a–c. This is a case of a 48-year-old male with a known history of progressive low-grade astrocytoma (LGA) who died from complications secondary to a generalized tonic-clonic seizure. **a** Gross analysis of a coronal brain section demonstrates an infiltrative white matter lesion of the basal frontal lobe (*arrow*). Note that the gray–white matter junction is obscured with relative preservation of the deep gray matter. **b** Histologic micrograph of a sample from this region reveals a hypercellular background of near-normal appearing astrocytes. Little destruction of the underlying white matter architecture is evident. **c** A cortical specimen reveals tumor cells clustered around neurons (e.g., satellitosis, *arrows*) which is not seen in reactive astrocytosis

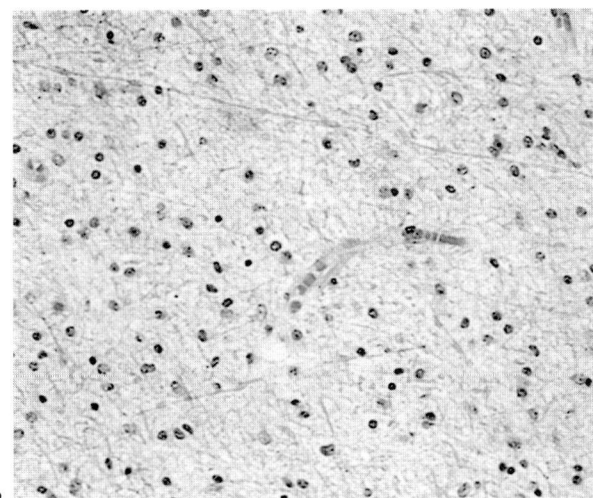

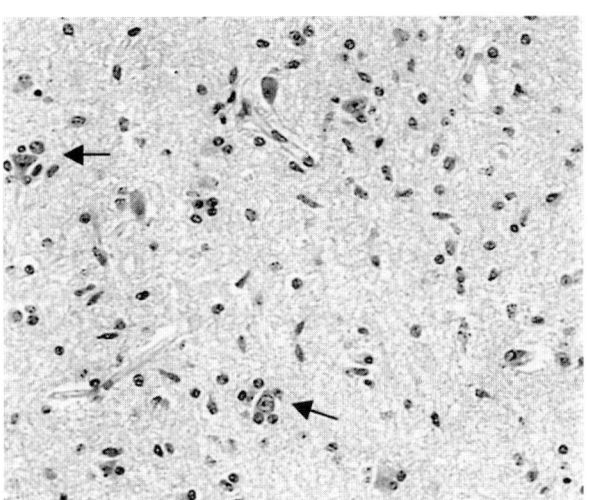

cortical gray–white matter interface may be obscured as well (RUSSELL and RUBINSTEIN 1989).

Special variant groups have also been described including the pilocytic or juvenile astrocytoma, the subependymal giant cell astrocytoma, and the pleomorphic xanthoastrocytoma. In addition to their characteristic histologic appearance, pilocytic astrocytomas demonstrate a unique clinical behavior that carries an excellent outcome and survival regardless of the surgical and radiation extent (PALMA and GUIDETTI 1989). Patients with pilocytic astrocytomas enjoy 10-year survival rates of 80% or more following complete or even incomplete resection (GARCIA and FULLING 1985). Like the pilocytic lesions, most authors feel that the distinguishing features of the giant cell and pleomorphic variants warrant their consideration as separate entities (BLOOM 1982; KEPES et al. 1979; DAUMAS-DUPORT et al. 1988). Aside from the above caveats, the use of descriptive terminology for astrocytomas has been shown to have little prognostic significance.

To provide a more clinically meaningful yard-rule of the biological potential of LGAs, new grading schemata were devised to categorize these lesions including those of Kernohan (grade 1 and 2), Ringert (astrocytoma), Daumas-Duport (grade II), Rubinstein (astrocytoma), and the World Health Organization (grade 1) (KERNOHAN et al. 1949; RINGERTZ 1950; DAUMAS-DUPORT et al.1984; SHAW et al.1989). Subsequent studies have since validated these classifications by positively correlating tumor grade with outcome survival (DAUMAS and DUPORT 1988; KIM et al. 1991). A review of these heuristic systems provides a general histologic gestalt of LGAs. They are comprised primarily of astrocytes with moderate hypercellularity, an infiltrative growth pattern with a broad transition zone to normal tissue, a near normal cell morphology with rare or absent anaplasia, no mitoses, minimal endothelial proliferation, and, importantly, no necrotic areas. Intratumoral heterogeneity and interobserver variability, however, are common and can cause confusion as to the exact grade of a lesion

(PAULUS and PEIFFER 1989). Although impractical, we should thus be mindful of RUSSELL's and RUBINSTEIN's (1989) admonition that „grading, if used at all, should be restricted to autopsy material when the whole tumour can be sampled."

Microscopic examination of protoplasmic lesions reveals engorged tumor cells that possess fewer and shorter processes than their normal cousins. The cells are typically suspended in a fine network of an eosinophilic matrix. The cells force apart the usually orderly white matter array of nonmyelinated nerve fibers. Penetrating blood vessels are rare and may result in the characteristic microcystic degeneration and calcification (15%–30% of cases) that is often found in the deeper aspects of the tumor. On the other hand, the neuroglial extensions of the fibrillary astrocytoma can achieve a significant length and form a woven matrix within which the tumor cell bodies are unevenly clustered. Although separated by the tumor cells, the cortical neurons are otherwise normal in appearance.

Cytologically, diffuse astrocytomas possess a fair amount of nuclear pleomorphism with slightly larger and more coarsely textured nuclei. This nuclear irregularity typically exceeds that of oligodendrogliomas and can aid in diagnosis (BURGER et al. 1991). The cell bodies may be also concentrated in the subpial zone below areas of infiltrated cortical tissue. In the cortex itself, tumor cells often accumulate around neurons (satellitosis), which is a useful diagnostic feature not seen in reactive gliosis (OKAZAKI et al. 1988). Some authors have correlated the presence of these secondary structures (i.e., satellitosis and subpial growth) with active dedifferentiation of the tumor (SCHERER 1938). Extensive multivariate analysis on the prognostic value of these histologic features in 165 cases has revealed that cell density, endothelial hyperplasia, mitoses, and vessel frequency are amongst the most highly significant findings ($p<0.0001$). Nuclear polymorphism, microcysts and vessel size were also important ($p<0.01$).

Interestingly, the presence of early anaplastic or "malignant" changes had more prognostic significance than any of the clinical variables (i.e., Karnofsky score or extent of resection) (SCHIFFER et al. 1987).

Normal astrocytes engage in the formation of cytoplasmic processes with a variable amount of constituent cytoplasmic filaments. Electron microscopy reveals these filaments to be bundles of intermediate filaments ranging from 7 nm to 11 nm in diameter. Whereas these fibrils are abundant in fibrillary astrocytomas, they are sparse or absent in protoplasmic tu-

mors. This accounts for the usually negative staining for GFA (glial fibrillary acidic) protein in protoplasmic varieties and the uniformly positive staining in fibrillary astrocytomas. Immunopositivity of LGAs for vimentin, S-100 protein, glutamine synthetase, and aldolase C isoenzyme is also useful for confirmation (RUSSELL and RUBENSTEIN 1989).

15.3.2
Molecular Biology

With the notable exception of the phakomatoses, there has been little clinical evidence to suggest an inherited genetic component in the pathogenesis of LGAs. WARNICK et al. (1994) noted that low-grade gliomas associated with cases of neurofibromatosis behave in a more aggressive and malignant manner. Low-grade astrocytomas in neurofibromatosis occur predominantly along the optic pathway but can occur at the brainstem, cortex, and cerebelleum in approximately 15% of cases. Tuberous sclerosis patients will similarly develop subependymal giant cell astrocytomas in up to 6% of cases (MORANTZ 1996).

On a contemporary front, modern molecular biology techniques have begun to delineate the oncogenetic changes behind these tumors and to provide valuable clinical prognostic information. In a study of 134 astrocytomas, low-grade (grade II) astrocytomas demonstrated no aneuploid DNA as compared to glioblastoma specimens which had an 80% aneuploid fraction. Additionally, a low S-phase fraction was seen in the majority of well-differentiated tumors. Cox regression data analysis confirmed the clinical prognostic significance of these two variables (VAVRUCH et al. 1996). Based on clinical data, many physicians have postulated that well-differentiated astrocytomas have a very slow growth rate. Growth kinetic and cytogenetic studies of these lesions have since corroborated these conclusions (HOSHINO et al. 1986; SHITARA et al. 1983).

Numerous techniques are also in development to identify intracellular molecular markers that may herald increased growth and a potentially more malignant behavior. The use of monoclonal antibodies for Ki-67 and PCNA (proliferating cell nuclear antigen) have demonstrated good correlation between clonal growth and immunoreactivity (ZUBER et al. 1988). Other significant techniques include in vivo labeling with tritiated thymidine (HOSHINO et al. 1988) and 5-bromodoexyuridine (BUdR; LABROUSSE et al. 1991). For well-differentiated astrocytomas, BUdR and Ki-67 immunoreactivity are seen in less than 1% of tumor cells (BURGER et al. 1991). Patients whose LGAs have a high BudR labeling index tend to progress earlier and die sooner than those who have a low level of immunoreactivity (ITO et al. 1994). HARA et al. (1990) have also described a morphological means of predicting biological potential by quantifying the nucleolar organizing regions of astrocytoma cells. A great deal of recent interest has also been focused on the p53 tumor suppressor gene. A recent study found mutations in the p53 gene in 0% of LGAs, 36% of anaplastic astrocytomas, and 28% of glioblastomas. Additionally, chromosome 10 abnormalities were noted in 61% of glioblastomas but no grade II tumors (FULTS et al. 1992). Other authors have suggested that clonal expansion of p53 expression in astrocytomas carries with it an increased chance of recurrence and malignant progression (SIDRANSKY et al. 1992). Similarly, as gemistocytic LGAs are known to carry a poorer clinical prognosis, they are also most likely to be p53-positive as well. It is important to note, however, that subsequent work on the p53 epitope has yielded mixed results regarding grade and malignancy. After extensive multivariate analysis of p53, Ki-67, and PCNA immunoreactivity in 120 cases of LGA, no prognostic utility could be demonstrated after adjusting for patient age and tumor grade (CUNNINGHAM et al. 1997). Thus placing too much emphasis on any one means of assessing proliferative potential in astrocytomas should be avoided. Nonetheless, these exciting new avenues of research are providing a much needed look into the actual biology underlying gliomas. Whereas LGAs had been previously lumped together based on arbitrary histologic criteria, it is now clear that they are actually a heterogeneous group with a diverse genetic potential.

15.3.3
Natural History

One of the greatest obstacles to treating LGAs has been the inability to accurately define their natural history. As these tumors are frequently quiescent for long periods prior to diagnosis, it is very difficult to gain a clear picture of their prototypical behavior. From historical series, we find that LGA patients often have vague symptoms for 2–3 years prior to their presentation (ELVIDGE et al. 1937). Furthermore, the amount of time it takes for an LGA to manifest such nonspecific symptoms has also never

been established. Even after becoming symptomatic and diagnosed, LGAs can go on to have prolonged periods of latency with little to no growth. Figure 15.2 demonstrates just such a case of a 37-year-old woman whose LGA remain unchanged for nearly 17 years before progressing at age 54. Whereas patients in the past have typically presented with a high proportion of compressive symptoms and increased intracranial pressure, modern day patients are generally diagnosed much earlier after having only an episode of altered consciousness (MORANTZ 1996). Given this observation, it is reasonable to assume that LGAs, left to their own devices, will eventually progress to the point where they will require treatment. The time it takes to reach this symptomatic threshold remains undefined.

To further complicate matters, there are also numerous reports in the literature demonstrating that many LGAs will become more malignant over time (APUZZO 1995). Although we do not know how long it takes for an LGA to become symptomatic, we do know that anywhere from 30%–90% of these tumors will demonstrate evidence of malignant progression at 22–60 months after diagnosis (Table 15.1). This observation has been consistently documented by virtually all large series for both treated and untreated tumors. Although it may be reasonable to conservatively observe some LGAs during their latent period, this overall propensity for malignant progression must be taken into account when formulating a management plan. As such, earlier treatment for LGAs may be warranted on the basis of reducing the risks of such dedifferentiation. A more detailed discussion of this ominous phenomena follows (see Sect. 15.10 Disease Progression).

15.4
Clinical Presentation

Space-occupying lesions of the cerebrum both intra- and extra-axial herald their clinical presence through one of three common pathways. The duration of quiescent growth that occurs before detection varies with the doubling time and growth characteristics of each individual tumor. First, the tumor may enlarge until it achieves a mass effect significant enough to cause a generalized increase in intracranial pressure. Hydrocephalus, papilledema, cognitive decline, headache, and sixth nerve findings are the late findings typically associated with this scenario.

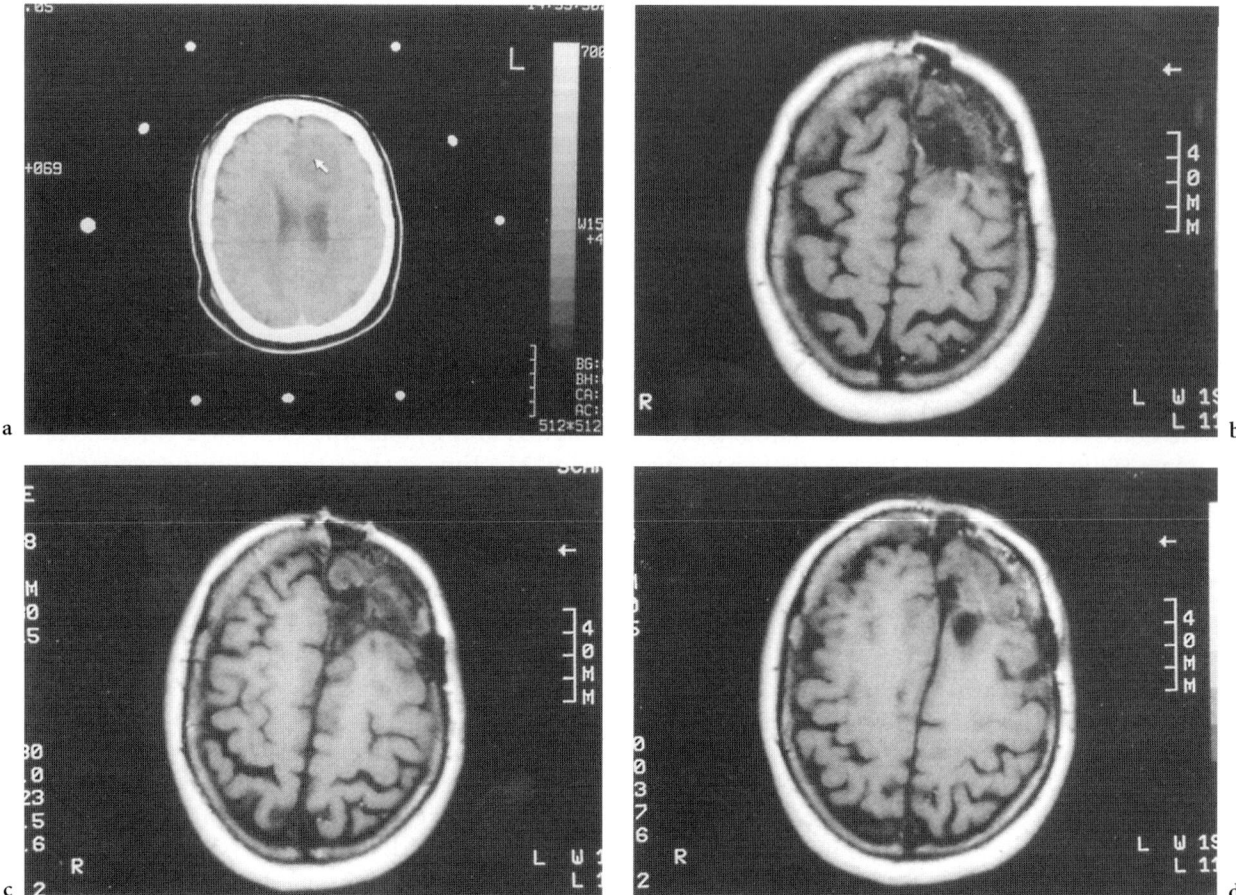

Fig. 15.2a–d. This 54-year-old woman presented with the return of seizures after being conservatively managed for over 17 years for a biopsy-confirmed low-grade astrocytoma (LGA). **a** Contrast-enhanced axial CT image demonstrates a hypodense left frontal mass with no clear areas of enhancement. Comparison with prior images revealed a slight increase in size. The Cosman-Roberts-Wells stereotactic frame's fiducials are evident in the surrounding ring of hyperdense points. Sequential axial images containing these fiducials define the three-dimensional stereotactic volume containing the biopsy target point (*arrowhead*). A gross total resection was achieved with no new post-operative deficits. **b–d** T-1 weighted axial MR images of the resection bed obtained at 5 months reveal no evidence of recurrent tumor

Second, the tumor may expand locally to compress adjacent vital or sensitive structures. In this case, the presenting signs and symptoms will vary according to the specific area of dysfunction (i.e., cranial nerve palsies or pituitary-hypothalamic insufficiency). Third, tumor cells may directly infiltrate and destroy the neural substance either locally or distally through metastases. This can produce site-specific neurological deficits and also, more commonly, seizure activity. Based on their morphology, LGAs have been similarly classified as well. DAUMAS-DUPORT (1984) classified these tumors on their pathological appearance into one of three broad categories. Type I lesions were typically well-circumscribed with a well-defined tumor volume. There was typically only a small surrounding area of edematous white matter.

Type II lesions still demonstrated a clear tumor mass but also had a significant surrounding perimeter or halo of infiltrated, swollen white matter. Type III lesions only contained a broad, ill-defined region of abnormal white matter with interspersed tumor cells and no clearly definable tumor mass. Figure 15.3 illustrates these different types of patterns.

For LGAs, epilepsy or seizure is by far the most common presenting symptom or sign at the time of diagnosis in 40%–78% of patients (LOTE et al. 1997). When one considers the gradual infiltrative nature of these tumors, it is not surprising that this is the case. Aside from seizures, the most common findings, in order, are headaches, focal motor or cranial nerve dysfunction, cognitive decline, nausea/vomiting, visual or speech difficulties, and lethargy. Table 15.2 summa-

Table 15.1. Incidence of low-grade astrocytoma recurrence and malignant transformation

Author/year	Total study (*N*)	Number of clinical recurrences (%)	Interval (months)	Number who had second look	Malignant at second look (%)[a]
Laws (1984)	461	79 (18)	30	79	50
Piepmeier (1987)	60	–	–	14	43
Soffietti (1989)	86	24 (29)	<60	7	79
Steiger (1990)	50	10 (20)	22	4	100
North (1990)	77	32 (48)	–	15	30
Vertosick (1991)	25	14 (56)	60	14	88
McCormack (1992)	53	24 (41)	54	7	86
Phillipon (1993)	179	76 (50)	52	25	72
Berger (1994)	53	10 (19)	38	7	46
Janny (1994)	58	33 (57)	38	16	57
Lote (1997)	379	–	25	66	45
Leighton (1997)	167	90 (54)	50	71	50

[a] Figure represents percent of patients with malignant changes at second look confirmation.

rizes the reported frequency of these signs and symptoms from three larger clinical series. Whereas data obtained from earlier this century contained a sizable number of patients with evidence of intracranial hypertension and focal compressive neurological deficits, contemporary series demonstrate a dramatic decrease in the proportion of such patients (Levy and Elvidge 1956; Horrax 1954; Laws et al. 1988). The drastic decrease in the percentage of patients with papilledema is a striking example of this trend. This observation underscores the tremendous impact that modern diagnostic imaging has had in altering the clinical course of such lesions. The slow insidious growth pattern of LGAs combined with inadequate radiographic imaging frequently led to misdiagnosis (i.e., idiopathic epilepsy) and prolonged delays in

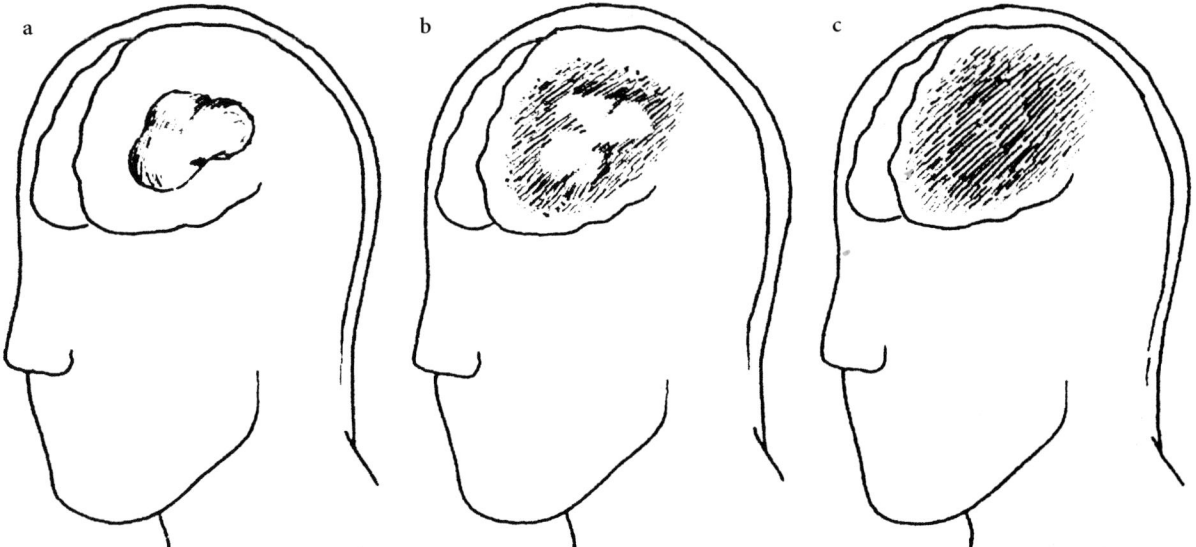

Fig. 15.3a–c. This figure graphically demonstrates the three broad morphological groups of low-grade astrocytomas (LGAs) as originally defined by Daumas-Duport (1984) and subsequently reconfirmed by Kelly (1987) using radiographic criteria. **a** Type I lesions are well circumscribed with a fairly distinct margin and little surrounding infiltrated white matter. **b** Type II lesions contain a distinct solid component but are surrounded by a more vague ring or halo of edematous, infiltrated white matter. **c** Type III lesions contain only such hypoattenuated, edematous white matter without a clearly definable central tumor lobule

Table 15.2. Signs and symptoms of low-grade astrocytomas at time of diagnosis

	Gol (1961)	Laws (1984)	Lote (1997)	Leighton (1997)
Number of patients	194	461	379	167
Period of treatment	Pre-1960	1915–1975	1980–1995	1979–1995
Seizures (%)	56	66	78	78
Nausea/vomiting (%)	31	10	15	–
Headache (%)	72	44	–	29
Lethargy (%)	22	7	10	9
Functional decline (%)	31	16	27	11
Visual dysfunction (%)	22	16	13	–
Speech dysfunction (%)	18	14	–	–
Motor deficit (%)	40–50	26	21	31
Papilledema (%)	59	43	–	9

treatment. Since then, the advent and ready availability of computerized tomography (CT) and magnetic resonance (MR) imaging has greatly expedited the early identification of these lesions (Piepmeier 1987). The largest series (*n*=176) of astrocytomas, from the early 1900s, described a surprisingly long median interval from the onset of symptoms (27–29.8 months) for non-pilocytic LGAs (Elvidge et al. 1937). Three decades later, Gol (1961) reported a 10–12 month median interval in his series. In contrast, Leighton et al. (1997) found a median delay of only 2 months in their retrospective review of patients treated in the contemporary era. It is important to keep this greatly shortened diagnostic „lag" effect in mind when considering the improved outcome data of modern series as compared to that of the traditional literature (Vertosick et al. 1991).

Despite such great diagnostic strides, however, patients harboring LGAs may still have focal symptoms and seizures for many years prior to being diagnosed. Indeed, the natural presymptomatic history of LGAs in toto may not at all be accurately represented by the literature data. Some authors have speculated that patients with more indolent or inactive tumors are often treated expectantly by their physicians and may not routinely be referred to brain tumor centers. As such, these cases with a better prognosis may have been „hidden" and thereby are underrepresented in the published data from these tertiary referral institutions (Cairncross et al. 1990). If the lag effect and early diagnosis account for the increased survival seen in contemporary outcome reports, then why have these same series consistently emphasized the fact that survival is better in patients with longer pre-treatment symptomatic periods (Laws et al. 1984)? Thus the possibility that

such an under-reported or more „benign" subgroup of LGAs exists cannot be dismissed.

Another important aspect of the initial clinical presentation is the functional state of the patient at the time of diagnosis. Fadul et al. (1984) found that of 213 patients with supratentorial astrocytomas, nearly 39% had Karnofsky performance scores greater than 70 and only 17% were severely impaired (KPS<60). Similarly, Phillipon et al. (1993) reported 37% of patients with KPS>70 and only 15% with an impaired score result. Paralleling the trend towards earlier diagnoses, Lote et al. (1997) recently reported only 9% of their 379 patients as having significant functional limitations at the time of presentation. Thus clinicians who choose to treat LGAs must also bear the additional responsibility of causing potential harm to a healthy and intact patient.

15.5
Diagnostic Imaging

Radioisotope scanning, plain skull radiographs, and cerebral angiograms formed the mainstay of imaging modalities earlier this century. Routine roentgenograms of the skull showed abnormalities in 48% of cases with well-differentiated astrocytomas due to the late presentation seen in older series. Clinoid erosion and pineal gland displacement were the most common findings whereas suture diastasis, inner table changes, and calcifications were detected less frequently (7%). Cerebral angiography was sensitive (80%) in identifying frontal hemispheric lesions, but was disappointing for tumors in other locations. Air ventriculograms were reportedly able to achieve a crude surgical localization of the lesion in over three-quarters of cases (ELVIDGE et al. 1956; GOL 1961). These modalities are now only of historical interest and are seldom of utility in visualizing LGAs. Like their histology, which is often merely a slight exaggeration of the normal white matter architecture, LGAs may possess only subtle structural differences from the surrounding brain parenchyma. As such, many low-grade tumors can only be visualized with MR imaging on the basis of their slightly increased tissue density, lower free dipole content, and surrounding edema (see Chap. 7). Most neuroradiologists would agree that MR imaging is the most sensitive test available today to diagnose LGAs (MORANTZ 1995).

The CT and MR imaging findings vary with the specific histology, biology, and invasiveness of each individual tumor. Low-grade astrocytomas are characterized by infiltration of the brain parenchyma with minimal mass effect relative to the size of the lesion, and either absent (60%–90%) or faint, homogenous (10%–40%) contrast enhancement (VERTOSICK et al. 1991; WEINGART et al. 1991). With larger lesions, impingement of ventricular structures is not uncommon. On standard CT axial images, the lesion is typically hypodense with respect to normal brain. On MR imaging, there is dark T1, bright T2 signal abnormality which is often larger than the area of abnormal density seen on CT (Fig. 15.4). This is due to the much greater sensitivity of MR imaging to changes in tissue water content than CT which is based primarily on absolute tissue density. Gadolinium usually does little to improve the diagnostic yield for small lesions, but may be helpful in ruling out higher grade tumors. Some LGAs are truly cystic and may contain fluid-filled portions. The presence of a tumor nodule may often be the only clue to differentiate a cystic astrocytoma from other fluid-filled collections such as an infection. For astrocytomas, the presence of a cyst on imaging was an unreliable correlate of tumor grade (LOFTUS et al. 1985). Neuraxis dissemination of LGAs is an uncommon occurrence and is seldom initially encountered. Current estimates have found evidence of radiographic and / or cerebrospinal fluid (CSF) metastases in 3.7%–5% of cases at the time of diagnosis (GAJJAR et al. 1995). From a cost-analysis standpoint, imaging of the entire neuraxis and sampling of the CSF for every patient with suspected low-grade tumors would thus be difficult to justify. However, the incidence of dissemination at the time of disease progression has been reported to be markedly higher and would thereby warrant a more aggressive diagnostic screening at that time (MAMELAK et al. 1994).

Although many of the neoplasms will appear low in intensity on T1 sequences with correspondingly bright T2 images, most will actually prove to be solid on gross inspection during surgery. Careful histologic exam will then reveal numerous characteristic microcysts as the cause of the increased relaxation time on the T2-weighted sequences. Correlation of the usually homogenous and well-circumscribed area of increased T2 signal with gross specimens usually demonstrates no evidence of hemorrhage, old blood, or necrosis (DRAYER et al. 1987). Other studies correlating serial stereotactic biopsies with these MR-defined abnormalities confirmed that there is almost always actual tumor infiltration in such areas in addition to edematous white matter. As such, it is virtually impossible to differentiate what is tumor and what is infiltrated normal parenchyma solely on the basis of static MR images (KELLY et al. 1987). The radiological term *microcystic astrocytoma* has been applied to lesions with such an appearance.

Whereas studies utilizing early generation CT scanners did not find any statistically significant correlation between contrast enhancement and outcome (SILVERMAN and MARKS 1981), a review of more recent retrospective series reveals inconsistent findings. PHILLIPPON et al. (1993), in their sizable review of 179 patients treated between 1978 and 1987 at the Hopital de la Salpetriere, also could not find any significant prognostic effect of contrast enhancement. Most other authors have, however, indicated that contrast enhancement of LGAs on CT scanning portends a poor biological and clinical course. As contrast enhancement generally connotes an active breakdown of the blood–brain barrier, it is thought that extravasation of dye material on CT indicates malignant invasion of the neurovascular interface. PIEPMEIER (1987), in his review of 60 cases, found that, irrespective of adjuvant radiation, patients with tumors marked by contrast on CT had a significantly shorter mean survival. The difference was still pronounced even after the data were adjusted for age, which is the strongest statistical predictor of outcome in LGAs (SOFFIETTI et al.1989; JANNY et al.1993). Similarly, MCCORMACK et al. (1992), in their analysis of 53 cases of supratentorial lesions, calculated an increased recurrence risk ratio of 6.8 for tumors demonstrating pre-treatment contrast enhancement. In their large series of 379 patients treated exclusively in the CT and MRI era, LOTE et al. (1997) reported a more conservative 2.0 hazards ratio for patients with initial CT tumor enhancement. Additionally, tumor enhancement was a

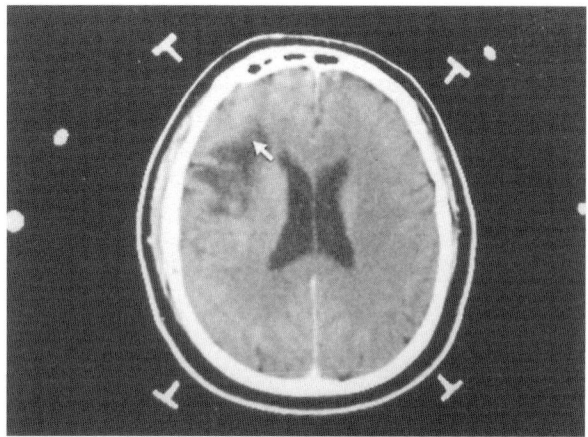

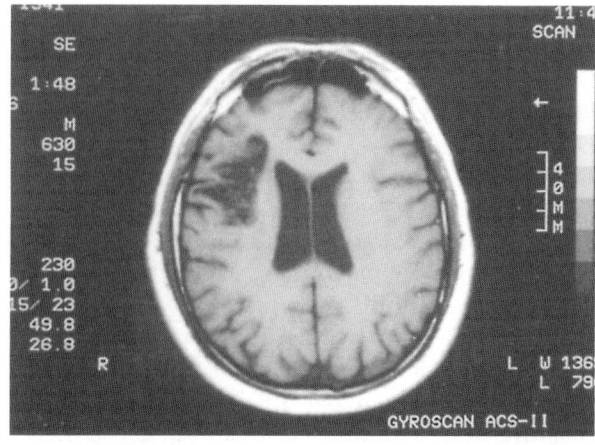

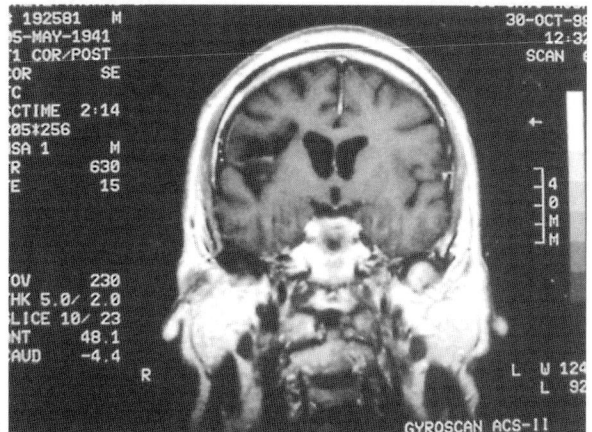

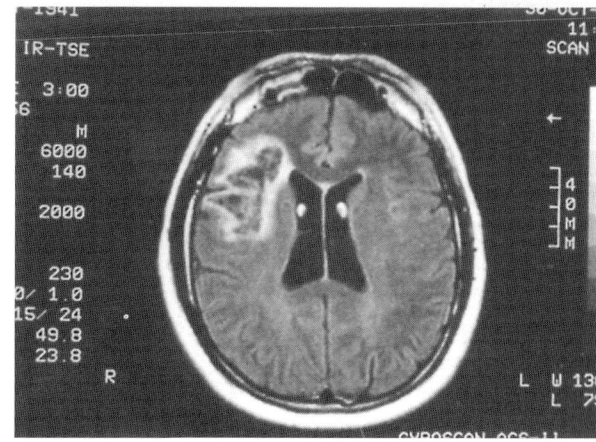

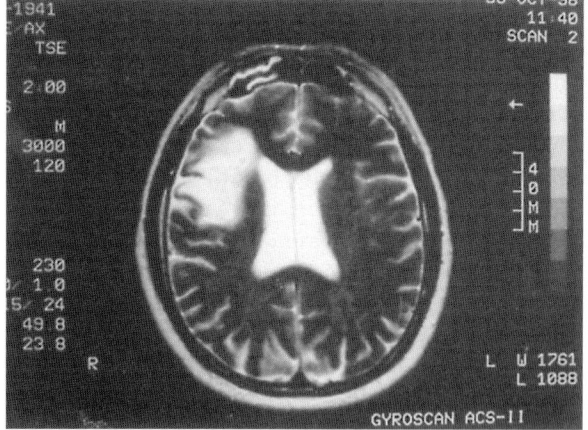

Fig. 15.4a–e. A 58-year-old left-handed male presented with a 2-year history of progressive cognitive decline, clumsiness, and difficulty writing. **a** Non-contrast-enhanced CT reveals a hypodense mass within the substance of the right frontal lobe. This image, taken at the time of stereotactic biopsy, shows the target point (*arrowhead*) from which tissue confirmed the presence of a low-grade glioma. **b, c** T1-weighted gadolinium-enhanced axial and coronal MR images reveal a low-attenuation lesion in the frontal white matter with relative preservation of the overlying cortical ribbon and little mass effect. **d, e** FLAIR sequence and T2-weighting of the area demonstrates a very limited amount of surrounding edema. Note that the FLAIR sequence is able to differentiate between the tumor and surrounding white matter infiltration whereas the T2 sequence reveals only a homogeneous bright signal

multivariate negative prognostic factor for survival in their analysis. Thus, the issue of contrast enhancement remains unresolved and will likely persist as newer data from patients treated in the era of MR imaging becomes available.

Laws et al. (1984) observed that „the proportion of patients treated by biopsy has fallen over time, reflecting an increased accuracy of neuroradiological diagnosis." As a result, many clinicians have treated solely on the basis of the radiographic diagnosis and forego tissue confirmation. Such an over-reliance on diagnostic imaging may prove questionable as some studies have since demonstrated a poor correlation between CT and MR grading of astrocytomas and the histopathological findings from the surgical specimen. For example, the use of contrast enhancement on CT to predict malignancy in astrocytic tumors has been advocated. However, 31% of biopsy-proven highly anaplastic astrocytomas and 54% of moderately anaplastic tumors showed no contrast enhancement whatsoever on CT (CHAMBERLAIN et al. 1988). In another analysis of 71 low-grade and anaplastic lesions, 36.1% of low-grade lesions enhanced and 28.6% of anaplastic tumor did not enhance (MCDERMOTT et al. 1992). Conversely, pilocytic astrocytomas routinely show striking homogeneous enhancement but demonstrate a relatively benign clinical course. KONDZIOLKA et al. (1993), in their review at the University of Pittsburgh found that MR imaging and CT had a 50% false-positive rate in predicting the histologic grade of astrocytomas. In their words, „providing conservative management of patients with anaplastic tumors because the imaging appearance seems typical for LGAs is inappropriate.“

With the recent innovations and improved resolution of functional imaging, neuroradiologists in conjunction with physiologists are now able to directly probe the metabolic, chemical, and electrical activity of a given cerebral volume and thereby gain an impression of its biological potential. For LGAs, a hint of these new technologies is evident in the work that has been done with positron emission tomographic (PET) and functional MR imaging scanning (HARSH 1999). By utilizing isotope-labeled 2- or 18-fluoro-deoxyglucose, PET is able to visualize the relative metabolic activity of a tumor in relation to the adjacent brain parenchyma. Purely low-grade lesions are hypometabolic or „cold“ on PET scanning (Fig. 15.5),

while actively growing malignant or dedifferentiating tumor areas appear hypermetabolic or „hot“ (FRANCAVILLA et al. 1989). Real-time information can thereby be provided as to the biological activity of a given lesion and thus serve as a potential predictor of prognosis (ALAVI et al. 1988). Similarly, functional diffusion and perfusion MR imaging techniques can estimate the actual amount of blood flow to an astrocytoma thus providing an index of growth (LE BIHAN et al. 1993). Ultimately, this type of information may be extremely valuable in determining the best site for stereotactic biopsy, the limits of surgical resection, and perhaps even which patients are most likely to benefit from adjuvant therapies (WORTHINGTON et al. 1987).

15.6
Clinical Decision Making

Clearly, the rapidity and accuracy with which intracerebral neoplasms are now diagnosed has increased at least a hundred-fold over the last century. What has not essentially changed, however, is the actual art of clinical decision making. Regardless of how quickly or elegantly a diagnosis is attained, there still ultimately comes a moment of truth when the physician and the patient must decide on what course of action to pursue. The innovations of medical tech-

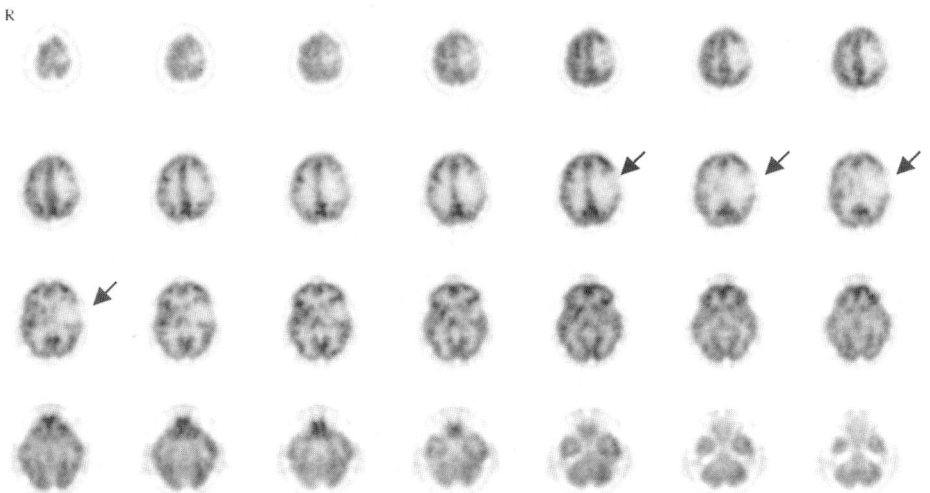

Fig. 15.5. Positron emission tomographic (PET) scan axial images demonstrating decreased fluorodeoxyglucose metabolism in the left posterior frontal region *(arrowheads)*. Upon correlation with the MR anatomical images, these areas corresponded with the location of a previously biopsied low-grade astrocytoma (LGA). Thus the tumor was felt to be „cold“ in metabolism and less likely to be associated with increased proliferation and anaplasia. The patient was observed after stereotactic biopsy for over 7 years to date without evidence of local progression or transformation

nology have only served to change the backdrop against which these crucial decisions must still be made. Earlier this century, patients with LGA were characteristically much farther along in their disease course when diagnosed. Frequently, they had suffered from „epileptic" fits for some time under the care of their personal physician and were not referred for treatment until they developed debilitating neurological deficits. The choice of whether or not to intervene was usually clear-cut at this juncture. Thus there was little question that these patients should undergo an open craniotomy for either biopsy, debulking, or attempted resection to relieve their symptoms Today, on the other hand, the modern neurosurgeon and oncologist are faced with a very different clinical picture (WILSON and PRADOS 1986). Aside from an initial stimulus such as a persistent headache or seizure which led to a positive CT or MR imaging scan, the overwhelming majority of patients will present with no neurological deficit or functional impairment. For them, anticonvulsant therapy, a brief course of glucocorticoids, mild analgesics, and some reassurance are often all that is initially required. As they are otherwise intact, the decision to intervene at this point and to thereby cause potential harm cannot be taken lightly – *Primum non nocere.*

To minimize any such unnecessary risks, all possible options should be reviewed to ensure an informed choice by all parties. Using basic, modern day oncological principles, the therapeutic possibilities at this point are usually: (1) conservative management and expectant observation, (2) limited biopsy (open or stereotactic) for tissue diagnosis, (3) craniotomy for surgical debulking and/or attempted resection, and (4) external beam irradiation of the tumor. From a Punnett square type analysis of these choices, a list of the viable initial management options is obtained:

1. Expectant observation only based on imaging diagnosis of LGA
2. Biopsy with confirmation of LGA and then observation only
3. Biopsy with confirmation of LGA and then surgical resection only
4. Biopsy with confirmation of LGA and then irradiation only
5. Biopsy followed by surgical resection and irradiation
6. Primary surgical resection of suspected LGA only
7. Primary surgical resection followed by irradiation
8. Empirical irradiation of suspected LGA on basis of imaging diagnosis

Each of these options has been and is being presently utilized by different brain tumor centers worldwide in the primary management of LGAs. Additionally, each of these institutions has also published their protocol's outcomes and they have all demonstrated varying degrees of success. Although no convincing, prospective randomized study has been done to date, it is important to familiarize oneself with the available literature to thereby make an educated „guess" as to which options (1–8) are most appropriate.

15.6.1
Conservative Management

Modern genetic and molecular analysis have proven the majority of LGAs to be anything but „benign", yet this descriptive term has heavily influenced the psyche of those caring for these patients. In the past, many physicians have recommended a period of cautious observation for patients after treating their presenting ictus. Most commonly, the diagnosis of LGA was based on a supposedly typical clinical history and „characteristic" radiographic findings. To many physicians, the risk of injuring a neurologically intact person by open surgery or radiotherapy was difficult to justify for what was presumed to be a very slow-growing or „benign" lesion. A sizable proportion of these patients would then undergo only a stereotactic biopsy for tissue confirmation. After being certain of the tumor's low-grade nature, a period of conservative follow-up thus ensued (option 2). For small lesions in eloquent tissue of the speech, motor, or sensory cortex, even the small risk of a limited biopsy seemed prohibitive and thus these patients would be only observed (option 1) (CAIRNCROSS and LAPERRIER 1990).

As radiographic grading of gliomas has been shown to be notoriously inaccurate (see Sect. 15.5 Diagnostic Imaging), the majority of academic centers have been reluctant to employ such a period of only „watchful waiting" without biopsy (option 1). As a result, little published outcome data for this pathway are available for review. In one of the only such studies, a group of 46 patients was retrospectively identified who had presented with a transient event and subsequent radiographic evidence strongly suggestive of a low-grade primary supratentorial neoplasm. Twenty-six of these patients had all therapy (except anticonvulsants) withheld for a variety of reasons including surgical inaccessibility, equivocal diagnosis, and patient/physician preference. Of this expectantly managed group, 15 (68%)

went on to require intervention at a median interval of 29 months for either progressive seizures, new neurological symptoms, or radiographic evidence of malignant transformation. The other 20 patients in the cohort had almost immediate surgical and/or radiation therapy and were used as a control. When compared, there were no statistical differences in performance scores, quality of life, amount of intratumoral anaplasia (at resection or autopsy), rate of malignant transformation, or overall survival between the two groups (RECHT et al. 1992). Of note is the fact that there were no grossly incorrect radiographic diagnoses with confirmation of the astrocytic lineage in all operated patients. As such, the merits of expectant management for LGAs (options 1 and 2), although seemingly counterintuitive to modern oncological thinking, should not be readily dismissed.

15.6.2
Resection vs Biopsy

As residual cells have a propensity for continued growth and/or malignant dedifferentiation, most centers have recommended either a radical or „gross total" resection whenever possible for cases of astrocytomas. Options 3, 5, 6, and 7 reflect this underlying tenet of surgical tumor reduction and will subsequently be discussed in detail (see Sect. 15.8 Cytoreductive Surgery). The overwhelming majority of surgical studies have thus focused on the degree of cytoreduction and compared the results of limited resections vs more aggressive extirpations. More recently, however, some authors have begun to question the actual need for surgical debulking. In a well-crafted review of 417 cases of astrocytomas, no survival advantage could be demonstrated between extensive surgical resection and limited open or stereotactic biopsy (SCANLON and TAYLOR 1979). VERTOSICK et al. (1991), in analyzing their experience with LGAs between 1978 and 1989, found a median survival of almost 8.2 years. When compared to comparable modern series employing surgical reduction (SHAW 1989: 4.5 years, PIEPMEIER 1987: 7.5 years, MEDBERRY 1988: 4.0 years, PHILLIPON 1993: 8.8 years), this figure represents a very reasonable if not excellent outcome. Importantly, over two-thirds of their patients underwent only closed stereotactic needle biopsy followed by external beam irradiation (option 4). Some have argued that comparing survival lengths from the earlier literature is biased by the higher morbidity associated with older

surgical techniques and the diagnostic lag effect. They have pointed out that, with improved diagnostic and operative techniques, outcome data from contemporary operative series would be more likely to demonstrate the benefit of radical surgical resection. From a very recent analysis of 379 patients with low-grade gliomas treated between 1980 and 1995 (LOTE et al. 1997), we find that this still may not be the case. When comparing their two groups (biopsy followed by irradiation, resection followed by irradiation), there was no statistically significant difference in the duration of survival. Subgroup analysis did, however, substantiate the use of surgical debulking for patients who presented with symptoms of increased intracranial pressure ($p<0.03$).

Should surgical debulking and/or resection be attempted for all patients with suspected LGA, or is a limited biopsy followed by irradiation as effective? Table 15.3 summarizes several of the major clinical reports that have addressed the effect of surgical resection in LGAs on outcome and survival. The studies are further subdivided into those which have found benefit with more aggressive resection and those which have not. Although without statistical relevance, a simple summation of the data reveals ten series with 1395 patients that show a benefit of aggressive resection and nine others with 1274 patients that do not. SALCMAN (1985), in his retrospective literature review of 603 patients, compared survival curves of patients after gross-total resection vs biopsy. Although, an overall increased survival was shown in the resected group early on, both curves converged after 24 months. Thus, for the moment, it would appear that there are no clear-cut answers to this pressing clinical dilemma. Perhaps more importantly, these conflicting data underscore the need to remain flexible when treating cases of LGA. Rather than blind dogmatic adherence to preset management protocols, it is best to take into account the specific needs of each individual patient and to tailor the treatment plan accordingly.

15.6.3
Primary Radiotherapy

Perhaps even more controversial than the benefits of aggressive resection is the role of radiotherapy in the management of LGAs (see Chap. 16). Many studies have retrospectively attempted to address this issue by looking for prolonged survival in irradiated vs non-irradiated patients. A brief summary (Table 15.4) of several such major series will be discussed

Table 15.3. Effect of surgical resection on survival: summary

Resection benefit?	N	Study period	Author(s)	Biopsy/partial			Subtotal			Gross		
				3 yr	5 yr	10 yr	3 yr	5 yr	10 yr	3 yr	5 yr	10 yr
No (na)[a]	53	1935–1950	Elvidge (1956)	–	–	–	100	100	43	100	91	28
No (na)[a]	417	1960–1969	Scanlon (1979)	–	–	–	–	64	–	–	–	–
No (na)[a]	88	1960–1985	Whitton (1990)	–	–	–	–	–	–	–	–	–
No (p>0.81)	167	1960–1982	Shaw (1995)	–	–	–	–	52	55	–	20	23
No (p>0.25)	50	1960–1986	Medberry (1988)	–	–	–	–	43	–	–	57	–
No (p>0.83)	60	1975–1985	Piepmeier (1987)	6.24*	–	7.22*	–	8.47*	–	–	–	–
No (na)[b]	25	1978–1988	Vertosick (1991)	90	62	35	–	–	–	–	–	–
No (p>0.70)	379	1980–1995	Lote (1997)	78	60	50	–	–	–	85	70	45
No (na)[b]	35	1982–1992	Lunsford (1995)	–	88	47	–	–	–	–	–	–
Yes (na)[a]	197	?	Gol (1961)	0.7*	–	–	–	–	–	2.2*	–	–
Yes (p<0.0001)	461	1915–1976	Laws (1986)	–	32	37	–	44	52	–	61	59
Yes (p<0.01)	85	1950–1982	Soffietti (1989)	21	–	–	56	24	3	79	51	11
Yes (na)[a]	68	1958–1974	Fazekas (1977)	–	–	–	57	40	27	90	90	27
Yes (p=0.03)	58	1970–1990	Janny (1994)	–	–	–	–	57	31	–	88	68
Yes (p=0.002)	77	1975–1984	North (1990)	50	43	–	80	64	–	85	85	–
Yes (na)[b]	53	1977–1988	McCorm(1992)	–	–	–	64	62	40	–	–	–
Yes (p<0.01)	179	1978–1987	Phillipon (1993)	–	45	–	–	50	–	–	80	–
Yes (p=0.006)	167	1979–1995	Leighton (1997)	–	–	–	–	64	41	–	82	59
Yes (p=0.09)	50	1984–1989	Steiger (1990)	–	–	–	50	–	–	70	–	–

[a] Paper compares groups based on amount of resection, but no statistical analysis done. Conclusions on benefit of surgical resection solely from authors' statements.

[b] Paper does <u>not</u> compare groups based on resection. Only one group primarily studied. Conclusions on benefit of surgical resection based solely from author's statements.

* Mean survival in years

Table 15.4. Effect of postoperative irradiation on survival: summary

Radiation benefit?	N	Study period	Author	Survival(%) 5 years		10 years		RT dose
				S	S+RT	S	S+RT	
Yes	152	1939–59	Bouchard (1960)	38	49	–	–	5000–6000 cGy
Yes	176	1940–49	Levy (1956)	26	36	–	–	?
Yes	108	1942–67	Leibel (1975)	19	46	11[a]	35	3500–5000 cGy
Yes (p=0.02)	86	1950–1979	Garcia (1985)	22	40	9	9	3500–6100 rads
No	83	1955–1959	Uihlein (1966)	65	54	–	–	2000–6000 cGy
Yes	45	1956–70	Stage (1974)	20	42	–	–	3500–6500 cGy
Yes	68	1958–1974	Fazekas (1977)	32	54	32	26	850–1400 rads
No(p>0.04)	461	1915–1976	Laws (1986)	34	49	18	20	4000–7900 rads
No (p>0.05)	86	1950–1982	Soffietti (1989)	30	9–25	–	–	4000–5500 cGy
Yes (p=0.04)	126	1960–1982	Shaw (1989)	32	54	11	27	600–6500 rads
Yes	119	1965–1989	Shibamoto (1993)	37	60	11	41	3000–6000 cGy
No (p>0.05)	58	1970–1990	Janny (1994)	50	67	26	25	2000–7000 cGy
No (p>0.05)	179	1978–1987	Philippon (1993)	65	55	50	40	5000–6000 cGy
No (p>0.05)	63	1974–1992	Bahary (1996)	66	67	50	42	4500–6000 cGy
No (p=0.83)	167	1979–1995	Leighton (1997)	84	62	70	35	5000–5500 cGy
Yes (p<0.05)	38	1980–1992	Hara (1995)	63	0	–	–	4700–5000 cGy
No (p=0.20)	379	1980–1995	Lote (1997)[b]	–	–	–	–	4500–7000 cGy

S, surgery; RT, radiotherapy.

[a] Fifteen-year survival data.

[b] Statistical analysis done, but exact survival data were not published.

(see Sect. 15.9 Adjuvant Radiotherapy and Chemotherapy) with a detailed analysis to follow in the next chapter. For the moment, it is sufficed to say that no clear consensus exists as to whether radiation therapy is of benefit in surgically resected patients. Furthermore, it is also unclear as to whether patients who have surgery and radiation have any improved survival over those who have only a biopsy and irradiation. As such, these findings thereby raise the interesting possibility of option 8 (primary irradiation after radiographic diagnosis of a LGA). There are essentially two broad arguments against this course of action. First, no tissue confirmation is obtained thus leaving great uncertainty as to exactly what is being irradiated. Although radiographic grading of astrocytomas has been shown to have significant error and variability, the data of RECHT et al. (1992) suggest that this may not necessarily have a negative impact on outcome. The second argument is that a lack of cytoreduction leaves some tumor cells protected within the core of the mass. However, as already discussed, the benefit of debulking is controversial at best for LGAs. Although empirically subjecting the cerebrum to the potentially harmful effects of irradiation would seem cavalier, there is no clear-cut evidence to reject the use of up-front radiotherapy (option 8). Indeed if biopsy plus irradiation yields similar outcomes to resection plus irradiation, would it be so unreasonable to postulate that irradiation alone would also be effective?

15.6.4
General Guidelines

At this point, one cannot help but wonder if any meaningful clinical decision making is possible in light of this conflicting information. Although an extensive, prospective multivariate analysis to identify an „ideal" or „optimal" care plan would be the ideal solution, the practical difficulties of such an undertaking render it wishful thinking at best. For the moment, we are thus left with the published data of these retrospective series upon which to base our decisions. From them, we can at least glean a few general principles, trends, and observations by which to formulate some management strategies.

For all patients who present with a suspected LGA appropriate symptomatic therapy should be initiated. Anticonvulsants such as phenytoin, neurontin, or carbamazepine should be initiated to prevent the injurious effects of further seizures. Mild analgesics and a brief course of glucocorticoids can be employed for patients with significant headache, compressive signs, or mass effect. Patients with hydrocephalus and increased intracranial pressure typically have developed their symptoms gradually over time and typically do not require acute intervention. Some initial diuretic therapy, perioperative steroids, and mild fluid restriction are generally adequate to stabilize most patients until therapy. For those who are in extremis, a ventriculostomy will sometimes be needed for several days before surgery with trial occlusions done to determine if permanent CSF diversion will be needed.

After this initial cluster of issues has been addressed, a full non-invasive diagnostic and radiological work-up of the patient should be completed. If not yet done, good-quality enhanced MR imaging and/or CT must be obtained and interpreted by an experienced neuroradiologist. A reasonable attempt should also be made to exclude other diagnostic possibilities. A broad differential would also include metastases, lymphoma, other glial tumors, vasculitis, recent stroke, venous hypertension, venous infarction, focal meningitis, viral infections, degenerative diseases of the white matter, post-traumatic edema, and toxin- or radiation-induced injury. Within the spectrum of low-grade gliomas, other tumors such as pilocytic astrocytomas, pleomorphic xanthoastrocytomas, dysembryonic neuroepithelial tumors, gangliogliomas, and oligodendrogliomas must also be considered. As the radiographic appearances of these lesions are often very similar, the definitive diagnosis must often be withheld until an adequate tissue sampling is obtained. If costs are not prohibitive, additional tests to assess the tumor's metabolic activity (i.e., PET or functional MR imaging) can provide further valuable insight into the biological potential of the lesion . If LGA continues to top the differential diagnosis, then the most important step at this point is a conference with the patient and the family. All the options (1–8) should be presented, with a detailed discussion of the pros and cons of each. For patients with neurological deficits and/or signs of increased intracranial pressure, early surgical debulking would seem to be a reasonable initial recommendation (options 6, 7). In patients who are too weak or ill to undergo any surgical procedure, early irradiation (option 8) may be the only choice aside from glucocorticoids and observation alone (option 1). Unfortunately, this still leaves the overwhelming majority of LGA patients who are intact. For those who wish to postpone any risk of intervention until absolutely necessary, a period of watchful waiting (option 1) is certainly not unreasonable in light of our previous discussion. However as the risk of the procedure is minimal (see Sect. 15.7 Stereotactic Biopsy), we would recommend that all medically eligible patients undergo an image-guided stereotactic tumor biopsy at this stage to confirm the astrocytic nature and grade of the lesion. A careful histologic analysis and proliferative index assessment can also provide helpful prognostic information. For tumors with radiological, histologic, and molecular findings suggestive of an increased risk of early growth or anaplasia, the neurosurgeon may wish to recommend earlier intervention (options 3, 4, or 5). For a well-differentiated lesion with a low-proliferative index and a cold PET scan appearance, postponing treatment until the disease progresses may also be appropriate (option 2). Lacking absolute guidelines, the „best" choice in therapy is often simply that which both the physician and patient can comfortably agree upon. Primary management for LGAs thus remains very much an „art" and should be tailored to meet the needs of each individual case.

15.7 Stereotactic Biopsy

Once the decision has been made to obtain a „definitive" tissue diagnosis, the surgeon is thus faced with the question of how to obtain a representative sample of tumor tissue while, at the same time, minimizing risk to the patient (Lote et al. 1997). Whereas open-biopsy was routinely performed as a result of inadequate pre-operative localization in the era before CT and MR imaging (Levy and Elvidge 1956), minimally invasive, image-guided stereotactic biopsy is now the mainstay of sampling techniques for intracerebral lesions.

15.7.1 Stereotactic Techniques

Traditionally, the technique begins with affixing a base ring rigidly to the patient's skull via an array of skull pins. A variety of systems are commercially available for this purpose (i.e., Cosman-Roberts-Wells (CRW) and Brown-Roberts-Wells (BRW) apparati; Radionics Inc., Burlington, Mass.; Lars Leksell apparatus, Eleckta Inc.). Then, with the use of thinly formatted contrast-enhanced CT or MR images, the surgeon chooses one or more tumor volumes thought to be representative of the entire neo-

plasm. By means of a mathematical rendering and triangulation, a set of three-dimensional coordinates is generated from the two-dimensional data set with the assistance of a computer workstation. Typically, these coordinates are referenced to fixed fiducial points within a localizer ring or box that has been applied to the base ring during the image acquisition process. These fiducial points define the three-dimensional volume that the computer and surgeon will work in (Fig. 15.2a). After imaging, the localizer setup is removed and the patient is then prepared for surgery. A second working stereotaxis frame that is adjustable in three dimensions is then applied to the base ring for the actual procedure. Prior to biopsy, additional planning is typically done in real-time with examination of the intended trajectory on the planning workstation to insure a safe and minimally invasive path.

Using only local anesthesia and mild intravenous sedation, a small scalp incision is made down to the bony calvarium. Using the series of rings and arcs on the stereotactic working frame, the entry site and direction of the predetermined trajectory is determined in relation to the patient's skull. A small, orthogonal twist drill hole is made down to the level of the dura which is then sharply penetrated with a sharp probe. Hemostasis of the dura and cortical surface is usually readily achieved through a combination of bipolar cautery and cool irrigation. Through an adapter attached to the frame's system, the surgeon is then able to pass an instrument (i.e., a needle core device, side-cutting aspirator, spiral needle, side-cutting needle or micro-cup forceps) through the predetermined trajectory to target for tissue sampling. A series of cylindrical 1–2 mm^3 biopsy specimens are thereby obtained with multiple samples often taken along a particular trajectory. Contrary to popular belief, the volume of tissue obtained from stereotactic biopsy, despite its small size, typically provides more representative material from a lesion than is obtained from an open-biopsy specimen, in which tissue is obtained without radiological guidance from the periphery of a grossly defined lesion (Chandrasoma et al. 1989). Through a small scalp incision and twist drill hole, the entire operation can be safely done with minimal risk to the patient under local anesthesia. For deep-seated lesions such as those around the third ventricle, deep gray matter, and medial temporal or parietal areas, stereotactic biopsy is particularly attractive as there is frequently no other safe or feasible means of obtaining tissue for diagnosis (Apuzzo et al.1983).

For cystic lesions or tumors with suspected ventricular involvement, it may be desirable to obtain a fluid sample during the course of the procedure. A standard 14-gauge probe with a Luer lock at its proximal end is typically adequate for this purpose. With a small syringe attached, fluid can be cautiously aspirated from either the tumor cyst or ventricle and sent for laboratory analysis (e.g., germ cell markers or tumor cells). For cyst walls or ependyma that appear to be thickened on the pre-operative images, a variety of cannulae with sharp, beveled tips are available to permit access to the cavity (RABB et al. 1995). Caution should be exercised to avoid overdrainage of fluid-filled spaces as a resulting subdural or epidural hematoma may result from cortical collapse. Stereotactic cyst aspiration may also be benefited by the concomitant use of endoscopy. A 6.2-mm diameter, fiber-optic rigid endoscope as well as a variety of third-generation, smaller flexible endoscopes have been employed for both cerebroscopy and ventriculoscopy (APUZZO et al. 1977). Direct visualization is also helpful for procedures adjacent to vascular and other critical structures.

The new generation of frameless systems has added a new dimension to stereotactic surgery. Through a series of simple fiducials applied directly to the scalp during image acquisition, the three-dimensional volume and data set can be defined without the use of the base ring. These can be applied to the scalp or directly to the skull depending on the degree of accuracy required for the procedure (ROBERTS et al. 1986). Intraoperatively, a stereotactic localizer ring is attached to the Mayfield head-rest away from the operative field. A fiber-optic digitizer camera array is positioned over the surgical area to track the movement of the localizer ring and specialized operative instruments which are embedded with either emitting diodes or passive reflectors. Via infrared light, the ring, fiducials and surgical instruments are tracked in space by the camera array. This is achieved through the use of a high-speed computer workstation that performs the necessary mathematical calculations (ADLER 1993). The fiducials and localizer ring are „registered" together to the computer thus defining the three-dimensional volume to be used in surgery. This process is in essence a modification of the traditional stereotactic technique that utilized a localizer frame or box placed on a base ring. A minimum of three points in the whole volume data set or volume of images rather than three points in each two-dimensional image is used for spatial cross-registration to a stereotactic frame. This use of spatial cross-registration

and transformation of the two-dimensional data set is referred to as „transformational stereotaxis" (HEILBRUN 1996). By using one of the „smart" instruments as a probe, the surgeon is then able to visualize, in real-time, where the tip of instrument is in relation to the image on the workstation. The workstation then reformats the image's data set to show the surgeon exactly where he or she is on the MR or CT image (BRODWATER et al. 1992). This ability to „navigate" within the cerebrum has opened many new possibilities. The lack of a bulky apparatus, up-to-the-minute information, and the freehand ability provided by such frameless systems greatly improve their utility in craniotomies and some cases of stereotactic biopsy. Frameless systems allow the surgeon to precisely plan the trajectory thereby allowing for a smaller craniotomy to be performed. Additionally, some surgeons utilize the navigation system to actually define the margins of the tumor on the cortical surface and also to guide resection of the lesion in real-time. This technique is, however, severely limited by the inevitable shifting of the cerebrum that occurs when the dura is opened. With the loss of CSF, iatrogenic brain relaxation, and violation of the ventricles, the anatomy of the cerebral hemispheres becomes increasingly distorted and no longer matches the relationships that were defined on the pre-operative images that were used for planning. As such, intraoperative, frameless stereotactic navigation should be used with great caution.

Since the early report of CONWAY (1973), a large body of experience has since accumulated with the use of stereotactic brain biopsy and has proven it to be safe, efficacious, and reliable. From the review of LUNDSFORD et al. (1995) of over 700 stereotactic biopsies performed on brain tumors, surgical morbidity remained at less than 1% with no cases of procedure-related death. Other independent, large clinical series have echoed this experience (APUZZO et al. 1987, COLOMBO et al. 1988). From a technical standpoint, experimental validation studies of fixed-frame stereotactic techniques have documented an accuracy of less than 1 mm of error between the predetermined radiological target and the actual biopsy site (CHANDRASOMA et al. 1989). Although initially not as accurate as traditional frame-based systems, newer generation, frameless stereotactic systems are now able to achieve working accuracies of 1.5 mm or less as well (BUCHOLZ et al. 1998). These accuracies diminish by several orders of magnitude, however, as brain shifting occurs intraoperatively.

Whereas little disagreement remains about the overall safety and technical efficacy of the stereotactic technique, significant questions persist regarding its clinical utility in predicting a tumor's actual histology and grade. There are four primary considerations in this controversy: (1) A large proportion of LGAs are histologically heterogeneous in nature. From this, the question of needing multiple specimens arises. (2) As tumors are heterogeneous, where then is the best place to target on the pre-operative imaging? (3) Does inter-observer variability exist regarding histologic grading of biopsy specimens? (4) Lastly, do stereotactic biopsies accurately predict the overall response and clinical outcomes of LGAs? A thorough understanding of these issues surrounding stereotactic biopsy is crucial as therapy of LGAs is nowadays based almost solely on its results.

15.7.2
Intratumoral Heterogeneity

Addressing the first point, SCHERER et al. (1940), in his classic manuscript, carefully sectioned the cerebral hemispheres of 18 patients with prior surgically diagnosed LGAs. In this group, he found 13 (72%) to have areas of significant anaplastic changes. RUSSELL and RUBENSTEIN (1989), in their subsequent work, corroborated these findings when they examined the autopsy material from 55 patients known to have harbored well-differentiated astrocytomas. They observed that nearly half had foci of anaplasia present. Conversely, in a series of 129 autopsies of patients with known glioblastoma multiforme, approximately 28% were felt to have arisen from low-grade tumors based on the histologic findings. Several have postulated that malignant transformation from the time of the initial biopsy was responsible for the large number of anaplastic features found during autopsy confirmation. To control for this phenomena, PAULUS and PEIFFER (1989) took en bloc specimens from 50 surgically resected supratentorial gliomas and punched multiple, small-sized needle-like samples from them to study the degree of tumor heterogeneity present. They discovered that 62% of the gliomas had both low-grade (grade 2) and malignant (grade 3) features. With respect to diagnosis, the greatest variability of diagnosis occurred at the breakpoint between the well-differentiated (grades 1, 2) and malignant (grades 3, 4) groups. Their findings echo a subsequent report suggestingd that small-sized needle biopsies may more frequently undergrade lesions than larger biopsy specimens (GLANTZ et al. 1991). As the number of samples and the individual punch size decreased, so

too did sampling error increase. From these data, they concluded that tissue should be sampled from as many different sites as possible during stereotactic biopsy. More recent work utilizing proliferation indices have further emphasized this intratumoral heterogeneity. Using Ki-67 labeling, serial biopsy specimens from LGAs were found to display markedly different amounts of intratumoral immunoreactivity and growth patterns (PARKINS et al. 1991).

A counterpoint to this seemingly one-sided argument against the validity of stereotactic biopsy is found in the work of CHANDRASOMA et al. (1989). From a series of 30 patients who had a history of stereotactic biopsy and subsequently underwent open resection of the mass, they reported histologically appropriate diagnoses in 28 of 30 patients. Overall, they found only one case of diagnostic error that was sufficient in magnitude to cause what was felt to be a clinically significant error in management. Additionally, they concluded that multiple points of biopsy were not essential in most cases, and that a single well-selected target point was able to provide a reliable pathological diagnosis. From another series of 34 stereotactically biopsied patients with follow-up surgical resection, only two cases of underdiagnosed astrocytoma grade were found (COLOMBO et al. 1988). Two, large comprehensive reviews of stereotactically biopsied gliomas with subsequent reconfirmation on open resection or autopsy revealed an overall 60% and 94% diagnostic accuracy of the initial biopsy (KEPES 1994; KLEIHUES et al. 1984). Like so many aspects of LGAs, the issue of stereotactic sampling error thus remains unresolved.

15.7.3
Target Selection

Regardless of the number of biopsies ultimately chosen, the question still remains: Where is the best and most representative area to target on the pre-operative planning image? Several studies have attempted to quantitatively examine serial sampling from a variety of CT-defined tumor regions and correlate them with their histologic yield. DAUMAS-DUPORT et al. (1984) separated tumors on the basis of their CT volumes into three groups. Fairly well-circumscribed tumors were designated as type I. Tumors with a solid component and surrounding edema on CT were classified as type II. Tumors containing only hypoattenuated areas on CT without a clear central area were labeled type III. When contras -enhancement (type II) was present, biopsies from the marginal zone typically corresponded to tumor tissue proper, adjacent infiltration of normal parenchyma, and a frequent increased vascularity. Additionally, sampling from low-attenuation areas (types II and III) without enhancement often yielded edematous white matter parenchyma infiltrated with tumor cells as well. However, a negative biopsy from hypodense targets (types I, II, III) cannot rule out the presence of tumor in these areas. Thus the concept of utilizing serial biopsies to establish a „negative" surgical margin or „gross" total resection in cases of LGA is a tenuous one at best (LUNDSFORD et al. 1995). A subsequent report from this Mayo Clinic group extended this analysis to MR imaging studies as well. Ultimately, these authors felt that biopsy of type II lesions was the most reliable as the border between tumor and parenchyma is clearly visualized. More tenuous in their minds, however, are the type I and III lesions for which no definitive radiological target „center" is defined on either T1 or T2 weighting. For these lesions, it is recommended that a second or multiple biopsy trajectories be taken around the involved volume to decrease the number of false negatives and to provide a more accurate spatial representation of the tumor. Additionally, targeting areas of different attenuation within a suspected lesion may help to improve the diagnostic yield (KELLY et al. 1987). Other caveats of targeting include avoiding areas with cystic volumes and areas suggestive of necrosis (COLUMBO et al. 1988; APUZZO et al. 1989).

15.7.4
Interpretation Errors

Like all biopsies, the interpretation of stereotactic samples is subject to the same inherent observer biases and variability that all clinical assessments are subject to. Whereas the issue of sampling error discussed above deals with the validity of the technique (e.g., is the biopsy actually reflective of the tumor), intra- and inter-observer differences are facets of a distinct and separate issue – reliability (e.g., does everyone grade the same slide the same way). MITTLER et al. (1996) reviewed 30 stereotactic biopsy specimens that were multiply interpreted by four, separate dedicated neuropathologists. Intra-observer agreement in one individual between his first and second readings of the same slide was 65.22% for LGAs and 74.73% for glioblastoma. Similarly, inter-observer correlation of the group was 57.14% for low-grade tumors and 62.41% for high-grade tumors. For both intra- and

inter-observer variability, the greatest degree of reliability was seen within the low- and high-grade groups. The highest variability thus occurred at the most critical clinical juncture – the border between grade 2 and grade 3 lesions. From their analysis, there seem to be no clear-cut solutions to this troublesome phenomenon. The development of a more subtle histologic grading scheme to better classify such „borderline" grade astrocytomas would help to reduce inter-observer disagreement, but would have little effect on intra-observer variability. PAULUS and PEIFFER (1989) arrived at the same conclusions as this study and recommended that group neuropathological evaluation would help to increase the confidence intervals of the final diagnosis. Although an attractive option, this may not be wholly practical as even the busiest tertiary neurosurgical referral centers typically have only one or two dedicated neuropathologists on staff.

A final point to consider in the interpretation of LGA biopsies is the difficulty of differentiating tumor from reactive gliosis. Whereas purely gliotic tissue will have a more heterogeneous population that includes fibrillary, gemistocytic, protoplasmic and inflammatory cells, LGAs typically contain a more uniform hypercellular picture. The presence of „satellitosis" with tumor cells clustered about normal neurons and subpial clustering are also helpful distinguishing features (OKAZAKI et al. 1988). When present, however, a diligent effort should also be made to rule out areas suggestive of malignancy or anaplasia. To improve the certainty of the reading, it is essential that the surgeon provide the pathologist with additional clinical and operative information (RABB et al. 1995).

15.7.5
Prognostic Utility

At this point, one would wonder if stereotactic biopsy should be used at all for LGAs given the many caveats and potential errors that are inherent in the technique itself. Like all assessment tools, however, the final judge of a given technique's utility is in its ability to accurately predict outcome. Thus if the results of stereotactic biopsies, as a whole, correlate with the clinical behavior of LGAs, then it is a useful tool despite whatever flaws it may possess. In their careful analysis of 419 image-guided stereotactic biopsies, REVESZ et al. (1993) found that there was an excellent overall correlation between the histologic Daumas-Duport grade and survival probability

($p<0.0001$) despite histologic heterogeneity and variability between the initial biopsy and subsequent follow-up data. They also noted a good correlation of survival in patients with both grade 2 and grade 3 tumors and a clear-cut difference in outcome between these two histologically defined groups. A further testimony to the prognostic utility of stereotactic biopsy was voiced by LUNSFORD et al. (1995), who in their review of 700 cases found no cases of clinical undergrading that resulted in inadvertent early disease progression. Thus despite its many inherent biases and technical limitations, we must conclude that stereotactic biopsy is a useful and valid means of categorizing LGAs regarding their overall clinical behavior. If one weighs the additional considerations of practicality, cost, and surgical risk, then image-guided stereotactic tumor sampling clearly sets the gold standard for methods to obtain a tissue diagnosis.

15.8
Cytoreductive Surgery

Despite the continuing controversy over its benefits, a large proportion of tertiary brain tumor referral centers presently advocate a radical or near-total resection whenever possible for patients with LGA. This philosophy stems from the often presumed, but not completely proven, oncological principle of always attempting a maximal reduction of tumor burden (DEVITA 1983). As the residual tumor cells are suspected of having an increased propensity to undergo further malignant transformations, most surgeons consider it prudent to attempt a „gross total" removal of the lesion to limit further spread and future recurrence. It is also thought that an initial cytoreduction optimizes subsequent adjuvant therapy by removing central ischemic tumor areas that are „protected" from the effects of chemotherapy and irradiation (SALCMAN 1990; SHAW 1990). One study recently utilized volumetric analysis to quantify the volume of tumor resection and subsequently correlated the data to recurrence and outcome. The authors noted that patients with less than 10 mm^3 of residual tumor had a decreased incidence of recurrence (14.8%) (Fig. 15.2b–d) and a shorter overall interval to recurrence (50 months) when compared to those patients with >10 mm^3 of the lesion remaining (46.2% recurrence at mean of 30 months; BERGER et al. 1994). From Table 15.3, we find several large retrospective studies that have

stratified the degree of surgical resection achieved and correlated it with long-term survival. Even in the early literature, GOL et al. (1961) concluded that patients who had a „gross total" resection fared far better, with a significantly increased median survival length of 18 months. Other series from the recent surgical literature have since corroborated these conclusions. From their multivariate analysis of outcomes in 461 LGA patients, LAWS et al. (1986) reported a striking two-fold increase in 5-year survival for patients in whom complete resection was felt to have been achieved ($p<0.0001$). Other studies of patients treated exclusively in the era of modern imaging (1975 on) have also observed similar life-table gains for aggressive resection at 5 years (45% vs 80%, PHILLIPON et al. 1993; 64% vs 82%, LEIGHTON et al. 1997). For retrospective clinical series in which resection (either partial or total) was used as the standard of care, the vast majority of authors have thus concluded that a more extensive surgical resection correlated with a longer survival.

Although tantalizing, *these statements must be viewed cautiously due to significant biases within the studies.* As they are all retrospective, there was no randomization as to which patients underwent partial vs „gross total" resections. As such, it is quite likely that these two study groups were not entirely comparable. LGAs that were larger, more diffuse, in more eloquent cortical areas, or in a deeper location likely precluded such patients from having a complete tumor extirpation. This selection of more „ideal" surgical lesions for „gross total" resection would naturally result in these patients having an improved median survival (MORANTZ et al. 1995, 1996). The majority of these clinical series have also focused only on outcome as it pertains to the degree of surgical resection. Few of these studies have addressed the possibility of using only a biopsy followed by either observation or irradiation (options 2 and 4). When one actually compares biopsy alone followed by irradiation (option 4) vs resection followed by irradiation (option 5), the supposed benefits of cytoreductive surgery become far less clear (SCANLON et al. 1979; WHITTON and BLOOM 1990; PIEPMEIER 1987; SHAW 1995; LOTE et al. 1997).

15.8.1
Pre-operative Considerations

Notwithstanding the above caveats, the decision to resect a LGA brings with it the inevitable risks of surgical complication and neurological deterioration. As such, meticulous attention to the operative details is an essential part of minimizing the risk of iatrogenic injury. Indeed, this focus on the surgery itself combined with careful peri-operative management are often the only tools that the neurosurgeon has to ensure a good clinical outcome. Important surgical considerations when planning a LGA resection include: thorough evaluation of the imaging studies, a full three-dimensional appreciation of the gross and microsurgical regional anatomy, careful positioning of the patient to optimize tumor visualization, a well-planned incision and subsequent osseous exposure, adequate neuroanesthetic brain relaxation and protection techniques, appropriate intraoperative electrical monitoring, and the need for adjunctive intraoperative resection guidance with imaging and or other techniques (OJEMANN 1995; CIRIC and ROSENBLATT 1993).

As with all surgery, cautious pre-operative evaluation and management are essential in minimizing operative-related complications. As the majority of patients with LGA do not require emergent surgery, it is best to optimize the medical condition of the patient prior to surgery (GROSSMAN 1993). Any potentially adverse medications (e.g., coumadin, aspirin, insulin). should be held for an adequate length of time before the operation. Appropriate screening and control of pre-existing cardiovascular, hematologic, pulmonary, metabolic, renal, and infectious disorders must be routinely performed. When in doubt, consultations from respective specialists are obtained to help further minimize potential risks (ALLEN and JOHNSTON 1990). Upon arrival in the operating suite, careful induction of anesthesia should be accomplished to avoid large swings in arterial blood pressure. Additionally, hypercapnia should be guarded against to avoid inadvertent increases in the intracranial pressure. The importance of proper positioning of the patient cannot be stressed enough. We recommend that the cranium be rigidly fixed with a Mayfield-Kees or similar type apparatus with attention paid to place the pins perpendicular to the skull to avoid slippage. The surgeon must then determine which position is the best to gain an optimal exposure of the lesion. Positioning should allow vital structures to fall away naturally from the lesion thus minimizing the amount of retraction needed to see the tumor. Although proper surgical alignment of the neck and cranium is important for the operative exposure, secondary attention to the rest of the patient is perhaps even more crucial (TEW and SCODARY 1993). Extreme positions of the neck must be avoided to prevent jugular and venous compression which can induce more vigorous venous bleeding and increased intracranial pressure. Inadequate padding of the pressure points and eyes can also lead to pressure ulcers, corneal abrasions, neuropathies, and potentially devastating compartment syndromes. Alternating thigh-high air compression boots or stockings should also be placed on the legs to prevent venous stasis and secondary complications of thrombotic occlusion.

For most cases of craniotomy for LGA, we recommend at least the following retinue of intraoperative monitoring: electrocardiogram, intra-arterial (radial) blood pressure monitoring line, non-invasive blood pressure cuff, cutaneous oxygen saturation probe, urinary Foley catheter, and an end-tidal pCO_2 monitor. When a heavier amount of bleeding is suspected or the patient is a higher anesthetic or surgical risk, it is also prudent to obtain central venous access in addition to the prerequisite large-bore intravenous lines. We do not routinely employ the use of Swan-Ganz monitoring except in patients with a serious pre-existing cardiac history. When the semi-sitting position is used or the head is well above the heart, a precordial Doppler monitor and a specialized central venous line capable of aspiration should be in place. Beyond this basic panel, it is the responsibility of the surgeon to decide if any additional specialized monitoring is indicated (OJEMANN et al. 1995). For tumors located within or adjacent to eloquent cortex, cortical electrical stimulation should be considered to limit the resection. For inferior parietal or high temporal lesions, awake mapping may also be needed for language and speech localization. Electrocorticography may also be helpful for patients with a seizure disorder to ensure resection of the primary electrical loci. Finally, infratentorial tumors adjacent to critical structures (i.e., cerebellopontine lesions) should be monitored with appropriate cranial nerve- and brainstem-evoked signals as well (OJEMANN and MARTUZA 1990). Information provided by such intraoperative electrical monitoring helps to prevent neurological injury from over-aggressive resection and to avoid secondary medicolegal issues.

Prior to incision, several maneuvers should be undertaken to decrease surgical morbidity by reducing the amount of traction-, edema-, infectious-, and seizure-related complications (STEWART and KRAWCHENKO 1985). Most patients are given a moderate dose of furosemide or similar loop diuretic initially. Soon thereafter, an additional 20% solution of mannitol is given in a dosage of 1–1.5 g/kg body weight over 20–30 min. This diuretic regimen aids greatly to minimize intraoperative brain retraction and maximize the operative exposure. Mild intraoperative hyperventilation to induce hypocapnia is also useful in this regard. For lesions such as those in the frontal lobe, where adequate cerebrospinal fluid (CSF) drainage may be difficult, we often place a lumbar drain before the patient is in the final surgical position. The drain is subsequently opened during the procedure to decompress the cisterns and to further relax the cerebrum. Short-course peri-operative glucocorticoids (e.g., 10–20 mg of dexamenthasone q 2–6 h followed by tapering dosages) are helpful, in our experience, in reducing iatrogenic edema, traction injury and stress-related systemic phenomena. Intravenous antibiotic prophylaxis should be given up front and then periodically through the course of the procedure (e.g., a second-generation cephalosporin or vancomycin) to prevent infectious complications. Seizures should be adequately controlled by anti-epileptics before surgery with a therapeutic blood level obtained. Intra-operatively, additional doses of the antiseizure medications can be given to prevent breakthrough ictal activity.

15.8.2
Surgical Approaches

A large proportion of the operative time is spent not so much on resecting the tumor itself but instead on exposing the surgical corridor to the lesion. A poorly planned exposure can lead to injury of vital structures along the way and to increased morbidity from an inadequately visualized removal. Thus, prior to the actual incision, the optimal surgical exposure and craniotomy type should have already been decided by the surgeon. This decision is based not only on the location of the tumor but on other important considerations as well: (1) finding the shortest trajectory that places the fewest neurovascular structures at risk, (2) picking an approach through the least eloquent cortex, (3) choosing a corridor that will provide the widest visualization of the tumor and its borders without extensive brain retraction, and (4) the handedness of the surgeon and his/her comfort during the case (RHOTON 1990). The specific exposures used for LGA resection span the entire spectrum of classical, supratentorial neurosurgical techniques. These include the bifrontal, middle frontal, frontotemporal (pterional), extended temporal, orbitozygomatic, temporal, temporopolar, infratemporal, frontoparietal, occipital, temporal suboccipital, and suboccipital (lateral, far lateral, and midline)

approaches. For unusually located tumors, specialized skull base approaches are used on rare occasion as well (SEKHAR and JANECKA 1993). Although a detailed analysis of these techniques is beyond the scope of this discussion, some of the more commonly employed approaches are summarized.

Bifrontal and Middle Frontal Approaches. Given their predilection for the abundant white matter of the frontal lobes, the bifrontal and middle frontal craniotomies are among the most common of the approaches used for LGA resection. The bifrontal approach provides excellent exposure of the superior and medial aspects of both frontal lobes initially. With a generous bone flap and adequate brain relaxation, good visualization of the inferomedial frontal lobes can be obtained as well. The patient is placed supine with the head in mild to moderate extension. For medial lesions, the head is typically turned towards the tumor to allow the frontal lobe to fall away from the falx on that side. For more laterally located tumors, the head is turned away, with a middle frontal approach often being better. A coronal incision is then made behind the anterior hairline with careful preservation of the underlying pericranium and the temporalis muscle and fascia laterally. The pericranial flap is valuable for patching dural leaks and for exenteration of the bony frontal sinus to prevent mucoceles or encephaloceles. Burr holes are placed in the anatomic „keyholes" inferior and posterior to the anterior temporal line and zygomatic arch. Importantly, burr holes should be placed on either side of the midline sagittal sinus to prevent inadvertent venous injury during elevation of the craniotomy flap. The burr holes are connected with a craniotome and an inferior cut is then made from side to side just above the supraorbital ridge. A crescent-shaped flap is thus removed to expose the bilobed dural covering of the frontal lobes (Fig. 15.6a). The bony frontal sinus is almost inevitably violated and will require mucosal stripping and packing with subsequent coverage by the pericranial flap.

The middle frontal approach is similar in nature except that the bone flap is made only on one side. It is best for more laterally placed convexity lesions of one frontal lobe. Typically, lesions of the far inferolateral and posterior frontotemporal region will require other types of approaches for adequate visualization. The head is positioned such that the apex of the tumor is at the highest point. An inferiorly based U-shaped skin incision is made to the frontal floor laterally and slightly across the sagittal suture. A burr hole is placed only in the ipsilateral

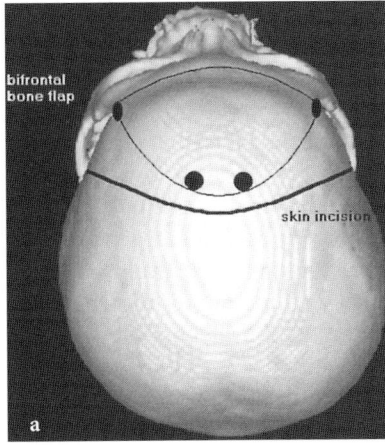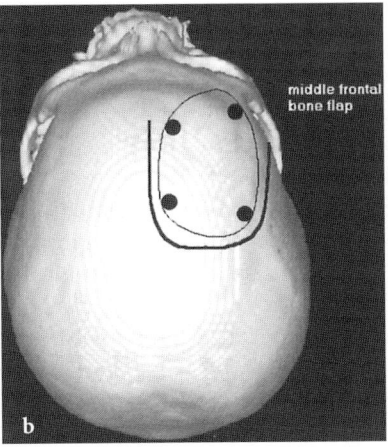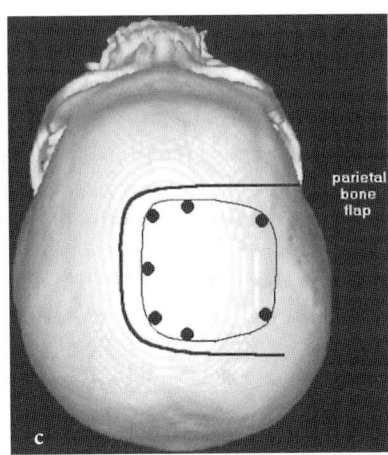

Fig. 15.6a–c. Examples of common surgical approaches for low-grade astrocytomas (LGAs) of the frontal and parietal areas. **a** Bifrontal craniotomy with a coronal skin incision (*dark line*) and a bilateral frontal bone flap. Burr holes bridge the sagittal sinus to prevent inadvertent premature venous injury. **b** Middle frontal craniotomy with a more limited unilateral bone flap with burr holes placed on the ipsilateral border of the sagittal sinus. **c** Frontoparietal or vertex approach requires the placement of additional burr holes to bridge the sagittal sinus, as injury in the middle third of its course carries far greater clinical consequences

keyhole and connected to burr holes placed on the ipsilateral side of the sagittal sinus and posterior frontal bone. In this fashion, an oval-shaped bone flap is removed to expose only the involved frontal lobe (Fig. 15.6b).

For both approaches, the dural opening is then tailored to maximize the exposure of the tumor and at the same time to minimize the amount of brain retraction needed. With adequate neuroanesthetic cerebral relaxation and the gentle use of fixed retractors, a generous view of the tumor bed can usually be obtained (GREENBERG 1985). Particular attention should be paid to the posterior and inferior aspects of the resection bed during either a bifrontal or middle frontal approach. As visualization of the inferolateral and posterior frontal lobe, anterosuperior temporal lobe and sylvian fissure, and anterior parietal lobe is often limited by the dural opening and bony exposure, inadvertent injury to the motor and somatosensory cortices can occur. Injury to the deep and medial vascular structures (e.g., internal cerebral veins, sylvian vessels, pericallosal arteries) are also of concern.

Frontoparietal (Vertex) Approaches. Many LGAs will extend along the white matter of the centrum semiovale to involve both the substance of the frontal and parietal lobes. A posterior frontoparietal approach will provide the broad exposure needed to safely resect such extensive lesions. The patient is usually placed in a semi-lateral, semi-sitting position

with the head positioned such that the coronal suture is the highest point of the cranium. A laterally based horseshoe incision is made such that the medial limb is 2–3 cm across the midline. The anterior and posterior limbs should be far enough to allow visualization beyond the limits of the tumor. For this approach, sagittal sinus injury will occur in the middle-third of its course, thus carrying with it much more serious consequences than a more anteriorly located violation. Thus, a generous number of burr holes should be placed to bridge and free the sagittal sinus from the overlying bone before attempting to raise the craniotomy flap (Fig. 15.6c). The dural separation and the craniotomy cut over the sinus should be made last such that immediate hemostasis can be achieved in case of sinus injury. A combination of surgicel gel foam impregnated with thrombin and cottonoids should be used to control bleeding over the sinus. After adequate hemostasis, the dura is then opened in a medially based C-shape to expose the parietal convexity. Careful attention to avoid injury to bridging and cortical veins will help to reduce the risk of thrombotic occlusion and subsequent venous infarction. Overly aggressive resection in this area carries a serious risk of neurological deficit as the somatosensory and motor areas are immediately adjacent to or directly infiltrated by the lesion itself.

Frontotemporal (Pterional and Extended Temporal) Approaches. This classic neurosurgical approach described by YASARGIL et al. 1987 provides an excellent visualization of lateral, inferolateral, posterolateral frontal tumors. The patient is placed supine with the head turned away from the lesion and the ipsilateral shoulder elevated. Mild extension to assist the frontal lobe falling away from the orbital roof is helpful for subsequent tumor visualization. A C-shaped incision is made behind the hairline from the zygomatic arch just anterior to the tragus (to prevent injury to the more anteriorly located frontalis branch of the facial nerve) to a point slightly beyond the midline. A flap consisting of the skin, temporalis muscle, and pericranium is then turned anteriorly and inferiorly to expose the inferolateral frontal and anterior temporal bones. Burr holes are placed in the ipsilateral keyhole, anterior temporal bone above the zygomatic arch, and over the frontoparietal region according to the surgeon's preference. A craniotome is then used to raise the oval-shaped bone flap to expose the dura of the frontotemporal region (Fig. 15.7a). The dura is usually opened in an inferior based C-shape. The exposure of this approach is typically limited in the inferior posterior frontal and anterior temporal regions. As such, accidental injury to the anterior temporal tip veins, motor and somatosensory cortex, Broca's area, carotid artery, optic nerve, third nerve, and sylvian vessels are all possible.

Several additional maneuvers and modifications can extend the utility and visualization afforded by the frontotemporal approach. Drilling and flattening of the sphenoid wind and anterior temporal bone can provide better exposure of the inferolateral frontal and anterior temporal skull base. Additionally, the skin incision can be carried below the zygoma with the temporalis muscle incised to expose the bony root of the arch. The arch can then be transected and removed with the temporalis then turned inferiorly to provide an even larger corridor to the frontotemporal region. More extensive variants such as the orbito-zygomatic, fronto-orbital zygomatic, and extended temporal approaches have also been described for use in radical resections (HAKUBA et al. 1986; IKEDA et al. 1991). By curving the pterional incision around the top of the ear and extending it more medially and anteriorly, a more extensive exposure of the temporal squama can also be accomplished. This extended temporal approach allows greater exposure of the anterior and medial temporal areas along the sphenoid ridge and for greater retraction of both the anterior temporal and frontal lobes (OJEMANN et al. 1988).

Temporal and Temporopolar Approaches. For lesions contained within the temporal and inferoparietal regions, a more limited lateral exposure can be accomplished through the classic temporal approach. The patient is placed either in a semi-lateral or lateral position with the ipsilateral shoulder well-mobilized up and away from the operative area. The head is

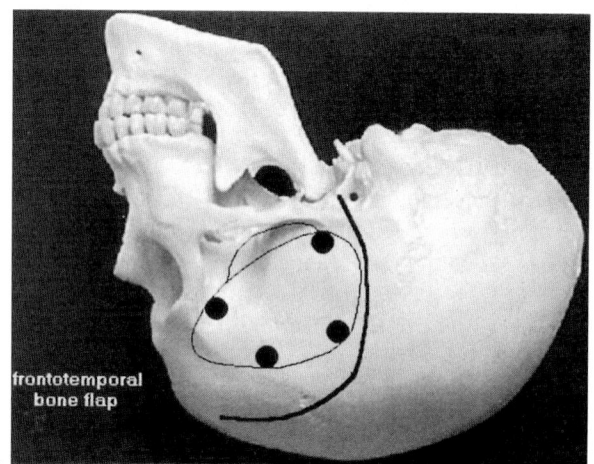
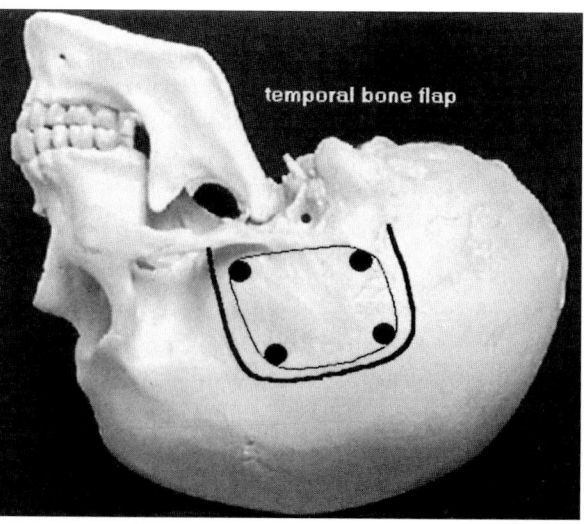

a b

Fig. 15.7a, b. Surgical approaches for tumors of the frontotemporal and temporal regions. **a** Frontotemporal or pterional craniotomy with a curvilinear skin incision extending from the root of the zygoma to the frontal midline. Burr holes are placed in the anatomic keyhole, low-temporal and frontal regions to form the oval bone flap centered over the pterion. Additional craniectomy of the area drawn in the temporal region can provide additional exposure of the middle fossa floor. **b** Temporal approach with an inferiorly based U-shape or horseshoe flap. The small rectangular-shaped bone flap provides excellent exposure of the temporal and temporoparietal areas

thus turned such that the ipsilateral side is nearly parallel to the floor. The vertex is dropped slightly away from the tumor to help the temporal lobe fall away from the middle fossa floor. The incision is begun anterior to the tragus along the zygomatic arch and follows a U-shape superiorly and posteriorly to end near the mastoid tip. An inferiorly based horseshoe-shaped scalp flap is thereby raised along the floor of the middle fossa. Burr holes are placed along the floor of the temporal squama and in the inferior part of the parietal bone. A rectangular-shaped bone flap is raised with additional exposure of the middle fossa base accomplished by further craniectomy (Fig. 15.7b). The dura is then opened in either a Y-shape or curvilinear fashion to expose the lateral aspects of the temporal and inferior parietal lobes. Additional exposure of the anterior and anteriomedial temporal lobe can be accomplished by a few modifications of the temporopolar technique (SANO 1980). As with the above approaches, injury to structures at the limits of the surgical exposure must be avoided. Structures particularly prone to injury via the temporal approach include several venous structures (Labbe, Roland, internal cerebral, sylvian, anterior temporal tip), the middle cerebral artery and its branches, the temporal portions of the ventricular system, speech areas, lateral somatosensory and motor cortex, and the underlying cranial nerves and brainstem.

15.8.3
Operative Technique and Morbidity

Once adequate surgical exposure of the lesion has been achieved, the surgeon is then faced with the additional challenge of how much to resect. As discussed earlier, there is literature to support both a radical and a conservative approach to tumor cytoreduction. Given this uncertainty, we generally approach the resection of LGAs with the underlying principle of avoiding new neurological deficits. Although many lesions will seemingly extend to the surface on the pre-operative images, it is our experience that there will often be a bulging, gliotic „cap" of cortical tissue over the tumor. As such, we typically begin our corticotomy directly over the most superficial aspect of the tumor with the important caveat of avoiding eloquent tissue such as the motor or somatosensory strip. Using bipolar forceps and Surgicel to obtain hemostasis in the pial layer, the cortical incision is gradually extended and deepened until the tumor itself is encountered. Preservation of

as many superficial cortical arteries and draining veins as possible is important in averting the delayed vascular sequelae of ischemia and venous congestion. As with other intrinsic brain tumors, LGAs should initially be entered as close to the center as possible. The debulking process can then proceed in a centrifugal fashion towards the periphery of the tumor. It is here, at the interface between tumor and normal brain parenchyma, that the risk of neurological injury is the greatest (GUTHRIE and LAWS 1990).

For smaller or more deeply seated lesions, it is often difficult to precisely pinpoint the location of the tumor. Visual landmarks or guides are frequently not available to identify what is tumor and what is not. To avoid a large craniotomy and an excessive cortical opening, the use of stereotactic guidance is extremely helpful (MORANTZ 1996). The center of the tumor is identified on the pre-operative images and used as the target. With traditional frame-based systems, a thin catheter is then passed from the desired entry site to the tumor. The trajectory of the catheter can also be checked beforehand on the computer workstation to ensure that eloquent brain parenchyma and vital neurovascular structures are avoided. At the time of the craniotomy, the surgeon simply centers the craniotomy on the catheter's entrance site. After the dura is opened, the corticotomy is extended along the path of the catheter down to the tumor. This ensures not only the safest possible surgical corridor but also that the tumor itself is being removed. Modern, frameless transfomational stereotactic systems not only facilitate this procedure by removing the bulky frame and catheter, but also provide the added benefit of allowing real-time intraoperative neuronavigation (HEILBRUN 1996). As previously detailed, the surgeon is able to check and recheck the location of the tumor in relation to the stereotactic probe. After the osseous and dural exposure, the „smart" probe can be used to define the exact margins of the tumor in relation to the cortical surface. Intraoperative displacement of the cortical anatomy resulting from resection, dehydration, traction, shift, loss of CSF, and diuresis limit navigational accuracy as the resection proceeds. Nevertheless, the frameless stereotaxy probe is still helpful in delimiting the deeper margins of the resection.

Safe removal of the tumor is facilitated by slow extensive internal decompression using a combination of bipolar coagulation, sharp dissection, and controlled suctioning. Use of the Cavitron ultrasonic aspirator (CUSA) is helpful as LGAs can often be firm and tenacious in character (MORANTZ et al.

1995). When present, gentle traction of the tumor capsule away from the surrounding parenchyma minimizes the need for brain retraction and can allow for separation of vascular and arachnoid attachments. Cottonoids are used to protect normal boundaries of the surrounding tissue. Excessive manipulation of surrounding brain tissue is a frequent but unwarranted cause of surgical morbidity (SALCMAN 1990). More commonly, however, such a clear interface between the tumor and the brain is lacking. The infiltrative nature of most LGAs and the edematous nature of the white matter often result in a vague transition zone both macro- and microscopically. Histologic analysis of tissue from these regions have confirmed the lack of a clear boundary at a cellular level (KELLY et al. 1987). It is thus critical to exercise extreme caution at the periphery of a low-grade tumor. As the lesion is often bordered by vital cortical tissue, overly aggressive resection can lead to devastating neurological compromise in a previously intact patient. Intraoperative ultrasound visualization of the tumor and its boundaries can often help avoid such sequelae. The sterile ultrasound probe is placed on the cortical surface prior to incision and during the debulking process to keep track of the tumor–brain interface, which often displays a more distinct border echogenically than to the naked eye (DOHRMANN and RUBIN 1985; EPSTEIN 1985; LEROUX et al. 1992). Intraoperative, cortical somatosensory evoked-potentials, electrocorticography, and awake language mapping are additional technical adjuncts that can help to safely delimit a resection. These techniques can actually facilitate a more extensive resection in many cases by revealing the relationship of the site of cortical traverse and of the subsequent subcortical dissection in eloquent brain (BERGER et al. 1990). At the end of what is felt to be the safe limit of resection, several authors have recommended the use of serial biopsies from the margin from the surrounding edematous brain to verify the absence of tumor. Although attractive in theory, the infiltrative nature of LGAs and the amorphous transition area to normal, vital tissue often makes such a practice difficult. Meticulous attention to hemostasis by filling the cavity with saline in conjunction with a brief, gentle Valsalva maneuver will help reduce the incidence of post-operative bleeding and hematoma. Caution to avoid episodes of hypertension during the peri-operative period is also crucial in this respect. The resection bed is typically lined with resorbable Surgicel as an extra precautionary hemostatic measure and filled again with irrigation. Hyperventilation should be discontinued at this point along with the initiation of gentle rehydration to permit expansion of the brain during closure. A careful, watertight closure of the dura and galea is time well spent to avoid the troublesome complications of wound breakdown and infection. This is especially true for patients who are likely to receive radiation through the operative site.

At the beginning of this century, Harvey CUSHING (1932) reported an overall operative mortality for intracranial gliomas of 11% over the last decade of his 30 years of experience. With the advent of modern neuroanesthetic techniques, peri-operative steroids, prophylactic antibiotics, and the operating microscope, this mortality rate has diminished significantly, to 0.7%–3% (SALCMAN 1985). In the modern era, however, it is the morbidity of surgery that ultimately defines its clinical utility and indications. A contemporary surgical series of patients with LGAs revealed no significant difference between pre- and post-operative neurological status thus implying a minimal surgical morbidity (PHILLIPON et al. 1993). In a series of 140 patients with supratentorial gliomas, it was found that, of patients with pre-operative Karnofsky scores of 70 or greater, 7.8% experienced a post-surgical deterioration to a KPS of less than 60 (FADUL et al. 1988). Overall, 13% who were completely normal beforehand developed a new neurological deficit after surgery. Of those who had pre-existing deficits, 16% experienced worsened or new neurological abnormalities. Bilateral and deep midline tumor location and an age greater than 55 were the two strongest predictors of post-operative functional deterioration. Most interesting, however, was the observation that the extent of resection, as determined by CT, had no statistical effect on the degree of postoperative functional impairment. McCORMACK et al. (1992) found that 5.6% of their 56 patients who were intact before surgery developed new postoperative neurological deficits. Other studies of functional outcome after LGA resection have demonstrated similar statistics regarding post-surgical functionality (RANSOHOFF et al. 1986; AMMIRATI et al. 1987).

Whereas modern neurosurgical techniques have greatly reduced the incidence of post-operative neurological deterioration, the resultant morbidity, as reported in the literature, is nonetheless not insignificant. For a patient who is otherwise intact prior to surgery, even a 5%–8% chance of impairment can be unacceptable. As there is no clear-cut evidence in support of radical debulking, we generally advocate conservative resection for lesions that are adjacent to or within eloquent neural parenchyma.

15.9
Radiation and Adjuvant Therapy

Even after the most aggressive „gross-total" resections, it is now widely accepted that there will still be a significant number of LGA cells left behind In accordance with modern oncological philosophy, many treatment centers have advocated an attempt at early control and eradication of this residual load. Through adjuvant therapies such as ionizing external beam radiation and chemotherapy, the goals of these treatment regimens are local control, decreasing recurrence, and preventing malignant transformation. Thus it is not surprising that radiotherapy has been internationally employed in the management of LGAs for nearly three-quarters of a century. Despite this long and widespread clinical experience, the effects of irradiation on the natural history of treated LGAs is even more controversial than the effects of surgical resection. This debate over radiation stems from the fact that no multi-center, randomized, controlled prospective clinical trial has been completed to either support or refute its use. Although one such study of LGAs conducted by the European Organization for Research and Treatment of Cancer (EORTC) has recently closed to patient registration, its outcome data will not be available for many years (KARIM et al. 1996). A review of the published retrospective clinical data reveals many obstacles that prevent a comparison of their results. These include heterogeneous patient subgroup characteristics (i.e., Karnofsky score), multiple classification schemes used to grade LGAs, different timings of treatment, lack of uniform radiation dosages and field sizes, a frequent absence of a non-irradiated control group, and the different types of surgery performed (MORANTZ 1987,1995).

Despite this lack of class I evidence, many neurosurgeons, medical oncologists, and radiation oncologists consider the use of adjuvant irradiation as the standard of care for LGAs (LEIGHTON et al. 1997). This practice is based on the recommendations of several well-respected retrospective LGA series demonstrating that overall and progression-free survival times were enhanced by immediate post-operative radiation (LAWS et al. 1986; SHIBAMOTO et al. 1993; GARCIA et al. 1985; SHAW et al. 1989). In one of the more striking outcomes, LEIBEL et al. (1975) was able to show nearly a 2.5-fold increase in survival at 5 and 10 years for resected patients treated early with 35–50 Gy of radiation. Other authors have reported more conservative findings with a benefit demonstrated only in patients who had incompletely resected tu-

mors. In these studies, radiation had no effect on long-term outcome in those who had gross-total resections (FAZEKAS 1977; SHELINE 1986; WARA 1985). The presence or absence of a relationship between survival and dose in irradiated patients is also disputed. Whereas some series have suggested an improved outcome for higher radiation doses (SOFFIETTI et al. 1989, MEDBERRY 1988), other more recent and larger series have failed to demonstrate any such dose–response effect on survival (KARIM et al. 1996; LOTE et al. 1997). Interestingly, this disagreement is present even at the institutional level. SHAW et al., in their 1987 report, found no advantage for doses greater than 5200 cGy, whereas they did observe a better outcome for patients receiving greater than 5300 cGy in a subsequent 1989 series.

Of those in support of post-operative radiotherapy, the primary point of contention is the actual timing of adjuvant treatment. One school of thought has advocated immediate post-surgical irradiation in the hope of capitalizing on the vulnerability of tumor cells immediately after surgery. Treatment at this point would seem to offer the best chance of greater cytoreduction and long-term prevention of recurrence (SHAW 1990; ERYE 1993). Others favor delaying treatment until there is evidence of progression as many LGAs demonstrate an indolent growth pattern. Furthermore, radiation may have deleterious long-term effects that are difficult to predict (CAIRNCROSS and LAPERRIERE 1989; MULHERN and KUN 1991). Serious consequences of radiotherapy include endocrine dysfunction, intellectual impairment, radionecrosis, retarded development in children, and the risk of secondary malignancies (SKLAR and CONSTINE 1995; SCHULTHEISS et al. 1995; BRADA et al. 1992). The risk of such potentially devastating sequelae has also been correlated with the amount of radiation delivered. From a review of 371 patients treated for cerebral tumors, radiation necrosis was seen in only 1.5% of patients at 55 Gy, 4% at 60 Gy, and much more frequently at higher doses (MARKS and WONG 1985). Since the advent of MR imaging, radiation changes in such patients are being detected with even greater frequency due to the increased sensitivity of the modality to the white matter composition. The effect of radiation on cognitive development must also not be disregarded as up to 50% of children irradiated for LGAs between 1975 and 1984 had mental retardation at 5-year follow-up (NORTH et al. 1990). As much of this outcome data was gathered from the era of whole-brain and wide-field radiation techniques, many have suspected that modern conformal radiotherapy techniques would be associated with a decreased incidence and spectrum of toxicities. TAPHOORN et al. (1994) evaluated cognitive function and mood in patients with low-grade glioma and a control group of patients with low-grade hematologic malignancies. Although there were many more intellectual and psychological difficulties in the LGA group, they could not demonstrate any such differences between irradiated and non-irradiated glioma patients at 3 years. More remarkably, another similar study examining cognitive function in two groups of LGA patients could not demonstrate significant differences between those who had been simply observed and those who had received surgical resection and conformal irradiation (VIGLIANIS et al. 1996). Nevertheless, as there is no overwhelming evidence to support the use of higher doses, most radiation oncologists advocate the use of less than 6000 cGy as adjuvant therapy for LGAs (JANNY et al. 1993; MORANTZ 1996).

In contrast to the data supporting the notion that with radiation comes increased survival, findings from more recent clinical reports have failed to corroborate any such advantage. Table 15.4 summarizes some of these series that have compared the survival outcomes of radiated and non-irradiated patients after surgical resection. Salient features of this summary include the quite heterogeneous radiation dosages used in the protocols (600–7900 cGy) and a general trend towards increased survival for all groups in recent series. From our review, the majority (>70%) of large contemporary studies have not been able to demonstrate an overall survival benefit to radiation over surgery alone . If we limit the discussion to patients treated solely in the modern era (after 1970), this lack of statistical radiation benefit in the literature is further underscored. Some studies have even reported a survival disadvantage and a poorer prognosis for patients treated with adjuvant radiation (STEIGER et al. 1990). However, multivariate analysis in these studies have potentially identified specific subgroups that may statistically benefit from irradiation. These include patients who have significant residual tumor burden after resection and patients who are older than 40 years of age (PHILLIPON et al. 1993; LAWS et al. 1986). Interestingly, SHAW et al. (1989) made the same observation in their series which supported the use of adjuvant radiation. The fact that both studies for and against the use of adjuvant radiation have identified this subset of partially resected patients as more likely to benefit from its use is significant.

Even more so than radiation, experience with chemotherapy for LGAs has been extremely limited. Most institutions have employed various combinations of lomustine (CCNU), carmustine (BCNU), vincristine and procarbazine(PCV) to this end (DJERASSI et al. 1985; EAGAN et al. 1982). A recent analysis compared the use of such a regimen after radiation in 75 patients to radiation only in 57 other patients. This study appeared to demonstrate a longer survival for those treated with the aggressive chemotherapy regimen. Of note, however, was the lack of statistical significance of this difference and the number of side effects related to the cytotoxic drugs (WATNE et al. 1992). In the largest single-institution retrospective study to date, LOTE et al. (1997) found that neither the PCV nor the CCNU protocols used in 175 patients conferred any survival advantage over the 204 patients who did not receive chemotherapy. Whereas there is no class I data regarding surgical resection and radiation, a prospective randomized trial conducted by the Southwest Oncology Group has shown that there was no benefit to adding CCNU to radiation for LGA patients (EYRE et al. 1993). Modern cytometric analysis of LGAs has revealed that the majority of cells within a LGA are noncycling, thus making these tumors likely to be more resistant to cell cycle-specific drugs. Furthermore, such cells often rapidly develop biochemical means of resistance to such chemotherapeutic regimens as well (HOSHINO et al. 1988; KORNBLITH and WALKER 1988).

From this jumbled body of information, we can assemble a few general guidelines on adjuvant therapy for LGAs. In patients who have had „gross" resection of a LGA, radiation can be postponed until disease progression without fear of withholding beneficial therapy. It is reasonable to recommend adjuvant radiotherapy for patients with partially resected lesions and/or for those over 40 years of age as these are the only populations in which consistent benefit has been shown. Similarly, patients too frail to have surgery should probably undergo radiation for lack of any other strategies. High doses greater than 60 Gy should be avoided and the treatment field should be limited to avoid secondary complications of the radiation itself. Ionizing radiation should also be used extremely judiciously in children due to its potentially damaging effects on cognitive development. Modern conformal techniques of radiotherapy (i.e., Gamma Knife and Linac) may be associated with a decreased toxicity to surrounding brain tissue. As such, clinicians may now recommend adjuvant radiation for patients with LGA with significantly less trepidation than before. Based on existing chemotherapeutic regimens, there is currently no evidence to support their use in the management of LGAs.

15.10
Disease Progression

One of the most worrisome aspects of LGAs is their tendency to recur locally at an often higher histologic and clinical grade. From the extensive Mayo Clinic experience, only 79 of 461 (18%) patients had evidence of tumor recurrence at the time of reoperation or autopsy (LAWS et al. 1984). As these patients were treated from 1915 to 1975, before the advent of modern imaging techniques, such a low incidence of clinical progression is not surprising. As CT and MR imaging have aided in the diagnosis of LGAs, so too have they had an impact on surveillance for recurrence. In their recent study of 167 patients, LEIGHTON et al. (1997) observed tumor progression in 90 (54%) of 167 patients at a median interval of 50 months. No difference in recurrence between the post-operative irradiation group and the non-irradiated group was found. This finding was echoed in a similar contemporary series that demonstrated a 50% radiographic recurrence rate at a mean interval of 52 months (PHILLIPON et al. 1997). The most common clinical correlate of these radiographic findings is the return of epilepsy for patients who had been seizure-free after their initial operation. Almost without exception, the radiological pattern of disease progression is that of local recurrence and extension at the original tumor location (NORTH et al. 1989). Non-contiguous, contralateral progression and distal metastatic seeding is extremely rare and typically associated with highly malignant lesions. For deep-seated or near-midline lesions, this pattern of regional expansion can lead to an earlier symptomatic recurrence and decline (median survival 2 years) with usually no evidence of anaplastic transformation (MCCORMACK et al. 1992).

Enlarging low-grade tumors often resemble the original lesion radiographically, but can sometimes demonstrate new contrast enhancement at the time of disease progression (Fig. 15.8). As previously discussed, enhancement has been variably correlated with anaplasia malignancy in the tumor (see Sect. 15.5 Diagnostic Imaging). Low-grade tumors that enhance at the time of diagnosis are 2.0–6.8 times more likely to recur after surgery than non-enhancing ones (LOTE et al. 1997). Most commonly, new malignant growth in a previously non-enhancing glioma enhances thus facilitating the diagnosis. Whereas only 30% of LGAs enhance initially, this number climbs to over 90% for the same lesions at the time of disease progression (MCCORMACK et al. 1992). This finding should be used cautiously for prognostic decisions as nearly one-third of anaplastic astrocytomas and one-fifth of glioblastomas do not enhance with contrast on CT (MCDERMOTT et al. 1992). Just as a tissue confirmation is needed to definitively grade a LGA at the time of diagnosis, so too does the same caveat apply at the time of recurrence.

When low-grade gliomas regrow after therapy, approximately one-half will remain non-anaplastic tumors, while the remaining half will have progressed to a more malignant form on re-biopsy, reoperation, or autopsy (HARSH 1999). This startling phenomena was studied extensively in 137 patients who had an initial tissue-confirmed diagnosis of LGA. At the time of clinical or radiographic disease progression (mean 31 months), a second biopsy or reoperation was performed to resample the recurrent lesion. Whereas 14% of the tumors remained grade I or grade II lesions, 55% were now anaplastic in nature, and 30% met criteria for glioblastoma multiforme. From this work, it was concluded that up to two-thirds of treated LGAs may dedifferentiate to a more malignant state over time (MÜLLER et al. 1977).

Since this landmark work, subsequent authors have reiterated this observation to varying degrees. A representative sample of this data is presented in Table 15.1, which demonstrates a wide variation in the clinical course of LGAs. From an average follow-up interval of 9.2 years from these series, the percentage of recurrent cases ranges from a low of 18% to as high as 57%. Such recurrences were typically diagnosed on the basis of radiographic and/or clinical evidence at a mean interval of 22–60 months. Of the patients who recurred, over 60% overall had some form of tissue reconfirmation via either reoperation, rebiopsy, or autopsy. Excluding the high and low extremes of the cohort, recurrent LGAs have a 45%–88% likelihood of malignant dedifferentiation at second look.

Numerous hypotheses have been put forth to explain this ominous facet of the LGAs' clinical behavior. One or a combination of several pathophysiological mechanisms have been postulated (DIRKS et al. 1994):

1. Some LGA subtypes may undergo spontaneous malignant transformation as part of their natural history.

2. A second tumor may have developed as a result of irradiation therapy.

3. Several of the LGAs were undergraded at the time of diagnosis due to sampling error and were actually higher grade lesions.

4. The patients may have a genetic predilection for malignant progression.

5. Radiation therapy may have induced an accelerated dedifferentiation of a previously low-grade tumor.

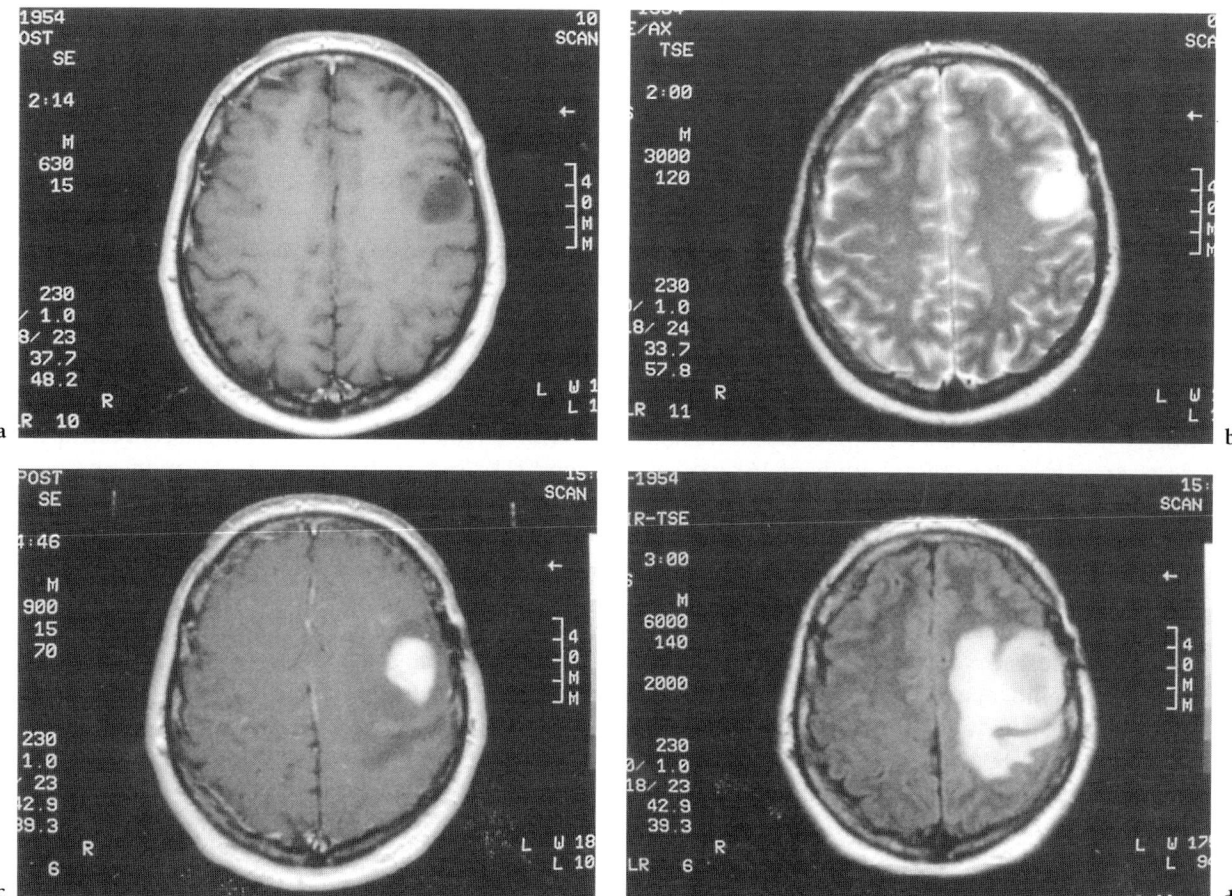

Fig. 15.8a–d. This is a 44-year-old male who had been treated for chronic seizures for over 4 years before having a diagnostic MR imaging scan. **a** T1-weighted gadolinium-enhanced axial image demonstrates a low-attenuation cortical mass of the left frontal lobe with no contrast enhancement and minimal mass effect. **b** T2-weighting of the same axial image confirms the increased water content of the mass with little surrounding white matter edema. A stereotactically guided biopsy of the mass was performed and confirmed the low-grade nature of the astrocytoma. Except for anticonvulsants, no other therapy was given. After 15 months, his seizure disorder became medically intractable. **c** Repeat T1-weighted gadolinium-enhanced axial MR image reveals new contrast enhancement with increased mass effect and mild midline shift. **d** FLAIR-weighted MR image confirms the striking change in white matter edema surrounding the mass. A left middle frontal craniotomy was performed and confirmed the presence of anaplastic features on histologic analysis

Whereas the natural history of LGAs remains poorly defined, clinical data have suggested that there may be subtypes with more aggressive or more indolent propensities (RUSSELL and RUBINSTEN 1989). KROUWER et al. (1991) reported that the presence of at least 20% gemistocytes in a glial tumor was a poor prognostic sign irrespective of the rest of the pathological background. Sampling error has been discussed in detail and may account for up to a 70% heterogeneity in low-grade tumors. From the earlier discussion, multivariate analysis of LGA histology has identified features that are prognostic of malignant progression. Additionally, molecular techniques have confirmed the heterogeneous prolifera-

tion indices of histologically similar tumors. The presence of any of these findings in a patient's tumor may warrant more aggressive surveillance and early treatment to prevent upgrading.

Of cerebral radiation-induced malignancies, astrocytomas are the third most common after sarcoma and meningioma. The behavior of such iatrogenic lesions has been debated. Some authors have observed a more anaplastic and aggressive course for radiation-induced anaplastic astrocytomas than their spontaneous counterparts (BERNSTEIN and LAPERRIERE 1991). Others, however, have come to the opposite conclusion. WINGER et al. (1989), in their study of 285 consecutive adults diagnosed with supratentorial anaplastic glioma, identified 28 patients with a previously documented LGA. After multivariate analysis, they noted that this preceding history of LGA was a positive clinical prognostic variable in terms of survival and KPS outcome. DIRKS et al. (1994) presented six children who developed anaplastic astrocytomas from a cohort of 55 children with a history of prior low-grade glioma resection. They noted that only the children who received radiation therapy developed spontaneous transformation, at a mean of 6.4 years (50–52.5 cGy). No unradiated child had evidence of anaplastic dedifferentiation. Whether this phenomenon is the result of sudden dedifferentiation of normal astrocytes or progressive dedifferentiation of the LGA cells remains unclear. Since TARLOV's suggestion, in 1937, that radiation may cause secondary neoplasms, modern oncological research has identified the role of progressive environmentally related genetic „hits" in the stepwise evolution of low-grade tumors to malignant lesions. Taking a different tack, MULLER et al. (1977) exquisitely analyzed 137 cases of recurrent supratentorial astrocytomas and crafted probability models of anaplastic transformation. From their analysis, they did not find evidence to support a definitive role for either radiotherapy or surgery in the earlier recurrence or malignant transformation of LGAs. Instead, they postulated an inherent tendency of astrocytoma tumor tissue towards malignant transformation.

Based on these observations, it is prudent to obtain serial surveillance imaging of patients on a yearly basis to screen for local recurrences and malignant transformation. When discovered, radiographic recurrence, in and of itself, does not necessarily imply intervention. For the stable or asymptomatic patient, continued observation is a perfectly reasonable course of action. Most reports have, however, suggested that radiographic findings such as contrast enhancement typically herald an accelerating clinical course and a poor clinical prognosis (MORANTZ 1996). As such, a repeat biopsy for tissue reconfirmation should be considered for patients who develop such changes on their follow-up imaging. In cases with histologic confirmation of anaplastic transformation or those with symptoms of a mass effect, repeat resection and debulking may be warranted for palliation. Since the interval between the initial treatment and recurrence can be lengthy, re-irradiation for some patients is also a viable option and has occasionally yielded good results (SELBERGELD et al. 1992). As definitive salvage protocols are heterogeneous, the exact treatment

plan for recurrent LGAs should be tailored to the specific wishes and needs of each individual patient.

Given the large body of evidence on the propensity of LGAs to progress toward malignancy, it is important to factor this into the management decision process.

After obtaining a tissue diagnosis to confirm the low-grade nature of an astrocytoma, there is often no emergent or pressing need for intervention (RECHET et al. 1992). This is especially true today as most patients are relatively asymptomatic at the time of diagnosis. Herein, however, lies the difficulty. Whereas it is perfectly reasonable to observe such patients for awhile, the surgeon must always be mindful of the eventual likelihood of disease progression. As the natural history of LGA remains undefined, the time interval for such malignant change to occur is also unclear. From our experience as well as that of many other authors, LGAs once identified will sooner or later progress and require treatment (APUZZO 1995). Although there are many reports of prolonged latency periods with no growth, there have been no reports to our knowledge of tumor involution. For the majority of patients who have a diagnosed LGA, the need for eventual intervention thus seems to be an unavoidable certainty. The only question is when. When we consider the 30%–88% likelihood of malignant progression during this „observation" period (Table 15.1), the need for earlier intervention becomes more evident. Based on this premise, our protocol is to attempt a gross resection earlier on for patients with LGAs in noneloquent cortex who are amenable to and safe for surgery. As empirical data to support this or any other strategy are still lacking however, the decision to either operate or not must ultimately be based on the decision of the individual patient.

15.11
Outcome

Without a doubt, modern medical advances have brought much-needed hope to patients suffering from LGAs. As few therapeutic options were available in the past, many of these patients were frequently overcome by a sense of despair and hopelessness. Contemporary oncological techniques have thus empowered both patients and clinicians by affording them viable therapeutic choices. In their review of patients treated in the pre-modern era (1940–1950), LEVY and ELVIDGE (1956) reported a 5-year survival of approximately 30% for all treatment groups. Since that time, the reported survival periods have significantly improved for most modern series. From a review of Table 15.4, we can estimate approximate overall survival rates at 5 years of 42% (surgery) and 49% (surgery and radiation) and at 10 years of 28% (surgery) and 30% (surgery and radiation). If we examine only recent series after 1970, these numbers are seemingly even more optimistic, with a mean 5-year survival of 70% (surgery) and 60% (surgery and radiation) and a 10-year survival of 54% (surgery) and 40% (surgery and radiation).

Table 15.5 succinctly summarizes these dramatic improvements in the reported median survival of patients with LGAs. Average survival estimates of over 100 months have been simultaneously reported by the three largest contemporary series (PHILLIPON et al. 1993; LEIGHTON et al. 1997; LOTE et al. 1997). When compared to the median survivals from earlier this century of 30–40 months, this would seemingly represent over a 200% increase in longevity for patients treated in the modern era. Although it would be tempting to attribute such dramatic improvements to the advances made in tumor oncology, it is also important to factor in the diagnostic lag effect. From our earlier discussion, ELVIDGE and LEVY (1937) reported an average symptomatic period of 27–29 months before diagnosis in their series of LGAs. Modern imaging and

clinical practice has greatly shortened this interval to an average of 1–2 months in the contemporary literature. Subtracting this estimated diagnostic lag interval from the modern estimates leaves us with a corrected figure of 71–73 months of average survival. These figures are similar to those reported for patients treated from the 1960s to the 1980s, before the era of modern diagnostic imaging. From this analysis, it would appear that LGA patients have benefited from approximately an 80% improvement in overall survival over the last century. Modern microsurgical techniques, improved sterile surgical methods, antibiotic prophylaxis, and peri-operative glucocorticoid use are some of the likely underlying causes of this improvement.

15.12
Conclusion

As one of the clinician's most difficult duties, the ability to provide prognostic information to the patient is at once crucial and yet troublesome. The results of our previous discussion on postponing therapy, biopsy alone, surgical resection, and radiation emphasize the difficulty in giving any definitive guidance. To aid in this task, numerous authors have analyzed their patient data to search for additional factors and variables that may affect prognosis. Limiting our review to only studies that have utilized the Cox variable hazards regression model for simultaneous analysis of multiple variables (Table 15.6), we find that few clinical and surgical variables seem to have any statistical outcome advantage. Factors only associated with prolonged survival include a shorter pre-operative symptomatic period, a history of cognitive or personality changes, pre-operative neurological deficit, evidence of increased intracranial pressure, tumor cyst, and nausea or vomiting. However, none of these variables reach a significant level after multivariate analysis. Only a younger age at diagnosis, pre-operative performance scores, and tumor grade 1 on initial histology seem to have any consistent statistical effect on survival ($p < 0.01$). Nonetheless, even this information should be used cautiously as these studies are neither prospective nor controlled in their clinical and surgical patient selection.

Table 15.5. Reported median survival of low-grade astrocytoma patients

Author (year)	Period studied	N	Median survival (months)
LEVY (1956)	1940–1949	176	36–60
GOL (1961)	–	194	23–32
STAGE and STEIN (1974)	1956–1970	45	40
LEIBEL (1975)	1942–1967	108	24–36
WEIR (1976)	1960–1970	107	31
PIEPMEIER (1987)	1975–1985	60	76
SOFFIETTI (1989)	1950–1982	85	60
SHAW (1989)	1960–1982	167	36–48
VERTOSICK (1991)	1978–1988	25	96
McCORMACK (1992)	1977–1988	53	88
PHILLIPON (1993)	1978–1987	179	108
JANNY (1994)	1970–1990	58	64
LEIGHTON (1997)	1979–1995	167	110
LOTE (1997)	1982–1992	379	100

Table 15.6. Cox proportional hazard regression multivariate analysis of prognostic factors on survival (p values)

	Laws[a]	Shaw	Soffietti	Lote	Leighton
Year	1984	1989	1989	1997	1997
N (patients)	461	167	85	379	167
Younger age (<40)	<0.0001	<0.01	ns[b]	<0.0001	<0.883
Sex (male vs female)	–	<0.009	ns	–	<0.397
Shorter symptom period	<0.03	–	ns	ns	<0.088
Seizures at diagnosis	<0.4	–	ns	ns	<0.012
Preoperative neurological deficit	<0.2	–	ns	<0.04	–
Cognitive personality change	<0.06	–	ns	<0.0001	–
Headache	<0.9	–	ns	<0.03	–
Nausea/vomiting	<0.3	–	ns	ns	–
Papilledema	<0.8	–	ns	–	–
Visual changes	<0.3	–	ns	–	–
Preoperative performance score	<0.1	–	ns	<0.0006	<0.834
Preoperative tumor size	<0.4	<0.7	ns	–	–
Presence of tumor cyst	<0.05	–	ns	–	–
Tumor grade (1 vs 2)	<0.04	<0.19	–	<0.014	<0.001
Postoperative neurological deficit	<0.2	–	–	–	–
Postop erative performance score	<0.4	–	<0.006	–	–
Radiotherapy	<0.01	<0.07	ns	ns	ns

ns, Not significant.

[a]Based on analysis of 5-year survival data.

[b]Data analyzed but reported only as not significant ($p>0.01$).

References

Alavi JB, Alavi A, Chawluk J, et al. (1988) Positron emission tomography in patients with gliomas: a predictor of prognosis. Cancer 62:1074–1078

Adler JR (1993) Image-based frameless stereotactic radiosurgery. In: Maciunas RJ (ed) Interactive image-guided neurosurgery. American Association of Neurological Surgeons, Park Ridge, Illinois, pp 81–89

Allen MB Jr, Johnston KW (1990) Preoperative evaluation: complications, their prevention and treatment. In: Youmans JR (ed) Neurological Surgery. WB Saunders, Philadelphia, pp 833–896

Ammirati M, Vick N, Liao Y, Ciric U, Mikhael M (1987) Effect of the extent of surgical resection on survival and quality of life in patients with supratentorial glioblastomas and anaplastic astrocytoma. Neurosurgery 21:201–206

Apuzzo MLJ (ed) (1995) Neurosurgical topics: benign cerebral glioma, vols. I, II. American Academy of Neurological Surgeons, Park Ridge, Illinois

Apuzzo MLJ, Heifetz MD, Weiss MH, Kurze T (1977) Neurosurgical endoscopy using the side-viewing telescope. Technical note. J Neurosurg46:398–400

Apuzzo MLJ, Sabshin JK (1983) Computed tomographic guidance stereotaxis in the management of intracraial mass lesions. Neurosurgery 12:277–285

Apuzzo MLJ, Chandrasoma PT, Cohen D, Zee CS, Zelman V (1987) Computed imaging stereotaxy: Experience and perspective related to 500 procedures applied to brain masses. Neurosurgery 20:930–037

Bahary JP, Villemure JG, Choi S, et al (1996) Low-grade pure and mixed cerebral astrocytomas treated in the CT era. J Neurooncol 27:173–179

Berger MS, Deliganis AV, Dobbins J, et al. (1994) The effect of extent of resection on recurrence in patients with low grade cerebral hemisphere gliomas. Cancer 74(6):1784–1791

Berger MS, Ojemann GA, Lettich E (1990) Neurophysiological monitoring during astrocytoma surgery. Neurosurg Clin North Am 1:65–80

Bernstein M, Laperriere N (1991) Radiation induced tumors of the nervous system. In: Gutin PH, Leibel SA, Sheline GE (eds) Radiation injury to the nervous system. Raven, New York, pp 455–472

Bloom HJG (1982) Intracranial tumors: Response and resistance to therapeutic endeavors, 1970–1980. Int J Rad Onc Biol Phys 8:1083–1113

Bouchard J, Peirce BC (1960) Radiation therapy in the management of neoplasms of the central nervous system with a special note in regard to children: twenty years' experience 1939–1958. Am J Rad 84:610–628

Brada M, Ford D, Ashley S, et al (1992) Risk of second brain tumour after conservative surgery and radiotherapy for pituitary adenoma. Br Med J 304:1343–1346

Brodwater B, Roberts D, Nakajima T, et al. (1992) Extracranial application of the frameless stereotactic operating microscope: Experience with the lumbar spine. Neurosurgery 32:209–213

Burger PC, Scheithauer BW, Vogel FS (1991) Surgical pathology of the nervous system and its coverings. Churchill Livingstone, New York, pp 196–208

Cairncross JG, Laperriere NJ (1990) Low-grade gliomas: to treat or not to treat? A reply. Arch Neurol 47:1139–1140

Chamberlain MC, Murovic JA, Levin VA (1988) Absence of contrast enhancement on CT brain scans of patients with supratentorial malignant gliomas. Neurology 38:1371–1374

Chandrasoma PT, Smith MM, Apuzzo MLJ (1989) Stereotactic biopsy in the diagnosis of brain masses: Comparison of results of biopsy and resected surgical specimen. Neurosurgery 24(2):160–165

Ciric IS, Rosenblatt S (1993) Supratentorial craniotomies. In: Apuzzo MLJ (ed) Brain surgery complications avoidance and management. Churchill Livingstone, New York, pp 51–60

Colombo F, Casentini L, Zanusso M, et al. (1988) Validity of stereotactic biopsy as a diagnostic tool. Acta Neurochirurgica Suppl 42:152–156

Conway LW (1973) Stereotaxic diagnosis and treatment of intracranial tumours, including an initial experience with cryosurgery for pinealomas. J Neurosurg 38:453–60

Cunningham JM, Kimmel DW, Scheithauer, et al. (1997) Analysis of proliferation markers and p53 expression in gliomas of astrocytic origin: relationships and prognostic value. J Neurosurg 86:121–130

Cushing H (1932) Intracerebral tumors: notes upon a series of two-thousand verified cases with surgical-mortality percentages pertaining thereto. Thomas, Springfield, Illinois

Daumas-Duport C, Monsaingeon V, Nguyen JP (1984) Some correlations between histological and CT aspects of cerebral gliomas contributing to the choice of significant trajectories for stereotactic biopsies. Acta Neurochir, Suppl 33:185–194

Daumas-Duport C, Scheihauer B, O'Fallon J et al. (1988) Grading of astrocytomas. Cancer 62:2152–2165

DeVita VT (1983) The relationship between tumor mass and resistance to chemotherapy. Cancer 51:1209–1220

Dirks PB, Jay V, Becker LE (1994) Development of anaplastic changes in low-grade astrocytomas of childhood. Neurosurgery 34: 68–78

Djerassi I, Kim JS, Rigger A (1985) Response of astrocytomas to high dose methotrexate with citrovorum factor rescue. Cancer 55:2741–2747

Dohrmann GJ, Rubin JM (1985) Intraoperative diagnostic ultrasound. In: Wilkins RH, Rengachary SS (eds) Neurosurgery. McGraw-Hill, New York, pp 457–460

Drayer BP, Johnson PC, Bird CR (1987) Magnetic resonance imaging and glioma. Barrow Neurol Inst Q 3:44–55

Eagan RT, Dinapoli RP, Herman RC et al (1982) Combination carmustine (BCNU) and dihydrogalactiol in the treatment of primary brain tumors recurring after irradiation. Cancer Treat Rep 66:1647–49

Elvidge AR, Penfield W, Cone W (1937) The gliomas of the central nervous system. A study of 210 verified cases. Res Nerv Ment Dis 16:107–181

Elvidge AR, Martinez-Coll A (1956) Long term follow-up of 106 cases of astrocytoma. J Neurosurg 13:318–331

Epstein F (1985) Ultrasound dissection. In: Wilkins RH, Rengachary SS (eds) Neurosurgery. McGraw-Hill, New York, pp 476–483

Erye H, Crowley J, Townsend J, et al (1993) A randomized trial of radiotherapy versus radiotherapy plus CCNU for incompletely resected low-grade gliomas: A Southwest Oncology Group study. J Neurosurg 78:909–914

Fadul C, Wood J, Thaler H, et al. (1988) Morbidity and mortality of craniotomy for excision of supratentorial gliomas. Neurology 38:1374–1379

Fazekas JT (1977) Treatment of grades i and ii brain astrocytomas. The role of radiotherapy. Int J Radiation Oncology Biol Phys 2:661–666

Francavilla TL, Miletich RS, DiChiro G et al. (1989) Positron emission tomography in the detection of malignant degeneration of low-grade gliomas. Neurosurgery 26:1–5

Fults D, Brockmeyer D, Tullous MW (1992) P53 mutation and loss of heterozygosity on chromosome 17 and 10 during human astrocytoma progression. Cancer Res 52:674–679

Gajjar A, Bhargava, Jenkins, et al. (1995) Low-grade astrocytoma with neuraxis dissemination at diagnosis. J Neurosurg 83:67–71

Garcia DM, Fulling KH (1985) Juvenile pilocytic astrocytoma of the cerebrum in adults. J Neurosurg 63:382–386

Garcia DM, Fulling KH, Marks JE (1985) The value of radiation therapy in addition to surgery for astrocytomas of the adult cerebrum. Cancer 55:919–927

Glantz MJ, Burger PC, Herndon JE, Friedman AH, et al (1991) Influence of the type of surgery on the histologic diagnosis in patients with anaplastic gliomas. Neurology 41:1741–44

Gol A (1961) The relatively benign astrocytomas of the cerebrum: A clinical study of 194 verified cases. J Neurosurg 18:501–506

Grossman RG (1993) Preoperative and surgical planning for avoiding complications. In: Apuzzo MLJ (ed) Brain surgery complications avoidance and management. Churchill Livingstone, New York, pp 99–109

Guthrie BL, Laws ER (1990) Supratentorial low-grade gliomas. Neurosurg Clin N Amer 1:37–48

Hakuba A, Liu S, Nishimura S (1986) The orbitozygomatic infratemporal approach: a new surgical technique. Surg Neurol 26: 271–276

Hara A, Hirayoma H, Sakai N (1990) Correlation between nucleolar organizer region staining and Ki-67 immunostaining in human gliomas. Surg Neuro 33:320–324

Hara A, Nishimura Y, Sakai N, et al. (1995) Effectiveness of intraoperative radiation therapy for recurrent supratentorial low grade glioma. J Neurooncol 25:239–243

Harsh GR (1999) Management of recurrent gliomas. In: Berger MS, Wilson CB (eds) Gliomas. WB Saunders, Philadelphia, pp 649–659

Heilbrun MP (1996) Frameless stereotactic localization and guidance. In Youmans JR (ed) Neurological surgery: a comprehensive reference guide to the diagnosis and management of neurosurgical problems, 4th edn. WB Saunders, Philadelphia, pp 786--794

Helseth A, Mork S (1989) Neoplasms of the central nervous system in Norway. III. Epidemiological characteistics of intracranial gliomas according to histology. APMIS 97:547–555

Horrax G (1954) Benign (favorable) types of brain tumor: The end results (up to twenty years) with statistics of mortality and useful survival. NEJM 250(23):981–984

Hoshino T, Rodriguez LA, Cho KG et al. (1988) Prognostic implications of the proliferative potential of low-grade astrocytomas. J Neurosurg 69:839–842

Hoshino T, Nagashima T, Murovic J, et al. (1986) In situ cell kinetic studies on human neuroectodermal tumors with bromodeoxyuridine labeling. J Neurosurg 64:453–459

Ikeda K, Yamashita J, Hashimoto M, et al (1991) Orbitozygomatic temporopolar approach for a high basilar tip aneurysm associated with a short intracranial internal carotid artery: A new surgical approach. Neurosurgery 28:105–110

Ito S, Chandler KL, Prados MD, et al. (1994) Proliferative potential and prognostic implication of low-grade astrocytoma. J Neurooncol 19:1–9

Janny P, Cure H, Mohr M, et al. (1994) Low grade supratentorial astrocytomas: management and prognostic factors. Cancer 73(7):1937–45

Karim ABMF, Maat B, Hatlevoll R, et al (1996) A randomized trial on dose-response in radiation therapy of low-grade cerebral glioma: European Organization for Research and Treatment of Cancer (EORTC) study 22844. Int J Radiat Oncology Biol Phys 36:549–556

Kelly PJ, Daumas-Duport C, Scheithauer BW, et al. (1987) Stereotactic histologic correlations of computed tomography- and magnetic resonance imaging-defined abnormalities in patients with glial neoplasms. Mayo Clin Proc 62:450–459

Kepes JJ, Rubinstein LJ, Eng LV (1979) Pleomorphic xanthoastrocytoma: a distinctive meningocerebral glioma of young subjects with relatively favorable prognosis. Cancer 44:1839–1852

Kepes JJ (1994) Pitfalls and problems in the histopathologic evaluation of stereotactic needle biopsy specimens. Neurosurg Clin North Am 5:19–33

Kernohan JW, Mabon RF, Svien HJ, et al. (1949) A simplified classification of gliomas. Proc Staff Meetings Mayo Clin 24:71–75

Kim TS, Halliday AL, Hedley-Whyte ET, Convery K (1991) Correlates of survival and the Daumas-Duport grading system for astrocytomas. J Neurosurg 74(1):27–37

Kleihues P, Volk B, Anagnostopoulos J, Kiessling M (1984) Morphological evaluation of stereotactic brain tumour biopsies. Acta Neurochir S33:171–181

Kondziolka D, Lunsford LD, Martinez AJ (1984) Unreliability of contemporary neurodiagnostic imaging in evaluating suspected adult supratentorial (low-grade) astrocytoma. J Neurosurg 79:533–536, 1993

Kornblith PL, Walker M (1988) Chemotherapy of gliomas. J Neurosurg 68:1–17

Krouwer HG, Davis RL, Silver P et al. (1991) Gemistocytic astrocytomas: a reappraisal. J Neurosurg 74:399–406

Krouwer HG, Prados MD (1995) Infiltrative astrocytomas of the thalamus. J Neurosurg 82(4):548–57

Labrousse F, Daumas-Duport C, Batorski L, Hoshino T (1991) Histological grading and bromodeoxyuridine labeling index of astrocytomas. Comparative study in a series of 60 cases. J Neurosurg 75(2):202–205

Laws ER, Taylor WF, Clifton MB (1984) Neurosurgical management of low-grade astrocytoma of the cerebral hemispheres. J Neurosurg 61:665–673

Laws ER, Taylor WF, Bergstralh, et al. (1986) The neurosurgical management of low-grade astrocytoma. Clin Neurosurgery 33:575–588

Le Bihan D, Douek M, Argyropoulou M, et al. (1993) Diffusion and perfusion magnetic resonance imaging in brain tumors. Top Magn Reson Imaging 5:25–31

Leibel SA, Sheline GE, Wara WM, et al. (1975) The role of radiation therapy in the treatment of astrocytomas. Cancer 35:1531–1557

Leighton C, Fisher B, Bauman G, et al. (1997) Supratentorial low-grade glioma in adults: an analysis of prognostic factors and timing of radiation. J Clin Onc 15(4):1294–1301

LeRoux PD, Berger MS, Wang K et al. (1992) Low-grade gliomas: comparison of intraoperative ultrasound characteristics with preoperative imaging studies. J Neurooncol 13:189–198

Levy LF, Elvidge AR (1956) Astrocytoma of the brain and spinal cord: a review of 176 cases, 1940–1949. J Neurosurgery 13: 413–443

Loftus CM, Coperland BR, Carmel PW (1985) Cystic supratentorial gliomas: natural history and evaluation of modes of surgical therapy. Neurosurgery 17:19–24

Lote K, Egeland T, Hager B, et al. (1997) Survival, prognostic factors, and therapeutic efficacy in low-grade glioma: A retrospective study in 379 patients. J Clin Oncol 15(9):3129–3140

Lunsford LD, Somaza S, Kondziolka D, et al: (1995) Survival after stereotactic biopsy and irradiation of cerebral nonanaplastic, nonpilocytic astrocytoma. J Neurosurg 82:523–529

Mamelak AN, Prados MD, Obana WG, et al. (1994) Treatment options and prognosis for multicentric juvenile pilocytic astrocytomas. J Neurosurg 81:24–30

McCormack BM, Miller DC, Budzilovich GN, et al (1992) Treatment and survival of low-grade astrocytoma in adults: 1977–1988. Neurosurgery 31(4):636–642

Mcdermott MW, Krouwer HGJ, Asai A, et al. (1992) Comparison of CT contrast enhancement and BUDR labeling indices in moderately and highly anaplstic astrocytomas of the cerebral hemispheres. Can J Neurol Sci 19:34–39,1992

Medbery CA, Straus KL, Steinberg SM, et al. (1988) Low-grade astrocytomas: Treatment results and prognostic variables. Int J Rad Onc. Biol. Phys. 15:837–841

Mittler MA, Walters BC, Stopa EG (1996) Observer reliability in histological grading of astrocytoma stereotactic biopsies. J Neurosurg 85:1091–1094

Morantz RA (1995) Low grade astrocytomas. In: Kaye AH, Laws ER (eds) Brain tumors: an encyclopedic approach. Churchill Livingstone, Edinburgh, pp 433–448

Morantz RA (1996) Low-grade astrocytomas. In: Wilkins RH, Rengachary SS (eds) Neurosurgery. McGraw-Hill, New York, pp 789–798

Mulhern RK, Kun LE (1991) Changes in intellect associated with cranial radiation therapy. In: Gutin PH, Sheline GE (eds) Radiation injury to the nervous system. Raven, New York, pp 325–340

Müller W, Afra D, Schroder R (1977) Supratentorial recurrences of gliomas. Morphological studies in relation to time intervals with astrocytomas. Acta Neurochirurgica 37:75–91

North CA, North RB, Epstein JA, et al. (1990) Low-grade cerebral astrocytomas: survival and quality of life after radiation therapy. Cancer 66:6–14

Ojemann RG (1995) Surgical principles in the management of brain tumors. In: Kaye AH, Laws ER (eds) Brain tumors: an encyclopedic approach. Churchill Livingstone, Edinburgh, pp 293–303

Ojemann RG, Heros RC, Crowell RM (1988) Surgical management of cerebrovascular disease. Williams & Wilkins, Baltimore

Ojemann RG, Martuza RL (1990) Acoustic neuromas. In: Youmans JR (ed) Neurological surgery. WB Saunders, Philadelphia, pp 3316

Okazaki H, Scheithauer BW (1988) Atlas of neuropathology. JB Lippincott, Philadelphia, pp 59–65

Palma L, Guidetti B (1985) Cystic pilocytic astrocytomas of the cerebral hemispheres. J Neurosurg 62:811–815

Parkins CS, Darling JL, Gill SS, Revesz T, Thomas DG (1991) Cell proliferation in serial biopsies through human malignant brain tumors: measurement using Ki-67 antibody labelling. Br J Neurosurg 5:289–98

Paulus W, Peiffer J (1989) Intratumoral histological heterogeneity of gliomas: aquantitative study. Cancer 64:442–447

Philippon JH, Clemenceau SH, Fauchon FH, et al. (1993) Supratentorial low-grade astrocytomas in adults. Neurosurgery 32(4):554–559

Piepmeier JM (1987) Observations on the current treatment of low-grade astrocytic tumors of the cerebral hemispheres. J Neurosurg 67:177–181

Rabb CH, Apuzzo MLJ (1995) Stereotaxis in the diagnosis and management of brain tumors. In: Kaye AH, Laws ER (eds) Brain tumors: an encyclopedic approach. Churchill Livingstone, Edinburgh, pp 433–448

Radhakrisnan K, Bohnen NI, Kurland LT (1993) Epidemiology of brain tumors. In: Morantz RA, Walsh J (eds) Brain tumors: a comprehensive text. Dekker, New York

Ransohoff J, Kelly P, Laws E (1986) The role of intracranial surgery for the treatment of intracranial gliomas. Semin Oncol 13:27–37

Recht LD, Lew R, Smith TW (1992) Suspected low grade glioma: Is deferring treatment safe? Ann Neurol 31:431–436

Revesz T, Scaravilli F, Coutinho L, et al. (1993) Reliability of histological diagnosis including grading in gliomas biopsied by image-guided stereotactic technique. Brain 116:781–793

Ringertz N (1950) Grading of gliomas. Acta Pathol Microbiol Scand 27:51–64

Roberts D, Strohbehn J, Hatch J, et al (1986) A frameless stereotactic integration of computerized tomographic imaging and the operating microscope. J Neurosurg 65:545–549

Russell DS, Rubinstein LJ (1989) Pathology of tumors of the nervous system, 5th edn. Williams & Wilkins, Baltimore, pp 126–225

Salcman M (1990) Radical surgery for low-grade glioma. Clin Neurosurg 36:353–366

Salcman M (1985) Supratentorial gliomas: clinical features and surgical therapy. In: Wilkins RH, Rengachary SS (eds) Neurosurgery. McGraw-Hill, New York, pp 579–590

Sano K (1980) Temporopolar approach to aneurysms of the basilar artery at and around the distal bifurcation: technical note. Neurol Res 2: 361–367

Scanlon PW, Taylor WF (1979) Radiotherapy of intracranial astrocytomas: analysis of 417 cases treated from 1960 through 1969. Neurosurgery 5:301–308

Scherer JH (1938) Structural development in gliomas. Am J Cancer 34:333–351

Scherer JH (1940) Cerebral astrocytomas and their derivatives. Am J Cancer 40:159–198

Schiffer D, Chio A, Giordana MT, et al. (1988) Prognostic value of histologic factors in adult cerebral astrocytoma. Cancer 61:1386–1393

Schultheiss TE, Kun LE, Ang KK, et al (1995) Radiation response of the central nervous system. Int J Radiat Oncol Biol Phys 31:1093–1112

Sekhar LN, Janecka IP (1993) Surgery of cranial base tumors. Raven, New York

Shaw EG (1995) The low-grade glioma debate: Evidence defending the position of early radiation therapy. Clin Neurosurg 40:488–494

Shaw EG (1990) Low-grade gliomas: to treat or not to treat? A radiation oncologist's viewpoint. Arch Neurol 47:1138–1139

Shaw EG, Daumas-Duport C, Scheithauer BW, et a (1989) Radiation therapy in the management of low-grade supratentorial astrocytomas. J Neurosurg 70:853–861

Sheline GE (1986) The role of radiation therapy in the treatment of low-grade gliomas. Clin Neurosurg 33:533–74

Shibamoto Y, Kitakabu Y, Takahashi M, et al (1993) Supratentorial low-grade astrocytoma. Correlation of computed tomography findings with effect of radiation therapy and prognostic variables. Cancer 72:190–195

Shitara N, McKeever PE, Whang-Peng J, et al: Flow-cytometric and cytogenetic analysis of human cultured cell lines derived from high- and low-grade astrocytomas. Acta Neuropathol 60:40–48

Sidransky D, Mikkelsen T, Schwechheimer K et al. (1992) Clonal expansion of p53 mutant cells is associated with brain tumor progression. Nature 355:846–847

Silverman C, Marks JE (1981) Prognostic significance of contrast enhancement in low-grade astrocytomas of the adult cerebrum. Radiology 139:211–213

Sklar CA, Constine LS (1995) Chronic neuroendocrinological sequelae of radiation therapy. In J Radiat Oncol Biol Phys 31:1113–1121

Sofietti R, Chio A, Giordana MT, et al. (1989) Prognostic factors in well-differentiated cerebral astrocytomas in the adult. Neurosurgery 24(5):686–692

Stage WS, Stein JJ (1974) Treatment of malignant astrocytomas. Am J Rad 120:7–18

Steiger HJ, Markwalder RV, Seiler RW, et al. (1990) Early prognosis of supratentorial grade 2 astrocytomas in adult patients after resection or stereotactic biopsy. Acta Neurochir 106:99–105

Stewart DH Jr, Krawchenko J (1985) Patient positioning. In: Wilkins RH, Rengachary SS (eds) Neurosurgery. McGraw-Hill, New York, pp 452–460

Taphoorn MJB, Schiphorst AK, Snoek FJ, et al. (1994) Cognitive functions and quality of life in patients with low-grade gliomas: the impact of radiotherapy. Ann Neurology 36:48–54

Tarlov IM (1937) Effect of roentgenotherapy on gliomas. Arch Neurol Psychiatry 38:513–536

Tew JM Jr, Scodary DJ (1993) Supratentorial procedures – basic techniques and surgical positioning. In: Apuzzo MLJ (ed) Brain surgery complications avoidance and management. Churchill Livingstone, New York, pp 31–50

Uihlein A, Colby MY, Layton DD et al. (1996) Comparison of surgery and surgery plus irradiation in the treatment of supratentorial gliomas. Acta Radiologica 5:67–78

Vavruch L, Nordenskjold B, Carstensen J, Enestrom S (1996) Prognostic value of flow cytometery and correlation to some conventional prognostic factors: a retrospective study of archival specimens of 134 astrocytomas. J Neurosurg 85(1):146–151

Vertosick FT, Selker RG, Arena VC (1991) Survival of patients with well-differentiated astrocytomas diagnosed in the era of computed tomography. Neurosurgery 23:496–501

Vigilanis MC, Sichey N, Poisson M, et al (1996) A prospective study of cognitive function following radiotherapy for supratentorial gliomas in young adults: 4 year results. Int J Radiat Oncol Biol Phys 35: 527–533

Wara WM (1985) Radiation therapy for brain tumors. Cancer 55:2291–2295

Watne K, Hannisdal E, Nome O (1992) Combined intra-arterial chemotherapy followed by radiation in astrocytomas. J Neurooncol 14:73–80

Warnick RE (1993) Tumors associated with phakomatoses. In: Morantz RA, Walsh J (eds) Brain tumors: a comprehensive text. Dekker, New York

Weingart J, Olivi A, Brem H (1991) Supratentorial low grade astrocytomas in adults. Neursurg Q 1:141–159

Weir B, Grace M (1976) The relative significance of factors affecting post-operative survival in astrocyomas, grades I and II. Can J Neuro Sci 3:47–50

Whitton AC, Bloom HJG (1990) Low grade glioma of the cerebral hemispheres in adults: A retrospective analysis of 88 cases. Int J Rad Onc Biol Phys 18:783–786

Wilson CB, Prados MD (1986) Surgery for low-grade glioma: Rationale for early intervention. Clin Neurosurgery 33:383–390

Winger MJ, MacDonald DR, Cairncross JG (1989) Supratentorial anaplastic gliomas in adults. J Neurosurg 71:487–493

Worthington C, Tyler JF, Villemare JG (1987) Stereotactic biopsy and positron emission tomography correlation of cerebral gliomas. Surg Neuro 27:87–92

Yasargil MG, Reichmann MV, Kubik S (1987) Preservation of the frontotemporal branch of the facial nerve craniotomy. Technical article. J Neurosurg 67:463–466

Zuber P, Hamou M, de Tribolet N (1988) Identification of proliferating cells in human gliomas using the monoclonal antibody Ki-67. Neurosurgery 22:364–368

Zülch KJ (1986) Brain tumors: their biology and pathology, 3rd edn. Springer-Verlag, Berlin Heidelberg New York pp 210–213

16 Radiotherapy in the Management of Low-Grade Gliomas

Rolf Dieter Kortmann, Branislav Jeremic, and Michael Bamberg

CONTENTS

16.1 Introduction

Low-grade gliomas account for approximately 10%–15% of all primary brain tumours in adults (Burger et al. 1982). The tumours are slowly progressing and are therefore often considered "benign". They affect the brain by two mechanisms: (1) infiltration of tumour cells may alter neurological function; (2) this is usually accompanied by a space-occupying effect leading to compression of adjacent neural tissue and subsequently causing increased intracranial pressure. Due to the different locations within the brain of the disease, the clinical symptoms and signs vary considerably and many patients have a long medical history at the time of diagnosis. The most common features are seizures (66%), focal deficits (51%), headache (44%), neuropsychological disorders (16%) and visual deterioration (16%) (Laws et al. 1984). According to the histological criteria of the World Health Organization (WHO) gliomas are classified into grades I and II (Zulch 1979). In the most recent WHO classification of gliomas (Kleihues et al. 1993), low-grade tumours are subdivided into "ordinary" astrocytoma (fibrillary, protoplasmic, gemistocytic); oligodendroglioma; mixed oligoastrocytomas displaying features of diffuse infiltration; and the circumscribed pilocytic astrocytoma. Less common variants include pleomorphic xanthoastrocytoma, subependymal giant astrocytomas, and subependymomas, the latter group being related to the pilocytic astrocytomas. In all of these systems, oligodendrogliomas are mostly considered as low-grade gliomas, although their histology and clinical course can vary from that of other low-grade gliomas. The hallmark of the histological picture of low-grade glioma is the absence of necrosis, while there is some overlap between anaplastic astrocytoma, the intermediate grade of the three-tiered system (Ringertz 1950; Burger et al. 1991), and grades 2 and 3 of the four-tiered classification (Kernohan and Sayre 1952; Daumas-Duport et al. 1988) regarding vascular proliferation. In order to improve uncertainties in classification, attempts have been made to identify distinct subgroups of patients with low-grade glioma. A labelling index of <1% was associated with a lower recurrence rate than a labelling index of >1% (Hoshino et al. 1988). It was also found that chromosome number and structure abnormalities may adversely influence survival (Jenkins et al. 1992).

A vast majority of gliomas are located supratentorially (Fig. 16.1). The therapeutic strategy basically consists of surgery and radiotherapy, but also of watchful waiting. The choice and time of treatment are a matter of debate. There is agreement that the decision as to when to treat should be based on how much improvement in the clinical course can be expected thereby. Extent of disease, site of tumour, patient age, clinical performance and additional histological subtypes should be considered. The options are surgery alone – biopsy or resection; radiotherapy alone; or postoperative radiotherapy treatment (only in cases of progressive disease; see Chap. 15). Numerous reports published on this subject have favoured one or another approach, identified possible prognostic factors and suggested "optimal" treat-

R.D. Kortmann, MD; M. Bamberg, MD; B. Jeremic, MD
Department of Radiology–Radiotherapy, Hoppe-Seyler-Strasse 3, 72076 Tübingen, Germany

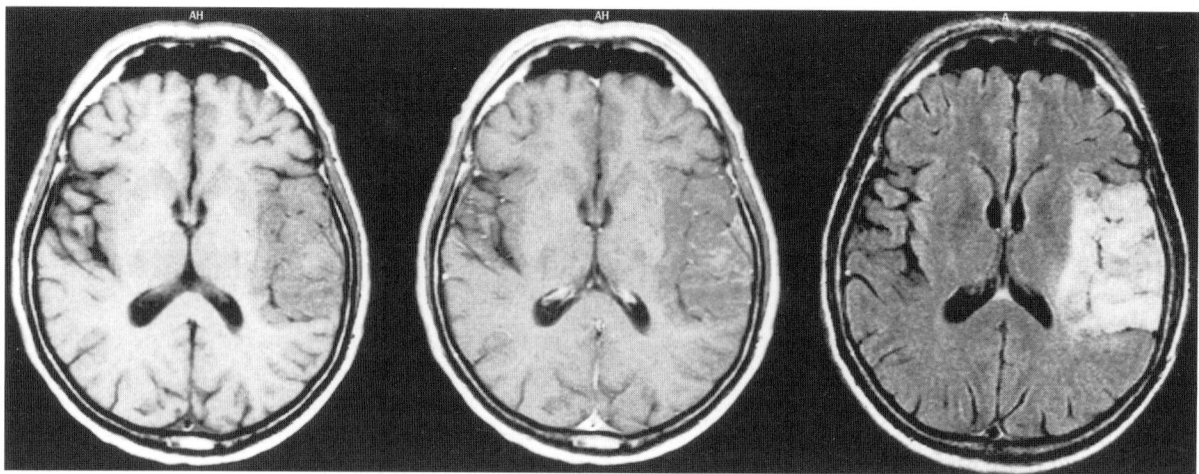

Fig. 16.1. Axial magnetic resonance image of a left parietal low-grade glioma (astrocytoma WHO grade II). Low signal intensity on T1-weighted image (*left*), no contrast enhancement (*centre*), FLAIR (flow attenuation inversion recovery) sequence (*right*); gadolinium DTPA. (We thank Dr. M. Skalej, Dept. of Neuroradiology, University of Tübingen)

ment approaches based on these factors. Unfortunately, all of these studies were retrospective, covering long time periods during which diagnostic and therapeutic variables differed substantially. Also, in some studies data on all treatment parameters were not always available. It is, invariable, therefore, that the discussion in this chapter will be influenced by such shortcomings in the literature.

16.2
Role of Radiotherapy

One of the most controversial decisions is whether or not to use radiation therapy. Relevant issues include the natural history of disease, early (at time of diagnosis) vs delayed (at time of recurrent disease) radiotherapy, expected outcome with postoperative radiation therapy, which radiation treatment fields to use (whole-brain vs tumour site), radiation dose and toxicity of radiotherapy.

Low-grade "non-pilocytic" glioma are frequently only subtotally resected; however, due to infiltration of surrounding normal neural tissue, postoperative radiotherapy is a substantial adjuvant treatment. The past three decades have provided increasing evidence that postoperative radiotherapy improves survival in subtotally resected low-grade glioma, although no prospective randomised study has provided clear evidence.

16.2.1
Astrocytoma and Oligoastrocytoma

Table 16.1 summarises the outcome of surgery alone vs surgery plus radiation therapy, including patients treated between 1956 and 1998. BOUCHARD and PIERCE (1960) reported on 20 years of experience. The use of postoperative radiotherapy was associated with a 5-year survival of 49% compared to 38% with surgery alone. LEIBEL et al. (1975) reported on 122 consecutive patients with astrocytoma, 108 of whom underwent an incomplete tumour resection. Of these, 71 were treated with postoperative radiotherapy (50–55 Gy in 1.8 Gy fractions), while 37 did not receive postoperative radiotherapy. The extent of tumour removal was similar between these two groups. The addition of postoperative radiotherapy improved 5-year survival compared to the surgery-only patients (46% vs 19%). The 10-year survivals were 35% and 11%, respectively. When childhood cases were excluded, 5-year survival was 32% and 10%, respectively, favouring postoperative radiotherapy. This advantage was seen during a follow-up of 20 years. In several other series consisting of varying patient numbers and in which postoperative radiotherapy was retrospectively compared with no further treatment, overall survival rates were between 49% and 54% after radiotherapy and were superior to those obtained by a "wait and see" policy, with overall survivals ranging from 21% to 32% at 5 years (Table 16.1). SHAW et al. (1989a) showed that, in pa-

Table 16.1. Treatment outcome in patients with low-grade astrocytomas

Author	Year	Patients (*n*)	5-year S	5-year S+RT	10-year S	10-year S+RT
LEVY/ELVIDGE	1956	87	26	36		
BOUCHARD	1966	149	26	49		
STAGE/STEIN	1974	28	20	40		
LEIBEL et al.	1975	108	19	46	11	35
MARSA et al.	1975	40		41		20
FAZEKAS	1977	68	32	54	32	26
OLMSTED/PLANK	1978	5	0	50		
SCANLON/TAYLOR	1979	417		58–76		
RUTTEN et al.	1981	27		35		
SILVERMAN/MARKS	1981	22		58–65 (4-yr)		
LAWS et al.	1984	326	34	49	18 (15-yr)	20 (15-yr)
GARCIA et al.	1985	86	21	50	10	25
MEDBERY et al.	1988	50		45		32
SOFFIETTI et al.	1989	86	30	9–25		
SHAW et al.	1989a	167	32	54	11	27
SHAW et al.	1989b	121		40–83		
NORTH et al.	1990	129		55		43
WHITTON/BLOOM	1990	88		36		26
McCORMACK et al.	1992	53		64		48
PHILLIPON et al.	1993	179	65	55		
SHIBAMOTO et al.	1993	119	37	60	11	41
PIEPMEIER et al.	1996	55		90		77
KARIM et al.	1996	343		59		
LEIGHTON et al.	1997	90		62		39
JEREMIC et al.	1998	37		75		

S, surgery; RT, radiotherapy.

tients with ordinary astrocytomas and mixed oligoastrocytomas, those who received "high-dose" radiotherapy (≥ 53 Gy) had a significantly better survival than patients treated with surgery alone (5- and 10-year survival rates of 68% and 39% vs 32% and 11%, respectively). MEDBERY et al. (1988) compared 50 patients who underwent postoperative radiotherapy and ten patients treated with surgery alone. Of the latter, four underwent incomplete tumour resection and all died of recurrent tumours within 6 years. The 5- and 10-year survival for the postoperative radiotherapy group was 45% and 30%, respectively. In a small study of VERTOSICK et al. (1991), of 25 patients with well-differentiated astrocytomas, 18 (22%) received immediate postoperative radiotherapy while seven did not. The median time to dedifferentiation, used as a parameter for progression, was 5.9 years for immediate radiotherapy vs 3.7 years for surgery alone ($p=0.18$). However, it should be noted that the total dose was unknown in five cases, while eight patients received 54–56 Gy. BERGER et al. (1994) reported on 53 patients, 40 of whom received postoperative radiotherapy with doses between 45 and 60 Gy. Postoperative radiotherapy did not influence the risk for recurrence and time to progression when analysed with respect to either postoperative residual tumour volume or percent of resection. However, the mean follow-up in this study was only 48.7 months (range: 24–172 months). After 25 years of follow-up of 119 patients from Kyoto with resected supratentorial low-grade glioma, SHIBAMOTO et al. (1993) observed that the 5- and 10-year survival rates for the 101 patients in the irradiated group were significantly better (60% and 41%, respectively) than those for the 18 patients treated with surgery alone (37% and 11%, respectively; $p=0.048$).

16.2.2
Timing of Postoperative Radiotherapy

The optimal timing of postoperative radiotherapy in incompletely resected low-grade glioma is an unsettled issue. Although not specifically addressing the problem, several studies have indicated an advantage for immediate postoperative radiotherapy regarding overall survival and progression-free survival (Garcia et al. 1985; Laws et al. 1984; Leibel et al. 1975; Shaw et al. 1989a; Shibamoto et al. 1993). However, there are also reports that did not find such a relationship. Piepmeier et al. (1996) reported on 21 patients with supratentorial low-grade astrocytomas. Ten patients received immediate postoperative radiotherapy, while in 11 patients radiotherapy was administered at time of recurrence. The timing of radiotherapy influenced neither time to tumour recurrence nor survival (median time to tumour recurrence: 7 vs 5 years; median survival time: 9 years vs not achieved yet at the time of report). Bahary et al. (1996) put special emphasis on the timing of radiotherapy. In 20 patients radiotherapy was given at the time of recurrence, in 43 patients immediate postoperative radiotherapy was administered. There was no difference in survival at 5 years (66% vs 67%), although there was a higher early mortality rate in the postoperative radiotherapy group. The extent of surgery was a prognostic factor in the delayed radiotherapy group and significantly influenced survival favouring patients with gross total tumour resection and subtotal tumour resection over biopsy only ($p=0.002$). Leighton et al. (1997) found a survival benefit in a group of 156 patients in whom radiotherapy was deferred. The 5- and 10-year survival rates were 84% and 70% as compared to 62% and 35% in 96 patients who underwent immediate postoperative radiotherapy. In a univariate analysis these difference were statistically significant but timing could not be identified as an independent prognostic variable on multivariate analysis. In addition, those patients who underwent immediate radiotherapy showed "unfavourable" prognostic factors. This was because they had a higher rate of bulky residual disease and their tumours were predominantly astrocytomas. Most recently, preliminary results of an EORTC/MRC study (Karim et al. 1998) have shown that immediate postoperative radiotherapy in low-grade glioma improved progression-free survival over that seen with observation only (5-year progression-free survival: 44% vs 37%, $p=0.02$). Unfortunately, this advantage was not translated into an improvement in overall survival. However, the follow-up is presently too short (median: 4.6 years) to allow us come to definite conclusions.

16.3
Impact of Modern Imaging Methods

The advantage of contemporary (CT era) over earlier (pre-CT era) studies seems to lie in better imaging. Delineation of the tumour is "more adequate", allowing a higher degree of precision in tailoring treatment fields. Medbery et al. (1988) found a significant improvement in survival in patients treated in the CT era (starting in their 1978 analysis). Survival advantage in recent series was largely limited to patients treated with partial-brain radiotherapy only and may suggest a possible effect of a better definition of tumour site, which may have led to fewer marginal misses. Shibamoto et al. (1993) found that survival rates tended to be higher for patients treated in the post-CT era than in the pre-CT era ($p=0.061$). Also, in the study of Shimizu et al. (1993) on oligodendrogliomas, the use of CT was associated with significantly better 5-year survival when compared to the pre-CT era (76% vs 41%, $p>0.05$), although the use of CT was associated with the use of higher radiotherapy doses. In contrast to these findings, Westergaard et al. (1997) did not find an advantage for patients having oligodendroglioma histology who were treated in the CT era (Table 16.2). Since 60%–70% of all low-grade gliomas may be non-enhancing on CT (Shaw et al. 1993), it is to be expected that MR imaging would lead to better and earlier diagnosis and that it may also be used for treatment planning. Finally, a precise definition of target volume and delineation of organs at risk are a prerequisite for a successful dose escalation and lower incidence of radiotherapy-induced toxicity, such as brain necrosis (Hohweiler et al. 1986; Marks and Wong 1985). Additionally, the radiological appearance (contrast-enhanced vs non-enhanced tumour) may be of prognostic significance and may have an impact on the therapeutic decision. Piepmeier et al. (1996) observed that patients with contrast-enhancing low-grade astrocytomas have a shorter survival time than those with non-contrast-enhanced low-grade astrocytomas. Furthermore, one study has shown that the addition of radiotherapy/chemotherapy to the treatment protocol increased the survival of patients with contrast-enhanced low-grade astrocytomas to 70% at 7 years (Levin et al. 1995).

Table 16.2. Treatment outcomes in patients with oligodendroglioma

Author	Year	Patients (n)	5-year S	5-year S+RT	10-year S	10-year S+RT
CHIN et al.	1980	54	82	100		
REEDY et al.	1983	48	67	63		
BULLARD et al.	1987	71	47	60		
LINDEGAARD et al.	1987	170	27	36		
WALLNER et al.	1988	42	55	80	18	56
NIJAAR et al.	1993	72		66		30
SHIMIZU et al.	1993	41[a]	25	74		
CELLI et al.	1994	105	36	57		
GANNETT et al.	1994	41	51	83	36	46
LEIGHTON et al.	1997	156		84		52

S, surgery; RT, radiotherapy.
[a] Includes eight patients with high-grade tumours.

16.4
Treatment Fields

For those patients receiving radiotherapy, a decision must be made with regard to the optimal treatment fields. Although it has been shown, using stereotactic biopsies, that tumour cells can extend beyond imaging abnormalities (DAUMAS-DUPORT et al. 1987; LAWS et al. 1984), which may suggest wider radiotherapy treatment fields, data accumulated over decades support the use of localised fields to treat supratentorial low-grade gliomas. BULLARD et al. (1987) performed both univariate and multivariate analyses and demonstrated that the use of larger treatment fields, including whole-brain irradiation with a tumour volume boost, offered no survival benefit over limited field radiotherapy. Furthermore, SHAW et al. (1989a) found no influence of irradiated volume on patient survival, while SCANLON et al. (1979) found a detrimental effect of large or whole-brain fields on treatment outcome. In the series of SHAW et al. (1989b), consisting of 20 patients, all failures occurred locally. In a corresponding analysis by NORTH et al. (1990) 15 out of 15 recurrences were local. In another series using treatment fields confined to the primary tumour site, 91% of recurrences

occurred locally (within the radiotherapy field), while only one case was marginal and without out-of-field recurrences (JEREMIC et al. 1998). In summary, the observation that tumour relapse occurs predominantly at the site of the primary tumour within the irradiated treatment volume implies that treatment fields encompassing the tumour are appropriate (SHAW et al. 1989; PU et al. 1995). With the identification of isolated tumour cells beyond the margin of a tumour on a T2-weighted MR image (MRI), the appropriate clinical target volume should include the MRI-indicated extent of the tumour with a 2–3 cm margin of surrounding brain tissue with respect to anatomical boundaries. PU et al. (1995) used three-dimensional, conformal, external-beam radiotherapy to treat 46 patients. Initial target volume included the tumour plus a 1–3 cm margin treated with a dose of 45–50.4 Gy and a boost that encompassed the tumour plus a 0–2 cm margin treated with a total of 54–59–4 Gy. Only 11 (24%) failures were observed at a median follow-up of 32.7 months. Limiting the high-dose volume did not cause an increased marginal or out-of-field failure rate. With the widespread use of sophisticated technologies affecting treatment planning and delivery, it is reasonable to assume that future strategies will be developed. Conformal treatment preserving normal tissue and organs at risk will allow delivery of high doses of radiotherapy and, therefore, achieve a better outcome in terms of tumour control and reduction of side effects.

16.5
Influence of Histology

Several studies have addressed the different behaviours and outcomes of various histological subtypes (low-grade astrocytomas, oligodendrogliomas and mixed gliomas). MARSA et al. (1975) were the first to provide information on the possible differences among the various histological subtypes of low-grade glioma. In their series, patients with oligodendroglioma had better overall and median survivals than patients with either mixed low-grade glioma or low-grade astrocytomas. In addition, patients with mixed low-grade glioma had a better median survival time than those with low-grade astrocytomas, but no difference could be seen 7 years after treatment. Similarly, WHITTON and BLOOM (1990) found improved survival for patients with oligodendrogliomas as compared to those with astrocytomas, although this difference was less pronounced after 10 years of follow-up (oligodendroglioma vs astrocytoma: 5-year survival, 64% vs 36%; 10-year survival, 35% vs 26%). Recently, LEIGHTON et al. (1997) documented longer overall and progression-free survivals for patients with an oligodendroglioma or mixed glioma than with astrocytoma (5- and 10-year survivals: 84% and 62% vs 62% and 39%, respectively; median 13 vs 7.5 years, p=0.003; progression-free, 5.6 vs 4.4 years, p=0.054). In the study of JEREMIC et al. (1998), patients with mixed gliomas tended to have a survival/progression-free survival similar to those with oligodendrogliomas, but not with ordinary astrocytomas (7-year survival: 78% and 80% vs 59%, respectively; 7-year progression-free survival: 79% and 81% vs 61%, respectively).

16.6
Progression to a High-Grade Glioma

Malignant transformation of low- into high-grade glioma was found in recurrent or autopsied cases. MÜLLER et al. (1977) used a three-tiered system to find progression towards a higher grade in 33% of their patients, with an additional 38% of patients progressing to glioblastoma multiforme. The tumours of the remaining 29% patients were described as progressing from grade I to grade II. These findings were confirmed by SHAW et al. (1989a) and JEREMIC et al. (1998). In the series of LAWS et al. (1984), 79 patients with recurrent tumours were analysed. A progression to astrocytoma grade III or IV occurred in 39 (49%) patients. A higher incidence of progression was noted in several other series, but mainly in those with up to only 25 patients (MARSA et al. 1975; PIEPMEIER et al. 1996; PHILLIPON et al. 1993; VERTOSICK et al. 1991; Table 16.3). McCORMACK et al. (1992) observed a contrast enhancement of low-grade gliomas in CT studies in 22 of 24 patients (92%) suggesting malignant transformation. Of seven re-operated recurrences in this series, six (86%) had progressed to high grade malignancy. In the study of GANNETT et al. (1994), progression was observed in five of eight cases (63%). Low-grade oligodendroglioma show the same tendency to malignant transformation. In the series of WALLNER et al. (1988), six out of ten patients with pure oligodendrogliomas who underwent either surgical re-resection or post-mortem sampling, had progressed to high-grade malignancy, while in the series of NIIJAR et al.

(1993), progression of oligodendroglioma to glioblastoma multiforme occurred in eight of 22 (36%) patients. A summary of these reports is given in Table 16.3.

Table 16.3. Progression of a low-grade glioma to a high-grade glioma

Author	Year	Number of patients re-operated or autopsied	Number of patients with progression (%)
MARSA et al.	1975	16	10 (62)
MÜLLER et al.	1977	137	52 (38)
LAWS et al.	1984	79	39 (49)
WALLNER et al.	1988	10	6 (60)
SHAW et al.	1989a	10	4 (40)
VERTOSICK et al.	1991	25	14 (56)
McCORMACK et al.	1992	7	6 (86)
PHILLIPON et al.	1993	25	18 (72)
NIIJAR et al.	1993	22	8 (36)
GANNETT et al.	1994	8	5 (63)
PIEPMEIER et al.	1996	17	11 (65)
JEREMIC et al.	1998	8	3 (38)
Total		364	176 (48)

16.7
New Approaches/Quality of Life

Various approaches to improve the results obtained with surgery and postoperative radiotherapy have been tested in recent years. The addition of chemotherapy was investigated by EYRE et al. (1993) from the Southwest Oncology Group. Sixty adult patients with incompletely resected low-grade glioma were treated with postoperative radiotherapy (55 Gy in 32 daily fractions over a total of 6.5–7 weeks), with or without CCNU (100 mg/m^2 every 6 weeks), beginning 2 days prior to the onset of radiotherapy. CCNU was continued for a total period not exceeding 2 years in patients having either a complete or partial response. No statistically significant difference in survival time was seen between the two treatment groups. The median survival time was 4.5 years for the radiotherapy alone group and 7.4 years for the combined radiotherapy/chemotherapy group. The impact of additional chemotherapy on tumour control and survival is currently under investigation by the Radiation Therapy Oncology Group (RTOG).

Patients with unfavourable prognostic factors will be randomised to receive radiotherapy alone or radiotherapy followed by six cycles of PCV.

Interstitial radiosurgery was performed by KRETH et al. (1995) using ^{125}I either as a permanent or a temporary implant. A total of 455 patients with low-grade glioma were treated; 97 had pilocytic astrocytoma. The 5- and 10-year survival rates in patients with pilocytic astrocytoma were 85% and 83%, and in patients with WHO grade II astrocytomas (250 patients) 61% and 51%, respectively. Five-year survival rates for patients with oligoastrocytomas (60 patients) and oligodendrogliomas (27 patients) were 49% and 50%, respectively, and were not different from patients with grade II astrocytomas. The poorest survival (32%) was seen in cases of gemistocytic astrocytomas (21 patients). SCERRATI et al. (1994) also used either ^{192}Ir or ^{125}I sources as permanent or temporary implants. A mean peripheral dose of 89.7 Gy for permanent implants and 42.8 Gy for the temporary implants was administered in 36 patients (2 pilocytic astrocytoma, 23 astrocytoma, 11 oligodendroglioma). The survival estimates were 83% at 5 years and 39% at 10 years.

Stereotactic external-beam radiotherapy has also been used, with promising results. POZZA et al. (1989) reported on initial results from 14 patients with inoperable low-grade astrocytomas treated with a multiple, noncoplanar arc irradiation. A total dose of 16–50 Gy was administered either in one fraction or in two fractions 8 days apart. Twelve out of 14 patients had a partial or complete response, with an overall survival ranging between 11 and 48 months (median 27.5 months). This approach was also successfully combined with endocavitary (cystic) radiation using ^{186}Re to treat case of pilocytic astrocytoma in children (PROUST et al. 1998).

Hyperfractionation combined with three-dimensional treatment planning may be a method to improve outcome. It exploits differences in repair capacity between early-reacting tissues (tumours) and late-reacting normal tissues (neural structures). The use of smaller fraction sizes should theoretically result in reduced late-normal tissue toxicity, thereby permitting higher total doses than those allowable in conventionally fractionated regimens. In a prospective phase II study, hyperfractionated radiotherapy was investigated in a total of 37 adults with histologically proven, supratentorial, low-grade (grade II) glioma after incomplete resection (JEREMIC et al. 1998); 55 Gy were given in 50 fractions on 25 treatment days over 5 weeks, 1.1 Gy b.i.d. fractions. The results of this study compare favourably to those of other contemporary studies (7-year survival: 69%; 7-year progression-free survival: 70% at median follow-up of 74 months). Subsequent studies with larger patient numbers and longer follow–up intervals are needed before testing hyperfractionated radiotherapy against standard fractionated radiotherapy and could also include conformal radiotherapy as a method allowing further dose escalation.

Additionally, the quality of life of the long-term survivors is of increasing concern and plays an important role when deciding on treatment. TAPHOORN et al. (1994) investigated 41 patients with low-grade glioma who underwent surgery, 20 of whom received additional, immediate postoperative radiotherapy. The patients were compared with a control group with haematological malignancies. None of the survivors had significant neurological impairment when compared to control subject. The patients with low-grade glioma had significantly more cognitive disturbances, but no difference could be seen between patients with and without radiotherapy (TAPHOORN et al. 1994). These observations were confirmed by VIGLIANI et al. (1996), who evaluated the effects of limited-field irradiation on cognitive functions in 17 patients as compared to 14 patients without radiotherapy. Neurocognitive dysfunctions were present in both groups suggesting that the deficits are mainly tumour- or surgery-related, but radiation-induced late toxicity or neurological deficits may occur by the alteration of small blood vessels in the treatment area.

16.8
Conclusions

Treatment of low-grade glioma is still a challenging issue in neuro-oncology. The presumed "benign" histological character of low-grade glioma is in sharp contrast to its biologically aggressive manner, despite surgery and radiotherapy and the absence of a plateau in survival figures observed at long follow-up intervals. Additionally, a considerable number of patients experience malignant transformation, including glioblastoma multiforme. These facts may require a more aggressive, but carefully balanced therapeutic approach to optimise treatment outcome. While surgery is generally accepted as an important initial treatment, the role of post-operative radiotherapy is the subject of ongoing controversy.

The role of post-operative radiotherapy now appears clearer following a report from the EORTC study showing that an improvement in progression-free but not overall survival is obtained after immediate post-operative radiotherapy. However, a reliable identification of prognostic factors supporting the use of immediate postoperative radiotherapy is still lacking. Although another EORTC study and the preliminary results of the RTOG study did not indicate an advantage for higher doses of irradiation over lower doses, local dose escalations may carry a benefit for subsets of patients. With the introduction of CT/MR imaging into diagnosis and planning, it is expected that new generations of sophisticated, computerised systems for treatment planning and delivery will allow successful dose escalations confined to tumour and immediate brain parenchyma only, and will result in lower toxicity of radiotherapy. The combination of these advantages and the advantages of hyperfractionation or interstitial radiotherapy may be the next logical step in an attempt to define an "optimal" treatment approach to these tumours.

References

Bahary JP, Villemeure JG, Choi S, Leblanc R, Olivier A, Bertrand G, Souhami L, Tampieri D, Hazel J. (1996) Low-grade pure and mixed cerebral astrocytomas treated in the CT scan era. J Neuro-Oncol 27:173–177

Berger MS, Deliganis AV, Dobbins J, Keles GE. (1994) The effect of extent of resection on recurrence in patients with low-grade cerebral hemisphere gliomas. Cancer 74:1784–1791

Bernstein JJ, Goldberg WJ, Laws ER, Jr. (1989) Immunohitochemistry of human malignant astrocytoma cell xenografted to rat brain: apolipoprotein E. Neurosurgery 24:541–546

Bouchard J, Pierce CB. (1960) Radiation therapy in the management of neoplasms of the central nervous system with a special note in regard to children: twenty years experience, 1930–1958. AJR 84:610–628

Bouchard J (1966) Effects of irradiation in treatment of intracranial gliomas – treatment results by histologic groups. In Bouchard J (ed) Radiation therapy of tumors and diseases of the nervous system. Lea & Febiger, Philadelphia, pp 78–118

Bullard DE, Rawlings, CE, Philips B, Cox EB, Schold SC, Burger P, Halperin EC. (1987) Oligodendroglioma. An analysis of the value of radiation therapy. Cancer 60:2179–2188

Burger PC, Scheithauer BW, Vogel FS. (1991) Brain tumors. In: Burger PC, Scheithauer BW, Vogel FS (eds) Surgical pathology of the central nervous system and its coverings, Churchill Livingstone, New York, pp 193–437

Cairncross JG, Laperriere NJ. (1989) Low-grade glioma. To treat or not to treat? Arch Neurol 46:1238–1239

Celli P, Nofrone I, Palma L, Cantore G, Fortuna A. (1994) Cerebral oligodendroglioma: prognostic factors and life history. Neurosurgery 35:1018–1035

Chin HW, Hazel JJ, Kim Th, Webster JR. (1980) Oligodendrogliomas – a clinical study of cerebral oligodendrogliomas. Cancer 45:1448–1466

Daumas-Duport C, Scheithauer B, Kelly P. (1987) A histologic and cytologic method for the spatial definition of gliomas. Mayo Clin Proc 62:435–449

Daumas-Duport C, Scheithauer B, O'Fallon J, Kelly P. (1988) Grading of astrocytomas: A simple and reproducible method. Cancer 62:2152–2165

Donahue B, Scott BC, Nelson JS, Rotman M, Murray KJ, Nelson DF, Banker FL, Earle JD, Fischbach JA, Asbell SO, Gaspar LE, Markoe AM, Curran W. (1997) Influence of oligodendroglial component on the survival of patients with anaplastic astrocytomas: A report of Radiation Therapy Oncology Group. Int J Radiat Oncol Biol Phys 38:911–914

Elvidge A, Penfield W, Cone W. (1937) The gliomas of the central nervous system. A study of 210 verified cases. Res Nerv Ment Dis 16:107–181

Eyre HJ, Crowley JJ, Townsend JJ, Eltringham JR, Morantz RA, Schulman SF, Quagliana JM, Al-Sarraf M. (1993) A randomized trial of radiotherapy versus radiotherapy plus CCNU for incompletely resected low-grade gliomas: a Southwest Oncology Group study. J Neurosurg 78:909–914

Fazekas JT. (1977) Treatment of grades I and II brain astrocytomas. The role of radiotherapy. Int J Radiat Oncol Biol Phys 2 et al. 661–666

Gannett DE, Wisbeck WM, Silbergeld DL, Berger MS. (1994) The role of postoperative irradiation in the treatment of oligodendroglioma. Int J Radiat Oncol Biol Phys 30:567–573

Garcia D, Fulling K, Marks J. The value of radiation therapy in addition to surgery for astrocytomas of the adult cerebrum. Cancer 55:919–927, 1985

Griffin BR, Silbergeld DL, Berger MS. (1992) Oligodendrogliomas: postoperative radiotherapy increases survival. Int J Radiat Oncol Biol Phys 24 (Suppl. 1): 142

Guthrie BL, Laws ER, Jr. (1990) Supratentorial low-grade gliomas. Neurosurg Clin N Am 1:37–48

Hirsch JF. (1990) Treatment and prognosis of benign hemispheric gliomas in children. Ann Pediatr Paris 37:614–616

Hohweiler ML, Lo TC, Silverman ML, Friedberg SR. (1986) Brain necrosis after radiotherapy for primary intracerebral tumor. Neurosurgery 18:68–74

Horrax G, Wu WQ. (1951) Postoperative survival of patients with intracranial oligodendroglioma with special reference to radical tumor removal et al. a study of 26 patiernts. J Neurosurg 8:472–479

Hoshino T, Rodriguez LA, Cho KG, Lee KS, Wilson CB, Edwards MSB, Levin VA, Davis RA. (1988) Prognostic implciations of the proliferazive potential of low-grade astrocytomas. J Neurosurg 69:839–842

Jenkins CA, Long PP, Carson BS, Brem H. (1992) Chromosome abnormalities in low-grade central nervous system tumors. Cancer Genet Cytogenet 60:67–73

Jeremic B, Shibamoto Y, Grujicic D, Milicic B, Stojanovic M, Nikolic N, Dagovic A. (1998) Hyperfractionated radiation therapy for incompletely resected supratentorial low-grade glioma. A phase II study. Radiother Oncol 49:49–54

Karim ABMF, Maat B, Hatlevoll R, Menten J, Rutten EHJM, Thomas DGT, Mascarenhas F, Horiot JC, Parvinen LM, van Reijn M, Jager JJ, Fabrini MG, van Alphen AM, Heamers

HP, Gaspar L, Noordman E, Pierart M, van Glabbeke M.. A randomized trial on dose-response in radiation therapy of low-grade cerebral glioma: European Organization for Research and Treatment of Cancer (EORTC) study 22844. Int J Radiat Oncol Biol Phys (1996) 36:549–556

Karim ABMF, Cornu P, Bleehan N, Afra D, De Witte O, Schraub S, Darcel F, Brucher JM, Bolla M, Vecht C, Stenning S, Pierart M, Van Glabbeke M. (1998) Immediate postoperative radiotherapy in low-grade glioma improves progression free survival, but not overall survival: Preliminary results of an EORTC/MRC randomized phase III study. J Neurooncol 39:101 (Abstract O-11)

Kelly PJ, Daumas-Duport C, Scheithauer BW, Kall BA, Kispert DB. (1987) Stereotactic histologic correlations of computed tomography- and magnetic resonance imaging-defined abnormalities in patients with glial neoplasms. Mayo Clin Proc 62: 450–459

Kernohan JW, Sayre GP. (1952) Tumors of the central nervous system. In: Atlas of tumor pathology, Sec. 10, Fasc. 35 and 37. Armed Forces Institute of Pathology, Washington DC, pp 17–42

Kleihues P, Burger PC, Scheithauer BW. (1993) Histological typing of tumors of the central nervous system, 3rd edn. Springer-Verlag, Berlin Heidelberg New York

Kreth FW, Faist M, Warnke PC, Robner R, Volk B, Ostertag CB. (1995) Interstitial radiosurgery of low-grade gliomas. J Neurosurg 82:418–429

Laws ER Jr., Taylor WF, Clifton MB, Okazaki H. (1984) Neurosurgical management of low-grade astrocytoma of the cerebral hemispheres. J Neurosurg 61:665–673

Laws ER, Taylor WF, Bergstrahl EJ, Okazaki H, Clifton MB. (1985) The neurosurgical management of low-grade astrocytoma. Clin Neurosurg 33:575–588

Leibel SA, Sheline GE, Wara WM, Boldrey EB, Nielsen SL. (1975) The role of radiation therapy in the treatment of astrocytomas. Cancer 35:1551–1557

Leighton C, Fisher B, Bauman G, Depiero S, Stitt L, Macdonald D, Cairncross G. (1997) Supratentorial low-grade glioma in adults: An analysis of prognostic factors and timing of radiation. J Clin Oncol 15:1294–1301

Levin VA, Prados MR, Wara WM, Davis RL, Gutiin PH, Phillips TL, Lamborn K, Wilson CB. (1995) Radiation therapy with bromodeoxyuridine followed by CCNU, procarbazine, and vincristine (PCV) chemotherapy for the treatment of anaplastic gliomas. Int J Radiat Oncol Biol Phys 32:75–83

Levy LF, Elvidge AR. (1956) Astrocytoma of the brain and spinal cord. J Neurosurg 13:413–443

Lindergaard K-F, Mork SJ, Eide GE, Halvorsen TB, Hatlevoll R, Solgaard T, Dahl O, Ganz J. (1987) Statistical analysis of clinicopathological features, radiotherapy, and survival in 170 cases of oligodendroglioma. J Neurosurg 67:224–230

Macdonald DR. (1994) Low-grade gliomas, mixed gliomas, and oligodendrogliomas. Semin Oncol 21:236–248

Marks JE, Wong I. (1985) The risk of cerebral radionecrosis in relation to dose, time, and fractionation: a follow-up study. Prog Exp Tumor Res 29:210–218

Marsa GW, Goffinet DR, Rubinstein LJ, Bagshaw MA. (1975) Megavoltage irradiation in the treatment of gliomas of the brain and spinal cord. Cancer 36:1681–1689

McCormack B, Miller DC, Budzilovich GN, Voorhees GJ, Ranshoff J. (1992) Treatment and survival of low-grade astrocytoma in adults – 1977–1988. Neurosurgery 31:636–642

Medbery CA III, Straus KL, Steinberg SM, Cotelingam JD, Fisher WS. (1988) Low-grade astrocytomas: treatment results and prognostic variables. Int J Radiat Oncol Biol Phys 15:837–841

Morantz RA. (1987) Radiation therapy in the treatment of cerebral astrocytoma. Nuerosurgery 20:975–982

Muller W, Afra D, Schroder R. (1977) Supratentorial recurrences of gliomas. Morphological studies in relation to time intervals with astrocytomas. Acta Neurochir. 37:75–91

Mundinger F, Braus DF, Krauss JK, Birg W. (1991) Long-term outcome of 89 low-grade brain-stem gliomas after interstitial radiation therapy- J Neurosurg 75:740–746

Nijaar TS, Simpson WJ, Gadalla T, McCartney M. (1993) Oligodendroglioma. Cancer 71:4002–4006

North CA, North RB, Epstein JA, Piantadosi S, Wharam MD. (1990) Low-grade cerebral astrocytomas. Survival and quality of life after radiation therapy. Cancer 66:6–14

Olmsted CM, Plank H. (1978) Radiation therapy of astrocytomas grades I-IV. Int J Radiat Oncol Biol Phys 4 (Suppl.):229 (Abstract)

Palma L, Guidetti B. (1985) Cystic pilocytic astrocytomas of the cerebral hemispheres. Surgical experience with 51 cases and long-term results. J Neurosurg 62:811–815

Philippon JH, Clemenceau SH, Fauchon F, Foncin JF. (1993) Supratentorial low-grade astrocytomas in adults. Neurosurgery 32:554–559

Piepmeier J, Christopher S, Spencer D, Byrne T, Kim J, Knisel JP, Lacy J, Tsukerman L, Makuch R. (1996) Variations in the natural history and survival of patients with supratentorial low-grade astrocytomas. Neurosurgery 38:872–879

Pollack IF, Claassen D, Al-Shboul Q, Janosky JE, Deutsch M. (1995) Low-grade gliomas of the cerebral hemispheres in children: an analysis of 71 cases. J Neurosurg 82:536–547

Pozza F, Colombo, F, Chierego G, Avanzo RC, Marchetti C, benedetti A, Casentini L, danieli D. (1989) Low-grade astrocytomas: Treatment with unconventionally fractionated external beam stereotactic radiation therapy. Radiology 171:565–569

Proust F, Coche-Dequeant B, Carpentier P, Laquerriere A, Derlon J-M, Blond S, Christiaens J, Freger P. (1998) Traitement combine d'un astrocytome pilocytique: radiochirurgie stereotaxique et radiotherapie endocavitaire. Neurochirurgie 44:50–54

Pu A T, Sandler HM, Radany EH, Blaivas M, Page MA, Greenberg HS, Junck L, Ross DA. (1995) Low-grade gliomas: Preliminary analysis of failure patterns among patients treated using 3D conformal external beam irradiation. Int J Radiat Oncol Biol Phys 31:461–466

Recht LD, Law R, Smith TW. (1992) Suspected low-grade glioma: Is deferring treatment safe? Ann Neurol 31:431–436

Reedy DP, Bay JW, Hahn JF. (1983) Role of radiation therapy in the treatment of cerebral oligodendroglioma: An analysis of 57 cases and a literature review. Neurosurgery 13:499–502

Ringertz N (1950) Grading of gliomas. Acta Pathol Microbiol Scand 27:51–64

Roberts M, German WJ. (1966) A long-term study of patients wit oligodendrogliomas: Follow-up of 50 cases, including Dr. Harvey Cushing's series. J Neurosurg 24:697–700

Rutten EHJM, Kazem I, Slooff JL, Walder, AHD. (1981) Postoperative radiation therapy in the management of brain astrocytomata – retrospective study of 142 patients. Int J Radiat Oncol Biol Phys 7:191–195

Scanlon PW, Taylor WF. (1979) Radiotherapy of intracranial astrocytomas: Analysis of 417 cases treated from 1969 through 1969. Neurosurgery 5:301–307

Scerrati M, Montemaggi, Iacoangeli M, Roselli R, Rossi GF. (1994) Interstitial brachytherapy of low-grade cerebral gliomas: Analysis of results in a series of 36 cases. Acta Neurochir (Wien) 131:97–105

Shaw EG, Daumas-Duport C, Scheithauer B, Gilbertson DT, O'Fallon JR, Earle JD, Laws ER, Jr, Okazaki H. (1989a) Radiation therapy in the management of low-grade supratentorial astrocytomas. J Neurosurg 70:853–861

0Shaw, E., Scheithauer, B. W., Gilbertson, D. T, Nicols DA, Laws ER, Earle JD, Daumas-Duport C, O'Fallon JR, Dinapoli RP. (1989b) Postoperative radiotherapy of supratentorial low-grade gliomas. Int J Radiat Oncol Biol Phys 16:663–668

Shaw EG, Scheithauer BW, O'Fallon JR. (1991)Management of supratentorial low-grade gliomas. Semin Radiat Oncol 1:23–31

Shaw E, Scheithauer B, O'Fallon J. (1993) Management of supratentorial low-grade gliomas. Oncology 7:97–107

Shaw E, Arusell R, Scheithauer B (1998) A prospective randomized trial of low- versus high dose radiation therapy in adults with supratentorial low-grade glioma: initial report of NCCTG-RTOG-ECOG study Proceedings of ASCO 17:401A

Sheline GE, Boldrey E, Karlsberg P, Phillips TL. (1964) Therapeutic considerations in tumors affecting the central nervous system: oligodendrogliomas. Radiology 82:84–89

Shenkin HA, Grant FC, Drew JH. (1947) Postoperative period of survival in patients with oligodendroglioma of the grain. Arch Neurol Psych 58:710–715

Shibamoto Y, Kitakabu Y, Takahashi M, Yamashita J, Oda Y, Kikuchi H, Abe M. (1993) Supratentorial low-grade astrocytomas. Correlation of computed tomography findings with effect of radiation therapy and prognostic variables. Cancer 72:190–195

Shimizu KT, Tran LM, Mark RJ, Selch MT. (1993) Management of oligodendrogliomas. Radiology 186:569–572

Silverman C, Marks JE. (1981) Prognostic significance of contrast enhancement in low-grade astrocytomas of the adult cerebrum. Radiology 139:211–213

Smith MT, Ludwig CL, Godfrey AD, Ambrustmacher VW. (1983) Grading of oligodendrogliomas. Cancer 52:2107–2114

Soffietti R, Chio A, Giordana MT, Vasario E, Schiffer D. (1989) Prognostic rfactors in well-differentiated cerebral astrocytomas in the adult. Neurosurgery 24:686–692

Stage WS, Stein JJ. (1976) Treatment of malignant astrocytomas. AJR 120:7–18

Taphoorn MJB, Schiphorst AK, Snock FJ, Lindeboom J, Wolbers JG, Karim ABMF, Huijgens PC, Heimans JJ. (1994) Cognitive function and quality of life in patients with low-grade gliomas: The impact of radiotherapy. Ann Neurol 36:48–54

Vertosick FT, Selker RG, Arena VC. (1991) Survival of patients with well – differentiated astrocytomas diagnosed in the era of computed tomography. Neurosurgery 28:496–501

Vigliani MC, Sichez N, Poisson M, Delattre JY. (1996) A prospective study of cognitive functions following conventional radiotherapy for supratentorial gliomas in young adults: 4-year results. Int J Radiat Oncol Biol Phys 35(3):527–533

Wallner KE, Gonzalez M, Sheline GE. (1988) Treatment of oligodendrogliomas with or without postoperative irradiation. J Neurosurg 68:684–688

Weingart J, Olivi A, Brem H. (1991) Supratentorial low-grade astrocytomas in adults. Neurosurg Q1:141–159

Westergaard L, Gjerris F, Klinken L. (1997) Prognostic factors in oligodendrogliomas. Acta Neurochir (Wien) 139:600–605

Whitton AC, Bloom HJG. (1990) Low-grade glioma of the cerebral hemispheres in adults: a retrospective analysis of 88 cases. Int J Radiat Oncol Biol Phys 18:783–786

Zulch KJ. (1979) Histologic typing of the tumors of the central nervous system. International histological classification of tumors, No. 21. World Health Organization, Geneva

17 Surgical Therapy and Problems in the Treatment of Private Malignant Gliomas

Michael Salcman

CONTENTS

17.1
Introduction

Surgery remains an essential therapeutic modality in the contemporary management of malignant gliomas. In appropriate patients, extent of surgical resection can be shown to be an important determinant of length of survival. Resection removes cells that are otherwise inherently resistant to other therapeutic modalities, improves or stabilizes neurologic function, potentiates the effects of other therapies and facilitates their delivery. Some patients would not survive to receive further treatment without the beneficial effects of craniotomy. The safety and efficacy of open resection have been greatly improved through the application of microsurgical techniques and image-based localization. In patients who are neurologically intact and have lesions smaller than 2 cm in critical locations, image-guided stereotactic biopsy is a reasonable alternative. Image-guided stereotaxy can also be used to deliver interstitial chemotherapy, immunotherapy, hyperthermia and

M. SALCMAN, MD
Head, Division of Neurological Surgery, Sinai Hospital, 9101 Franklin Square Drive, Suite 310, Baltimore, MD 21237-3928, USA

brachytherapy. Hybrid techniques, in which image-based stereotactic localization is used to guide microsurgical resection, are becoming increasingly important in reducing neurologic morbidity and patient length of stay. Within the context of an aggressive multimodality therapy program, technological advances in the safety and efficacy of open resection have increased the indications for repeat surgery.

The role of the surgeon in the management of patients with malignant gliomas is to establish a diagnosis, preserve life and function, and effect a cure if possible. Since virtually no malignant glial tumor can be treated by surgical resection alone, the type and extent of surgery offered to a patient should be considered in the context of other therapeutic options and should be consistent with the technical resources of the physician and the psychosocial resources of the patient and his or her family. In the majority of cases, some combination of open resection or stereotactic surgery can produce a diagnosis, ameliorate symptoms, decrease the intracranial pressure, improve the neurologic status, remove most of the tumor, and deliver other therapeutic agents. Proliferating non-surgical treatment options and recent technical advances that increase the safety and efficacy of surgery only serve to increase the complexity of the surgeon's decision-making process. It is within this process that the art of medicine resides.

The surgical treatment of high-grade gliomas, especially malignant astrocytoma and glioblastoma multiforme, has been an issue of controversy since the earliest days of neurology and neurosurgery (SALCMAN 1999). Periods of great enthusiasm for the surgical treatment of malignant brain tumors have alternated with periods of despair and pessimism. I believe we have now entered an era in which these debates can be set aside, at least for the great majority of patients. Technical limitations are now a secondary issue and the proper role of surgery in any given situation should be determined by the nature of the tumor and the situation of the patient. The surgeon should determine whether the goal of the operation is to be a chance for cure, a prolongation of survival, an amelioration of symptoms or the potentiation of other therapies (Table 17.1). In setting goals, a proper appreciation of the biology of the tumor, the age and condition of the patient, and the nature of prior or concurrent therapies is indispensable. Prior to describing a few technical aspects of craniotomy for malignant glioma, a brief review of the rationale for such procedures is presented.

Table 17.1. Rationale for extensive resection in glioma patients

Surgery	Benefits
Mechanical cytoreduction	Provide rapid 2-log cell kill
	Remove resistant cells
	Prolong survival
Surgical decompression Or facilitate	Decrease intracranial hypertension
	Improve neurologic function
	Resection may potentiate
	Radiation Therapy
	Chemotherapy
	Immunotherapy
	Brachytherapy and hyperthermia
Extensive tissue sampling	

17.2
Tumor Resection and Length of Survival

In general, patients undergo craniotomy for the purposes of diagnosis and treatment. As indicated in Table 17.1, it is hoped that excision will have a positive effect on both the length and quality of survival. That the length of survival in patients with malignant tumors is directly affected by the surgical stage of disease is a basic tenet of oncology and has been demonstrated on many occasions both inside and outside the nervous system (SALCMAN 1985,1994). Wide excision of solid malignancies of the lung, breast, colon and skin is carried out according to this principle and the extent of resection evaluated from the surgical specimen. Unfortunately, a true cancer operation only rarely can be achieved within the intracranial cavity, and much of the literature on surgery for brain tumors has been based on the surgeon's impression of the amount of tumor resected rather than a careful measurement of the volume of residual tumor imaged on the postoperative scan.

The effectiveness of surgery has thereby been obscured and the results of multicenter trials have sometimes been contaminated by the variability of the surgery offered in different institutions. Nevertheless, carefully analyzed retrospective studies and controlled clinical trials have demonstrated a positive correlation between length of survival and extent of resection for a wide variety of intracranial lesions, including meningioma (ADEGBITE et al. 1983; MIRIMANOFF et al. 1985), medulloblastoma (PARK et al. 1983), pilocytic astrocytoma (ILGREN et al. 1986), ependymoma, ordinary astrocytoma (LAWS et al. 1984; HOSHINO 1984; SALCMAN 1996) and metastatic brain tumors (PATCHELL et al. 1990). In these lesions, it would appear that a total removal of the tumor is at least as effective as the combination of a smaller operation and radiation (SALCMAN 1990).

For a variety of reasons, it has been difficult to establish a similarly unequivocal relationship between the extent of resection and the length of survival in patients with high-grade gliomas such as malignant astrocytoma or glioblastoma multiforme. Most of the studies are retrospective in nature, contaminated by the effects of other treatments, and the extent of tumor removal is almost exclusively based on the surgeon's intraoperative impression; the latter has been shown to be three times as inaccurate as postoperative imaging (Albert et al. 1994). When only CT or MR-controlled data are used in analyzing this problem, the results are perfectly consistent with what is known about solid tumors outside the central nervous system (Albert et al. 1994; Andreou et al. 1983; Ammirati et al. 1987; Wood et al. 1988). Furthermore, a retrospective analysis of 603 glioblastoma patients drawn from the literature who were subjected only to biopsy, partial excision or radical resection without subsequent radiation or chemotherapy also supports the conclusion of more recent clinical trials. This analysis indicates a general relationship between the extent of resection and the length of survival (Salcman 1985). Andreou et al. (1983) were probably the first to correlate the residual tumor burden present on the postoperative CT scan with the length and quality of survival. They found that the amount of postoperative tumor was inversely related to the length of useful survival ($p<0.01$), defined as a Karnofsky rating of greater than 30. In particular, a residual tumor diameter of less than 45 mm was associated with a 70% chance of long-term (more than 700 days) survival, and this rose to 78% if the residual tumor volume was less than 30 mm in diameter.

In a more recent series of 42 cases of supratentorial gliomas, a gross- total or nearly total clearing, as observed on postoperative CT scan, was possible in 86% of patients with an improved or stable neurologic status in 97% and no operative mortality (CIRIC et al. 1987). The rate of neurologic morbidity after partial resection was 40%. In a series of 31 consecutive patients, the extent of resection was quantified by an early, enhanced postoperative CT scan; the difference in the survival curves between the gross total removals and the subtotal tumor resections was significant at $p<0.001$ (AMMIRATI et al. 1987; Fig. 17.1). A significant difference in the quality of survival could be discerned at the $p=0.007$ level by determining the amount of time the patient spent living independently, as defined by the Karnofsky performance scale (Fig. 17.2). These data confirm the observation of SHAPIRO (1982), that preoperative neurologic abnormalities are almost always significantly improved or stable ($p<0.05$) after glioma surgery rather than made worse. In the study by AMMIRATI et al. (1987), an improvement in the postoperative functional status was seen only after a gross total removal ($p=0.006$), and the median survival of 90 weeks in this group compares with a median survival of 43 weeks in the subtotal resection group. The relationship between postoperative residual tumor volume and survival has been analyzed in 510 patients from the trial 80-01 of the Brain Tumor Study Group (WOOD et al. 1988). The postoperative tumor area as measured by CT scan was significantly related to survival ($p<0.0001$), whereas preoperative tumor

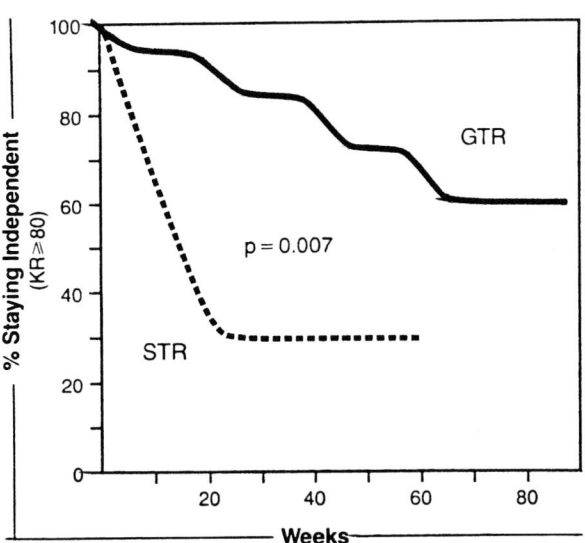

Fig. 17.2. Extent of resection and length of functional survival. Note that the length of time spent in an independent status (Karnofsky score >80) is dependent on the extent of resection at the $p=0.007$ level. *GTR*, gross total resection; *STR*, subtotal resection. (From AMMIRATI et al. 1987)

size was not (Fig. 17.3); this effect was independent of patient age, performance status or histology.

Other contemporary studies have also substantiated the importance of surgery, even when this issue was not the original focus of the investigation. In a report of the Radiation Therapy Oncology Group, the extent of surgery was relatively more important to patient prognosis than the performance status (NELSON et al. 1985). Patients with malignant astrocytoma survived a median of 46.8 months after a partial or complete excision and only 15.2 months after a biopsy ($p<0.001$). In another study, surgically treated patients had a longer survival than patients treated with biopsy ($p<0.002$); quite naturally, strong statistical correlations were discovered between operability and the age and performance status of the patient (COHADON et al. 1985). Multivariate analysis of survival in another group of patients indicated six important prognostic variables, two of which were the number of operations and the amount of tumor removed (HIRAKAWA et al. 1984). In a reappraisal of the clinical behavior of gemistocytic astrocytoma, all four patients originally undergoing a gross total removal were still alive while all five who had received only biopsy had already died (KROUWER et al. 1991). Lobectomy does not appear to add to the survival benefit conferred by complete excision and has been found to actually worsen the early outcome and total survival time in patients with incompletely re-

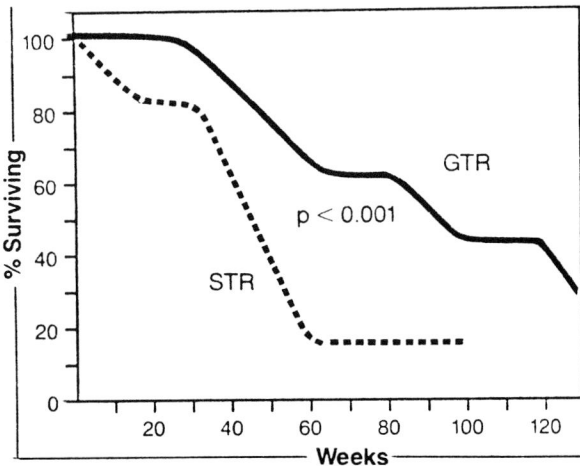

Fig. 17.1. Extent of resection and length of survival. Note that survival after gross total resection (*GTR*) is significantly longer than that after subtotal resection (*STR*) at the $p<0.001$ level. (From AMMIRATI et al. 1987)

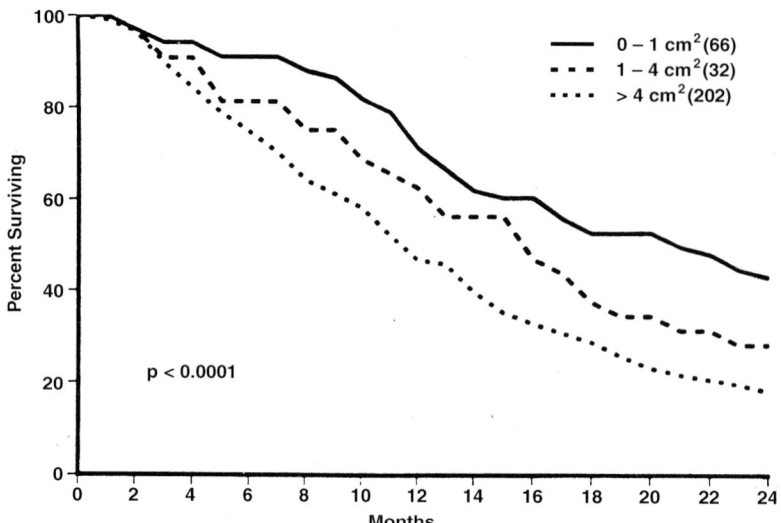

Fig. 17.3. Survival related to size of residual tumor on postoperative CT scan. In the Brain Tumor Cooperative Group, total survival was dependent on the amount of residual tumor measured on the post-operative CT scan; a similar relationship was found for the amount of residual tumor observed on the post-radiation therapy scan. (From WOOD et al. 1988)

sected glioblastoma (HOLLERHAGE et al. 1991). Contemporary studies that deny the association between the extent of resection and the length of survival in patients with gliomas are compromised by the small number of patients enrolled, the lack of postoperative imaging analysis, and the uncontrolled application of other therapies (COFFEY et al. 1988; PIEPMEIER 1987). The overall results reported in these papers are inferior to those of other series and are peculiar in a number of other respects, including the lack of an observed effect of age or performance status on survival, relationships that are consistently observed in other series large and small (KROUWER et al. 1991; SALCMAN et al. 1982; WALKER et al. 1980).

In the 1990s, six of nine radiographically controlled series demonstrated superior survival for patients subjected to resection in comparison to patients undergoing partial resection or stereotactic biopsy (HESS 1999; VECHT et al. 1990; DEVAUX et al. 1993; BERGER 1994). In one series of anaplastic astrocytoma and glioblastoma patients, the difference in 3-month survival between patients undergoing stereotactic biopsy and those undergoing more than 95% resection was 41% and 87% respectively, (VECHT et al. 1990). In another study, the difference in 1-year survival between the two procedures was 29% and 51.1% respectively (DEVAUX et al. 1993). In particular, in recurrent glioblastoma, patients with less than a 25% resection had a median survival of 32 weeks; this increased to 63 weeks for resections of 50%–74% and 93 weeks for gross total resections (BERGER 1994). From a methodological point of view, however, each of these modern studies contains statistical flaws, particularly in relation to patient se-

lection factors (HESS 1999). Nevertheless, the general trend should not be ignored; in a small prospective study in which confounding factors were statistically adjusted, the survival advantage of gross total resection was significant at the $p=0.0002$ level (ALBERT et al. 1994).

17.3
Tumor Resection and Multimodality Therapy

As indicated above, resection of high-grade glial tumors not only may result in cure or prolonged survival but may also improve neurologic function and performance status. Raised intracranial pressure or emotional despondency over a neurologic disability may not allow an otherwise salvageable patient to receive radiation or life-enhancing rehabilitation therapy. Surgical amelioration of mass effect sometimes promotes neurologic recovery when mild deficits are secondary to the proximity of peritumoral edema and not due to direct invasion by tumor. Improvement in cerebral blood flow and glucose metabolism may occur at sites distant from the craniotomy, at times even in the contralateral hemisphere (BEANEY et al. 1985). The probability of functional recovery can be enhanced through the use of intraoperative mapping of eloquent cortex (ROSTOMILY et al. 1991).

Surgery can also be used to potentiate the efficacy of other therapies especially by decreasing the tumor burden encountered by any particular agent or the host's own defensive mechanisms. It is known that the immunocompetence of glioma patients is compromised, and laboratory studies have shown that surgery can potentiate the efficacy of immunotherapy (Brooks et al. 1980; Young et al. 1991). In addition to decreasing the number of clonogenic cells, surgery alters vascular permeability and may remove some of the blocking factors produced by the tumor. Some of these mechanisms may help to explain experimental demonstration of the potentiation of chemotherapy by surgical manipulation (Tel et al. 1980). In addition to improved vascular access, surgery removes many of the cells that are inherently resistant to radiation and chemotherapy, especially cells in the more central portions of the tumor with poor vascular supply, low oxygen tension, and low mitotic or metabolic states (Salcman 1988, 1990, 1996). The combination of resection and interstitial chemotherapy via implantable biodegrable wafers has been shown to be an effective rescue therapy for recurrent lesions (Brem et al. 1995). A decrease in population pressure and the removal of resistant tissue may stimulate non-dividing cells to enter the cell cycle and thus become more sensitive to radiation and chemotherapy (Hoshino 1984). Of course, craniotomy can also be used to immediately implement phototherapy, interstitial radiation, chemotherapy or immunotherapy to follow resection during the same procedure. In all of these ways, surgical resection can be viewed as an important component of multimodality therapy. It has long been my view that the heterogeneity of the cell populations within any single glial tumor requires the near simultaneous application of a variety of treatment modalities to address a diversity of metabolic, kinetic and vascular factors (Salcman 1996b).

17.4
Planning for Tumor Resection

All successful operations begin with proper patient selection and preoperative planning. The decision to offer excision rather than biopsy and the selection of an approach that is the most appropriate for that particular patient and his or her tumor are the initial steps in surgical technique (Salcman 1989, 1990; Toms et al. 1999). As a rule, patients selected for craniotomy should have solitary lesions that are well-defined on contrast-enhanced CT or MR scans and a functional status or social situation sufficient to support them through subsequent therapy. In general, small poorly defined lesions located in critical

regions in neurologically intact patients are more appropriately dealt with by stereotactic means (Salcman 1989, 1990; Kondziolka and Lunsford 1999). Since surgery for gliomas almost always takes place through a transcortical incision, it is of the utmost importance that this incision be planned beforehand and that the appropriate localization methods and instrumentation be available to facilitate the trajectory of the approach. In general, the craniotomy should be planned so as to provide the shortest possible working distance between the tumor and the surface of the brain, even if that surface includes eloquent cortex.

Three-dimensional planning is just as important to the surgeon as to the radiation oncologist. The surgeon should carefully measure the tumor in all three major axes on the contrast-enhanced MR or CT scan and determine which side of the tumor is nearest the motor strip, a language area, the visual cortex or the thalamus. The most useful internal landmarks to note are the sphenoid wing, tentorial edge and portions of the ventricular system, while the coronal suture, pterion and external ear are the most important external aids to localization. Because the majority of high-grade gliomas are located in the frontoparietal region, the probable relationship of the tumor to the motor strip is usually the most important preoperative determination in planning the approach and the degree of resectability.

The most widely available method for preoperative planning is the enhanced MRI scan. The location of the motor cortex can be inferred from the axial cut, on which the premotor sulcus is seen to meet the superior frontal sulcus (Berger et al. 1990). Similarly, on the midline sagittal view, the location of the motor area for the lower extremity is demarcated by the point at which the supramarginal sulcus stops following the line of the corpus callosum and turns upwards towards the surface. Although the scan can provide the surgeon with a good idea of the proximity of the tumor to the motor cortex, it is still necessary to use intraoperative measurements to confirm the probable location of the motor strip. In this regard, a number of anatomical clues remain useful. The Taylor-Haughton lines can be used to approximate the location of the motor strip on the lateral aspect of the skull, with the topmost point usually about 2 inches posterior to the coronal suture. This technique was known to Cushing and involved sectioning into quadrants a line running from the inion to the nasion. From well behind the coronal suture, the sensorimotor gyri run at approximately a 45° line relative to the anterior skull base until they reach the pterion; the inclination and location of this line is very similar to the course taken by the initial segment of the posterior branch of the middle meningeal artery (Salcman 1985).

Of course, the most definitive localization of eloquent areas of cortex is provided by intraoperative electrophysiologic mapping (Rostomily et al. 1991). When such specialized techniques are not available or thought inappropriate, stereotactic frames can be used to guide the craniotomy or to implant preoperative markers in the field. Frameless stereotaxy via robotic arms can also be used to point out the location of important anatomical landmarks that have been visualized on the CT or MR planning scan. Since the accuracy of measurements on CT scans is superior and the majority of procedures are carried out under CT guidance, a technique („image fusion") for cross-registration of the anatomical details of an archived MRI scan on the intraoperative CT study has proved to be most useful.

In addition to anatomical details, some idea of the tightness of the brain and the degree of cortical swelling can also be obtained from the preoperative scans. This information may prove useful in discussing the case with both the patient and the anesthesiologist. Peak increases in intraoperative intracranial pressure (ICP) have been shown to correlate with semiquantitative estimates of tumor edema on the preoperative study (Bedford 1983). When the location of the tumor is such that brain cannot be excised in the face of an intraoperative emergency, preoperative planning for untoward swelling is essential. Ideally, patients should receive corticosteroids for several days in preparation for surgery (e.g. 4–6 mg of dexamethasone or its equivalent every 4–6 h) and mannitol (0.5–1.0 g per kg body weight i.v.) during induction if there is any question. A prophylactic antibiotic should be administered at least 1 h prior to the skin incision (1.0 g of cefazolin sodium i.v.).

Induction must be achieved without a major increase in ICP or blood pressure (Bedford 1983). The patient should be positioned with the intended operative field parallel to the floor of the operating theater. For most transcranial approaches this means that the tumor is kept superiorly, and gravity is used to facilitate gentle retraction of the brain downwards. Care should be taken to avoid extreme rotation of the neck with possible kinking of the vessels and impairment of venous drainage from the head. In surgery for temporal or parietal lesions, it is often safer to put the patient in a true lateral position. Almost all frontal and anterior temporal tumors can be

approached with the patient supine and the head rotated away from the operative side. The majority of tumors near the midline can be reached from above with the head elevated 30° and the patient in a lounging position. Most occipital tumors should be approached with the patient in a three-quarter prone or completely prone position. For glial tumors in the posterior fossa, alternatives to the sitting position include fully prone with the surgeon midline at the top of the patient's head, a Concord variant that allows the surgeon to stand or sit at the patient's side, a park bench or three-quarter prone position ordinarily used for trigeminal neuralgia and supine with a large roll and the head sharply turned as in retromastoid surgery. Good head position keeps the tumor topmost, facilitates gravity retraction of the brain, promotes good venous drainage, and does not restrict the size or site of the craniotomy.

17.5
The Operative Procedure

Although this is not primarily a surgical text, a few general technical points are in order. Operations for brain tumors are generally carried out through craniotomies that are considerably larger than those employed in microsurgical procedures for aneurysms and other perisellar lesions. The flap must be large enough to allow for contingencies such as mislocalization, untoward brain swelling, emergency lobectomy, and the use of multiple large instruments such as the laser, ultrasonic aspirator, stereotactic frame and intraoperative ultrasound, in addition to the usual self-retaining retractors and operating microscope. Before the scalp incision is drawn, the position of the tumor relative to the external landmarks of the skull is reviewed and the position of appropriate structures such as the midline, the coronal suture, the pterion or the zygomatic arch are marked. The intended bone flap should have the center of the tumor in the center of the craniotomy. For small lesions, this may require the use of stereotactic guidance or a robotic arm (see later). It is also possible to label the site preoperatively by aligning the lesion with the aiming laser of the CT scanner positioned at right angles to the slice containing the longest axis of the tumor.

In general, the use of preoperative marking and intraoperative localization technology make it safe to reduce the size of the craniotomy if the tumor is in a non-eloquent area and if the preoperative scan indicates relatively little peritumoral edema and shift. Once the appropriate flap has been planned, it is a cardinal mistake of tumor surgery to progressively decrease the size of the operative field at each successive stage of the procedure (i.e., when retracting the scalp flap, or making the burr holes and saw cuts). Mannitol, if needed, should have been started with the skin incision and half the dose given by drip in the first 15–20 min; completion of mannitol administration should be timed to coincide with elevation of the bone flap. Once complete hemostasis has been established, the self-retaining retractor is secured in the field and attention is turned to the dural incision.

A correctly designed bone flap should place the tumor in the center of the exposed dura; this can be confirmed through gentle palpation of the cortical surface, or the use of a stereotactic probe or intraoperative ultrasound for deeper lesions. The dura should be examined for the presence of respiratory and circulatory pulsations and the anesthesiologist notified if the brain is still „tight". Elevation of the head, uncoiling of the neck, hyperventilation, or additional mannitol may all be necessary. The patient's head position, urinary output, arterial pCO_2 and endotracheal tube are checked. The incision should be delayed until the brain is relaxed. If the brain swells or becomes tight *during* the dural incision, speed in completing the incision is of the utmost importance since, as Dandy knew, incarceration of the brain in a small dural opening is sure to cause further swelling and cerebrovascular disturbance in the as yet unexposed tissues.

Most dural incisions are horseshoe-shaped and the initial segment should be made over the least critical area in the exposure. The incision is then carried towards the site of a major vessel, eloquent cortex or the tumor itself. In other words, the sagittal sinus, the middle cerebral artery or the motor strip should run along the base of the dural flap.

Microsurgical techniques permit the removal of relatively large tumors (5–8 cm diameter) through relatively short cortical incisions (1.5–3 cm) with good functional results so long as certain anatomical principles are applied. The incision must be oriented perpendicular to the long axis of the sensorimotor cortex so as to cut across the motor homunculus at but a single point. The incision must be kept as short as possible without producing subpial hemorrhage through undue retraction at its edges and corners. Self-retaining retractors should be employed to gently retract the edges of the incision, with the tapered blades kept flat against the brain so as to avoid cut-

ting into the tissue with their sides. The subcortical tissues must be gently spread in the long axis of the incision until the tumor is reached; white matter is *never* resected in order to create the transcortical tunnel. Microsurgical techniques also can be used to reach the tumor through dissections carried out in a naturally occurring fissure or sulcus (Fig. 17.4) so as to shorten the distance and avoid the crown of a gyrus (PIA 1986; SALCMAN 1993). If the surface of the brain looks and feels unremarkable, the use of intraoperative ultrasound or a stereotactic probe can be invaluable and is far preferable to blind needling of the brain in eloquent regions. In the frontal or temporal lobes, it is often possible to sacrifice some tissue and uncap the lesion from anterior to posterior.

The cortex and white matter are spread (not resected) in the long axis of the incision with a bayonet forceps and a large microfreer dissector. Self-retaining retractors are positioned on opposite sides of the incision (never at its corners) over cottonoid strips placed perpendicular to the surface. Use of the microscope depends on the size and location of the tumor as well as the length of the transcortical approach (Fig. 17.4). The tumor is recognized by its coloration and texture. Low-grade gliomas are slightly grayer or pinker than the surrounding white matter, while high-grade tumors often display a variety of red, gray, yellow and purple discoloration. Necrotic tissue in the center is cheesy-soft and iseasily removed by suction. Peripheral areas of the tumor may be very vascular and quite firm if composed of a high density of fibrillary astrocytes and their processes. This type of tissue can be rubbery and sometimes must be peeled out of the surrounding brain with a microfreer and a two-point suction cautery almost as if there were a distinct macroscopic plane. In critical areas, firm tumor is resected with the aid of a surgical laser or an ultrasonic aspirator.

Normal-appearing white matter on the periphery of the tumor can be seen to glisten with edema fluid under the illumination of the microscope and is covered and protected with cottonoid strips. At the conclusion of the macroscopic removal, the major axes of the resection cavity are measured and compared to the preoperative measurements on the enhanced MR or CT scan. If the measurements match and the surface of the cavity everywhere is white and smooth, soft and glistening, then the resection can be terminated or an extra few millimeters safely shaved down with the laser or a fine aspirator. Prior to closure, perfect hemostasis must be achieved at a normal or slightly elevated systolic blood pressure.

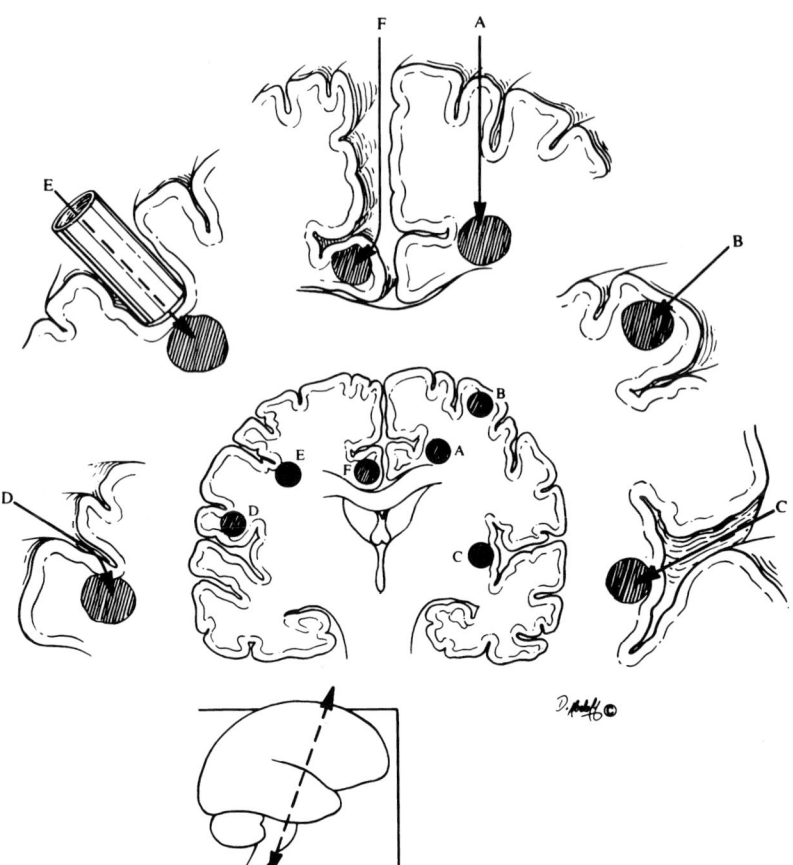

Fig. 17.4A–F. General microsurgical approaches to hemispheric tumors. Transcortical approaches can be made through a white matter tunnel (**A**), at the apex or crown of a gyrus (**B**), through a fissure (**C**), through a sulcus along its side (**D**) or at its deepest portion (**E**). Paramedian approaches are neither subarachnoid nor transcortical but may require a transcortical tunnel at their termination (**F**). (Modified from SALCMAN, 1993a)

17.6
Technology and Instrumentation

No amount of sophisticated technology can substitute for the care and wisdom that the surgeon utilizes in the selection of the patient and operative approach, or for the gentleness of touch and respect that he or she shows in the handling of tissues. Since the ultimate goal is to remove the maximum amount of tumor with minimum resection and physiologic disturbance of the surrounding brain, the use of technology should be tailored to those situations in which this goal cannot be achieved without such assistance. Use of the operating microscope promotes gentle handling of tissues, improves visualization of the apparent tumor–tissue interface, provides illumination for deep approaches and permits removal of large tumors through small incisions (SALCMAN et al. 1982; PIA 1986). The microscope can also be used as a stage for the precise use of the carbon dioxide laser, a microinstrument capable of removing very firm tissue without mechanical disturbance of the brain (SALCMAN et al. 1986). For most tumors, however, piece-

meal removal with a microaspirator and bipolar cautery allows the surgeon to morcellate, cauterize and aspirate away all but the firmest of tumors. The ultrasonic aspirator is useful for the gentle removal of tissues intermediate in firmness between those requiring laser resection and those susceptible to ordinary microdissection.

The use of intraoperative electrocorticography and stimulation has certainly allowed some surgeons to carry tumor resections right to the very edge of functional areas (ROSTOMILY et al. 1991; BERGER et al. 1990). For example, it is difficult to predict where the language areas are located in the dominant hemisphere; intraoperative electrical recordings can locate eloquent cortex and have demonstrated that resections within 1 cm of a primary language area cortex are likely to produce permanent postoperative deficits (MATZ et al. 1999). However, it is not known whether the time and effort involved in the resection of small additional portions of malignant tumor can be shown to improve length of survival. It is likely that this technology will prove more useful in the removal of low-grade tumors, especially in patients who present with seizures, since the safety and precision of surgery can be improved with the use of intraoperative recording. Similarly, the use of computer-controlled, stereotactic laser resection of intraaxial neoplasms has improved safety without demonstrating an oncologic advantage in patients with deep-seated glioblastomas (KELLY et al. 1986, 1987). Since it is impossible to predict whether the future development of more effective non-surgical treatments for glial tumors will increase or decrease the requirement for complete macroscopic resection, the further refinement of surgical techniques must be encouraged. Recently, a novel method was described in which a stereotactically guided craniotomy was further refined through functional mapping obtained by noninvasive magnetoencephalography (REZAI et al. 1996). The advent of hybrid technology and stereotactic frames to guide all stages of the craniotomy has lessened the use of intraoperative ultrasound for brain tumor localization, but it remains a useful technique for judging the extent of resection (TOMS et al. 1999).

17.7
Treatment Results and Complications

Post-operatively, patients are usually maintained on corticosteroids and prophylactic anticonvulsants (NORTH et al. 1983). If all has gone well, the best time to perform a post-operative enhanced CT or MRI scan to gauge the amount of residual tumor is in the first 2–3 days; *no patient should be allowed to leave the hospital or undergo subsequent therapy without such a study.* The surgeon's intraoperative assessment of the amount of tumor resected is unreliable (ALBERT et al. 1994). It is impossible to analyze the results of treatment or to recommend subsequent therapy without such radiographic control.

Over the last 50 years, there has been a progressive decline in the morbidity and mortality associated with craniotomy carried out in patients with malignant astrocytomas (Table 17.2). A similar phenomenon has been observed in the operative treatment of low-grade gliomas (LAWS et al. 1984). Thirty-day operative mortality rates of 20%–40% were common

Table 17.2. Morbidity and mortality of craniotomy for glioma

Series and year	Tumor	N	Mortality (%)	Morbidity (%)
CUSHING 1932	Glioma	1173	17.2	–
DAVIS et al. 1949	GBM	187	41.1	–
GRANT 1956	Astro	279	20.0	–
	GBM	350	38.0	–
	Oligo	48	19.0	–
FRANKEL and GERMAN 1958	GBM	183	18.5	–
ROTH and ELVIDGE 1960	GBM	399	21.5	–
LEY et al. 1962	Astro	37	16.2	–
	GBM	207	31.4	–
	Oligo	40	30.0	–
HITCHCOCK and SATO 1964	GBM	222	19.0	–
JELSMA and BUCY 1967[a]	GBM	122	27.9	–
	GBM	35	2.9	–
LEIBEL et al. 1975	Astro	147	17.0	–
SALCMAN et al. 1982	GBM	74	0.7	–
AMMIRATI et al. 1987	GBM/AA	31	0.0	16.0 (t)
CIRIC et al. 1987	Glioma	42	0.0	7.0
FADUL et al. 1988	Glioma	104	3.3	19.7
HOLLERHAGE et al. 1991	GBM	118	3.4*	–
			17.0	
VECHT et al. 1991	GBM/AA	243	20.0	
SALCMAN et al. 1994[b]	GBM	509	2.7	8.0
	GBM	220	3.5	8.0

One-month mortality rates except as noted (*=1 week); morbidity rates are neurologic except as noted (t=total); GBM, glioblastoma; astro, astrocytoma; oligo, oligodendroglioma; glioma, all glial tumors; AA, anaplastic astrocytoma.
[a] First series is 1948–1961; second is 1962–1964.
[b] First series is all cases; second is reoperations only.

prior to the introduction of corticosteroids and modern anesthesia (JELSMA and BUCY 1967). Contemporary mortality rates in the hands of experienced operators have generally ranged from 0%–3.5% but can be higher depending on the mix of patients. In our series of 509 procedures carried out during the last decade, the 30-day mortality was 2.7% (SALCMAN 1996). Mortality and morbidity are increased in older patients and in those with deeply seated tumors of higher grade (FADUL et al. 1988). A recent review indicates an overall complication rate of 6%–21% in patients undergoing craniotomy (VIVES and PIEPMEIER 1999). The authors emphasized the high incidence of deep vein thrombosis (DVT)in patients with high-grade glioma; significant risk factors for DVT include a paretic limb, a history of thromboembolism or the use of chemotherapy. The neurologic morbidity rate is generally about 8% (SALCMAN 1996; CIRIC et al. 1987) but can be as high as 20%. Post-operative infections occur in 0%–11% of patients and are more frequent after reoperation (TENNEY et al. 1985). The combined neurologic and medical morbidity after conventional craniotomy may reach 31% (FADUL et al. 1988).

The type of surgical procedure *does* appear to influence post-operative recovery and morbidity (Table 17.3). In one series, no patient who underwent a complete resection suffered either a post-operative hemorrhage requiring reoperation or cerebral herniation (Fadul et al. 1988). Patients undergoing complete resections are more likely to have an improved functional status ($p=0.006$ vs $p>0.05$) than patients with incomplete resections ($p=0.002$) and spend significantly longer time in a functionally independent state (185 weeks vs 12.5 weeks; $p=0.007$) than patients with partial resections (Ammirati et al. 1987). In incompletely resected tumors, lobectomy further worsens the early results (Hollerhage et al. 1991). In one series of hemispheric lesions, the CT scan was cleared of all tumor in 86% of cases and 97% of these patients demonstrated either a stable or improved

neurologic status (Ciric et al. 1987). The rate of neurologic morbidity after a partial resection was 40%. Hence the interest in microsurgery and in computer-based stereotactic laser resection, methods that decrease operative morbidity by permitting extensive tumor resection with minimal manipulation of the surrounding brain even in the basal ganglia and thalamus (Pia 1986; Kelly et al. 1986, 1987). In a series of 118 patients, the longer survival observed after microsurgery was actually due to the improved early results and the increased proportion of patients who could undergo further therapy (Hollerhage et al. 1991). Microsurgery patients spent less time in the intensive care unit (mean 1.8 days vs 3.7) and had a much lower 1-week mortality rate (0 vs 5%).

In matched patients with malignant astrocytoma and glioblastoma, the extent of surgery was significantly related to the length of survival at the $p<0.001$ level (AMMIRATI et al. 1987). Patients with total and subtotal tumor resections had median survivals of 90 and 43 weeks respectively. In patients with gemistocytic astrocytoma, only those receiving gross total resection were still alive at the time of the report (KROUWER et al. 1991). The beneficial effect of complete tumor resection is probably due to the improved early functional status of the patient as well as the reduced post-operative tumor burden (SALCMAN 1996). For more than a decade, we have attempted to carry out a complete excision in every patient referred to our neuro-oncology service, either initially or at the time of reoperation (SALCMAN et al. 1982). The impact of the routine use of an aggressive surgical approach within the context of a multimodality treatment plan can be inferred from the results presented in Fig. 17.5. These data are based on 289 adult patients with hemispheric glioblastoma and at least a 3-year follow-up (SALCMAN et al. 1994). As in most series, the survival of these patients was heavily dependent on age at diagnosis, histology, and radiation dose, and less so on response to chemotherapy. Pre- and postoperative performance status is also an important prognostic factor.

In addition to age, histology, performance status and treatment variables, tumor location not only influences the choice of procedure (i.e. resection vs biopsy) but also helps determine the length of survival. Patients with midline tumors do less well than those with lobar lesions, frontal lobe tumors have a better prognosis than those in other sites, and cortical tumors are more favorable than deeper ones (Vives and Piepmeier 1999). Lesions in which the enhanced T1 MRI image is the same size as the T2 signal change are more amenable to a gross total resection.

Table 17.3. Rate of neurologic stability or improvement by the type of operation

Series	N	Incomplete resection (%)	Complete resection (%)
CIRIC 1987	42	60	96
FADUL 1988	138	61–70	80
HOLLERHAGE 1991	118	50–91[a]	74–77

[a]Partial resections with and without lobectomy.

Probability Survival

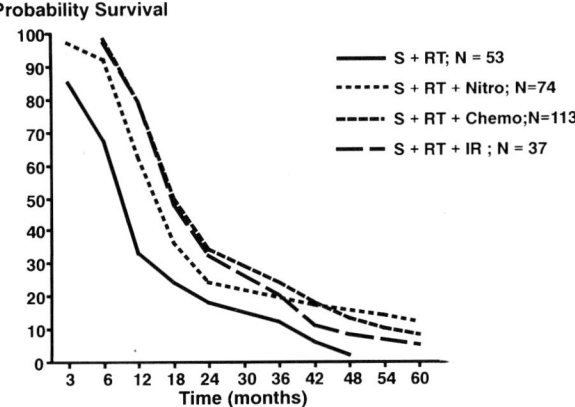

Fig. 17.5. Survival after aggressive surgery and multimodality therapy. These Kaplan-Meier survival curves are based on 289 patients with malignant astrocytoma entered into a multimodality treatment program employing extensive resection on an aggressive and repetitive basis with a minimum 36-month follow-up. Survival in patients less than 40 years of age was unrelated to the type of therapy received beyond surgery and external radiation (S+RT). Patients were prospectively assigned to different experimental protocols. The majority received a nitrosourea in addition to surgery and radiation (S+RT+Nitro) while others received experimental chemotherapy or biologic response modifiers in addition to or in place of nitrosoureas (S+RT+Chemo). Finally, some patients underwent interstitial brachytherapy at the time of recurrence (S+RT+IR), usually without concomitant microwave hyperthermia. (From SALCMAN et al. 1994)

In surgical series, each of these prognostic factors is a potential source of selection bias; nevertheless, a recent review of seven series from the past decade reveals a significant survival advantage based on the extent of tumor resection (Vives and Piepmeier 1999).

17.8
Stereotactic Surgery

Contemporary neurosurgery has greatly benefited from two important technical revolutions; the first was the advent of the operating microscope (already discussed), and the second, the introduction of CT- and MR-compatible image-based stereotactic instrumentation (SALCMAN 1999). In image-based stereotaxy, a mechanical device is rigidly attached to the patient's head and an MR or CT scan is obtained in the usual fashion. The computer in the scanner is then utilized to determine the three-dimensional coordinates of any point inside the head in relation

to the stereotactic space delimited by the frame. It is important to understand that this space is not equivalent to the radiographic space of pixels within the scanner nor to the conventional anatomical space used to relate structures within the brain to external landmarks during open craniotomy. Hence, it is necessary to use simple calculations to convert the radiographic coordinates used in the scanner to the coordinate system employed by any particular stereotactic system or frame. In addition, because the physical relationship of the frame to the target is visible on the scan, there is no need to precisely align the attachment of the frame to any individual landmark such as the anatomical midline (SALCMAN et al. 1989). Once the coordinates are obtained, they are entered into micrometers attached to the frame in the operating room and probes of various types can be directed to the target through small twist-drill holes. These probes are usually biopsy instruments to obtain tissue (OSTERTAG et al. 1980) but may be endoscopes for use within the ventricular system (APUZZO et al. 1987) or afterloading catheters for the delivery of interstitial radiation (GUTIN et al. 1987; SALCMAN 1993) or microwave hyperthermia (SALCMAN 1991).

The procedures have the great advantage that they are carried out under local anesthesia and often employ small puncture holes produced by stereotactic drills so as to avoid further compromising devitalized tissue (Salcman et al. 1989). Entry sites and trajectories must avoid the known locations of major fissures, arteries, sinuses and bridging veins. The single most useful entry point for deep targets is just in front of the coronal suture and 3 cm off the midline (i.e. the same as for ventricular puncture); from here, one can reach the ipsilateral basal ganglia, thalamus and central portions of the brain stem. For many brain stem targets lateral to the tentorial edge or elsewhere in the posterior fossa, a direct transcerebellar approach can be taken. In general, MR guidance for posterior fossa stereotactic surgery is preferable to CT.

Relative indications for the use of stereotactic surgery in glioma patients are outlined in Table 17.4. As previously indicated, neurologically intact patients with small, ill-defined tumors in critical locations are the ideal candidates for stereotactic biopsy. Small or non-enhancing tumors with shaggy or ill-defined borders on CT or MR are almost impossible to distinguish from the surrounding brain at open surgery, and the risks of attempted extirpation from a central or critical location clearly outweigh the potential benefits. Some of these tumors are picked up inci-

Table 17.4. Relative indications for stereotactic surgery

Tumor:	Is centrally located
	Is poorly defined by CT or MR
	Is smaller than 2 cm
	Is primarily cystic
	Has changed character
Patient:	Is too ill for craniotomy
	Is neurologically intact
Therapy:	Deliver brachytherapy
	Interstitial hyperthermia
	Interstitial phototherapy
	Stereotactic radiosurgery
	Requires repeat tissue sampling

dentally or after a seizure and their natural history is not completely understood (Salcman 1990). On the other hand, deeply placed enhancing tumors almost always turn out to be high-grade astrocytomas and complete excision by computerized techniques from the basal ganglia and thalamus does not appear to influence survival above and beyond that obtained by stereotactic biopsy and radiation (Coffey et al. 1988; Kelly et al. 1986,1987). Some tumors with large cysts can be treated with stereotactic aspiration and the instillation of a radiopharmaceutical. Stereotactic techniques can also be used to deliver a wide variety of adjunctive therapies such as brachytherapy, hyperthermia and photoactivated chemotherapy. The relative frequency of different stereotactic procedures constituted 20% of all operations carried out for brain tumors in our hospital (Salcman 1990).

Tissue biopsy remains the most frequent indication for stereotactic surgery. Tissue can be safely obtained from the thalamus, the basal ganglia and the brain stem with less than a 2.3% mortality, a 3% risk of hemorrhage and a 1% morbidity rate (Apuzzo et al. 1987; Ostertag 1980). In a series of 300 patients, the overall complication rate was 6.3% (Bernstein and Parent 1994). All the mortalities occurred in patients with glioblastoma multiforme and were usually due to raised intracranial pressure. Transient deficits occurred in 3.3% (Bernstein and Parent 1994). The small pieces of tissue are usually diagnostic in more than 90% of cases and, if not, the procedure can safely be repeated in debilitated patients and through compromised tissue. Difficulty in histologic interpretation is most frequently encountered in the differential diagnosis of low-grade astrocytoma from reactive gliosis and in poorly differentiated primary tumors from metastatic lesions (Taratuto et al. 1991). In these two circumstances, cytologic examination by smear techniques and immunocytochemistry may prove essen-

tial. It is important for the surgeon to provide the neuropathologist with an adequate tissue specimen based on serial sampling techniques. The trajectory of the biopsy should be chosen in such a way that samples are obtained from brain adjacent to tumor on both sides of the mass, at both edges of the enhancing margin and in the center. Obtaining a sample only from the center is frequently non-diagnostic in malignant lesions with large areas of necrosis. Use of a side-cutting aspiration cannula or the Backlund spiral biopsy needle is safer than a punch or microalligator forceps. Suction is gently applied to the side-cutting cannula to draw the tissue into a slot where it is then separated from the surrounding brain by rotation of an internal tube acting as a guillotine. In this way a 1+10-mm sample can be obtained, sufficient in size even for kinetic studies performed with the Ki-67 monoclonal antibody.

Technical considerations involved in handling tissue samples and intraoperative bleeding are discussed elsewhere (Salcman 1996; Kondziolka and Lunsford 1999). Stereotactic biopsy is a remarkably safe procedure even in elderly and debilitated patients. Some authors feel that stereotactic biopsy should be performed in all patients with a suspected intrinsic tumor for whom acute cytoreductive surgery is not required and in all patients in whom infectious etiologies may be confused with neoplastic disorders (Kondziolka and Lunsford 1999). Reoperation necessitated by hemorrhage is rare and almost all intracerebral bleeding is discovered incidentally on the postoperative check scan and is usually without clinical consequence. In a series of 403 patients, only one (0.25%) required postoperative evacuation (Kondziolka and Lunsford 1999). On the dry scan, a drop of air is often present at the biopsy site and offers a visual clue as to whether the intended target has been reached. In our experience of studying several hundred such target points on postoperative scans, the accuracy of image-based stereotaxy is remarkable and targets are missed only when the cannula or the catheter is deflected by bone or the tentorium. Such problems are invariably noted by the surgeon during the procedure.

17.9
Hybrid Techniques

For a growing number of glioma patients, the optimum surgical approach consists of some combination of techniques such as an open surgical implant or a stereotactically guided craniotomy (SALCMAN 1990; MOORE et al. 1989). In the latter approach, a stereotactic frame is applied to the patient's head and a scan is performed to obtain the geometric coordinates of the tumor. The patient is then returned to the operating theater and the electrode holder or the probe carrier of the frame is attached. A blunt probe is then stereotactically lowered to the surface of the scalp and used as a guide to outline a relatively small scalp incision. A similar maneuver is utilized in designing the bone flap and in opening the dura. The stereotactic probe is then used to select the appropriate gyrus or sulcus for microsurgical incison and the probe can be used as a guide to orient a transcortical tunnel all the way down to the target. When the tumor has been reached, the operating microscope is moved into place and the stereotactic arc removed. Variations on this theme include the use of a robotic arm to mark the incision points, so-called frameless stereotaxy, and computer-directed vaporization of the tumor by a laser attached to the stereotactic frame and guided by a stacked-slice reconstruction of the tumor volume stored in the computer's memory (KELLY 1988; WATANABE et al. 1991). This technique, when applied to a wide variety of lesions, can have an overall morbidity and mortality as low as 9.3 and 1% respectively. Through the use of such combined approaches, it is possible to remove small tumors in relatively dangerous or poorly demarcated locations, lesions which formerly would have been subjected to stereotactic biopsy alone.

These techniques depend on surgical navigation systems in which three-dimensional digitizers are used to link a volume of image data with a volume of space in the operating room that includes the intended surgical region. As indicated above, three-dimensional surgical navigation permits minimal-access craniotomy, optimally defines a trajectory for the transcortical approach, and can be used to guide and judge the extent of resection (Barnett 1999). Conventional MR and CT images can be coupled to data obtained from positron emission tomography (PET), functional magnetic resonance imaging (fMRI), magnetic encephalography (MEG), magnetic source imaging (MSI) and transcutaneous magnetic stimulation (Barnett 1999).

Some non-enhancing large lesions with ill-defined margins, otherwise acceptable for open resection, can be more safely removed after the stereotactic placement of visual markers (Hassenbusch et al. 1991). Dummy radiation seeds and catheters can be placed during a separate stereotactic operation and the tumor resected down to these margins during the subsequent craniotomy. Alternatively, the markers can be deposited by stereotactic techniques through the craniotomy window; except for the multiplicity of probes, this technique more nearly resembles the combined approach discussed above.

As previously indicated, stereotactic catheters can be used to deliver other treatment modalities such as radiation and hyperthermia to any tumor volume defined by the scan. Experimental techniques being developed include the stereotactic delivery of laser light for photoactivation of chemotherapy (Popovic et al. 1996), endoscopic laser ablation of intraventricular masses and catheter deposition of immunological reagents and other biologicals. A recent development has been the application of stereotactic radiosurgery to the treatment of malignant gliomas (Coffey et al. 1991; Alexander and Loeffler 1998). In this technique, the stereotactic frame and target calculation are carried out in the usual fashion, but instead of a probe being delivered to the tumor, the target is positioned at the intersection of multiple cobalt beams in the gamma knife or at the isocenter of rotation of a linear accelerator. Stereotactic radiosurgery has achieved some success in the treatment of benign tumors; it is too early to know what its role will be in the therapy of glial lesions. Results with radiosurgery are now approaching those of interstitial brachytherapy (Alexander and Loeffler, 1998). This is important because, next to reoperation, stereotactic brachytherapy has proven itself to be the single most useful rescue technique in the treatment of patients with recurrent malignant glioma (Gutin et al. 1987; Salcman 1990). Unfortunately, limitations due to tumor size and patient condition restrict the use of stereotactic techniques to less than 20%–30% of patients with malignant glioma, and it remains to be seen whether the addition of hyperthermia, chemotherapy or other modalities will widen the applicability of either interstitial brachytherapy or radiosurgery. Since the full extent of infiltrative glial neoplasms is not revealed by present imaging technology, it is unlikely that regionally based therapies alone can be used to cure patients with malignant tumors (Kelly et al. 1987; Burger 1983; Salcman 1991).

17.10
The Role of Repeat Surgery

Prior to the advent of modern neurosurgical techniques and more effective adjuvant therapies, reoperations for glioma patients were only infrequently and selectively performed (Salcman 1985; Salcman et al. 1982; Jelsma and Bucy 1967). Historically, reoperated patients tended to be younger and to have longer intervals to recurrence than non-reoperated patients. Of course, intensive therapy of any kind is more likely to be offered to healthier patients, and this has been shown to occur even in randomized brain tumor trials (i.e. the concept of the „valid study group") and in patients selected for brachytherapy (Winger et al. 1989). It is only recently that extensive use of reoperation has become an accepted part of malignant glioma management and this trend appears to be growing (Salcman et al. 1982, Salcman 1996, 1988; Young et al. 1981; Ammirati et al. 1987b; Harsh et al. 1987). In each major series, reoperation has been shown to add an additional median survival of 36–37 weeks from the time of the second operation until either a third procedure or death, so long as surgery is followed by further adjuvant therapy. Reoperation also appears to improve performance status, confirming the early data of Shapiro (1982) on the general effect of surgery in glioma patients. In one study, 46% of reoperated patients demonstrated improved Karnofsky scores while 25% became worse (Ammirati et al. 1987b).

Since 1978, we have prospectively used reoperation prior to the administration of any new therapy for malignant astrocytoma in patients with either radiographic or clinical evidence of recurrence (Salcman et al. 1982). We have reviewed 289 adult patients with hemispheric lesions for whom a 3-year follow-up was available (Salcman et al. 1994). In the entire series, 509 craniotomies were performed, with a neurologic morbidity rate of 8% and a mortality of 2.7%. Reoperations were carried out in 168 of the 289 patients (58%) with a similar morbidity and mortality (Table 17.2). There were 1.3 reoperations per patient or 220 in total. Reoperated patients had a mean age of 48 years, a male:female ratio of 1.53 and nearly 80% had grade 4 tumors; in all these respects, they resembled the patients who did not undergo reoperation. The median survival for all 168 patients after the second operation was 9 months (Fig. 17.6) and was age and histology dependent. Grade 3 patients had a longer postoperative survival (median 12 months) than grade 4 patients (median 8 months) and grade 4 patients under 40 years of age had a longer postoperative survival (median 11 months) than patients over 40 (median 6 months; $p<0.001$). Age did not appear to influence the length of surviv-

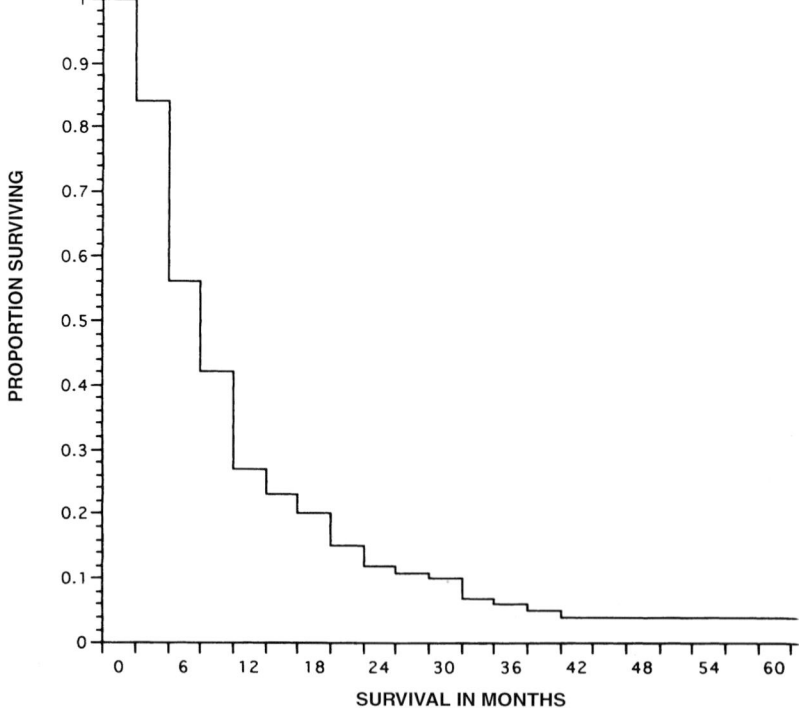

Fig. 17.6. Survival after reoperation and multimodality therapy. The Kaplan-Meier survival curve measures the length of survival from the time of a reoperation until the time of a third procedure or death in 168 patients with malignant astrocytoma and at least a 3-year follow-up. The median additional survival time was 9 months. (From Salcman et al. 1994)

al in patients with grade 3 tumors. Reoperation was more frequently used in males and in patients with grade 4 tumors as rescue therapy. The total survival of reoperated patients with both grade 3 and grade 4 tumors (median 24 and 17 months respectively) was longer than that of non-reoperated patients (median 13 and 8 months). In the entire series of 289 patients, 20% lived more than 36 months and the use of reoperation was disproportionately represented among these long-term survivors ($p<0.001$). Therefore, reoperation carried out within the context of a multimodality treatment program appears to confer a distinct survival benefit and can be performed with minimal morbidity and mortality (Salcman et al. 1994). In addition to ameliorating symptoms and reducing tumor burden, reoperation often improves performance status and makes some patients eligible for further therapy that they would not otherwise receive. Repeat stereotaxy is also a useful approach, especially to document response to therapy or when the radiographic picture is indeterminate and radiation necrosis rather than tumor recurrence is a distinct possibility.

17.11
Future Directions

Partially in response to evolving technology and partially because of a change in treatment philosophy, surgical resection and surgically based therapies are likely to remain the linchpin of glioma management for the foreseeable future. The imperative to increase the amount of tumor resected while at the same time avoiding any disturbance of the surrounding brain will further increase the popularity of stereotactically guided craniotomies and microsurgical approaches. Gentleness of technique and precision are especially important during reoperation on previously compromised or traumatized tissues. The desire by patients and surgeons alike for minimally invasive procedures means that frameless stereotaxy and the application of space-age technology are likely to become integral components of routine brain tumor procedures. Computer-generated images of the tumor in relation to any superficial or deep structure as well as other useful information from monitoring systems and surgical atlases can be exported to the lenses of the microscope or to a „virtual reality" helmet worn by the surgeon. The latter technology is presently available for fighter pilots and can also be used to control the movements of a laser or any other automatic dissecting and resection tool. Stereotactic coordinates can be generated in relation to the four corners of the operating room by using an acoustical or microwave link or in relation to superficial landmarks inputted to the computer by a robotic arm, thus eliminating the need to apply a frame to the patient's head or the requirement that the surgeon perform even simple calculations to obtain the target points. By such means, a mixture of computer- and image-guided procedures will be carried out through the microscope on a semi-automated basis in the near future.

The biological diversity of glial neoplasms, the inherent resistance of some cell compartments within the tumor to a variety of other therapies, and delivery and activity problems regarding a number of the newest adjuvant agents will continue to insure a prominent role for surgical resection and delivery (Salcman 1995). Polymer implants of pharmaceuticals and monoclonal antibodies are already being investigated and are typically placed in the resection cavity at the conclusion of craniotomy. Similarly, the most efficient and effective way to deliver radiation or photochemotherapy may be through intraoperative exposure at the conclusion of resection. Stereotactic techniques will continue to be used for the delivery of interstitial brachytherapy and hyperthermia, perhaps in combination with systemic or local administration of radiolabeled monoclonal antibodies directed at genes and growth factors.

References

Adegbite AB, Khan MI, Paine KWE, et al. (1983) The recurrence of intracranial meningioma after surgical treatment. J Neurosurg 58:51–56

Albert FK, Forsting M, Sartor K, et al. (1994) Early postoperative magnetic resonance imaging after resection of malignant glioma: objective evaluation of residual tumor and its influence on regrowth and prognosis. Neurosurgery 34:45–61

Alexander E, Loeffler JS (1998) Clinical experience with Linac radiosurgery. In: Gildenberg P, Tasker,R (eds) Textbook of stereotactic and functional neurosurgery. McGraw-Hill, New York, pp 745–756

Ammirati M, Galicich JH, Arbit E, et al. (1987a) Reoperation in the treatment of recurrent intracranial malignant gliomas. Neurosurgery 21:601–614

Ammirati M, Vick N, Liao Y, et al. (1987b) Effect of the extent of surgical resection on survival and quality of life in patients with supratentorial glioblastomas and anaplastic astrocytomas. Neurosurgery 21:201–206

Andreou J, George AE, Wise A, et al. (1983) CT prognostic criteria of survival after malignant glioma surgery. Am J Neuroradiol 4:488–490

Apuzzo MLJ, Chandrasoma PT, Cohen D, et al. (1987) Computed imaging stereotaxy: Experience and perspective related to 500 procedures applied to brain masses. Neurosurgery 20:930–937

Barnett, GH (1999) The role of image-guided technology in the surgical planning and resection of gliomas. J. Neurooncol 42:247–258

Beaney RP, Brooks DJ, Leenders KL, et al. (1985) Blood flow and oxygen utilization in the contralateral cerebral cortex of patients with untreated intracranial tumors as studied by positron emission tomography, with observations on the effect of decompressive surgery. J. Neurol Neurosurg Psychiatry 48:310–319

Bedford RF (1983) Anesthetic management for supratentorial tumor surgery. J Neurooncol 1:319–326

Berger MS (1994) Malignant astrocytomas: Surgical aspects. Semin Oncol 21:172–185

Berger MS, Cohen WA, Ojemman GA (1990) Correlation of motor cortex brain mapping data with magnetic resonance imaging. J Neurosurg 72:383–3877

Bernstein M, Parent AG (1994) Complications of stereotactic biopsy for intra-axial brain lesions. J Neurosurg. 81:165–168

Brem H, Piantadosi S, Burger PC, et al. (1995) Placebo-controlled trial of safety and efficacy of intraoperative controlled delivery by biodegradable polymers of chemotherapy for recurrent gliomas. Lancet 345:1008–1012

Brooks WH, Roszman TL (1980) Cellular immune responsiveness of patients with primary intracranial tumors. In: Thomas DGT, Graham DI (eds) Brain tumors: scientific basis, clinical investigation, and current therapy. Butterworth, London, pp 121–132

Burger PC (1983) Pathologic anatomy and CT correlations in the glioblastoma multiforme. Appl Neurophysiol 46:180–187

Ciric I, Ammirati M, Vick N, et al (1987) Supratentorial gliomas: Surgical considerations and immediate postoperative results. Gross total resection versus partial resection. Neurosurgery 21:21–26

Coffey RJ, Lunsford D, Flinkinger JC (1991) The role of radiosurgery in the treatment of malignant brain tumors. Neurosurgery Clinics of North America 3(1):231–244

Coffey RJ, Lunsford LD, Taylor FH (1988) Survival after stereotactic biopsy of malignant gliomas. Neurosurgery 22:465–473

Cohadon F, Aouad N, Rougier A, et al. (1985) Histologic and non-histologic factors correlated with survival time in supratentorial astrocytic tumors. J. Neurooncol 3:105–111

Devaux BC, O'Fallon JR, Kelly PJ (1993) Resection, biopsy and survival in malignant glial neoplasms. A retrospective study of clinical parameters, therapy, and outcome. J Neurosurg 78:767–775

Fadul C, Wood J, Thaler H, et al. (1988) Morbidity and mortality of craniotomy for excision of supratentorial gliomas. Neurology 38:1374–1379

Gutin PH, Leibel SA, Wara WM, et al. (1987) Recurrent malignant gliomas: Survival following interstitial brachytherapy with high-activity iodine-125 sources. J Neurosurg 67:864–973

Harsh GR IV, Levin VA, Gutin PH, et al. (1987) reoperation for recurrent glioblastoma and anaplastic astrocytoma. Neurosurgery 21:615–621

HASSENBUSCH SJ, Anderson JS, Pillay PK (1991) Brain tumor resection aided with markers placed using stereotaxis guided by magnetic resonance imaging and computed tomography. Neurosurgery 28:801–806

Hess KR (1999) Extent of resection as a prognostic variable in the treatment of gliomas. J Neurooncol 42:227–231

Hirakawa K, Suzuki K, Ueda S, et al. (1984) Multivariate analysis of factors affecting postoperative survival in malignant astrocytoma. J Neurooncol 2:331–340

Hollerhage H-G, Zumkeller M, Becker et al. (1991) Influence of type and extent of surgery on early results and survival time in glioblastoma multiforme. Acta Neurochir (Wien) 113:31–37

Hoshino T (1984) A commentary on the biology and growth kinetics of low grade and high grade gliomas. J Neurosurg 61:895–900

Ilgren EB, Stiller CA (1986) Cerebellar astrocytomas: therapeutic management. Acta Neurochir (Wien) 81:11–26

Jelsma R, Bucy PC (1967) The treatment of glioblastoma multiforme of the brain. J Neurosurg 27:388–400

Kelly PJ (1988) Volumetric stereotactic surgical resection of intra-axial brain mass lesions. Mayo Clin Proc 63:1186–1198

Kelly PJ, Daumas-Duport C, Kispert DB, et al. (1987) Imaging-based stereotaxic serial biopsies in untreated intracranial glial neoplasms. J Neurosurg 66:865–874

Kelly PJ, Kall BA, Goerss S, et al. (1986) Computer-assisted stereotaxic laser resection of intra-axial brain neoplasms. J Neurosurg 64:427–439

Kondziolka D, Lunsford LD (1999) The role of stereotactic biopsy in the management of gliomas. J Neurooncol 42:205–213

Krouwer HGJ, Davis RL, Silver P, et al. (1991) Gemistocytic astrocytomas: a reappraisal. J. Neurosurg 74:399–406

Laws ER, Taylor WF, Clifton MB, et al. (1984) Neurosurgical management of low grade astrocytoma of the cerebral hemispheres. J Neurosurg 61:665–673

Matz PG, Cobbs C, Berger MS (1999) Intraoperative cortical mapping as a guide to the surgical resection of gliomas. J Neurooncol 42:233–245

Mirimanoff RO, Dosoretz DE, Linggood RM, et al. (1985) Meningioma: Analysis of recurrence and progression following neurosurgical resection. J Neurosurg 62:18–24

Moore MR, Black PMcl, Ellenbogen R, et al. (1989) Stereotactic craniotomy: methods and results using the Brown-Roberts-Wells stereotactic frame. Neurosurgery 25:572–578

Nelson DF, Nelson JS, Davis DR, et al. (1985) Survival and prognosis of patients with astrocytoma with atypical or anaplastic features. J Neurooncol 3:99–103

North JB, Penhall RK, Hanieh A, et al. (1983) Phenytoin and postoperative epilepsy. A double blind study. J Neurosurg 58:672–677

Ostertag CB, Mennel HD, Kiessling M (1980) Stereotactic biopsy of brain tumors. Surg Neurol 14:275–283

Park TS, Hoffman HJ, Hendrick EB, et al. (1983) Medulloblastoma: Clinical presentation and management: Experience at the Hospital for Sick Children, Toronto, 1950–1980. J. Neurosurg 58:543–552

Patchell RA, Tibbs PA, Walsh JW, et al. (1990) A randomized trial of surgery in the treatment of single metastases to the brain. N Engl J Med 322:494–499

Pia HW (1986) Microsurgery of gliomas. Acta Neurochir 80:1–11

Piepmeier JM (1987) Observations on the current treatment of low-grade astrocytic tumors of the cerebral hemispheres. J Neurosurg 67:177–181

Popovic EA, Kaye AH, Hill JS (1996) Current status of photodynamic therapy for brain tumors. In: Salcman M (ed) Current techniques in neurosurgery, 2nd edn. Current Medicine/Churchill Livingstone, Philadelphia, pp 124–140

Rezai AR, Hund M, Kronberg E, et al. (1996) The interactive use of magnetoencephalography in stereotactic image-guided neurosurgery. Neurosurgery 39:92–102

Rostomily RC, Berger MS, Ojemann GA, et al (1991) Postoperative deficits and functional recovery following removal of tumors involving the dominant hemisphere supplementary motor area. J Neurosurg. 75:62–68

Salcman M (1985) Resection and reoperation in neurooncology. Rationale and approach. Neurol Clin 3:831–842

Salcman M (1985b): Supratentorial gliomas: Clinical features and surgical therapy. In: Wilkins RH, Rengachary SS (eds) Neurosurgery. McGraw-Hill, New York, pp 579–550

Salcman M (1988) The role of surgical resection in the treatment of malignant brain tumors: Who benefits? Oncology 2:47–59

Salcman M (1989) Surgical decision-making for malignant brain tumors. Clin Neurosurg 35:285–313

Salcman M (1990) Malignant glioma management. Neurosurgery Clinics of North America 1(1):49–63

Salcman M (1990b) Radical surgery for low-grade glioma. Clin. Neurosurg 36:353–366

Salcman, M (1991) Hyperthermia. In: Salcman M (ed) The neurobiology of brain tumors, vol. 4. Concepts in Neurosurgery, Williams and Wilkins, Baltimore, pp 359–373

Salcman M (1991b) In vivo estimates of kinetic parameters. In: Thomas GT, Salcman M (eds) The neurobiology of brain tumors, vol. 4. Concepts in Neurosurgery, Williams and Wilkins, Baltimore, pp 229–249

Salcman M (1993a) Intrinsic cerebral glioma. In: Apuzzo MLJ (ed) Brain surgery, complication avoidance and management. Churchill Livingstone, New York, pp 379–390

Salcman M (1993b) Recent advances and future directions in interstitial brachytherapy. In: Salcman M (ed) Current techniques in neurosurgery, 1st edn. Current Medicine, Philadelphia, pp 4.1–4.14

Salcman M (1994) The value of cytoreductive surgery. Clinical Neurosurgery 41:464–488

Salcman M (1995) Glioblastoma and malignant astrocytoma. In: Laws ER, Kaye, AH (eds) Encyclopaedia of brain tumors. Churchill Livingstone, New York, pp 449–477

Salcman M (1996a) The surgical management of gliomas. In: Tindall GT, Cooper PR, Barrow DL (eds) The practice of neurosurgery. William and Wilkins, Baltimore, pp.649–670

Salcman M (1996b) The therapeutic implications of the natural history of low grade glial tumors. Current Techniques in Neurosurgery, 2nd edition, Salcman M (ed.), Churchill Livingstone/Current Medicine, Philadelphia, pp.109–122

Salcman M (1999) Historical development of surgery for glial tumors. J Neurooncol 42:195–204

Salcman M, Bellis EH, Sewchand W, et al. (1989) Technical aids for the flexible use of the Leksell stereotactic system. Neurol Res 11:89–96

Salcman M, Kaplan RS, Ducker TB, et al. (1982) Effect of age and reoperation on survival in the combined modality treatment of malignant astrocytoma. Neurosurgery 10:454–463

Salcman M, Robinson W, Montgomery E (1986) Laser microsurgery: A review of 105 intracranial tumors. J Neurooncol 3:363–371

Salcman M, Scholtz H, Kaplan RS, Kulik S (1994) Long term survival in patients with malignant astrocytoma. Neurosurgery 34:213–220

Sawaya R (1999) Extent of resection in malignant gliomas: a critical summary. J Neurooncol 42:303–305

Shapiro WR (1982) Treatment of neuroectodermal brain tumors. Ann Neurol 12:231–237

Taratuto AL, Sevlever G, Piccardo P (1991) Clues and pitfalls in stereotactic biopsy of the central nervous system. Arch Pathol Lab Med 115:596–602

Tel E, Hoshino T, Barker M, et al. (1980) Effect of surgery on BCNU chemotherapy in a rat brain tumor model. J Neurosurg 52:529–532

Tenney JH, Vlahov D, Salcman M, et al. (1985) Wide variation in risk of wound infection following clean neurosurgery: Implications for perioperative antibiotic prophylaxis. J Neurosurg 62:243–247

Vecht, CJ, Avezaat, CJ, van Putten, WL, et al (1990) The influence of extent of surgery on the neurological function and survival in malignant glioma. A retrospective analysis in 243 patients. J Neurol Neurosurg Psychiat 53:466–471

Vives KR, Piepmeier JM (1999) Complications and expected outcome of glioma surgery. J Neurooncol 42:289–302

Walker MD, Green SB, Byar DP, et al. (1980) Randomized comparisons of radiotherapy and nitrosoureas for the treatment of malignant glioma after surgery. N Engl J Med 303:1323–1329

Watanabe E, Mayanagi Y, Kosugi Y, et al. (1991) Open surgery assisted by the neuronavigator, a stereotactic, articulated, sensitive arm. Neurosurgery 28:792–800

Winger M, Macdonald DR, Schold SC, et al. (1989) Selection bias in clinical trials of anaplastic glioma. Ann Neurol 26:531–534

Wood JR, Greene SB, Shapiro WR (1988) The prognostic importance of tumor size in malignant gliomas: a computed tomographic scan study by the Brain Tumor Cooperative Group. J Clin Oncol 6:338–343

Young B, Oldfield EH, Markesbery WR, et al. (1981) Reoperation for glioblastoma. J Neurosurg 55:917–921

Young HF, Merchant RE, Apuzzo MLJ (1991) Immunocompetence of patients with malignant glioma. In: Salcman M (ed) Neurobiology of brain tumors. Williams and Wilkins, Baltimore, pp 211–227

18 Radiation Therapy Principles for High-Grade Gliomas

Curtis Miyamoto

CONTENTS

18.1 Introduction

Gliomas are the most common primary brain tumors, comprising 40–60% of all primary brain tumors. The most frequent types are glioblastoma multiforme, astrocytoma, and oligodendroglioma. Radiation therapy is one of the most important treatment modalities for gliomas, mainly because these tumors are usually localized. The patient's head can be immobilized, allowing for good targeting of the tumor. As a result of technological advances, the range of treatment options using radiation therapy has increased. Photon, electron, neutron and proton radiation beams are all in clinical use. The accuracy of the treatment delivery has also improved, with the development of three-dimensional techniques and image fusion. Our understanding of both the radio sensitivity of gliomas, and the tolerance of normal brain tissue is better, allowing the design of novel fractionation schemes. Radiation is being combined with both local and systemic chemotherapy, offering hope for patients in terms of improved local and overall control, as well as improved tolerance to treatment while maintaining a good quality of life. This chapter will discuss the indications, techniques and outcomes for the radiation therapy of high-grade gliomas in adults.

18.1.1 Historical Background

In 1966, one of the first studies examining the long-term results of radiation therapy of intracranial tumors was published (BOUCHARD 1966). Two studies were published in 1978 where combined management, which included surgery, radiation therapy and chemotherapy, was examined. In a study by WALKER et al. (1978), patients were randomized into four treatment groups: surgery alone, surgery and BCNU, surgery and radiotherapy, and surgery combined with irradiation and chemotherapy. The median survival time was best in the groups that included radiation therapy (14–19 weeks vs. 35–36 weeks). That same year, the European Organization for Research and Treatment of Cancer (EORTC) Brain Tumor Group (BTG) published a study evaluating late and early administration of CCNU with surgery and irradiation (EORTC 1978). The median survival time in the irradiated group was between 43 and 62 weeks, superior to the above mentioned 14 to19 weeks median survival seen without irradiation. Another of

C. MIYAMOTO, MD
Associate Professor and Clinical Service Chief, Department of Radiation Oncology, The Brain Tumor Center, M.S. 200, MCP Hahnemann University, 216 North Broad Street, Philadelphia, PA 19102-1192, USA

the early landmark studies in the use of radiation therapy for high-grade gliomas was performed by the Brain Tumor Cooperative Group (WALKER et al. 1980). In this study, patients with malignant gliomas were randomly selected to receive post-operative irradiation or to be observed. Ninety percent of the 222 patients had glioblastoma multiforme. The median survival time for the supportive-care group was 14 weeks and for the post-operative irradiation group was 36 weeks, *P*=0.001. The 1-year actuarial survival was 3% for the non-irradiated group and 24% for the post-operative irradiation group. It is easy to see how radiation therapy has become one of the mainstays of the management of high-grade gliomas (Fig. 18.1).

Since these original studies, many new techniques have been developed in an attempt to both improve local control and to decrease normal tissue toxicity. In this chapter, most of the major developments in radiation therapy for high-grade gliomas will be presented.

18.2
Mechanisms of Radiation Effects and Normal Tissue Tolerance

18.2.1
Radiation Effects

The exact mechanism for the effectiveness of radiation therapy is still relatively poorly understood (see Chap. 4 for relevant details). Ionizing radiation is thought to produce secondary electrons, which results in damage to the cellular DNA and the cell membrane by the production of hydroxyl radicals. These hydroxyl radicals are probably more effective in oxygenated tissues. Many forms of DNA damage can occur, including double- and single-strand breaks, base damage and DNA-protein cross-linkages. The double-strand breaks have the greatest corre-

lation with human tumor cell line death (KELLAND et al. 1988; SCHWARTZ et al. 1988; WLODEK and HITTELMAN 1987). How ionizing radiation destroys tumor cells more efficiently than normal cells is not clear, but it is widely believed that the reason for the sensitivity of tumor cells to radiation is because of their characteristic of replicating more rapidly than normal tissues. This, although true, only partially explains the effect. There are many normal tissues such as endothelial, epithelial and hematopoetic cells that replicate as quickly as tumor cells do but yet sustain less damage. It is likely that anticancer agents induce p53 protein-dependent apoptosis, thereby leading to the elimination of radiation damaged cells (GUPTA et al. 1996).

18.2.2
Complications of Radiotherapy

The deleterious clinical effects of radiation therapy on normal brain tissues are well known. In some early studies, when the whole brain, or large portions of the brain, were treated with a high radiation dose, significant morbidity occurred. Clearly, the effect is multi-factorial. Patient characteristics such as age, history of previous cerebral vascular events, presence of dementia, and the region of the brain irradiated, affect the tolerance to radiotherapy. There are also treatment-related factors, which include dose per fraction, overall length of treatment, total dose, and volume of brain tissue being treated. Radiation side effects are divided into acute, subacute and chronic or late. With a daily dose of 1.8–2 Gy per fraction (standard fractionation) and a total dose approaching 70–80 Gy, acute changes during the treatment course are very uncommon. Administration of a large single dose of 35 Gy in monkeys is known to produce increased cerebral edema after 18–36 weeks (CAVENESS 1977). Neuronal changes are followed by breakdown of the myelin, and proliferative and degenerative changes in astrocytes and oth-

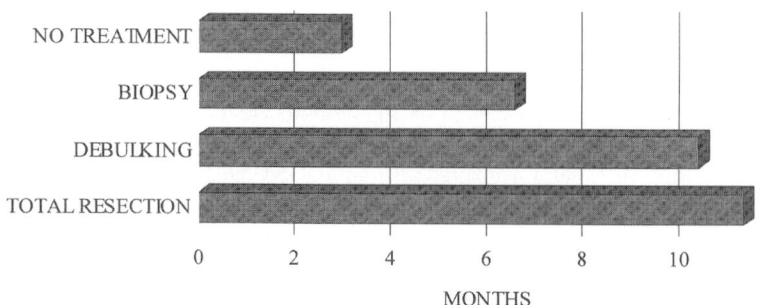

Fig. 18.1. Survival rates of patients managed with standard radiation therapy

er glial elements after 12–20 weeks. Symptoms include nausea, vomiting, headache, neurological deterioration and sleepiness. The effects occur during the first 6 months after irradiation, and include breakdown or decreased production of myelin due to damage to the oligodendroglial cells. This usually occurs approximately 2 months after irradiation and is generally reversible. The symptoms are similar to the acute effects and include somnolence, anorexia, lassitude, irritability and emotional lability (FREEMAN et al. 1973). The resulting demyelination is usually visible on MRI and CT imaging. Enhancement is seen in the irradiated areas on T2-weighted MRI scans and slowing may be observed in the region, on EEG (GROOTHUIS et al. 1980). Other objective findings include pleocytosis or mild protein elevation in the cerebrospinal fluid.

Effects occurring after 6 months are considered to be chronic or of late toxicity. This late toxicity is generally permanent and may progress. There can be significant vascular damage with thickening of the vascular walls, endothelial proliferation, fibrinoid necrosis, perivascular fibrosis and thrombosis (BURGER et al. 1979). This vascular damage results in necrosis, which in turn produces edema and mass effect, and often it is very difficult to distinguish between progression of disease and radiation necrosis. There is an increase in contrast enhancement in both circumstances, on MRI and CT images, and patients may be symptomatic. Thallium SPECT imaging and positron emission tomography (PET) scanning can be equivocal. In one study however, LOBERBOYM et al. (1997) prospectively performed thallium-201 uptakes on 60 post-surgical patients with either primary brain malignancies or metastatic lesions, 6–12 weeks after treatment with conventional radiotherapy and/or radiosurgery. Abnormally increased ^{201}Tl uptake was observed in 40 (67%) of 60 patients. In all patients with positive results, the diagnosis of residual tumor was confirmed at biopsy or by clinical follow-up sequential imaging studies. In the 20 patients with negative findings, there was no abnormal ^{201}Tl uptake, despite suspicious findings on CT and/or MRI scans. Ten of the negative ^{201}Tl studies were true-negatives, while the remaining ten were false-negatives. This may in part be due to the fact that six of these patients had lesions <1 cm in maximum diameter, and three patients had low-grade astrocytoma. Tumor-to-background ratio of ^{201}Tl uptake did not distinguish between tumor types or predict clinical outcome. The authors concluded that thallium-201 scintigraphy had a very high specificity (100% in this cohort) for detecting viable residual tumors.

Changes in ^{201}Tl retention after radiation therapy seemed to have prognostic value.

A PET scan with ^{18}F-fluoro-2-deoxy-D-glucose (FDG) is currently considered to be the non-invasive gold standard for distinguishing brain tumor recurrence from radiation necrosis. Hypermetabolism of FDG has been associated with inflammatory necrotic changes following radiation of meningioma (FISCHMAN et al. 1997). In another study, RICCI et al. (1998) evaluated the ability of PET to differentiate recurrent tumor from post-therapy radiation necrosis in 84 consecutive patients where recurrent tumor or radiation necrosis had been suggested by clinical or MRI findings. Metabolic activity of the PET abnormality was compared qualitatively with the normal contralateral gray and white matter. The findings from PET were confirmed histologically in 31 patients. With contralateral white matter as the standard of comparison, the PET scan sensitivity and specificity were found to be 86% and 22%, respectively. With contralateral gray matter as the standard reference, the sensitivity and specificity became 73% and 56%, respectively. Overall, nearly one-third of the patients would have been treated inappropriately in either scheme had the PET scan been the sole determinant of therapy.

Positron emission tomography does not always provide reliable information. For example, in one case report, a patient had a history of atypical meningioma and was treated with surgical resection and post-operative proton-beam radiation therapy (the biological effect of protons on the target volume is the same as that of photons) (SHIBAMOTO et al. 1997).

Approximately 16 months after completion of therapy, MRI demonstrated two new regions of enhancement, and an FDG-PET study was performed to characterize further these lesions. FDG-PET revealed an area of intense hypermetabolism, and a wide surgical resection was performed. Histological examination of the surgical specimen revealed reactive changes and areas of necrosis. There was no evidence of either recurrent or radiation-induced tumor.

Dynamic MRI and proton magnetic resonance imaging (MRS) have also been employed to differentiate between recurrent tumor and radiation necrosis. HAZLE et al. (1977) used dynamic MRI in 95 patients with intracranial mass lesions, using T1-weighted fast spin-echo (FSE) MRI at 1.5 T. Histological findings included treatment-related changes (n=32), primary tumors (n=41), metastatic tumors (n=5), meningiomas (n=4), and mixed primary/treatment related changes (n=13). Based on maximal enhancement rates, treatment- related changes could be differentiated from primary tumors, meta-static tumors, and meningiomas ($P<0.05$). Lesions of mixed tumor and treatment-related change had intermediate values. The study investigators concluded that dynamic MRI could be used to distinguish treatment-related changes from primary tumors in previously treated patients based on maximal enhancement rates.

A new emerging test to differentiate radiation necrosis from tumor recurrence is MRS. CHONG et al. (1999) compared MR spectroscopic scans from 13 healthy individuals and from 18 patients with radiographic temporal lobe necrosis, and found that N-acetyl-aspartate (NAA) levels were reduced in all but one spectrum (96%). Choline level was increased in 11%, was normal in 14% and was reduced in 75% of patients. Creatine (Cr) concentration was normal in 29% and reduced in 71%. Most notable was the finding that four patients with normal imaging findings had abnormal MR spectroscopy results. Primary and recurrent tumors generally show markedly elevated choline levels with reduced or absent NAA (Table 18.1).

The normal brain tolerance was suggested to be 52 Gy with 2 Gy per fraction (SHELINE et al. 1980). The necrosis rate at this dose level was estimated to be 0.04–0.4%. The authors concluded that a dose of 60 Gy using 2 Gy per fraction was reasonably safe to use in clinical practice. This is still considered to be the case. Different fractionation schemes have been used. The effects of these various fractionation schemes can theoretically be determined by using a formula calculating the biological equivalent dose or BED. This formula is based on what is termed the a/b ratio, which is different for early (high) and late (low) reacting tissues. The brain is considered to be a late reacting tissue and therefore has a ratio of 3. The ratio is used in the formula BED in Gy=D[1+d/[a/b], where "D" is the total dose and "d" is the dose per fraction (the amount given at each treatment). This formula can be used to determine the biological equivalence between different treatment programs.

18.3
Neurocognitive Effect of Irradiation

The neurocognitive effects of irradiation are poorly understood, and there are still no comprehensive studies available on this subject. In one study, the effects of post-operative radiotherapy in patients with glioma was examined (Scheibel et al. 1996). Neuropsychological testing showed no correlation with tumor grade. There was a relationship with tumor lateralization and treatment type. Scores on a test of graphomotor speed were lowest for patients who had received radiation or a combination of radiation and chemotherapy, regardless of lesion location. Patients with left hemispheric lesions had lower verbal scores, while those with right-sided lesions had lower scores for a test of facial recognition.

18.4
Treatment with Radiation

18.4.1
Standard Fractionation

The most widely used form of treatment is external beam photon irradiation. Photon beams can be either X-rays (artificially produced) or gamma rays

Table 18.1. Late effects: diagnostic studies

Modality	Finding with tumor	Finding with necrosis	Sensitivity	Specificity
CT scan	Enhancement with mass effect and edema	Enhancement with mass effect and edema	–	–
MRI	Enhancement with mass effect and edema	Enhancement with mass effect and edema	–	–
PET	Increased activity	Decreased activity	73–86%	22-56%
Thallium SPECT	Increased activity	Decreased activity	–	100%
MR spectroscopy	Reduced metabolites especially NAA	Elevated choline levels	96%	–

NAA, N-acetyl-aspartate.

(produced from radioactive decay). Linear accelerators are the most widespread of the treatment devices and artificially produce radiation. Commonly, radiation is delivered in multiple fractions in order to decrease toxicity to the normal tissue, while maintaining the same tumor response.

Standard fractionation consists of the daily delivery of 180 to 200 cGy fractions of radiation (Table 18.2). The time interval between fractions allows for "repair" of sublethal radiation damage, which is the first of what has been termed the four "R's" of radiation biology. These are repair of sublethal damage, reassortment, reoxygenation, and repopulation. The mechanism of repair in sublethal radiation damage is not well understood, but may possibly be related to the integrity of the cell cycle checkpoints in normal tissue, where normal checkpoints, e.g., p21, arrest the cell cycle in radiation damaged tissue, allowing time for repair to take place. Given the prevalence of checkpoint defects in tumors (WALDMAN et al. 1997), radiation-damaged malignant cells may proceed through cell cycle and probably into an apoptosis (programmed cell death) pathway.

Standard radiation therapy increases survival for patients with glioblastoma multiforme by 3–6 months or roughly doubles the survival time from surgery alone. This was demonstrated early on by the Brain Tumor Study Group (WALKER et al. 1978, 1980), who showed an increase of median survival from 14 weeks for surgery alone, to 36 weeks, with post-operative radiation treatment. The 1-year survivals were 3% and 24%, respectively. Standard of care today for glioblastoma multiforme, anaplastic astrocytoma and malignant oligodendroglioma requires the delivery of a total dose of 5,000–7,000 cGy, using standard fractionation. There has been no proven survival benefit from increased total radiation doses over 60 Gy.

18.4.2
Hyperfractionation

Typically, this is a delivery of two doses of radiation daily, separated by 4 to 6 hours. It has the theoretical advantage of delivering a higher total dose of radiation to the tumor, while reducing the normal tissue toxicity. The overall length of the treatment is the same as that for standard fractionation. Again, the rationale behind this treatment schedule is to irradiate the maximum number of tumor cells at vulnerable times in the cell cycle. The time between the radiation treatments allows for the repair of suble-

Table 18.2. Results of standard fractionation

Investigator	Treatment	Median survival time
WALKER et al.	Supportive care	14–19 weeks
	RT + chemotherapy	35–36 weeks
EORTC	RT + CCNU	43–62 weeks
BRAIN TUMOR COOPERATIVE GROUP	Supportive care	14 weeks
	Post-operative RT	36 weeks
BLEEHEN	RT-45 Gy	9 months
	RT-60 Gy	12 months

RT, standard radiation therapy; EORTC, European Organization for Research and Treatment of Cancer; CCNU,

thal damage in the normal tissue. In some clinical studies, the utilization of this technique has resulted in an improved local control rate and survival (EDWARDS et al. 1989). In one study, total doses of 64.8, 72.0, 76.8 and 81.6 Gy were delivered using 1.2 Gy per fraction twice a day (MURRAY et al. 1995). The median survival time for anaplastic astrocytoma patients at 72.0 Gy was 49.9 months. Inferior survival outcome was observed at the highest hyperfractionated total dose of 81.6 Gy. With hyperfractionated radiotherapy, an increased incidence of necrosis requiring surgery was reported, compared with standard fractionation.

18.4.3
Accelerated Fractionation

Another schedule of radiation delivery is accelerated fractionation, the use of standard-sized fractions given twice daily. Accelerated fractionation reduces the overall number of treatment days by half (THAMES et al. 1992; PETERS et al. 1982; FOWLER 1984). The potential late-term effects should theoretically be the same, since the total number of fractions is unchanged. This should result in an increased probability of tumor control and possibly survival, because of a reduction in repopulation in rapidly proliferating tumors, however, this has yet to be tested in a prospective randomized trial (WANG 1988). In another study, no dose-response correlation was noted for patients treated for malignant glioma between accelerated hyperfractionated (1.6 Gy per fraction) radiotherapy with total doses of 48.0 and 54.4 Gy (MURRAY et al. 1995). The acute effects of radiation are increased, which can result in a need for interruption of the treatment course. In a clinical trial, it was noted that the rate of disease progression during the course of treatment was much lower than that for standard fraction radiotherapy (NELSON 1990), though in some cases contrast-enhanced tumor-negative lesions mimicking a brain tumor, consisting of necrosis and reactive gliosis, were observed on MRI after a total dose of 60 Gy (VAN TASSEL et al. 1995).

18.5
Brachytherapy

This form of radiotherapy is also known as interstitial implantation, and involves the direct placement of one or multiple radioactive sources in the area of the tumor, most frequently performed by a minimally invasive neurosurgical procedure. This allows the delivery of high doses of radiation to the target volume while minimizing radiation exposure to the surrounding structures. The radiation sources can be implanted directly into the tumor cavity, either for a short time or indefinitely, depending on the desired effect. This is limited by tumor size (the larger the tumor the more difficult to implant the treatment volume completely and uniformly), and location, i.e., accessibility to treatment (Schupak et al. 1995). Relatively few newly-diagnosed patients are candidates for this procedure. Iodine-125 is the most commonly employed isotope, but other isotopes such as iridium-192 have also been implanted. Scharfen et al. (1991), implanted 307 patients with high-activity removable iodine-125 interstitial implants at the University of California in San Francisco. Patients treated primarily also underwent external beam irradiation. The median survival time for patients with primary glioblastoma multiforme was 88 weeks. For high-grade (non-glioblastoma) glioma this increased to 142 weeks. For recurrent glioblastoma multiforme the median survival time from the date of implant was 49 weeks. The corresponding time for recurrent high-grade non-glioblastoma tumors was 52 weeks. Forty percent of patients with high-grade glioma required reoperation, with a median time of 33 weeks after implantation. The authors concluded that interstitial implantation is a well-tolerated procedure that prolongs survival in patients with primary and recurrent glioblastoma multiforme, as evidenced by the 3-year survival rates of 22% and 15%, respectively. In one study (Ostertag and Kreth 1992), permanent and temporary implants were compared. Three hundred and forty-five patients received temporary implants, and 194 patients were treated with permanent implants. The 2-year survival rate was 36% for anaplastic glioma and 16% for glioblastoma patients. Patients with World Health Organization (WHO) grade II astrocytoma had a significantly improved outcome if they had temporary implants rather than permanent implants. Sneed et al. (1996), reviewed their patients with glioblastoma multiforme with temporary iodine-125 implants. Dose volume histograms were able to be obtained from 97 patients. In this group, a quadratic relationship was found between a total biologically effective dose and survival, with a trend toward optimal survival probability at 47 Gy minimum brachytherapy dose (corresponding to about 65 Gy to 95% of the tumor volume); survival decreased with lower or higher radiation doses.

In spite of the benefits reported by some investigators, the use of implants remains controversial. This is due to other published reports, which showed little or no gain in survival. A recently published report, with results of a randomized trial of brachytherapy as part of the initial management for malignant astrocytoma, is of interest (LAPERRIERE et al. 1998). The study-patients had to have biopsy-proven malignant astrocytoma less than or equal to 6 cm in maximum dimension, not crossing midline, not involving the corpus callosum, and with a Karnofsky performance status (KPS) of greater than or equal to 70. Patients were randomly selected to receive 50 Gy of external beam irradiation with or without a stereotactic temporary iodine-125 implant delivering a minimum peripheral tumor dose of 60 Gy. The median survival times of the patients randomly assigned to brachytherapy vs. no brachytherapy were 13.8 and 13.2 months, respectively. The authors therefore concluded that there was no significant survival benefit with the use of interstitial implants.

Some clinical trials with stereotactic placement of iodine-125 and iridium-192, combined with chemotherapy, have shown improved survival for patients with glioblastoma multiforme (SCHARFEN et al. 1991). FONTANESI et al. (1993), treated 28 patients interstitially with iodine-125 (60 Gy over 6 days), concomitantly with cisplatin administration and hyperfractionated irradiation (110 cGy twice a day to a total dose of 66 Gy). There were 18 patients with glioblastoma multiforme, and ten patients with anaplastic astrocytoma. The overall local control was 77% and the median survival time was 15 months. The Northern California Oncology Group (NCOG) study 6G-82-2, examined 107 patients with unifocal, circumscribed malignant glioma treated with iodine-

125 implant boosts (50–60 Gy) and six courses of procarbazine, lomustine and vincristine, after a standard course of definitive radiotherapy consisting of 60 Gy (Gutin et al. 1991). Of the 101 evaluable patients, 63 (62%) received implants. The median survival time was 157 weeks for the patients receiving implants and 88 weeks for those patients receiving implants and who had received a diagnosis of glioblastoma multiforme. Of the 34 patients with glioblastoma multiforme, nine were alive after 2 years and three after 3 years. Almost half of the patients receiving implants later required reoperation after a median time of 46.1 months (Table 18.3). Other studies have shown a significant rate of failure, requiring reoperation (Hopkins et al. 1995).

Implants with high linear energy transfer (LET) isotopes have also been performed. This technique has the advantage of being able to kill malignant cell clones resistant to the conventional radiation (low LET). Patchell et al. (1997), conducted a phase I trial to test the feasibility of neutron brachytherapy using californium-252 (Cf-252). The study was an open-ended dose-escalation trial, and no external beam irradiation was given. Ten of the 33 patients developed scalp necrosis. It was not until a dose of 1,300 ncGy was reached that two out of three patients (the end point) developed radiation necrosis of the brain. The authors concluded that Cf-252 as the sole source of radiation was a feasible treatment. The recommended interstitial neutron dose was felt to be 1,200 ncGy.

Table 18.3. Brachytherapy

Investigator	Treatment time	Median survival
Scharfen et al	Temporary I-125 implant + RT	GBM=88 weeks Non-GBM=142 weeks
Fontanesi et al.	Temporary I-125 implant + cisplatin	GBM + AA=15 months
NCOG	I-125 implant + 60 Gy RT + chemotherapy	157 weeks (88 weeks for GBM)
Laperriere	50 Gy + Temporary I-125 implant	RT only=13.2 months
?	RT + implant=13.8 monthsY	

RT, standard radiation therapy; GMB, glioblastoma multiforme; AA, anaplastic astrocytoma; NCOG, Northern California Oncology Group.

18.6
Stereotactic Radiosurgery

Stereotactic irradiation is the delivery of a single high-dose radiation fraction to a limited volume of tissue, using multiple arcs or beams from different directions. There are three conventionally used stereotactic radiosurgery methods. They include the gamma knife, a linear accelerator based stereotactic radiosurgery and proton beam stereotaxy (See chapter 6). The gamma knife consists of multiple collimators in a helmet with 201 cobalt-60 sources, while the linear accelerator utilizes multiple sweeps or arcs. Both techniques are designed to deliver radiation from multiple directions to a targeted focus, thus sparing the surrounding normal tissue. Three-dimensional reconstruction of target areas is employed in both techniques. A similar dose-delivery can be obtained with the proton beam stereotactic system (Table 18.4).

Although the exact radiobiology of single high dose fractions is still poorly understood, the outcome is expected to be more cytotoxic than the multi fraction doses. Stereotactic radiosurgery is usually used as an adjunct therapy to surgical debulking and conventional radiotherapy. Clinical studies have shown consistent improvement in 2-year survival rates with the use of stereotactic boost (Hall et al. 1995). Sarkaria et al. (1995), published a report evaluating the impact of stereotactic radiosurgery on the survival of patients treated for malignant glioma. A total of 115 patients from three medical centers were treated with a combination of surgery, external beam radiation therapy, and linear accelerator (linac)-based radiosurgery (Joint Center for Radiation Therapy, $n=75$; University of Wisconsin, $n=30$; University of Florida, $n=10$). The actuarial 2-year and median survival time for all patients analyzed was 45% and 96 weeks, respectively. In comparison with the results from a previously published analysis of 1,578 patients entered on three Radiation Therapy Oncology Group external beam radiotherapy protocols from 1974 to 1989, those patients treated with radiosurgery had a significantly improved 2-year and median survival time ($P=0.01$). Only the Karnofsky score was a significant predictor of outcome, on multivariate analysis. Median and 2-year survival for patients with a Karnofsky score >or=70 were 106 weeks and 51%, respectively, compared with 38 weeks and 0% for patients with a Karnofsky score <70% ($P=0.001$). The authors concluded that the addition of radiosurgery to conventional treatment (surgery and external beam radiotherapy) of malignant glioma appeared to improve survival when compared with his-

Table 18.4. General comparison of linear accelerator-based versus gamma knife stereotactic irradiation

	Linear accelerator	Gamma knife
Source	Linear accelerator	Cobalt-60
Field arrangement	Multiple arcs and static fields	Multiple static fields
Field blocking	Multileaf collimators, cerrobend Independent jaws	Not conventionally employed
Time to treat average isocenter	Long	Short
Field shaping	Blocking, multiple isocenters, addition of static fields, differential weighting of fields	Multiple isocenters
Fractionation	Commonly done	Not commonly done
Availability	Commonly available	At select centers
Collimator sizes	50–55 mm	4–18 mm
Imaging for planning	CT is mandatory. Image fusion with angiography and MRI	MRI has been the standard. Now CT and angiography compatible

torical reports. Kondziolka et al. (1997), compared their results from treating 64 patients with glioblastoma multiforme and 43 patients with anaplastic astrocytoma, with historical controls. The median survival time after initial diagnosis was 26 months, with median survival after radiosurgery of 16 months. For the 45 patients who underwent adjuvant radiosurgery, the median survival time was 20 months. The authors concluded that there was a survival benefit for patients with both anaplastic astrocytoma and glioblastoma multiforme. Shrieve et al. (1999), reviewed their use of stereotactic radiosurgery (SRS) as an adjunct therapy for glioblastoma multiforme. Seventy-eight patients were treated between June 1988 and January 1995. All patients were treated with surgery and standard radiotherapy followed by SRS. The median survival time for all patients was 19.9 months. The 1- and 2-year actuarial survival rates were 88.5% and 35.9%, respectively. An age of less than 40 years was the only significant prognostic factor, on multivariate analysis. Acute complications were unusual and no new neuropathies secondary to the radiosurgery were reported. Thirty-nine (50%) patients underwent reoperation for radiation necrosis or recurrent tumor. Single-dose radiosurgery and fractionated radiotherapy for recurrent high-grade glioma was compared in a recently published study (Cho et al. 1999). Forty-six patients were treated with radiosurgery and 25 were treated with radiotherapy. A median dose of 17 Gy was delivered to patients treated with radiosurgery (SRS) and 37.5 Gy in 15 fractions to

those in the external beam radiotherapy group. The median survival time for the SRS group was 11 months and for the radiotherapy group it was 12 months. The authors concluded that SRS may be a better option due to an equivalent survival in spite of worse prognostic factors and a lower incidence of late complications. Stereotactic radiotherapy has also been used as a concomitant boost during standard fractionated irradiation. Treatment outcome in a pilot study was reported in 12 patients with malignant glioma following a biopsy or a debulking procedure (Cardinale et al. 1998). An external beam irradiation dose of 44 Gy was given together with three, weekly, stereotactic radiotherapy boosts of 12 Gy. Three patients with anaplastic astrocytoma and 9 patients with glioblastoma multiforme had median survival times of 33 months and 16 months, respectively. The benefit from either stereotactic radiotherapy (SRT) or radiosurgery in part is due to the selection bias. Patients who are candidates for SRT or SRS are already in a more favorable group, as was evident in a report of an RTOG study (Shrieve et al. 1999) (Table 18.5).

18.7
Intraoperative Radiation Therapy

Intraoperative radiotherapy (IORT) is the delivery of a single large dose of radiation during surgery. A special cone is placed directly over the tumor or

Table 18.5. Stereotactic radiosurgery and radiotherapy

Investigators	Treatment	Median survival time
SAKARIA et al.	S+RT+SRS	96 weeks
KONDZIOLKA et al.	S+RT+SRS	After diagnosis=26 months After SRS=16 months SRS as adjuvant=20 months
SHRIEVE et al.	S+RT+SRS	GBM
CHO et al. (Recurrent high-grade astrocytomas)	S+RT+SRS S+RT+SRT	11 months 12 months
CARDINALE et al.	S+RT+SRT	AA=33 months GBM=16 months

S, surgery; RT, standard radiation therapy; SRS, stereotactic radiosurgery; GMB, glioblastoma multiforme; SRT, stereotactic radiotherapy; AA, anaplastic astrocytoma.

tumor-bed under direct visualization and a dose of radiation using electron beam or superficial X-rays is given. Occasionally, low energy photon irradiation (orthovoltage) has also been employed. This modality is available in only a limited number of institutions. For obvious reason, it is applicable only for more superficial tumors. A preliminary report on ten patients treated with IORT at the time of wide excision for primary resection or salvage resection has been published (CHUNG et al. 1995). In this study, the IORT doses ranged from 15–25 Gy, depending on the tumor volume and previous radiation therapy. After IORT, the Karnofsky performance status improved in four patients and was unchanged in the remaining six patients. There were several complications after IORT including: radiation necrosis, communicating hydrocephalus, wound infection, and abnormal CT findings (i.e., a diffuse low-density area in and around the operation site). Radiation necrosis was pathologically confirmed in a recurrent meningioma patient 12 months after IORT. At the last follow-up, ranging from 1 to 16 months, there were no deaths. Another study was reported on 19 patients with various brain tumors (SHIBAMOTO et al. 1994), when IORT was given as primary treatment in two patients with malignant glioma, and for recurrent tumor in another 17 patients. The two subjects who received no prior treatment had 33 Gy by IORT alone, and 30 Gy by IORT in combination with 50 Gy of external beam. They survived for 12 and 9 months, respectively. The 17 patients with recurrent disease received external beam radiation therapy 4–12 months before IORT. In this group, single doses of 23–40 Gy were delivered by IORT after maximum tumor debulking.

The median survival time after IORT was 12 months for the nine patients with glioblastoma or anaplastic astrocytoma, and 51 months for the eight patients with less invasive tumors (ependymoma, anaplastic ependymoma, and anaplastic oligodendroglioma). One patient with ependymoma and another with anaplastic ependymoma are currently alive with no evidence of disease at 7 and 11 years respectively, after IORT. Symptomatic brain necrosis occurred in three patients following IORT. The symptoms were resolved in two patients after removal of necrotic brain tissue. It was concluded that IORT combined with extensive tumor removal has an acceptable toxicity in previously irradiated patients and can be effective for selected patients with recurrent malignant brain tumors. ORTIZ DE URBINA et al. (1995) treated 17 patients with primary, n=8 or recurrent, n=9 high-grade malignant glioma. Four patients had anaplastic astrocytoma, six had anaplastic oligodendroglioma and seven had glioblastoma multiforme. Patients underwent surgical resection and a single dose of 10–20 Gy IORT delivered to the tumor-bed. Fourteen patients received either pre-operative, n=8 or post-operative, n=6 external beam radiation therapy. There was a 56% incidence of survival at 18 months (range: 1–21 months) for primary glioma with the median survival time not yet having been reached. Four patients developed tumor progression with a median time to tumor progression of 9 months. Recurrent glioma had an 18-month actuarial survival rate and median survival time of 47% and 13 months (range: 6–32+ months), respectively. The median time to tumor progression was 11 months. No IORT-related mortality was observed.

18.7
Combination of
Radiation Therapy and Chemotherapy

Combination therapy involving radiation and chemotherapy has been used in a variety of configurations (KIU et al. 1995; KYRITSIS et al. 1996; BRANDES and FIORONTINO 1996; FOUTZILAS et al. 1997; BOIARDI et al. 1997). One of the earliest studies of randomized trials combining chemotherapy and radiation therapy was published in 1980 (WALKER et al. 1980). There were four treatment arms: semustine, radiotherapy, carmustine and radiotherapy, and semustine and radiotherapy. No statistically significant benefit in survival was found for the combined treatment groups as compared with the radiotherapy-only group. In 1993, a large meta-analysis was published, reviewing the results from 16 randomized trials involving more than 3,000 patients (FINE et al. 1993). The survival of patients treated with radiation therapy alone was compared with the survival of patients treated with radiation therapy and any single or combination chemotherapy regimen. The estimated increase in survival for patients treated with combination radiation and chemotherapy was 10.1% at 1 year and 8.6% at 2 years. A phase I study was conducted to determine the safety, toxicity, and maximum tolerated dose of pre-irradiation chemotherapy using carmustine (BCNU) and cisplatin in the treatment of high-grade glioma. Patients that had newly diagnosed high-grade glioma received BCNU (40 mg/m^2 BCNU on days 1 through 3 before irradiation, and 200 mg/m^2 BCNU once every 8 weeks for four cycles after irradiation) and cisplatin (30 mg/m^2 cisplatin on days 1 through 3 and 29 through 31 before irradiation) after surgery, both before and during definitive radiation therapy (RAJKUMAR et al. 1999). Radiation therapy consisted of 160 cGy fractions administered twice daily for 15 days, for a total dose of 48 Gy. Dose escalation of BCNU only, was planned. The dose of cisplatin was to be held constant and BCNU dose escalated to 50 mg/m^2 on days 1 through 3. There was a total of 18 patients in this study, and the median survival time was 14 months. Objective responses occurred in 45% of the patients evaluable for response. The authors concluded that this schedule of pre-irradiation administration of BCNU and cisplatin with accelerated hyperfractionated radiation therapy for the treatment of high-grade glioma provided a less toxic alternative to that of previous studies of pre-irradiation chemotherapy with these agents.

The combination of vincristine, etoposide and procarbazine was looked at in the phase II Eastern Cooperative Oncology Group (ECOG) study E2392 (HELLMAN et al. 1998). This was added to post-operative radiation therapy for patients with either glioblastoma multiforme ($n=27$) or anaplastic astrocytoma ($n=6$). The toxicity was manageable (no lethal toxicities) and the median overall survival time was 14.2 months. Radiation therapy and hydroxyurea followed by a combination of 6-thioguanine and BCNU for the treatment of primary malignant brain tumors was studied at the University of California San Francisco (PRADOS et al. 1998). The intention was to evaluate a combined modality treatment for malignant glioma using a radiosensitizer and an adjuvant chemotherapy regimen. All patients were treated primarily with 60 Gy of external beam irradiation with concurrent administration of hydroxyurea. This was followed by BCNU and 6-thioguanine. The median survival time for 135 study-patients with glioblastoma multiforme was 56 weeks and for the 110 patients with anaplastic glioma (anaplastic astrocytomas, $n=103$ and high-grade mixed oligoastrocytoma, $n=7$) the median survival rate had not been reached at the time of the report. This regimen was therefore found to be equivalent to other regimens for glioblastoma multiforme. For anaplastic glioma it was felt to be an equivalent to the combination of procarbazine, CCNU and vincristine (PCV).

Combined SRT with radiation sensitizing weekly doses of cisplatin (40 mg/m^2) was used in a study of patients with high-grade glioma (GLASS et al. 1992). Of the 20 study-patients, one had a partial response, 11 had stable disease and eight had tumor progression. The median duration of response was 18.5 weeks and the median survival time was 55 weeks. A treatment recently approved by The Food and Drug Administration involves the application of BCNU (carmustine)-impregnated biodegradable wafers in the tumor bed at the time of surgical resection (SIPOS et al. 1997). Clinical studies have shown some improvement in increased post-operative survival (VALTONEN et al. 1997).

The feasibility of intraarterial application of chemotherapeutic agents, i.e., infusion into the arteries that feed the tumor, is under study (NAKAGAWA et al. 1994).

18.8
Three-Dimensional Conformal Radiotherapy

In recent years, techniques have been developed to deliver radiation therapy in a much more conformal way (see chapter 5). This has the great advantages of improving the localization of the target volume, as well as decreasing the dose to the normal structures. Three dimensional (3-D) treatment planning has become accessible to most patients, and the methods are analogous to those employed in stereotactic irradiation. The differences between these two treatment delivery systems are diminishing. As with stereotactic irradiation, patients are placed in an immobilization frame attached to a localization device. No targeting technique will be of any use if the patient is not prevented from moving during treatment delivery. The brain is as one of the better parts of the human body for immobilization. Unlike other parts of the body where there is a lot of internal movement, the brain is fairly fixed within the skull; therefore, immobilization of the skull results in immobilization of the brain. There are many techniques that have been designed over the years. In earlier times, most methods were invasive, employing pins or screws which were placed into the periosteum. These were attached to a ring which in turn was attached to a CT or MRI scanner to target imaging, followed by attachment to the treatment table for irradiation. Today, in addition to the invasive frames, there are variety of non-invasive frames (repeat localizers), which in general, are less uncomfortable for patients, and allow for repeated fractionation (the giving of multiple fractions of irradiation). There is likely to be less precision with the use of these frames, compared with the invasive frames, although this is debated. Immobilization is obtained by form fitting facial molds attached to base plates, dental impression mouth molds and occipital plates, nose clips and external auditory canal inserts, and so on. The main goal is accuracy and reproducibility of the treatment position. A CT, or MRI scan, or both are obtained and a 3-D reconstruction is performed. This imaging allows for good definition of target volumes, and normal structures can also be well visualized. The use of this technique, means that multiple fields from many different angles, beam modifiers (materials placed in the beam to make the distribution of radiation in the treatment volume more uniform), and custom blocking of normal tissues (blocking the radiation in the fields to limit normal tissue exposure, utilizing poured cerrobend blocks or multiple leaf collimators) can be better employed. This treatment planning technique also allows for generation of dose-volume histograms, isodose volumes and surface wash. A dose-volume histogram gives the quantitative graphic representation of the dose compared with the volume of interest, normal structure or target volume. The isodose volume is the computerized representation of the volume receiving a certain dose. This allows for a visual reference of the doses to structures in the volume. The surface wash shows the dose to the surfaces of any defined structures. This is especially useful when doses need to be very restricted to areas close to the treatment volume (i.e. optic chiasm, optic nerve, and so on.). Treatment cannot consist only of multiple coplanar and non-coplanar fields but also includes the use of beam modification known as dose intensity modulated radiation therapy (IMRT), which permits partial or complete blocking of the fields, allowing variable amounts of radiation to be delivered within a given area. This results in an improved conformation of the high-dose area to the target volume. It also minimizes the dose to the surrounding normal structures.

These techniques have allowed for renewed efforts at dose escalation to the tumor, as well as for retreatment of persistent or recurrent tumors. Two-dimensional (2-D) techniques (orthogonal films) were compared with CT planning in a recently published study (CROSBY et al. 1998). Twenty consecutive adult patients with high-grade astrocytoma were treated with radiotherapy planned with conventional techniques (2-D) and CT planning, using post-operative, contrast-enhanced CT scans to define the tumor volume. A total of 19 of these 20 patients had a reduction in planning target volumes when CT planning was used. This represented a 25% reduction in volume, which was statistically significant, $P<0.001$. The planning target volumes were reduced in 18 of the 20 patients (mean 24 cm^3, 23%, $P<0.001$). This led to appreciable reductions in the size of the planning target areas and volumes receiving therapeutic doses of radiation. Additionally, it reduced significantly, the amount of normal brain tissue being irradiated and was more accurate in terms of tumor localization.

A study on retreatment of 20 patients was reported by the group from the University of Michigan (KIM et al. 1997). All patients had previously received a full course of irradiation (51 to 65 Gy). The mean target dose of re-irradiation was 36 Gy. The median survival time was 9 months and the 1-year actuarial survival rate was 26%. Radiographic evidence of regression or disease stabilization was seen in 68% of the treated patients. The failure pattern was reported in patients treated with high dose conformal radiotherapy (LEE et al. 1999). Seventy-one patients were entered into a dose escalation trial using standard fractionation (1.8–2 Gy per fraction) given until a total dose of 70 or 80 Gy was reached). As of October 1995, 47 (66%) patients showed CT or MR evidence of recurrence, at which time 36 scans were obtained and analyzed. In 29 (41%) patients a solitary lesion was seen on the scans. Twenty-six of the recurrences were in the central portion of the field, and three were marginal; therefore, none were outside the field. One patient did have a failure considered mainly to be outside the high-dose region. At MCP Hahnemann University all primary high-grade gliomas are treated by the use of 3-D techniques. Often the field arrangements vary from the standard two to four field techniques. Patients with residual or recurrent tumors who are not candidates for brachytherapy or stereotactic irradiation are routinely considered for re-irradiation with 3-D conformal radiotherapy.

18.8
Other Treatment Modalities

The high failure rate of conventional treatments has lead to the development of numerous novel treatment techniques. Some are directed at making the treatment more specific while others are aimed at making it more tumoricidal. The less conventional treatment modalities are at different stages of laboratory and clinical trials and are too numerous to review exhaustively in this article; thus we concentrate on a few of the methods, all promising for the future treatment of brain tumors, that have progressed into human clinical trials. Some of these techniques are already being considered as part of conventional management in a few select programs.

18.8.1
Boron-Neutron Capture Therapy

As mentioned above, neutrons differ from most other forms of external beam irradiation in that they have a high LET, thus depositing larger amounts of energy per length of tissue penetrated. High LET radiation is less affected by sublethal damage repair (the repair that occurs between fractions of radiation), hypoxia, and cell cycle effects, which makes neutron beam extremely effective at killing both the normal and tumor cells. This fact has greatly reduced the therapeutic ratio of neutron radiation. One method of increasing the efficacy of neutron beam capture therapy is to concentrate the radiation dose to the tumor versus normal brain, and this is accomplished by the administration of boron to the patient prior to irradiation. Multiple methods have been employed to increase the concentration of boron in tumor cells, one major effort being the synthesis of boron-containing compounds with greater selectivity for neoplastic cells than for normal cells. One method includes the use of monoclonal antibodies (Hawthorne et al. 1972). One possible target is the epidermal growth factor receptor which is a 53-amino-acid-containing polypeptide whose receptor is frequently overexpressed in glioblastoma multiforme. Recently, bispecific antibodies have been explored (Liu et al. 1996). Boron-containing porphyrins (tetrakis-carbirabe-carborane ester of deuteroporphyrin) have been synthesized (Hill et al. 1995), which are taken up in large amounts by tumor cells and appear to have in vivo localizing properties. Some of the most intensely studied compounds include sodium borocaptate (disodium undechydromercapto-closo-dode-

caborate), p-dihydroxyborylphenylalanine (p-boronophyenylalanine) and ^{10}B-sodium-mercaptoundecahydrododecaborate (Barth et al. 1996). These have been employed in clinical trials with moderate success (Barth et al. 1999; Laramore and Spence 1996). In one study, 18 (21%) of 87 patients treated for malignant brain tumors received intraarterial ^{10}B-sodium-mercaptoundecahydrododecaborate and neutrons and survived for longer than 5 years (Hatanaka and Nakagawa 1994). Other compounds include caboranylalanine, and pyrimidines and purines (taken up by the cells using the salvage pathway for incorporating nucleic acid precursors). Boron accumulates to a much greater degree in tumor tissue, allowing a greater differentiation in dose. Clinical trials are under way to evaluate this radiation method.

18.8.2
Proton Beam Irradiation

Protons are positively charged particles produced by a cyclotron. Proton beam irradiation has some potential advantages due to what is termed the Bragg peak effect (see Chap. 6), which denotes that the proton beam has a very specific range. This allows the proton beam to be used for the irradiation of tumors adjacent to critical normal structures (i.e., the brain stem or optic chiasm). The biological effect of protons is the same as for photons (X-rays and gamma rays) or electrons, which are low LET radiation. These are available only in select locations around the world. There is little clinical information on intracranial tumors, though there are several theoretical models, especially for pediatric CNS malignancies.

18.9
Radioimmunotherapy

The advent of specific monoclonal antibodies directed against cell surface molecules has allowed for the definition of a number of glial epitopes associated with gliomas, and has opened a new era in the treatment of cancers in general, and brain tumors in particular (Kohler and Milstein 1975). Antibodies raised against the neural cell adhesion molecules (Patel et al. 1989), epidermal-growth factor receptors (Brady et al. 1990) and tenascin-C (Natali et al. 1991) are of interest for treatment of malignant gliomas (see chapter 25). The rationale for this treatment is that the antibodies bind to the tumor tissue and cause disruption of neoplastic cell function by blocking receptors to trophic factors and/or other epitopes. Furthermore, these monoclonal antibodies can be coupled with toxins (Press et al. 1986) or radioactive sources (Miyamoto et al. 1995), causing further selective destruction of tumor cells.

Monoclonal antibodies against epidermal growth factor receptors (EGFR) for treatment of brain tumors have been studied extensively and have progressed to phase II clinical trials. These receptors are overexpressed in malignant gliomas (Reifenberger et al. 1989), whereas their expression is low in normal brain tissue. There may be a role for EGFR in oncogenesis and tumor growth (Lieberman et al. 1985), where theoretically, the blocking of these receptors could inhibit proliferation of tumor cells (Faillot et al. 1996). Preliminary clinical studies have shown substantial in vivo tumor binding and concentration of one type of these antibodies, (EMD55900), after intravenous administration of a single 200 mg dose. In a study in this medical center (Miyamoto et al.1995), 60 patients with clinical and radiological diagnosis of glioblastoma multiforme were pre-operatively treated with an average of three intravenous or intraarterial infusions of I-125-labeled murine anti-EGFR monoclonal antibodies. The study revealed that repeated administration of these antibodies is safe and may have some benefit in the management of glioblastoma multiforme, especially for those patients who do not qualify for other forms of more aggressive management (Miyamoto et al. 1995). This method of administration of antibodies is of particular interest, as it treats not only the tumor core, but also the radiographically and histologically silent advancing edge of malignant gliomas.

18.10
Treatment by Tumor Type

18.10.1
Anaplastic Astrocytoma and Glioblastoma Multiforme

Radiation therapy is almost always indicated when a diagnosis of anaplastic astrocytoma or glioblastoma multiforme is made. The majority of these tumors progress locally making them good targets for radiation therapy. Today, the standard of care remains as resection followed by post-operative irradiation.

When resection is not possible due to tumor location, size, and overall medical condition or because of patient preference, definitive or palliative irradiation should be considered. Anatomical imaging with CT and MRI has become routine for treatment planning. These modalities, however, remain unable to distinguish tumor enhancement from that caused by other etiologies (principally post-operative changes and radiation necrosis). Contrast-enhanced post-operative MRI scanning must be done within 3 days of resection to be able to define what is unresected tumor versus post-operative changes. After this time the image findings become progressively less reliable. In a limited fashion, MRI spectroscopy can distinguish radiation necrosis from recurrent or persistent tumor, but this is still not widely available and is considered by many radiologists as an investigational modality. Tumor volumes cannot be defined with this technique, therefore it is of little value for tumor targeting. Functional brain imaging with PET and thallium SPECT scanning can help determine whether changes seen on anatomical scans represent recurrent tumor, post-operative changes or radiation necrosis. Image fusion allows integration of these imaging modalities.

The total dose and the target volume for irradiation have been closely studied over the past three and a half decades. These results need to be taken in context. What we are able to accomplish today is much different from what occurred even just 10 years ago. Today's standard of care, however, remains essentially based on the older techniques. The target volume usually initially consists of a larger volume designed to include the actual tumor, as well as the surrounding area felt to contain microscopic tumor spread that could result in failure. Until 15–20 years ago this generally meant whole-brain irradiation. This was based on several studies that demonstrated that many high-grade gliomas, especially glioblastoma multiforme were multifocal, that is to say, tumor cells could be found away from the primary tumor. In autopsy studies of patients with known high-grade glioma, over 25% of cases were demonstrated to have implants away from the primary lesion (Packer et al. 1985; Erlich et al. 1978). Three fourths will have tumor cells in the hypodense area surrounding the CT contrast-enhancing tumor (Burger 1987) and up to one fourth will have tumor crossing the corpus callosum (Alazar et al. 1976). Antibody studies show that a significant number of patients will have tumor cells >2 cm beyond the CT and MRI enhancing volumes (Kelly et al. 1987). A standard radiation portal arrangement starts with a large field (tumor and edema with a 2–2.5 cm margin). This large field is treated up to a total dose of 40–45 Gy by standard fractionation, followed by a boost of an additional 15–25 Gy to the tumor and a 2–3 cm margin.

The pioneering work of Jean Bouchard laid the foundation for the modern management of patients with high-grade glioma (BOUCHARD 1966). This work was continued and expanded, with the addition of chemotherapy to surgery and radiotherapy, in important studies published in 1978 and 1980 (WALKER et al. 1978, 1980). The outcome of studies of a similar importance was reported during the same time by the EORTC Brain Tumor Group (EORTC 1978). All of the above studies showed relatively poor patient survival, and the importance of the addition of radiotherapy to surgery.

In a more recent report, 64 patients in and around Olmsted County, Minnesota, USA, who were diagnosed with high-grade astrocytoma (81% with glioblastoma multiforme) were managed with a variety of treatments (60% underwent surgical resection, 80% had radiotherapy, and 50% had chemotherapy) (SILVERSTEIN et al. 1996). After the initial treatment, 75% of patients had a stable disease period lasting for a median duration of 198 days. The overall median survival time was 323 days. As expected, younger patients with lower-grade astrocytoma did better than older patients with glioblastoma multiforme (1,493 days vs. 205 days). The mean total direct medical expense for the treatment of a patient in this study was $67,887. Therefore, although there was a significant period of stable disease, it came at a relatively high financial cost.

The timing of response to irradiation was addressed in a study published in 1993 (GASPER et al. 1993). The authors looked at the frequency, timing, and clinical significance of radiographic response to radiation treatment in a retrospective study of 71 patients with supratentorial malignant gliomas. Twenty tumors had a response by the end of the radiation therapy course including 17 (24%) who had a complete response. As expected, a larger proportion of patients with anaplastic astrocytoma responded to radiation than those with glioblastoma. Protracted or delayed responses were observed only in patients with anaplastic glioma. Patients who responded to radiation did not live significantly longer than nonresponders. Tumor progression in the first 6 to 8 weeks after irradiation was associated with a significantly shorter survival time.

The addition of a higher boost after standard radiation therapy has been shown to have a potentially beneficial effect on both local control and survival as outlined above. Survival time can potentially be doubled for glioblastoma multiforme with the addition of either an implant or stereotactic irradiation; whether by stereotactic radiosurgery or radiotherapy is still unknown. Radioactive implants offer at least the same beneficial effect. There are, however, fewer candidates for this latter procedure. Tumors need to be small and in a location accessible for an interstitial implant. Whether permanent implants or temporary implants are superior is again unknown, and even the optimum radioactive isotope still needs to be determined.

The role of chemotherapy added to radiation therapy is controversial as discussed above. Today, most patients with malignant glioma will receive some form of systemic therapy in addition to surgery and irradiation. FINE et al. (1993) published a meta-analysis using the results from 16 randomized clinical trials involving over 3,000 patients with malignant glioma, and comparing the survival times of irradiated patients with and without chemotherapy. The estimated increase in survival for patients treated with chemo-radiotherapy combination was 10.1% at 1 year and 8.6% at 2 years. In an early report from the Northern California Oncology Group, patients with anaplastic astrocytoma seemed to benefit from the addition of BudR, given during the course of irradiation, followed by procarbazine, CCNU, and vincristine (PCV) chemotherapy (LEVIN et al. 1995). In a recently published results of a phase III randomized trial, patients undergoing radiotherapy received also PCV with or without BudR (PRADOS et al. 1999). The authors concluded that the addition of BudR was unlikely to result in a survival benefit for patients with anaplastic glioma.

Most recently, an increasing number of patients are treated with BCNU-impregnated wafers placed in the tumor bed. These wafers slowly release the chemotherapy agent over approximately a 2-week period. Standard radiation therapy, more and more, is being administered with these wafers in place. At MCP Hahnemann University, no increased morbidity has been observed during the management of these patients (unpublished data). Their ultimate outcome is still being determined.

Also controversial is the need for either systemic corticosteroids (dexamethasone, hydrocortisone, etc.) or the use of anticonvulsants to prevent seizures. There is no absolute need in most patients to use either. Although it is true that most patients with high-grade glioma will have some cerebral edema, and that irradiation may make this worse, many patients are able to remain relatively asymptomatic. Patients can be placed on corticosteroids at any time should it become necessary. A dose of dexamethasone of between 8–16 mg per day is usually sufficient. Care must be taken to control possible adverse reactions to the steroid therapy. This includes Stevens-Johnson syndrome, hyperglycemia, peripheral edema, weight gain, proximal muscle atrophy, mood changes and striae. Patient may undergo such strong and long lasting adrenocortical suppression that a level of exogenous steroids may need to be maintained indefinitely.

18.10.2
Anaplastic Oligodendroglioma

These tumors behave similarly to malignant astrocytoma, and the treatment is almost identical. The major difference is in their chemosensitivity, especially for the lower-grade lesions which tend to be more chemosensitive. High response rates have been observed after the administration of PCV chemotherapy. Nijjar et al. (1993) published treatment results from 68 patients with oligodendroglioma, malignant oligodendroglioma and mixed oligodendroglioma. Eighty-five percent of the patients received external beam irradiation, consisting usually of 50 Gy. Five- and 10-year survival rates were 66% and 30%, respectively. Specifically, patients with malignant oligodendroglioma had a 5-year survival of 32%. Jeremic et al. (1999) published results of a phase II trial using a combination of PCV chemotherapy and irradiation in 23 adult patients with pure anaplastic oligodendroglioma or mixed anaplastic oligoastrocytoma, given post-operative radiotherapy consisting of 60 Gy given at 2.0 Gy daily fractions. Two weeks following completion of this radiotherapy, adjuvant 'modified' PCV (mPCV) was administered every 6 weeks up to six cycles or until progression occurred. The median survival time has not been attained as yet, while 2- and 5-year survival rates are 100% and 52%, respectively. They concluded that this combination was effective in the management of patients with anaplastic glioma and there was an acceptable toxicity noted. Of interest is a report on a study where 32 patients were treated for mixed oligodendroglial and astrocytic tumors with procarbazine, lomustine (CCNU), and vincristine (PCV) chemotherapy (Kim et al. 1996). Of these, 19 patients were treated prior to radiation therapy and 12 following irradiation (one patient received concurrent radio-

therapy and chemotherapy). Ninety-one percent of the 32 patients responded to the therapy. There were ten (31%) complete responses and 19 (59%) partial responses. The median time to progression was 15.4 months for all patients and 23.2 months for those with grade III tumors. The median time to progression for patients with grade III oligoastrocytoma was 13.8 months and for those with grade IV oligoastrocytoma was 12.4 months. For those with anaplastic oligodendroglioma the median time to progression was 63.4 months. These patients survived from the start of chemotherapy for a median period of 49.8, 16, and 76 months, respectively, (*P*=0.0154).

KRYITSIS et al. (1993) evaluated the treatment outcome in 17 patients with anaplastic oligodendroglioma and 17 patients with anaplastic mixed oligodendroglioma-astrocytoma. In the anaplastic oligodendroglioma group, eight patients were treated primarily with radiotherapy and adjuvant chemotherapy, and nine were treated with salvage chemotherapy at the time of recurrence. Three patients who failed primary chemo-irradiation were given salvage chemotherapy. In the initial group, there was one complete response, three partial responses, and four patients who had stable disease. All except one patient progressed within 10 months. Of the 12 patients who received chemotherapy for recurrence, there was one complete response, two partial responses, and six patients with stable disease. There was a long duration of response and survival (15–132+ months). In the anaplastic mixed oligodendroglioma-astrocytoma group, 12 patients were treated primarily and six patients were treated at the time of recurrence. The initial treatment resulted in two complete responses, three partial responses, and seven stable diseases, with most responses lasting longer than 12 months. Patients treated at the time of recurrence had one partial response and five stable disease cases, with a median time to progression of 6 months. The authors concluded that aggressive treatment is beneficial for recurrent anaplastic oligodendroglioma and mixed glioma, as well as for primarily treated mixed glioma but has only a minimal advantage over conventional radiotherapy for the initial treatment of patients with anaplastic oligodendroglioma. CAIRNCROSS et al. (1994) examined the rate and duration of response, in patients with anaplastic oligodendroglioma, to a dose-escalated combination chemotherapy regimen consisting of procarbazine, lomustine (CCNU), and vincristine (PCV). In this single-arm multicenter phase II study, patients with measurable, newly-diagnosed or recurrent, contrast-enhancing anaplastic oligoden-

drglioma were treated with up to six cycles of PCV.
Eighteen of the 24 eligible patients (75%) responded,
nine completely (38%), four had stable disease (SD),
and two progressed during the first cycle of PCV. Responses were observed in nine of ten patients (90%)
with a pre-existing low-grade oligodendroglioma
and ten of 15 (67%) with necrotic tumors. Previously
irradiated patients were as likely to respond to PCV
as those newly-diagnosed. The median time to progression was at least 25.2 months for complete responders, 14.2 months for partial responders and 6.8
months for stable patients. The authors concluded
that anaplastic oligodendroglioma is a chemosensitive tumor. Currently, RTOG 94-02 is investigating
patients treated with irradiation alone or PVC chemotherapy followed by radiation therapy after four
cycles. These results will be very helpful in determining the effectiveness of chemotherapy in this important group of tumors.

References

Barth RF, Soloway AH, Brugger RM (1996) Boron neutron
capture therapy of brain tumors: past history, current status, and future potential. Cancer Invest 14(6):534–550

Barth RF, Soloway AH, Goodman JH, Gahbauer RA, Gupta N,
Blue TE, Yang W, Tjarks W (1999) Boron neutron capture
therapy of brain tumors: an emerging therapeutic modality. Neurosurgery 44(3):433–450; discussion 450–451

Bleehen NM, Wiltshire CR, et al. (1981) A randomized study
of misonidazole and radiotherapy for Grade 3 and 4 cerebral astrocytoma. Br J Cancer 43: 436–442

Boiardi A, Silvani A, Pozzi A, Farinotti M, Fariselli L, Broggi G,
Salmaggi A (1997) Advantage of treating anaplastic gliomas with aggressive protocol combining chemotherapy
and radiotherapy. J Neurooncol 34(2):179–185

Bouchard J (1966) Radiation therapy of intracranial tumors –
long term results. Acta Radiol Ther Phys Biol. 5:11–16

Brady LW, Markoe AM, Woo DV, Rackover MA, Koprowski H,
Steplewski Z, Peyster RG (1990) Iodine125 labeled anti-
epidermal growth factor receptor-425 in the treatment of
malignant astrocytomas. A pilot study. J Neurosurg Sci.
34(3–4):243–249

Brandes AA, Fiorentino MV (1996) The role of chemotherapy
in recurrent malignant gliomas: an overview. Cancer Invest: 14 (6):551–559

Burger, PC (1987): The anatomy of Astrocytomas (editorial).
Mayo Clin Proc 62:527–529

Burger PC, Mahaley MS Jr, Dudka L, Vogel FS (1979) The
morphologic effects of radiation administered therapeutically for intracranial gliomas. Cancer 44: 1256–1272

Cairncross G, Macdonald D, Ludwin S, Lee D, Cascino T,
Buckner J, Fulton D, Dropcho E, Stewart D, Schold C Jr, et
al. (1994) Chemotherapy for anaplastic oligodendroglioma. National Cancer Institute of Canada Clinical Trials Group. J Clin Oncol 12(10):2013–2021

Cardinale RM, Schmidt-Ullrich RK, Benedict SH, Zwicker RD,
Han DC, Broaddus WC (1998) Accelerated radiotherapy regimen for malignant gliomas using stereotactic concomitant
boosts for dose escalation. Radiat Oncol Investig 6(4):175–181

Caveness WF (1977) Pathology of radiation damage to the
normal brain of the monkey. Natl Cancer Inst Monogr
46:57–76

Cho KH, Hall WA, Gerbi BJ, Higgins PD, McGuire WA, Clark
HB (1999) Single dose versus fractionated stereotactic radiotherapy for recurrent high-grade gliomas. Int J Radiat
Oncol Biol Phys 45(5):1133–1141

Chong VFH, Rumpel H, Aw YS, Ho GL, Fan YF, Chua EJ (1999)
Temporal Lobe Necrosis Following Radiation Therapy for
Nasopharyngeal Carcinoma: 1H MR Spectroscopic Findings. Int J Radiation Oncology Biol Phys 45(3): 699–705

Chung YG, Kim CY, Lee HK, Lee KC, Chu JW, Choi MS (1995)
Preliminary experiences with intraoperative radiation
therapy (IORT) for the treatment of brain tumors. J Korean Med Sci 10(6):449–452

Crosby TD, Melcher AA, Wetherall S, Brockway S, Burnet NG
(1998) A comparison of two planning techniques for radiotherapy of high grade astrocytomas. Clin Oncol (R
Coll Radiol) 10(6):392–398

Edwards MS, Wara WM, Urtasun RC, Prados M, Levin VA,
Fulton D, Wilson CB, Hannigan J, Silver P (1989)
Hyperfractionated radiation therapy for brain-stem
glioma: a phase I-II trial. J Neurosurg. 70(5):691–700

EORTC Brain Tumour Group (1978): Effect of CCNU on survival rate of objective remission and duration of free interval in patients with malignant brain glioma – final
evaluation. Eur. J. Cancer 14: 851–856

Erlich, SS and Davis, RL (1978) Spinal subarachnoid metastasis from primary intracranial glioblastoma multiforme.
Cancer 42: 2854–2864

Faillot T, Magdelenat H, Mady E, Stasiecki P, Fohanno D,
Gropp P, Poisson M, Delattre JY (1996) A phase I study of
an anti-epidermal growth factor receptor monoclonal antibody for the treatment of malignant gliomas. Neurosurgery 39(3):478–483

Fine HA, Dear KBG, Loeffler, JS, Black, PM, Canellos, GP
(1993) Meta-Analysis of Radiation Therapy With and
Without Adjuvant Chemotherapy for Malignant Gliomas
in Adults. Cancer 71: 2585–2597

Fischman AJ, Thornton AF, Frosch MP, Swearinger B,
Gonzalez RG, Alpert NM (1997) FDG hypermetabolism
associated with inflammatory necrotic changes following
radiation of meningioma. J Nucl Med. 38(7):1027–1029

Fontanesi J, Clark WC, Weir A, Barry A, Kumar P, Miller A,
Eddy T, Tai D, Kun LE (1993) Interstitial iodine 125 and
concomitant cisplatin followed by hyperfractionated external beam irradiation for malignant supratentorial
glioma. Preliminary experience at the University of Tennessee, Memphis. Am J Clin Oncol 16(5):412–417

Fountzilas G, Karavelis A, Makrantonakis P, Selviaridis P,
Tzitzikas J, Kalogera-Fountzila A, Hatzibaloglou A,
Karkavelas G, Foroglou G, Tourkanotonis (1997) Concurrent
radiation and intracarotid cisplatin infusion in malignant
gliomas: a feasibility study. Am J Clin Oncol 20(2): 138–142

Fowler JF (1984) Non-standard fractionation in radiotherapy.
Int J Radiat Oncol Biol Phys. 10(5):755–759

Freeman JE, Johnston PGB, Voke JM (1973) Somnolence after
prophylactic cranial irradiation in children with acute
lymphoblastic leukaemia. Br Med J 4: 523–525

Gaspar LE, Fisher BJ, et al. (1993) Malignant Glioma–Timing of Response to Radiation Therapy. Int J Radiat Oncol Biol Phys 25(5):877–879

Glass J, Hochberg FH, Gruber ML, Louis DN, Smith D, Rattner B. The treatment of oligodendrogliomas and mixed oligo-dendroglioma-astrocytomas with PCV chemotherapy. J Neurosurg 76(5):741–745

Groothuis DR, Vick NA (1980) Radionecrosis of the central nervous system: the perspective of the clinical neurologist and neuropathologist. In: Gilbert HA, Kagan AR (Eds), Radiation Damage to the Nervous Sustem. A Delayed Therapeutic Hazard, 93--106, Raven Press, New York

Gupta N, Vij R, Haas-Kogan DA, Israel MA, Deen DF, Morgan WF (1996) Cytogenetic damage and the radiation-induced G1-phase checkpoint. Radiat Res 145(3):289–298

Gutin PH, Prados MD, Phillips TL, Wara WM, Larson DA, Leibel SA, Sneed PK, Levin VA, Weaver KA, Silver P, et al. (1991) External irradiation followed by an interstitial high activity iodine-125 implant "boost" in the initial treatment of malignant gliomas: NCOG study 6G-82-2. Int J Radiat Oncol Biol Phys 21(3):601–606

Hall WA, Djalilian HR, Sperduto PW, Cho KH, Gerbi BJ, Gibbons JP, Rohr M, Clark HB (1995) Stereotactic radiosurgery for recurrent malignant gliomas. J Clin Oncol 13(7):1642–1648

Hatanaka, H, Nakagawa, Y (1994) Clinical Results of Long-Surviving Brain Tumor Patients Who Underwent Boron Neutron Capture Therapy. Int J Radiat Oncolo Biol Phys 28(5): 1061–1066

Hawthorne MF, Wiersema RJ, Takasugi M (1972) Preparation of tumor-specific boron compounds. 1. In vitro studies using boron-labeled antibodies and elemental boron as neutron targets. J Med Chem 15(5):449–452

Hazle JD, Jackson EF, Schomer DF, Leeds NE (1997) AJNR Am J Neuroradiol 18(9):1753–1761

Hellman R, Neuberg DS, Wagner H, Grunnet M, Robins HI, Karp D, Flynn P, Adams G (1998) A therapeutic trial of radiation therapy with Vincristine, etoposide, and Procarbazine (VVP) in high grade intracranial gliomas–an Eastern Cooperative Oncology Group Study (E2392). J Neurooncol 37(1):55–62

Hill JS, Kahl SB, Stylli SS, Nakamura Y, Koo MS, Kaye AH (1995) Selective tumor kill of cerebral glioma by photodynamic therapy using a boronated porphyrin photosensitizer. Proc Natl Acad Sci USA 92(26):12126–12130

Hopkins K, Chandler C, Bullimore J, Sandeman D, Coakham H, Kemshead JT (1995) A pilot study of the treatment of patients with recurrent malignant gliomas with intratumoral yttrium-90 radioimmunoconjugates. Radiother Oncol 34(2):121–131

Jeremic B, Shibamoto Y, Gruijicic D, Milicic B, Stojanovic M, Nikolic N, Dagovic A, Aleksandrovic J (1999) Combined treatment modality for anaplastic oligodendroglioma: a phase II study. J Neurooncol 43(2):179–185

Kelland LR, Edwards SM, Steel GG (1988) Induction and re-joining of DNA double-strand breaks in human cervix carcinoma cell lines of differing radiosensitivity. Radiat Res 116(3):526–538

Kelly PJ, Duport CD, Scheithauer BW, Kall BA and Kespert DB (1987) Stereotactic histologic correlations of computed tomography and magnetic resonance imaging-defined abnormalities in patients with glial neoplasms. Mayo Clin Proc 62;450–459

Kim L, Hochberg FH, Thornton AF, Harsh GR 4th, Patel H, Finkelstein D, Louis DN (1996) Procarbazine, lomustine, and vincristine (PCV) chemotherapy for grade III and grade IV oligoastrocytomas. J Neurosurg 85(4):602–607

Kiu MC, Chang CN, Cheng WC, Lin TK, Wong CW, Tang SG, Leung WM, Chen LH, Ho YS, Ng KT, et al. (1995) Combination chemotherapy with Carmustine and cisplatin before, during, and after radiotherapy for adult malignant gliomas. J Neurooncol 25(3):215–220

Kohler G, Milstein C (1975) Continuous cultures of fused cells secreting antibody of predefined specificity. Nature 256(5517):495–497

Kondziolka D, Flickinger JC, Bissonette DJ, Bozik M, Lunsford LD (1997) Survival benefit of stereotactic radiosurgery for patients with malignant glial neoplasms. Neurosurgery 41(4):776–783

Kyritsis AP, Yung WK, Jaeckle KA, Bruner J, Gleason MJ, Ictech SE, Flowers A, Levin VA (1996) Combination of 6-thioguanine, procarbazine, lomustine, and hydroxyurea for patients with recurrent malignant gliomas. Neurosurgery 39(5):921–926

Laperriere NJ, Leung PM, McKenzie S, Milosevic M, Wong S, Glen J, Pintilie M, Bernstein M (1998) Randomized study of brachytherapy in the initial management of patients with malignant astrocytoma. Int J Radiat Oncol Biol Phys 41(5):1005–1011

Laramore GE, Spence AM (1996) Boron neutron capture therapy (BNCT) for high-grade gliomas of the brain: a cautionary note. Int J Radiat Oncol Biol Phys 36(1):241–246

Lee SW, Fraass BA, Marsh LH, Herbort K, Gebarski SS, Martel MK, Radany EH, Lichter AS, Sandler HM (1999) Patterns of failure following high-dose 3-D conformal radiotherapy for high-grade astrocytomas: a quantitative dosimetric study. Int J Radiat Oncol Biol Phys 43(1):79–88

Levin VA, Prados MD, Wara WM, Davis RL, Gutin PH, Phillips TL, Lamborn K, Wilson CB (1995) Radiation therapy and bromodeoxyuridine chemotherapy followed by procarbazine, lomustine, and vincristine for the treatment of anaplastic gliomas. Int J Radiat Oncol Biol Phys 32:75–83

Libermann T, Nusbaum H, Razon N, Kris R, Lux I, Soreq H, Whittle M, Waterfield M, Ullrich A, Schlessinger J (1985) Amplification and overexpression of the EGF recceptor gene in primary human glioblastomas. J Cell Sci Suppl 3:161–172

Liu L, Barth RF, Adams DM, Soloway AH, Reisfeld RA (1996) Critical evaluation of bispecific antibodies as targeting agents for boron neutron capture therapy of brain tumors. Anticancer Res 16(5 A):2581–2587

Lorberboym M, Mandell LR, Mosesson RE, Germano I, Lou W, DaCosta M, Linzer DG, Machac J (1997) The role of thallium-201 uptake and retention in intracranial tumors after radiotherapy, J Nucl Med 38(2):223–226

Miyamoto C, Brady LW, Rackover M, Emrich J, Class, R, Bender H, Dadparvar S, Woo D, Young T, Eshleman J, Dilling T, Micaily B, Steplewski Z, Koprowski H, Black P, Nair S, McCormack T (1995) Utilization of 125 I Monoclonal Antibody in the Management of Primary Glioblastoma Multiforme. Radiation Oncology Investigations 3:126–132

Murray KJ, Nelson DF, Scott C, Fischbach AJ, Porter A, Farnan N, Curran WJ Jr (1995) Quality-adjusted survival analysis of malignant glioma. Patients treated with twice-daily radiation (RT) and carmustine: a report of Radiation Therapy Oncology Group (RTOG) 83-02. Int J Radiat Oncol Biol Phys 31(3):453–459

Nakagawa H, Fujita T, Kubo S, Tsuruzono K, Yamada M, Tokiyoshi K, Miyawaki Y, Kanayama T, Kadota T, Hayakawa T (1994) Selective intra-arterial chemotherapy with a combination of etoposide and cisplatin for malignant gliomas: preliminary report. Surg Neurol 41(1):19–27

Natali PG, Nicotra MR, Bigotti A, Botti C, Castellani P, Risso AM, Zardi L (1991) Comparative analysis of the expression of the extracellular matrix protein tenascin in normal human fetal, adult and tumor tissues. Int J Cancer 47(6):811–816

Nelson DF, Yuh WT, Wen BC, Ryals TJ, Cornell SH (1990) Cerebral necrosis simulating an intraparenchymal tumor. AJNR Am J Neuroradiol 11(1):211–212

Nijjar TS, Simpson WJ, Gadalla T, et al. (1993) Oligodendroglioma: the Princess Margaret Hospital experience (1958–1984). Cancer 71:4002–4006

Ortiz de Urbina D, Santos M, Garcia-Berrocal I, Bustos JC, Samblas J, Gutierrez-Diaz JA, Delgado JM, Donckaster G, Calvo FA (1995) Intraoperative radiation therapy in malignant glioma: early clinical results. Neurol Res 17(4):289–294

Ostertag CB, Kreth FW (1992) Iodine-125 interstitial irradiation for cerebral gliomas. Acta Neurochir (Wien) 119(1–4):53–61

Packer RJ, Siegel KR, Schut L, Gruce DA, Sutton LN and Litmann P (1985) Central nervous system spread of childhood brain tumors at diagnosis or at initial disease recurrence, Concepts Pediatr. Neurosurg 6:16–24

Patchell RA, Yaes RJ, Beach L, Kryscio RJ, Davis DG, Tibbs PA, Young B (1997) A phase I trial of neutron brachytherapy for the treatment of malignant gliomas. Br J Radiol 70(839):1162–1168

Patel K, Rossell RJ, Pemberton LF, Cheung NK, Walsh FS, Moore SE, Sugimoto T, Kemshead JT (1989) Monoclonal antibody 3F8 recognizes the neural cell adhesion molecule (NCAM) in addition to the ganglioside GD2. Br J Cancer 60(6):861–866

Peters LJ, Withers HR, Thames HD Jr, Fletcher GH (1982) Tumor radioresistance in clinical radiotherapy. Int J Radiat Oncol Biol Phys 8(1):101–108

Prados MD, Larson DA, Lamborn K, McDermott MW, Sneed PK, Wara WM, Chang SM, Mack EE, Krouwer HG, Chandler KL, Warnick RE, Davis RL, Rabbitt JE, Malec M, Levin VA, Gutin PH, Phillips TL, Wilson CB (1998) Radiation therapy and hydroxyurea followed by the combination of 6-thioguanine and BCNU for the treatment of primary malignant brain tumors. Int J Radiat Oncol Biol Phys 40(1):57–63

Prados MD, Scott C, Sandler H, Buckner JC, Phillips T, Schultz C, Uratsun R, Davis R, Gutin P, Cascino TL, Greenberg HS, Curran WJ (1999) A phase 3 randomized study of radiotherapy plus Procarbazine, CCNU, and Vincristine (PVC) with or without BudR for the treatment of anaplastic astocytoma: a preliminary report of RTOG 9404. Int. J. Radiation Oncology Biol Phys 45(5):1109–1115

Press OW, Vitetta ES, Farr AG, Hansen JA, Martin PJ (1986) Evaluation of ricin A-chain immunotoxins directed against human T cells. Cell Immunol 102(1):10–20

Rajkumar SV, Buckner JC, Schomberg PJ, Pitot HC 4th, Ingle JN, Cascino TL (1999) Phase I evaluation of preirradiation chemotherapy with carmustine and cisplatin and accelerated radiation therapy in patients with high-grade gliomas. Neurosurgery 44(1):67–73

Reifenberger G, Prior R, Deckert M, Wechsler W (1989) Epidermal growth factor receptor expression and growth fraction in human tumours of the nervous system. Virchows Arch A Pathol Anat Histopathol 414(2):147–155

Ricci PE, Karis JP, Heiserman JE, Fram EK, Bice AN, Drayer BP (1998) Differentiating recurrent tumor from radiation necrosis: time for re-evaluation of positron emission tomography? AJNR Am J Neuroradiol 19(3):407–413

Salazar OM and Rubin P (1976) The spread of glioblastoma multiforme as a determining factor in the radiation treated volume. Int J Radiat Oncol Biol Phys1:627–637

Sarkaria JN, Mehta MP, Loeffler JS, Buatti JM, Chappell RJ, Levin AB, Alexander E rd, Friedman WA, Kinsella TJ (1995) Radiosurgery in the initial management of malignant gliomas: survival comparison with the RTOG recursive partitioning analysis. Radiation Therapy Oncology Group. Int J Radiat Oncol Biol Phys 32(4):931–941

Scharfen CO, Sneed PK, Wara WM, Larson DA, Phillips TL, Prados MD, Weaver KA, Malec M, Acord P, Lamborn KR, et al. (1992) High activity iodine-125 interstitial implant for gliomas. Int J Radiat Oncol Biol Phys 24(4):583–591

Schupak K, Malkin M, Anderson L, Arbit E, Lindsley K, Leibel S (1995) The relationship between the technical accuracy of stereotactic interstitial implantation for high grade gliomas and the pattern of tumor recurrence. Int J Radiat Oncol Biol Phys 32(4):1167–1176

Schwartz JL, Rotmensch J, Giovanazzi S, Cohen MB, Weichselbaum RR (1988) Faster repair of DNA double-strand breaks in radioresistant human tumor cells. Int J Radiat Oncol Biol Phys 15(4):907–912

Scheibel RS, Meyers CA, Levin VA (1996) Cognitive dysfunction following surgery for intracerebral glioma: influence of histopathology, lesion location, and treatment. J Neurooncol 30(1):61–69

Shibamoto Y, Nishimura Y, Tsutsui K, Sasai K, Takahashi M, Abe M (1997) Comparison of accelerated hyperfractionated radiotherapy and conventional radiotherapy for supratentorial malignant glioma. Jpn J Clin Oncol 27(1):31–36

Shibamoto Y, Yamashita J, Takahashi M, Abe M (1994) Intraoperative radiation therapy for braintumors with emphasis on retreatment for recurrence following full-dose external beam irradiation. Am J Clin Oncol 17(5):396–399

Sheline GE, Wara WM, Smith V (1980) Therapeutic irradiation and brain injury. Int J Radiat Oncol Biol Phys 6(9):1215–1228

Shrieve DC, Alexander E 3rd, Black PM, Wen PY, Fine HA, Kooy HM, Loeffler JS (1999) Treatment of patients with primary glioblastoma multiforme with standard post-operative radiotherapy and radiosurgical boost: prognostic factors and long-term outcome. J Neurosurg 90(1):72–77

Silverstein MD, Cascino TL, Harmsen WS (1996) High-grade astrocytomas: resource use, clinical outcomes, and cost of care. Mayo Clin Proc 71(10):936–944

Sipos EP, Tyler B, Piantoadosi S, Burger PC, Brem H (1997) Optimizing interstitial delivery of BCNU from controlled release polymers for the treatment of brain tumors. Cancer Chemothera Pharmacol 39(5):383–389

Sneed PK, Gutin PH, Larson DA, Malec MK, Phillips TL, Prados MD, Scharfen CO, Weaver KA, Wara WM (1994) Patterns of recurrence of glioblastoma multiforme after external irradiation followed by implant boost. Int J Radiat Oncol Biol Phys 29(4):719–727

Thames HD, Schultheiss TE, Hendry JH, Tucker SL, Dubray BM, Brock WA (1992) Can modest escalations of dose be detected as increased tumor control? Int J Radiat Oncol Biol Phys 22(2):241–246

Valtonen S, Timonen U, Toivanen P, Kalimo H, Kivipelto L, Heiskanen O, Unsgaard G, Kuurne T (1997) Interstitial chemotherapy with carmustine-loaded polymers for high-grade gliomas: a randomized double-blind study. Neurosurgery41(1):44–48; discussion 48–49

Van Tassel P, Bruner JM, Maor MH, Leeds NE, Gleason MJ, Yung WK, Levin VA (1995) MR of toxic effects of accelerated fractionation radiation therapy and carboplatin chemotherapy for malignant gliomas. AJNR Am J Neuroradiol 16(4):715–726

Waldman T, Zhang Y, Dillehay L, Yu J, Kinzler K, Vogelstein B, Williams J (1997) Cell-cycle arrest versus cell death in cancer therapy. Nat Med 3(9):1034–1036

Walker MD, Alexander E Jr, Hunt WE, MacCarty CSW, Mahaley MS, Mealey J, Norrel HA, Owens G, Ransohoff J, Wilson CB, Gehan EA, Strike A (1978): Evaluation of BCNU and/or radiotherapy in the treatment of anaplastic gliomas. A cooperative clinical trail. J Neurosurg 49: 333–343

Walker MD, Green SB, Byar DP, Alexander E, Batzdorf U, Brooks WH, Hunt WE, MacCarty CS, Mahaley MS, Healey J, Owens G, Ransohoff J, Robertson JT, Shapiro WR, Smith KR, Wilson CB, Strike TA (1980) Randomized comparisons of radiotherapy and nitrosoureas for the treatment of malignant glioma after surgery. N Engl J Med 303(23):1323–1329

Wang CC (1988) Local control of oropharyngeal carcinoma after two accelerated hyperfractionation radiation therapy schemes. Int J Radiat Oncol Biol Phys14(6):1143–1146

Wlodek D, Hittelman WN (1987) The repair of double-strand DNA breaks correlates with radiosensitivity of L5178Y-S and L5178Y-R cells. Radiat Res 112(1):146–155

19 The Role of Stereotactic Radiosurgery in the Management of Primary Brain Tumors

David Huang, Joseph Chen, Cheng Yu, and Zbigniew Petrovich

CONTENTS

D. Huang, MD
Senior Resident, Department of Radiation Oncology, University of Southern California School of Medicine, 1441 Eastlake Avenue G34, Los Angeles, CA 90033, USA
J. Chen, MD, PhD
Fellow, Department of Neurosurgery, University of Southern California School of Medicine, 1441 Eastlake Avenue, Los Angeles, CA 90033, USA
C. Yu, PhD
Assistant Professor, Department of Radiation Oncology-Physics, University of Southern California School of Medicine, 1441 Eastlake Avenue, Los Angeles, CA 90033, USA
Z. Petrovich, MD
Professor and Chairman, Department of Radiation Oncology, University of Southern California School of Medicine, 1441 Eastlake Avenue G34, Los Angeles, CA 90033, USA

19.1 Introduction

Stereotactic radiosurgery (SRS) is a sophisticated form of radiotherapy that usually delivers a large single-fraction dose of irradiation to small, well-defined intracranial targets. This is accomplished with a high degree of accuracy (± 1 mm). Stereotactic guidance is provided by the use of modern imaging modalities, notably computed tomography (CT), magnetic resonance imaging (MRI), or cerebral angiography. Noninvasive, bloodless delivery of a tumoricidal dose to a selected intracranial target-volume, with concurrent sparing of adjacent normal tissue, can be accomplished by various modalities, but is generally done by the cross-firing of photon radiation-beams through a precise target point from different angles, based on stereotactic localization with the aforementioned imaging techniques.

The technique of SRS was introduced to clinical practice by a Swedish neurosurgeon, Lars Leksell, in the 1950s (Leksell 1951). Over the past half-century, the technology has evolved and the indications for its use have expanded (Leksell 1983; Lunsford et al. 1993; Backlund 1992). Its roots in the neurosurgical management of functional disorders, including trigeminal neuralgia, behavior and movement disorders, which were the initial interests of Leksell, have now led to the branching out to the therapy of various multiple benign and malignant lesions. Vascular lesions such as arteriovenous malformations (AVMs) were common indications for radiosurgery through the early 1980s and 1990s, but they have been recently overshadowed by the increasing use of radiosurgery for tumor ablation, which has now become the most common use for SRS.

The size limitation imposed on SRS allows for the treatment of relatively small, noninvasive, circumscribed lesions, generally less than 35 mm in greatest dimension. Candidates include patients with small primary benign and malignant brain tumors and metastatic lesions (see Chap. 21 for details on the management of metastatic tumors).

Stereotactic radiosurgery is a technique which provides, in carefully selected patients, a viable alternative to craniotomy. Patients with lesions that are not readily accessible to conventional neurosurgical procedures or with poor surgical risk may benefit from this type of treatment. It is recommended that the use of SRS should be limited to only major medical centers with an experienced multidisciplinary team. This is required for optimal treatment outcome and safety. Such a team should include:

- A neurosurgeon with special expertise in stereotaxy
- A radiation oncologist
- A radiation physicist
- A neuroradiologist
- A neuropathologist
- A neuroanesthesiologist
- Specially trained nurses and radiation therapy technologists

Evaluation of patients should be done by this team, with careful selection of patients to fit criteria of medical indication, lesion size, and probability of benefit from such labor-intensive treatment.

19.2
History

In 1949, a prototype stereotactic guiding device was developed (Leksell 1949). Subsequently, in 1951, Leksell introduced a term of radiosurgery for such a stereotactic guidance technique (Leksell 1951). He was able to couple an orthovoltage X-ray tube (300 kVp) to a semicircular stereotactic frame and rotate this tube along an arc around a point target. The treatment of this target was accomplished via multiple small, stationary portals. The initial report on the use of radiosurgery described the relief of pain in patients receiving the treatment for trigeminal neuralgia, through the point irradiation of the gasserian ganglion.

19.2.1
Particle-Beam SRS

Throughout the 1950s and 1960s, Leksell and his radiobiologist associate Borje Larsson experimented with the use of proton beams for neuroradiosurgery (Larsson 1962; Larsson and Leksell 1968). Others were interested in such charged-particle radiotherapy, which had the characteristic of the Bragg peak that potentially delivers high radiation doses to a point with a rapid falloff distally. The physics of this is discussed in further detail in Chap. 6. During the same period, others were conducting clinical experiments with particle-beams in the United States at Harvard and Berkeley, as well as in the Soviet Union (Kirn 1988). Raymond Kjellberg began the SRS program using the Harvard cyclotron in 1962 (Kjellberg et al. 1983). They reported very good clinical results in a large number of patients treated with a 160 MeV proton beam. Because of the very high cost of building such facilities, particle-beam centers for SRS are few around the world.

19.2.2
Gamma Knife

Leksell and Larsson eventually developed a dedicated SRS device called a "gamma knife" in 1968 (Leksell 1968; Backlund 1992). The prototype consisted of 179 sources of cobalt-60 radioisotope. The gamma rays from the cobalt-60 provided greater penetration and better skin sparing characteristics than the previously used orthovoltage X-rays. The beams from the multiple sources are collimated to point towards a common intersection, so that there is a three-dimensional dose-distribution about this isocenter. The first gamma knife procedure was performed on a patient with craniopharyngioma in 1968. However, Leksell's original priority in indications focused on functional disorders, such as intractable pain (Backlund 1992). This gamma unit model eventually evolved into the modern gamma knife which uses 201 cobalt sources (see Chap. 6 for relevant details).

Imaging advances along with computer hardware and software development in the 1970s and 1980s paved the way for modern high quality images from CT and MRI scans. The ability to compile data from multiple image planes has allowed the reconstruction of images in three-dimensions. Volumes of objects of interest could be localized more accurately than with previous two-dimensional imaging techniques. Along with this evolution of imaging and computer technology, the gamma knife was redesigned as well, based on the original 1968, 179-source model. Production and use of the modern gamma knife, which uses 201 cobalt sources, expanded in the 1980s. In 1991, there were 17 gamma knife units in use worldwide. By December 1998, there were 114 such units, which corresponded to the expanding indications for the use of SRS.

19.2.3
Linear Accelerator-Based SRS

In the 1980s, standard radiotherapy linear accelerators were modified for use in SRS (Colombo et al. 1985). The first report on this was by Betti and Derechinsky (1983) in France. Linear accelerator-generated X-rays are directed at a target isocenter with several moving arcs at different angles. Throughout the past decade, as the most financially affordable type of radiosurgery facility, the use of linear accelerator-based SRS has expanded to several hundred facilities worldwide, and is the most common type of SRS system (see Chap. 6). However, many of these systems are not necessarily a part of dedicated SRS centers.

19.3
Radiobiological Considerations

19.3.1
Single High-Dose Fraction Effect

Radiobiological issues are covered in detail in chapter 4. However, there are certain issues pertaining specifically to radiosurgery that are briefly readdressed here.

The principle behind SRS is the delivery of large doses of radiation in a single fraction to relatively small lesions, usually in or near the brain. Radiobiologically, the large single fractions of radiation have a greater damaging effect in the slow-growing, late-responding tissues (Hall and Brenner 1993). This is contrasted with its lesser effect on rapidly growing, early-responding tissues. Examples of tumors of late-responding tissues which are considered to be radiobiologically ideal for SRS are acoustic neuromas, meningiomas, and pituitary adenomas. Arteriovenous malformations are also considered to be such tissues, and have had a long history of being successfully controlled by SRS (Scheneider et al. 1997). The effects of SRS are to stop the growth of these tumors and subsequently to decrease their size.

Low-dose multiple fraction radiotherapy, as with conventional radiotherapy, has a different effect radiobiologically (Hall and Brenner 1993). With fractionated radiotherapy, there is more of a damaging effect to early-responding tissues such as malignant tumors, and less of an effect on late-responding tissues. According to Hall's radiobiological data, the use of single-fraction treatment is useful for some tumors but probably not as useful for others. Hall believed that SRS was useful for benign tumors and AVMs but questioned its use for the treatment of malignant tumors.

Larson described four categories of radiosurgical targets based on the radiobiological effects of the abnormal and normal tissues within the target (Larson et al. 1993). These categories attempted to define the appropriateness of radiosurgical management based on the target composition and the radiobiological effects.

Category I includes abnormal and normal tissues which are both late-responders to radiation. An example of this is AVM, in which the abnormal tissue is embedded within normal tissue. High-dose fractions have a large effect on both tissues. Category II includes abnormal tissues which are late-responders, but without normal tissues within the target volume. An example is meningioma, which is generally a well-circumscribed tumor. The large radiobiological effect would affect only the tumor and not the surrounding brain. Category III consists of early-responding abnormal tissues, and late-responding normal tissues. An example is low-grade glioma. The normal tissues experience a larger effect than abnormal tissues, and single-fraction radiosurgery may be suboptimal treatment. Fractionated regimens may be more beneficial. Category IV consists of early-responding abnormal tissues, but with no normal tissues within the target. Examples would be metastatic carcinomas or high-grade gliomas. The abnormal tissue would experience a moderately large effect. This suggests that fractionated radiotherapy may be preferable, since the tumor cells become more radiosensitive with reoxygenation and redistribution within the cell cycle between fractions (Larson et al. 1993).

19.3.2
Complications

The dose limitations imposed on SRS are due to the risks of toxicity, including brain necrosis and cranial neuropathy. Such toxicity depends on the total radiation dose, the region of the brain treated, the volume of tissue irradiated, and the fractionation scheme.

A Radiation Therapy Oncology Group (RTOG), study 90–05, examined this in a phase I dose escalation trial, which established maximum tolerable doses for various tumor diameters. Maximum tolerable doses for tumors with diameters of less or equal to 20 mm, 21–30 mm, and 31–40 mm were 21 Gy, 18 Gy, and 15 Gy, respectively (Shaw et al. 1996).

Immediate side effects due to stereotactic radiotherapy and radiosurgery were studied in 78 patients treated with a linear accelerator (Werner-Wasik et al. 1999). A total of 27 (35%) patients experienced side effects within the first 2 weeks after the procedure. Most of these were mild, usually nausea, dizziness/vertigo, seizures, or new headaches. There were two episodes of worsening neurological deficit and two of orbital pain which were considered moderate. Such side effects occurred less in those taking corticosteroids prophylactically. These side effects were all self-limited.

Major complications of SRS in properly selected patients are uncommon. Such problems may include necrosis and edema which may be manifested as increased intracranial pressure, increased seizure frequency, and focal neurological deficits (most commonly motor weakness). Complications were analyzed by the Harvard Group who identified important variables predicting a higher incidence of complications in patients treated with linear accelerator-based SRS (Nedzi et al. 1991). These were:
- tumor dose inhomogeneity ($P<0.00001$)
- maximum tumor dose ($P<0.00002$)
- number of isocenters ($P<0.00002$)
- maximum normal tissue dose ($P<0.00005$)
- tumor volume ($P<0.0001$)

The authors concluded that SRS is associated with a low incidence of complications in patients with the following tumor and treatment parameters:
- treatment volume <10 cc
- the use of a single isocenter
- maximum tumor dose <25 Gy
- tumor dose inhomogeneity <10 Gy

Fewer than a third of the patients treated with SRS exhibit late complications, manifested by evidence of local edema on imaging. This can appear as a low-density area on CT imaging, and high-signal area on T2-weighted MR images. About 75% of patients with these findings remain clinically asymptomatic. In the remaining quarter of patients, neurological symptoms may occur, but respond quite well with simple medical management. Symptoms may occur between 3 and 18 months (mean 10 months) post-treatment. Resolution occurs within 6 to 12 months in most patients (Hall 1995).

Cranial nerve neuropathies may occur as a result of radiosurgery, particularly in view of an increased use of SRS for the treatment of cavernous sinus and pituitary lesions. The optic nerves and chiasm are particularly sensitive to radiation damage, which may result in the devastating sequel of vision loss. Fractionated radiotherapy with greater than 2.2 Gy per day to the optic chiasm results in a higher incidence of chiasm damage than do lower doses (Aristizabal et al. 1977). Larger, single fractions of radiosurgery greater than 8 to 10 Gy may likewise cause such injury, so cautious planning to avoid overdose to this area should be undertaken (Tishler et al. 1993).

Other cranial nerves may also be damaged, especially if previous external beam irradiation has already been given. Otherwise, they generally have a greater tolerance to SRS. Treatment of acoustic neuromas have been reported to cause neuropathies in cranial nerves V and VII in 5–15% of patients, but most of these are self limited and resolve within 12 months.

19.4
Technical Considerations

The process of SRS involves the initial placement of a ring-like stereotactic headframe on the skull. This will establish a three-dimensional coordinate system with highly accurate fiducial landmarks. After placement of this device, neuroimaging is obtained with CT, MRI, or in the case of AVMs, also with cerebral angiography. The intracranial targets can be identified and localized accurately on an X,Y,Z coordinate system with respect to the stereotactic frame (Verhey and Smith 1995). The target-volume is outlined and prescribed a dose of radiation. The treatment planning software calculates how the machine will deliver this prescribed dose. The patient is brought to the SRS suite and the headframe is immobilized with respect to the treatment machine. Once the treatment plan and prescription are finished, and the patient is precisely positioned, the treatment may be delivered. As there is a known relationship between the radiation source and this three-dimensional coordinate system, accurate delivery of radiation to the planned target is achieved.

19.5
Radiosurgical Systems

A radiosurgical system consists of a stereotactic frame, a radiation delivery system, treatment planning computer hardware and software, and an imaging system. There are currently three general methods by which SRS is delivered: gamma knife, modified linear accelerator, and proton beam. Details of the physical properties of each system are described in chapter 6 of this text. Each system contains these components and produces similar outcomes.

19.5.1
Gamma Knife

Leksell originally developed the gamma knife in 1968 at the Karolinska Institute in Stockholm, Sweden. The basic design of this device has remained unchanged over the past three decades, and consists of a large metallic hemisphere which houses 201 radioactive Co-60 sources. The sources are positioned radially, and produce beams which point at the same target (isocenter) located in space within the metallic hemisphere, equidistantly 40 cm from the source positions. The target accuracy is 0.1 mm.

Several financial drawbacks are associated with the gamma knife system. One is the initial capital investment required for a device dedicated only to SRS, amounting to approximately $3.5 million, along with maintenance costs, including the required replacement of the 201 cobalt sources every 5 years. However, a major benefit of a dedicated SRS system is available. At the end of 1998, there were 114 gamma knife facilities worldwide.

19.5.2
Linear Accelerator-Based Systems

Linear accelerators can be modified for SRS at a fraction of the cost of purchasing a new gamma knife unit. Financially, this is a much more affordable alternative, even with the purchase of a new linear accelerator. It provides a target size of 10 to 50 mm, which can be obtained, with an accuracy of 0.1 to 1 mm. Radiation delivery entails the use of dynamic moving portals during treatment. During treatment, the gantry is rotated through an arc around a target isocenter for each of several stationary couch angles (see Chap. 6 for details). Other techniques involve moving the couch simultaneously with the gantry arc rotation, for "dynamic" SRS to avoid overlap by the entrance and exit beams, and the use of a rotating chair with a stationary radiation beam. These systems are not necessarily dedicated, as the linear accelerators may still be utilized for other types of radiotherapy.

19.5.3
Particle-Beam Radiosurgery

The Bragg peak principle allows for an intense power deposition within the precisely defined target-volume for particle-beam radiosurgery. This principle may substantially decrease radiation dose outside the target-volume (LYMAN et al. 1986; PHILLIPS et al. 1990). Also, the radiobiological effect of proton beam therapy may be slightly greater than that of photons (URANO et al. 1983). However, the extremely high cost of building the necessary facility is about fifteen times that of a gamma knife and a hundred times that of a linear accelerator system.

The three modalities of SRS have been compared by several authors (LUXTON et al. 1993). The authors concluded that there may be physical and biological advantages to proton radiosurgery which may be useful with larger lesions, but these have not yet been demonstrated clinically. Equally effective clinically are gamma knife and linear accelerator-based photon systems, although the linear accelerator may have an advantage in terms of flexibility and individualized beam control as well as the lowest financial cost. Some investigators (VERHEY et al. 1998) found that proton beams had some dose distribution advantages for large and peripheral tumors, and that gamma knife was the most successful for conforming to highly irregular shapes.

19.6
Trends

Much of the reported earlier experience with SRS has been with the treatment of vascular malformations, due to the ability to image vascular lesions with angiography, which had been available prior to CT or MRI imaging techniques. However, with the advent of these imaging technologies and advancement in computer hardware and software, the accurate localization of benign and malignant tumors has permitted radiosurgical treatment of these entities. Up to the early 1990s, AVMs were the predominant lesions treated, with extensive experience supporting their indication. Obliteration of such lesions occurs in greater than 80% of cases treated with SRS (FRIEDMAN and BOVA 1992; LUNSFORD et al 1993). Some data supported the treatment of a few types of benign tumors such as pituitary adenomas and acoustic neuromas (LEKSELL 1983). Unfortunately, the early available retrospective data did not support the treating of other types of lesions. However, in the past decade, the use of radiosurgery for other lesions has been evolving, and there is now a greater number of data supporting indications for management of benign and malignant tumors, both primary and metastatic.

Tables 19.1 through 19.4 demonstrate data on gamma knife treatments, from most of the known dedicated centers worldwide. Of the 114 units at 112 sites, 91 centers reported data. These data were compiled by the Leksell Gamma Knife Society and provide some insight into the trends of this principal SRS modality. Because the gamma knife is provided by a single supplier, Elekta Systems, data are easier to obtain than with other treatment modalities, whose

systems are varied and less organized. Particle-beam and linear accelerator data have not been compiled in the same way.

In the past decade, there has been an obvious, exponential increase in the number of facilities offering gamma knife treatment, as well as in the number of patients treated. Table 19.1 illustrates this sharp increase well, with about 20% of the total number of gamma knife patients being treated in each of the past few years. In 1996, 17.7% (17,666 of 99,981) of the total number of gamma knife patients were treated. In 1997, 20.4% (20,395 of 99,981) were treated, and in 1998, 21.5% (21,520 of 99,981) were treated. By 1990, only 4,710 patients had been treated with gamma knife at 13 sites. By 1994, 26,673 patients had been treated at 56 sites. The total number of patients treated since 1968 approached 100,000 at 112 sites in 1998. Table 19.2 describes the cumulative indications for the use of gamma knife for vascular disorders, benign and malignant tumors, and functional disorders. Of all patients treated, 74% have had tumors, about half of which are benign, the other half malignant. This is in contrast to earlier in the last decade, when tumors were uncommonly treated.

Tables 19.3 and 19.4, respectively, display the breakdown of types of benign and malignant tumors treated with radiosurgery. The most common benign tumors treated have been acoustic neuromas, meningiomas, and pituitary tumors. The most common malignant tumors treated have been brain metastases, which constitute nearly two-thirds of cancer indications (see Chap. 21 for details). Malignant gliomas in recent years have also been commonly treated with SRS.

Table 19.1. Distribution of patients, by treatment-year, from 1968 to 1998[a]

Period	Number of patients	%	Number of medical centers
1968–1986	1,320	1.3	2
1987	370	0.4	5
1988	500	0.5	5
1989	950	1.0	10
1990	1,570	1.6	13
1991	2,268	2.3	22
1992	4,326	4.3	32
1993	5,437	5.4	46
1994	9,932	9.9	56
1995	13,727	13.7	70
1996	17,666	17.7	78
1997	20,395	20.4	89
1998	21,520	21.5	112
Total	99,981	100.0	112

[a]Modified from data provided by Leksell Gamma Knife Society, Elekta Radiosurgery, Atlanta, Georgia, USA.

Table 19.2. Distribution, by treatment indication, of patients treated with gamma knife 1968–1998[a]

Indication for therapy	Number of patients	%
Vascular lesions	21,064	21.1
Total tumors	74,115	74.1
Benign tumors	38,147	38.1
Malignant tumors	35,968	36.0
Functional disorders	4,802	4.8
Total	99,981	100.0

[a]Modified from data provided by Leksell Gamma Knife Society, Elekta Radiosurgery, Atlanta, Georgia, USA.

19.7
Clinical Results

Radiosurgery has become an increasingly popular treatment modality for the management of both benign and malignant tumors, as evidenced by the above data. Generally, for benign tumors, surgical resection is attempted, although, in some instances it may be difficult due to anatomic constraints, and risks to morbidity and mortality. Radiosurgery is generally indicated for residual disease, recurrent disease, medically inoperable patients, elderly patients, or those who refuse surgery.

The majority of malignant tumors treated with SRS are metastases. The other principle type of cancerous lesion treated is glioma. Historically, because of the tumor's infiltrative and microscopic nature, radiobiological considerations, high cost, and questionable benefit of radiosurgical treatment, SRS was not considered to be an option for such tumors. Evidence has accumulated to suggest that SRS may play an important part in the management of selected patients with malignant gliomas (SHRIEVE et al. 1999). Increased tumor dose to gliomas, delivered by SRS or interstitial brachytherapy, may stave off tumor growth for a period of time, to delay progression of disease (LOEFFLER et al. 1992; SHRIEVE et al. 1995; KONDZIOLKA et al. 1997; SHRIEVE et al. 1999). The other malignant tumors are rare and are not covered in this text.

Table 19.3. Distribution of gamma knife patients with benign tumors[a]

Tumor	Number of patients	% Of benign tumors	% Of all tumors
Acoustic neuroma	10,138	26.6	13.7
Meningioma	12,643	33.1	17.1
Pituitary	9,790	25.7	13.2
Pineal	1,391	3.6	1.9
Craniopharyngioma	1,296	3.4	1.7
Hemangioblastoma	544	1.4	0.7
Chordoma	586	1.5	0.8
Trigeminal Neuroma	598	1.6	0.8
Schwannoma	534	1.4	0.7
Other	627	1.6	0.8
Total benign	38,147	100	51.5
Total tumors	74,115	–	100

[a]Modified from data provided by Leksell Gamma Knife Society, Elekta Radiosurgery, Atlanta, Georgia, USA.

Table 19.4. Distribution of patients with malignant tumors[a]

Tumor	Number of patients	% Of malignant tumors	% Of all tumors
Metastasis	23,712	65.9	32.0
Glial	9,509	26.4	12.8
Chondrosarcoma	120	0.3	0.2
Glomus	302	0.8	0.4
Ocular melanoma	441	1.2	0.6
NPH carcinoma	550	1.5	0.7
Hemangiopericytoma	369	1.0	0.5
Other	965	2.7	1.3
Total malignant	35,968	100	48.5
Total tumors	74,115	–	100

[a]Modified from data provided by Leksell Gamma Knife Society, Elekta Radiosurgery, Atlanta, Georgia, USA.

19.7.1
Pituitary Tumors

The principle means of treatment of pituitary adenomas remains transsphenoidal surgery, as only this modality is able to accomplish an immediate relief of symptoms due to compression of adjacent structures or hypersecretion of hormones (see Chap. 8). Irradiation has a delayed effect, and clinical problems that require immediate results (such as with compression of the optic nerves or chiasm by tumor mass) are not appropriate for such therapy. However, conventional radiotherapy of 45–50 Gy with 1.8 Gy fractions daily, has historically been used in the adjuvant setting for recurrent or residual tumor, or as definitive therapy for those who are medically inoperable or refuse to have surgery (see Chaps. 8 and 9 for details). Stereotactic radiosurgery is another treatment option which has become more popular in recent years as the technology and treatment outcomes have become more widely available. It reportedly controls pituitary hypersecretion more rapidly than does conventional radiotherapy and also diminishes the amount of irradiation to normal structures (JACKSON and NOREN 1999). It may also be used to ablate tumors with invasion into the cavernous sinus. Unsatisfactory control of hormonal secretion by microsurgical management has led to the increased use of adjuvant SRS.

Pituitary adenomas were among the first tumors to be treated with SRS (BACKLUND 1992). Since the 1950s, a handful of centers, Harvard, Berkeley, Moscow, and St. Petersburg, utilized charged-particle beams for pituitary irradiation for adenomas, as well as for conditions responsive to pituitary suppression (LEVY et al. 1993; KJELLBERG et al. 1968; KJELLBERG and ABBE; 1988). Kjellberg's series from Harvard University has been the largest reported on the treatment of patients with pituitary tumors. Leksell's gamma knife series also included this indication among the initial group of patients treated. Stereotactic radiosurgery has been used for the treatment of such tumors as acromegaly, Cushing's disease, prolactinoma, Nelson's syndrome, and nonsecreting tumors. Successful radiation hypophysectomy was achieved in patients at these and other centers, for the management of both secreting and nonsecreting adenomas as SRS has gained in worldwide popularity. As of 1998, a quarter of the benign tumors that have been treated with gamma knife have been pituitary adenomas.

Kjellberg's series utilizing proton beam, at Harvard University, showed clinical improvement of acromegaly in 90% of 600 patients at 24 months, with 60% of patients achieving normalized hormone levels (KJELLBERG and KLIMAN 1979). Linfoot also reported successful outcomes with the use of helium-particle irradiation at Berkeley, in which a cohort of 65 patients with residual or recurrent pituitary adenoma with excess growth hormone was treated with SRS (LINFOOT 1979). Hormone levels normalized in 30% of patients within 2 years, 68% of patients within 6 years, and 95% of patients within 8 years. Another group used gamma knife for the management of acromegaly (THOREN et al. 1991). The authors used a dose of 40-70 Gy for up to three treatments as a definitive therapy while 30–50 Gy was given to those patients who received prior external beam radiotherapy. With follow up of 1 to 21 years, clinical improvement was demonstrated in 48% of patients, whereas 52% of patients showed no change.

Control of Cushing's disease has been successful as well. Kjellberg's series with proton beam use on such patients resulted in 85% clinical improvement, and only 15% without response (KJELLBERG and KLIMAN 1979). Linfoot's series at Berkeley also reported significant clinical and biochemical improvement in 89% of 83 patients treated (LINFOOT 1979). A report of gamma knife results in 39 patients from the University of Virginia demonstrated a 58% remission rate at 1 year following SRS (LAWS and VANCE 1999).

Stereotactic radiosurgery has also had success in the control of nonsecreting adenomas. The greater effect is the halting of further growth, although in some cases, the tumor has decreased in size. A report from the University of Virginia on the follow up of a series of nine patients with such tumors, showed that two adenomas decreased in size, six remained stable, and in one patient, treatment failed with resulting increase in the tumor size (STEINER et al. 1988).

Stereotactic radiosurgery has an important role in treating patients with Nelson's syndrome and prolactinomas. Successful treatment outcomes were reported by the Berkeley group, with the use of particle-beam SRS (LINFOOT 1979). Nearly all patients had significant decrease of hormone levels, in both diseases. The University of Virginia group was less encouraged with their results with gamma knife, with only one in 13 patients in remission after SRS treatment for prolactinoma, and with one in nine patients in remission after SRS for Nelson's syndrome (STEINER et al. 1998).

The potential complications that may result from high-dose single fraction radiosurgery is of particular concern in pituitary tumors. The optic chiasm and optic nerves are very sensitive to high radiation doses, and visual field deficits and visual loss may ensue. Also, other vital structures, including the contents of the cavernous sinus, such as the cranial nerves III, IV, VI and the carotid artery, and surrounding brain parenchyma are nearby, and subject to toxicity such as radionecrosis. Care in treatment planning is required to minimize the probability of treatment complications. Treatment plans should encompass the tumor tightly with the prescribed radiation isodose line which excludes optic chiasm and optic nerves. In general, patients selected for SRS should have a tumor to chiasm distance of no less than 5 mm. Those with adenoma in a closer proximity to the chiasm should be considered for conformal fractionated external beam radiotherapy. At the University of Southern California (USC), we generally limit our doses to the optic chiasm to 8 Gy and no more than 10 Gy to the optic nerve, while the dose to the adenoma is 15 Gy prescribed to the 50% isodose line.

19.7.2
Craniopharyngiomas

Craniopharyngiomas are slow-growing suprasellar tumors which may compress the optic chiasm, pituitary, the third ventricle, and surrounding brain. The main treatment in the management of craniopharyngiomas is surgical resection, although complete resection has been a difficult goal to achieve without risking significant morbidity with respect to endocrine and visual function (see Chap. 10 for details). Conventional radiotherapy using 1.8 Gy per fraction to 50.4 to 54 Gy is reserved for treatment of recurrent, residual, and inoperable disease (see Chap. 11). Combined planned partial resection followed by adjuvant radiotherapy has resulted in good long term control rates (THOMSETT et al. 1980; HETELEKIDIS et al. 1993). Cyst drainage with intracystic injection of a radioisotope has also been used to control the cystic component of the tumor (KOBAYASHI et al. 1981). Stereotactic radiosurgery is an alternative approach which may minimize radiation toxicity such as optic neuropathy, endocrine dysfunction, and radionecrosis in such a clinical setting.

Treatment results with SRS have been reported in several small series. The University of Virginia reported on SRS in nine craniopharyngioma patients, with eight (89%) of these patients with stable disease after gamma knife therapy (Prasad et al. 1995). There was no associated visual or endocrine toxicity in these patients. Another report on 36 patients initially treated for the cystic component with radionuclide yttrium-90, followed by SRS consisting of 20 to 50 Gy, resulted in 100% response rate (Steiner 1988). The University of Pittsburgh group reported on two of three craniopharyngioma patients who had stable disease after gamma knife SRS (Coffey and Lunsford 1990).

Published data suggest that SRS is an effective treatment modality in the management of selected patients with craniopharyngioma. However, due to this tumor's anatomic location in the parasellar region, care needs to be taken to avoid excessive irradiation to sensitive structures, similar to that in the case of pituitary tumors. Unfortunately, visual impairment occurred in two of the three patients studied by the University of Pittsburgh group, although toxicities in the other published reports were minimal or transient.

The optimal doses are unknown, although Steiner suggested a minimum peripheral dose of 10 Gy (Steiner 1988). At USC, for patients with craniopharyngioma treated with gamma knife, we use a dose of radiation of 15 Gy defined usually to the 50% isodose line. The dose limitations are similar to those described in patients with pituitary adenomas. It is apparent that only carefully selected patients with craniopharyngioma can be considered for the treatment with SRS.

19.7.3
Cavernous Sinus Tumors

Meningiomas and pituitary adenomas may invade into the cavernous sinus, with other tumors only occasionally seen at this site. As tumors of the cavernous sinus progress, patients may present with diplopia, retroorbital pain and problems resulting from compression of the internal carotid artery. The management of cavernous sinus tumors presents a major challenge to neurosurgeons. Surgical resection is rarely attempted due to a well-known treatment toxicity particularly evident in patients with more advanced lesions. In recent years SRS has become an attractive treatment alternative for the management of patients with these tumors.

The University of Pittsburgh experience consisted of gamma knife SRS in the treatment of cavernous sinus meningiomas in 34 patients (Duma et al. 1993). A dose of from 10 to 20 Gy was given, with a maximum dose to the optic nerve or tract of 9 Gy in 31 patients. There was 100% tumor control during a median follow up of 26 months. Tumor regression was seen in 56% of patients imaged at an average of 18 months. Of the 31 patients treated, eight (26%) improved clinically. There were four (13%) patients who developed new or worsened cranial nerve deficits. Two of these patients subsequently showed complete resolution of their symptoms. There was no endocrinopathy or new extraocular muscle paresis.

A study on the tolerance of cranial nerves in 62 patients treated with SRS for tumors in the cavernous sinus was reported by Harvard University and the University of Pittsburgh (Tishler et al. 1993). The maximum dose to the cavernous sinus ranged from 10 to 40 Gy. In a follow-up period of 3 to 49 months after SRS, new cranial nerve neuropathies developed in 12 (19%) patients. In four (6%) patients there were complications affecting the optic system, and eight (13%) had an injury to the sensory or motor nerves crossing the cavernous sinus. There was no clear relationship between the maximum dose to the cavernous sinus and complications for cranial nerves III–VI. For cranial nerve II, there was an increased incidence of complications with the increase in the radiation dose. Four of the 17 (24%) patients receiving 8 Gy or more to any part of the optic apparatus, developed visual complications. None of the 35 patients who received less than 8 Gy developed these complications. In this study, a radiation dose of 8 Gy appears to be a threshold dose beyond which the optic apparatus is at an increased risk of neuropathy.

Of interest is a report on a series of 88 patients treated with gamma knife for skull base meningiomas (Morita et al. 1999). Median treatment volume was 10 cm^3, and the median dose to the tumor margin was 16 Gy. The 5-year progression-free survival rate was 95%. Functioning optic nerves received a median dose of 10 Gy, and no treatment-related vision loss occurred.

We have recently evaluated our early experience with gamma knife SRS for patients with cavernous sinus tumors (unpublished data). A total of 62 patients were treated in a 5-year period, with a median follow up time of 22 months. There were 30 (48%) patients with meningioma including one with malignant meningioma, 27 (44%) with pituitary adenoma, four (6%) with neuromas, and one (2%) had melanoma. A majority (56%) of patients had locally advanced lesions (Grades III–V). Mean tumor volume was 6.5 cm^3 and the mean radiation dose was 15.4 Gy defined to the 50% isodose line. Stereotactic radiosurgery was very well-tolerated by these patients, and complications were uncommon. A total of two (3%) patients had cranial nerve deficit following therapy. The first patient with surgical grade III pituitary adenoma developed VIth nerve palsy 25 months following SRS. This problem resolved spontaneously 7 months later. The second patient with bilateral cavernous sinus pituitary adenoma developed VIth nerve palsy 3 months after SRS, which remained unchanged during 15 months of observation. Four patients who presented with cranial nerve dysfunction experienced resolution of this problem or substantial improvement in their deficit. One female patient with prolactin-secreting adenoma following gamma knife SRS experienced normalization of endocrine function with return of menstrual cycle. During the period of observation, one (2%) patient with malignant meningioma died of tumor progression, while the remaining 61 (98%) patients had stable disease. Based on these data, we believe gamma knife SRS is an important treatment for patients with cavernous sinus tumors. Figure 19.1 demonstrates gamma knife SRS for a patient with left cavernous sinus meningioma. Due to the patient's poor general condition SRS was the only viable treatment option.

Utmost care needs to be taken in the management of tumors of the cavernous sinus, to protect the normal structures which are very sensitive to a single large-fraction radiotherapy. Effective treatment may be given with radiosurgery, but avoidance of doses greater than 8 Gy to the optic chiasm is imperative in order to prevent loss of vision.

19.7.4
Acoustic Tumors

Acoustic neuromas are benign tumors of the VIIIth cranial nerve, which arise in the cerebello-pontine angle. Microsurgical resection is considered to be the standard management for healthy patients with unilateral acoustic neuromas. This procedure is a safe and effective treatment modality for patients with these tumors (WALLNER et al. 1987; POLLOCK et al. 1995; KONDZIOLKA et al. 1998b) (see Chap. 12 for details on surgical therapy).

The first acoustic neuroma treated with SRS was irradiated with a gamma knife in 1969 (LEKSELL 1969). Leksell subsequently reported on a series of 94 patients with acoustic neuromas, in which he was able to obtain good tumor control rates as well as good treatment tolerance (LEKSELL 1983).

A series of 669 patients with acoustic neuromas treated with SRS, followed from 1969 to 1997, is of major interest (NOREN 1998). Long-term tumor control was achieved in 95% of unilateral lesions. Patients treated early in this series had a significant risk of facial weakness (38%) and numbness (33%). This high incidence of complications of SRS was reduced to less than 2% during the 1990s. Preservation of hearing was achieved in nearly 70% of patients. There was a small risk (1.4%) of peritumoral reaction causing blockage of CSF circulation which required shunting. The sharp reduction in the incidence of treatment toxicity was primarily due to radiation dose reduction.

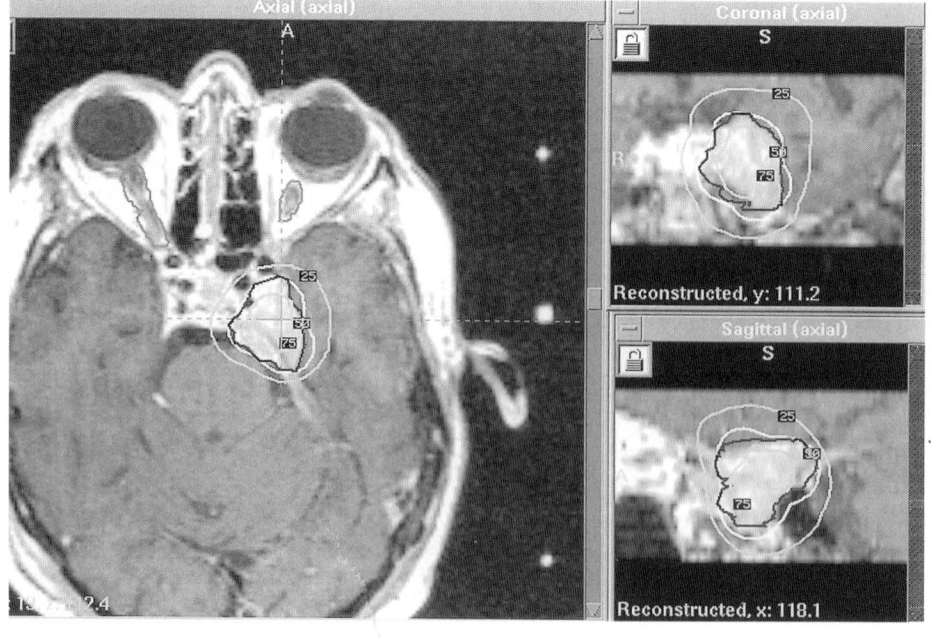

Fig. 19.1a. This is illustrates the case of a 90-year-old female patient with several months' history of severe pain in the left trigeminal nerve distribution. On MRI a 24+25+28.5 mm lesion was noted, extensively invading the left cavernous sinus. A diagnosis of meningioma was made. Gamma knife stereotactic radiosurgery was the only viable treatment option for this patient. A dose of 16 Gy was given to the tumor periphery, defined to the 50% isodose line. Six isocenters were treated

Histogram

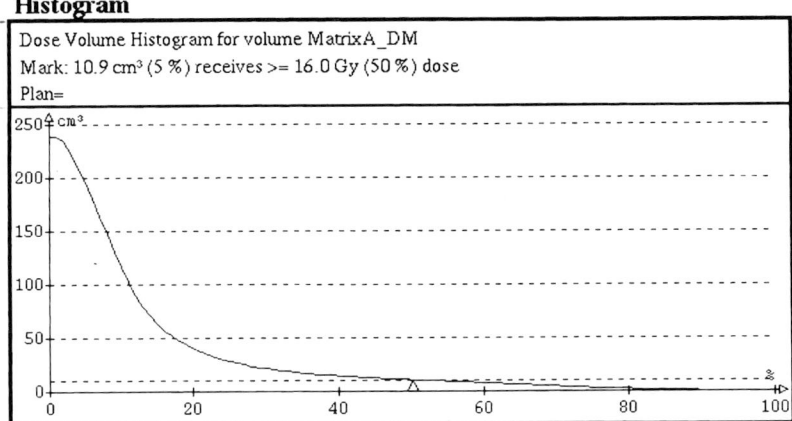

Dose Volume Histogram for volume MatrixA_DM
Mark: 10.9 cm³ (5 %) receives >= 16.0 Gy (50 %) dose
Plan=

Histogram

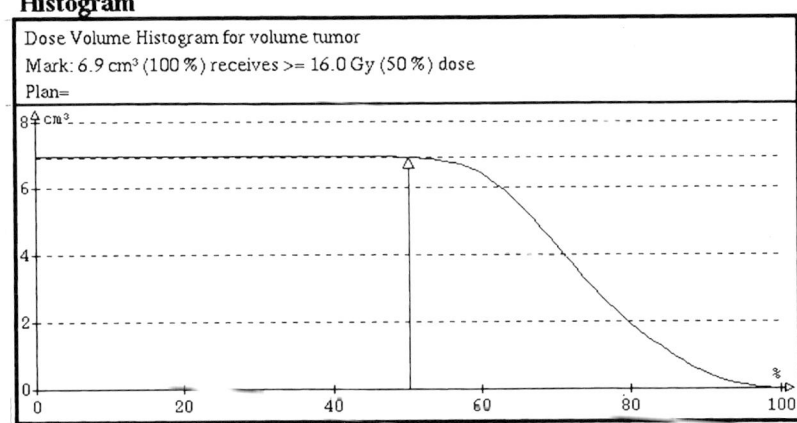

Dose Volume Histogram for volume tumor
Mark: 6.9 cm³ (100 %) receives >= 16.0 Gy (50 %) dose
Plan=

b

Fig. 19.1b. Dose-volume histogram shows tumor volume of 6.9 cm³ and treated volume of 10.9 cm³

The group from the University of Pittsburgh reported treatment results in 162 patients with acoustic neuromas treated with gamma knife, using an average dose of 16 Gy to the tumor margin (KONDZIOLKA et al. 1998b). The authors were able to achieve a tumor control rate of 98%, with 62% of tumors decreasing in size, 33% remaining unchanged, and 6% becoming slightly larger. Only four (2%) patients within 4 years of SRS required a tumor resection. Facial nerve function was preserved in 79% of patients and trigeminal nerve function was preserved in 73%. Hearing was preserved in 51% of patients.

A comparison of microsurgical management and SRS in patients with acoustic neuromas <3 cm in diameter, demonstrated SRS as having similar rates of tumor control, a better rate of preservation of nerve function, lower morbidity, and lower treatment cost (POLLOCK et al. 1995).

Based on the published data and our clinical experience at USC, we tend to treat larger lesions surgically, reserving SRS for the treatment of residual tumor. Smaller lesions are treated well with gamma knife SRS. In the past 12 months, based on the University of Pittsburgh data, we have decreased radiation dose to periphery of tumor from 16 to 14 Gy. Figure 19.2 shows gamma knife SRS for right-sided acoustic neuroma.

19.7.5
Meningiomas

Complete microsurgical resection of the tumor and its dural base is the management of choice for meningiomas. It is not uncommon, however, for the tumor to invade an important vascular structure, cranial nerves, and/or brain parenchyma, making complete tumor removal difficult, without a loss of function. An incomplete tumor resection will lead to a high incidence of recurrence (SIMPSON 1957). Conventional external beam radiotherapy up to a dose of 55 Gy for benign meningiomas, or 56 to 60 Gy for the less common malignant meningiomas, is delivered to residual disease in the adjuvant setting. Surgical

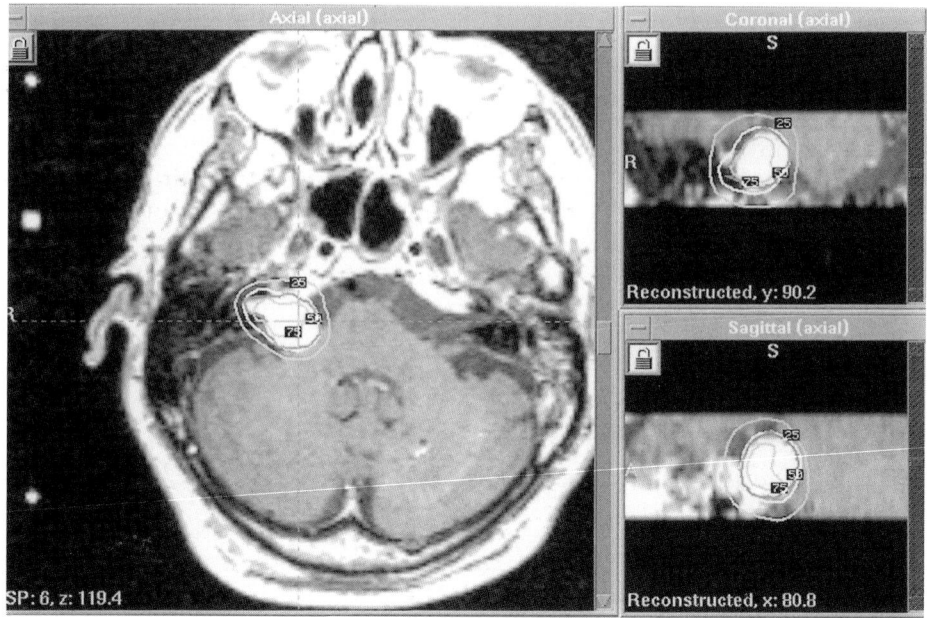

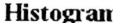

Histogram

Dose Volume Histogram for volume MatrixA_DM

Mark: 3.6 cm³ (3 %) receives >= 12.0 Gy (50 %) dose

Plan=

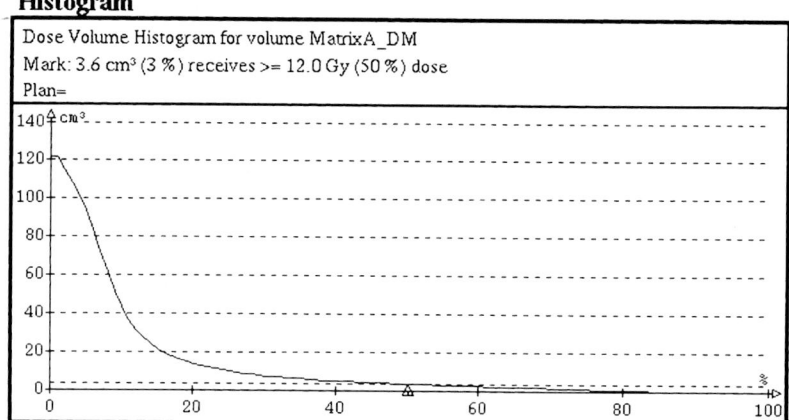

Histogram

Dose Volume Histogram for volume tumor

Mark: 2.4 cm³ (100 %) receives >= 12.0 Gy (50 %) dose

Plan=

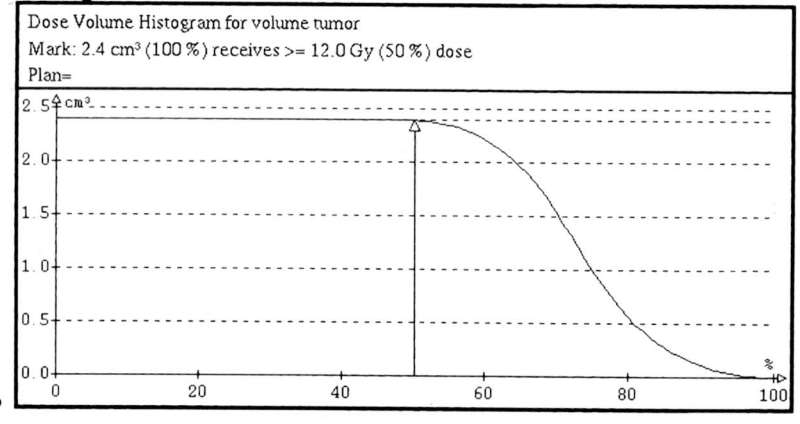

Fig. 19.2. a This represents the case of a 75-year-old male with 13 years' history of progressive loss of hearing in the right ear, and dizziness. MRI showed a 22.5+16+14 mm lesion in the right cerebello-pontine angle with characteristics of acoustic neuroma. The patient was a poor surgical risk and he was recommended to undergo gamma knife SRS. The patient was treated with 12 Gy to the 50% isodose line using six isocenters. **b** Dose-volume histogram shows tumor volume of 2.4 cm³ and treated volume of 3.6 cm³

and conventional radiotherapeutic management of meningiomas are described in chapters 13 and 14 respectively.

In recent years radiosurgery has become an acceptable primary treatment modality in the management of small (<3 cm) and previously untreated meningiomas. These tumors are well suited to SRS. They are usually well circumscribed, rarely invasive and easily visualized by CT or MRI. Primary SRS is particularly useful in patients with tumors of the skull base, cerebello-opontine angle, and cavernous sinus, where conventional surgery may result in a higher incidence of complications (MAYBERG and SYMON 1986). Additionally, SRS is indicated for the treatment of recurrent or residual disease following surgical resection.

The University of Pittsburgh Group reported a multicenter study of 203 patients with benign parasaggital meningiomas, who underwent resection with or without external beam radiotherapy or radiosurgery (KONDZIOLKA et al. 1998). A total of 66 (32%) patients received SRS as a primary treatment. The mean tumor volume was 10 cm^3. The overall 5-year tumor control rate was 93% in patients who received SRS alone. There was no treatment failure in patients with small tumors (<7.5 cm^3) or in those without a previous surgical resection. It has been shown that in patients with previous resection, the control rate was only 60%, while the control rate for the radiosurgery-treated volume was 85%. The authors suggested that in cases of small parasagittal tumors, SRS may be utilized as the procedure of choice. Those with larger tumors or with neurological progression should receive surgery first, and additional radiosurgery for residual and/or recurrent tumor.

In a study of 72 SRS-treated patients with middle fossa meningiomas, 17 (24%) were treated with SRS after incomplete surgical resection, 21 (29%) had tumor recurrence, and 34 (47%) had SRS as a primary treatment (VALENTINO et al. 1993). Doses delivered ranged from 15 to 45 Gy. Treatment was well-tolerated, without complications. Fifty (69%) patients showed regression of tumor from 24 to 91% of the initial tumor volume, 18 (25%) showed stable tumor, two (3%) had tumor progression, and two (3%) patients showed tumor recurrence after an initial decrease in tumor size. The authors concluded that SRS is preferable to reoperation in recurrent meningiomas and its use is indicated after incomplete surgical removal, or for those patients with high risk for surgery.

Another study analyzed treatment outcomes following SRS in 127 patients with 155 meningiomas (HAKIM et al. 1998). Stereotactic radiosurgery was performed in 48 (31%) lesions as the initial treatment, and in 107 (69%) lesions as an adjuvant therapy. On follow up from 1.2 to 80 months, there was an 84% rate of freedom from progression. In the remaining 16%, tumor progressed. The 5-year tumor control rate was 89% for benign meningiomas. However, for atypical and malignant tumors, the 4-year survival rate was only 21.5%.

Radiosurgery in patients with meningioma is an effective treatment modality, with tumor growth control obtained in 80 to 95% of patients. This includes approximately one-half who demonstrate significant tumor regression (VALENTINO et al. 1993; DUMA et al. 1993). At USC our policy is to treat surgically, patients with larger (>3 cm) meningiomas, and follow with planned SRS for those who have an incomplete resection or recurrent tumor. Smaller tumors are treated with primary SRS. Radiation dose to tumor periphery is 16 Gy, usually defined to the 50% isodose line. Tumor control has been obtained in all benign meningiomas (unpublished data). Figure 19.3 shows the treatment of a large and aggressive meningioma which was invading the pons. Contrary to some reports, we have not observed substantial tumor shrinkage during the period of observation (VALENTINO et al. 1993). In meningiomas, we define tumor control as a lack of tumor growth rather than tumor regression.

19.7.6
Pineal Tumors

Tumors in the region of the pineal gland are uncommon. They include pineocytomas, pineoblastomas, germinomas, astrocytomas, ependymomas, and meningiomas. These tumors may produce symptoms by causing pressure on the adjacent structures including the lateral geniculate nuclei, superior colliculi, and 3rd ventricle. Parinaud's ophthalmoplegia is a symptom associated with pineal tumors and hydrocephalus may occur with larger lesions. Due to their location, pineal tumors are difficult to remove surgically without causing morbidity. Surgery is utilized mainly for biopsy and shunting, although in recent years, microsurgery has much improved the morbidity and mortality rates. External beam radiotherapy is often used for definitive treatment, usually with a dose of 45 to 50 Gy delivered to the primary tumor in 1.8 Gy fractions.

Stereotactic radiosurgery has become another viable treatment option in the management of patients with pineal tumors. Gamma knife was first used in Sweden for the treatment of pinealocytoma in 1974 (BACKLUND 1974). The reported treatment outcome was good and the author recommended the use of SRS for this indication. Backlund later reported on a series of pineal-region tumors treated with gamma knife with a dose of 20 to 75 Gy (BACKLUND 1979). Patients with pineocytomas showed an excellent response to SRS therapy. Of the five patients with astrocytoma and ependymomas who were treated, three responded well to SRS while two showed tumor progression. In a study of six patients treated by linear accelerator-based SRS, early and good response was reported in patients with germinoma (CASENTINI et al. 1990).

A study reported treatment outcomes in 11 patients with pineal-region tumors treated with SRS and given a dose of 12 to 20 Gy to tumor periphery (MANERA et al 1996). Histological diagnosis in these patients was: pinealocytoma, tectal astrocytoma, germinoma, pinealoblastoma, and meningioma. All tumors responded to the treatment well and disappeared or ceased growing. Of the 11 patients treated, eight showed substantial tumor volume reduction while in three patients the tumors completely disappeared. Treatment was well-tolerated by all patients, with no major complications. One patient had a headache and a transient worsening of an abducent nerve palsy, which were controlled by the administration of corticosteroids.

Stereotactic radiosurgery has become a valuable alternative to conventional surgery in the treatment of pineal-region tumors. Results of treatment are excellent, especially in cases of pineocytomas, where complete regression of tumor is often achieved.

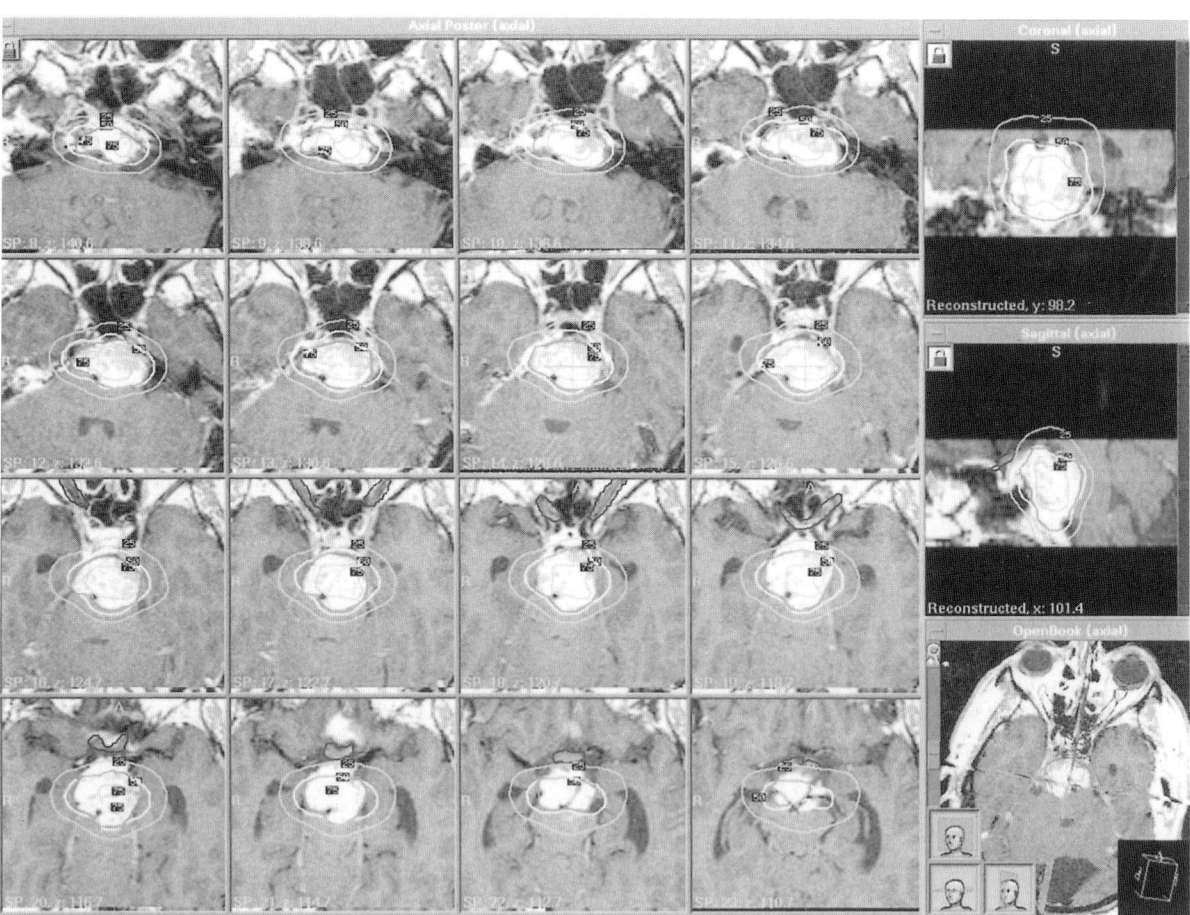

Fig. 19.3. Illustration of the case of a 60-year-old male with a 2-year history of left VIth nerve palsy. Two months prior to gamma knife SRS, he underwent partial surgical resection. Histological diagnosis was atypical or malignant meningioma. At this time MRI showed a large residual mass of the clivus, measuring 35.4+31.1+40.2 mm. In spite of a large (18.9 cm³) tumor volume, gamma knife was the only viable treatment option. The total volume treated was 27 cm³, and the patient received 15 Gy defined to the 50% isodose line using eight isocenters

19.7.7
Low-grade Gliomas

Low-grade gliomas are relatively uncommon primary brain tumors, with about 3,000 patients being diagnosed per year in the United States (Laws and Thapan 1993). Management of low-grade gliomas usually entails surgical resection and adjuvant external beam radiation therapy particularly in patients with grade II tumors. Administration of postoperative irradiation reduces the incidence of tumor recurrence in this group of patients. Alternatively, patients may undergo a stereotactic biopsy and receive definitive external beam radiotherapy. Treatment of low-grade gliomas is discussed in chapters 15 and 16. Stereotactic radiosurgery for many years has been used in the management of low-grade gliomas. A study of nine patients with inoperable tumors treated with a linear accelerator-based system reported a good treatment tolerance without major toxicity (Colombo et al. 1985). The treated tumors were relatively small ranging from 7 to 25 mm in diameter. On initial follow-up of 6 to 18 months, six (67%) of these nine patients had shrinkage of tumor on CT imaging, and four (44%) had clinical improvement. On further follow up after 18 to 43 months, seven (78%) patients showed tumor response, and six (67%) had clinical improvement.

A second report by the same group of investigators described 14 patients with nonoperable low-grade astrocytomas who were treated with fractionated stereotactic radiotherapy (Pozza et al. 1989). Doses of 16 to 50 Gy were delivered in one or two fractions 8 days apart, and patients were followed from 11 to 48 months after. Of the 14 patients treated, 12 (86%) had a partial or complete response to treatment, demonstrated on CT imaging.

A report on the use of fractionated stereotactic radiotherapy in eight patients with low-grade astrocytomas recommended radiation doses from 37.8 to 42 Gy delivered in seven equal fractions every other day (Souhami et al. 1991). Treatment was well tolerated without complications. Major clinical improvement was noted in seven (88%) of the eight patients treated. This included three (38%) who became asymptomatic, four (50%) who had improvement of symptoms, and two (25%) who experienced improvement in their seizures.

At USC, we have used SRS for the treatment of low-grade gliomas since 1985, initially with a linear accelerator-based system, and since 1994 also with a gamma knife. Stereotactic radiosurgery was used first for the treatment of selected patients with recurrent low-grade gliomas following definitive external beam radiotherapy. Patients accepted for the treatment had lesions <35 mm in greatest dimension. A dose of from 16 to 18 Gy was given, usually defined to the 80% isodose line, in those treated with a linear accelerator stereotactic system and to the 50% isodose line in patients treated with a gamma knife. Based on good treatment tolerance, low incidence of clinically significant toxicity and encouraging results in terms of tumor control, the use of SRS in patients with low-grade gliomas was expanded (Petrovich et al. 1996; Petrovich et al. 1997). At the present time we use the following indications for SRS in this group of patients: 1. Treatment of postradiation recurrences in patients with lesions <35 mm in diameter, delivering a dose of 18 Gy to the 50% isodose line; 2. A planned SRS boost consisting of 16 Gy in patients receiving 54 Gy involved fields external beam radiotherapy; 3. SRS as the only therapy in patients with central neurocytomas or pilocytic astrocytomas following stereotactic biopsy. Figure 19.4 demonstrates treatment of a pediatric patient with a third recurrence of a posterior fossa pilocytic astrocytoma. A dose of radiation depends to a large extent on tumor location. Patients with tumors in midbrain or in the vicinity of optic chiasm or other particularly radiosensitive structure receive no more than 16 Gy to the periphery of a lesion. Figure 19.5 shows SRS with gamma knife in a patient with grade II astrocytoma but with the clinical behavior of a malignant glioma.

At the present time, the use of SRS in patients with low-grade gliomas is in the process of being defined. Caution needs to be exercised with SRS to minimize the probability of potentially significant late complications in patients with low-grade gliomas who are expected to survive for a long period of time.

19.7.8
High-Grade Gliomas

High-grade gliomas including anaplastic astrocytomas and glioblastoma multiforme, are the most common primary brain tumors (Laws and Thapan 1993). They are characterized by their aggressive behavior and wide infiltration into the surrounding brain parenchyma. Despite gross tumor resection, local failure nearly always is the cause of death (Wallner et al. 1989). Standard management includes surgical resection of the tumor, despite the

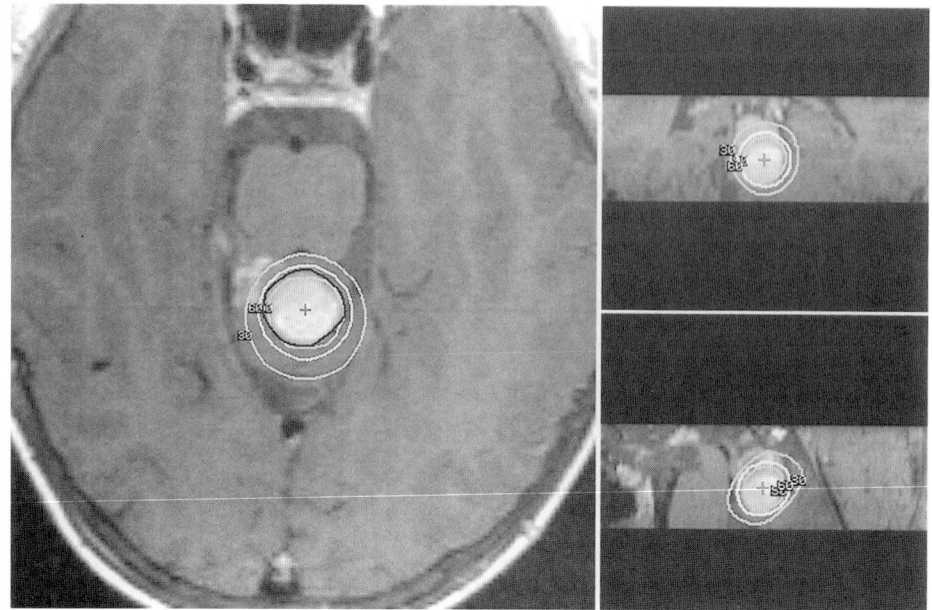

a

Histogram

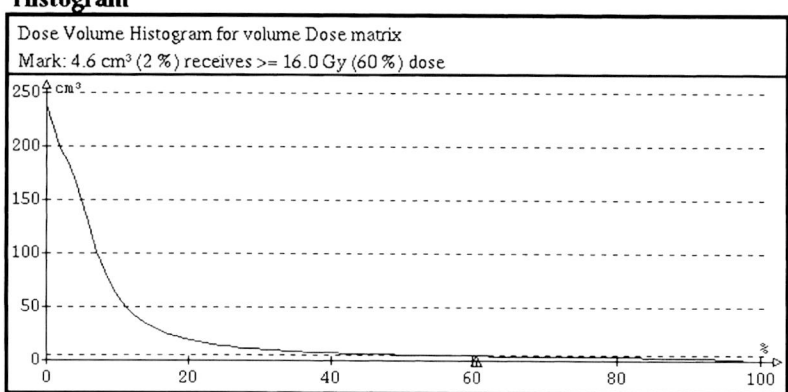

Dose Volume Histogram for volume Dose matrix

Mark: 4.6 cm³ (2 %) receives >= 16.0 Gy (60 %) dose

Histogram

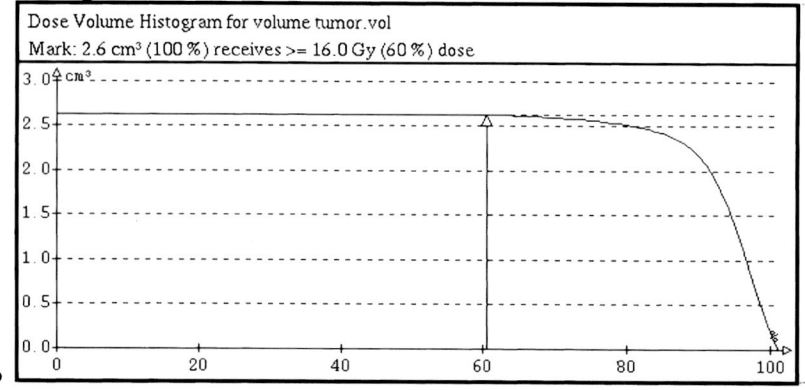

Dose Volume Histogram for volume tumor.vol

Mark: 2.6 cm³ (100 %) receives >= 16.0 Gy (60 %) dose

b

Fig. 19.4. a This represents the case of a 9-year-old male who had undergone two resections for posterior fossa pilocytic astrocytoma. The tumor measured 18.2+17.5+20.3 mm, with a volume of 2.6 cm³. The patient was treated in early 1996, with 16 Gy delivered, defined to the 50% isodose line using a single isocenter. There was no evidence of tumor growth in over 3 years of observation. b Dose-volume histogram demonstrating a good tumor volume coverage. Total volume treated was 4.6 cm³

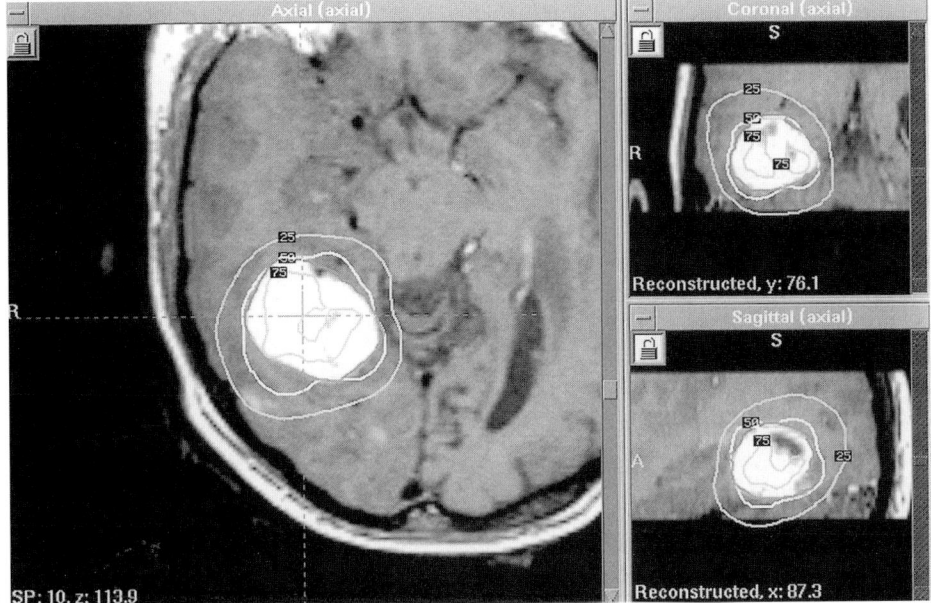

a SP: 10, z: 113.9

Histogram

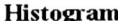

Dose Volume Histogram for volume Matrix A_DM

Mark: 23.6 cm³ (10 %) receives >= 18.0 Gy (50 %) dose

Plan=

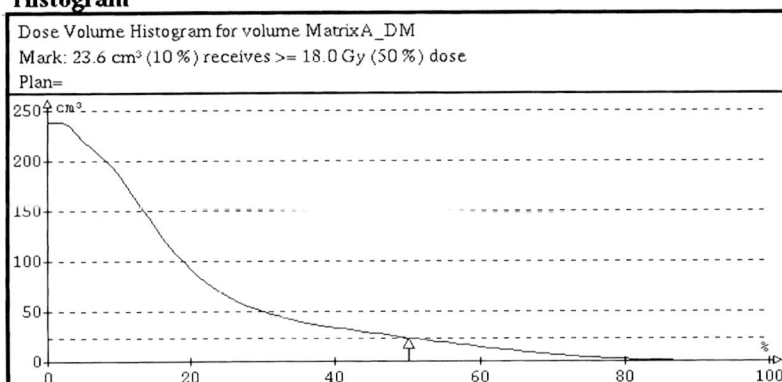

Histogram

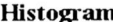

Dose Volume Histogram for volume tumor

Mark: 15.7 cm³ (99 %) receives >= 18.0 Gy (50 %) dose

Plan=

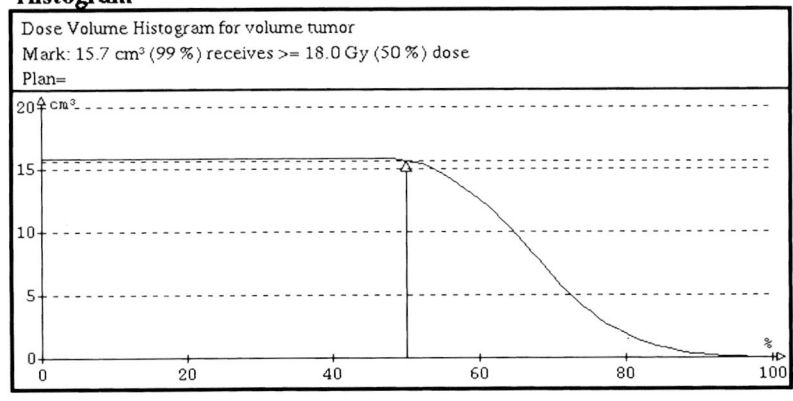

b

Fig. 19.5. a This represents the case of a 42-year-old female who in July 1996 presented with seizures. Subsequent astereotactic biopsy demonstrated grade 2 astrocytoma. The patient was treated at another medical center with external beam radiotherapy, up to a total dose of 57.6 Gy. One year following radiotherapy, she developed a recurrent tumor. On MRI the tumor was noted in the right posterior temporal lobe, and measured 36.0+35.0+30.8 mm. The patient received 18 Gy, to the 50% isodose line using seven isocenters. Several months later the patient developed a second lesion in the left parietal lobe. The SRS-treated lesion remained under control for the duration of the follow-up period. **b** Dose-volume histogram shows tumor volume of 15.7 cm³ and treated volume of 23.6 cm³

knowledge that microscopic disease remains adjacent to the tumor bed (see Chap. 17). Adjuvant external beam radiotherapy to 60 Gy is indicated in order to maintain local control for as long as possible and to maintain a good quality of life and to extend survival (see Chap. 18). Currently, with the best available management, patients with anaplastic astrocytomas may expect a median survival time of approximately 30 months and those with glioblastoma multiforme, approximately 9 months.

A study on the analysis of important prognostic factors influencing survival in 1,578 patients with high-grade gliomas treated in three RTOG trials is of interest (CURRAN et al. 1993). The pretreatment prognostic factors adversely affecting survival were as follows: patient age >50 years, glioblastoma multiforme histology and performance status. Favorable treatment characteristics influencing survival included: more extensive surgery, radiation dose >54.4 Gy, treatment with carmustine and with semustine and decarbazine. The survival gain of more extensive surgery and higher radiation doses needs to be carefully weighed against possible decrease in the quality of life which may be associated with a more aggressive treatment.

Increased radiation doses may lead to an improved local control and extended survival. Interstitial brachytherapy has been used to deliver boost doses of irradiation to the areas at high risk of a tumor recurrence, while limiting radiation doses to the surrounding brain (LEIBEL et al. 1989; SHRIEVE et al. 1995). The median survival time of patients with glioblastoma multiforme receiving brachytherapy boost was 11.5 months. At the present time, the use of brachytherapy boost is not common due to the invasive nature of this procedure, its high cost and a significant risk of radiation necrosis requiring repeated craniotomies. Based on our clinical experience with stereotactic brachytherapy at USC, we discontinued the use of this procedure in 1990 (LUCAS et al. 1991).

Stereotactic radiosurgery as a less invasive procedure than stereotactic brachytherapy, has become an increasingly more commonly used treatment modality to boost radiation dose following external beam radiotherapy, in selected patients with high-grade gliomas. Additionally, SRS is being used to treat patients with recurrent disease following external beam therapy.

A study was reported on a group of 64 patients with glioblastoma multiforme and 43 patients with anaplastic astrocytoma who received SRS either before disease progression, or at the time of recurrence (KONDZIOLKA et al. 1997). In the 64 glioblastoma patients, median survival time was 26 months from diagnosis and 16 months from radiosurgery. For the 43 anaplastic astrocytoma patients, the median survival time was 32 months from diagnosis, and 21 months following radiosurgery. These survival times reflect an improvement on published series where SRS was not a part of treatment. Direct comparison with other published reports is difficult due to selection of patients with smaller tumors, for radiosurgery.

A study of 23 patients with glioblastoma multiforme treated with 59.4 Gy external beam radiotherapy followed by a planned radiosurgery boost with a linear accelerator-based stereotactic system giving an additional 10 to 20 Gy, showed a median survival time of 26 months (LOEFFLER et al. 1992).

An interesting RTOG study on 115 patients with malignant gliomas treated with surgery, external beam radiotherapy, and linear accelerator-based radiosurgery showed a very good treatment outcome (SARKARIA et al. 1995). The 2-year actuarial survival rate was 45% with a median survival time of 96 weeks. This represented an improvement in survival when compared with the RTOG historical database of patients treated similarly but without the addition of SRS. The survival improvement was demonstrated best in patients with the worse prognosis factors.

The value of SRS in patients with glioblastoma multiforme was recently studied at Harvard (SHRIEVE et al. 1999). A total of 78 patients received standard external beam radiotherapy following stereotactic biopsy or subtotal tumor resection. Stereotactic radiosurgery was performed with a dedicated 6 MV linear accelerator. Radiation doses ranged from 6 to 24 Gy with a median dose of 12 Gy and a median tumor volume of 9.4 cm^3. The 1- and 2-year actuarial survival rates were 88.5% and 36%, respectively, with a median survival time of 20 months. In multivariate analysis, patient age <40 years was the only important factor influencing survival. This study is of obvious importance, clearly demonstrating improved survival in patients with glioblastoma multiforme treated with SRS-external beam combination. A major problem in this study is a surprisingly high (50%) incidence of reoperations following SRS. Symptomatic brain necrosis requiring reoperation was reported in 20 (26%) while in the remaining 19 (24%) patients there was necrosis with tumor being present. The reason for this high incidence of brain necrosis is not readily apparent since the radiation dose and tumor volume were relatively low. At USC, the incidence of symptomatic brain necrosis requiring a reoperation is <5% and we use higher (16–18 Gy) radiation doses (PETROVICH et al. 1996; PETROVICH et al. 1997 data).

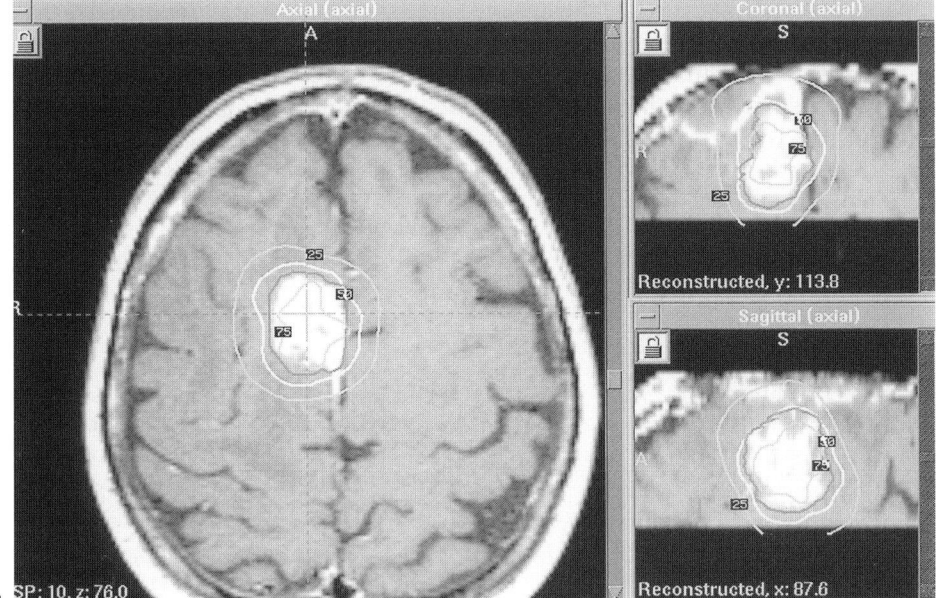

Histogram

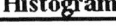

Dose Volume Histogram for volume MatrixA_DM

Mark: 19.4 cm³ (8 %) receives >= 16.0 Gy (50 %) dose

Plan=

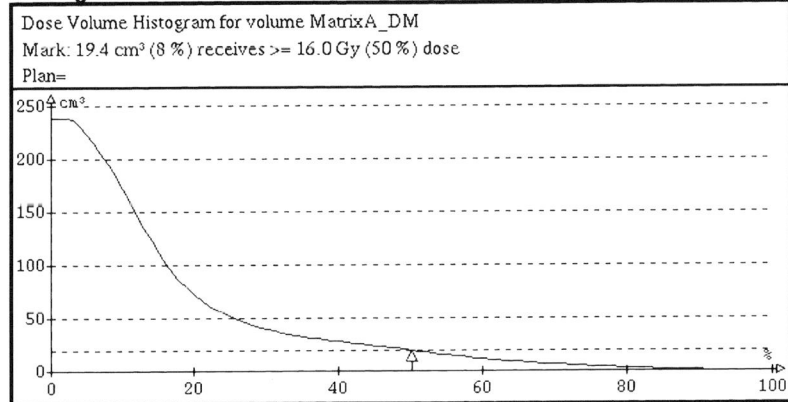

Histogram

Dose Volume Histogram for volume tumor

Mark: 11.0 cm³ (100 %) receives >= 16.0 Gy (50 %) dose

Plan=

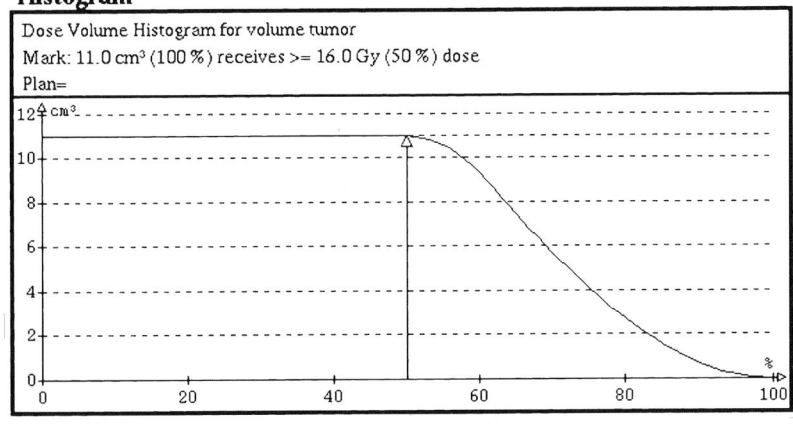

Fig. 19.6. a This represents the case of a 60-year-old female with a sudden onset of left hemiparesis. MRI demonstrated a right parasagittal, posterior frontal mass. A partial tumor resection was performed, with histological diagnosis of glioblastoma multiforme. Tumor measurements were: 26.0+29.4+37.7 mm with a tumor volume of 11.0 cm³. The patient was treated with involved fields external beam radiotherapy consisting of 60 Gy given at 2.0 Gy daily fractions followed by gamma knife SRS consisting of 16 Gy, to the 50% isodose line using six isocenters. **b** Dose-volume-histogram demonstrating tumor volume coverage and total volume (19.4 cm³) treated

The role of SRS in the management of 38 recurrent brain tumors following the administration of 60 Gy external beam radiotherapy was examined (Shaw et al. 1996). Patients with tumors <4 cm in the greatest dimension and lower (<18 Gy) radiation doses had a low incidence of severe treatment toxicity, while those with larger tumors and/or receiving higher radiation doses had an unacceptable incidence of complications.

At the present time we use SRS on selected patients with glioblastoma multiforme following external beam radiotherapy which consists of 60 Gy given at 2 Gy daily fractions. Figure 19.6 shows gamma knife SRS in a patient with glioblastoma multiforme. This patient received prior planned 60 Gy external beam radiotherapy, and SRS dose ranges from 16 to 18 Gy depending on the tumor volume and location. Patients treated with SRS-external beam combination are generally those with tumors <35 mm in diameter. Similar criteria for patient selection and SRS radiation doses are used in the management of patients with postradiation recurrences. This treatment is given on an outpatient basis under conscious sedation. Stereotactic radiosurgery is well-tolerated with a low incidence of severe treatment toxicity.

19.8
Conclusions

By December 1998, nearly 100,000 patients had been treated with gamma knife SRS worldwide (Leksell Society December 1998). This treatment has been applied to a wide variety of intracranial tumors and other conditions. Nearly three quarters of these patients were treated for tumors.

In the past, there had been strong evidence to support the use of radiosurgery for the treatment of AVMs and a few other conditions. During the 1990s, the indications shifted towards the management of multiple types of tumors, both benign and malignant, and an exponential increase in utilization of SRS was seen. Results of therapy with all modalities of radiosurgery have demonstrated efficacy in the treatment of many tumors, although there are some critics who say that the proof has yet to be established in randomized controlled trials. (Brada and Cruickshank 1999).

In theory, the higher the dose of radiation delivered to a tumor, the higher the probability of control. Radiosurgery allows maximization of this radiation dose and control rate, although it becomes limited by the dose to surrounding structures. Supportive evidence for the use of SRS is now seen in published reports, where there are long-term follow up times for various tumors such as acoustic neuromas and pituitary adenomas, and evidence is accumulating for other indications, as follow up periods lengthen.

References

Aristizabal S, Caldwell WL, Avila J (1977) The relationship of time-dose fractionation factors to complications in the treatment of pituitary tumors by irradiation. Int J Rad Oncol Biol Phys 2:667–673

Backlund EO, Rahn T, Sarby B (1974) Treatment of pinealomas by stereotaxic radiation surgery. Acta Radiol: Ther Phys Biol 13:4,368–76

Backlund EO (1979) Stereotactic radiosurgery in intracranial tumours and vascular malformations. In: Krayenbuhl HA, (ed) Advances in Technical Standards in Neurosurgery. Springer-Verlag, New York, pp 3–37

Backlund EO (1992) The history and development of radiosurgery. In: Lunsford LD (ed) Stereotactic Radiosurgery Update. Elsevier, New York, pp 3–9

Betti O, Derechinsky V (1983) Irradiation Stereotaxique Multifasceaux. Neurochirurgie 29:295–298

Brada M, Cruickshank G (1999) Radiosurgery for brain tumours. BMJ 318:411–412

Casentini L, Colombo F, Pozza F, et al. (1990) Combined radiosurgery and external radiotherapy of intracranial germinomas. Surg Neurol 34:79–86

Coffey RJ, Lunsford LD (1990) The role of stereotactic techniques in the management of craniopharyngiomas. Neurosurg Clin North Am 1:161–172

Colombo F, Benedetti A, Pozza F, et al. (1985) Stereotactic radiosurgery utilizing a linear accelerator. Appl Neurophysiol 48:133–145

Curran WJ, Scott CB, Horton J, et al. (1993) Recursing partitioning analysis of prognostic factors in three Radiation Therapy Oncology Group malignant glioma trials. J Natl Cancer Inst 85:704–710

Duma CM, Lunsford LD, Kondziolka D, et al. (1993) Stereotactic radiosurgery of cavernous sinus meningiomas as an addition or alternative to microsurgery. Neurosurg 32:699–704

Friedman WA, Bova FJ (1992) Linear accelerator radiosurgery for arteriovenous malformations. J Neurosurg 77:832–841

Hakim R, Alexander E, Loeffler JS, et al. (1998) Results of linear accelerator based radiosurgery for intracranial meningiomas. Neurosurg 42:446–454

Hall EJ, Brenner DJ (1993) The radiobiology of radiosurgery: Rationale for different treatment regimes for AVMs and malignancies. Int J Rad Oncol Biol Phys 25:381–385

Hall WA (1995) Stereotactic radiosurgery in perspective. In: Cohen AR, Haines SJ (eds) Concepts in Neurosurgery: Minimally invasive techniques in neurosurgery. Williams and Wilkins, Baltimore pp 104–117

Hetelekidis S, Barnes PD, Tao ML, et al. (1993) Tarbell NJ 20-year experience in childhood craniopharyngioma. Int J Rad Oncol Biol Phys 27:189–195

Jackson IM, Noren G (1999) Role of gamma knife therapy in the management of pituitary tumors. Endocrinol Metabolism Clin N Am 28:133–142

Kirn TF (1988) Proton radiotherapy: some perspectives. JAMA 259:787–788

Kjellberg RN, Shintani A, Frantz AG, et al. (1968) Proton beam therapy in acromegaly. N Engl J Med 278:689–695

Kjellberg RN, Kliman B (1979) Lifetime effectiveness-a system of therapy for pituitary adenomas, emphasizing Bragg peak proton hypophysectomy. In: Linfoot JA (ed) Recent advances in the diagnosis and treatment of pituitary tumors. Raven Press, New York, pp 268–269

Kjellberg RN, Hanamura T, Davis KR, et al. (1983) Bragg peak proton beam therapy for arteriovenous malformations of the brain. N Engl J Med 309:269–274

Kjellberg RN, Abbe M (1988) Stereotactic Bragg peak proton beam therapy. In: Lunsford LD (ed) Modern Stereotactic Neurosurgery. Martinus Nijhoff, Boston pp 463–470

Kobayashi T, Kageyama N, Ohara K (1981) Internal irradiation for cystic craniopharyngioma. J Neurosurg 55:896–903

Kondziolka D, Flickinger JC, Bissonette DJ, et al. (1997) Survival benefit of stereotactic radiosurgery for patients with malignant glial neoplasms. Neurosurg 41:776–785

Kondziolka D, Flickinger JC, Perez B (1998a) A Judicious resection and or radiosurgery for parasaggital meningiomas and or radiosurgery for parasaggital menigiomas. Neurosurg 43:405–414

Kondziolka D, Lunsford LD, McLaughlin MR, et al. (1998b) Long term outcomes after radiosurgery for acoustic neuromas. N Engl J Med 339:1426–1433

Larson DA, Flickinger JC, Loeffler JS (1993) The radiobiology of radiosurgery. Int J Rad Oncol Biol Phys 25:557–561

Larsson B, Leksell L (1958) The high energy proton beam as a neurosurgical tool. Nature 182:1222–1223

Larsson B (1962) On the application of a 185 MeV proton beam to experimental cancer therapy and neurosurgery: a biophysical study. Acta Univ Upsal 9:7–23

Laws ER, Thapan K (1993) Brain tumors. Ca Cancer J Clin 43:263–271

Laws ER, Vance ML (1999) Radiosurgery for pituitary tumors and craniopharyngiomas. Neurosurg Clin N Am 10:327–336

Leibel SA, Gutin PH, Wara WM, et al. (1989) Survival and quality of life after interstitial implantation of removable high-activity iodine-125 sources for the treatment of patients with recurrent malignant gliomas. Int J Rad Oncol Biol Phys 17:1129–1139

Leksell L (1949) A stereotactic apparatus for intracerebral surgery. Acta Chir Scand 99:229–233

Leksell L (1951) The stereotactic method and radiosurgery of the brain. Acta Chir Scand 102:316–319

Leksell L (1968) Cerebral radiosurgery I. Gammathalamotomy in two cases of intractable pain. Acta Chir Scand 134:585–595

Leksell L (1969) A note on the treatment of acoustic tumors. Acta Chir Scand 137:763–765

Leksell L (1983) Stereotactic Radiosurgery. J Neurol Neurosurg Psychiatry 46:797–803

Levy RP, Fabrikant JI, Frankel KA (1993) Particle irradiation of the pituitary gland. In: Alexander E III (ed) Stereotactic Radiosurgery. McGraw Hill, New York, pp 157–165

Linfoot JA (1979) Heavy ion therapy: Alpha particle therapy of pituitary tumors. In: Linfoot JA (ed) Recent advances in the diagnosis and treatment of pituitary tumors. Raven Press, New York, pp 268–269

Loeffler JS, Alexander E III, Shea WM, et al. (1992) Radiosurgery as part of the initial management of patients with malignant gliomas. J Clin Oncol 10:1379–1385

Lucas GL, Cohen D, Apuzzo ML, et al. (1991) Treatment results of sterotactic interstitial brachytherapy for primary and metastatic brain tumors. Int J Rad Oncol Biol Phys 21:715–721

Lunsford LD (1993) The role of SRS in the management of brain vascular malformations. In: Alexander E III, Loeffler JS, Lunsford LD (eds) Stereotactic Radiosurgery, McGraw-Hill, New York, pp 111–121

Lunsford LD, Alexander E III, Loeffler JS (1993) History of radiosurgery. In: Alexander E III, Loeffler JS, Lunsford LD (eds) Stereotactic Radiosurgery. McGraw-Hill, New York, pp 1–4

Luxton G, Petrovich Z, Joszef G, et al. (1993) Stereotactic radiosurgery: principles and comparison of treatment methods. Neurosurg 32:241–259

Lyman JT, Kanstein L, Yeater F (1986) A Helium ion beam for stereotactic radiosurgery of central nervous system disorders. Med Phys 13:695–699

Manera L, Regis J, Chinot O, et al. (1996) Pineal region tumors: the role of stereotactic radiosurgery. Stereotact Funct Neurosurg 66(Suppl):164–173

Mayberg MR, Symon L (1986) Meningiomas of the clivus and apical petrous bone. Report of 35 cases. J Neurosurg 65:160–167

Morita A, Coffey RJ, Foote RL, et al. (1999) Risk of injury to cranial nerves after gamma knife radiosurgery for skull base meningiomas: experience in 88 patients. J Neurosurg 90:42–49

Nedzi LA, Kooy H, Alexander E III, et al. (1991) Variables associated with the development of complications from radiosurgery of intracranial tumors. Int J Rad Oncol Biol Phys 21:591–599

Noren G (1998) Long-term complications following gamma knife radiosurgery of vestibular schwannomas. Stereotact Funct Neurosurg 70(Suppl):65–73

Petrovich ZP, Luxton G, Formenti SC, et al. (1996) Stereotactic radiosurgery for primary and metastatic brain tumors. Cancer Invest 14:445–454

Petrovich ZP, Luxton G, Formenti SC, et al. (1997) Sterotactic radiosurgery for benign and malignant diseases of the brain. In: Kornblith PL, Walker MD (eds) Advances in Neuro-Oncology II, Futura Publishing Co., Armonk, pp 219–258

Phillips MH, Frankel KA, Lyman JT (1990) Comparison of different radiation types and irradiation geometries in stereotactic radiosurgery. Int J Rad Oncol Biol Phys 18:211–220

Pollock BE, Lunsford LD, Kondziolka D, et al. (1995) Outcome analysis of acoustic neuroma management: a comparison of microsurgery and stereotactic radiosurgery. Neurosurg 36:215–224

Pozza F, Colombo F, Chierego G, et al. (1989) Low-grade astrocytomas: treatment with unconventionally fractionated external beam stereotactic radiation therapy. Radiology 171:565–569

Prasad D, Steiner M, Steiner L (1995) Gamma knife surgery for craniopharyngioma. Acta Neurochir 134:167–176

Sarkaria JN, Mehta MP, Loeffler JS (1995) Radiosurgery in the initial management of malignant gliomas: survival comparison with RTOG recursive partitioning analysis. Int J Rad Oncol Biol Phys 32:931–941

Schneider BF, Eberhard DA, Steiner LE (1997) Histopathology of arteriovenous malformations after gamma knife radiosurgery. J Neurosurg 87:352–357

Shaw E, Scott C, Souhami L, et al. (1996) Radiosurgery for the treatment of previously irradiated recurrent primary brain tumors and brain metastases: initial report of Radiation Therapy Oncology Group Protocol (90–05) Int J Rad Oncol Biol Phys 34:145

Shrieve DC, Alexander E III, Wen PY, et al. (1995) Results of radiosurgery vs. brachytherapy in the treatment of recurrent glioblastoma multiforme. Neurosurg 36:275–284

Shrieve DC, Alexander E, Black PML, et al. (1999) Treatment of patients with primary glioblastoma multiforme with standard postoperative radiotherapy and radiosurgical boost: prognostic factors and long-term outcome. J Neurosurg 90:72–77

Simpson D (1957) The recurrence of intracranial meningiomas after surgical treatment. J Neurol Neurosurg Psychiatry 20:22–39

Souhami L, Olivier A, Podgorsak EB (1991) Fractionated stereotactic radiation therapy for intracranial tumors. Cancer 68:2101–2108

Steiner L (1988) Stereotactic radiosurgery with the Cobalt-60 Gamma unit in the surgical treatment of the intracranial tumors and arteriovenous malformations. In: Schmidek HH, Sweet WH (eds) Operative Neurosurgical Techniques. Grune and Stratton, New York, pp 515–523

Steiner L, Prasad D, Lindquist C, et al. (1998) Clinical aspects of gamma knife stereotactic radiosurgery. In: Gildenberg P (ed) Textbook of stereotactic and functional neurosurgery. McGraw-Hill, New York, pp 763–803

Thomsett MJ, Conte FA, Kaplan SL, et al. (1980) Endocrine and neurologic outcome in childhood craniopharyngioma: review of effect of treatment in 42 patients. J Pediatrics 97:728–735

Thoren M, Rahn T, GuoWY, et al. (1991) Stereotactic radiosurgery with the cobalt-60 gamma unit in the treatment of growth hormone producing pituitary tumors. Neurosurg 29:663–668

Tishler RB, Loeffler JS, Lunsford LD, et al. (1993) Tolerance of cranial nerves of the cavernous sinus to radiosurgery. Int J Rad Oncol Biol Phys 27:215–221

Urano M, Goitein M, Verhey L, et al. (1983) Relative biological effectiveness of modulated proton beams in various murine tissues. Int J Rad Oncol Biol Phys 10:509

Valentino V, Schinaia G, Raimondi AJ (1993) The results of radiosurgical management of 72 middle fossa meningiomas. Acta Neurochir(Wien) 122:60–70

Verhey LJ, Smith V (1995) The physics of radiosurgery. Semin Rad Oncol 5:175–191

Verhey LJ, Smith V, Serago CF (1998) Comparison of radiosurgery treatment modalities based on physical dose distributions. Int J Rad Oncol Biol Phys 40:497–505

Wallner KE, Pitts LH, Wara WM, et al. (1987) Efficacy of irradiation for incompletely excised acoustic neurilemmomas. J Neurosurg 67: 858–863

Wallner KE, Galicich JH, Krol G, et al. (1989) Patterns of failure following treatment for glioblastoma multiforme and anaplastic astrocytoma. Int J Rad Oncol Biol Phys 16:1405–1409

Werner-Wasik M, Rudoler S, Preston PE, et al. (1999) Immediate side effects of stereotactic radiotherapy and radiosurgery. Int J Rad Oncol Biol Phys 43:299–304

20 Frameless Stereotactic Radiosurgery

Steven D. Chang, Martin J. Murphy, David P. Martin and John R. Adler, Jr.

CONTENTS

S. D. Chang, MD
Cerebrovascular Surgery Fellow, Department of Neurosurgery, Stanford University School of Medicine, 300 Pasteur Drive, Stanford, CA 94305, USA
M. Murphy, PhD
Radiation Physicist, Department of Radiation Oncology, Stanford University School of Medicine, 300 Pasteur Drive, Stanford, CA 94305, USA
D. P. Martin, MD
Clinical Assistant Professor, Department of Neurosurgery, Stanford University School of Medicine, 300 Pasteur Drive, Stanford, CA 94305, USA
J. R. Adler, Jr., MD
Professor and Director of Radiosurgery and Stereotactic Neurosurgery, Departments of Neurosurgery and Radiation Oncology, Stanford University School of Medicine, 300 Pasteur Drive, Stanford, CA 94305, USA

20.1
Introduction

Stereotactic radiosurgery combines stereotactic localization with multiple cross-fired beams from a highly collimated high-energy radiation source. Over the last three decades, this method of noninvasive ablation has proven to be an effective alternative to conventional neurosurgery, cranial irradiation, and brachytherapy, for selected small cranial tumors and arteriovenous malformations. Current stereotactic techniques rely on a rigid frame fixed to the patient's skull for head immobilization and target localization. However, such a frame-based system results in numerous constraints which limit treatment options. Frameless stereotactic radiosurgery was conceived as a method to overcome these limitations of conventional systems.

20.1.1
Limitations of
Frame Based-Radiosurgical Systems

Stereotactic localization that relies on external frames and skeleton fixation has several inherent limitations. Existing cranial fixation systems only allow treatment of intracranial or, at most, high cervical lesions. Although a modified linear accelerator system has been used to treat 19 patients with spine metastases, this method utilizes a body-frame, attached to the patient through open surgery, using clamps affixed to bony processes (Takacs et al. 1999). Such surgery, along with the necessary prolonged anesthesia, subjects the patient to potential complications (two wound infections noted in the above 19 patients) and, when combined with radiosurgery itself, to a very long procedure. Furthermore, a fixed frame limits the treatment degrees of freedom, while the metal components of current frames produce imaging artifacts on CT and MRI. Finally, the discomfort associated with skeletal fixation makes treatment of children difficult and fractionation cumbersome.

A fixed isocenter, where all beams converge on a well-defined point, is the basis for standard radiosurgery instruments such as the Gamma Knife, and conventional linear accelerators (Linacs). This system works well with spherical targets but is not ideal for complex or irregular shapes. To treat intricately shaped tumors, these radiosurgery methods rely on multiple overlapping spherical dose volumes, a method which results in intralesional dose heterogeneity. A system that achieves shape matching without significantly compromising dose homogeneity could be particularly advantageous for treating many intracranial lesions. Furthermore, a frameless stereotactic radiosurgery system with increased degrees of freedom would allow treatment of extracranial (and even nonneural) tumors.

A recently approved technology developed by Accuray, (Sunnyvale, Calif., USA) uses noninvasive image-guided localization, a lightweight high-energy radiation source, and a robotic delivery system, to address these limitations. This system, called the Cyberknife, has been used to treat patients with intracranial tumors and arteriovenous malformations (AVMs), and more recently, extracranial targets within the spine and abdomen.

20.2
Image-Guided Radiosurgery

The present design of image-guided radiosurgery (IGR) derives from the original concept of a frameless alternative to conventional intracranial radiosurgery. As with other forms of stereotaxy, the system presumes a fixed relationship between the target and the skull. The instrumentation for IGR is illustrated schematically in Fig. 20.1. A compact 130 kg, 6 MV X-ray Linac is carried by a robotic arm that can move and point the Linac with six degrees of freedom. Two X-ray imaging devices are positioned on either side of the patient's head and acquire real-time radiographs of the skull, at repeated intervals during treatment. The images are automatically registered to digitally reconstructed radiographs (DRRs) derived from the treatment planning CT. This registration process allows the position of the skull (and thus the treatment site) to be translated to the coordinate frame of the Linac. A control loop between the imaging system and the robotic arm adjusts the pointing of the Linac therapeutic beam to the observed position of the skull. If the patient moves, the change is detected during the next imaging cycle and the beam is adjusted and realigned with the target.

The Cyberknife delivery treatment follows a sequential step-and-shoot format. After the patient has been placed on the treatment table, the imaging system acquires a pair of alignment radiographs and determines the initial location of the treatment site within the robotic coordinate system. This information is sent to the robot to initialize the pointing of the Linac beam. The robotic arm then moves the Linac through a sequence of preset nodes surrounding the patient. At each node the Linac stops and a new pair of images is acquired, from which the position of the skull is redetermined. The position of the target is delivered to the robot, which adapts beam pointing to compensate for any movement, and the Linac delivers the preplanned dose of radiation for that direction. The complete process is repeated at each node, for a total of approximately 100 nodes.

20.2.1
Robotic Manipulator

A standard gantry-mounted Linac moves in a planar arc and always points at a fixed isocenter. In contrast, IGR can position and point the Linac anywhere in space. Because of this increased maneuverability, consideration of the robotic arm's "workspace" is necessary during treatment planning and delivery. The workspace is the total volume within which the

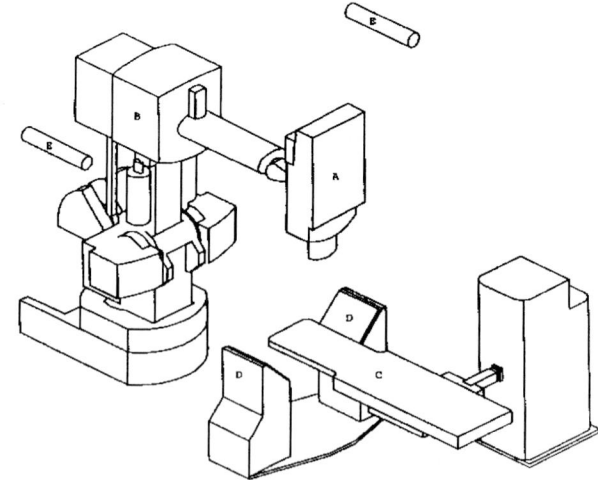

Fig. 20.1A–D. A schematic of the image-guided radiosurgery system, identifying the major system components. The 6 MV X-band Linac (**A**) is mounted on the arm (**B**) of the robotic manipulator. The treatment couch (**C**) is positioned between the two X-ray cameras (**D**) and their respective diagnostic X-ray tubes (**E**). Reprinted with permission from ADLER et al. (1999)

robot can maneuver without contacting any other object, or interfering with any lines of sight for the imaging instrumentation. Because the robot has no physical constraints on its motion, the workspace is defined by a three-dimensional computer model of all of the objects within its reach, including floor, ceiling, walls, and the patient. While in motion, the robot avoids collisions by continually comparing its position with the computer model.

The robot workspace for cranial radiosurgery occupies a hemispherical volume centered on a coronal plane through the patient's head. Portions of this hemisphere are excluded by the lines of sight between the X-ray sources and cameras and by the floor directly below the patient, resulting in a geometric coverage of about 1.6 p steridians for the beam directions. When moving from node to node, the robot follows planned trajectories, thus it is important not to reconfigure the workspace without updating the computer model.

20.3
Targeting Precision of Image-Guided Stereotactic Radiosurgery

The principal innovation embodied by IGR is the use of radiographic images of internal anatomical features to align the treatment beam with the target volume. This advancement eliminates the need for a stereotactic frame, but inevitably raises concerns about the spatial accuracy of dose placement when compared with existing frame-based systems. The overall IGR system has several sources of dose placement uncertainty comparable to conventional frame-based radiosurgery, beginning with the process of treatment planning.

20.3.1
Precision of the Treatment Planning

Image-guided radiosurgery requires DRRs generated from CT; therefore, CT or CT/MR coregistration is the necessary basis for treatment planning. A standard CT slice thickness of 1.5 to 3.0 mm introduces an uncertainty of approximately 0.75–1.5 mm in the inferior/superior coordinate of the treatment volume. Radiographic technical limitations, including edge softening from attenuation of the diagnostic X-rays, blurring from the reconstruction technique,

and other ambiguities in the delineation of structure within an image, introduce an uncertainty of about 0.5–1.0 mm in the other two planning coordinates. Frame-based radiosurgery has uncertainties in target localization which are nearly identical in magnitude (LEMIEUX et al. 1994).

20.3.2
Mechanical Accuracy of the Robot

The Linac beam is pointed by the robotic arm at an isocenter from each of about 100 different beam positions. The individual beams miss the isocenter with errors that are randomly distributed around a zero mean for each coordinate axis, with a net root mean square (rms) radial error of 0.7 mm (MURPHY and COX 1996). For a treatment that utilizes all beams, the effect of this source of error is to blur rather than offset the dose distribution. This rms radial pointing error of IGR is comparable to the deviation in the arc motion of a Linac moving along a gantry path, which has been reported in one instance to be 0.6 mm (WINSTON and LUTZ 1988).

20.3.3
Accuracy of Imaging System Calibration

For IGR to communicate the position of a patient's anatomy within the camera field of view into beam coordinates for the robot, the position of a fixed reference point must be established in both the robot and camera coordinate frames. This point is located in the camera coordinate frame by the attachment of a pointer to the Linac that is coaxial with the beam and holds an aluminum ball at the "isocenter." The camera system acquires pictures of the aluminum ball as the robot moves from node to node. Multiple measurements yield the position of the "isocenter" within the camera frame with a precision of approximately ±0.5 mm along each axis. This registration of camera and robot coordinate systems corresponds to the alignment of the frame-holding mechanism with a gantry arc or beam isocenter in conventional radiosurgery.

20.3.4
Precision of Image-to-Image Correlation

The location of the patient's anatomy within the coordinate frame of the camera relative to the position in the CT coordinate frame is measured by the image-guidance system. This is accomplished by registering a pair of digital radiographs acquired by the camera with two DRRs which are calculated from prior CT data in an exact emulation of the camera perspectives. Differences in the position and orientation of the anatomical images within the radiographs correspond to differences in the three-dimensional position and orientation of the anatomy between the camera and CT coordinate frames. Once this measurement has been completed, a lesion visualized on the treatment planning CT can be located within the workspace of the robot, and the beam directed at this target. The precision of this registration, which affects the apparent position of the target relative to the treatment beam, is analogous to the mechanical precision, stability, and stiffness of a stereotactic frame (MACIANUS et al. 1994). The imaging process presently used with IGR measures the three translational degrees of position with an rms precision of 0.3–0.6 mm per axis (MURPHY and COX 1996).

The four positioning errors described above combine to produce a net radial offset of the delivered dose from the targeted site. If the individual sources of error contribute randomly and independently, then the rms overall radial error is about 2.1 mm.

20.3.5
Measurements of Error

A series of trials using a dosimetric phantom suitable for radiographic imaging has been used to measure the actual radial offset of IGR. This phantom, made of polystyrene and Teflon, contains a cubic stack of GAF radiochromic films and is capable of forming a three-dimensional (3-D) image of dose distribution. In the trials, the assembled phantom, loaded with film, was imaged by CT, and the target was designated by standard planning procedures. Subsequently the phantom was irradiated with a dose distribution that simulated the treatment to be administered to the patient. The actual position of the dose center was compared to the intended (planned) center to obtain the offset along the three coordinate axes, and thus the net radial error. From 13 trials, the dose offsets were randomly scattered around a mean of zero for each axis. The rms radial error was 1.8 mm, which is consistent with the expectation of 2.1 mm based on the individual error sources.

When treating a patient, the Linac moves to each of 100 nodes and pauses, first to acquire radiographs that update beam pointing and then to deliver the prescribed increment of radiation. While each additional measurement is independent of the previous one, some components of the pointing error are not. A significant fraction of the targeting offset comes from systematic errors that do not vary during a particular treatment. As an example, planning errors in target localization are clearly fixed for a particular treatment. Meanwhile the inaccuracy associated with the image registration process depends mostly on systematic effects in matching the reference DRRs to the acquired radiographs; if the dosimetric phantom is kept in one position during a treatment simulation, then there is almost no fluctuation in its measured position from image to image. The offset of isocenter position in the camera coordinate frame is a fixed systematic error. Only the accuracy of robot pointing varies from node to node. Consequently, errors in beam pointing do not fluctuate appreciably from node to node, but rather maintain a fixed offset through the entire treatment, a situation that is similar to conventional forms of radiosurgery. This results in a dose distribution that is mostly offset rather than spread out. However, for each treatment, the various sources of error combine in changing ways, so that the dose placement error is distributed around a mean of zero in each directional axis.

The image correlation algorithm currently used with IGR cannot accurately measure and correct for rotational changes in the patient's position. Consequently it was necessary to minimize rotational movements by using some type of head restraint [the Laitinen stereoadapter (Laitinen et al. 1985) or a molded AquaPlast (Thornton et al. 1991) mask] during CT and treatment. These restraints also serve to confine the head to a small region (±10 mm) within which the imaging system is calibrated to measure translations. Even with the capacity to measure rotations, some form of nonrigid immobilization will remain useful for establishing and maintaining a "reasonable" position throughout treatment.

20.3.6
Patient Movement

Since frameless radiosurgery allows some motion, it introduces a fifth factor in the precision of dose placement. In the present IGR system, patient position is measured prior to the delivery of each dose, typically at intervals of approximately 20–40 s. If the patient moves while the beam is on, that portion of the dose will be misdirected. The patient's changed position will be detected and compensated for at the beginning of the next increment. With over 100 nodes, a single patient movement affects no more than about 1% of the total administered dose in a single-fraction treatment. Clinical experience with IGR has shown that in the vast majority of patients, movements are few in number and small in magnitude (Fig. 20.2).

20.3.7
Practical Considerations

Because IGR relies on DRRs, a CT of the patient is required prior to treatment, and provides the image basis for treatment planning. If MRI is to be used for planning, then such images must be fused with the CT. Additionally, the system acquires a pair of positioning images 100 or more times during the course of a typical radiosurgical treatment, each exposing the patient

to X-rays. The imaging system is presently limited to an exposure of less than about 5 cGy during a treatment, or 25 µGy per image. This is not a significant issue for cranial treatments, where the skull silhouette can be clearly imaged with an exposure of 1.5 µGy, but can become a limiting factor when the system is to be used to locate extracranial sites.

20.3.8
Treatment Planning

The Cyberknife can be programmed to administer either spherical single-isocenter or overlapping multiple-isocenter doses. However, as with other radiosurgical devices, the treatment of irregular tumor volumes with multiple isocenters can be quite time-consuming. The treatment planning system of the Cyberknife exploits the robot's six-degrees-of-freedom maneuverability, and allows an array of overlapping beams to be superimposed without an isocenter. An inverse planning procedure optimizes the set of beam directions and dose to be used on lesions of arbitrary shapes, and has been demonstrated to

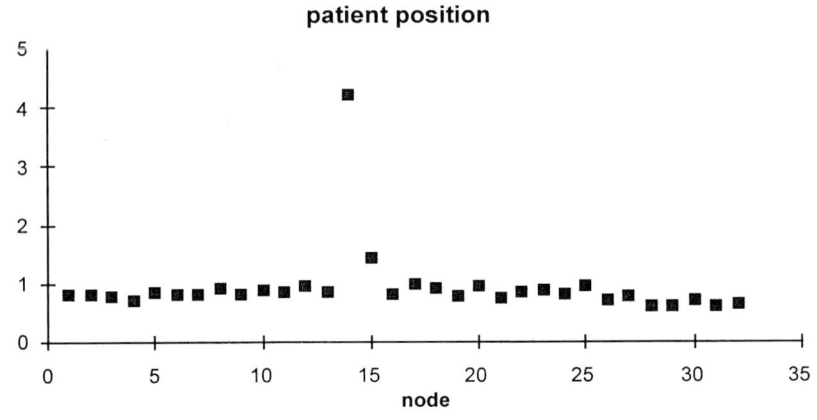

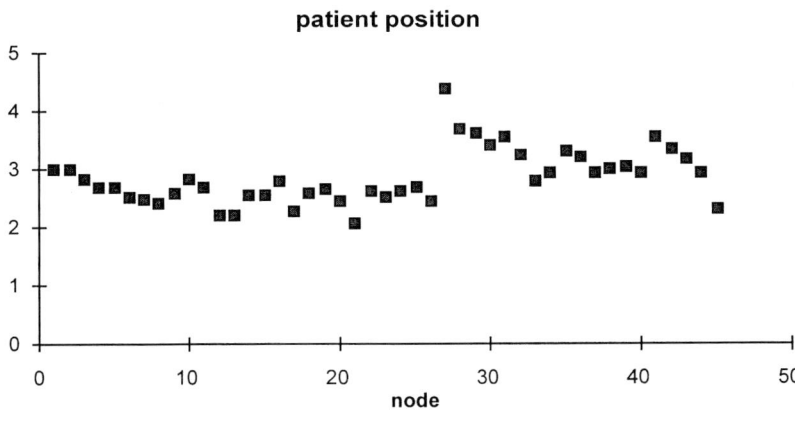

Fig. 20.2. Records of patient position during two treatments, showing typical degree of movement during treatment. The figures record the fluctuations in radial position of the treatment site from node to node. Importantly, the *absolute magnitude* of the position at each node is not a pointing error, because the robot corrects for it. The *change* in the position reveals the magnitude and frequency of patient movement, and illustrates the amount of misalignment of the beam if the patient moves between imaging updates, while the beam is on. In one case the fluctuations average 0.1 mm with a single significant (=1 mm) transient shift in position; in the second case the fluctuations average 0.5 mm and again show only a single significant shift of position. Reprinted with permission from ADLER et al. (1999)

deliver homogeneous dose distributions that closely conform to even highly irregular volumes (Sch-weikard et al. 1993, 1994).

IGR corrects for changes in patient position by preserving the pattern in which both the beams traverse patient anatomy and intersect within the target. If the patient's treatment position in the camera coordinate system is exactly the same as in the CT study, then the image-guidance system makes no positioning correction and the robot moves the Linac to the original workspace nodes specified by the treatment plan. If the patient moves during treatment or is displaced relative to the CT coordinates at initial setup, then the robot adjusts the spatial position and orientation of the nodal hemisphere in a way that keeps the position of the beams fixed with respect to the skull, thereby ensuring that all beams not only continue to point at the planned target, but also pass through the patient anatomy as prescribed.

Because IGR is not inherently isocentric, in contrast to other radiosurgical technologies, a rigorous quality assurance process is necessary, which relies on a thorough simulation of each treatment plan prior to delivery. After the designing of a treatment plan, the previously described phantom, containing radiochromic film, is scanned by CT and set up in the position of the patient's head within the Cyberknife treatment room. The entire treatment is then emulated – the phantom is located by the imaging system, the robot moves through its complete path, and the radiochromic film is exposed to the entire dose that will be administered. This process verifies that the dose distribution has the prescribed shape, the guidance system places it at the right position within the phantom, and the robotic arm moves through the entire treatment sequence uneventfully.

20.4
Improvements to Frameless Stereotactic Radiosurgery: Six-Dimensional Tracking

The first generation IGR system could not detect and accommodate rotational changes in the position of the radiographic features that are used to locate a radiosurgical target. While it has required the use of head restraints to restrict rotational movements, this situation has not affected the system's usefulness in performing radiosurgery within the cranium, nor has it compromised dose placement accuracy. However, a new image registration

process has been designed to measure all six degrees of freedom (6-D) in the position and orientation of patient anatomy (Murphy 1997). This method also allows complete flexibility in adapting the image field of view and magnification to a particular subject. This algorithm is presently implemented on the Cyberknife in the image-guided facility at Stanford Medical Center where it has undergone clinical testing for nearly 1 year.

Phantom-tests of the 6-D positioning algorithm revealed that the CT slice thickness has a significant influence on overall accuracy. This is illustrated in Fig. 20.3, which shows translation and rotation measurements made with a skull phantom. The measurements were first made using DRRs generated from a CT using 3.0 mm thick slices, and then repeated using a CT of 1.5 mm slices. All components of error showed a factor-of-two improvement at higher CT resolution, and the new 6-D process achieved translational rms accuracy of 0.1 mm and rotational rms precision of 0.4 deg per axis. This level of translational tracking precision is significantly better than the above-described 3-D measurement process.

20.5
Amorphous Silicon Detectors

The Cyberknife localization method can in principle be used wherever radioopaque features are associated with an anatomic target, a concept that would allow the extension of radiosurgical technique to extracranial sites. IGR has already been used to treat sites within the cervical spine (Chang et al. 1998a–c), but the extension of this technique to the thorax and abdomen has not been possible previously because of limitations in imaging, a restriction which can be overcome by improvements to the X-ray detectors.

20.5.1
Limitations of Current Cameras

There are multiple shortcomings to the first generation imaging system used by the Cyberknife. As currently configured, the X-ray sources used with the Cyberknife are positioned 365 cm from the cameras to allow the robot a large workspace. Because this is approximately three times the conventional distance for diagnostic imaging, there is a resulting nine-fold reduction in X-ray level at the patient's head. The

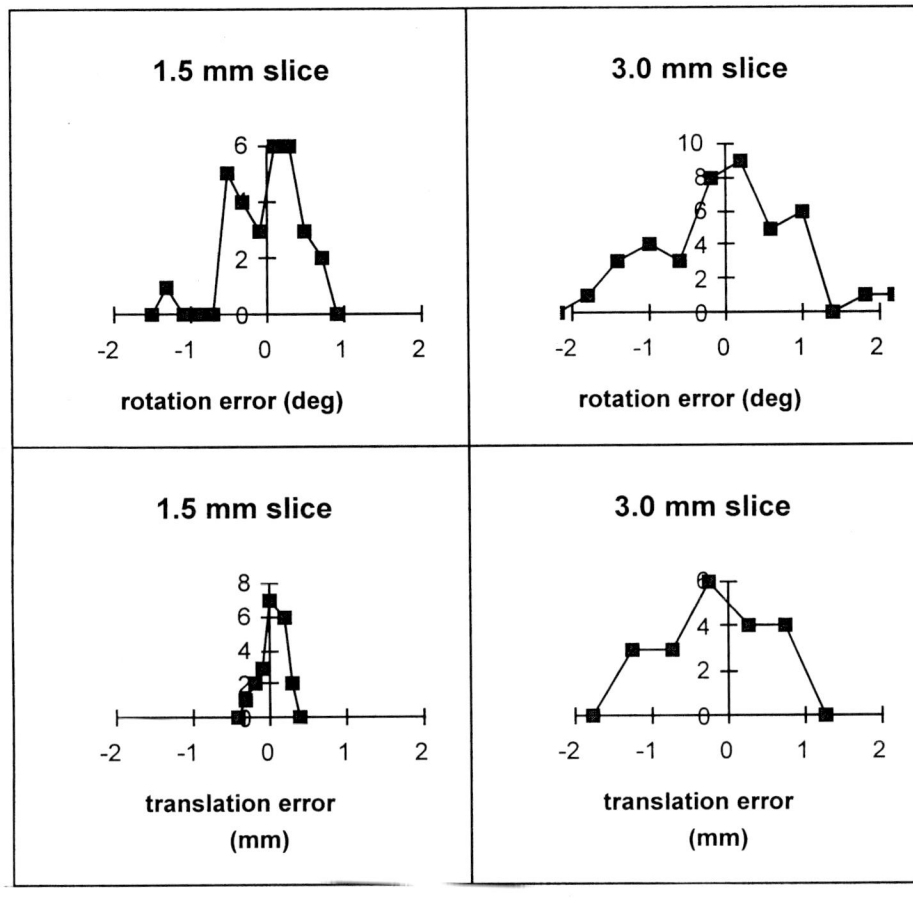

Fig. 20.3. Errors in measuring translations and rotations with a six-degrees-of-freedom image registration algorithm, from tests using an anthropomorphic skull phantom. The tests used CT studies with two different slice thicknesses to generate the digitally reconstructed radiographs (DRRs) used by the registration algorithm. Reprinted with permission from ADLER et al. (1999)

present X-ray cameras are fluoroscopes consisting of a gadolinium oxysulfide screen viewed by a light-amplified video CCD. Lens optics require that the CCD be 60 cm from the screen, which results in (1) poor signal-to-noise ratios at low exposure levels, (2) low contrast, and (3) significant veiling glare. This design has made it difficult to obtain good-quality images of the skeletal anatomy within and around the thorax and abdomen.

The present imaging system used in the Cyberknife limits the pixel size to 1.25 mm, which gives poor spatial resolution. When locating a target in the cervical spine, for example, experience has demonstrated that the vertebrae are better imaged with a pixel size of 0.25–0.5 mm. Furthermore, a higher degree of spatial resolution allows for superior imaging of small fiducial markers implanted near soft-tissue targets.

The registration of DRRs (generated from CT) with images taken by the Cyberknife camera system, requires an accurate representation of the camera imaging geometry. To accomplish this, the distortion caused by the CCD camera lenses must be measured and modeled in the DRRs. Any imprecision in quan-

tifying this optical arrangement has a direct impact on registration accuracy, which in turn affects the dose placement accuracy.

20.5.2
Advantages of the Amorphous Silicon Detectors

To overcome the above limitations, the previous cameras in the Cyberknife have been replaced with flat-panel amorphous silicon X-ray cameras (dpiX, Palo Alto, Calif., USA) (ANTONUK et al. 1995; WEISFIELD et al. 1997). Figure 20.4 illustrates the Cyberknife with two amorphous silicon sensors at the facility in Stanford Medical Center. These devices have a pixel pitch of 0.125 mm and acquire flat images that avoid the distortions inherent in lensed or X-ray image intensifier techniques. When images from these sensors are processed by the new 6-D registration software, it will be possible to achieve a ten-fold improvement in spatial resolution. The new imaging software and hardware have been specifically designed to provide variable fields of view and magni-

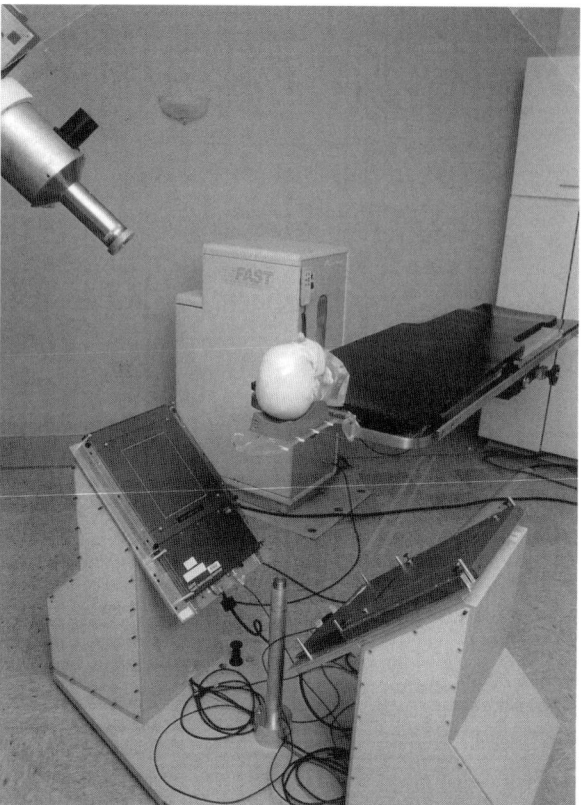

Fig. 20.4. A picture of the Cyberknife, showing the Linac, the robotic arm, the treatment couch, and the amorphous silicon X-ray cameras (mounted on the floor)

fication ranges that can be adapted to multiple anatomic locations. For example, amorphous-silicon X-ray sensors create a high-quality image of the lumbar spine using the typical Cyberknife imaging geometry (10 mAs, 75 kV X-ray exposure (ANTONUK et al. 1995). Such an exposure corresponds to a dose per image of approximately 25 μGy, which is within the limits discussed earlier.

20.6
Clinical Experience with Intracranial Lesions

As of August 1999, more than 300 patients with benign and malignant intracranial tumors have been treated with the Cyberknife at Stanford Medical Center and six other sites worldwide. In addition to the intracranial treatments, six cervical lesions, including four intramedullary spinal cord tumors or vascular malformations, have been treated at Stanford under a

company-sponsored IDE. Radiosurgery of the cervical region has been performed by using the vertebral bodies as points of radiographic reference and spatial location. To date, the outcome for all lesions as defined clinically and radiographically appears to mirror that achieved with standard radiosurgery. Food and Drug Administration (FDA) approval of the Cyberknife in July 1999 will allow expanding use of IGR.

20.7
Clinical Experience with Extracranial Lesions

A primary objective behind the development of IGR was the ability to treat extracranial lesions. With the implementation of an amorphous silicon camera system, achieving this goal has become feasible. Since most extracranial lesions within the thorax and abdomen typically move with respiration, i.e. are not fixed with respect to bony structures, a system for target localization has been developed which relies on implanted fiducials.

20.7.1
Targeting with Fiducials

Several metal implantable fiducials have been identified, with the requisite characteristics of being readily imaged by the Cyberknife. For example, gold spheres 2 to 3 mm in diameter can be successfully sutured to soft tissue within the abdomen, allowing the targeting of abdominal cancers. Alternatively, smaller gold balls can be implanted with a 14 gauge needle (SANDLER et al. 1993), and gold wires (1 mm diameter) have also been used (CROOK et al. 1995). Meanwhile, small bone-screws can be anchored to the spine through stab incisions and provide an acceptable level of contrast relative to bone. While fiducials fixed to bone can be assumed to maintain their relative position, it is unclear whether or not, and if so over what time interval, markers attached to soft tissue can migrate. Studies are under way to investigate the issue of fiducial migration within soft tissue.

20.7.2
Clinical Experience with Extracranial Cases

To date, two patients with thoracolumbar lesions have been treated with the Cyberknife. One patient had a schwannoma of the lumbar nerve roots (located anterior to the cord at T9) treated with three fractions, while another patient had a bony spine metastasis successfully treated with two fractions. Both of these patients had had 4 mm screw fiducials implanted in the spine through stab incisions. In contrast, a pancreatic tumor patient underwent implantation of gold fiducial balls during a laparotomy for pancreatic carcinoma. This patient was treated with a highly conformal single fraction of 15 Gy using breath-holding throughout the procedure. This treatment, administered as part of a dose escalation protocol, provided significant relief from pretreatment symptoms.

20.8
Conclusion

Stereotactic neurosurgery has been evolving towards frameless technology that is both less invasive and more flexible. However, nearly all widely available radiosurgical systems continue to use stereotactic frames for localization and immobilization. While such frame-based radiosurgical systems can be adapted to fractionated treatment, some compromise in precision is necessary. These devices are also not amenable to treatment outside the cranium, and typically require prolonged general anesthesia when used in children. Image-guided radiosurgery was developed in an attempt to overcome these restrictions, and although the initial clinical system has been limited by the hardware used for imaging and the software used in targeting, most of the original design objectives have been accomplished. Although the Cyberknife does not use skeletal fixation, its overall accuracy compares favorably with that achieved by conventional Linac and Gamma Knife systems that rely upon invasive stereotactic frames. In addition, treatment planning and delivery software has been shown to allow delivery of homogeneous conformal dose distribution to targets of irregular shape. Perhaps most importantly, this technology is finally making it possible to consider performing radiosurgery at almost any location within the body.

References

Adler JR, Murphy MJ, Chang SD, et al (1999) Image-guided robotic radiosurgery. Neurosurgery 44:1299–1307

Antonuk LE, Yorkston J, Huang W et al (1995) A real time, flat panel, amorphous silicon, digital x-ray imager. Radiographics 15:993–1000

Chang SD, Adler JR, Murphy MJ (1998a) Stereotactic radiosurgery of spinal lesions. In: Maciunas RJ (eds) Advanced Techniques in Central Nervous System Metastasis. American Association of Neurologic Surgeons, Park Ridge, Illinois, pp 269–276

Chang SD, Murphy M, Geis P et al (1998b) Clinical experience with image-guided robotic radiosurgery (the Cyberknife) in the treatment of brain and spinal cord tumors. Neurol Med Chir (Tokyo) 38:780–783

Chang SD, Murphy MJ, Tombropoulos R et al (1998c) Robotic radiosurgery. In: Alexander E, Maciunas R (eds) Advanced Neurosurgical Navigation. Thieme, New York, pp 443–449

Crook JM, Raymond Y, Salhani D et al (1995) Prostate motion during standard radiotherapy as assessed by fiducial markers. Radiother and Oncol 37:35–42

Laitinen LV, Liliequist B, Fagerlund M et al (1985) An adapter for computed tomography-guided stereotaxis. Surg Neurol 23:559–566

Lemieux L, Kitchen ND, Hughes SW et al (1994) Voxel-based localization in frame-based and frameless stereotaxy and its accuracy. Med Phys 21:1301–1310

Maciunas RJ, Galloway RL, Jr., Latimer JW (1994) The application accuracy of stereotactic frames. Neurosurgery 35:682 694; discussion 694–685

Murphy MJ (1997) An automatic six-degree-of-freedom image restoration algorithm for image-guided frameless stereotaxic radiosurgery. Med Phys 24:857–866

Murphy MJ, Cox RS (1996) The accuracy of dose localization for an image-guided frameless radiosurgery system. Med Phys 23.2043–2049

Sandler HM, Bree RL, McLaughlin PW et al (1993) Localization of the prostatic apex for radiation therapy using implanted markers. Int J Radiat Oncol Biol Phys 27:915–919

Schell MC, Bova FJ, Larson DA et al (1995) Stereotactic Radiosurgery. AAPM Task Group 42 Report 54 :6–8

Schweikard A, Adler JR, Latombe JC (1993) Motion planning in stereotaxic radiosurgery. Proc. IEEE Int. Conf. Robotics and Automation :1909–1916

Schweikard A, Tombropoulos RZ, Adler JR et al (1994) Treatment planning for a radiosurgical system with general kinematics. Proc. IEEE Conf. Robotics and Automation :1720–1727

Takacs I, Hamilton AJ, Lulu B et al (1999) Frame based stereotactic spinal radiosurgery: Experience from the first 19 patients. Presented at the 1999 Quadrennial Meeting of the American Soceity for Stereotactic and Functional Neurosurgery

Thornton AF, Ten Haken RK, Weeks KJ et al (1991) A head immobilization system for radiation simulation, CT, MRI, and PET imaging. Medical Dosimetry 16:51–56

Weisfield RL, Street RA, Apte R et al (February 1997) An improved page size 127 mm pixel amorphous-silicon image sensor for x-ray diagnostic medical imaging applications. SPIE International Symposium on the Physics of Medical Imaging

Winston KR, Lutz W (1988) Linear accelerator as a neurosurgical tool for stereotactic radiosurgery. Neurosurgery 22:454–464

21 Treatment of Brain Metastasis

Zbigniew Petrovich, Cheng Yu and Michael L. J. Apuzzo

CONTENTS

21.1 Introduction

Metastatic brain tumors present major management problem in patients with cancer. The incidence of brain metastases is increasing with the increase in our ability to control with surgery or radiotherapy, disease at the primary site, and with chemotherapy, systemic extracranial disease. In the 1970s, approximately 18% of patients dying of cancer were found at autopsy to have brain metastases (POSNER 1977). In a national survey of US hospitals on patients admitted during 1973 to 1974, nearly equal numbers of patients were diagnosed as having primary and metastatic brain tumors (WALKER et al. 1985). Several years later, it has been estimated that 30% of patients with metastatic tumors develop brain metastases (CAIRNCROSS and POSNER 1983). The incidence of primary malignant brain tumors is increasing, however the incidence of brain metastases is increasing at a higher rate. At the present time, the ratio of metastatic to primary brain tumor is nearly 6:1 (LAWS and THAPAR 1993). It has been estimated that from 100,000 to 170,000 new patients with metastatic disease are diagnosed per year in the United States (PATCHELL et al. 1990; POSNER 1992; LAWS and THAPAR 1993).

The presence of brain metastases is of major importance, due to a well-known severe disability resulting from progression of brain disease, which decreases patient quality of life, and sharply reduces patient survival (DEANGELIS 1994; CAIRNCROSS et al. 1980; BREGA et al. 1989). In view of the above implications, it is imperative to make an early diagnosis, with timely application of an appropriate therapy. In recent years, real progress was made in establishing an early diagnosis of brain metastasis. At the present time, patients with primary tumors with a known high incidence of brain metastasis, such as those with melanoma or small-cell carcinoma of the lung, undergo periodic brain imaging which allows an early diagnosis in asymptomatic patients to be made. At the University of Southern California (USC) more than one-half of patients with metastases are asymptomatic, and are diagnosed on routine screening with magnetic resonance imaging (MRI) (LEVINE et al. 1999).

Z. PETROVICH, MD
Professor and Chairman, Department of Radiation Oncology, University of Southern California School of Medicine, 1441 Eastlake Avenue G34, Los Angeles, CA 90033, USA
C. YU, PhD
Assistant Professor, Department of Radiation Oncology–Physics, University of Southern California School of Medicine, 1441 Eastlake Avenue, Los Angeles, CA 90033, USA
M. L.J. APUZZO, MD
Professor, Neurological Surgery, University of Southern California School of Medicine, LAC+USC Medical Center, 1200 North State Street, Room 5046, Los Angeles, CA 90033, USA

21.2 Natural History

21.2.1 Incidence

Brain metastasis is a common manifestation of distant disease, with the reported incidence of 30% in patients with solid tumors (CAIRNCROSS and POS-

NER 1983). In the United States, from 100,000 to 170,000 patients are diagnosed with metastatic brain disease each year (PATCHELL et al. 1990; LAWS and THAPAR 1993; JOHNSON and YOUNG 1996; POSNER 1992). Some primary tumors are known to have a high incidence of brain metastasis. Patients with small-cell carcinoma of the lung have been reported to have a 70% incidence of brain metastasis, while those with melanoma have an incidence of 10–60% (WEN and LOEFFLER 1999; NUGENT et al. 1979). The incidence of brain metastasis in some common primary tumors is shown in Table 21.1.

Table 21.1. Incidence of brain metastasis in solid tumors

Primary tumor	% Brain metastasis
Lung cancer	50–63
Melanoma	10–60
Breast carcinoma	15–20
Unknown primary	10
Genitourinary	6
Colon carcinoma	5

Data from LAWS and THAPAR (1993), WEN and LOEFFLER (1999), and WALKER et al. (1985)

21.2.2
Clinical Presentation

It has been widely assumed that most patient with brain metastases present with multiple lesions. In fact, 50% of patients present with a solitary metastasis, 20% of patients have two lesions and 10% have more than five lesions at the time of diagnosis (DELATTRE et al. 1988; ZIMM et al. 1981; CAIRNCROSS et al. 1980). These data may be modified, based on the more recent period, when modern imaging techniques have been used for diagnostic work up of brain metastases. It is likely that based on MRI the proportion of patients with solitary metastases will decrease, and those with multiple lesions will increase. These data are of an obvious importance in the design of treatment strategy. Most (90%) metastatic lesions are supratentorial, with posterior fossa tumors seen primarily in patients with cancer of the prostate, uterus and renal cell carcinoma (DELATTRE et al. 1988). In recent years, due to a routine use of imaging modalities such as MRI in the screening of patients at a high risk of developing brain metastases, more and more patients are diagnosed with asymptomatic disease. In a report based on a large number of patients, symptoms caused by increased intracranial pressure predominated, with seizures

being next in frequency (Table 21.2) (LAWS and THAPAR 1993).

Table 21.2. Symptoms and signs of brain metastasis at diagnosis

Symptom or sign	%
Headache	65
Seizures	30
Visual symptoms	30
Personality change	15
Nausea and vomiting	10

Modified from LAWS and THAPAR (1993)

21.2.3
Prognosis

Diagnosis of brain metastasis requires prompt management, since the median survival time of untreated patients is approximately 1 month, which is extended to a median survival time of 2 months in those receiving corticosteroid therapy (ZIMM et al. 1981; HAZRA et al. 1972). Important prognostic signs for patients with brain metastasis are shown in Table 21.3 (LAWS and THAPAR 1993). A similar list of favorable prognostic factors was published by investigators from the National Cancer Institute (ZIMM et al. 1981). It has been well documented in the literature, that the primary cause of deaths in patients with brain metastasis is CNS disease, while some investigators reported systemic disease progression as being the main cause of death in these patients (LEVINE et al. 1999). In that study, 45 patients with metastatic melanoma to the brain were treated with gamma knife stereotactic radiosurgery. Of the 26 patients who are known to have died, only in two (8%) was disease progression in the brain the cause of death.

Table 21.3. Important prognostic factors in patients with brain metastasis

Prognostic factor	Favorable	Unfavorable
Patient age	<50	+50
Number of lesions	1	>1
Systemic disease	Controlled	Uncontrolled
Karnofsky performance status	+70	<70
Increased intracranial pressure	None	Present
Primary cancer	Unknown	Melanoma

Modified from LAWS and THAPAR (1993)

21.3
Prophylactic Cranial Irradiation

In view of the serious impact of brain metastases on quality of life and survival, it is of importance to prevent development of brain metastases in patients who are known to have a high incidence of this disease. It has been well documented that patients with small-cell lung cancer treated with chemo-radiotherapy combination, have up to 70% incidence of brain metastases (NUGENT et al. 1979). Prophylactic cranial irradiation (PCI) has been shown to be an effective treatment in the prevention of development of brain metastases in 987 patients with small-cell carcinoma (AUPERIN et al. 1999). In that report, the incidence of brain metastases was reduced by nearly 50% (58% vs. 33.3%). Patients receiving higher radiation doses (30, 36 and 40 Gy) had a reduced risk of subsequent brain metastases when compared with those who received lower radiation doses (8, 24, 25 Gy), $P=0.02$. An improved overall and disease-free survival was noted in patients receiving PCI. There was a 5.4% increase in survival rates at 3 years post-treatment in PCI patients compared with those in the control group. No additional survival benefit was recorded in PCI patients receiving higher radiation doses.

In a randomized trial reported by the Radiation Therapy Oncology Group (RTOG) on 187 patients with large-cell carcinoma and adenocarcinoma of the lung, no statistically significant difference was noted in the incidence of brain metastases in patients receiving PCI, when compared with those in the control group (RUSSEL et al. 1991). PCI patients received 30 Gy in ten equal fractions. It is apparent that more prospective randomized trials need to be conducted to establish the place of PCI in the prevention of clinical brain metastasis. PCI should be considered only for patients with stable or controlled extracranial disease.

21.4
Surgical Therapy

Surgery is an important treatment modality in properly selected patients with brain metastases. Stereotactic biopsy is a commonly used and safe procedure, frequently essential in patients who require for their management, histological confirmation of diagnosis. Craniotomy with tumor resection is imperative in patients who present with larger (>35 mm) lesions with significant mass effect, which may result in acute or even life-threatening signs and symptoms.

Surgical treatment in such patients rapidly improves their quality of life and allows them to return to the state of well being. If there is any residual tumor after open surgery, patients can be successfully treated with stereotactic radiosurgery. Most patients with smaller (<35 mm) solitary lesions or few metastases can be successfully managed with stereotactic radiosurgery (LEVINE et al. 1999).

A retrospective analysis on 17 patients with melanoma who underwent 18 craniotomies for solitary brain metastases showed resolution of symptoms in 14 (82%) patients (WORNOM et al. 1986). There was, however, a high incidence of significant toxicity reported as well as a surprisingly long (16 days) average hospital stay. Two (12%) patients died within 30 days of surgery, and a further patient died 34 days after surgery. Another study on 25 surgically treated patients with metastatic melanoma of the brain, showed that 20 (80%) had solitary lesions and five (20%) had multiple lesions (HAFSTROM et al. 1980). Complete relief of symptoms was recorded in 17 (68%) and partial relief in two (8%) patients. Of the 25 patients treated, three (12%) died following surgery. The median survival time was 5 months. In two other reports on surgical treatment of patients with metastatic melanoma of the brain, no treatment mortality was noted and relief of symptoms was reported in two-thirds of the patients (GUAZZO et al. 1989; BREGA et al. 1980).

An interesting study on 56 patients with cerebral metastases was reported by the group from MD Anderson Cancer Center (BINDAL et al. 1993). Patients were divided into three treatment groups (Table 21.4). Group 1 consisted of 30 patients, who had one or more lesions left unresected. Group 2 con-

Table 21.4. Histological diagnosis in surgically treated patients

Diagnosis	Multiple lesions	Group 1	Group 2	Group 3
Melanoma	25	13	12	12
Breast cancer	11	6	5	5
Lung cancer	7	4	3	3
Sarcoma	5	3	2	3
Colon cancer	3	1	2	2
Renal cell cancer	2	1	1	1
Ovarian cancer	1	0	1	0
Unknown primary	2	2	0	0
Total	56	30	26	26

Data from BINDAL et al. (1993)

tained 26 patients, who had all lesions resected, and group 3 comprised 26 patients, each presenting with a solitary metastasis, which was resected. Median survival time for the patients in groups 1, 2 and 3 was 6, 14 and 14 months, respectively. Tumor recurrence in the brain occurred in 31% of group 2 and in 35% of group 3 patients. Symptom-improvement was recorded in 65% of group 1, 84% of group 2 and in 85% of group 3 patients. A worsening of symptoms was seen in 13%, 6% and 0% of groups 1, 2 and 3 patients, respectively. The mortality rate was <4% and complication rate was 9%. In multivariate analysis, the only important factor affecting survival was the presence or absence of systemic disease ($P<0.05$). Based on their experience, the authors recommended surgical removal of all brain metastases in selected patients.

In a recent review of surgical management of patients with brain metastases, the group from MD Anderson Cancer Center stated, " The presence of multiple brain metastases does not automatically contraindicate surgery because in properly selected patients, resection of multiple metastases can extend survival and enhance the quality of life" (LANG et al. 1998). We disagree with this statement, as a less invasive treatment modality such as stereotactic radiosurgery, can produce treatment results similar to those of open craniotomy (LEVINE et al. 1999; PETROVICH et al. 1996; KONDZIOLKA et al. 1999).

21.4.1
Surgery–Radiotherapy Combination

Due to somewhat disappointing treatment results in patients with brain metastases managed with surgery, the use of postoperative whole brain irradiation (WBI) was explored in a number of studies. A group from Memorial Sloan-Kettering Cancer Center reported a study of 104 patients with solitary metastasis in non small-cell carcinoma of the bronchus (MANDELL et al. 1986). Of the 104 study-patients, 35 (34%) were treated with surgery (S) followed by WBI and 69 (64%) were treated with WBI alone. The two groups were dissimilar with WBI alone compared with S-WBI combination, having the following differences: (1) The initial treatment to the primary site was less aggressive (64% vs 28%); (2) In 12%, brain stem or basal ganglia involvement was present vs. none in the combined treatment group; (3) Extracranial disease was present in 74% in WBI alone vs. 49% in S-WBI patients; (4) Distant metastases were present in 49% WBI patients vs. 6% in those treated with S-WBI. The 69 WBI patients had a subjective and objec-

tive treatment response in 83% and 72%, respectively, while it was 80% and 87%, respectively for those treated with S-WBI combination. Median survival was also different, with WBI patients having a median survival time of 4 months vs. 16 months for S-WBI patients, $P<0.0001$. The 5 year actuarial survival rate was 0% for the former and 22% for the latter group, $P<0.0001$. It is of interest to analyze the cause of death in the 104 study-patients. Death, in 50%, was due to an intracranial relapse in the 69 WBI patients, compared with 9% in the 35 S-WBI group. The authors believed that the use of a more aggressive treatment approach in patients with brain metastases improves survival. This conclusion is difficult to support, due to the selection process favoring patients in a better general condition with lesion(s) accessible to surgical resection in patients treated with S-WBI vs. acceptance of almost unselected patients with brain metastases for radiotherapy alone.

21.4.2
Randomized Trials

An important prospective randomized study was reported on the value of postoperative WBI in patients with solitary metastatic lesions treated with a total tumor removal (PATCHELL et al. 1990, 1998). From 1989 through 1997, 95 patients with solitary brain metastasis were treated with total tumor removal. Of the 95 study-patients, 49 (52%) were randomly selected to receive postoperative WBI and 46 (48%) received no further treatment. The pattern of failure in the brain was different for the two treatment groups. Tumor relapse in the brain was less common in S-WBI patients than in those treated with surgery alone (18 vs. 70%, $P<0.001$). Local recurrence was reported in 10% of S-WBI and in 46% of surgery-alone patients, $P<0.001$. Central nervous system-related cause of death was seen in six (14%) of the 43 S-WBI patients who are known to have died in this group and in 17 (44%) of the 39 patients who died in the surgery-alone group, $P=0.003$. There was no difference between the two treatment groups in overall survival and in the duration of the ambulatory status.

A prospective randomized trial in 63 patients with solitary brain metastasis, comparing S-WBI with WBI alone was reported from the Daniel den Hoed Cancer Center from Rotterdam (VECHT et al. 1993). Patients treated with S-WBI had longer overall survival and median survival times (12 vs. 7 months) than did those treated with WBI alone, $P=0.04$ and had a longer duration of functionally independent survival,

P=0.06. The superiority of the combined treatment over radiotherapy alone was demonstrated for younger (<60 years of age) and older (>60 years of age) patients. As expected, older patients in both treatment groups had a hazard ratio of dying of 2.74, P=0.001, when compared with the younger patients. The authors recommended a more aggressive (S-WBI) treatment approach in patients with solitary brain metastasis and stable peripheral disease.

21.5
External Beam Radiotherapy

External beam radiotherapy was the first successful treatment modality used in the management of patients with metastatic brain disease. At the present time, WBI remains the most frequently applied therapy in these patients. In a large number of published reports, WBI consistently resulted in overall symptom-improvement in over two-thirds of treated patients (CAIRNCROSS et al. 1980; ZIMM et al. 1981; CHOI et al. 1985; POSNER 1977; DEANGELIS 1994; WEN and LOEFFLER 1999; BORGELT et al. 1980). This improvement was independent of histological diagnosis, number of metastatic lesions, total radiation dose and radiation schedule. Symptom-improvement was of a relatively short duration, since the median survival time of treated patients ranged from 3 to 6 months (Table 21.5). WBI is a widely available and relatively easy to administer treatment. WBI in combination with surgery, is discussed in sections 21.4.1 and 21.4.2, and WBI combined with stereotactic radiosurgery (SRS) is discussed in section 21.6.

During the past 25 years, various radiation schedules have been used in WBI for metastatic brain tu-

mors. The largest experience with the management of brain metastases was reported by the RTOG (BORGELT et al. 1980). The first RTOG study consisted of 900 patients randomly selected to receive: 30 Gy in 2 weeks, n=233 patients; 30 Gy in 3 weeks, n=217; 40 Gy in 3 weeks, n=233; and 40 Gy in 4 weeks, n=227. The second study was randomized into three groups as follows: 20 Gy in 1 week, n=447 patients, 30 Gy in 2 weeks, n=228; and 40 Gy in 3 weeks, n=227. There was no significant difference in median survival time, the degree of palliation, and time to tumor progression in patients treated with these five radiotherapy schedules. The overall improvement in neurological function was 47% and 52% in patients in the first and second studies respectively. Relief of neurological symptoms such as headache, was reported in 82% while seizures were controlled in 90% of patients. Median survival time ranged from 14 to 20 weeks depending on the radiation schedule. These differences in survival were not statistically significant. The incidence of death due to brain metastases ranged from 46 to 54% in the first study and 25 to 33% in the second study.

Outcomes similar to those obtained by RTOG in patients with brain metastasis treated with WBI alone, were reported by other investigators in nonrandomized trials (POSNER 1977; CAIRNCROSS et al. 1980; ZIMM et al. 1981; HOSKIN et al. 1990; RYAN et al. 1994; WEN and LOEFFLER 1999). There was no improvement in the incidence of tumor control or median survival time in a study of 194 patients treated with accelerated fractionation radiotherapy reported by the group from MD Anderson Cancer Center (CHOI et al. 1985).

We believe that WBI may be an over-utilized treatment in the management of patients with brain metastases. Patients with solitary metastases should be considered first for SRS, and WBI should be reserved for those with multiple metastatic lesions. This is of particular importance for patients who are expected to survive for more than 6 months, where the toxicity of WBI in the lowering of quality of life may become apparent. In patients who receive WBI and are expected to be long-term survivors, caution needs to be exercised to use lower radiation fraction, as this may reduce the incidence of late toxicity.

Table 21.5. Treatment outcome in selected reports on whole brain irradiation in patients with brain metastases

Investigator(s)	Number of patients	Survival time	
		Median (months.)	1 Year
HENDRICSON 1975	1000	3.8	–
YOUNG et al. 1974	162	3	3
ZIMM et al. 1981	156	3.3	12
HOSKIN et al. 1990	209	3.5	15
HAIE-MEDER et al. 1993	216	4.2	–
RYAN et al. 1994	416	3.3	–
BORGELT et al. 1980	900	4–5	–
	901	3.5–3.75	–

21.6
Stereotactic Radiosurgery

Stereotactic radiosurgery is a treatment modality which is growing in importance in the management of patients with brain metastasis. There are no readily available data on the number of patients with brain metastasis who are being treated with linear accelerator-based SRS systems or proton beam therapy. There are, however, data maintained by, and available from, the Leksell Gamma Knife Society, on patients treated worldwide with gamma knife SRS. This treatment in the past was applied infrequently in the management of patients with brain metastasis, but in recent years has become the most common treatment used in patients treated with gamma knife. Until December 1998, a total of 99,981 patients had been treated at 112 gamma knife facilities worldwide. This number included 23,712 (24%) patients treated for metastatic disease (courtesy of Leksell Gamma Knife Society). Recently, based on favorable reports on the use of gamma knife SRS in patients with brain metastasis, there was a steep increase in the number of patients managed with this treatment modality.

A study reported by the group from Stanford University, on the treatment of brain metastases with a linear accelerator-based SRS system, evaluated the influence of number of metastatic lesions on survival (JOSEPH et al. 1996). A total of 120 patients were treated in a 4 year period, with a mean dose of 26.6 Gy to the 80% isodose line and a mean target volume of 5.31 cm^3. WBI was given to 100 (83%) of these patients. The median survival time was 32 weeks. In 24% of patients who died, death was due to progressive disease in the brain. Patients with >three lesions had a shorter survival time than did those with fewer lesions, $P<0.002$. Focal brain necrosis at the treated site developed in 20 (17%) patients.

A study on 248 consecutive patients with 421 metastatic lesions treated over a 7 year period with a linear accelerator SRS-based system was reported by Harvard Medical School (ALEXANDER et al. 1995). Single metastases were present in 69%, recurrent brain disease in 76%, and 69% had systemic disease. The median tumor volume was 3 cm^3, and the median radiation dose was 15 Gy, with WBI having been given to those without prior radiotherapy. Median survival time was 8.5 months and depended on: the absence of systemic disease, age of patients <60 years, female patients and the presence of one or two lesions, $P<0.05$. Local tumor control at 1 year was 85%, and was 65% at 2 years post-treatment. Decreased local control was reported in patients with larger lesions, infratentorial locations and in those with recurrent lesions, $P<0.05$. The authors concluded that SRS is an effective, minimally invasive therapy with tumor control rates equivalent to those obtained with surgical resection. Stereotactic radiosurgery is superior to surgery, since it can suc-cessfully manage patients with lesions which are not accessible to surgical removal.

The importance of radiation dose on the incidence of tumor control in 119 evaluable patients with 219 lesions treated with gamma knife SRS was reported by the University of California San Francisco (SHIAU et al. 1997). The median tumor volume was 1.3 cm^3 and the median dose was 18.5 Gy. The actuarial freedom from tumor progression for all lesions was 82% at 6 months and 77% at 1 year. This incidence was 93% and 90%, respectively, in 145 lesions receiving higher radiation doses (>18 Gy). There was no significant difference in freedom from progression in patients with previously irradiated lesions, and in those treated with SRS alone.

The routine use of WBI, prior to or following SRS, has been a subject of controversy (CHANG et al. 1998; BOYD and MEHTA 1999; LEVINE et al. 1999). Recently-reported studies favor the use of SRS alone as the initial treatment in patients with few metastatic lesions (LEVINE et al. 1999; SNEED et al. 1999). It is apparent that there is need for prospective randomized trials to answer this important question. Another important dilemma in the management of patients with brain metastasis, is what treatment should be used first, WBI alone, SRS alone, or SRS as a planned combined treatment with WBI? A recently published study randomly selected patients with two to four metastases, of 25 mm or less in diameter, to receiving WBI alone (30 Gy in 12 fractions) vs. WBI-SRS combination (KONDZIOLKA et al. 1999). A total of 27 patients were randomly chosen, 14 to WBI alone and 13 to WBI combined with SRS. This study was stopped, following interim analysis at 60% of intended accrual. The incidence of local failure at 1 year was 100% in WBI group vs. 8% in the combined treatment group. The median time to local failure was 6 months for the former and 36 months for the latter group, $P=0.0005$. The median survival time of WBI-treated patients was 7.5 months compared with 11 months for those receiving WBI-SRS combination, $P=0.22$. Survival depended on the extent of systemic disease but did not depend on tumor histology or number of brain metastatic lesions.

RTOG Protocol 90-05 examined the value of SRS in patients with recurrent and previously irradiated brain metastases (SHAW et al. 1996). As expected, greater (8.2 cm^3) tumor volume and higher radiation doses were associated with a higher incidence of unacceptable toxicity, which included radionecrosis. On the other hand, SRS was very well-tolerated without severe toxicity in those patients with smaller (<40 mm) lesions treated to a dose of 18 Gy.

An interesting report examining cost effectiveness of SRS compared with surgical resection, in patients with solitary brain metastasis, was published by the group from the University of Wisconsin (MEHTA et al. 1997). Patients treated with surgical resection alone and SRS alone had better survival, and functional independence, than those treated with WBI alone. There was very little difference in important outcomes between patients treated with surgery alone and SRS alone. Surgical resection had 1.8 times greater cost than SRS. SRS had superior cost outcomes on all measured parameters, even with sensitivity analysis of up to 50%. In order for surgery to become as equally cost effective as SRS, its cost should decrease by 48%, or median survival would have to improve by 108%. This study estimated a mean cost per week of survival per treatment. It was $310 for WBI, $524 for surgery combined with radiotherapy, and $270 for SRS and WBI. The authors recommended a more aggressive use of SRS in patients with solitary brain metastases.

The SRS experience at USC consists of 150 patients treated between 1985 and 1994 with a linear accelerator-based SRS system and 729 patients treated with gamma knife SRS between 1994 and 1999. All of the SRS patients were treated with the use of conscious sedation under the supervision of a neuroanesthesiologist. We believe this approach increased the safety of the procedure, reduced patient anxiety, and improved treatment tolerance. Details on stereotactic procedures have been published (PETROVICH et al. 1996, 1997). Patients with metastatic brain tumors were infrequently treated at USC with a linear accelerator-based SRS system, while brain metastasis have commonly been treated with gamma knife SRS. A total of 239 patients with brain metastasis received 340 separate gamma knife treatment sessions. Table 21.6

shows distribution of these patients by histological diagnosis. It is of interest to note that, at USC, melanoma is the number one diagnosis for patients with brain metastases treated with gamma knife SRS.

It has been our policy to treat solitary metastases >35 mm in diameter, in patients with symptoms and signs of increased intracranial pressure, with surgical resection. Patients with smaller (<35 mm in diameter) lesions are treated with SRS.

The following case report illustrates well this policy. This is a case of a 37-year-old patient, who was diagnosed with cutaneous melanoma in 1997. This lesion was treated with complete surgical excision and no further therapy. The patient did very well until 18 months later, when he developed progressively severe headache, nausea and vomiting. MRI of the brain revealed a large (7+5+4 cm) ring enhancing lesion in the right frontal lobe, extending to the corpus callosum and crossing the midline. Extensive peritumoral edema was present with evidence of hemorrhage. A similar but smaller lesion was present in the left frontal lobe. The patient was treated at an outside medical center with corticosteroids and received WBI consisting of 30 Gy in two weeks. His symptoms and signs improved for a short period, followed by a recurrence. The patient was referred to USC for further management. His left frontal lesion measured 19.8+21.8+22.3 mm with tumor volume of 4.1 cm^3, and was treated with gamma knife SRS consisting of 18 Gy to the 50% isodose line (Fig. 21.1). The following day, the patient underwent a right frontal craniotomy with tumor resection. This treatment program was very well tolerated without complications. He was discharged on the 4th postoperative day and he remains asymptomatic 3 months after his therapy.

Radiation doses used in the treatment of our patients were: for soft tissue sarcomas, melanomas and renal cell carcinomas a mean dose of 21 Gy usually defined to the 50% isodose line, other previously untreated metastatic tumors received a mean dose of 20 Gy. In patients with lesions in particularly sensitive parts of the brain such as the pons, a dose of 14–16 Gy was given. The following patient history illustrates such a treatment. A 25-year-old male patient with well-documented metastatic melanoma presented with diplopia and difficulty in walking. MRI demonstrated a metastatic lesion in the pons measuring 16.5+15+20 mm. The patient was treated with gamma knife SRS to a dose of 16 Gy to the 50% isodose line. His condition rapidly improved following this therapy and he was able to lead a normal life, which included full-time employment. He died due to progressive systemic disease with tumor control in the brain (Fig. 21.2). Treatment

Table 21.6. Distribution, by primary site, of patients with brain metastases in University of Southern California (USC) study

Primary tumor	Number of patients	%	Number of treatment sessions	%
Melanoma	121	51	166	49
Lung cancer	48	20	78	23
Renal cell cancer	17	7	26	8
Breast cancer	16	7	25	7
Gastrointestinal cancer	14	6	16	5
Other sites	23	10	29	8
Total	239	100	340	100

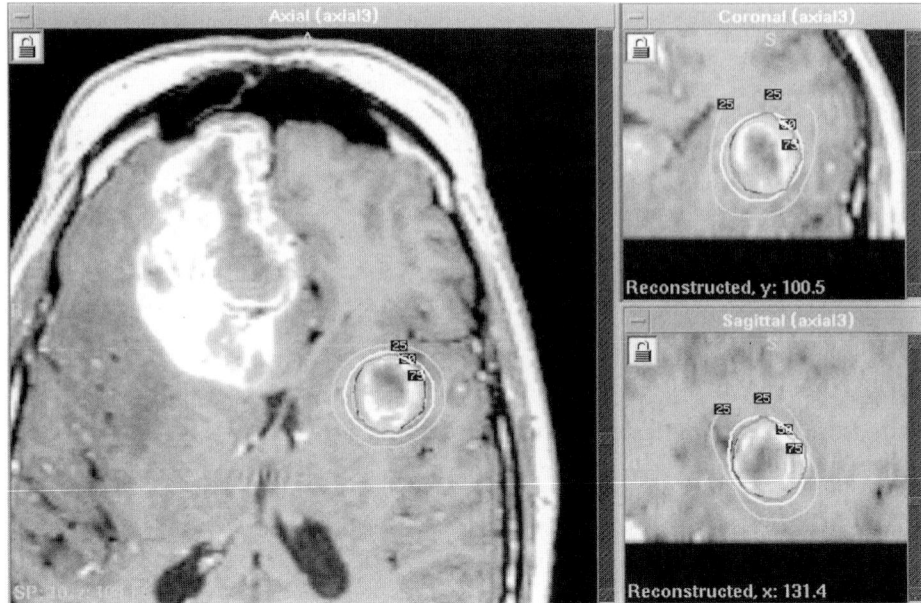

a

Histogram

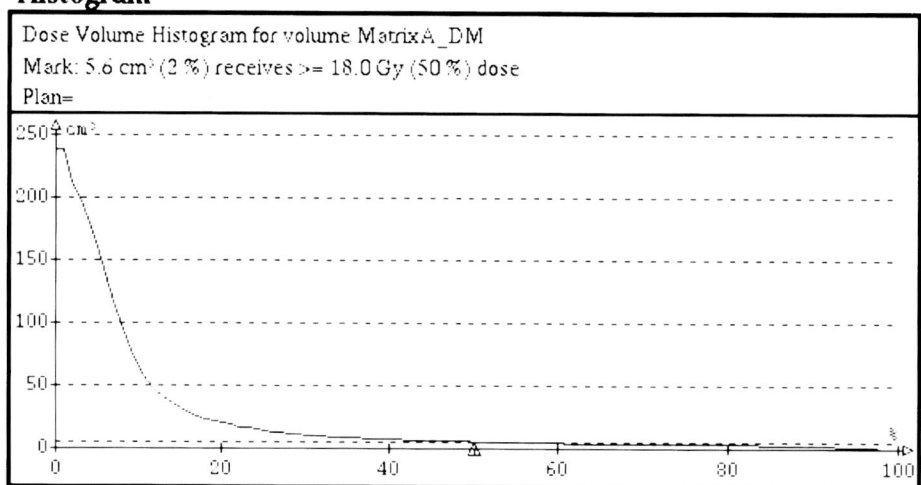

Dose Volume Histogram for volume MatrixA_DM

Mark: 5.6 cm³ (2 %) receives >= 18.0 Gy (50 %) dose

Plan=

Histogram

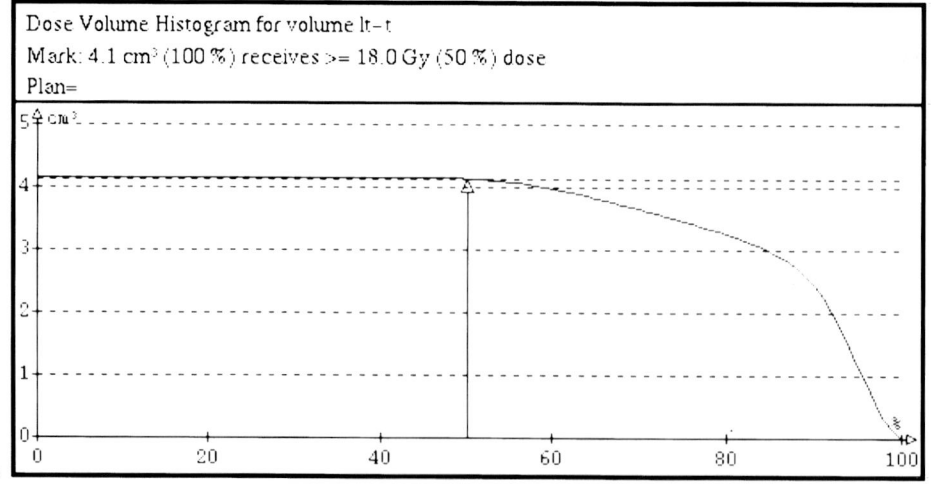

Dose Volume Histogram for volume lt–t

Mark: 4.1 cm³ (100 %) receives >= 18.0 Gy (50 %) dose

Plan=

b

Fig. 21.1. a Axial image demonstrating a large right frontal lesion, which was treated with surgery, and a smaller left frontal lesion shown with iso-dose lines resulting from gamma knife SRS. **b** Dose-volume histograms showing tumor volume of 4.1 cm³ and treated volume of 5.6 cm³

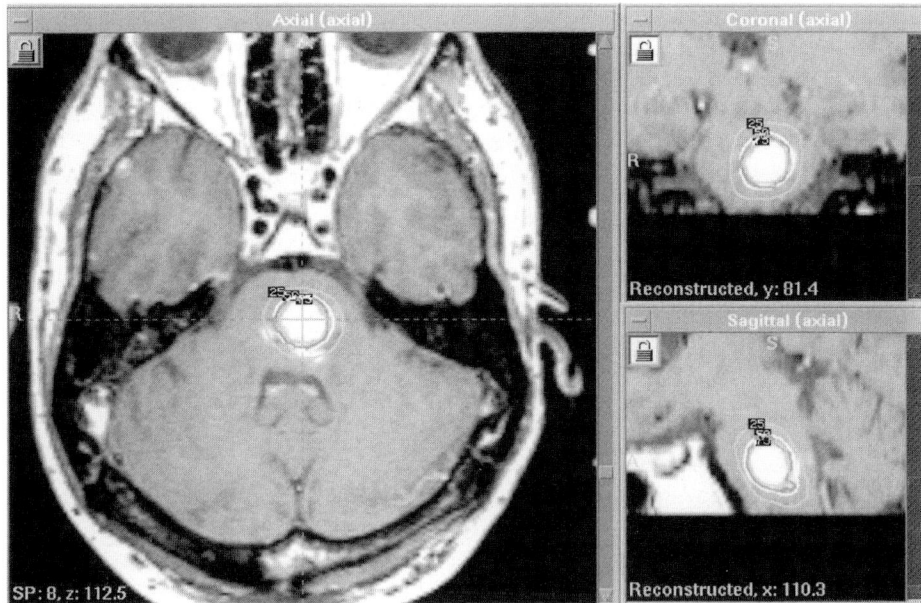

Histogram

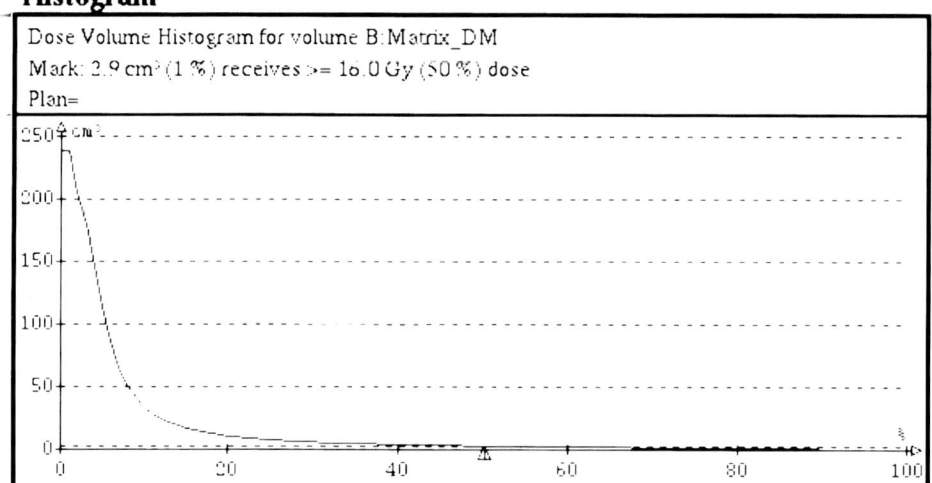

Histogram

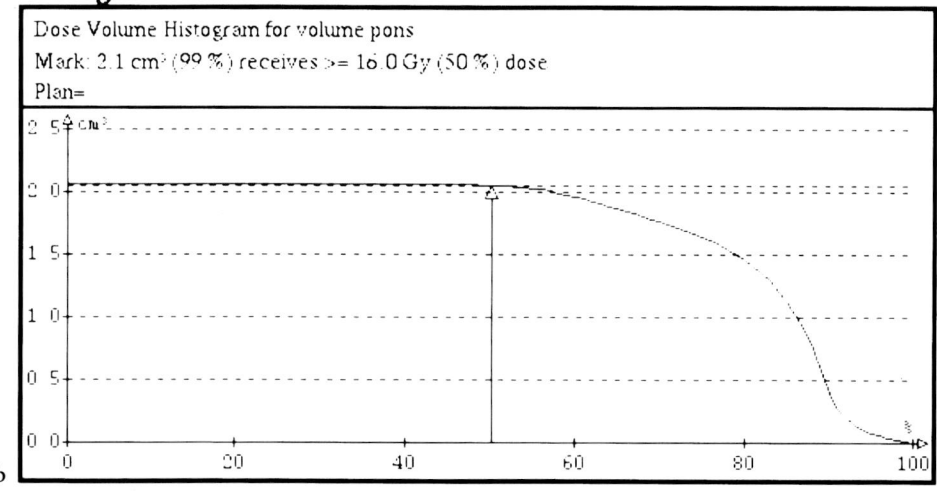

Fig. 21.2. a Axial MR images showing a large pontine metastatic lesion with isodose lines. Tumor volume was 2.1 cm^3 and treated volume was 2.9 cm^3, with three isocenters being used for this treatment to deliver 16 Gy. b Dose-volume histograms for this patient

of a patient with breast carcinoma, with a solitary lesion in the left side of cerebellum is shown in Fig. 21.3, and treatment of a patient with small-cell carcinoma of the lung extensively involving the pons is shown in Fig. 21.4.

We have reviewed our experience with brain metastasis treated at USC with gamma knife SRS over a 54 month period (unpublished data). A total of 190 consecutive patients with 434 metastatic lesions received their treatment in 263 sessions. Diagnoses were: melanoma in 88 (46%), lung cancer in 45 (24%), renal cell and breast carcinoma in 12 (6%) patients each, and other tumors in 33 (17%) patients. Mean lesion volume was $3.31 cm^3$, mean radiation dose was 19.8 Gy with a mean of 2.4 isocenters being treated. A total of 70 (37%) patients received WBI either before or after SRS. Our policy was not to give routine WBI in this group of patients. A majority of patients who received WBI were treated in outside medical centers. When we recommended WBI in patients with multiple brain lesions, 40 Gy in 4 weeks was advised. Mean follow-up time was 36 weeks.

Median survival from the time of SRS was 34 weeks. Non-melanoma patients had a median survival time of 38 weeks while the median survival for melanoma patients was 28 weeks, $P=0.01$. Controlled systemic disease had an important influence on survival, $P=0.002$. There was no significant difference in survival by the number of metastatic lesions from one to four, $P=0.24$. No survival benefit could be demonstrated in patients receiving WBI. Radiographically determined control of lesions was obtained in 89% of patients. A total of 132 (69%) study-patients are known to have died. Of the 88 melanoma patients, death due to systemic disease occurred in 31 (35%), due to CNS causes in 29 (33%), and to causes unknown in 6 (7%). Of the 102 non-melanoma patients, death due to systemic disease occurred in 45 (44%), due to CNS problems in 17 (17%), and to causes unknown in 4 (4%) patients.

SRS was well tolerated, and clinically significant toxicity was uncommon (<5%). Based on this experience, we concluded that SRS is an important treatment in selected patients with brain metastasis. Controlled systemic disease and non-melanoma histology had a favorable influence on survival.

We have also analyzed the incidence of tumor relapse in the brain (unpublished data). Of the 190 patients treated, 45 (24%) had a relapse outside the previously SRS-treated volume. A single salvage SRS was performed in 34 (76%), ten (22%) had two procedures and one (2%) patient had three salvage procedures. Systemic disease was present in 26 (58%) while 19 (42%) patients had only CNS involvement. A total of 80 lesions was treated in the first SRS salvage procedure and the mean time from the initial SRS was 26 weeks. Mean lesion volume was $2.47 cm^3$ and mean radiation dose was 20 Gy.

Median survival time from the initial SRS was 50 weeks and median survival time from the salvage procedure was 28 weeks. Tumor control verified by MRI was obtained in 90% of the treated patients. Of the 45 patients treated, 33 (73%) are known to have died, with 19 (58%) having died from systemic disease, 13 (39%) from CNS causes, and in one (3%) patient the cause of death was unknown. Salvage SRS was well tolerated by these 45 patients and there was no severe acute or late toxicity. SRS salvage represents a valuable means of treatment for CNS-caused recurrence in patients who have previously undergone SRS for metastatic disease to the brain. SRS offers distinct advantages over WBI salvage by virtue of providing effective treatment, even for tumors poorly responding to radiotherapy such as melanoma or renal cell carcinoma.

In a study of 45 patients with metastatic melanoma to the brain 59 gamma knife SRS treatment sessions were given (LEVINE et al. 1999). Median time from the original diagnosis to brain metastasis was 27.5 months. Active systemic disease was present in 35 (78%), seizure disorder in five (11%), and 16 (36%) patients had neurological symptoms. A total of 54 gamma knife SRS sessions was used to treat 31 (57%) patients with solitary lesions, 13 (24%) with two lesions, and five (9%) with three lesions, while the remaining five (9%) sessions were for those with>three lesions. It was relatively common to find during the process of treatment planning, more lesions than were visible on the pretreatment MRI. The mean treatment volume was $5.6 cm^3$ with a mean radiation dose of 21.6 Gy prescribed to a mean of 56% isodose line. Median survival from the time of diagnosis was 43 months, and was 8 months from gamma knife SRS. Treatment resulted in 35 (78%) patients with either stable or improved CNS symptoms at the time of last follow up or at the time of death. Of the 45 patients treated, 26 (58%) are known to have died, with tumor progression in the brain being a cause of death in two (8%). MRI of the brain demonstrated local tumor control in 97% of the treated lesions, with 28% lesions not identifiable on follow-up scans. New lesions in the brain outside the SRS-treated volume were seen in six (13%) patients who were treated with a second SRS procedure. SRS was well tolerated by the study-patients, without clinically significant toxicity.

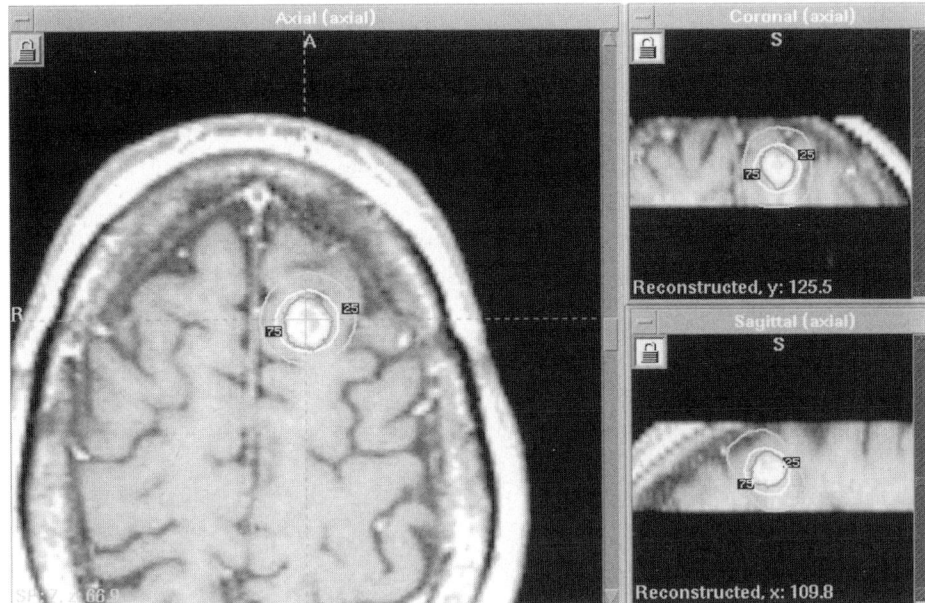

a

Histogram

Dose Volume Histogram for volume MatrixA_DM

Mark: 1.8 cm³ (3 %) receives >= 22.0 Gy (75 %) dose

Plan=

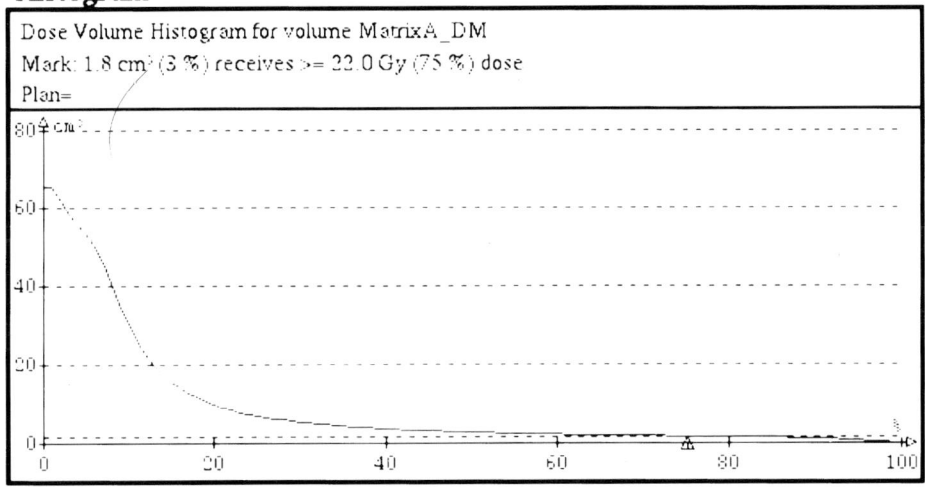

Histogram

Dose Volume Histogram for volume tumor

Mark: 758.8 mm³ (100 %) receives >= 22.0 Gy (75 %) dose

Plan=

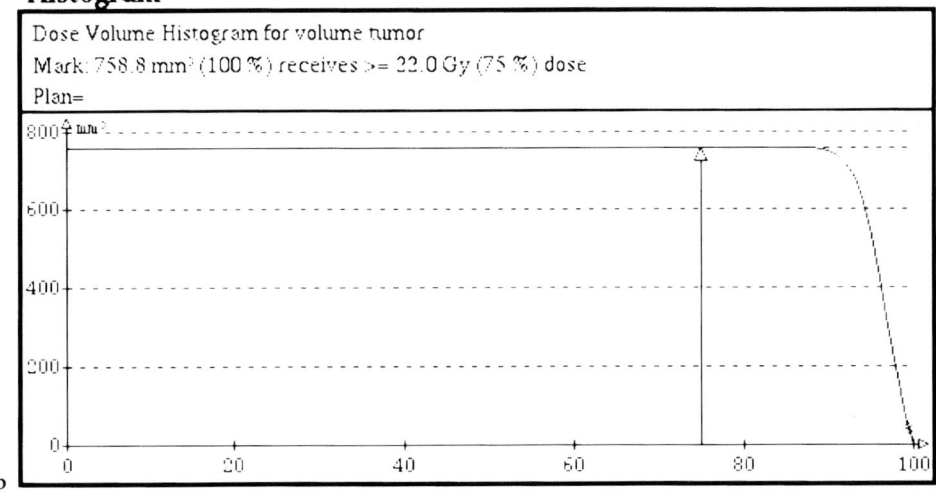

b

Fig. 21.3. a A 47-year-old female patient with a well-documented metastatic carcinoma of the breast developed a symptomatic recurrent metastatic lesion to the left cerebellum measuring 26+27.4+27.6 mm. Axial images are shown with the lesion, which received only 16 Gy due to the prior WBI. The dose was defined to the 50% isodose line. **b** Dose-volume histogram showing tumor volume of 8.6 cm³ and the treated volume of 14.1 cm³

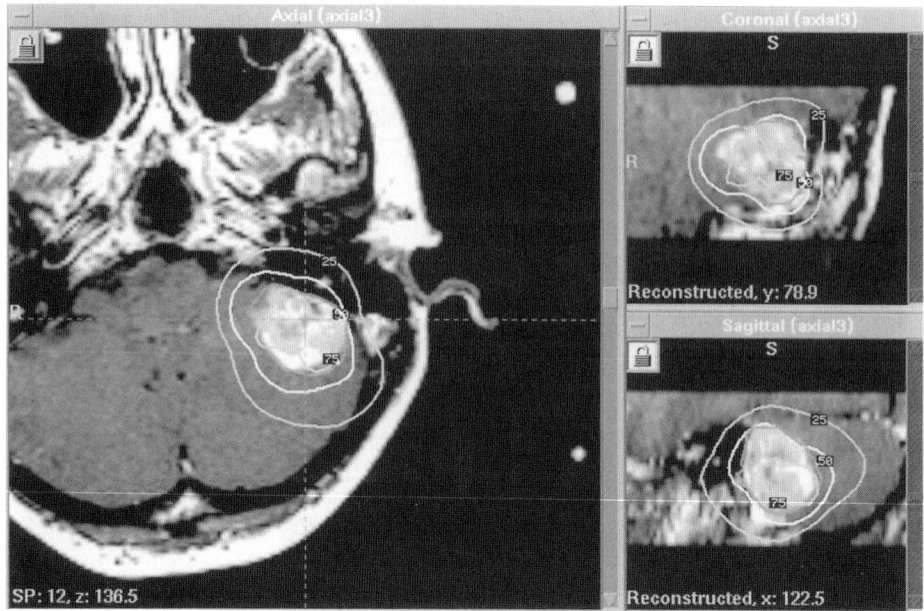

Histogram

Dose Volume Histogram for volume A:Matrix_DM

Mark: 14.1 cm³ (6%) receives >= 16.0 Gy (50%) dose

Plan=

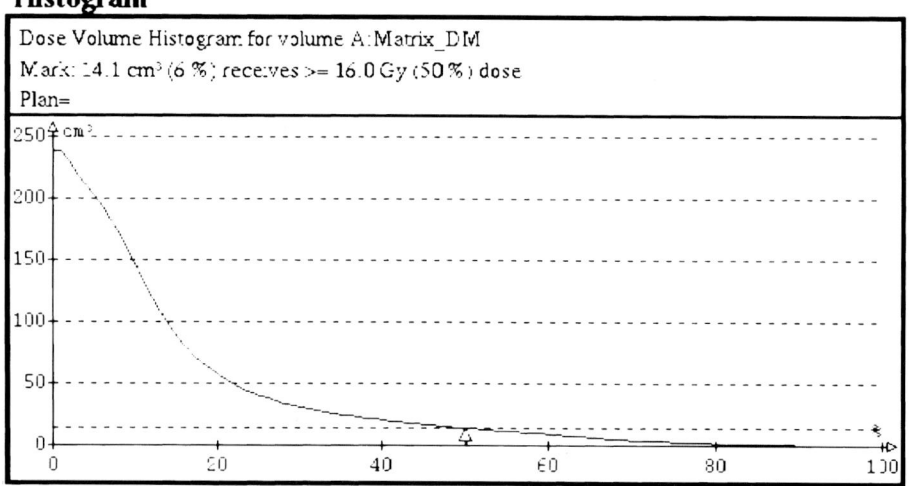

Histogram

Dose Volume Histogram for volume lt-c

Mark: 8.5 cm³ (99%) receives >= 16.0 Gy (50%) dose

Plan=

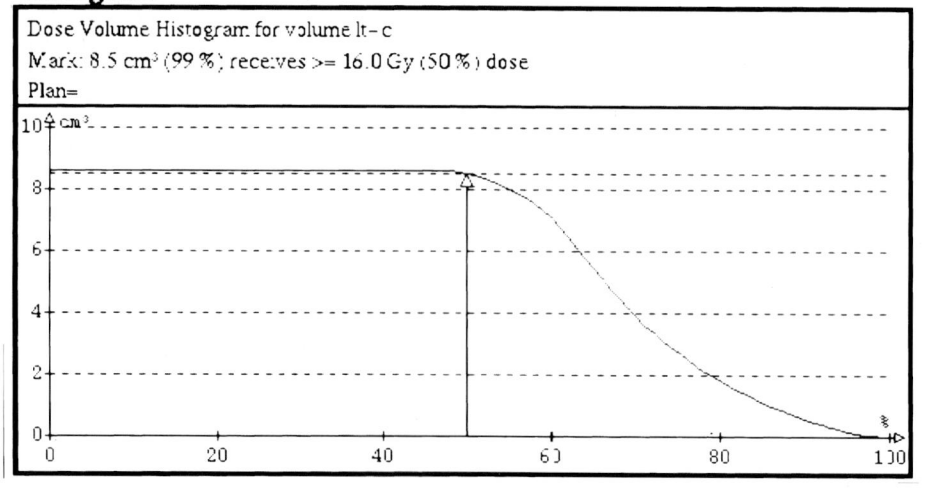

Fig 21.4. a Axial images of a 47-year-old female patient with small-cell carcinoma of the bronchus, with multiple metastases. The patient received, at an outside medical center, WBI consisting of 40 Gy in 4 weeks. A 29+19+27 mm, severely symptomatic lesion is invading the pons. A total dose of 14 Gy, to the 50% isodose line, was given together with SRS. This patient died 4 months later due to progressive widespread metastases. **b** Dose-volume histogram showing tumor volume of 5.5 cm³ and treated volume of 6.4 cm³

21.7
Treatment Complications

Details of treatment toxicity in the management of patients with brain metastasis are addressed in Chap. 33.

21.7.1
Surgery

Complications in contemporary neurosurgery in patients treated for metastasis to the brain are limited to <10%. They include common complications of any surgical procedure, such as bleeding, infection, and delayed healing of surgical incision. Mortality rates for craniotomy are low in the currently reported series (BINDAL et al. 1993) but a mortality rate >10% was also reported (HAFSTROM et al. 1980; WORNOM et al. 1986). Neurological deficit, or reduced quality of life of surgically treated patients should be uncommon in properly selected patients. Postoperatively, patients are expected to return rapidly to the state of well being following a short (3–4 days) hospital stay.

21.7.2
External Beam Radiotherapy

21.7.2.1
Whole Brain Irradiation

Whole Brain Irradiation is a well-tolerated treatment, even in those who are in a poor general condition. Typically, during the course of radiotherapy, patients experience only mild fatigue, with headache or dizziness being an uncommon problem. A common misconception is that there is a routine need for corticosteroid therapy during WBI. There is no need for this therapy, with the exception of patients who present with signs and symptoms of increased intracranial pressure. Temporary hair loss and skin dryness in the treated area occur in all patients. Temporary decrease in hearing is seen in patients undergoing WBI and is due to radiation-induced otitis. This problem usually resolves itself spontaneously, shortly following the course of radiotherapy.

The brain is very sensitive to radiotherapy. Tolerance to radiation depends on a number of factors, which are patient and treatment related. Patient-related factors adversely affecting treatment tolerance include the following: age >65, prior surgery, non-ambulatory status, neurological dysfunction and the presence of systemic diseases such as diabetes mellitus. Treatment-related factors are total radiation dose, size of daily radiation fraction, with 1.8–2.0 Gy being the optimum, brain volume within the target area, administration of prior or concurrent chemotherapy. Whole brain tolerance is from 15–25 Gy if given as a single dose or 60–70 Gy given in 2.0 GY fraction (RUBIN 1989). The most important and irreversible complication of radiotherapy is brain necrosis. Patients treated with WBI and receiving a total dose of 50 Gy given over 5 weeks at a daily dose of 2.0 Gy have an approximately 5% probability of brain necrosis (FAJARDO 1982; MARKS et al. 1981). In a study of 139 patients, treated for primary brain tumors with a dose of at least 45 Gy given at 1.8–2.0 Gy daily fractions, seven (5%) developed histologically-confirmed brain necrosis (MARKS et al. 1981). Median time from completion of radiotherapy to brain necrosis was 14 months. A higher incidence of this event is expected among those who receive a dose of 54 Gy at a standard fraction size. Necrotic focus may be present near or remote from the radiation-treated tumor area. Focal brain necrosis may respond well to the administration of corticosteroid therapy. If there is no response to this treatment and the patient remains symptomatic, surgical treatment to remove the necrotic focus may be required. Most of the patients so treated, following surgery, rapidly return to the state of well being.

It is of interest to review the importance of the size of the radiation daily fraction on the incidence of treatment complications. At Memorial Sloan-Kettering Cancer Center, 370 patients were treated with WBI for cerebral metastases during a 6 year period (DEANGELIS et al. 1989). A group of 12 patients including six with carcinoma of the lung and six with lesions of other primary sites, had solitary metastases. Median age was 64 years with two patients presenting with hypertension and two with diabetes mellitus. In eight of these patients, radiotherapy was combined with surgical resection and in four patients WBI was the only therapy. WBI consisted of 25 to 39 Gy given in 3 to 6 Gy fractions. With a median time of 14 months (range 5–36 months) from radiotherapy, patients developed progressive dementia. Median survival time in these 12 patients was 4.5 years. There were other symptoms present including: decreased recent memory, disabling ataxia, dysarthria, diffuse hyperreflexia and urinary incontinence, which developed in six patients. Imaging studies demonstrated no recurrent tumor, diffuse atrophy and extensive white matter changes. A total dose of radiation used in the treatment of these 12 patients should not have resulted in brain necrosis except for the high daily radiation fraction. A similar observation on the importance of radiation fraction size was made by other investigators (ASAHI et al. 1989). As it was stated above, brain tolerance is optimal with the use of 1.8 to 2.0 Gy fractions. In the Sloan-Kettering study, the reason for brain necrosis in those 12 patients was most likely to have been an unconventional radiation fraction size, although other factors such as diabetes mellitus, severe hypertension and advanced patient age might have contributed to the reported complications (DEANGELIS et al. 1989). Progressive and severe intellectual deterioration was well-documented in pediatric patients who were treated with radiotherapy for medulloblastoma or other tumors (HOPPE-HIRSCH et al. 1990; DUFFNER et al. 1985). Complications of radiotherapy in pediatric patients are discussed in Chap. 27.

21.7.3
Stereotactic Radiosurgery

Stereotactic radiosurgery is generally a well-tolerated treatment for patients with brain metastases (KONDZIOLKA et al. 1999). In a recent report on the treatment 45 consecutive patients with metastatic melanoma to the brain who received 59 gamma knife sessions, there was no mortality and the procedure-related morbidity was low (LEVINE et al. 1999). Seizures were reported in 6% of patients who were not receiving anti-seizure prophylactic therapy. Following introduction of the routine use of anti-seizure medications in patients treated with SRS, this problem was eliminated. Transient nausea within 24 h of the procedure was recorded in 3%, and transient increase in pretreatment paresis was found also in 3% of patients. Focal peritumoral edema, which occurred with a median time of 3 months of SRS, was noted in 20% of patients who responded well to corticosteroid therapy. Following a few weeks' course of corticosteroid therapy three (5%) patients with focal peritumoral edema failed to respond to this treatment and required craniotomy and removal of the necrotic focus. There were no further complications in these three patients. This finding of low toxicity in patients undergoing SRS was confirmed in another USC study on 190 patients with brain metastases treated in 263 SRS sessions (unpublished data).

21.8
Conclusions

Metastatic brain tumors are diagnosed in progressively larger number of patients with solid cancers. There is a consensus on the management of patients with multiple lesions, where WBI is the treatment of choice. Only a small number of medical centers recommend an aggressive therapeutic approach with surgical treatment with or without postoperative WBI in selected patients with multiple brain metastases. There is no consensus on the management of solitary metastases. Some medical centers use surgery alone for the treatment of these patients while others add postoperative WBI. A rapidly-growing number of investigators recommend the use of SRS alone or followed by WBI, in most of the patients presenting with solitary metastases. Based on our experience and information from published reports, at USC we developed the following treatment options for patients with metastatic brain disease: (1) Patients with large (>35 mm) solitary lesions with acute symptoms of increased intracranial pressure are treated with craniotomy, which may be followed by SRS for residual tumor; (2) Patients with smaller (<35 mm) solitary lesions are treated with SRS and their progress carefully followed with MRI; WBI is given to those who show several (> three) recurrent lesions, otherwise SRS is repeated; (3) Patients with multiple (> three) brain metastases receive WBI, with SRS being given to dominant lesion(s) in patients with melanoma, renal cell carcinoma and sarcoma. Patients with multiple lesions treated with WBI who show evidence of tumor recurrence are treated with SRS.

References

Asahi A, Matsutani M, Kohno T, et al. (1989) Subacute brain atrophy after radiation therapy for malignant brain tumor. Cancer 63:1962–1974

Auperin A, Arriagada R, Pignon JP, et al. (1999) Prophylactic cranial irradiation for patients with small-cell lung cancer in complete remission. N Engl J Med 341:476–484

Bindal RK, Sawaya R, Leavens ME, et al. (1993) Surgical treatment of multiple brain metastases. J Neurosurg 79:210–216

Borgelt B, Gelber R, Kramer S, et al. (1980) The palliation of brain metastases: final results of the first two studies of the Radiation Therapy Oncology Group. Int J Radiat Oncol Biol Phys 6:1–9

Brega K, Robinson WA, Winston K, et al. (1990) Surgical treatment of brain metastases in malignant melanoma. Cancer 66:2105–2110

Cairncross JG, Kim JH, Posner JB (1980) Radiation therapy for brain metastases. Ann Neurol 7:529–541

Cairncross JG and Posner JB (1983) The management of brain metastases. In: Walker MD (ed) Oncology of the central nervous system: cancer treatment and research. Vol. 12, Martinus Nijhoff, Boston, pp 341–377

Chang SD, Adler JA, Hancock SL (1998) Clinical uses of radiosurgery. Oncol 12:1181–1191

Choi KN, Withers HR, Rotman M (1985) Intracranial metastases from melanoma. Clinical features and treatment by accelerated fractionation. Cancer 56:1–9

DeAngelis LM, Delattre JY, Posner JB (1989) Radiation-induced dementia in patients cured of brain metastases. Neurology 39:789–796

DeAngelis LM (1994) Management of brain metastases. Cancer Invest 12:156–165

Delattre JY, Krol G, Thaler HD, et al. (1988) Distribution of brain metastases from systemic cancer. Arch Neurol 45:741–744

Duffner PK, Cohen ME, Thomas PRM, et al. (1985) The long-term effects of cranial irradiation on the central nervous system. Cancer 56:1841–1846

Fajardo LF (1982) Nervous System In: Fajardo LF (ed) Pathology of radiation injury. Masson Monographs in Diagnostic Radiology, New York, pp 216–230

Guazzo EP, Atkinson RL, Weidmann M, et al. (1989) Management of solitary metastasis of the brain. Aust N Z J Surg 59:321–324

Hafstrom L, Jonsson PE, Stromblad LG (1980) Intracranial metastases of malignant melanoma treated by surgery. Cancer 46:2088–2090

Haie-Meder C, Palleae-Cosset B, Laplanche A, et al. (1993) Results of a randomized clinical trial comparing two radiation schedules in the palliative treatment of brain metastases. Radiother Oncol 26:111–116

Hazra T, Mullins GM, Lott S (1972) Management of cerebral metastasis from bronchogenic carcinoma. Johns Hopkins Med J 130:377–383

Hendricson FR (1975) Radiation therapy of metastatic tumors. Semin Oncol 2:43–46

Hoskin PJ, Crow J, Ford HT (1990) The influence of extent and local management on the outcome of radiotherapy for brain metastases. Int J Radiat Oncol Biol Phys 19:111–115

Hoppe-Hirsch E, Renier D, Lellouch-Tubiana A, et al. (1990) Medulloblastoma in childhood: progressive intellectual deterioration. Childs Nerv Syst 6:60–65

Johnson JD and Young B (1996) Demographics of brain metastasis. Neurosurg Clin North Am 7:337–344

Joseph J, Adler JR, Cox RS, et al. (1996) Linear accelerator-based stereotactic radiosurgery for brain metastasis: the influence of number of lesions on survival. J Clin Oncol 14:1085–1092

Kondziolka D, Patel A, Lunsford LD, et al. (1999) Stereotactic radiosurgery plus whole brain radiotherapy versus radiotherapy alone for patients with multiple brain metastases. Int J Radiat Oncol Biol Phys 45:427–434

Lang FF, Wildrick DM, Sawaya R (1998) Management of cerebral metastases: the role of surgery. Cancer Control 5:124–129

Laws ER and Thapar K (1993) Brain Tumors. Ca Cancer J Clin 43:263–271

Levine SD, Cohen-Gadol AA, Morton DL, et al. (1999) Gamma knife radiosurgery for metastatic melanoma: an analysis of survival, outcome and complications. Neuro-surg 44:59–66

Marks JE, Baglan RJ, Prassad SC, et al. (1981) Cerebral radionecrosis: incidence and risk in relation to dose, fractionation and volume. Int J Radiat Oncol Biol Phys 7:243–252

Mehta M, Noyes W, Craig B, et al. (1997) A cost-effectiveness and cost-utility analysis of radiosurgery vs. resection for single-brain metastases. Int J Radiat Oncol Biol Phys 39:445–454

Nugent JL, Bunn PA, Matthews MJ, et al. (1979) CNS metastases in small cell bronchogenic carcinoma: increasing frequency and changing pattern with lengthening survival. Cancer 44:1885–1893

Patchell RA, Tibbs PA, Walsh JW, et al. (1990) A randomized trial of surgery in the treatment of single metastases to the brain. N Engl J Med 322:494–500

Patchell RA, Tibbs PA, Regine WF, et al. (1998) Postoperative radiotherapy in the treatment of single metastases to the brain. A randomized trial. JAMA 280:1485–1489

Posner JB (1977) Management of central nervous system metastases. Sem Oncol 4:81–91

Posner JB (1992) Management of brain metastases. Rev Neurol 148:477–487

Petrovich ZP, Luxton G, Formenti SC, et al. (1996) Stereotactic radiosurgery for primary and metastatic brain tumors. Cancer Invest 14:445–454

Petrovich ZP, Luxton G, Formenti SC, et al. (1997) Sterotactic radiosurgery for benign and malignant diseases of the brain. In: Kornblith PL, Walker MD (eds) Advances in Neuro-Oncology II, Futura Publishing Co., Armonk, pp 219–258

Rubin P (1989) The law and order of radiation sensitivity, absolute vs. relative. In: Vaeth JM, Meyer JL, (eds) Radiation tolerance of normal tissues. Frontiers of Radiation Therapy and Oncology, Vol. 23, Karger, Basel, Switzerland, pp 7–40

Russell AH, Pajak TE, Selim HM, et al. (1991) Prophylactic cranial irradiation for lung cancer patients at high risk for development of cerebral metastasis: results of a prospective randomized trial conducted by the Radiation Therapy Oncology Group. Int J Radiat Oncol Biol Phys 21:637–643

Ryan GF, Ball DL, Smith JG (1994) Treatment of brain metastases from primary lung cancer. Int J Radiat Oncol Biol Phys 31:273–278

Saha S, Meyer M, Krementz ET, et al. (1994) Prognostic evaluation of intracranial metastasis in malignant melanoma. Ann Surg Oncol 1:38–44

Shaw E, Scott C, Souhami L, et al. (1996) Radiosurgery for the treatment of previously irradiated recurrent primary brain tumors and brain metastases: initial report of Radiation Therapy Oncology Group Protocol 90–05. Int J Radiat Oncol Biol Phys 34:647–654

Shiau CY, Sneed PK, Shu HKG, et al. (1997) Radiosurgery for brain metastases: relationship of dose and pattern of enhancement to local control. Int J Radiat Oncol Biol Phys 37:375–383

Sneed PK, Lamborn KR, Forstner JM, et al. (1999) Radiosurgery for brain metastases: is whole brain radiotherapy necessary? Int J Radiat Oncol Biol Phys 43:549–558

Vecht CJ, Haaxma-Reiche H, Noordijk EM, et al. (1993) Treatment of single brain metastasis: radiotherapy alone or combined with neurosurgery? Ann Neurol 33:583–590

Walker AE, Robins M, Weinfeld FD (1985) Epidemiology of brain tumors: the National survey of intracranial neoplasms. Neurology 35:219–226

Wen PY and Loeffler JS (1999) Management of brain metastases. Oncology 13:941–961

Wornom IL, Smith JW, Soong SJ, et al. (1986) Surgery as palliative treatment for distant metastases of melanoma. Ann Surg 204:181–185

Young DF, Posner JB, Chu F, et al. (1974) Rapid course radiation therapy of brain metastases: results and complications. Cancer 34:1069–1076

Zimm S, Wampler GL, Stablein D, et al. (1981) Intracerebral metastases in solid-tumor patients: natural history and results of treatment. Cancer 48:384–394

22 Management of Skull Base Tumors

J. Diaz Day and Rick A. Freidman

CONTENTS

22.1
Introduction

The treatment of skull base tumors has undergone a tremendous change within the past decade. This change has been largely technology driven, but also secondary to advances in surgical technique and instrumentation. A new subspecialty has been created, bringing neurosurgeons together with otologists, head and neck surgeons, and plastic surgeons to specifically address these very complex problems with a level of expertise not seen before. Teams of skull base surgeons have been formed dedicated to helping patients with problems previously thought to harbor little hope of recovery. The surgical techniques which have been de-

J. D. Day, MD
Neurological Surgery, House Neurological and Skull Base Surgery Associates, House Ear Clinic, Inc., 2100 W. 3rd St., Los Angeles, CA 90057, USA
R. A Freidman, MD
Neuro-otologist, House Ear Clinic, Inc., 2100 W. 3rd St., Los Angeles, CA 90057, USA

veloped to treat such lesions are without question of the highest level of complexity and sophistication in modern medicine. Likewise, adjuvant therapies for these patients also take advantage of the latest technology. In particular for skull base tumors, stereotactic radiosurgery plays a major adjuvant role in many cases. Despite the demonstrated successes of conventional radiotherapy in limiting further tumor growth, lesions at the skull base have mandated a different approach. This is largely owing to the complex anatomy involved and the relative inability to completely shield adjacent structures, such as sensitive cranial nerves or the brainstem. The importance of the different elements of the treatment strategy mean that an optimal outcome is more likely to be achieved when treatment is delivered by a multidisciplinary team who treat such lesions frequently.

22.2
Evaluation

Patients are evaluated by the members of the skull base surgical team in order to determine the best management strategy. It is important that all members of the team are involved in this initial process. The complexity of these lesions mandates the input of all the various specialists involved. Particularly important in these cases is careful evaluation of the various imaging studies. For this reason, a neuroradiologist is a particularly important asset to the skull base surgical team. Precise definition of the anatomy involved and a complete differential diagnosis are critical to sound decision-making in this arena. Depending upon the lesion site, preoperative neurophysiological testing may also be important.

Numerous factors must be taken into account in the decision-making process for treatment of skull base neoplasms. The age and general medical condition of the patient are critical factors in terms of surgical strategy. Advanced age and/or the presence of multiple medical conditions certainly affects any decision for aggressive surgical intervention prior to radiation or chemotherapy. Many such patients are only candidates for palliative therapy because of these selection factors. The supposed pathology based upon imaging and location is also a factor that directs therapeutic strategy. Some anatomical locations make surgical intervention difficult or ill advised based upon pathology. Whether the lesion is metastatic or primary is also considered. Available data are also an important consideration as many of these tumors are relatively rare. It is uncommon for any one center to have a wide experience with the wide breadth of neoplasms which may affect the skull base.

22.3
Anatomical Considerations

The skull base can be considered to be composed of four main regions: anterior, middle, central, and posterior. The anterior skull base is mainly composed of the frontal fossa, which extends from the anterior margin of the frontal bone posteriorly to the sphenoid ridge. The middle skull base is delineated by the middle cranial fossa from the temporal squama laterally to the lateral wall of the sellae medially. The middle fossa contains the superior portion of the petrous bone and is considered to contain the cavernous sinus. The central cranial base is that region around the sella turcica containing the pituitary gland. The central cranial base posterior limit is essentially the dorsum sellae, and it extends anteriorly to and including the tuberculum sellae. It is laterally limited by the lateral walls of the sella turcica. The posterior skull base is considered to be the posterior fossa. The bony boundaries are the occipital bone, petrous bone, and clivus.

Many skull base tumors spill over from one anatomical region to another. Determining the exact location of a lesion based upon imaging studies is the important first step in determining the treatment strategy. Each anatomical region can be accessed by a finite set of skull base surgical approaches. Each case is considered individually, and a tailored surgical approach is determined. This all depends not only on location but on the differential diagnosis for the lesion.

22.4
Imaging Considerations

At present, the vast majority of patients are diagnosed with a skull base tumor by way of magnetic resonance imaging (MRI). MRI technology is rapidly changing, providing much finer anatomical detail than was previously available. MRI of the head, neck, brain, and temporal bones tends to provide the bulk of presurgical information. However, under certain circumstances other imaging modalities are of use. It is frequently helpful to the surgeon to obtain a computed tomography (CT) scan, specifically with viewing the bone at the cranial base in mind. MRI continues to be a poor imaging modality with regard to delineating bony detail. For this reason, lesions which appear to be involving the bone, such as chordomas, chondrosarcomas, and the like, benefit in terms of developing surgical strategy from preoperative CT scanning. In selected tumors it is also helpful to obtain four-vessel cerebral angiography as a part of the presurgical decision-making process. These studies are especially helpful in cases where the tumor clearly involves the carotid artery and there is evidence on the MRI scan of narrowing or invasion of the adventitial wall. Some lesions require consideration of a cerebrovascular bypass procedure as a component of the overall strategy. At the present time, the angiogram remains the gold standard for viewing the cerebrovasculature as compared with magnetic resonance angiography, which remains an inadequate modality for such planning purposes.

In cases in which bypass of one of the major vessels is a consideration, the angiogram also allows determination of the cerebrovascular reserve by means of balloon test occlusion (BTO). BTO is performed at the time of angiography. A catheter equipped with a balloon is advanced into the internal carotid artery or the vertebral artery. At the appropriate location, the balloon is inflated. The patient is awake for the procedure and is continuously monitored neurologically. EEG monitoring is a frequent adjunctive monitoring method during this type of procedure in addition to neurological examination. In general, if the patient tolerates at least 20–30 min of occlusion with no neurological or EEG changes, then he or she is considered to have passed. In such cases there is reasonable, though not absolute, certainty that the patient will tolerate sacrifice of the vessel which was occluded. Patients who fail BTO require revascularization via a bypass procedure. Preoperative angiography also allows the delineation of blood supply to the tumor. For many tumors located at the skull base, a thorough and intimate knowledge of cerebrovascular anatomy allows the surgeon to infer the tumor's blood supply. Therefore, angiography is not always employed in our practice to determine the blood supply. One of the critical questions is whether preoperative embolization of the tumor will be of help. In selected circumstances, such as skull base meningiomas and large glomus jugulare tumors, this certainly is a helpful adjunct. However, in those tumors where the blood supply to the lesion will be exposed as a consequence of the surgical approach, we have not found preoperative embolization to be of help. We in fact feel that the potential morbidity of the procedure causes a failure in the risk/benefit ratio analysis.

Selected cases also require determination of the venous anatomy involved by the lesion. This is important in terms of avoiding the potentially disastrous consequences of venous insufficiency. Cerebral angiography with filming of the venous phase is the gold standard test. With the continued refinement of MRI, venograms of sufficient quality are now possible in many centers. Certainly, tumors involving the major venous sinuses and jugular bulb should have consideration given to the venous anatomy prior to any intervention. This is, of course, of paramount importance in cases where surgery is an element of the treatment strategy.

22.5
Surgical Strategies

When surgery is a part of the treatment strategy, the surgical team must make a determination of the best approach for the situation. As already indicated, many factors are considered, including patient age, medical condition, pathology, prognosis, and anatomical factors. Ideally, the surgical approach is tailored for each individual patient. With the wide range of techniques currently available to the contemporary skull base surgical team, options are essentially without limit. A basic overview of these strategies will be outlined in this section.

Prior to surgery all patients should undergo a routine general medical examination including routine preoperative laboratory studies to identify intercurrent systemic illness. A careful neurological examination, accurately documented, is very important to allow precise determination of improvement or morbidity postoperatively. A full radiological work-up is imperative to adequately image the offending lesion and develop surgical strategy. In cases in which a metastatic lesion is included in the differential diagnosis, a full metastatic workup is important in terms of decision-making.

Medications which are initiated prior to surgery include anticonvulsants, corticosteroids, and calcium channel blockers in the event of subarachnoid hemorrhage. All patients who will have the supratentorial compartment breached are started on Dilantin with the goal in mind of attaining a therapeutic level prior to the procedure. This is not critical, however, and patients may be started just prior to induction of general anesthesia with an intravenous loading dose of 15 mg/kg. Corticosteroids are initiated in the operating room for the purpose of limiting postoperative swelling and for their putative cerebroprotective effect against ischemia. Perioperative antibiotics are routinely utilized. Prophylaxis against the gastrointestinal complications of steroids is strictly practiced with the use of H-2 blockers and antacids. Sequential pneumatic compression boots are applied and their function initiated in the operating room.

22.5.1
Anterior Approaches

The anterior approaches to the skull base are appropriate for a wide variety of lesions. They can be used not only for tumors involving the anterior cranial fossa but also for those located at the central and posterior skull base, as well as the air sinuses and pharynx. There is a wide variety of these approaches which include, but are not limited to, the transoral approach, the transbasal approach, and the transmaxillary approach (DEROME 1988; UTTLEY 1989). There are many variations and permutations of the standard approaches to the anterior skull base. Many of these surgical techniques have been employed for many years. As the methods and techniques advance in cranial base surgery, there has been a resultant refinement in the basic techniques. Continuous refinements in these and the other techniques which will be discussed have resulted in the past years in a reduction in surgical morbidity and mortality secondary to these very complicated methods.

The classic anterior skull base approach is generally termed the anterior transbasal approach. DEROME (1988) is credited with refining and popularizing this now common approach. This involves making a bicoronal scalp incision and a rather large scalp flap which is retracted anteriorly to expose the frontal bone. Typically, a large pericranial graft is also fashioned as a part of this scalp elevation. This vascularized pericranial graft is a critical element of the later reconstruction of the skull base. As a general principle, large defects left in the base of the skull are closed with vascularized tissue. The next step in the transbasal approach is a bifrontal craniotomy. There are many different permutations of the technique. Generally, a generous bifrontal bone flap is removed with the inferior margin being the supraorbital rims and the glabella medially. The bony opening can be extended in various ways with the goal of removing the supraorbital ridge. This added bone removal is typically termed the extended or extensive transbasal approach. The result is a reduced need for brain retraction and an increased view both in the lateral directions and in the cephalocaudad dimension. Some authors have utilized a technique whereby the olfactory nerves are preserved by making an osteotomy around the cribriform plate and elevating this area with its preserved nasal mucosa with the subfrontal dura (SPETZLER 1993). This has met with some success in reducing the morbidity of loss of olfactory nerve function.

The dura is then typically elevated from the frontal fossa floor. The frontal sinus is opened and exenterated. The bony floor of the frontal fossa is opened to expose the ethmoid sinuses, and the planum sphenoidale is also opened to permit access to the sphenoid sinus. The procedure also typically employs skeletonization of the optic canals bilaterally, and thinning or complete removal of the superior aspect of the bony orbits. The resultant view after bone drilling extends from the nasal bones to the pituitary fossa. In some cases the clivus is removed. In this circumstance, the inferior extent of exposure is down to the base of the clivus and the anterior arch of C1. Anteriorly and inferiorly, complete access is gained to the nasal cavity and turbinates, down to the floor of the nasal cavity. This technique is typically utilized, for example, for juvenile angiofibromas, esthesioneuroblastomas, frontal meningiomas, and clival chordomas or chondrosarcomas, to name a few. It is also a strategy employed for malignant histopathology in the region.

22.5.2
Approaches to the Central Skull Base

The lesions involving the central skull base can be exposed through a variety of surgical approaches. These lesions tend to spill over into the frontal, middle, or posterior fossa; therefore, they are, in general, surgically attacked via one of the anterior, lateral, or posterior skull base approaches. One of the more typical central skull base lesions is the pituitary ad-

enoma. This is commonly exposed via a transsphenoidal exposure. Currently, methods of endoscopy are also being employed, which provide a minimally invasive strategy for adequate exposure of the tumor and its subsequent removal. Malignancies involving the sphenoid sinus are also among the more common lesions, and are approached through a variety of methods. Generally, however, there is extension into the paranasal sinuses, and these lesions require an anterior transbasal or a transmaxillary type of combined approach. Other lesions involve the parasellar region and cavernous sinus, and these are generally exposed via a frontotemporal type of exposure. In this context there are many different variations in terms of exposure of the cavernous sinus. Some lesions require nothing more than a simple frontotemporal bone flap. However, others are more easily and comfortably exposed via a transzygomatic or an orbitozygomatic type of approach because of various extensions. In the transzygomatic exposure, osteotomies are made anteriorly and posteriorly in the zygomatic arch in order to either temporarily remove it or hinge it inferiorly on the masseter muscle, clearing a path to the floor of the middle fossa. The orbitozygomatic approach similarly allows a wider exposure of the frontal and middle skull base through removal of the superior and lateral orbital rim along with the zygomatic arch. These two strategies are also useful in the case of a central skull base tumor which extends high above the level of the dorsum sellae. This allows a better inferior to superior viewing angle while requiring less brain retraction for this added exposure.

A landmark innovation in exposure of lesions of the central and middle skull base was the combined epi- and subdural exposure of the parasellar region proposed by DOLENC (1983). This method employs a significant degree of extradural bony removal at the middle and central skull base, which then allows a mostly extradural exposure of the cavernous sinus region. This represents a major advance in technique, which has led to a significant reduction in surgical morbidity when operating in this region.

22.5.3
Approaches to the Lateral and Posterior Skull Base

This group constitutes some of the more complex skull base approaches. These most frequently require the participation of a team of surgeons, commonly involving a neurotologist, in addition to the neurosurgeon. The approaches to the lateral skull base mostly involve resection of various portions of the petrous bone or its entirety. These approaches are typically utilized for lesions of and around the petrous bone, the petroclival region, and the clivus. The lateral approaches are also the means of exposure of infratemporal fossa lesions. These various exposures can all be combined for a global exposure of the cranial base from the posterior aspect of the frontal fossa through the central and middle skull base to the posterior skull base.

The posterior approaches are fewer in number and permutations. Certainly, the simplest posterior skull base approach is the classic midline suboccipital approach to the craniocervical junction. A more lateral suboccipital approach can also be employed for lesions that are lateralized at the posterior foramen magnum region. A more complex approach, which was first proposed in the 1970s by Seeger (Bertalanffy 1996), has been further refined and increasingly utilized in the past 10 years. This approach is termed variously the transcondylar approach or the extreme lateral inferior transtubercular approach. It involves a quite far lateral suboccipital craniotomy with drilling anteriorly to expose the sigmoid sinus and the undersurface of the jugular bulb. The exposure is carried further anteriorly by limited removal of the posterior aspect of the occipital condyle. The bone between the condyle and the inferior surface of the jugular bulb is removed to expose the hypoglossal canal. Between the hypoglossal canal and the undersurface of the jugular bulb, the bone is further removed, which results in reduction of the jugular tubercle. The result of this complicated bone removal is an entirely flat access across the front surface of the brainstem. This is especially critical in the case of vascular lesions such as those located at the origin of the posterior inferior cerebellar artery or the vertebral basilar junction. Certainly, the brainstem does not tolerate even a modicum of retraction, and this is the rationale behind the design of this surgical approach.

Major contributions to the development of the more lateral approaches have been made by Ugo Fisch (1984). Professor Fisch has developed several permutations of the lateral skull base approach to the temporal bone and infratemporal fossa (Fisch 1984). These various permutations of the Fisch approach allow increasing exposure from posterior to anterior. They are generally used for malignancies at the skull base, as well as large glomus jugulare tumors.

Less extensive approaches than some of those introduced by Fisch involve progressive removal of portions of the temporal bone. These are variously termed the retrolabyrinthine, translabyrinthine, transcochlear, and petrosal approaches (Al-Mefty 1988; Hakuba 1988; Harsh 1992; Hitselberger 1993; House 1976; Kawase 1991; Samii 1989; Spetzler 1992). The transtemporal approaches are most frequently employed for petroclival meningiomas and acoustic neuromas. A popular approach, which has been developed by a number of different surgeons over the past 20 years, has been what is generally termed the combined petrosal approach. This involves a variable amount of removal of the petrous bone from a posterior trajectory combined with an "L"-shaped craniotomy around the ear. In some permutations of this technique, the petrous apex is removed via an extended middle fossa type of exposure extradurally. This technique generally provides a wide panoramic view of the petroclival region and also allows access to the cavernous sinus above and the foramen magnum region below. This combined petrosal approach is currently widely employed for both vascular and neoplastic lesions in these regions.

22.5.4
Reconstruction of the Skull Base

A critical element in determining the outcome in patients undergoing a contemporary skull base surgical approach is the prevention of complications related to leakage of cerebrospinal fluid. For this reason, proper reconstruction of the anatomical layers of the skull base is of paramount importance. In general, defects left by a skull base surgical approach are reconstructed with vascularized tissue if available. Various adipose and muscular grafts are also frequently employed along with sealants such as fibrin glue for complete re-establishment of the barrier between the cerebrospinal fluid space and the outside environment. For large lesions located in an area that is in contact with the air sinuses or the nasopharynx or oral pharynx, a more complex reconstruction is typically required. This usually necessitates placement of a free vascularized graft. A common donor for such purposes is the rectus abdominis free flap. Without the use of such vascularized tissue, the subsequent infection rate due to cerebrospinal fluid leakage is extremely high, as are the resultant morbidity and mortality.

22.6
Management of Specific Tumors

Several skull base locations and pathological types are problematic in terms of treatment strategy. Some tumors can be treated in a number of ways and there is no shortage of controversy generated between different groups treating these patients. Selected tumors in this category are discussed individually below. Many of the common tumors affecting the skull base, such as squamous cell carcinoma, are covered elsewhere in this publication.

22.6.1
Esthesioneuroblastoma

Esthesioneuroblastoma was first described by BERGER and Luc in 1924. These are very uncommon tumors which arise from olfactory epithelium and may extend to involve not only the upper nasal cavity, but the intracranial compartment as well. Small, localized tumors have historically carried a good prognosis with combined treatment regimens of surgery and radiotherapy. Larger, more extensive tumors, however, have a poor prognosis for long-term disease-free survival. Some management protocols have also included chemotherapy as part of their regimen, with mixed results. Because of the rarity of these tumors, insufficient experience at any one center has contributed to the controversy surrounding their optimal management. Only in recent years have large enough groups of patients been reported from which any solid conclusions may be drawn.

These tumors are assigned a clinical grade, which is based upon imaging study determination of the anatomical extent of the tumor. This "Kadish" grading scale assigns the designation of "A," "B," or "C" (KADISH 1976). Stage A tumors are those confined to the nasal cavity. Tumors confined to the nasal cavity and one or more paranasal sinuses are designated as stage B. When tumor extends beyond the nasal cavity, including involvement of the orbit, skull base, intracranial cavity, cervical lymph nodes, or distant metastatic sites, it is designated as stage C. This classification has been shown to be predictive of prognosis. Tumors are also assigned a histological grade (HYAMS 1988). Interestingly, in some series the histological grade has not seemed to have any effect on outcome (POLIN 1998).

Multidisciplinary management of these tumors has led to satisfactory outcomes, as evidenced by several series of patients from single institutions. At UCLA, 26 patients were treated over 20 years with combined surgical and radiation therapy. A 92% recurrence-free rate was reported over the follow-up period (DULGUEROV and CALCATERRA 1992). Combined radical surgical resection and radiotherapy was also utilized over a 10-year period at the University of Toronto in 12 patients (IRISH et al. 1997). Seventy-five percent were free of disease with an average follow-up time of 54 months. The complication rate was 25%, the complications consisting of one myocardial infarction, one pulmonary embolus, and one cerebrospinal fluid leak with meningitis. Of the 12 patients, ten were treated with radiation therapy, in nine cases postoperatively. The other two patients in the series were treated with adjuvant chemotherapy.

Pre- or postoperative chemotherapy has been another element explored for its efficacy, mainly in patients with stage C disease. The experience with preoperative chemotherapy and radiation therapy has been reported by the group at the University of Virginia (POLIN et al. 1998). Thirty-four consecutive patients over an 18-year period were reviewed. The majority of patients (31 of 34) received preoperative radiation averaging 51.1 Gy. Seven patients also received postoperative radiation therapy at an average of 45 Gy. Sixteen patients received a combination of cyclophosphamide and vincristine prior to surgery. In 14 of these adriamycin was added to the protocol. Another seven patients received chemotherapy after surgery. Five of these patients had to subsequently undergo bone marrow transplantation. With an average follow-up of 71 months, 22 patients were alive with no evidence of disease. Three survived with disease. Five patients were dead as a result of their esthesioneuroblastoma, and four more died of unrelated causes. Three of these four had evidence of active disease at autopsy. None of the disease-related deaths were in patients with stage A or B tumors. Most patients in this series showed radiographic response to preoperative adjunctive therapies. Those who did not respond at all had Kadish stage C disease. Fourteen patients with stage A or B disease showed a partial or minor response. Conclusions from this group of patients were that the Kadish stage is predictive of disease-free survival and that advanced age is also a predictor of poor outcome. Those patients responding to preoperative adjuvant therapy had a better chance of long-term disease-free survival. Presumably, this is because reduction of the tumor burden improves the chance of gross total surgical resection. Five-year disease-free survival in stage A and B patients was 86%, and in stage C 60%. These results were updated and reconfirmed by LEVINE (1999).

Patients with stage C disease have also been treated with chemotherapy alone with some prolongation of survival (McELROY 1998). Ten such patients were treated with various chemotherapeutic regimens at the Mayo Clinic. There was a significant difference in response to chemotherapy depending upon the histological grade of the tumor. Patients with low-grade tumors survived an average of 44.5 months (range 3–130 months). However, those with high-grade tumors only survived an average of 26.5 months (range 2–67 months). The authors concluded that patients with high-grade tumors are candidates for cisplatin-based chemotherapy and have a reasonable chance of prolongation of survival.

A treatment strategy which mostly excludes surgical resection of tumor has been applied which combines chemotherapy with proton radiation with promising results (BHATTACHARYYA et al. 1997). Nine patients with either esthesioneuroblastoma or neuroendocrine carcinoma were given combination therapy consisting of cisplatin and etoposide, followed by radiation therapy. Radiotherapy consisted of combined photon therapy and stereotactic proton beam therapy. Patients were then given another two cycles of chemotherapy. One patient failed to demonstrate a radiographic response to the initial chemotherapy and had a craniofacial resection. The other eight had such a dramatic response that surgery was not deemed necessary prior to radiation. No recurrences were seen at an average of 14 months utilizing this protocol. Such strategies, utilizing preoperative adjunctive therapies, seem to provide the best chance for long-term disease-free survival in these patients. The above study also demonstrates that radical surgical resection may not always be a necessary element of the treatment strategy.

22.6.2
Petroclival Meningiomas

Meningiomas located at the junction of the petrous bone and clivus remain one of the quintessential technical challenges for neurosurgeons. Their central location in the posterior fossa, anterior to the brainstem, places them in a locale where a number of cranial nerves are interposed between surgeon and tumor. Surgical removal invariably involves working through restricted operative corridors bounded by unforgiving nervous structures. Lesions such as these provided the impetus for the development of contemporary cranial base operative techniques. Difficulty in obtaining a total resection, or the inability to completely eradicate the attachment region of the tumor, often necessitates adjuvant radiotherapy. This has been performed using either focused beam fractionated radiotherapy or stereotactic radiosurgery (SUBACH et al. 1998), with a high success rate as regards long-term control of tumor growth.

The first line of therapy in these patients is surgical resection. The typical contemporary surgical technique is generically termed a "combined petrosal approach" (AL-MEFTY et al. 1988). This technique derives from several essential approach elements, used singly or in combination, depending upon exposure requirements. In essence, an "L"-shaped craniotomy flap is cut around the mastoid, composed of temporal and occipital bone. At minimum, a partial mastoidectomy is performed. Depending upon a number of factors, including tumor size, age and condition of the patient, and pre-existing neurological deficits (i.e., hearing loss), the labyrinth may be partially preserved (SEKHAR et al. 1999) or wholly removed. In some circumstances complete petrous bone resection may be performed. In others, removal of the petrous apex is performed via the middle fossa trajectory, sparing the hearing. The details of approach selection are beyond the scope of this chapter.

A review of the literature demonstrates the improvement in surgical outcomes witnessed in the past 10 years (COULDWELL et al. 1996). Cranial nerve morbidity has certainly been reduced, in addition to overall morbidity and mortality. The addition of radiotherapy in cases where a subtotal resection is performed has demonstrated benefit in reducing recurrence rates and further growth of residual tumor (CONNELL et al. 1999). In 1966, CHERRINGTON and SCHECK reported a series of 32 petroclival meningiomas operated on by a traditional suboccipital approach. A gross total resection was achieved in only 3% of patients with an operative mortality rate of 55%. Subsequently, YASARGIL et al. (1980) and MAYBERG and SYMON (1986) reported 20 and 35 patients, respectively, who were operated on by a combined supra and infratentorial type of approach and in whom a surgical microscope was utilized. The mortality rate in these patients was 10% and 9%, respectively. The use of the surgical microscope thus had a dramatic effect on surgical mortality. Subsequent authors have reported mortality rates of 0% in the past decade (COULDWELL et al. 1996; AL-MEFTY et al. 1988; SAMII et al. 1989). All have utilized a combined petrosal type of strategy. In fact, if the mortality figures of surgical series of the past decade are combined, the mortality rate is less than 5%. The operative morbidity is approximately 40% when considering new cranial nerve deficits. The combined rate of new motor deficits after surgical resection is roughly 15%. These figures are admittedly high; however, they represent the best we can currently offer patients with these very difficult lesions.

Total resection is not possible in all patients. The use of postoperative stereotactic radiosurgery to the remaining tumor mass has been documented to be of benefit. A recent report presented the results in 62 patients in whom stereotactic radiosurgery was employed either after subtotal surgical resection or as primary therapy (SUBACH et al. 1998). As would be expected, the majority of patients suffered no additional cranial nerve morbidity after radiosurgery. Tumor volume decreased in only 23% after radiosurgery, with 68% remaining stable over the average follow-up period of 37 months. Five patients (8%) suffered new cranial nerve deficits after radiosurgery, all in a delayed fashion. The conclusion of the authors was that stereotactic radiosurgery is a safe therapy method in patients with small (<3 cm diameter) petroclival meningiomas, as either primary or adjuvant treatment. However, its role as primary therapy is debatable. When considering the surgical results in small tumors achieved by experienced surgeons, the complication rates are seen to be correspondingly low and recurrence rates are also low (COULDWELL 1996). Until very long term data in a sufficient number of patients become available, we continue to recommend surgical resection in all patients soon after diagnosis, with stereotactic radiosurgery used postoperatively should there be a small residual tumor. In cases where a large residual tumor is present, fractionated conventional radiotherapy is prescribed.

In summary, petroclival meningiomas are extremely challenging lesions to treat surgically. Newer skull base approach methods have helped to dramatically lower surgical complication rates and mortality. The addition of focused beam radiotherapy and/or stereotactic radiosurgery is of benefit in limiting growth of residual tumor mass in these cases.

22.6.3
Clival and Foramen Magnum Meningiomas

The tight confines of the foramen magnum region and the posterior fossa create a tenuous situation for the medulla when the limited available space is occupied by meningioma. These lesions typically cause a significant degree of medullary distortion and com-

pression prior to diagnosis. This is, of course, owing to the classically slow-growing nature of the tumor. Meningiomas at this location tend to be an almost exclusively surgical disease. In only a limited number of cases will adjuvant radiotherapy be necessary or even advisable.

The site of origin of these lesions is important in terms of the expected surgical outcome. Lesions located ventrally are the most challenging to manage. Ventral foramen magnum tumors tend to displace the medulla posteriorly and the lower cranial nerves are draped over the lateral aspect. The vertebral artery may be encased by these lesions, or simply displaced posteriorly against the medulla. Ventral foramen magnum tumors require a far lateral approach with a variable degree of removal of the occipital condyle and jugular tubercle for adequate exposure. Foramen magnum lesions which arise laterally or posteriorly are an entirely different entity in terms of the potential surgical morbidity and chances of total resection. These tumors require a less complex and more routine posterior or lateral suboccipital surgical approach. The location of the cranial nerves on the medial side of the mass tends to make total tumor removal with lower morbidity more feasible. Laterally placed tumors, however, may encase the vertebral artery. The artery is not always separable from the tumor, resulting in a subtotal resection.

Several recent series published in the microsurgical era have presented the results achieved utilizing a contemporary skull base surgical approach. Results in a series of 40 patients presented by GEORGE et al. (1997) showed that a total resection is possible in almost all cases with very low morbidity. In cases of purely intradural meningioma, they were able to attain a 94% rate of total resection. The more aggressive tumors with extradural extension could only be resected 50% of the time. In this rather large series from Paris, 90% of patients improved clinically after surgery. Only 7.5% developed worsening of symptoms. Similar excellent results were presented in 19 patients with ventral meningiomas, all treated by the far lateral transcondylar surgical strategy (BERTALANFFY et al. 1996). All patients underwent total resection of tumor with no major complications. In the same year SAMII et al. (1996) presented their experience with 38 patients harboring these lesions. Their patients underwent total resection in 63% of cases. Complications were observed in 30% of patients, mostly those with very difficult recurrent or infiltrative or en plaque meningiomas. The authors further observed that patients tended to have an improvement in preoperative ataxia or motor deficits, whereas cranial nerve deficits were more likely to remain unchanged after surgery. Only an occasional patient in any of the above-mentioned series underwent any kind of radiation therapy as an adjunct. It was quite unusual in any of the aforementioned surgical series to observe a recurrence of tumor after surgical resection.

One recent paper from Pittsburgh has suggested that stereotactic radiosurgery can be used as an alternative or an adjunctive treatment in patients who are not able to undergo surgical resection of a ventral foramen magnum meningioma (MUTHUKUMAR 1999). This group reported five patients with advanced age, complicated medical conditions, or residual meningioma at the foramen magnum. The age range of these patients was 73–84 years. The follow-up interval was 1–5 years with a median of 3 years. There was no further growth in four patients. One patient died of intercurrent illness. This study's findings are very hard to interpret due to the very slow growing nature of meningiomas, especially in the elderly population. It is impossible to tell exactly what positive effect the treatment had in such a patient population. Our group does not recommend stereotactic radiosurgery even in this difficult-to-manage group, owing to the difficulty in targeting and the uncertain benefit of the technique.

When presented with a patient with a foramen magnum meningioma it is our recommendation to proceed with surgical treatment without significant delay. There is little reason to simply follow these tumors in this location owing to the significant increase in surgical morbidity that accompanies increased size of the tumor. A recent report demonstrated the relationship between preoperative Karnofsky score and outcome in a series of 18 patients with ventral foramen magnum meningiomas (ARNAUTOVIC et al. 2000). A Karnofsky score lower than 60 was a poor prognostic indicator. Therefore, early diagnosis and treatment are recommended to prevent such poor outcomes.

22.6.4
Chordoma and Chondrosarcoma

Chordomas, which arise from the notochordal remnants, are usually histologically benign but malignant in behavior. These tumors are rare, constituting no more than 1% of all intracranial neoplasms (MIZERNY et al. 1995). Males are more often affected than females. The fourth decade of life is the most likely age at diagnosis. While the majority of chordomas

are histologically benign, some are capable of metastasis. Recurrence of tumor is extremely common and there are few long-term survivors even with aggressive treatment.

Chordomas have been shown in the past to be relatively resistant to conventional radiation therapy. This has resulted in a treatment strategy that has been largely surgical, with repeated resection offered for recurrent disease. Some centers have administered postoperative fractionated radiotherapy with disappointing results. MIZERNY and KOST (1995) presented the experience at the Montreal Neurologic Institute over a 13-year period with 11 patients. Ten patients had surgery followed by fractionated radiation therapy. One patient had surgery only. Five patients died of disease at an average of 4.4 years after surgical treatment. Another five patients had recurrent or progressive disease from 2–6 years after treatment. The remaining patient was treated with surgery only and was alive with no evidence of disease 6 months post surgery. Early in this experience, radiation dose was rather low, presumably owing to the inherent anatomical constraints of location. A dose-response relationship was found by PEARLMAN and FRIEDMAN (1970) in chordomas treated by high-dose photon radiation. They found that their patients who received more than 80 Gy had an 80% local control rate. By contrast only a 20% success rate was observed in patients receiving 40–60 Gy. Clival chordomas are surrounded by sensitive cranial nerve structures and the brainstem, making high-dose conventional radiotherapy a high-risk undertaking (HUG and MUNZENRIDER 1994).

Because of the difficulties of administering high-dose radiation to residual tumor in this location, the role of proton beam therapy has been elucidated in recent years. AUSTIN-SEYMOUR et al. (1989) reported their experience in 63 patients with skull base chordomas and chondrosarcomas treated with proton beam therapy. The actuarial local control rate in these patients was 85%. Complications were limited to visual in 4.4% and pituitary insufficiency in 13.2%. Only six patients experienced a local recurrence at a median time of 53 months. Further experience has been reported more recently by HUG et al. (1999) with fractionated proton beam radiation therapy in 58 patients, including 33 with chordoma and 25 with chondrosarcoma. Of these 58 patients, 91% had residual tumor after various surgical procedures. Actuarial 5-year survival rates were 79% for patients with chordoma and 100% for patients with chondrosarcoma. Factors affecting local control rates were found to be tumor volume of greater than

25 ml and brainstem involvement. Patients with brainstem involvement had a necessary reduction in dose which resulted in only a 53% local control rate.

Another radiation therapy modality has been utilized with success, namely charged-particle irradiation with helium. BERSON et al. (1988) reported their experience with 45 patients with chordomas and chondrosarcomas of the skull base and cervical spine, treated by initial surgical resection followed by such irradiation. The 5-year actuarial survival rate was 62%, with a disease-free survival rate of 59%. Tumor volume was also found to have an effect on outcome. A residual tumor volume of less than 20 cm^3 resulted in a 5-year actuarial control rate of 80%, whereas tumors greater than this volume had a control rate of only 33%.

These series confirm that the best treatment strategy currently is initial optimal surgical resection, followed by fractionated proton beam therapy. This offers the best chance for tumor control and survival in the majority of patients with chordoma.

Chondrosarcomas are more common than chordomas, but share their general treatment strategy. Chondrosarcomas are more often located in a more lateral location, generally occupying the petroclival region rather than the more midline clival location that is common in chordoma. Chondrosarcomas are cartilaginous tumors that constitute 11%–19% of primary bone tumors of the skull base (WEBER et al. 1995). Clinical symptomatology depends upon location. Sixth nerve palsy is a frequent finding owing to compression of the nerve in Dorello's canal. Patients may also exhibit a jugular foramen syndrome secondary to common involvement of this region. Treatment of chondrosarcomas is initial radical surgical resection, followed by proton beam radiotherapy. The 5-year control rate following fractionated proton irradiation has been demonstrated to be 95%, versus 62% for chordoma (MUNZENRIDER et al. 1993).

22.6.5
Glomus Jugulare and Vagale Tumors

Numerous classification schemes have been devised for the clinical characterization of paragangliomas. These schemes are largely based upon anatomical location and tumor extent. The classification described by DE LA CRUZ has been extremely useful in the treatment planning for these tumors (GREEN et al. 1994). In this classification scheme, tumors are described by their anatomical extent and each group of tumors has a corresponding operative approach.

Tympanic tumors are those arising in the middle ear and confined entirely to the mesotympanum. The complete extent of the tumor is visible through the tympanic membrane; hence, tumor excision can be performed through a transcanal approach. In contrast, a *tympanomastoid* tumor arises from the middle ear but has extended into the posterior tympanum or the hypotympanum beyond the visible confines of the tympanic annulus. Radiographically, these tumors do not involve the jugular bulb, and they can be excised through a mastoid-extended facial recess approach.

Jugular bulb tumors are confined to this region and may extend to the middle ear and mastoid. They do not involve the carotid artery or the intracranial compartment. These tumors are excised through the mastoid-neck approach. Large tumors may require limited rerouting of the facial nerve. *Carotid artery* and *transdural* tumors are far more extensive and require an infratemporal fossa approach and excision of the intracranial component.

22.6.5.1
Tympanicum Tumors

O'LEARY et al (1991) reviewed 64 cases of tympanicum tumors treated at the House Ear Clinic between 1957 and 1990. Eighty percent of these tumors were removed through a mastoid-extended facial recess approach. The preoperative mean air-bone gap was reduced from 10 dB to a postoperative mean of 4 dB. There were only five complications including two tympanic membrane ruptures, one cholesteatoma, and one transient facial palsy that resolved to a House grade II/VI after decompression.

22.6.5.2
Jugulare Tumors

GREEN et al. (1994) reviewed the surgical outcome in 52 previously untreated jugulare tumors managed at the House Ear Clinic between 1980 and 1991. The surgical approach most commonly used was the infratemporal fossa approach (83%). Twenty-nine percent of the tumors extended intradurally, and 21% involved the internal carotid artery. Complete surgical removal was possible in 85%, and there were no surgical mortalities. Of the eight patients with incomplete removal, three had involvement of the internal carotid artery and five had significant intraoperative blood loss prohibiting complete tumor removal in a single stage.

Postoperative complications are infrequent. Long-term facial nerve function was good (House grade I/

VI or II/VI) in 95% of the patients treated. Approximately 19% of the patients required vocal cord augmentation, and four required enteric feeding due to aspiration. No patient required immediate postoperative tracheotomy and, overall, 85% of the patients were able to resume the preoperative level of activity.

22.6.5.3
Radiation Therapy

The role of radiation therapy in the treatment of jugulotympanic paragangliomas is quite controversial. Many reports have appeared in the old and recent literature reporting tumor control rates of 70%–90% with radiation as primary, adjunctive, or salvage therapy (PARKIN 1981; PATEL et al. 1994; PENSAK and JACKLER 1997). The doses given in these studies are between 35 and 50 Gy. The primary effect of radiation therapy appears to be on the vascular and stromal elements of the tumor, with little effect on the tumor cells (PETERMAN et al. 1991). Viable tumor cells remain after radiation, and tumors have been known to recrudesce after more than a decade (PENSAK and JACKLER 1997). With the advent of microsurgical techniques, we have identified few specific indications for radiation therapy. We recommend this form of treatment for elderly patients with symptomatic tumors or for patients who are unsuitable or unwilling to undergo surgical resection.

22.6.6
Trigeminal Schwannomas

Schwannomas arising from the trigeminal nerve are rare tumors that may occupy the cavernous sinus, parasellar region, posterior fossa, or extracranial compartment. These tumors typically cause a variable degree of trigeminal dysfunction. They may also present with other cranial nerve signs, especially diplopia (DAY and FUKUSHIMA 1998). This condition has traditionally been a surgically treated disease. Contemporary techniques of cranial base surgery have led to improved outcomes with a very low rate of recurrence (DAY and FUKUSHIMA 1998). Despite data from experienced surgeons demonstrating low complication rates and very low chances of recurrence, stereotactic radiosurgery has recently been used in a limited number of patients. Safety of this technique has been demonstrated in a small number of cases from one institution; however, there has been no demonstrated long-term efficacy (HUANG et al. 1999).

These tumors are divided into four different types, classified by their location. Tumors arising from the trigeminal nerve root, contained within the posterior fossa, are the first type. These are best approached via a retrosigmoid type approach. A second type of tumor, the *dumbbell* type, spans the posterior and middle fossae. These masses involve both the nerve root and the ganglion, and, when very large, may extend peripherally. This type of tumor usually requires a combined petrosal type of strategy. The large majority of ganglion type tumors may be approached via an entirely extradural, temporopolar approach (DAY et al. 1994). Ganglion tumors located laterally may also be approached via an extradural subtemporal transpetrosal approach. Peripheral type neurinomas are also handled by one of these extradural strategies, or a variation thereon. The key concept is that these latter two types of schwannoma are located extradurally and that a contemporary cranial base strategy can result in total resection with low morbidity (DAY and FUKUSHIMA 1998; DOLENC 1994).

DOLENC (1994) reported his results in 35 patients undergoing initial operation for trigeminal schwannoma utilizing a frontotemporal epidural approach. All patients in the series were reported to have had a total resection of the lesion. There was no mortality or major surgical morbidity. Five patients had abducens palsy preoperatively, which in all cases resolved after surgery. Trigeminal hypesthesia improved in 11, was unchanged in 9, and slightly worsened in 10 patients. DAY and FUKUSHIMA (1998) published a similar experience in 38 patients with 39 trigeminal schwannomas. A total resection was achieved in 75% of patients. Three patients who had subtotal resection had malignant histology, which required postoperative radiation therapy. No recurrences were observed over an average follow-up time of 6.4 years (range =–15 years). The complication rate was also very low. One patient developed new diplopia, and one patient required a shunt for hydrocephalus. Otherwise, other complications were related to trigeminal hypesthesia or anesthesia. There was no major surgical morbidity in this series.

In summary, trigeminal schwannomas are rare tumors that have been treated surgically in the past with good results. There is a high likelihood of resolution of cranial nerve-related symptoms after surgical removal. The recurrence rate after a gross total resection is very low over a long period of time. Stereotactic radiosurgery may be offered as an alternative in patients who are poor surgical candidates with small tumors. However, the long-term efficacy of this treatment modality is unknown at this time for these tumors.

22.6.7
Cavernous Sinus Tumors

The "cavernous sinus," so named by Winslow in the eighteenth century, has historically been a neurosurgical "no man's land." Uncontrollable, excessive bleeding, postoperative cranial nerve deficits, and potential damage to the intracavernous carotid artery have been effective deterrents to widespread attempts at directly approaching lesions of the region. BROWDER (1937) is credited with the first report of a direct approach to the cavernous sinus in 1937, describing the obliteration of a carotid-cavernous fistula by packing muscle through the roof of the cavernous sinus. The neurosurgical literature was devoid of reference to a successful direct approach into the region until 1965. In that year, PARKINSON (1965) reported his successful direct repair of a traumatic carotid-cavernous fistula under the anesthetic conditions of hypothermia and cardiac arrest. No major series of direct cavernous sinus operations was subsequently reported until 1983, when DOLENC published his innovative combined epi- and subdural approach for cavernous sinus lesions (DOLENC 1983). A few neurosurgeons followed with reports of their own experience with Dolenc's technique in the late 1980s (DAY and FUKUSHIMA 1996; HAKUBA 1989; SEKHAR 1993).

Masses within the cavernous sinus have typical presentations that in general follow the original patterns described by JEFFERSON (1938) in his classic paper. Patients usually can be placed within the categories of an anterior versus middle versus posterior cavernous sinus syndrome. The presence of one of these symptom complexes, however, does not itself constitute an indication for operation. Many factors must be taken into account, including imaging characteristics, adjacent structures involved, the time course of the process, and the functional severity of symptoms. Patients presenting with painful ophthalmoplegia or rapid onset of visual compromise with a mass clearly involving the cavernous sinus tend to be offered an operation immediately. The main goal in these cases is decompression of the neural structures and establishment of a diagnosis. Total resection is performed if the circumstances favor such an attempt. Patients who are experiencing cerebral ischemia from embolic phenomena, secondary to carotid thrombosis from tumor invasion or compression, are similar-ly offered an urgent operation. This circumstance invariably involves a revascularization procedure.

Difficult decisions are made in cases of cavernous sinus involvement by extensions of malignant processes from the paranasal sinuses and pharynx. These procedures are palliative in nature because of the characteristically aggressive nature of these tumors, such as squamous cell carcinoma. En bloc resection of the cavernous sinus and adjacent areas may represent a merely heroic effort on the patient's behalf, with little realistic chance of long-term survival. Localized malignancies are an entirely different prospect in most circumstances. While chordomas and chondrosarcomas are incurable tumors, a reasonable long-term outcome can be achieved in cases of local invasion by means of subtotal resection and subsequent radiation therapy. Regardless of the nature of the malignant process, surgery in cases of cavernous sinus involvement is a formidable undertaking. As experience with these lesions grows, the indications will change according to technological developments and improved surgical capabilities.

Experience has demonstrated a disparity in outcome between meningiomas and other benign tumors surgically resected from the cavernous sinus (DAY and FUKUSHIMA 1996). Several authors have illustrated the uniformly favorable outcome of direct surgical removal of benign tumors such as trigeminal schwannoma, pituitary adenoma, cavernous angioma, dermoid and epidermoid tumors, and the like (SEKHAR 1993; DAY and FUKUSHIMA 1996; EISENBERG et al. 1999). DAY and FUKUSHIMA (1996) reported that only 6 of 62 patients (9.7%) with benign intracavernous lesions suffered postoperatively from permanent deficits involving oculomotor paresis or trigeminal nerve hypesthesias. Four patients in this group (6.5%) had a hemiparesis postoperatively that was not pre-existing. This contrasts with the results in 76 patients with intracavernous meningiomas as reported by the same authors. Of these patients, 68% suffered permanent oculomotor palsies, with 84% having trigeminal nerve complaints. Eight patients had a hemiparesis after surgery. Other complications, such as cerebrospinal fluid leakage, infection, seizures, and diabetes insipidus, were seen in less than 10%, and were uniformly temporary.

EISENBERG and colleagues (1999) reported a similar experience in 40 patients with mostly pituitary adenomas and trigeminal schwannomas. In these patients, total resection was achieved in 82.5%. Stable or improved extraocular muscle function was reported in 89.7%, with 40% showing improvement after surgery. Overall, cranial nerve deficits were improved in 51.5% postoperatively, while 42.2% demonstrated no change in function. Only 6.3% of patients fared worse. This can be compared with the results of aggressive removal of cavernous sinus meningioma by the same group (DeMonte et al. 1994). Forty-one patients with cavernous sinus meningioma were treated surgically, with a total resection rate of 76%. Cranial nerve deficits that were pre-existing improved in only 14% of patients, while 80% remained unchanged from their preoperative status. Permanent worsening was seen in 6%. Three patients died secondary to postsurgical complications. Two patients suffered permanent hemiparesis from vascular injuries. These data from different groups demonstrate the difficulties with surgical removal of meningiomas in the cavernous sinus. These problems have prompted the utilization of adjunctive treatment methods along with less aggressive surgery to try and improve results.

Radiotherapy and radiosurgery have been utilized with great success in limiting further growth of skull base meningiomas after surgery (Goldsmith et al. 1992; Duma et al. 1993). Reports with external beam radiotherapy have demonstrated tumor control rates of more than 90% over variable follow-up periods.

22.7 Conclusion

Tumors located at the base of the skull remain challenging lesions to eradicate while minimizing morbidity and mortality. In the last decade of the twentieth century, great strides were made in skull base surgery. Improvements have been driven by the formation of specialized multidisciplinary teams and advances in technology. These tumors are clearly best left in the care of such teams at centers where case volume is sufficient for meaningful outcome statistics to be generated. With concentration of these patients at such specialized centers, improvements in outcome for the various lesions at the skull base can be expected at an accelerated pace in the coming decade.

References

Al-Mefty O, Fox JL, Smith RR (1988) Petrosal approach for petroclival meningiomas. Neurosurgery 22:510–517

Arnautovic KI, Al-Mefty O, Husain M (2000) Ventral foramen magnum meningiomas. J Neurosurg(Spine 1)92:71–80

Austin JP, Urie MM, Cardenosa G, et al. (1993) Probable causes of recurrence in patients with chordoma and chondrosarcoma of the base of skull and cervical spine. Int J Radiat Oncol Biol Phys 25:439–444

Austin-Seymour M, Munzenrider J, Goitein N, et al. (1989) Fractionated proton radiation therapy of chordoma and low-grade chondrosarcoma of the base of skull. J Neurosurg 70:13–17

Berger L, Luc R (1924) L'esthesioneroepitheliome olfactif. Bull Assoc Fr Etude Cancer 13:410–421

Berson AM, Castro JR, Petti P, et al. (1988) Charged particle irradiation of chordoma and chondrosarcoma of the base of skull and cervical spine: the Lawrence Berkeley Laboratory experience. Int J Radiat Oncol Biol Phys 15:559–565

Bertalanffy H, Gilsbach JM, Mayfrank L, Klein HM, Kawase T, Seeger W (1996) Microsurgical management of ventral and ventrolateral foramen magnum meningiomas. Acta Neurochir Suppl (Wien) 65:82–85

Bhattacharyya N, Thornton AF, Joseph MP, Goodman ML, Amrein PC (1997) Successful treatment of esthesioneuroblastoma and neuroendocrine carcinoma with combined chemotherapy and proton radiation. Arch Otolaryngol Head Neck Surg 123:34–40

Browder J (1937) Treatment of carotid artery-cavernous sinus fistula. Report of a case. Arch Ophthal 18(supp. 2):95–102

Cherington M, Scheck SA (1966) Clivus meningiomas. Neurology 16:86–92

Connell PP, Macdonald RL, Mansur DB, Nicholas MK, Mundt AJ (1999) Tumor size predicts control of benign meningiomas treated with radiotherapy. Neurosurgery 44:1194–1200

Couldwell WT, Fukushima T, Giannotta SL, Weiss MH (1996) Petroclival meningiomas: surgical experience in 109 cases. J Neurosurgery 84:20–28

Day JD, Fukushima T (1996) Cavernous Sinus Neoplasms. In Youmans JR (ed), Neurological Surgery, 4th ed., WB Saunders, Philadelphia, pp.2862–2881

Day JD, Fukushima T (1998) The surgical management of trigeminal neuromas. Neurosurgery 42:233

Day JD, Giannotta SL, Fukushima T (1994) Extradural temporopolar approach to lesions of the upper basilar artery and infrachiasmatic region. J Neurosurg 81:223–235

DeMonte F, Smith H, Al-Mefty O (1994) Outcome of aggressive removal of cavernous sinus meningiomas. J Neurosurg 81:245–251

Derome PJ (1988) The transbasal approach to tumor invading the base of the skull, in Schmidek HH, Sweet WH (eds): Operative Neurosurgical Technique. W.B. Saunders, Philadelphia, pp 619–633

Dolenc V (1983) Direct microsurgical repair of intracavernous vascular lesions. J Neurosurg 58:824–831

Dolenc VV (1994) Frontotemporal epidural approach to trigeminal neurinomas. Acta Neurochir (Wien) 130:55–65

Dulguerov P, Calcaterra T (1992) Esthesioneuroblastoma: the UCLA experience 1970–1990. Laryngoscope 102:843–849

Duma CM, Lunsford LD, Kondziolka D, Harsh GR, Flickinger JC (1993) Stereotactic radiosurgery of cavernous sinus meningiomas as an addition or alternative to microsurgery. Neurosurgery 32:699–705

Eisenberg MB, Al-Mefty O, De Montebt F, Burson GT (1999) Benign nonmeningeal tumors of the cavernous sinus. Neurosurgery 44:949

Fisch U, Fagan P, Valvanis A (1984) The infratemporal fossa approach for the lateral skull base. Otolaryngol Clin North Am 17:513–552

George B, Lot G, Boissonet H (1997) Meningioma of the foramen magnum: a series of 40 cases. Surg Neurol 47:371–379

Goldsmith B, Wara W, Wilson C, Larson D (1992) Post-operative external beam irradiation for subtotally resected meningiomas. Int J Radiat Oncol Biol Phys 24(Suppl 1):126–127

Green JD, Brackmann DE, Nguyen CD, Arriaga MA, Telischi FF, De la Cruz A (1994) Surgical management of previously untreated glomus jugulare tumors. Laryngoscope 104:917

Hakuba A, Nishimura S, Jang BJ (1988) A combined retroauricular and preauricular transpetrosal-transtentorial approach to clivus meningiomas. Surg Neurol 30:108–116

Hakuba A, Tanaka K, Suzuki T, Nishimura S (1989) A combined orbitozygomatic infratemporal epidural subdural approach for lesions involving the entire cavernous sinus. J Neurosurg 71:699–704

Hitselberger WE, Horn KL, Hankinson H, Brackmann DE, House WF (1993) The middle fossa transpetrous approach for petroclival meningiomas. Skull Base Surgery 3:130–135

House WF, Hitselberger WE (1976) The transcochlear approach to the skull base. Archives of Otolaryngology 102:334–342

Huang CF, Konziolka D, Flickinger JC, Lunsford LD (1999) Stereotactic radiosurgery for trigeminal schwannomas. Neurosurgery 45:11–16

Hug EB, Loredo LN, Slater JD, De Vrics A, Grove RI, Schaefer RA, Rosenberg AE, Slater JM (1999) Proton radiation therapy for chordomas and chondrosarcomas of the skull base. J Neurosurg 91:432–439

Hug EB, Munzenrider JE (1994) Charged particle therapy for base of skull tumors: past accomplishments and future challenges. Int J Radiat Oncol Biol Phys 29:911–912

Hyams VJ (1988) Tumors of the upper respiratory tract and ear. In Hyams VJ, Batsakis JG, Michaels L, eds. Atlas of Tumor Pathology. Washington DC, Armed Forces Institute of Pathology, 2nd series, part 25, pp.240–248.

Irish J, Dasgupta R, Freeman J, et al. (1997) Outcome and analysis of the surgical management of esthesioneuroblastoma. J Otolaryngology 26:1–7

Jefferson G (1938) On the saccular aneurysms of the internal carotid artery in the cavernous sinus. Br J Surg 26:267–301

Kadish S, Goodman M, Wang CC (1976) Olfactory neuroblastoma: a clinical analysis of 17 cases. Cancer 37:1571–1576

Kawase T, Shiobara R, Toya S (1991) Anterior transpetrosal-transtentorial approach for sphenopetroclival meningiomas: surgical method and results in 10 patients. Neurosurgery 28:869–876

Levine PA, Galagher R, Cantrell RW (1999) Esthesioneuroblastoma: reflections of a 21-year experience. Laryngoscope 109:1539–1543

Mayberg M, Symon L (1986) Meningiomas of the clivus and apical petrous bone. Report of 35 cases. J Neurosurgery 65:160–167

McElroy EA, Buckner JC, Lewis JE (1998) Chemotherapy for advanced esthesioneuroblastoma: the Mayo Clinic experience. Neurosurgery 42:1023–1028

Mizerny BR, Kost KM (1995) Chordoma of the Cranial Base:The McGill experience. J Otolaryngol 24:14–19

Munzenrider JE, Liebsch NJ, Efird JT (1993) Chordomas and chondrosarcomas of skull base: treatment with fractionated x-ray and proton radiotherapy. In Johnson JT, Didolkar MS(eds), Head and Neck Cancer, New York, Elsevier Science

Muthukumar N, Kondziolka D, Lunsford LD, Flickinger JC (1999) Stereotactic radiosurgery for anterior foramen magnum meningiomas. Surg Neurol 51:268–273

O'Leary MJ, Shelton C, Giddings NA, Kwartler J, Brackmann DE (1991) Glomus tympanicum tumors: A clinical perspective. Laryngoscope 101:1038

Parkin JL (1981) Familial multiple glomus tumors and pheochromocytomas. Ann Otol 90:60

Parkinson D (1965) A surgical approach to the cavernous portion of the carotid artery; anatomical studies and case report. J Neurosurg 23:474–483

Patel SJ, Sekhar LN, Cass SP, Hirsch BE (1994) Combined approaches for resection of extensive glomus jugulare tumors. J Neurosurg 80:1026–1038

Pearlman AW, Friedman M (1970) Radical radiation therapy of chordoma. AJR 108:333–341

Pensak ML, Jackler RK (1997) Removal of jugular foramen tumors: the Fallopian bridge technique. Otolaryngol Head Neck Surg 17:586–591

Peterman SB, Taylor A, Hoffman JC (1991) Improved detection of cerebral hypoperfusion with internal carotid balloon test occlusion and ^{99m}Tc-HMPAO cerebral perfusion SPECT imaging. AJNR 12:1035

Polin RS, Sheehan JP, Chenelle AG, et al. (1998) The role of preoperative adjuvant treatment in the management of esthesioneuroblastoma: the University of Virginia experience. Neurosurgery 42:1029–1037

Samii M, Ammirati M, Mahran A, Bini W, Sepehrnia A (1989) Surgery of petroclival meningiomas: Report of 24 cases. Neurosurgery 24:12–17

Samii M,Klekamp J, Carvalho G (1996) Surgical results for meningiomas of the craniocervical junction. Neurosurgery 39:1086–1094

Sekhar LN, Ross DA, Sen C (1993) Cavernous sinus and sphenocavernous neoplasms. In Sekhar LN, Janecka IP (eds), Surgery of Cranial Base Tumors. New York, Raven Press, pp.521–604

Sekhar LN, Schessel DA, Bucur SD, Raso JL, Wright DC (1999) Partial labyrinthectomy petrous apicectomy approach to neoplastic and vascular lesions of the petroclival area. Neurosurgery 44:537–552

Spetzler RF, Daspit CP, Pappas CTE (1992) The combined supra and infratentorial approach for lesions of the petrous and clival regions: experience with 46 cases. J Neurosurgery 76:588–599

Spetzler RF, Fukushima T, Martin N, Zabramski JM (1990) Petrous carotid-to-intradural carotid saphenous vein graft for intracavernous giant aneurysm, tumor, and occlusive cerebrovascular disease. J Neurosurg 73:496–501

Spetzler RF, Herman JM, Beals S, et al. (1993) Preservation of olfaction in anterior craniofacial approaches, J Neurosurg 79:48–52

Subach BR, Lunsford LD, Kondziolka D, Maitz AH, Flickinger JC (1998) Management of petroclival meningiomas by stereotactic radiosurgery. Neurosurgery 71:705–710

Uttley D, Moore A, Archer DJ (1989) Surgical management of midline skull base tumors: a new approach. J Neurosurgery 71:705–710

Weber AL, Brown EW, Hug EB, Liebsch NJ (1995) Cartilaginous tumors and chordomas of the cranial base. Otol Clin N Am 28:453–470

Yasargil MG, Mortara RW, Curcic M (1980) Meningiomas of basal posterior cranial fossa, in Krayenbuhl H (ed): Advances and Technical Standards in Neurosurgery, Springer, Wien, pp 3–115

23 Treatment of CNS Lymphomas

Silvia C. Formenti and Anna Bettini

CONTENTS

23.1
Introduction

Non-Hodgkin's lymphomas that develop and remained limited to the CNS (and the eye) are classified as primary CNS lymphomas (PCNSL). They arise from the brain, the spinal cord, leptomeninges, or eyes. Originally described as perithelial sarcoma, microglioma, or reticulum sarcoma, most PCNSL proved to be of B cell origin following the introduction of immunohistochemical studies of surface markers (Burstein et al. 1963; Rubinsten 1972; Taylor et al. 1978).

PCNSL are often associated with immunodeficiencies, either congenital, such as the Wiskott-Aldrich syndrome and ataxia telangiectasia; iatrogenic, like after renal transplant; or acquired, as in association with AIDS (Edgar et al. 1961; Gunderson et al. 1971; Hoover et al. 1973; Schneck et al. 1971; Guinan et al. 1986; Snider et al. 1983; Welch et al. 1984; Ziegler et al. 1982).

S. C. Formenti, MD
Associate Professor, Departments of Radiation Oncology and Medicine, University of Southern California School of Medicine, 1441 Eastlake Avenue, Los Angeles, CA 90033-0804, USA
A. Bettini, MD
Research Fellow, Departments of Radiation Oncology and Medicine, University of Southern California School of Medicine, 1441 Eastlake Avenue, Los Angeles, CA 90033-0804, USA

During the past 10 years, an increase in the incidence of PCNSL has been recorded. Prior to this period, PCNSL were relatively rare, accounting for only 0.5–1.2% of all intracranial tumors (Jellinger et al. 1975; Zimmerman 1975). Today, they represent between 2% and 6% of all primary brain neoplasms and more than 1% of all non-Hodgkin's lymphomas (Camilleri et al. 1998). While the AIDS epidemic accounts for most of this increase in the incidence (Rosenblum et al. 1988; Welch et al. 1984), a clear increase among immunocompetent patients has also emerged. Data from the 1973–1984 National Cancer Institute Surveillance Epidemiology and End Results program (SEER) suggest a threefold increase in the incidence of PCNSL that can not be totally explained by improved diagnostic, nosologic, or epidemiologic considerations (Eby et al. 1988; Greig et al. 1990).

23.2
Etiology

The pathogenesis of PCNSL is still unknown. A strong association of the tumor with endogenous or exogenous immunosuppression suggests that a decreased immune surveillance might be a determinant factor for the transformation of polyclonal B cells into a monoclonal population. Moreover, PCNSL among immunocompetent subjects display a peak in the sixth and seventh decades of life, possibly reflecting the diminished immune surveillance of the elderly. In this population, it is easier to demonstrate chromosomal abnormalities that can correlate with B cell proliferation (DeAngelis et al. 1987).

The T-cell-mediated immunoregulation seems to have a key role in the development of PCNSL. The induction of T cell depletion with cyclosporine and/or monoclonal antibodies, to reduce graft-versus-host disease after allogenic transplantation, has resulted in an increased incidence and earlier occurrence of PCNSL than usually expected after this procedure (Swinnen et al. 1990). The HIV-induced

T cell deregulation might be the cause of the association between AIDS and PCNSL. This commonly occurs in the symptomatic phase of the infection when deregulation becomes clinically significant. Furthermore, in the immunocompromised patient, the presence of Epstein-Barr virus (EBV) has been detected in 90–100% of the cases affected by PCNSL, suggesting a possible pathogenetic role of this infection (AUPERIN et al; 1994, CHANG et al. 1993; DEANGELIS et al. 1992; GEDDES et al. 1992; HAMILTON-DUTOIT et al. 1993; IRONSIDE 1992; MURPHY et al. 1990; ROUAH et al. 1990). B-cell-tropic EBV is supposed to induce polyclonal B cell proliferation with chromosomal breaks and recombinations. These transforming proprieties have been related to the latent gene-encoded proteins (LMP-1 and 2) and to the EBV-encoded nuclear antigens (EBNA 1–6) (CRAIG et al. 1993; KARP et al. 1992). EBNA-5 in particular is capable of forming a complex with normal p53 protein interfering with G_1 phase DNA repair mechanism (SZEKELY et al. 1993). Additionally, EBNA-2 increases transcription of lymphocyte proliferation antigens CD21 and CD23 (KARP et al. 1992). Lymphocyte EBV infection is associated with the translocation of the growth-promoting oncogene c-myc to the immunoglobulin locus and with the upregulation of the bcl-2 oncogene, responsible for prolongation of the cell life (HENDERSON et al. 1991; SHIRAMIZU et al. 1991). Conversely, the correlation between EBV infection and PCNSL in immunocompetent patients is less understood. DEANGELIS et al. (1992) detected the EBV genome in 7 of the 13 non-immunodeficiency-related PCNSL using a standard PCR technique with EBV-specific primers. On the other hand, KROGH-JENSEN et al. (1998) have recently shown a lack of the EBV genome in 41 non-immunodeficiency-related PCNSL, using RNA in situ hybridization.

23.3
Clinical Characteristics

PCNSL can affect immunocompetent patients with peak incidence in the sixth and seventh decade of life and it occurs in younger immunocompromised patients (DEANGELIS et al. 1987). In the group of AIDS patients, more than 90% are men, but in the group of immunocompetent patients, there is only a slight male predominance, with a 3:2 male to female ratio (So et al. 1988).

CNSL are aggressive and rapidly growing tumors. At diagnosis it is common to document dissemination within the cerebrospinal axis. Headache is a common initial symptom, often accompanied by other symptoms and signs of an intracranial mass, such as: focal cerebral deficit (47%), change in mental status (37%), increased intracranial pressure (34%), or seizures (11%) (MURRAY et al. 1986). PCNSL show a predilection for the frontal lobes and the deep periventricular structures, with common symptoms of personality changes and reduction of alertness. The presence of malignant cells in cerebrospinal fluid (CSF) is common.

Ocular lymphoma is often associated with PCNSL and 50–59% of the patients with ocular lymphoma already have or will soon develop PCNSL (WOODMAN et al. 1985). Sometimes, eye involvement is present at the time of relapse. The ocular spread of PCNSL is considered a direct tumor extension from the brain and it does not imply the presence of a systemic tumor dissemination. Ocular lymphoma may present itself as chorioretinitis, vitreitis, and non-specific uveitis with blurred vision or floaters, but it can also be clinically silent. Invasion of the optic nerve has rarely been seen. Uveitis can be unilateral or bilateral with asymmetric features. Slit-lamp examination allows one to see a cellular infiltrate of the vitreous and it is recommended to stage PCNSL. Additionally, indirect ophthalmoscopy helps to detect lesions of the choroid and retina. Definitive diagnosis can be made by vitreous biopsy or aspirate. A high risk of false negative specimens should be suspected in patients previously treated with corticosteroids (WHITCUP et al. 1993; PETERSON et al. 1993).

Meningeal involvement associated with PCNSL is found in 30% of patients at the time of diagnosis, but primary leptomeningeal involvement, without parenchymal lesions, is present in only 7% of patients (WOODMAN et al. 1985; LA CHANCE et al. 1991; SCOTT et al. 1990; HOCHBERG et al. 1988). Primary spinal cord involvement is also rare and has been reported in less than 5% of patients at the time of autopsy.

23.4
Diagnosis and Staging

The initial differential diagnosis includes cerebral metastases and other primary brain tumors, which are more common causes of increased intracranial pressure than PCNSL.

Magnetic resonance imaging (MRI) is a very important diagnostic tool for PCNSL. In 90% of patients, there is a characteristic radiographic appearance of multiple lesions usually localized deep in the brain with prominent and diffuse enhancement, blurred borders, and a mild to moderate surrounding edema (DeAngelis et al. 1990; Schwaighofer et al. 1989). A lack of ring enhancement on an imaging study tends to exclude malignant gliomas and brain metastasis. However, in AIDS patients, the MRI appearance of PCNSL is less characteristic with occasional ring enhancing lesions (due to necrosis) that are almost indistinguishable from the MRI features of toxoplasmosis (Ciricillo et al. 1990). When suspected, a positive toxoplasmosis serology study followed by a reduction in size of the lesions after specific treatment against Toxoplasma confirms presumptive diagnosis of active toxoplasmosis and rules out PCNSL.

Corticosteroid treatment can dramatically affect PCNSL. In addition to the relief of symptoms it is possible to see shrinkage of the masses, which, in rare occasions, may completely disappear. While this feature is suggestive of PCNSL it is not specific, since brain lesions of multiple sclerosis or sarcoidosis may also respond well to corticosteroid therapy. Moreover, ocular involvement of lymphoma indicated by slit-lamp examination needs to be confirmed by a vitreous biopsy prior to initiation of corticosteroid therapy. The administration of corticosteroid therapy may convert patients to false negative status.

Abdominal computerized axial tomography (CT) and chest radiography are used as part of the initial staging to rule out systemic dissemination of lymphoma and to confirm a diagnosis of PCNSL. HIV antibody titers are routinely examined in consideration of the strong association between PCNSL and AIDS.

Lumbar puncture may help to obtain the diagnosis while sparing more invasive investigative procedures. It is of importance to document presence or absence of leptomeningeal involvement. Typically, CSF may only show increased proteins (Littman et al. 1987) and/or reactive lymphocytes sometimes associated with malignant cells (Murray et al. 1986). In spite of normal cytologic appearance, a monoclonal population of lymphocytes can be easily detected by the use of immunofluorescence (Levine et al. 1991). Glucose levels are usually normal, but they can be reduced at the presence of extensive meningeal involvement. Meningeal involvement of lymphoma is also associated with elevated levels of b_2-microglobulin, lactic acid dehydrogenase and b-glucoronidase.

In the absence of CSF involvement, a diagnostic test of choice is a stereotactic biopsy. Positive pathological findings usually show a monoclonal population of diffuse large cells, consistent with diffuse large-cell lymphoma or diffuse large-cell immunoblastic lymphoma. These findings represent the vast majority of AIDS-related PCNSL, but small non-cleaved lymphomas also occur among non-AIDS-related PCNSL patients (Levine et al. 1991; Raphael et al. 1991; Gill et al. 1985). The growth pattern is typical vasocentric. In the past, this feature determined its morphologic classification as "perivascular or perithelial sarcoma". Cell proliferation starts within the wall of the blood vessels, followed by a secondary infiltration of the surrounding parenchyma. Necrotic or hemorrhagic components are not commonly seen.

Monoclonal immunoglobulin heavy or light chain production is demonstrated by immunohistochemistry to document B monoclonality (Taylor et al. 1978; Hochberg et al. 1988; Nakhleh et al. 1989). Similar to systemic B cell lymphomas, most PCNSL show p53 and bcl-2 mutations which are not important prognostic factors (Krogh-Jensen et al. 1998). No specific molecular markers have been identified as characteristic of PCNSL (Jellinger et al. 1995). Primary T cell lymphomas of the CNS are rarely observed. Recent studies, however, (Morgello et al. 1989; Marsh et al. 1983; Grant et al. 1986; Ferracini et al. 1995) demonstrated a rise in their incidence possibly related to the recent introduction of better immunohistochemical diagnostic techniques. T cell PCNSL are characterized by leptomeningeal involvement (Marsh et al. 1983; Grant et al. 1986), and a more favorable prognosis (Ferracini et al. 1995). A common diagnostic pitfall is encountered when the tissue is obtained after corticosteroid therapy, when the B cell malignant population is no longer present, leaving only the reactive T cell component (Ng et al. 1989). B- or T cell origin of lymphoma does not influence treatment options.

23.5
Prognosis and Management

The staging criteria used for systemic non-Hodgkin's lymphomas (SL) are not applicable to describe PCNSL since their natural history is different from that of SL. In fact, PCNSL are typically localized within the CNS, an extranodal organ, making them stage I_E in the clinical staging for SL. Systemic lymphomas presenting as stage I_E are highly curable with approximately 70% survival at 10 years (VOKES et al. 1985). In contrast, median survival for PCNSL following whole brain irradiation (WBI) is 12–18 months and the 5-year survival is 4%, similar to that of glioblastoma multiforme (HOCHBERG et al. 1988; LITTMAN et al. 1987; DEANGELIS 1995; HENRY et al. 1974).

In spite of their prompt response to treatment, PCNSL have a high rate of early relapse within the CNS, usually at a different site, frequently in an area included within the radiation fields. The eye and leptomeninges are favorite sites of tumor recurrence. PCNSL rarely spread systemically, but 7–8% of PCNSL patients have metastases outside of the CNS at autopsy (LITTMAN et al. 1987; DEANGELIS 1995).

The poor treatment outcome of this disease has stimulated research. The current therapeutic approach consists of a combination of multiple chemotherapeutic agents with radiotherapy. Most studies of combination treatment involved immunocompetent patients since immunocompromised patients have a lower level of tolerance to an aggressive cytotoxic treatment (KAPLAN et al. 1997).

23.6
Therapy in Immunocompetent Patients

Historically, surgical removal of PCNSL provided disappointing results, with slightly improved survival rates over those achieved by supportive care only (BURSTEIN et al. 1963; JELLINGER et al. 1975; HENRY et al. 1974). Moreover, since PCNSL are often multifocal and deep within the brain, surgical excision is accompanied by significant neurological side effects (DEANGELIS et al. 1990). As a result, the only invasive procedure currently used in this disease is stereotactic biopsy when it is required to establish a diagnosis.

Consistent with the in vivo findings of steroid receptors in mouse lymphoma cells (GAMETCHU 1987), corticosteroids continue to be used in the management of PCNSL. As already mentioned, this treatment induces a dramatic, albeit short-term tumor response. In addition, the use of corticosteroids almost always induces a subjective improvement in patients' condition regardless of the objective reduction in size of the lesion(s). In spite of anecdotal reports of cure following corticosteroid therapy (SINGH et al. 1982), the initial improvement is consistently followed by early tumor progression.

External beam radiotherapy has traditionally played a key role in the management of CNS lymphoma patients. Since PCNSL commonly present as multifocal disease, WBI has been the treatment of choice. Recommended doses of radiotherapy are from 40 to 50 Gy. Lower radiation doses are less effective in controlling the tumor (HOCHBERG et al. 1988, DEANGELIS 1995). A recent prospective study conducted by the Radiation Therapy Oncology Group (RTOG) (NELSON et al. 1992) and another study by the Memorial Sloan-Kettering Cancer Center (MSKCC) (DEANGELIS et al. 1992) suggest a lack of benefit from the addition of a radiation boost to the tumor area. In both studies, the WBI dose was 40 Gy, but the boost dose in the RTOG protocol was 20 Gy while it was 14 Gy in the MSKCC study. The same rate of recurrence occurred in the volume receiving additional radiation dose as in the other parts of the brain. Median survival with WBI is 12–18 months, and its use at the present time as the only modality is limited to immunocompromised patients with a poor performance status.

The natural history of PCNSL inevitably includes a tumor spread to the leptomeninges. Almost all patients show meningeal metastases at autopsy. Craniospinal irradiation has been followed by an improved median survival compared with those treated with WBI alone (RAMPEN et al. 1980). Currently, total spinal cord irradiation is not recommended because of its myelosuppressive effects. The use of intrathecal chemotherapy is better tolerated and of comparable effectiveness to that of radiotherapy. This was shown in a recent multivariate analysis of 50 publications between 1980–1995 regarding therapeutic management of PCNSL in 1408 immunocompetent patients (RENI et al. 1997).

Radiotherapy represents the primary treatment for ocular involvement (WHITCUP et al. 1993; ROCKWOOD et al. 1984; MARGOLIS et al. 1980). An accepted treatment consists of 35–45 Gy radiotherapy to both eyes. Common side effects of this therapy include: dry eyes, conjunctivitis, vitreous hemorrhages, and cataract formation.

Chemotherapy combinations proven successful in treating systemic lymphoma, such as cyclophosphamide, doxorubicin, vincristine, prednisone (CHOP); cyclophosphamide, doxorubicin, vincristine, dexamethasone (CHOD); and methotrexate, adriamycin, cyclophosphamide, vincristine, prednisone, and bleomycin (MACOP-B), have been tested in PCNSL, given before radiation therapy. The rationale for these studies is that the blood–brain barrier (BBB) is disrupted at the PCNSL site allowing for drug penetration. The sequencing of treatment is based on the need to assess the chemotherapy effect. The RTOG 88–06 trial tested the CHOD regimen in 54 patients accrued from 1988 to 1992. A median survival of 16 months and a 2-year survival of 42% was reported (Schultz et al. 1996). No significant survival difference was detected when outcomes of the above study were compared to those of RTOG 83–15 in which 41 patients were treated with radiation doses greater than 50 Gy, without chemotherapy. Similarly, O'Neil et al. (1995) studied CHOP in 46 patients. The authors reported a median survival of 9.5 months. Finally, Brada et al. (1990) found a median survival of 14 months among eight PCNSL treated by MACOP-B. In these early polychemotherapy studies the survival of patients treated with a combination of chemotherapy and radiotherapy was not significantly different from that of those treated with radiotherapy alone.

The use of lipophilic drugs, like procarbazide, which can penetrate the BBB or the administration of high-dose methotrexate (MTX), which can reach intracranial therapeutic levels, have shown to be more promising. In 31 patients treated with systemic MTX (1 g/m^2 delivered by an intracranial Ommaya catheter), therapeutic levels of MTX in the CSF that persisted for 48 h were demonstrated (DeAngelis et al. 1992). Noticeably, recent follow-up analysis of the original cohort of patients treated with this regimen (Abrey et al. 1998) has shown a median cause-specific survival of 42 months with an impressive 5-year survival of 22.3%. Improved survival using high-dose MTX has also been observed by Gabbai et al. (1989) who tested an MTX dose of 3.5 g/m^2 for three cycles given prior to WBI in 13 patients.

Currently, the RTOG and the South West Oncology Group (SWOG) are testing the combination of high-dose MTX (2.5 g/m^2) procarbazine, and vincristine prior to radiotherapy, versus pre-irradiation single-agent MTX. This study was designed to assess whether the combination of drugs is more effective than the treatment with a single agent.

Chamberlain et al. (1992) and Levine et al. (1991) studied the effect of administering chemotherapy after WBI. In a pilot study of 16 patients, they used procarbazine, lomustine, and vincristine (PCV) combinations and achieved a median survival of 41 months.

The patient's age is a significant prognostic factor as shown by univariate analysis conducted by the RTOG (Schultz et al. 1996) and MSKCC (Abrey et al. 1998). In the MSKCC study, age less than 50 years was correlated with longer survival (P=0.01), while age more than 60 years predicted for substantially higher risk of late treatment-related toxicity (P<0.0001). In the group of patients older than 60 years of age, 69% suffered significant late side effects, versus 6% among patients younger than 50 years of age. Neurotoxicity was the main late treatment toxicity, characterized by a progressive dementia, gate ataxia, urinary incontinence, and significant decline in Karnofsky performance score that required custodial care in a few patients (Abrey et al. 1998). These data justified the design of a subsequent study testing chemotherapy alone in 13 patients older than 60 years of age. Ten complete responses were achieved, with six patients being alive from 12 to 35 months after treatment. No severe neurological toxicity was reported in this study (Freilich et al. 1996).

Encouraging results were obtained by Strauchen et al. (1989), who treated six primary ocular lymphomas with high doses of cytarabine, achieving four partial responses and one complete response. Similarly, Valluri et al. (1995), who used MTX plus high-dose cytarabine in three patients obtained a remission in all three, which persisted at 24 months of follow-up.

23.7
Therapy in Immunocompromised Patients

Immunocompromised patients with PCNSL have a lower tolerance to aggressive treatments, and are generally less responsive to therapy than immunocompetent patients. Treatment benefits are also of a shorter duration than in immunocompetent patients. We conducted a study (Formenti et al. 1989) at the University of Southern California (USC) on ten AIDS patients affected by PCNSL to check the efficacy of WBI in this patient population. Radiation doses ranged from 22 to 50 Gy, delivered to the whole brain. The median survival was 5.5 months (range from 2 to 16 months). We found that the duration of response of AIDS-related PCNSL to radiation therapy was short. The cause of death in these patients was recurrent disease and systemic opportunistic infections. At the present time, WBI associated with corticosteroids is still the cornerstone of therapy for this patient population. A median survival of only 2–5 months was obtained (Gill et al. 1985; So et al. 1986; Baumgartner et al. 1990; Ling et al. 1994).

Intrathecal administration of MTX is indicated when a positive CSF cytology test suggests leptomeningeal involvement. Generally, in this patient population, chemotherapy is reserved to treat recurrence after radiotherapy.

Results of combining WBI with chemotherapy have been reported. At MSKCC, among ten AIDS patients treated by chemoradiation, two patients were alive at 12 months and one was alive at 5 years (FORSYTH et al. 1994). GILL et al. (1985) used WBI and chemotherapy (bleomycin, doxorubicin, cyclophosphamide, vincristine, and prednisone) in two patients: one patient was alive at 16 months and the other was alive at 28 months after treatment. This anecdotal experience suggests that there might be a subpopulation of AIDS patients, with a good performance status, who could benefit from a more aggressive therapeutic approach.

23.8
Conclusions

During the past 15 years, clinical research has produced a better understanding of primary CNS lymphomas in spite of the limited progress achieved in their cure rate. WBI therapy remains the main treatment modality, and a radiation dose of at least 40 Gy is necessary, with no advantage being derived from a boost to the original tumor area. While the addition of polychemotherapy to WBI has failed to prove superior to radiation alone, better results can be achieved by the combination of single-agent high-dose MTX before WBI, resulting in a remarkably good 5-year survival rate of 22.3%.

Subset analysis suggests that a better prognosis can be expected among immunocompetent patients under 50 years of age. The use of intrathecally administered chemotherapy instead of craniospinal irradiation has proven as effective and safer, especially when chemotherapy is planned as part of the general management.

Experience in immunocompromised patients has discouraged the generalized use of aggressive treatment, but some anecdotal reports in selected cases with a good performance status support the use of chemoradiation combinations. For the majority of immunocompromised patients, WBI and steroids remain the treatment of choice.

In view of the noticeable increase in incidence of this disease and of the fact that it remains generally incurable, all patients should be strongly encouraged to enter clinical trials.

References

Abrey LE, DeAngelis LM, Yahalom J (1998) Long-term survival in primary CNS lymphoma. J Clin Oncol 16:3, 859–863

Auperin I, Mikol TJ, Oksenhendler E, Thiebaut JB, Brunet M, Dupont B, Morinet F (1994) Primary central nervous system malignant non-Hodgkin's lymphomas from HIV-infected and non-infected patients: expression of cellular surface proteins and Epstein-Barr viral markers. Neuropathol Appl Neurobiol 20:3, 243–252

Baumgartner JE, Rachlin JR, Beckstead JH, Meeker TC, Levy RM, Wara WM, Rosenblum ML. (1990) Primary central nervous system lymphomas: natural history and response to radiation therapy in 55 patients with acquired immunodeficiency syndrome. J Neurosurg 73:2, 206–211

Brada M, Dearnaley D, Horwich A, Bloom HJ (1990) Management of primary cerebral lymphoma with initial chemotherapy: preliminary results and comparison with patients treated with radiotherapy alone. Int J Rad Oncol Biol Phys 18:4, 787–792

Burstein SD, Kernohan JW, Uihlein A (1963) Neoplasms of the reticuloendothelial system of the brain. Cancer 289:16

Camilleri-Broet S, Martin A, Moreau A, Angonin R, Henin D, Gontier MF, Rousselet MC, Caulet Maugendre S, Cuilliere P, Lefrancq T, Mokhtari K, Morcos M, Broet P, Kujas M, Hauw JJ, Desablens B, Raphael M (1998) Primary central nervous system lymphomas in 72 immunocompetent patients: pathologic findings and clinical correlations. Am J Clin Pathol 110:5, 607–612

Chamberlain MC, Levin VA (1992) Primary central nervous system lymphoma: a role for adjuvant chemotherapy. J Neurooncol 14:3, 271–275

Chang KL, Flaris N, Hickey WF, Johnson RM, Meyer JS, Weiss LM (1993) Brain lymphomas of immunocompetent and immunocompromised patients: study of the association with Epstein-Barr virus. Mod Pathol 6:4, 427–432

Ciricillo SF, Rosenblum ML (1990) Use of CT and MR imaging to distinguish intracranial lesions and to define the need for biopsy in AIDS patients. J Neurosurg 73:5, 720–724

Craig FE, Gulley ML, Banks PM (1993) Posttransplantation lymphoproliferative disorders. Am J Clin Pathol 99:3, 265–276

DeAngelis LM (1995) Current management of primary central nervous system lymphoma. Oncology 9:1, 63–71

DeAngelis LM, Wong E, Rosenblum M, Furnaux H (1992) Epstein-Barr virus in acquired immune deficiency syndrome (AIDS) and non-AIDS primary central nervous system lymphoma. Cancer 70:6, 1607–1611

DeAngelis LM, Yahalom J, Heinemann MH, Cirrincione C, Thaler HT, Krol G (1990) Primary CNS lymphoma: combined treatment with chemotherapy and radiotherapy. Neurology 40:1, 80–86

DeAngelis LM, Yahalom J, Rosenblum M, Posner JB (1987) Primary CNS lymphoma: managing patients with spontaneous and AIDS related-disease. Oncology 1:6, 52–62

DeAngelis LM, Yahalom J, Thaler HT, Kher U (1992) Combined modality treatment for primary CNS lymphoma. J Clin Oncol 10:4, 635–643

Eby NL, Grufferman S, Flannelly CM, Schold SC Jr, Vogel FS, Burger PC (1988) Increasing incidence of primary brain lymphoma in the US. Cancer 62:11, 2461–2465

Edgar R, Dutcher TF (1961) Histopathology of the Bing-Neel syndrome. Neurology 11: 239–245

Ferracini R, Bergmann M, Pileri S, Rigobello L, Azzolini U, Manetto V, Poggi S, Sabattini E, Frank G, Spagnolli F (1995) Primary T-cell lymphoma of the central nervous system. Clin Neuropathol 14:3, 125–129

Formenti SC, Gill PS, Lean E, Rarick M, Meyer PR, Boswell W, Petrovich Z, Chak L, Levine AM (1989) Primary central nervous system lymphoma in AIDS. Results of radiation therapy. Cancer 63:6, 1101–1107

Forsyth PA, Yahalom J, DeAngelis LM (1994) Combined-modality therapy in the treatment of primary central nervous system lymphoma in AIDS. Neurology 44:8, 1473–1479

Freilich RJ, Delattre JY, Monjour A, DeAngelis LM (1996) Chemotherapy without radiation therapy as initial treatment for primary CNS lymphoma in older patients. Neurology 46:2, 435–439

Gabbai AA, Hochberg FH, Linggood RM, Bashir R, Hotleman K (1989) High-dose methotrexate for non-AIDS primary central nervous system lymphoma. Report of 13 cases. J Neurosurg 70:2, 190–194

Gametchu B (1987) Glucocorticoid receptor-like antigen in lymphoma cell membranes: correlation to cell lysis. Science 236:4800, 456–461

Geddes JF, Bhattacharjee MB, Savage K, Scaravilli F, McLaughlin JE (1992) Primary cerebral lymphoma: a study of 47 cases probed for Epstein-Barr virus genome. J Clin Pathol 45:7, 587–590

Gill PS, Levine AM, Meyer PR, Boswell WD, Burkes R, Parker JW, Hofman FM, Dworsky RL, Lukes RJ (1985) Primary central nervous system lymphoma in homosexual men. Clinical, immunologic and pathologic features. Am J Med 78:5, 742–748

Grant JW, Gallagher PJ, Jones DB (1986) Primary cerebral lymphoma. A histologic and immunohistochemical study of six cases. Arch Pathol Lab Med 110:10, 897–901

Greig NH, Ries LG, Yancik R, Rapoport SI (1990) Increasing annual incidence of primary malignant brain tumors in the elderly. J Natl Cancer Inst 82:20, 1621–1624

Guinan ME, Hardy A (1981 through 1986) Epidemiology of AIDS in women in the United States. JAMA 257: 2039–2042

Gunderson CH, Menry J, Malamud N (1971) Plasma globulin determinations in patients with microglioma. Report of five cases. J Neurosurg 35:4, 406–415

Hamilton-Dutoit SJ, Raphael M, Audouin J, Diebold J, Lisse I, Pedersen C, Oksenhendler E, Marelle L, Pallesen G (1993) In situ demonstration of Epstein-Barr virus small RNAs (EBER 1) in acquired immunodeficiency syndrome-related lymphomas: correlation with tumor morphology and primary site. Blood 82:2, 619–624

Henderson S, Rowe M, Gregory C, Croom Carter D, Wang F, Longnecker R, Kieff E, Rickinson A (1991) Induction of bcl-2 expression by Epstein-Barr virus latent membrane protein 1 protects infected B cells from programmed cell death. Cell 65:7, 1107–1115

Henry JM, Heffner RR Jr, Dillard SH, Earle KM, Davis RL (1974) Primary malignant lymphomas of the central nervous system. Cancer 34:4, 1293–1302

Hochberg FH, Miller DC (1988) Primary central nervous system lymphoma. J Neurosurg 68:6, 835–853

Hoover R, Fraumeni Jr JF. (1973) Risk of cancer in renal-transplant recipients. Lancet 2: 7820, 55–57

Ironside JW (1992) Epstein-Barr virus gene expression in CNS lymphomas. Clin Neuropathol 11:210 (abstr)

Jellinger K, Radaskiewicz TH, Slowik F (1975) Primary malignant lymphomas of the central nervous system in man. Acta Neuropathol (Berlin) Suppl 6: 95–102

Jellinger KA, Paulus W (1995) Primary central nervous system lymphomas: new pathological developments. J Neurooncol 24:1, 33–36

Kaplan LD, Straus DJ, Testa MA, Von Roenn J, Dezube BJ, Cooley TP, Herndier B, Northfelt DW, Huang J, Tulpule A, Levine AM (1997) Low-dose compared with standard-dose m-BACOD chemotherapy for non-Hodgkin's lymphoma associated with human immunodeficiency virus infection. National Institute of Allergy and Infectious Diseases AIDS Clinical Trials Group N Eng J Med. 336:23, 1641–1648

Karp JE, Broder S (1992) The pathogenesis of AIDS lymphoma: a foundation for addressing the challenges of therapy and prevention. Leuk Lymphoma 8:3, 167–188

Krogh-Jensen M, Johansen P, D'Amore F (1998) Primary central nervous lymphomas in immunocompetent individuals: histology, Epstein-Barr virus genome, Ki-67 proliferation index, p53 and bcl-2 gene expression. Leuk and Lymphoma 30:1–2, 131–142

Lachance DH, O'Neill BP, Macdonald DR, Jaeckle KA, Witzig TE, Li CY, Posner JB (1991) Primary leptomeningeal lymphoma: report of 9 cases, diagnosis with immunocytochemical analysis and review of the literature. Neurology 41:1, 95–100

Levine AM, Sullivan-Halley J, Pike MC, Rarick MU, Loureiro C, Bernstein-Singer M, Willson E, Brynes R, Parker J, Rasheed S, et al. (1991) Human immunodeficiency virus-related lymphom. Prognostic factors predictive of survival. Cancer 68:11, 2466–2472

Ling SM, Roach M 3rd, Larson DA, Wara WM (1994) Radiotherapy of primary central nervous system lymphoma in patients with and without human immunodeficiency virus. Ten years of treatment experience at the University of California San Francisco. Cancer 73:10, 2570–2582

Littman P, Wang CC (1975) Reticulum cell sarcoma of the brain. A review of the literature and a study of 19 cases. Cancer 35:5, 1412–1420

Margolis L, Fraser R, Lichter A, Char DH (1980) The role of radiation therapy in the management of ocular reticulum cell sarcoma. Cancer 45:4, 688–692

Marsh WL Jr, Stevenson DR, Long HJ (1983) Primary leptomeningeal presentation of T-cell lymphoma. Report of a patient and review of the literature. Cancer 51:6, 1125–1131

Morgello S, Maiese K, Petito CK (1989) T-cell lymphoma in the CNS: clinical and pathologic features. Neurology 39:9, 1190–1196

Murphy JK, Young LS, Bevan IS, Lewis FA, Dockey D, Ironside JW, OBrien CJ, Wells M (1990) Demonstration of Epstein-Barr virus in primary brain lymphoma by in situ DNA hybridisation in paraffin wax embedded tissue. J Clin Pathol 43:3, 220–223

Murray K, Kun L, Cox J (1986) Primary malignant lymphomas of the central nervous system. J Neurosurg 65:600–607

Nakhleh RE, Manivel JC, Hurd D, Sung JH (1989) Central nervous system lymphomas. Immunohistochemical and clinicopathologic study of 26 autopsy cases. Arch Pathol Lab Med 113:9, 1050–1056

Nelson DF, Martz KL, Bonner H, Nelson JS, Newall J, Kerman HD, Thomson JW, Murray KJ (1992) Non-Hodgkin's lymphoma of the brain: can high dose, large volume radiation therapy improve survival? Report on a perspective trial by the Radiation Therapy Oncology Group (RTOG): RTOG 83 15. Int J Rad Oncol Biol Phys 23:1, 9–17

Ng CS, Chan JK, Hui PK, Lau WH (1989) Large B-cell lymphomas with a high content of reactive T-cells. Hum Pathol 20:12, 1145–1154

O'Neill BP, O'Fallon JR, Earle JD, Colgan JP, Brown LD, Krigel RL (1995) Primary central nervous system non-Hodgkin's lymphoma: survival advantages with combined initial therapy? Int J Rad Oncol Biol Phys 33:3, 663–673

Peterson K, Gordon KB, Heinemann MH, DeAngelis LM (1993) The clinical spectrum of ocular lymphoma. Cancer 72:3, 843–849

Rampen FH, van Andel JG, Sizoo W, van Unnik JA (1980) Radiation therapy in primary non-Hodgkin's lymphomas of the CNS. Eur J Cancer 16:2, 177–184

Raphael M, Gentilhomme O, Tulliez M, Byron PA, Diebold J (1991) Histopathologic features of high-grade non-Hodgkin's lymphomas in acquired immunodeficiency syndrome. The French Study Group of Pathology for Human Immunodeficiency Virus-Associated Tumors. Arch Pathol Lab Med 115:1, 15–20

Reni M, Ferreri AJ, Garancini MP, Villa E (1997) Therapeutic management of primary central nervous system lymphoma in immunocompetent patients: results of a critical review of the literature. Ann Oncol 8:3, 227–234

Rockwood EJ, Zakov ZN, Bay JW (1984) Combined malignant lymphoma of the eye and CNS (reticulum-cell sarcoma). Report of three cases. J Neurosurg 61:2, 369–374

Rosenblum ML, Levy RM, Bredesen DE, So YT, Wara W, Ziegler JL (1988) Primary central nervous system lymphomas in patients with AIDS. Ann Neurol Suppl 23: S13–16

Rouah E, Rogers BB, Wilson DR, Kirkpatrick JB, Buffone GJ (1990) Demonstration of Epstein-Barr virus in primary central nervous system lymphomas by the polymerase chain reaction and in situ hybridization. Hum Pathol 21:5, 545–550

Rubinsten LJ (1972) Tumors of the cerebral nervous system: atlas of tumor pathology; second series, Fascicle 6. Washington, DC: Armed Forces Institute of Pathology 215

Schneck SA, Penn I (1971) De-novo brain tumors in renal-transplant recipients. Lancet 1:7707, 983–986

Schultz C, Scott C, Sherman W, Donahue B, Fields J, Murray K, Fisher B, Abrams R, Meis Kindblom J (1996) Preirradiation chemotherapy with cyclophosphamide, doxorubicin, vincristine, and dexamethasone for primary CNS lymphomas: initial report of radiation therapy oncology group protocol 88–06. J Clin Oncol 14:2, 556–564

Schwaighofer BW, Hesselink JR, Press GA, Wolf RL, Healy ME, Berthoty DP (1989) Primary intracranial CNS lymphoma: MR manifestations. Am J Neuroradiol 10:4, 725–729

Scott TF, Hogan EL, Carter TD, Garen PD, Brillman J, Kurent JE (1990) Primary intracranial meningeal lymphoma. Am J Med 89:4, 536–538

Shiramizu B, Barriga F, Neequaye J, Jafri A, Dalla Favera R, Neri A, Guttierez M, Levine P, Magrath I (1991) Patterns of chromosomal breakpoint locations in Burkitt's lymphoma: relevance to geography and Epstein-Barr virus association. Blood 77:7, 1516–1526

Singh A, Strobos RJ, Singh BM, Rothballer AB, Reddy V, Puljic S, Poon TP (1982) Steroid-induced remissions in CNS lymphoma. Neurology 32:11, 1267–1271

Snider WD, Simpson DM, Aronyk KE, Nielsen SL (1983) Primary lymphoma of the nervous system associated with acquired immune-deficiency syndrome. [letter]N Engl J Med 308:1, 45

So YT, Beckstead JH, Davis RL (1986) Primary central nervous system lymphoma in acquired immune deficiency syndrome: a clinical and pathological study. Ann Neurol 20:5, 566–572

So YT, Choucair A, Davis RL, et al. (1988) Neoplasm of the central nervous system in acquired immunodeficiency syndrome. In: Rosenblum ML, Levy RM, Bredesen DE, (ed) AIDS and the Nervous System. Raven Press, New York 285

Strauchen JA, Dalton J, Friedman AH (1989) Chemotherapy in the management of intraocular lymphoma. Cancer 63:10, 1918–1921

Swinnen LJ, Costanzo-Nordin MR, Fisher SG, O'Sullivan EJ, Johnson MR, Heroux AL, Dizikes GJ, Pifarre R, Fisher RI (1990) Increased incidence of lymphoproliferative disorder after immunosuppression with the monoclonal antibody OKT3 in cardiac transplant recipients. N Engl J Med 323:25, 1723–1728

Szekely L, Selivanova G, Magnusson KP, Klein G, Wiman KG (1993) EBNA-5, an Epstein-Barr virus-encoded nuclear antigen, binds to the retinoblastoma and p53 proteins. Proc Natl Acad Sci USA 90:12, 5455–5459

Taylor CR, Russell R, Lukes RJ, Davis RL (1978) An immunohistological study of immunoglobulin content of primary central nervous system lymphomas. Cancer 41:6, 2197–2205

Valluri S, Moorthy RS, Khan A, Rao NA (1995) Combination treatment of intraocular lymphoma. Retina 15:2, 125–129

Vaquero J, Martinez R, Rossi E, Lopez R (1984) Primary cerebral lymphoma: the "ghost tumor". Case report. J Neurosurg 60:1, 174–176

Vokes EE, Ultmann JE, Golomb HM, Gaynor ER, Ferguson DJ, Griem ML, Oleske D (1985) Long-term survival of patients with localized diffuse histiocytic lymphoma. J Clin Oncol 3:10, 1309–1317

Welch K, Finkbeiner W, Alpers CE, Blumenfeld W, Davis RL, Smuckler EA, Beckstead JH (1984) Autopsy findings in the acquired immune deficiency syndrome. JAMA 252:9, 1152–1159

Whitcup SM, de Smet MD, Rubin BI, Palestine AG, Martin DF, Burnier M Jr, Chan CC, Nussenblatt RB (1993) Intraocular lymphoma. Clinical and histopathologic diagnosis. Ophthalmology 100:9, 1399–1406

Woodman R, Shin K, Pineo G (1985) Primary non-Hodgkin's lymphoma of the brain. A review. Medicine 64:6, 425–430

Ziegler JL, Drew WL, Miner RC, Mintz L, Rosenbaum E, Gershow J, Lennette ET, Greenspan J, Shillitoe E, Beckstead J, Casavant C, Yamamoto K (1982) Burkitt's-like lymphoma in homosexual men. Lancet 2:8299, 631–633

Zimmerman HM (1975) Malignant lymphomas of the nervous system. Acta Neuropathol Suppl (Berlin) Suppl 6: 69–74

24 Chemotherapy in Adult CNS Tumors

Steven O'Day and Barbara Dykes

CONTENTS

tion/growth factors, mechanisms of glial cell invasion, angiogenesis), (2) mechanisms of tumor cell resistance, and (3) novel delivery systems. In addition to novel therapeutics, a more rigorous paradigm of clinical research has evolved with multidisciplinary participation. The more rigorous design of current and future clinical trials with clinically meaningful end points that account for cytostatic as well as cytotoxic drug properties are major accomplishments. In addition, an appreciation of the importance of brain tumor histologic subtypes and important prognostic variables will allow for more efficient and reliable testing of these new agents. In summary, scientific progress, improved clinical trial design, and novel therapeutics will give the neuro-oncologist of the twenty-first century an armamentarium of therapeutics that will complement the advances in surgery and radiation therapy in the pursuit of improving quality of life and survival of patients with CNS tumors.

24.1 Introduction

Historically, chemotherapy has played a limited role in the multidisciplinary treatment of adult patients with CNS tumors. However, as we begin the twenty-first century, a number of new cytotoxic and cytostatic drugs have entered the clinical arena. These drugs are the direct result of scientific research which has led to a better understanding of: (1) the molecular biology of CNS tumors (signal transduc-

S. O'Day, MD
Associate Director, Medical Oncology, John Wayne Cancer Institute at Saint John's Hospital, 2001 Santa Monica Boulevard, Suite 560W, Santa Monica, CA 90404, USA
B. Dykes
Research Associate, Division Medical Oncology, John Wayne Cancer Institute at Saint John's Hospital, 2001 Santa Monica Boulevard, Suite 560W, Santa Monica, CA 90404, USA

24.2 Malignant Gliomas

Neoplasms of glial origin are the most common primary CNS tumors presenting in adults, and malignant gliomas [glioblastoma multiforme (GBM) and anaplastic astrocytoma (AA)] are high grade, relatively chemoresistant to historical cytotoxic agents, and rapidly fatal. Median survival is approximately 10 months for patients with GBM and 2–3 years for AA (Pech et al. 1998; Burton and Prados 1999; Cokgor et al. 1999). Standard treatment at initial presentation is surgery, in efforts to maximally debulk the tumor, followed by focal, radiation therapy extending the margins of the surgery. Depending on the location of the tumor, stereotactic or interstitial brachytherapy has been added in attempts to improve locoregional control. Historically, patients with malignant gliomas have been treated with single-agent nitrosoureas (BCNU, CCNU), procarbazine, or nitrosourea-based combination chemotherapy regimens (PCV: procarbazine, CCNU, vincristine). Chemotherapy has been used in conjunction with surgery and radiation in the adjuvant or relapsed setting (COKGOR et al. 1999). Malignant glioma chemotherapy trials have suffered from small patient numbers and important clinical trial design deficiencies, non-rigorous pathologic review, and inconsistent criteria for reporting of response (FINE 1994). These inconsistencies have made it difficult to reach secure conclusions regarding efficacy of nitrosourea-based chemotherapy, although most neuro-oncologists accept a modest improvement in survival. More recently, a better understanding of subgroups of malignant glioma patients have been identified that potentially benefit from chemotherapy [young age, good performance status, anaplastic astrocytoma subgroup, maximal tumor debulking, early treatment (vs relapse)] and current clinical trials are now stratifying for these important variables (FINE 1994; EAGAN and SCOTT 1983; WONG et al. 1999). The major clinical challenge for the vast majority of malignant gliomas patients are microscopic metastases which exist well beyond the primary radiographic lesion resulting in locoregional and distant failure within the brain. This ultimately foils the best attempts at locoregional control with surgery and radiation. More effective systemic therapies that penetrate the entire CNS axis eradicating or preventing growth of tumor cells and preferentially sparing normal brain tissue are crucial for impacting the survival of patients with these aggressive tumors.

24.3
Oligodendrogliomas

Oligodendrogliomas (OD) and mixed gliomas (oligoastrocytomas) account for 5–15% of glial tumors, and are a fascinating subtype currently undergoing intensive research. These tumors are thought to arise from a precursor cell committed to oligodendroglial differentiation, and range from low- to high-grade histologies (anaplastic) with median survival of more than 10 years and 2–5 years, respectively. In the last decade, the majority of oligodendrogliomas have been noted to be remarkably chemosensitive. This is particularly true for anaplastic tumors, but a subgroup of low-grade tumors also appear to be chemosensitive (SHAW et al. 1992; PECH et al. 1998). This offers treatment alternatives to surgery and radiation therapy for recurrent low-grade tumors that

are symptomatic. In addition, a better appreciation for this histology as a component in mixed malignant glioma tumors (glioblastoma multiforme, anaplastic astrocytoma) may predict those patients most likely to benefit from adjuvant chemotherapy. More rigorous pathologic identification and standardization of oligodendroglioma histology, and the development of lineage specific markers is ongoing and will effect treatment strategies and the design of clinical trials for these patients in the near future. The allelic loss of chromosomes 1p and 19q are a molecular signature of these tumors and comprises 50–70% of anaplastic oligodendrogliomas (AOD) (REIFENBERGER et al. 1994). A recent study by CAIRNCROSS et al. (1998) demonstrated that 100% of AODs with chromosome 1p and 19q deletions were chemo-sensitive compared to only 25% of AODs with retained alleles. Survival at 5 years was 95% versus 25% in the two groups. The results of this study are provocative and need confirmation in a larger prospective study. A randomized trial of patients with AOD comparing postoperative irradiation with or without PCV is ongoing. All tumors will have chromosomal analysis prospectively in this trial. In the next decade, the treatment paradigm for patients with OD and mixed gliomas may change with more definitive identification of this subtype by molecular and lineage specific markers with minimally invasive surgery. This would allow up-front intensive induction combination chemotherapy for appropriate candidates and delay more aggressive surgery and postoperative radiation to those patients who relapse. This strategy would minimize long-term morbidity for a subgroup of patients that are expected to have excellent long-term survival.

24.4
Low-Grade Glial Tumors

Low-grade glial tumors without oligodendroglioma features are more common in young adults or children and traditionally present with seizures. Treatment consists of surgery with or without radiation therapy depending on the location of the tumors. These tumors have not been responsive to conventional chemotherapy; however, as the molecular biology of gliomas becomes better defined, even low-grade gliomas might respond to novel cytostatic or molecular-driven treatment strategies. This would be particularly important for recurrent tumors that are not amenable to further surgery or radiation therapy.

24.5
CNS Germ Cell Tumors

There is a rarer group of primary CNS tumors in adults that are markedly chemosensitive: (1) primary CNS lymphoma, (2) adult medulloblastoma (<1%), and (3) primary germ cell tumors of the CNS. CNS lymphoma and medulloblastoma (chemotherapy for pediatric tumors) are discussed in Chaps. 23 and 29 of this volume, respectively (HUBBARD et al. 1989).

Primary germ cell tumors of the CNS are infrequent and are categorized as germinomas or non-germinomas, similar to systemic germ cell tumors. Germinomas are exquisitely sensitive to radiation, while non-germinomas are less radiosensitive, similar to their systemic counterpart. Primary CNS germ cell tumors frequently seed the leptomeninges. Wide-local radiotherapy with or without spinal irradiation has been a standard treatment approach (PECH et al. 1998; KIDA et al. 1986; ALLEN 1991). Due to long-term sequelae of radiation therapy in these patients, combination chemotherapy, similar to treatment for testicular germ cell tumors (platinum compounds, bleomycin, and etoposide), is now being used for primary CNS germ cell tumors with excellent results (ALLEN et al. 1985; PATEL et al. 1992). Future treatment strategies for these tumors will be to diagnose patients with minimally invasive surgery and then use intensive induction chemotherapy with or without radiotherapy. High-dose chemotherapy with stem cell rescue has been evaluated with curative intent in efforts to overcome tumor resistance (PECH et al. 1998).

24.6
Historical Chemotherapy

24.6.1
Nitrosoureas and Combination Nitrosourea-Based Chemotherapy

In the late 1970s and early 1980s, postoperative irradiation was established as standard therapy for patients with high-grade gliomas (FINE 1994; WALKER et al. 1978; KRISTIANSEN et al. 1981). Inevitably, patients recurred and a variety of chemotherapy agents were tested in small clinical trials. Nitrosoureas (BCNU, CCNU) and procarbazine became the most commonly used drugs with response rates of 10–40% (BURTON and PRADOS 1999). In addition, cisplatin, carboplatin, cyclophosphamide, and vincristine were tested with modest activity (STEWART et al. 1983; GRUNBERG et al. 1987; LONGEE et al. 1990; LEVIN and PRADOS 1992). Unfortunately, single-agent or combination chemotherapy responses were of short duration (several months) in the relapsed setting and there was no significant impact on survival (COKGOR et al. 1999).

BCNU became the most commonly used single-agent chemotherapy for recurrent disease and was moved to the adjuvant setting after a randomized trial (BTSG 69–01) demonstrated BCNU and radiotherapy superior to radiotherapy alone. Similar results were obtained in studies using CCNU (BURTON and PRADOS 1999). In the 1980s, combination PCV (procarbazine) was developed and showed promise as a multidrug regimen. In 1990, LEVIN et al. (1990) published the results of a randomized trial comparing BCNU to PCV as post-radiation (whole-brain) treatment for patients with anaplastic gliomas, which was completed in 1983 (NCOG 6G61 Final Report). The survival advantage of PCV was restricted to patients with AA (157–82 weeks). However, the results of this study remain debatable. A recent retrospective analysis using the RTOG database was preformed by PRADOS et al. (1996), which included patients with newly diagnosed AA, treated with protocols including BCNU or PCV chemotherapy. The authors found no survival benefit of PCV chemotherapy. In addition, recent preliminary data from a large phase III Medical Research Council (MRC) trial in the UK have not demonstrated to date a survival advantage of PCV to radiation in either AA or GBM. Final analysis awaits longer follow-up (FINE et al. 1993).

A large meta-analysis of adjuvant chemotherapy for malignant gliomas was published by FINE et al. (1993). This study combined the results of 16 randomized adjuvant clinical trials involving more than 3000 patients over the past 15 years. The trials included single-agent nitrosoureas and only one trial included procarbazine, none with the PCV combination. The addition of chemotherapy to radiation improved 1-year survival by 10% and 2-year survival by 8.6%, with relative survival increases of 23% and 52% at 1 and 2 years, respectively. The survival benefit of chemotherapy appeared earlier in the AA patients. Since these absolute benefits were not impressive, it is understandable that smaller clinical trials would not have the statistical power to detect possible benefit.

24.6.2
Clinical Trial Design

It is difficult to evaluate the data from historical clinical trials for primary brain tumors due to deficiencies in clinical trial design. Three main factors have contributed to the lack of conclusive clinical data for the treatment of primary adult brain tumors: (1) small patient numbers, (2) heterogeneity of study patients, and (3) lack of uniform reporting criteria (FINE 1994). The first of these factors is a dearth of patient numbers on individual clinical trials. One explanation behind this is a lack of multi-institutional trials that ordinarily serve to overcome the problem of a small patient population. Primary brain tumor patients generally receive care from a variety of subspecialists, and in the past there has been a lack of coordinated clinical research programs. In addition, many physicians are reluctant to refer patients to clinical trials due to financial concerns and a low expectation that the patients will benefit from novel therapies. This reflects a national crisis in clinical cancer trial accrual.

Heterogeneity of patient populations comprising past studies is a critical factor that has made interpretation of historical data difficult. The generally accepted key prognostic factors in malignant brain tumors are: (1) tumor histology, (2) age, and (3) performance status. Data from several historical trials underscore the importance of histology as a prognostic factor. A review of data from the RTOG 7401 and ECOG 1374 trials suggested a much longer survival time for AA (36.2 months) than for GBM (8.6 months) (NELSON et al. 1983, 1985). A retrospective review of BTCG trials 7501, 7702, and 8001 showed the 2-year survival rate for AA patients to be 47%, compared to 10% for GBM patients (BURGER et al. 1985; SHELINE 1990). Unfortunately, many early trials did not stratify patient populations according to histology. In the cases where populations were divided according to pathology, the data are debatable due to the variability between the grading schemes used by neuropathologists as well as inter-observer variability. Among important prognostic factors, age has frequently been ignored in many previous clinical trials. Results of a phase III trial performed by the North Central Cancer Treatment Group suggest that age may in fact be even a more important factor than histology in predicting survival. The trial compared the effects of post-radiation BCNU vs PCNU. In the 40–59 years age group, regardless of treatment, histology was the chief survival predictor. AA patients lived significantly longer than GBM pa-

tients. However, in the 60 years-and-over age group, regardless of treatment, there was little difference in the survival time of AA and GBM patients (36 weeks vs 27 weeks) (DINAPOLI et al. 1993). Analysis of a BTCG as well as a RTOG/ECOG study confirms the improvement of survival in patients with superior performance status.

Lack of uniform response criteria is the third important factor contributing to the difficult nature of interpreting data from previous malignant brain tumor clinical trials. The variability in definition of response has been troubling in review of publications. MACDONALD et al. (1990) have suggested that radiographic response criteria similar to those used by medical oncologists in systemic tumors should be among the standard response criteria for evaluating malignant brain tumor treatments. Ultimately, clinical end points of progression-free survival, quality of life, and overall survival in more homogeneous patient populations will likely replace radiographic response as the critical end point. This will be especially true in testing the efficacy of novel cytostatic agents.

In summary, historical chemotherapy for recurrent malignant gliomas has not impacted survival. Its role in adjuvant therapy remains controversial, although a consensus has emerged that a modest survival advantage is likely. The superiority of PCV to BCNU, however, has not been clearly demonstrated and whether either of these regimens will be used in the control arm of future phase III trials is being hotly debated (PRADOS et al. 1999). More importantly, over the last two decades, a body of data has emerged demonstrating important prognostic factors (age, histology, performance status, and extent of surgery) that impact survival in patients with newly diagnosed malignant gliomas. Future phase II trials need to be interpreted with these factors in mind, and phase III trials will need to stratify up front for these factors.

24.7
Chemotherapy Resistance Modifiers

24.7.1
O⁶-BG

Although the nitrosoureas have shown significant activity in newly diagnosed gliomas, their effect against recurrent gliomas is minimal due to drug resistance acquired over the course of previous chemotherapy treatments. This is one of the single most important factors contributing to tumor progression and patient death due to malignant gliomas (DOLAN and PEGG 1997). Resistance to the methylating action of the drugs occurs via the activity of a cellular protein, O^6-alkylguanine-DNA alkyltransferase (AGT), which transfers the methyl group to a non-lethal position on the DNA. The drug O^6-benzylguanine (O^6-BG) combats the AGT resistance mechanism by inhibiting the DNA repair protein, thereby sensitizing the tumor cell to nitrosourea activity (FRIEDMAN et al. 1998). In a recently reported study, O^6-BG demonstrated promise for improving the therapeutic effect of nitrosoureas (specifically BCNU) (BELANICH et al. 1996). This study of 226 GBM and AA patients revealed low AGT levels directly correlated with a better response to BCNU treatment, and conversely, a high AGT level correlated with a poor response rate (BELANICH et al. 1996). Although the study population was small, similar results were obtained in a BCNU/O^6-BG study performed by the Southwest Oncology Group (SWOG). The 1998 study suggested that AGT level in the tumor cells be used as an independent prognostic factor (JAECKLE et al. 1998). FRIEDMAN et. al. (1998) performed an analysis of the response to temozolomide and correlation with AGT levels. As expected, responses to temozolomide correlated with tumor cells exhibiting low AGT levels. Few responses occurred in patients with high AGT expression. These data suggest that O^6-BG can induce improved chemo-sensitivity to alkylator therapy. A phase I trial conducted by FRIEDMAN et al. (1998) determined that 100 mg/m^2 of O^6-BG given before surgery reduced AGT activity to less than 10 fmol/mg protein for at least 18 h after drug administration. However, in conjunction with chemosensitization of tumor cells, toxicity resulted from the concurrent drug sensitization of hematopoietic stem cells as well as systemic organ cells which have a high AGT concentration. Reduction of alkylator doses may be necessary to reduce toxicity in future trials. Another possible means of circumventing this problem may be gene therapy with AGT mutant proteins, which are resistant to O^6-BG action and are found to occur naturally in a small number of cells. AGT mutant gene therapy in hematopoietic stem cells would have the dual beneficial effect of reducing nitrosourea toxicity during treatment, as well as decreasing the potential for the development of drug-related leukemias following treatment (DOLAN and PEGG 1997).

24.7.2
High-Dose Tamoxifen

Recent studies have demonstrated an important role of excessive activation of protein kinase C (PKC)-mediated signal transduction pathways in the proliferation of malignant gliomas (POLLACK et al. 1990a; COULDWELL et al. 1990, 1991). High-dose tamoxifen is a nonselective inhibitor of PKC (O'BRIAN et al. 1985) and has been studied in a series of phase I and II clinical trials of recurrent gliomas. Modest response rates and stabilization of disease (25–35%) have been reported with acceptable toxicity and safety in heavily chemotherapy-pretreated patients (VERTOSICK et al. 1992; BALTUCH et al. 1993; COULDWELL et al. 1996; BRANDES et al. 1999; CHAMBERLAIN and KORMANIK 1999). Plasma levels of 5–10 µmol/l have been achieved with 160–240 mg tamoxifen/day, which correlates with in vitro efficacy models (POLLACK et al. 1990b). High-dose tamoxifen has been shown to have two additional properties that may be useful clinically: (1) synergy with platinum chemotherapy compounds (MCCLAY et al. 1993) and (2) reversal of p-glycoprotein dependent drug efflux [multidrug resistance (MDR)] (STUART et al. 1992; TRUMP et al. 1992; FINE et al. 1990). MDR is an important mechanism of tumor cell resistance to several classes of chemotherapy drugs which have shown activity in gliomas including: (1) vinca alkaloids, (2) taxanes, and (3) etoposide (VP-16). Building on the independent and potential synergistic properties with chemotherapy, high-dose tamoxifen deserves further study in combination regimens for malignant gliomas.

24.8
New Cytotoxic Drugs

Historical cytotoxic chemotherapy (nitrosoureas predominately) has had minimal activity in malignant gliomas due to de novo and acquired resistance. Attempts at reversing drug resistance in vivo have been disappointing to date, although they continue to be an active area of translational research.

In the last several years a host of new cytotoxic chemotherapy drugs have been FDA (Food and Drug Administration) approved with novel mechanisms of action for a variety of systemic tumors. These drugs include temozolomide, CPT-11, Topotecan, Oxaliplatin, and the Taxanes, and are being intensively evaluated in malignant gliomas. These new generations of clinical trials are being performed with better clinical design, rigorous pathologic evaluation, and more standardized clinical end points of progression-free and overall survival.

24.8.1
Temozolomide

Temozolomide has recently received FDA approval for the treatment of adults with recurrent anaplastic astrocytoma following therapy with nitrosourea and procarbazine, and it also shows promising results for the treatment of other primary malignant gliomas. The drug is an oral agent which crosses the blood–brain barrier. It is an imidazotetrazine derivative of dacarbazine which spontaneously hydrolyses to its biologically active form, MTIC (5-(3-methyl-1-triazeno) imidazole-4-carb-oxamide). The mechanism of antitumor action is the disruption of DNA replication via methylation of DNA (AVGEROPOULOS and BATCHELOR 1999).

Phase I testing confirmed that the drug has excellent oral bioavailability and, using a 5-day schedule repeated every 4 weeks, clinical activity was detected in patients with high-grade astrocytomas which had recurred after radiotherapy (NEWLANDS et al. 1992). Temozolomide was given to 28 patients with primary brain tumors. Patients were treated with 150–200 mg/m^2 per day at 28-day intervals. Five of the ten patients with recurrent astrocytomas after radiation therapy had a major radiographic response and one other patient had a minor response. Four of the seven newly diagnosed high-grade astrocytomas responded prior to irradiation. Temozolomide was well tolerated with manageable toxicity (O'REILLY et al. 1993).

Recent clinical trials with Temozolomide involving recurrent high-grade gliomas (AA and GBM) have been published and offer new treatment options for patients. A large multicenter phase II trial involving 162 patients with anaplastic astrocytoma or grade 3 oligoastrocytomas treated with temozolomide at first relapse following surgery and radiotherapy was recently published by the Temodal Brain Tumor Group (YUNG et al. 1999a). Central pathologic and radiographic review for response was performed. Objective responses were observed in 35% of the patients (8% complete remission and 27% partial remission). An additional 26% of patients had stable disease. Of the patients, 46% reached the primary end point of 6-month progression-free surviv-

al and 24% were progression free at 12 months. Median survival was 13.6 months and 12-month survival was 56%. Importantly, there was no significant difference between 6-month progression-free survival in patients who had received prior chemotherapy (nitrosourea-based) versus chemotherapy naive patients (44% vs 50%). In a Cox regression analysis, only Karnofsky performance status was shown to be a significant independent predictor of progression-free or overall survival. Maintenance of progression-free status and objective responses were associated with quality of life benefits. The encouraging response and survival data in conjunction with the favorable toxicity profile compared to historical nitrosourea-based therapy has resulted in a new option for patients with high-grade astrocytomas at first relapse. Clinical trials are now focusing on adjuvant and neo-adjuvant treatment with temozolomide for high-grade astrocytomas and oligoastrocytomas.

Clinical trial results of temozolomide for recurrent GBM are equally promising. A large randomized phase II study was recently completed by the Temodal Brain Tumor Group (YUNG et al. 1999b) comparing temozolomide to procarbazine in glioblastoma multiforme at first relapse. Patients had histologically proven GBM with unequivocal evidence of relapse. In total, 225 patients (112 temozolomide, 113 procarbazine) were treated. Progression-free survival at 6 months and overall 6-month survival was significantly better in temozolomide-treated patients than with procarbazine, 21% vs 8% ($P<0.008$), and 60% vs 44% ($P<0.019$). As with the recurrent AA study, temozolomide demonstrated superior quality of life benefit at 3 and 6 months (OSOBA 1999). A second large multicenter phase II trial ($n=138$) was performed at 26 international sites for patients with recurrent GBM, confirming a progression-free survival of 19% at 6 months and similar overall response rate (CR, PR, SD) of 51% vs 46% (Schering Plough Corporation study 194–122).

In efforts to maximize increase dose density (AUC) and CNS penetration and decrease further toxicity, new doses and schedules of temozolomide are completing pilot trials. Continuous low-dosage daily temozolomide (75 mg/m^2 per day) for 6–7 weeks has been piloted by BROCK et al. (1998) with an excellent toxicity profile and a 41% response in glioma patients. A similar regimen has been piloted with concurrent radiation by STUPP et al. (1999) in patients with newly diagnosed GBM followed by six cycles of adjuvant temozolomide with the 5-day 200 mg/m^2 per day dose schedule. The regimen was well tolerated with encouraging preliminary results with an estimated 1-year survival of 75%. Plans for randomization of this approach are underway. In addition, schedules of 14-day or 21-day low-dosage (75–125 mg/m^2 per day) temozolomide with 1 week off are ongoing in phase I/II clinical trials (Schering Plough).

Since FDA approval for AA, temozolomide is being evaluated in multiple new clinical trials as a single agent or in combination for a variety of CNS tumors. FRIEDMAN et al. (1999a) are evaluating temozolomide in anaplastic oligodendroglioma and low-grade gliomas (FRIEDMAN et al. 1999a). The same group is evaluating temozolomide in combination with Gliadel wafers (BCNU) (FRIEDMAN et al. 1999c). Dr. Yung and colleagues have recently completed a phase II trial with temozolomide and interferon in recurrent malignant gliomas showing an apparent improvement in progression-free survival at 6 months compared to historical data with temozolomide alone (YUNG et al. 1999c). Rat models of intratumoral temozolomide via bulk flow microinfusion appear promising (A. Heimberger 1999, unpublished data) and may offer a novel delivery system to bypass the blood–brain barrier and deliver high concentrations of chemotherapy with less systemic toxicity.

24.8.2
CPT-11

CPT-11 (Irinotecan) is a water-soluble derivative of camptothecin. Given intravenously, carboxylesterases metabolize the drug to the 1000-times more potent molecule SN-38. This molecule acts by binding to topoisomerase I, a DNA replication protein, thereby inhibiting cell replication. CPT-11 is currently an approved drug for the treatment of colon cancer (ROTHENBERG 1996). A phase II trial conducted by FRIEDMAN et al. (1999d) involved 60 patients with histologically confirmed GBM given CPT-11 weekly [125 mg/m^2 per week+4, then off 2 weeks (1 cycle/6 weeks)]. Most patients had undergone extensive radiotherapy and chemotherapy. None of the 41 patients who had previously undergone chemotherapy had experienced objective responses as a result. Fifteen percent of patients had a partial response and 55% achieved a best response of stable disease lasting more than 12 weeks. The primary toxicities were infrequent neutropenia, nausea, vomiting, and diarrhea. CPT-11 and metabolites were noted to be only 25–40% of similar doses of CPT-11 given to colon cancer patients. This is likely related to the increased excretion rate of CPT-11 with concomitant hepatic enzyme-inducing dexamethasone and anticonvulsants. New pharmacokinetic dose-finding studies are underway with the weekly and 3-week CPT-11 regimens in efforts to maximize responses. The promising early results with CPT-11 are leading to the exploration of a number of new combinations with BCNU, temozolomide, and other active agents (FRIEDMAN et al. 1999a,d).

24.8.3
Topotecan

Topotecan, another specific inhibitor of topoisomerase 1, is a semisynthetic analogue of the alkaloid camptothecin, and demonstrates effectiveness against xenografts derived from high-grade gliomas grown in athymic nude mice. Based on statistically significant survival rates achieved with Topotecan treatment and xenografts, FRIEDMAN et al. (1999b) conducted a phase II trial with the drug for adults with newly diagnosed or recurrent malignant gliomas (histologically confirmed AA, GBM, or OA) to determine the drug's activity and toxicity. Patients were divided into groups consisting of either newly diagnosed (25 patients, 3 PR, 10 SD) or recurrent disease (38 patients, 3 PR, 10 SD). Although the results showed only modest drug activity, a small number of patients demonstrated partial responses and a larger cohort maintained stable disease, warranting further studies. As with CPT-11, dexamethasone and/or anticonvulsant drugs may reduce plasma levels of Topotecan and further dose escalation studies are warranted. A phase I trial of Topotecan and BCNU for adults with recurrent malignant gliomas is proceeding at Duke University (FRIEDMAN et al. 1999b).

24.8.4
Oxaliplatin

Oxaliplatin {[trans- (L-1, 2-diaminocyclohexane)] oxalatoplatinum (II)}, like cisplatin and carboplatin, is a platinum-based cytotoxic agent. It has demonstrated encouraging results in phase II and III clinical trials for treatment of colorectal cancer. Interestingly, oxaliplatin, unlike other platinum-based agents such as cisplatin, does not appear to cause ototoxicity, nephrotoxicity, cardiac toxicity, or alopecia in adults. These are commonly observed toxicities when treating brain tumors with platinum-based agents; thus oxaliplatin appears an ideal brain tumor treatment candidate. Data for treatment of malignant gliomas are currently sparse (AVGEROPOULOS and BATCHELOR 1999). SOULIE et al. 1997 report a complete response in one of nine patients with recurrent GBM. A phase II trial of neoadjuvant oxaliplatin will commence in the near future.

24.8.5
Paclitaxel

Currently approved for a variety of adult solid tumors (ovarian, breast, and non-small-cell lung cancer), paclitaxel exhibits antitumor activity by blocking cycling tumor cells at the G_2/M interface through promotion of microtubule assembly and inhibition of microtubule depolymerization (SCHIFF et al. 1979; PARNESS and HORWITZ 1981; MANFREDI et al. 1982). Arrest of tumor cells by paclitaxel in the most radiosensitive phase of the cell cycle makes it an excellent chemotherapy drug for radiosensitization (TISHLER et al. 1992; HEI et al. 1994). In vitro and in vivo activity against malignant gliomas has been established (CAHAN et al. 1994). Paclitaxel has been used in a variety of doses and schedules in a number of phase I and II clinical trials for malignant gliomas. Partial radiographic responses and disease stabilization has been observed in some of these patients indicating clinical activity. Most of the responses have been in patients with AA or OD features. Minimal response has been observed in GBM (CHAMBERLAIN and KORMANIK 1995, 1997; PRADOS et al. 1996; CHANG et al. 1998). The majority of these initial studies have been with traditional 3-week taxol regimens, and overall toxicity, particularly myelotoxicity, has been less than expected. Similar to trials with Topotecan and CPT-11, induction of hepatic enzymes (cytochrome P450) with anticonvulsants and dexamethasone has led to increased clearance of chemotherapy and reduced overall toxicity at equal doses. Pharmacokinetic data demonstrate that taxol clearance in patients receiving anticonvulsants and dexamethasone is twice as great as those not receiving these drugs with significant reduction in hematologic toxicity. Neurotoxicity has replaced hematologic toxicity at high doses of taxol given in 3-week schedules (CHAMBERLAIN and KORMANIK 1995; CHANG et al. 1998). Data from systemic solid tumors (breast and lung cancer) with weekly paclitaxel therapy (50–100 mg/m² per week) with or without concurrent radiation have demonstrated higher dose density,

equal or better efficacy, and significantly lower toxicity. Clinicians have noted prolonged disease stabilization in some patients with this dosage and schedule, and preliminary data suggest that weekly paclitaxel may have antiangiogenesis and antitumor invasion properties (KLAUBER et al.1997; TERZIS et al. 1997). Weekly paclitaxel schedules are appealing in malignant gliomas, particularly with concurrent radiation, and pilot studies have been performed with concurrent stereotactic radiosurgery with minimal toxicity (LEDERMAN et al. 1997, 1998;). Future studies of dose-dense weekly regimens of Taxol in combination with newer cytotoxic chemotherapy and novel agents, particularly in AA and OD, are warranted.

24.9
Blood–Brain Barrier: Drug Delivery

One of the major challenges to effective treatment of primary malignant gliomas with systemic agents has been the blood–brain barrier (BBB). Anatomically, tight junctions between endothelial cells in normal brain tissue and the junction of tumor and normal tissue prevents larger, water-soluble, highly protein-bound drugs from entering brain tissue. Most chemotherapy drugs have these properties. The BBB is less intact in the primary tumor mass due to aberrant or discontinuous tight junctions. However, long-term survival of patients with high-grade gliomas is dependent on control of micrometastatic disease outside the dominant tumor mass after surgery and localized radiation, precisely in areas of relative intact BBB. Strategies to circumvent the BBB include: the (1) use of osmotic agents to disrupt the BBB, (2) intra-arterial chemotherapy, and more recently, (3) interstitial chemotherapy with biodegradable chemotherapy-impregnated wafers. The first two strategies have been disappointing with increased toxicity and no improvement in response or survival of malignant glioma patients. Interstitial chemotherapy approaches have been more promising with recent FDA approval of BCNU wafers (FRIEDMAN et al. 1999c).

Interstitial therapy, inserting therapeutic-drug-impregnated biodegradable polymer wafers intratumorally, is currently showing promising results for treating newly diagnosed and recurrent malignant gliomas. Intratumoral insertion of the treatment agent both circumvents the blood–brain barrier and allows for high treatment doses delivered directly to the tumor without risk of systemic toxicity. Additionally, since 90% of malignant gliomas recur within 1–2 cm of the initial tumor site, interstitial therapy, like other localized treatments discussed in this book, is a practical means of treatment (AVGEROPOULOS and BATCHELOR 1999). A recent phase III randomized multi-institutional study with 222 patients tested the efficacy of BCNU-impregnated biodegradable wafers for the treatment of recurrent malignant brain tumors. Eight wafers composed of poly (carboxyphenoxy-propane/sebacic acid) anhydride with or without BCNU incorporated into the hydrophobic matrix of the polymer were inserted directly into the brain tumor at the time of surgery. The median survival time for the treatment group increased from 23 weeks to 31 weeks. In GBM patients, the 6-month mortality rate for the treatment group was 44% vs 64% in the placebo group. As a result of this trial, the FDA recently approved Gliadel for the treatment of recurrent malignant brain tumors (BREM and LAWSON 1999). A similar but much smaller study performed by VALTONEN et al. (1997) for the treatment of newly diagnosed malignant gliomas produced equally encouraging results. Patients underwent insertion of either BCNU or empty polymer wafers followed by external beam radiation. The median survival of the treatment group was 58 weeks as opposed to 40 weeks for the placebo group. Two years after implantation, 33% of the treatment group was still alive vs 6% of the placebo group (VALTONEN et al. 1997).

Delivery of other drugs by this method is currently under investigation. Initial rat tumor studies indicate that carboplatin, 4-hydroxycyclophosphamide, camptothecin, and paclitaxel can be effectively delivered intracranially (BREM and LAWSON 1995). A recent study by MENEI et al. (1999) tested the efficacy of 5-FU delivered via poly DL-lactide-co-glycolide (PLAGA) microspheres in newly diagnosed glioblastoma patients. In all eight patients, sustained concentrations of 5-FU were present in the CSF for 1 month with low concentrations of 5-FU in the blood. The median survival time for the group was an encouraging 98 weeks (MENEI et al. 1999). Further studies with 5-FU for the treatment of newly diagnosed and recurrent malignant gliomas are ongoing.

24.10
Molecular-Driven Therapeutics

Molecular-driven therapeutics target the cellular mechanisms which allow for tumor growth and invasion. In general, molecular-driven therapies and research efforts focus on cell cycle genes such as p53,

signal transduction pathways which are known to mediate growth and cellular migration (VEGF, protein kinase C), angiogenesis mechanisms, and matrix metalloproteinases, which play a role in cell growth and invasion (BURTON and PRADOS 1999).

To date, several molecular-driven therapies are undergoing phase II and III clinical trials. Marmistat, an MMP inhibitor by British Biotech, is currently being evaluated in a placebo-controlled phase III trial for newly diagnosed GBM after demonstrating positive results in phase I and II trials on several tumor types (BURTON and PRADOS 1999). SU-101, a signal pathway inhibitor, disrupts the platelet-derived growth factor pathway (PDGF), a tyrosine kinase family pathway. Several studies have reported the presence of both PDGF protein and receptor in tumor cells, a finding which suggests autocrine and paracrine stimulation for PDGF-related tumor cell growth. SU-101, Leflunomide, inhibits this pathway and in a phase I trial with malignant gliomas demonstrated objective responses in some patients (ECKHARDT et al. 1999). A multicenter phase III trial with SU-101 is currently underway to evaluate therapeutic activity in recurrent GBM. Studies are also being conducted combining SU-101 with procarbazine and BCNU, respectively. Other signal pathway disrupters under investigation are bryostatin, UCN-01, some farnesyl transferase inhibitors, hypericen, suramin, and SU-5271 (BURTON and PRADOS 1999).

Another mechanism for preventing tumor growth is to inhibit molecular pathways responsible for the tumor's vascularization. Thalidomide has been shown to inhibit angiogenesis by inhibiting the vascular endothelial growth factor pathway (VEGF), a pathway which is believed to be responsible for tumor neovascularization (BURTON and PRADOS 1999). A phase II trial of thalidomide for recurrent high-grade astrocytomas and mixed gliomas is currently underway. Preliminary results show low toxicity and promising biological activity (FINE 1997). Other antiangiogenesis drugs currently under clinical evaluation include SU-5416, which has demonstrated antiangiogenesis/antitumor activity by way of VEGF receptor inhibition, platelet factor 4, interleukin-12, interferon alpha, and TNP-470 (BURTON and PRADOS 1999).

24.11
Conclusion

After many years of slow clinical progress and lack of new drug options, chemotherapy for the treatment of adult CNS brain tumors is now beginning to show evidence of becoming a vital treatment tool for primary brain tumors, like surgery and radiation. The problems which stymied clinical progress in the past are now being overcome with improved understanding of the molecular mechanisms involved in neoplastic transformation and new knowledge concerning the important differences between brain tumor histology. These advances have opened the door for new drugs, different uses for old drugs, and clinical trials designed to evaluate these drugs according to more objective criteria than in the past. Some of these new drugs, specifically temozolomide, O6-BG, and BCNU used interstitially are already showing evidence of improving quality of life and progression-free survival times in adults with primary malignant gliomas. The historically poor prognosis for adult CNS tumors will undoubtedly continue to improve as clinical research moves forward.

References

Allen J (1991) Controversies in the management of intracranial germ cell tumors. Neurol Clin 9(2): 441–452

Allen J, Bosl G, Walker R, et al. (1985) Chemotherapy trials in recurrent primary intracranial germ cell tumors. J Neurooncol 3(2): 147–152

Avgeropoulos N and Batchelor T (1999) New treatment strategies for malignant gliomas. Oncologist 4(3): 209–224

Baltuch G, Shenouda G, Langleben A, et al. (1993) High dose tamoxifen in the treatment of recurrent high grade glioma: a report of clinical stabilization and tumour regression. Can J Neurol Sci 20(2): 168–170

Belanich M., Pastor M, Randall T, et al. (1996) Retrospective study of the correlation between the DNA repair protein alkyltransferase and survival of brain tumor patients treated with carmustine. Cancer Res 56(4): 783–788

Brandes A, Ermani M, Turazzi S, et al. (1999) Procarbazine and high-dose tamoxifen as a second-line regimen in recurrent high-grade gliomas: a phase II study. J Clin Oncol 17(2): 645–650

Brem H and Lawson H (1999) The development of new brain tumor therapy utilizing the local and sustained delivery of chemotherapeutic agents from biodegradable polymers. Cancer 86(2): 197–199

Brem H., Piantadosi S, Burger P, et al. (1995) Placebo-controlled trial of safety and efficacy of intraoperative controlled delivery by biodegradable polymers of chemotherapy for recurrent gliomas, The Polymer-brain Tumor Treatment Group. Lancet 345(8956): 1008–1012

Brock C, Newland E, Wedge S, et al. (1998) Phase I trial of temozolomide using an extended continuous oral schedule. Cancer Res 58(19): 4363–4367

Burger P, Vogel F, Green S, et al. (1985) Glioblastoma multiforme and anaplastic astrocytoma. Pathologic criteria and prognostic implications. Cancer. 56(5): 1106–1111

Burton E and Prados M (1999) New chemotherapy options for the treatment of malignant gliomas. Current Opinion in Oncology 11: 157–161

Cahan M, Walter K, Colvin O, et al. (1994) Cytotoxicity of taxol in vitro against human and rat malignant brain tumors. Cancer Chemother Pharmacol 33(5): 441–444

Cairncross J, Ueki K, Zlatesku M, et al. (1998) Specific genetic predictors of chemotherapeutic response and survival in patients with anaplastic oligodendrogliomas. J Natl Cancer Inst 90(19): 1473–1479

Chamberlain M and Kormanik P (1995) Salvage chemotherapy with paclitaxel for recurrent primary brain tumors. J Clin Oncol 13(8): 2066–2071

Chamberlain M and Kormanik P (1997) Salvage chemotherapy with paclitaxel for recurrent oligodendrogliomas. J Clin Oncol 15(12): 3427–3432

Chamberlain M and Kormanik P (1999) Salvage chemotherapy with tamoxifen for recurrent anaplastic astrocytomas. Arch Neurol 56(6): 703–708

Chang S, Kuhn J, Rizzo J, et al. (1998) Phase I study of paclitaxel in patients with recurrent malignant glioma: a North American Brain Tumor Consortium report. J Clin Oncol 16(6): 2188–2194

Cokgor I., Friedman H and Friedman A (1999) Chemotherapy for adults with malignant glioma. Cancer Invest 17(4): 264–272

Couldwell W, Antel J, Apuzzo M, et al. (1990) Inhibition of growth of established human glioma cell lines by modulators of the protein kinase-C system. J Neurosurg 73(4): 594–600

Couldwell W, Hinton D, Surnock A, et al. (1996) Treatment of recurrent malignant gliomas with chronic oral high-dose tamoxifen. Clin Cancer Res 2(4): 619–622

Couldwell W, Uhm J, Antel J, et al. (1991) Enhanced protein kinase C activity correlates with the growth rate of malignant gliomas in vitro. Neurosurgery 29(6): 880–887

Dinapoli R, Brown L, Arusell R, et al. (1993) Phase III comparative evaluation of PCNU and carmustine combined with radiation therapy for high-grade glioma. J Clin Oncol 11(7): 1316–1321

Dolan M and Pegg A (1997). O6-benzylguanine and its role in chemotherapy. Clin Cancer Res 3(6): 837–847

Eagan R and Scott M (1983) Evaluation of prognostic factors in chemotherapy of recurrent brain tumors. J Clin Oncol 1(1): 38–44

Eckhardt S, Rizzo J, Sweeney K, et al. (1999) Phase I and Pharmacologic Study of the Tyrosine Kinas Inhibitor SU101 in Patients with Advanced Solid Tumors. Journal of Clinical Oncology 17(4): 1095–1104

Fine H (1994) The basis for current treatment recommendations for malignant gliomas. J Neurooncol 20(2): 111–120

Fine H, Dear K, Loeffler J, et al. (1993) Meta-analysis of radiation therapy with and without adjuvant chemotherapy for malignant gliomas in adults. Cancer 71(8): 2585–2597

Fine H (1997) A Phase II trial of the anti-angiogenic agen thalidomide, in patients with recurrent high-grade gliomas. Proceedings ASCO (16), abstract #1372, pp. 385a

Fine R, Williams A, Jett P, et al. (1990) Tamoxifen potentiates the antitumor effect of vinblastine against instrinsically multi-drug resistant human renal carcinoma cell lines. Proc Am Assn Cancer Res 31: 359

Friedman A, Cokgor I, Kerby T, et al. (1999a) [abstract] Phase II Treatment of Anaplastic Oligodendro-Glioma and Low Grad Glioma with Temodal. Fourth Annual Meeting of French Society Neuro-Oncology, November 17–21, abstract #70, pp. 310

Friedman H, Kerby T, Fields S, et al. (1999b). Topotecan treatment of adults with primary malignant glioma. The Brain Tumor Center at Duke. Cancer 85(5): 1160–1165

Friedman H, Cokgor I, Kerby T, et al. (1999c) Phase I Clinical Trials of Gliadel Plus CPT-11 or Temodal. Fourth Annual Meeting of the Society for Neuro-Oncology, November 17–21, abstract #73, pp 311

Friedman H, Kokkinakis D, Pluda J, et al. (1998) Phase I trial of O6-benzylguanine for patients undergoing surgery for malignant glioma. J Clin Oncol 16(11): 3570–3575

Friedman H, McClendon R, Kerby T, et al. (1998) DNA mismatch repair and O6-alkylguanine-DNA alkyltransferase analysis and response to Temodal in newly diagnosed malignant glioma. J Clin Oncol 16(12): 3851–3857

Friedman H, Petros W, Friedman A, et al. (1999d) Irinotecan therapy in adults with recurrent or progressive malignant glioma. J Clin Oncol 17(5): 1516–1525

Grunberg S, Bertram M, McDermed J, et al. (1987) Treatment of astrocytoma with a 5-day cisplatin infusion. Cancer Drug Deliv 4(1): 47–53

Heimberger A, Archer G, Friedman H, et al. (1999) Intratumoral Temozolomide via Bulk Flow Microinfusion is Efficacious Against Intracranial Glioma. Fourth Annual Meeting of the Society for Neuro-Oncology, November 17–21, abstract #90, pp. 315

Hei T, Piao C, Geard C, et al. (1994) Taxol and ionizing radiation: interaction and mechanisms. Int J Radiat Oncol Biol Phys 29(2): 267–271

Hubbard J, Scheithauer B, Kispert D, et al. (1989) Adult cerebellar medulloblastomas: the pathological, radiographic, and clinical disease spectrum. J Neurosurg 70(4): 536–544

Jaeckle K, Eyre H, Townsend J, et al. (1998) Correlation of tumor O6 methylguanine-DNA methyltransferase levels with survival of malignant astrocytoma patients treated with bis- chloroethylnitrosourea: a Southwest Oncology Group study. J Clin Oncol 16(10): 3310–3315

Kida Y, Kobayashi T, Yoshida J, et al. (1986) Chemotherapy with cisplatin for AFP-secreting germ-cell tumors of the central nervous system. J Neurosurg 65(4): 470–475

Klauber N, Parangi S, Flynn E, et al. (1997) Inhibition of angiogenesis and breast cancer in mice by the microtubule inhibitors 2-methoxyestradiol and taxol. Cancer Res. 57(1): 81–86

Kristiansen K, Hagen S, Kollevold T, et al. (1981) Combined modality therapy of operated astrocytomas grade III and IV. Confirmation of the value of postoperative irradiation and lack of potentiation of bleomycin on survival time: a prospective multicenter trial of the Scandinavian Glioblastoma Study Group. Cancer 47(4): 649–652

Lederman G, Arbit E, Odaimi M, et al. (1998) Fractionated stereotactic radiosurgery and concurrent taxol in recurrent glioblastoma multiforme: a preliminary report. Int J Radiat Oncol Biol Phys 40(3): 661–666

Lederman G, Arbit E, Odaimi M, et al. (1997) Recurrent glioblastoma multiforme: potential benefits using fractionated stereotactic radiotherapy and concurrent taxol. Stereotact Funct Neurosurg 69(1–4): 162–174

Levin V and Prados M (1992) Treatment of recurrent gliomas and metastatic brain tumors with a polydrug protocol designed to combat nitrosourea resistance. J Clin Oncol 10(5): 766–771

Levin V, Silver P, Hannigan J, et al. (1990) Superiority of postradiotherapy adjuvant chemotherapy with CCNU, procarbazine, and vincristine (PCV) over BCNU for anaplastic gliomas: NCOG 6G61 final report. Int J Radiat Oncol Biol Phys 18(2): 321–324

Longee D, Friedman H, Albright R, et al. (1990) Treatment of patients with recurrent gliomas with cyclophosphamide and vincristine. J Neurosurg 72(4): 583–588

MacDonald D, Cascino T, Schold S, et al. (1990) Response criteria for phase II studies of supratentorial malignant glioma. J Clin Oncol 8(7): 1277–1280

Manfedi J, Parness J and Horwitz S (1982) Taxol binds to cellular microtubules. J Cell Biol 94(3): 688–996

McClay E, Albright K, Jones J, et al. (1993) Tamoxifen modulation of cisplatin sensitivity in human malignant melanoma cells. Cancer Res 53(7): 1571–1576

Menei P, Venier M, Gamelin E, et al. (1999) Local and sustained delivery of 5-fluorouracil from biodegradable microspheres for the radiosensitization of glioblastoma: a pilot study. Cancer 86(2): 325–330

Nelson D, Nelson J, Davis D, et al. (1985) Survival and prognosis of patients with astrocytoma with atypical or anaplastic features. J Neurooncol 3(2): 99–103

Nelson J, Tsukada Y, Schoenfeld D, et al. (1983) Necrosis as a prognostic criterion in malignant supratentorial, astrocytic gliomas. Cancer 52(3): 550–554

Newlands E, Blackledge S, Slack J, et al. (1992) Phase I trial of temozolomide (CCRG 81045: M&B 39831: NSC 362856). Br J Cancer 65(2): 287–291

O'Brian C, Liskamp A, Soloman D, et al. (1985). Inhibition of protein kinase C by tamoxifen. Cancer Res 45(6): 2462–2465

O'Reilly S, Newlands E, Glaser M, et al. (1993) Temozolomide: a new oral cytotoxic chemotherapeutic agent with promising activity against primary brain tumours [published erratum appears in Eur J Cancer 1993;29 A(10):1500]. Eur J Cancer 7: 940–942

Osoba D (1999) Proceedings ASCO (18) abstract #541, pp. 191a

Parness J, and Horwitz S (1981) Taxol binds to polymerized tubulin in vitro." J Cell Biol 91(2 Pt 1): 479–487

Patel S, Buckner J, Smithson W, et al. (1992) Cisplatin-based chemotherapy in primary central nervous system germ cell tumors. J Neurooncol 12(1): 47–52

Pech I, Peterson K, Cairncross J (1998) Chemotherapy for Brain Tumors. Oncology 1(12) #4, 537–543

Pollack I, Randall M, Kristofik M, et al. (1990a) Effect of tamoxifen on DNA synthesis and proliferation of human malignant glioma lines in vitro. Cancer Res 50(22): 7134–7138

Pollack I, Randall M, Kristofik M, et al. (1990b) Response of malignant glioma cell lines to activation and inhibition of protein kinase C-mediated pathways. J Neurosurg 73(1): 98–105

Prados M, Schold S, Spence A, et al. (1996) Phase II study of paclitaxel in patients with recurrent malignant glioma. J Clin Oncol 14(8): 2316–2321

Prados M, Scott C, Curran W, et al. (1999) Procarbazine, lomustine, and vincristine (PCV) chemotherapy for anaplastic astrocytoma: A retrospective review of radiation therapy oncology group protocols comparing survival with carmustine or PCV adjuvant chemotherapy [In Process Citation]. J Clin Oncol 17(11): 3389–3395

Reifenberger J, Reifenberger G, Liu L, et al. (1994) Molecular genetic analysis of oligodendroglial tumors shows preferential allelic deletions on 19q and 1p. Am J Pathol 145(5): 1175–1190

Rothenberg M (1996) CPT-11: an original spectrum of clinical activity." Semin Oncol 23(1 Suppl 3): 21–26

Schering Plough Corporation study 194–122 (1999) (Personal Contact)

Schiff P, Fant J, Horwitz S (1979) Promotion of microtubule assembly in vitro by taxol. Nature 277(5698): 665–667

Shaw E, Scheithauer W, O'Fallon J, et al. (1992) Oligodendrogliomas: the Mayo Clinic experience. J Neurosurg 76(3): 428–434

Sheline G (1990) Radiotherapy for high grade gliomas. Int J Radiat Oncol Biol Phys 18(4): 793–803

Soulie P, Raymond E, Brienza S, et al. (1997) Oxaliplatin: the first DACH platinum in clinical practice. Bull Cancer 84(6): 665–673

Stewart D, O'Bryan R, Al-Sarraf M, et al. (1983) Phase II study of cisplatin in recurrent astrocytomas in adults: a Southwest Oncology Group Study. J Neurooncol 1(2): 145–147

Stuart N, Philip P, Harris A, et al. (1992) High-dose tamoxifen as an enhancer of etoposide cytotoxicity. Clinical effects and in vitro assessment in p-glycoprotein expressing cell lines. Br J Cancer 66(5): 833–839

Stupp R, Ostermann S, Pica A, et al. (1999) Daily temozolomide and concomitant radiotherapy followed by adjuvant temozolomide for patients with newly diagnosed glioblastoma multiforme, a well tolerated and promising regimen. Thirteenth International Conference of Brain Tumor Research and Therapy, Sapporo, Japan. October 4–6

Terzis A, Thorsen F, Heese O, et al. (1997) Proliferation, migration and invasion of human glioma cells exposed to paclitaxel (Taxol) in vitro. Br J Cancer 75(12): 1744–1752

Tishler R, Schiff P, Geard C, et al. (1992) Taxol: a novel radiation sensitizer. Int J Radiat Oncol Biol Phys 22(3): 613–617

Trump D, Smith D, Ellis P, et al. (1992) High-dose oral tamoxifen, a potential multidrug-resistance-reversal agent: phase I trial in combination with vinblastine. J Natl Cancer Inst 84(23): 1811–1816

Valtonen S, Timonen U, Toivanen P, et al. (1997) Interstitial chemotherapy with carmustine-loaded polymers for high- grade gliomas: a randomized double-blind study. Neurosurgery 41(1): 44–49

Vertosick F, Selker R, Pollack I, et al. (1992) The treatment of intracranial malignant gliomas using orally administered tamoxifen therapy: preliminary results in a series of "failed" patients. Neurosurgery 30(6): 897–903

Walker M, Alexander E, Hunt W, et al. (1978) Evaluation of BCNU and/or radiotherapy in the treatment of anaplastic gliomas. A cooperative clinical trial. J Neurosurg 49(3): 333–343

Wong E, Hess K, Gleason M, et al. (1999) Outcomes and prognostic factors in recurrent glioma patients enrolled onto phase II clinical trials. J Clin Oncol 17(8): 2572

Yung A, Levin V, Albright R, et al. (1999a) Proceedings ASCO 18:abstract #532, pp. 139a

Yung W, Jaeckle K, Kyritsis A, et al. (1999b) [abstract] A combination of Temozolomide and Interferon-A in Recurrent Malignant Gliomas, A Phase II Study. Fourth Annual Meeting of the Society for Neuro-Oncology, November, abstract #217, pp. 347

Yung W, Prados M, Yaya-Tur R, et al. (1999c) Multicenter phase II trial of temozolomide in patients with anaplastic astrocytoma or anaplastic oligoastrocytoma at first relapse [In Process Citation]. J Clin Oncol 17(9): 2762

25 Immunotherapy for Primary Brain Tumors

JOHN E. LAHANIATIS and LUTHER W. BRADY

CONTENTS

25.1
Introduction

Tumors of the central nervous system (CNS) are represented by a wide spectrum of histological subcategories, which include: astrocytoma, oligodendroglioma, ependymoma, mixed glioma, choroid plexus tumors, neuronal and mixed neuronal-glial tumors, pineal tumors, and germinomas (see Chap. 2). The estimated incidence rate for all primary tumors including benign and malignant lesions in 1999 was 11.8 per 100,000 population, with malignant tumors accounting for 6.5 per 100,000 (LANDIS et al. 1999). This resulted in approximately 16,800 new cases of brain and other nervous system tumors in the United States (9500 males and 7300 females). Glioblastoma multiforme, high-grade oligodendroglioma, and anaplastic astrocytoma are among the most difficult primary brain tumors to control, with an annual incidence in the United States of over 10,000 patients. Their natural history is relatively short with rapid tumor progression leading to the patient's death. Even though longer survival times have been obtained using better surgical techniques, contempo-

J. E. LAHANIATIS, MD
Hahnemann University Hospital, Department of Radiation Oncology, Broad and Vine Streets, MS 200, Philadelphia, PA 19102, USA
L. W. BRADY, MD
Hahnemann University Hospital, Department of Radiation Oncology, Broad and Vine Streets, MS 200, Philadelphia, PA 19102, USA

rary radiotherapy, chemotherapy, or combinations thereof, no treatment is curative for a majority of these tumors.

25.2
Molecular Biology

The advances in molecular biology over the past decade have had a significant impact on our understanding of brain tumor biology. Similar to other tumors, CNS neoplastic lesions have a long process of development. Tumor genesis is a multistep process involving a number of interactions such as oncogene activation, tumor suppressor inactivation and oncogene overexpression, abnormalities in signal transduction pathways, alterations in cell cycle progression, and angiogenesis.

In astrocytic tumors, point mutations and deletions on chromosome 17p13 usually alter the P53 gene. This process can be found in about 30–40% of cases. The above gene plays a role in cell cycle regulation, response to DNA damage, and apoptosis. Oncogene amplification of the epidermal growth factor receptor, which is expressed in approximately 40% of glioblastoma multiforme, plays a role in cell proliferation and transformation. The epidermal growth factor receptor binds epidermal growth factor and transforming growth factor-alpha. When bound, it functions in signal transduction via a tyrosine kinase pathway. When transformed, the receptor is truncated lacking a functional ligand-binding domain, which results in a constitutively active transduction pathway continually stimulating tumor cell proliferation. Another tyrosine kinase receptor important in the carcinogenesis of astrocytoma is the platelet-derived growth factor receptor. Unlike the epidermal growth factor receptor, which is altered resulting in its being constitutively active, the platelet-derived growth factor receptor provides high signal transduction activity via two mechanisms. Astrocytomas express high levels of both platelet-derived growth factor receptors and ligands. Malignant gliomas also overexpress protein kinase C, which is an enzyme involved in signal transduction. Angiogenesis is an important factor in growth of primary CNS tumors. Hypoxia induces vascular endothelial growth factor, which functions as a mitogen thus inducing angiogenesis and vascular permeability, all of which aid in tumor growth.

Tumor cells express a wide range of antigens. Some of these antigens are similar to those found in nonmalignant host cells. Other antigens are overexpressed in tumors and thus have been termed tumor-associated antigens. A subset of tumor-associated antigens are tumor-associated transplantation antigens, which can induce a specific immunologic response. These tumor-associated transplantation antigens differ from normal cells of the individual host and can be recognized by the immune system through T cells or antibody mechanism. Tumor-associated transplantation antigen expression is high in viral-oncogene-associated tumors. It is important to recognize that not all tumors contain tumor-associated transplantation antigens.

25.3
Biologic Response Modifiers

Biologic response modifiers are natural substances that enhance host defenses against tumors. Strategies for the immunotherapy of cancer can generally be divided into active and passive approaches. Active immunotherapy refers to the immunization of the host with materials designed to elicit an immune reaction capable of eliminating or retarding tumor growth. Examples of active immunotherapy can be nonspecific in nature as is the case in BCG, *Corynebacterium parvum*, levamisole, and interferon or interleukin (IL)-2 therapy. Specific active immunotherapy involves immunization with tumor antigen vaccines. Passive immunotherapy can consist of: antibodies conjugated to toxins, chemotherapeutic agents or radiolabels, tumor infiltrating lymphocytes and LAK cells, or inhibition of growth factors.

Cells produce interferons in response to viral infection, antigens, or mitogens. They have a variety of biologic properties, including the following: immunomodulatory activities, antiviral properties, ability to interfere with cell cycle progression, inhibition of angiogenesis, regulation of differentiation, and ability to alter expression of cell surface antigens. IL-2 is a lymphokine produced by activated T cells, which in turn further activate T cells bearing IL-2 receptors, therefore stimulating an immune response.

Although quite intriguing, adoptive immunotherapy is not without its shortcomings and obstacles. Systemically administered IL-2 at therapeutic dose levels has produced potentially life-threatening pulmonary compromise, fever, and profound CNS effects. Fatigue and influenza-type symptoms are the most common toxicity of interferon-alpha. Treatment methods have been devised to eliminate a systemic administration of IL-2. In a phase I clinical trial, patients with recurrent malignant glioma were treated by repeated intracerebral injections of human recombinant IL-2 alone or in combination with systemic interferon-alpha (MERCHANT et al. 1992). A dose of rIL-2 of 50,000 IU triggered increased peritumoral edema with concomitant expression of increased intracranial pressure. Progressive debilitating fatigue was the most common side effect of interferon-alpha in doses ranging between 12 MIU and 18 MIU. The patient's clinical status returned to pretreatment level after immunotherapy was completed. The authors concluded that when this agent was administered 3 times per week, patients with malignant brain tumors could tolerate repeated intracerebral injections of 50,000 IU rIL-2 and subcutaneous injections of interferon-alpha of up to 12 MIU for at least 4 weeks.

IL-2 has been used alone or in conjunction with adoptive transfer of LAK cells. LAK cells are natural killer (NK) cells that possess high specificity towards a particular tumor cell line. They can be cultured in vitro and adoptively transferred to the tumor-bearing host. LAK cells are produced by incubating peripheral blood lymphocytes with IL-2. These cells show antitumor activity without destroying normal cells. It has been demonstrated that LAK cells can be produced in vitro from patients with glial tumors and can kill glial tumor cells (JACOBS et al. 1986). Mean and median survival of patients treated with LAK cells and IL-2 for malignant brain tumors was not prolonged beyond that which could be expected with the use of conventional treatment such as surgical resection combined with radiotherapy (MERCHANT et al. 1990; SANKHLA et al. 1996; BOIARDI et al. 1994).

An increased survival after reoperation with the use of intracavitary administration of IL-2 and LAK cells was demonstrated in a study of 15 glioblastoma multiforme patients (HAYES et al. 1995). The median survival for these 15 patients was 53 weeks after reoperation with a mean survival of 87.9±21.4 weeks SEM. Of the 15 patients studied, 2 (13%) were alive at

3.1 and 4.3 years, respectively. The 1-year survival was 53% (8 of 15 patients). It should be noted that some of the patients additionally received procarbazine chemotherapy and that contribution should be taken into account when evaluating response and increased survival.

Based on the published outcomes of phase I–II studies, a number of medical centers have abandoned adoptive immunotherapy in favor of using antibody-target killing or gene therapy (NITTA et al. 1990; RAM et al. 1993; OLDFIELD et al. 1993) (see Chap. 26 of this volume for relevant details).

25.4
Monoclonal Antibodies

Monoclonal antibodies against tumor antigens can be used therapeutically as: (1) biologic response modifiers (MILLER et al. 1983); (2) delivery systems for chemotherapeutic agents (EMBLETON et al. 1983; STAVROU 1990); (3) delivery systems for toxins (JANSEN et al. 1982; THORPE et al. 1985); and (4) delivery systems for radionuclides (BOURDON et al. 1984; BULLARD et al. 1986; HOPKINS et al. 1995; BRADY et al. 1990; EMRICK et al. 1996). Several pilot studies of radioimmunotherapy for primary brain tumors have been reported. A recently reported study used locoregional administration of ^{125}I-labeled monoclonal antibodies which recognize stromal and intracellular glycoprotein tenascin (RIVA et al. 1999). Tenascin is an antigen which is present particularly in glioblastoma multiforme. In the group of 74 glioblastoma multiforme patients, the clinical response was as follows: 10 (13.5%) had stable disease, 9 (12.2%) had partial response, 23 (31%) had no evidence of disease, and 1 (1.3%) patient had complete response. Patients with bulky lesions had a median survival of 17 months, whereas patients with small lesions had a median survival of 25 months. As expected, those with less aggressive disease had better outcomes.

Dose escalation studies were designed to determine the maximum tolerated dose of ^{131}I-labeled 81C6 monoclonal antibody (which binds to tenascin) injected into a cavity resulting from resection of a brain tumor (BIGNER et al. 1998; BROWN et al. 1996). Patients were selected with postsurgical cavities which did not communicate with the subarachnoid space. Dose-limiting toxicity was reached at 120 mCi of ^{125}I and was limited to neurologic or hematologic effects. Of the 11 patients who were treated at the 100-mCi dose level, none developed serious neurologic toxicity, although 1 developed neutropenia and thrombocytopenia. The major limitation when using ^{131}I is hematologic toxicity. It is of interest to note that disease stabilization occurred in 14 (42%) of the 33 study patients. The median survival following radiolabeled monoclonal antibody therapy for all patients was 60 weeks and for those with glioblastoma multiforme, 56 weeks. The authors of this study noted that none of the patients treated with ^{131}I-labeled 81C6 required reoperation for the treatment of symptomatic radionecrosis.

In another report, a total of 15 patients with primary brain tumors were treated with intratumoral injection of ^{90}Y-labeled ERIC-1 murine monoclonal antibody (HOPKINS et al. 1995). This monoclonal antibody binds to a surface of the neural cell adhesion molecule antigen. The median survival in this group of patients was 24 months. Pharmacokinetic analysis confirmed very high mean radiation doses and dose rates to the wall of the cavity in comparison to doses recorded in normal tissue and those measured in the bloodstream.

In one study, fractionated peripheral venous injection of epidermal growth factor receptor-425 monoclonal antibodies radiolabeled with ^{125}I was used in patients with high-grade glioma of the brain (MIYAMOTO et al. 1996; SNELLING et al. 1995). This study included 59 patients: 13 (22%) had astrocytomas with anaplastic foci and 46 (78%) had glioblastoma multiforme. Patients received the above-described radiolabeled antibody following the standard management. No significant life-threatening toxicity was observed during the trial. The median survival for both groups was 13.5 months with 34 (58%) of the study patients being alive at 1 year from treatment.

25.5
Gene Therapy

Malignant gliomas have not been greatly impacted by advances in newer surgical techniques, contemporary radiation therapy delivery, or new chemotherapeutic approaches. This is the main reason to pursue the newer experimental treatment protocols, which may have potential for high incidence of toxicity. Gene therapy offers the advantage of direct injection of the engineered vectors into the tumor cavity, thus overcoming limitations imposed by the blood–brain barrier, and sharply reduces a probability of systemic toxicity. A full discussion dealing with the vast and ever-expanding information which has been provided by molecular biology as it relates to malignant glioma would exceed the scope of this chapter (see Chap. 26). Suffice it to say that gene therapy has been applied to antiangiogenesis, defective gene repair, and suppression of genes regulating cell proliferation.

25.6
Conclusion

Even though our knowledge concerning the biologic behavior of malignant gliomas has vastly increased since the commonplace use of molecular techniques, investigators must continue the search for implementation of novel strategies to discover new molecular targets regulating cellular proliferation and to overcome current treatment limitations.

References

Bigner DD, Brown MT, Friedman AH, et al. (1998) Iodine-131-labeled antitenascin monoclonal antibody 81c6 treatment of patients with malignant gliomas: phase I trial results. J Clin Oncol 16(6):2202–2212

Boiardi A, Silvanni A, Ruffini PA, et al. (1994) Loco-regional immunotherapy with recombinant interleukin-2 and adherent lymphocyte activated killer cell (A-LAK) in recurrent glioblastoma patients. Cancer Immunol Immunother 39:193–197

Bourdon MA, Coleman RE, Blasberg RG, et al. (1984) Monoclonal antibody localization in subcutaneous and intracranial human glioma xenografts: Paired-label and imaging analysis. Anticancer Res 4:133–140

Brady LW, et al. (1990) Iodine-125-labeled anti-epidermal growth factor receptor-425 in the treatment of glioblastoma multiforme. A pilot study. Front Radiat Ther Oncol 24:151–160; discussion 161–165

Brown MT, Coleman RE, Friedman AH, et al. (1996) Intrathecal 131I-labeled antitenascin monoclonal antibody 81C6 treatment of patients with leptomeningeal neoplasms or primary brain tumor resection cavities with subarachnoid communication: phase I trial results. Clin Cancer Res 2(6):963–972

Bullard De, Adams CJ, Coleman RE, et al. (1986) In vivo imaging of intracranial human glioma xenografts comparing specific with nonspecific radiolabeled monoclonal antibodies. J Neurosurg 64:257–262

Embleton MJ, Rowland GF, Simmonds RG et al. (1983) Selective cytotoxicity against human tumor cells by a vindesine-monoclonal antibody conjugate. Br J Cancer 47:43–49

Emrich JG, Bender H, Class R et al. (1996) In vitro evaluation of iodine-125-labeled monoclonal antibody (Mab 425) in human high-grade glioma cells. Am J Clin Oncol 19(6):601–608

Hayes RL, Koslow M, Hiesiger EM, et al. (1995) Improved long term survival after intracavitary interleukin-2 and lymphokine-activated cell for adults with recurrent malignant gliomas. Cancer 76(5):840–852

Hopkins K, Chandler C, Bullimore J, et al. (1995) A pilot study of the treatment of patients with recurrent malignant gliomas with intratumoral ytrium-90 radioimmunoconjugates. Radiother Oncol 34(2):121–131

Jacobs SK, Wilson DJ, Kornblith PL, et al. (1986) In vitro killing of human glioblastoma by IL-2 activated autologous lymphocytes. J Neurosurg 64:114–117

Jansen FK, Blythman HE, Carriere D, et al. (1982) Immunotoxins: hybrid molecules combining high specificity and potent cytotoxicity. Immunol Rev 62: 185–216

Landis SH, Murray T, Bolden S, Wingo PA (1999) Cancer statistics 1999. CA Cancer J Clin 49:8–31

Merchant RE, Ellison MD, and Young HF (1990) Immunotherapy for malignant glioma using human recombinant interleukin-2 and activated autologous lymphocytes. A review of pre-clinical and clinical investigations. J Neurooncol 8:173+

Merchant RE, McVicar DW, Merchant LH, et al. (1992) Treatment of recurrent malignant gliomas by repeated intracerebral injection of human recombinant interleukin-2 alone or in combination with systemic interferon-alpha. A phase I clinical trial. J Neurooncol 12(1):75–83

Miller RA, Oseroff AR, Stratte PE, et al. (1983) Monoclonal antibody therapeutic trial in seven patients with T-cell lymphoma. Blood 62:988–995

Miyamoto CT, Brady LW, Rackover MA, et al. (1996) The use of epidermal growth factor receptor-425 monoclonal antibodies radiolabeled with iodine-125 in the adjuvant treatment of patients with high grade gliomas of the brain. Recent Results Cancer Res 141:183–192

Nitta T, Sato K, Yagita H, et al. (1990) Preliminary trial of specific targetting therapy against malignant glioma. Lancet 335:368–376

Oldfield EH, Ram Z, Culver KW, et al. (1993) Gene therapy for the treatment of brain tumors using intra-tumoral transduction with thymidine kinase gene and intravenous gancyclovir. Hum Gene Ther 4:39–69

Ram Z, Culver KW, Walbridge S, et al. (1993) Toxicity studies of retroviral-mediated gene transfer for the treatment of brain tumors. J Neurosurg 79:400–407

Riva P, Franceschi G, Frattarelli M, et al. (1999) 131I radioconjugated antibodies for the locoregional radio-immunotherapy of high-grade malignant glioma – phase I and II study. Acta Oncol 38(3):351–359

Sankhla SK, Nadkarni JS, and Bhagwati SN (1996) Adoptive immunotherapy using lymphokine-activated killer (LAK) cells and interleukin for recurrent malignant brain tumors. J Neurooncol 27(2):133–140

Snelling L, Miyamoto CT, Bender H, et al. (1995) Epidermal growth factor receptor 425 monoclonal antibodies radiolabeled with iodine-125 in the adjuvant treatment of high-grade astrocytomas. Hybridoma 14(2):111–114

Stavrou D (1990) Monoclonal antibodies in neuro-oncology. Neurosurg Rev 13(1):7–18

Thorpe PE, Brown ANF, Bremmer JAG Jr, et al. (1985) An immunotoxin composed of monoclonal anti-Thy-1.1 antibody and a ribosome inactivating protein from Saponaria officinalis: potent anti-tumor effects in-vitro. J Natl Cancer Inst 75:151–159

26 Prospects for Gene Therapy for Brain Tumors

Victor C.-K. Tse and Griff Harsh

CONTENTS

26.1
Introduction

Gliomas are the most common tumors originating in the brain. Most gliomas are malignant. They are the cause of death in almost all patients who harbor them. Even tumors that are originally relatively benign histologically, usually evolve into more malignant tumors and prove life-threatening. Current treatments for malignant gliomas include surgery, radiotherapy, chemotherapy, and immunotherapy, either singly or in combination. Transient control is

V. C.-K. Tse, MD, PhD
Assistant Professor, Department of Neurosurgery, Stanford University, School of Medicine, 300 Pasteur Drive, Boswell Building, A301, Stanford, CA 94305–5327, USA
G. Harsh, MD, MBA
Professor, Department of Neurosurgery, Stanford University, School of Medicine, 300 Pasteur Drive, Edwards Building, R227, Stanford, CA 94305–5327, USA

possible in many cases, yet recurrence is the rule. Possible reasons for tumor recurrence include failure to extirpate all infiltrating tumor cells, tumor resistance to chemotherapy and radiotherapy, and decreased immune response in the brain.

In the past decade, advancements in genetic engineering and increased understanding of the molecular biology of tumorigenesis have permitted development of gene therapy for brain tumors. Gene therapy is the transfer of genetic material into patients, to treat a disease. Strategies for the gene therapy of brain tumors involve transfer of genes intended to sensitize tumor cells to chemotherapeutic agents, to disrupt the cell-cycle of proliferating tumor cells, to induce apoptosis, to block tumor angiogenesis, or to enhance immunosurveillance and immunocytotoxicity (Chiocca and Harsh 1996). Some approaches employ multi-modal techniques to achieve complementary anti-tumor effects. This chapter reviews the basic concepts of gene transfer technology, recent experimental results from a variety of gene therapy approaches, and their clinical applications.

26.2
Current Gene Transfer Technology

The principal goal of gene therapy is functional expression of a therapeutic gene, or transgene, in target cells. The therapeutic gene is usually transferred into target cells by a carrier called a vector. Once inside target cells, this gene is transcribed, and its mRNA translated, by the host's cellular machinery. The resulting gene product then exerts its desired effect in the target cells. The expression of the transgene can be transient or permanent and regulated or unregulated.

This process of transfer of a therapeutic gene into target cells can occur ex vivo (in cell cultures) or in vivo (in the patient). The ex vivo approach requires the isolation of target cells from the patient, or the use of cultured cells from established cell lines.

These cells are genetically modified in cell culture such that they express the gene of interest and are then re-introduced into the patient. This approach is particularly useful for the delivery of genes encoding diffusible agents such as enzymes activating prodrugs, anti-angiogenic factors, and cytokines.

The in vivo approach involves transfer of the transgene into target cells remaining in the body. This is usually accomplished by injection of a gene-carrying vector. Viral vectors are most commonly employed. Other methods of in vivo delivery of therapeutic genes to target cells employ cationic liposomes, naked-plasmid DNA (gene gun and eletroporation), ribozymal antisense DNA, and hybrid systems, such as packaging cells and modified myoblasts or fibroblasts. All of these methods have been tried experimentally, but not all are applicable to brain tumor therapy.

26.3
Viral Vectors

Viral vectors are viruses modified for the delivery of transgenes. They contain a viral backbone of nucleic acid that encodes the genes required for viral entry into cells and subsequent viral replication. Selective deletion of genes from the virus both renders the virus incapable of replication and creates room within the virus for insertion of transgene sequences. There are three important components of a vector-inserted sequence: the expression cassette, the promoter element, and the reporter element. The transgene itself resides in the expression cassette.

The promoter element is designed to enhance selectively the transcription of the transgene. It is normally a very potent promoter able to propel downstream transcription both in vitro and in vivo. It may be either viral or non-viral in origin. The cytomegalovirus (CMV) promoter is an example of a viral promoter. Unfortunately, such viral promoters of a vector are eventually methylated by the host cell such that their activity is terminated.

Non-viral promoters may be universally or selectively active. The phosphoglycerate kinase (PGK) promoter is active in almost all cells, whereas cell-specific promoters such as the glial fibrillary acid protein promoter and the neuronal specific enolase promoter are selectively active, in astrocytes and neurons, respectively (ANDERSEN et al. 1992).

More sophisticated promoter systems, such as the tetracycline inducible promoter (Tet-on /Tet-off), permit control of the timing of transgene expression. The tet-inducible promoter contains genes encoding a fusion protein, the tet repressor-VP16 transactivated protein, and the tet operator linked to a CMV promoter. Expression of a transgene linked to this tet-inducible promoter (Tet-off) can be blocked by administering tetracycline and induced by removing tetracycline (PAULUS et al. 1996). Like all foreign promoters however, this tet-inducible promoter will eventually be silenced by the host cell. This results from both the lack of native enhancers of transcription and the anomalous 3-D configuration of the foreign promoter. Unless the host cell can recognize the transgene in an open configuration, expression will be terminated (TAMIYA et al. 1995).

The reporter element contains a gene encoding a protein whose product is histopathologically evident. LacZ and green fluorescence protein (GFP) are examples of reporter genes. Their expression signifies incorporation of the virus into the host cell.

There are at least six different types of viral vector systems currently available: retrovirus, adenovirus, adeno-associated virus, herpes virus, vaccina virus, and lentivirus. All have specific advantages and disadvantages for use in gene therapy. The first four have been used for the experimental gene therapy of brain tumors.

26.3.1
Retroviral Vectors

Retroviral vectors have been used more frequently in brain tumor therapy than other types. Retroviruses are RNA viruses. The retroviral genome is conveniently organized for its modification into a vector for gene therapy. The genes for virion structural proteins and enzymes (gag, pol, and env) are aligned and flanked at each end by genes responsible for integration and transcription (LTR) in the host cells. Encapsidation (packaging of the viral genome into the protein coat) is governed by the psi gene, which is located at the 5í end of the genome, adjacent to sequences specifying protein coating. In a recombinant retroviral vector, the genes encoding protein coating, but not the psi sequence, are deleted. This produces a viral backbone of approximately 14–20 kb able to accommodate up to 8 kb of foreign DNA inserted as a cassette of genes or a single transgene. The resultant recombinant retroviral vector cannot direct production of viable virus because it lacks the genes for protein coating.

Retroviral vectors are rapidly destroyed by a human host's immune system. Packaging cells are used to provide and maintain an effective concentration of retroviral vectors in tissue targeted by gene therapy. A packaging cell line is a cultured mouse fibroblast cell line stably transfected, with the genes encoding protein coating deleted from the recombinant retroviral vector. These do not include the psi sequence that directs encapsidation. When the recombinant retroviral vector carrying the transgene is introduced into these packaging cells, the packaging cells use the genes for the protein coating they possess, and the psi sequence in the recombinant vector to produce new viral particles. These new retroviral vectors carry the therapeutic transgene but lack the genes for protein coating. These replication-defective vectors are able to infect target cells and to effect integration and expression of the transgene, but they cannot propagate.

The retroviral vectors have the advantages of stable integration into target cells, integration and expression that is limited to dividing cells, and low toxicity to normal brain tissue. Moreover, because most cells of the body express on their surface the docking receptor for retroviruses, an ubiquitous phosphate transport protein, retroviruses have a broad host range (amphotropic).

Retroviral vectors have important limitations. The titers of virus stock produced by transduced target cells are generally low (107 PFU/ml) compared with those produced by other viral systems. The integration of the transgene into the host genome is random. Theoretically, this poses the threat of activation of potentially injurious genes or the inactivation of essential genes in the target cells. The expression of the transgene is dependent on an active viral promoter. Methylation and deletion of retroviral promoters limit the duration and magnitude of promoter activity and thus the amount of therapeutic protein produced in the target cell.

26.3.2
Adenoviral Vectors

The adenovirus is a double-stranded linear DNA virus. The backbone is approximately 38 kb in size. It can carry up to 35 kb of foreign DNA. Construction of recombinant adenoviral vectors is analogous to that for retroviral vectors. The replication region of the wild-type virus (E1, E3, and E4) is deleted and replaced by a cassette containing the transgene. The packaging cells provide the E1 protein required to produce a replication-deficient recombinant virus. Unlike retroviral vectors, however, adenovirus vectors do not integrate into the host's genome. They function episomally; consequently their expression is transient and they are not passed to the cell's progeny. Adenoviruses are tropic for a wide variety of tissues, and infect dividing as well as non-dividing cells. Adenoviruses can be designed to be replication competent or incompetent. The transfection rates and expression efficiency of adenoviral vectors are relatively high.

Adenoviral vectors have several disadvantages. Firstly, they are highly immunogenic. An immune response to viral antigens results in antigen-specific lymphocyte-mediated toxicity. This precludes repeated administration of adenovirus. Secondly, adenoviruses infect non-dividing as well as mitotic cells; there is no selectivity for proliferating tumor cells. Thirdly, adenovirus is a pathogenic virus, and "wild-type" adenoviral infection in humans is not uncommon. It is, therefore, theoretically possible that a recombinant adenovirus could back-mutate into a replication-competent virus of the pathogenic strain.

Several studies have shown repression of brain tumor growth in animal models following direct intratumoral injection of an adenovirus vector bearing the HSV-tk gene and systemic ganciclovir treatment (CHEN et al. 1994). The titres of adenovirus stock released by adenovirus transfected producer cell lines are five orders of magnitude higher than those from retrovirus producer cell lines.

6.3.3
Adeno-associated Viral (AAV) Vectors

The adeno-associated virus is a non-pathogenic single-stranded DNA virus. In vector construction, most of its genes are replaced by a cassette carrying the transgene. Large quantities of high quality virus can be produced through homologous recombination in E. coli (HE et al. 1998). The AAV construct containing the transgene is ligated to a wild-type adenovirus, the helper virus.

Although previously believed to integrate at a specific site in the target cell's genome, the recombinant AAV is actually episomal. This, and its small size (a capacity for less than 5 kb of foreign gene) are the main disadvantages of AAV vectors. Advantages of AAV vectors are the duration of transgene expression and the presence of a surface receptor for wild-type AAV on glioma cells. The latter raises the possibility of a higher uptake of viral particles into glioma cells than into surrounding normal glia (TENENBAUM et al. 1994).

26.3.4
Herpes Simplex Viral Vectors

Herpes simplex virus is a large, double-stranded DNA virus. It is a pathogenic virus that selectively infects non-mitotic neurons in the brain. Herpes virus is rendered replication-defective and less toxic by deleting one or more essential early regulatory genes and a gene that mediates neurovirulence (GLORIOSO et al. 1995). Advantages of this vector system include its large insert capacity (up to 50 kb of foreign DNA) and its stability. Knowledge of its complete sequence facilitates design of task-specific vectors by site-directed mutation (BREAKFIELD et al. 1995). For example, deletion of one or more of the genes for thymidine kinase, ribonucleotide reductase, and uridine triphosphate can make the vector more likely to replicate in tumor than in normal cells. Such replication-conditional vectors appear to be well suited for brain tumor therapy. Deletion of the gamma 34.5 locus makes the virus less toxic to neurons. Insertion of the cytochrome p450 gene into the transgene cassette makes target cells sensitive to cyclophosphamide. Other mutations lead to ganciclovir hypersensitivity and temperature-dependent activity (KRAMM et al. 1997).

Advantages of herpes virus vectors include high rates of infectivity and transgene expression. The expression of the transgene is prolonged and relatively stable, especially when the latency-based promoter (LATs) is used. The main disadvantages of the herpes virus vector are its potential neurotoxicity and the problems posed for delivery by its size. As with adenovirus, back-mutation with wild-type virus is of concern. However, this risk may be substantially reduced by the use of large deletions and other modifications.

26.4
Non-viral Vectors

Viral vectors have significant disadvantages. Most are unable to carry large fragments of foreign DNA. Multiple deletions reduce the viral titers produced. The limited range of a virus's tropism can preclude infection of certain cell types. The long-term expression of a transgene, dependent on both the presence of specific transactivating factors and a susceptible configuration of viral DNA, is highly variable. Viral vectors are also highly immunogenic; this limits the duration of effect and increases the risk of immune-induced injury. Non-viral systems have been developed to be less immmunogenic. The two most commonly used non-viral systems are cationic liposomes and polycation conjugates. Transfer of naked DNA into cells with a biolistic gene gun is another alternative.

26.4.1
Liposomes

Complexes of DNA and liposomes have been used to deliver therapeutic genes to diseased tissue. Recombinant DNA containing the therapeutic gene and regulatory sequences is mixed with synthetic, fusogenic lipid to form lipid-DNA vesicles. The DNA lies at the core of a positively charged complex 50–200 nm in diameter. These lipid vesicles fuse with the negatively charged cell membranes of target cells. They are internalized into the cells and release DNA which is expressed episomally.

Liposomes have multiple advantages. They are readily produced in bulk and are quite stable. They can transfer large amounts of DNA or RNA. They are neither immunogenic nor cytotoxic. Disadvantages include low rates of internalization and transduction (HSAIO et al. 1997a, ZERROUQI et al. 1996). Liposomes also lack specificity in binding; they may bind to cells other than the intended target cells. To improve the specificity of delivery to a targeted cell type and to improve the rate of internalization, viral cell-binding proteins have been incorporated into liposomes. The viral envelope proteins of these "virosomes" facilitate receptor-mediated endocytosis of lipid-bound DNA (HUG and SLEIGHT 1994).

26.4.2
Polycation Conjugates

Incorporating transgenic DNA in polycation conjugates is another method of delivering therapeutic genes to target cells. Conjugate vectors are designed to bind DNA and transport it into the target cells via receptor-mediated endocytosis (PERALES et al. 1994). The conjugates are bi-functional. One-half of the conjugate, usually polylysine, binds DNA. The cationic polylysine binds electrostatically with the recombinant DNA and condenses into a toroidal structure. The other half of the conjugate is covalently linked to a ligand for a surface receptor specific for the targeted cell. The receptor mediates internalization of the conjugate. Once inside the target cells, the entire conjugate fuses with an endosome. Transgenic DNA is subsequently translocated into the nucleus and expressed.

A low rate of translocation is the major barrier to transduction by polycation conjugates.

26.4.3
Ribozymes

Ribozymes have been used in gene therapy as an extension of strategies employing antisense RNA. Both are intended to block the translation of mRNA encoding proteins responsible for a tumor's malignant behavior. Antisense oligonucleotides are short nucleotides with a sequence complementary to the gene or mRNA that is to be negated (AHMED et al. 1994). They may be delivered to target cells by viral or non-viral vectors. Antisense oligonucleotides can be difficult to use. They require activation of RNase H, are unstable, and can be toxic to cells (CALABRETTE et al. 1993).

Therapeutic ribozymes, developed for gene therapy for HIV infection, circumvent these limitations. Ribozymes are short segments of RNA with secondary hairpin structure. They are designed to contain a nucleotide sequence complementary to a portion of the mRNA targeted for destruction. This gives them great specificity in binding the targeted mRNA species. The ribozyme catalyzes cleavage of the mRNA it binds at GUC tri-nucleotides within the mRNA. To be a suitable target for a therapeutic ribozyme, the targeted mRNA need contain only the nucleotide sequence GUC. In gene therapy protocols, the DNA template for a therapeutic ribozyme is cloned into a plasmid downstream from a promoter. The plasmid can be delivered into the cell by viral or non-viral vectors. Once produced inside the cell, the ribozyme will bind to and catalyze destruction of the targeted mRNA. For example, the ribozyme designed to cleave the GUC sequence located downstream from a mutated epidermal growth factor receptor, DDEG-FR, mRNA, specifically inhibits the expression of DDEGFR and reverses the DDEGFR-associated malignant phenotype of human glioblastoma cell line U-87MG (HALATSCH et al. 2000). The efficacy of ribozymes is limited by their sensitivity to nuclease degradation.

26.5
Hybrid Systems

Succesful in vivo gene transfer requires concentrated delivery of the vector throughout the targeted tissue, high rates of infection/transfection of targeted cells, and levels of transgene expression sufficient to induce the desired biological response. In that low rates of transfection of target cells is often the limiting process of this in vivo scenario, schemes using ex vivo transfection have been developed. In ex vivo approaches, such as that used to treat ADA deficiency, cells of choice are transfected with a vector or therapeutic transgene in cell culture and then implanted into the target tissue (BLAESE 1993). Creation of packaging cell lines used in retroviral-mediated HSV-tk / ganciclovir gene therapy for human brain tumors is another example (RAM et al. 1997).

Ex vivo transduction is often part of immuno-gene therapy strategies. One scheme of adoptive immuno-therapy of brain tumors transfects allogenic fibroblasts with the genes for IL-2 and IL-2/IFN-gamma prior to implantation in a tumor (GLICK et al. 1995). Local production of these cytokines enhances cell-mediated immunity and tumor cell death. The immunogenicity and limited in vivo life span of these modified cells may be advantageous or disadvantageous. An advantage is the low risk of their generating tumors. Disadvantages include the risk of neurotoxicity from too strong a local immune response and the waning of an effective immune response as cytokine secretion falls.

26.6
Gene Therapy for Brain Tumors

Over the past decade, many approaches to the gene therapy of brain tumors have been tried. These include replacing defective tumor suppressor genes, interrupting oncogene-driven growth factor signaling and cell-cycle pathways, blocking angiogenesis, enhancing the immune response, and delivering pro-drug-activating genes (Table 26.1).

26.6.1
Tumor Suppressor Genes

Loss of genes that control cell-cycle progression and effect DNA repair plays a major role in the genesis of brain tumors. Genes such as p53 and P-TEN have been identified as important. Replacing these deleted or defective genes has been a major focus of gene therapy (PIETSCH and WIESTLER 1997). Transfection of cells from tumors containing a defective p53 gene with the wild-type gene re-establishes the normal phenotype in cell culture and suppresses tumor

Table 26.1 Gene therapy strategies for brain tumors

Experimental strategy	Therapeutic genes	Mechanism of action
Tumor suppressor gene replacement	p53	Induces GI arrest or apoptosis Enhances radiosensitization and chemosensitization Inhibits angiogenesis
	p16	Induces GI arrest Inhibits tumor angiogenesis
Immune-enhancement	IL-2 IL-4 GM-CSF TNF	Enhances and modulates immune response
	Antisense TGF-beta	Inhibits tumor-induced immuno-suppression
Anti-angiogenesis	Dominant negative VEGF receptor	Inhibits angiogenic and mitigenic activity of VEGF
	Angiostatin and endostatin	Suppresses tumor growth and metastasis
	p53, p16	Inhibits angiogenesis
	Antisense VEGF	Inhibits expression of VEGF
	EGFR ribozyme	Inhibits expression of EGFR
Prodrug activation	HSV-tk	Activates ganciclovir, terminates DNA-synthesis
	E. coli gpt	Activates 6-thioquanine and 6-thioxanthine, inhibits purine-synthesis
	E. coli cytosine deaminase	Activates 5-fluorocytosine, inhibits DNA-synthesis

GM-CSF, granulocyte/macrophage colony-stimulating factor; TNF, tumor necrosis factor; TGF, transforming growth factor; VEGF, vascular endothelial growth factor; EGFR, epidermal growth factor receptor; gpt, guanine phosphoribosyl transferase; GI, growth inhibition

growth in vivo. In one study, an adenovirus was used to deliver a wild-type p53 gene into glioblastoma cell lines in vivo. This inhibited the growth of cells with endogenous wild-type p53 and induced apoptosis of cells with mutant p53 genes (GOMEZ-MANZANO et al. 1996). Restoration of p53 also potentiated the cytotoxicity of radiation and chemotherapy. (BADIE et al.1998, DORIGO et al. 1998) The effects of replacing other tumor suppressor genes, such as p16, p21, and Rb have also been studied. (HUNG et al. 2000, FUEYO et al. 1998, HSASIO et al. 1997b).

26.6.2
Anti-angiogenesis

Discovery of the importance of angiogenesis to tumor growth and the anti-tumor activity of inhibitors of angiogenesis has suggested angiogenesis as a target for gene therapy of solid tumors (O'REILLY et al. 1996). Angiogenic factors and their corresponding receptors include basic fibroblast growth factor (bFGF) and its receptor; vascular endothelial growth factor (VEGF) and its receptors (flk-1 and flk-2); tumor necrosis factor alpha (TNFaa) and its receptor; and human platelet factor 4 and its receptor. High-grade gliomas, such as glioblastoma multiforme (GBM), often have both high vascularity and necrosis. Glioblastomas also express high levels of VEGF and FGF which are essential to neovascular formation in tumors. Brain tumors are therefore good candidates for anti-angiogenic therapy.

Tumor angiogeneisis can be blocked by transferring dominant negative variants of VEGF receptors (flk-1) into tumor endothelial cells (MILLAUER et al. 1996). Antisense VEGF has been shown to inhibit tumor formation in nude mice (SALEH et al. 1996). Blocking angiogenesis by over-expressing p53 (an inducer of transactivation of thrombospondin-1, a naturally occurring glycoprotein inhibitor of angiogenesis) or p16 (a suppressor of VEGF expression) has also been tried (DAMERON et al. 1994, HARADA et al. 1999). Viral vector- mediated in vivo production of anti-angiogenic peptides such as angiostatin and endostatin is a strategy designed to counter the instability and short half-life of these peptides. It is, however, unclear whether blocking a particular angiogenic pathway will significantly disrupt the entire cascade of tumor angiogenesis.

26.6.3
Cytotoxic Agents

Viral vectors can have direct and indirect cytotoxic effects on tumors. Some viruses are intrinsically cytotoxic to rapidly dividing cells. Their use in gene therapy requires the balancing of the desirable abilities to replicate and lyse tumor cells, with the unwanted risk of injury to normal cells. This balance has been sought by attenuating the wild-type virus through mutations in genes for replication and neurovirulence. For instance, the genetically modified mutant of herpes simplex virus, HSV1, is able to replicate within tumor cells and cause cell lysis but is less toxic to the brain than wild-type virus (KRAMM et al. 1997). Replication-conditional adenovirus has been used to lyse tumor cells that are p53 deficient (BISCHOFF et al. 1996).

Viral vectors have been designed to be indirectly cytotoxic to tumor cells by increasing tumor sensitivity to radiation and chemotherapy. Transfection of tumor cells with the p53 or p21 gene enhances their radiosensitivity. Transfer of the bax gene promotes cell death in response to cytosine arabinoside (DONG et al. 1996, VOGELBAUM et al. 1998).

Increased sensitivity to chemotherapeutic agents can also be conferred to tumor cells by transfecting them with enzymes capable of activating prodrugs. This has the advantage of selective activation of the drug within tumor cells, and the corollary of reduced toxicity to surrounding normal cells. This approach is exemplified by the HSV-tk/ GCV system (RAM et al. 1993, 1994). In this therapeutic paradigm, the inactive prodrug, ganciclovir (GCV), is converted into its toxic metabolites by the thymidine kinase enzyme derived from herpes simplex virus. The cDNA encoding TK enzyme is delivered into the tumor cells by a retroviral vector secreted from packaging cells injected into the tumor.

Tumor cells expressing TK activate GCV when it is administered and die when they attempt to divide. Toxic metabolites produced in these tumor cells spread to adjacent, non-transfected tumor cells that also die in manifestation of the "bystander effect". This "bystander effect", also magnified by an immune response to dying tumor cells, compensates

somewhat for the limited spread of packaging cells and retroviral vector from the site of injection and the low rates of transduction and expression of the TK gene in tumor cells.

Other prodrug-activating enzymes effective in brain tumor models include the cytochrome product of CYP2b1 which activates cyclophosphamide and ifosfamide, cytosine deaminase that activates 5-fluorocytosine, and *Escherichia coli* guanine phosphoribosyl transferase (gpt) that activates 6-thioguanine. The gpt gene also activates 6-thioxanthine which is not normally active in mammalian cells (CONNORS 1995). Vectors carrying multiple enzymes capable of activating several components of combined chemotherapy are also being studied.

26.6.4
Immunotherapy

Strategies for using gene therapy to improve the immune response to brain tumors include immune enhancement with cytokines, and the reduction of immune suppression. Immune-surveillance and cytolysis can be increased by augmenting the function of cytotoxic lymphocytes. Activation of cytotoxic lymphocytes is a highly modulated process that requires the cooperation of CD4+ cells. Priming of CD4+ cells to evoke an antigen-specific response requires the interaction of its antigen-specific T-cell receptor with the MHC Class 2 molecules on the surface of antigen-presenting cells (APC). Granulocyte/macrophage colony-stimulating factor (GM-CSF) stimulates antigen-presenting activity. Vaccination with irradiated brain tumor cells transfected in vitro with the GM-CSF gene has enhanced anti-tumor immune response and provides long-term protection from tumor growth following rechallenge with tumor (DRANOFF et al. 1993). Other cytokines such as interleukin 2 and TNFg promote cell-mediated tumor lysis in similar investigational protocols (GLICK et al. 1995). Furthermore, dendritic cells, the body's premier APC, when primed with tumor-specific antigens derived from tumor homogenates and re-implanted into the host, promote immune-mediated tumor killing (LIAU et al. 1999).

The anti-tumor immune response is suppressed by several factors secreted by gliomas. These include insulin-like growth factor (IGF) and transforming growth factor beta (TGF-beta). IGF-1 and IGF-2 suppress the activity of CD8+ cells. Blockade of expression of IGF-1 enhances lymphocyte responsiveness to glioma cells (Trojan et al. 1993). TGF-beta inhibits the function of lymphocyte-activated killer cells. Gene therapy may facilitate disruption of this immune suppression. For instance, antisense mRNA for TGF beta enhances the immunogenicity of irradiated glioma cells in an animal model (Fakhrai et al. 1996).

26.7
Delivery of Gene Therapy

There are three basic routes by which gene therapy vectors can be delivered to tumors within the brain: through brain or tumor tissue (intraparenchymally), through cerebrospinal fluid (intrathecally), and through blood vessels (intravascularly) (Fig. 26.1). Intraparenchymal injection is the most commonly used route of delivery of viruses or their producing cells to brain tumors (Ram et al. 1997). In most protocols used thus far, injection is accomplished at the time of tissue harvest. Cells or vectors can be injected at the site of stereotactic biopsy or about the margins of resection after tumor removal. They can also be injected into the resection cavity postoperatively through an Ommaya reservoir left at the time of surgery. In that residual tumor cells are most dense at the resection margin, therapeutic vehicles are appropriately concentrated there. Unfortunately, the spread of packaging cells and non-replicating viral vectors from the site of injection is limited to several cell layers.

Convection-enhanced delivery is one method of increasing intraparenchymal dispersion of injected agents. Infusion of fluid through an intraparenchymal catheter establishes a pressure gradient conducive to bulk flow of fluid through the extracellular space away from the infusion site (Laske et al. 1997). Small molecules are widely distributed by infusions lasting several days. The dispersion of larger entities such as viral vectors and packaging cells is likely to be much more restricted.

Injection of therapeutic agents into the lumbar subarachnoid or intraventricular spaces takes advantage of CSF flow to achieve dispersion throughout the brain and spinal cord. Carcinomatous meningitis, in which disease is limited to the subarachnoid space, may be accessible by agents injected into the CSF. Effective treatment of intraparenchymal tumor, however, requires traverse of pial and ependymal barriers. Delivery to deeply situated tumors with limited surface presentation is likely to be very limited.

Intravascular injection of therapeutic agents requires that they traverse the blood-brain barrier to reach a targeted tumor. Although the blood-brain barrier is somewhat deficient in malignant gliomas, it is still relatively impermeable to virus-sized particles and cells. Hyperosmotic disruption of the blood-brain barrier increases delivery of chemotherapeutic agents such as carboplatin and methotrexate to parenchymal brain tumors. Mannitol transiently (5 to 15 min) increases capillary permeability to macromolecules by opening the tight junctions of

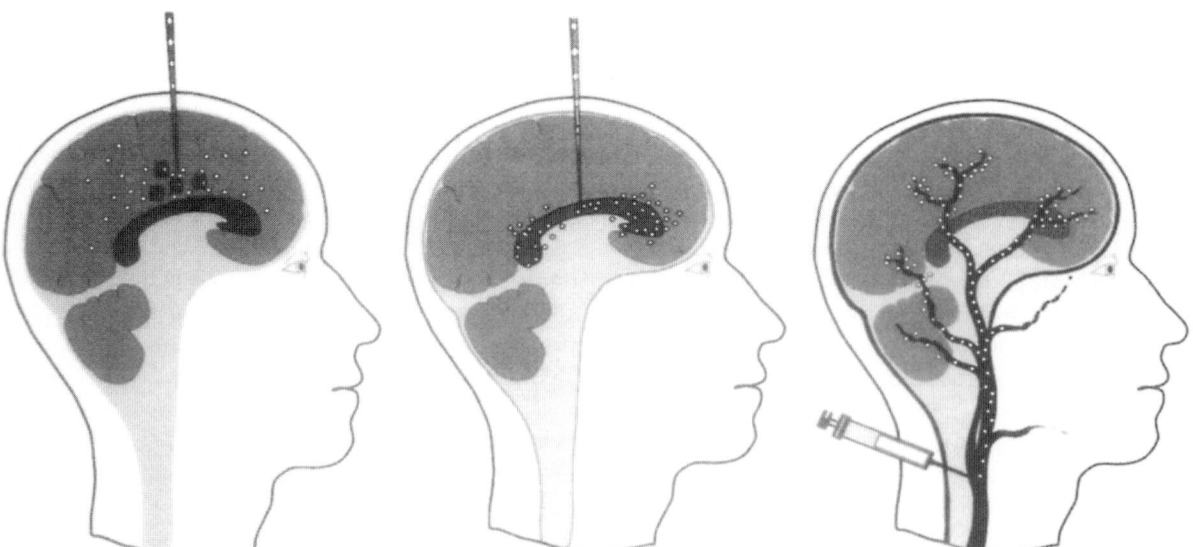

Fig. 26.1 Routes of delivery of gene therapy vectors to brain tumors (modified from Breakfield et al. 1995)

vascular endothelial cells. Similar blood-brain barrier disruption increases delivery of viral particles to brain parenchyma (NILAVER et al. 1995). The mode of viral uptake is unclear, since the pore size generated by osmotic disruption is only one-fourth the diameter of the viral particles. Penetration into the parenchyma is limited, as most viral particles are found in pericapillary cells.

RMP-7, an analogue of bradykinin, disrupts the blood-brain barrier pharmacologically by binding to a bradykinin receptor when injected intraarterially (MATSUKADO et al. 1996). Co-injection of viral vectors and RMP-7 significantly increases delivery to an intraparenchymal tumor over that achieved by injection of vector alone. Disadvantages of intravascular delivery include the need to inject the vector intraarterially and the risk of systemic toxicity from the large amount of vector not absorbed in the brain.

26.8
Clinical Trials: From Concept to Reality

In the past ten years, more than 300 experimental studies have investigated gene therapy for brain tumors. More than half a dozen clinical trials have been reported. Most have employed the tk-GCV paradigm. Both the initial study of 12 patients and a subsequent multi-centered trial of over 100 patients demonstrated that this form of retroviral gene therapy was safe but ineffective (RAM et al. 1997, KLATZMANN et al. 1998). Other studies have shown that this inefficacy reflects both limited dispersion of packaging cells and retroviral vectors from the site of injection, and low rates of tumor cell transduction and tk gene expression (HARSH et al. 2000). Further utilization of this and analogous paradigms must await improved methods of disseminated delivery of vector and more powerful promoters of transgene expression. Currently, there is enthusiasm for clinical trials of immuno-gene therapy in which genetic engineering techniques are used to modify cells used as anti-tumor vaccines so as to enhance the immune response they engender.

26.9
Conclusion

Gene therapy for brain tumors is in its infancy. Already, however, its tremendous potential is apparent.

The few clinical trials completed thus far have established the viability of the concept and its safety, when carefully applied, but not its efficacy.

In the near term, gene therapy approaches that circumvent the need for widespread delivery and high rates of in vivo transduction hold the most promise. That is, enhancement of the immune response by ex vivo modification of cells used for vaccination is currently more realistic than replacement of deleted tumor suppressor genes. In addition, chemosensitization paradigms requiring delivery and expression of genes for prodrug-activating enzymes will have significant anti-tumor activity only if an initial local effect is magnified and dispersed by the immune system.

In the longer term, improved methods of delivery and more specific targeting of transgenes to tumor cells, may make approaches requiring individual transfection of a high proportion of tumor cells more feasible. Intraparenchymal dispersion of therapeutic agents may be increased by the use of mobile neural stem cells as carriers, and by the pharmacological disruption of barriers not only between endothelial cells but also in the extraneural space. Identification of tumor-specific surface markers and glioma-associated extracellular matrix proteins, such as tenascin and vitronectin, should aid design of conjugates that can guide therapeutic vectors to the targeted tumor cells. Tumor-specific promoters, such as those for the E2F, TGF-alpha, and VEGF genes should help limit expression of potentially toxic therapeutic genes to tumor cells. And, as replication-competent oncolytic viruses are made more tumor-selective, they can be used with greater efficacy and less risk to the normal brain (MARTUZA et al. 1991).

In the future, gene therapy is likely to be part of a multi-modal approach to the treatment of gliomas, and gene therapy itself will be multi-modal. Surgery is likely to continue to be required for prompt reduction of tumor mass. Radiation therapy may be preceded by gene therapy designed to sensitize tumor cells and protect normal cells. Similarly, gene therapy may help increase the specificity of various chemotherapeutic agents for tumor cells. Oncolytic viruses targeted at tumor cells may be used to treat tumor remaining after a resection, either by direct cytolysis or by delivering genes to reverse the malignant phenotype. Other vehicles may deliver genes that restore tumor suppressor function, block tumor oncogenes, or induce apoptosis. Delivery methods, particularly for cytostatic therapies such as anti-angiogenesis, will need to allow repeated or even continuous therapy through indwelling infusion systems or slowly disintegrating polymers. Particularly for a diffusely invasive, commonly recurrent tumor such as malignant glioma, immune therapy will play a prominent role. Gene therapy techniques should prove tremendously valuable to efforts to increase anti-tumor immunity by enhancing the immune response at multiple levels (antigen recognition, antigen presentation, and cytokine production) and by diminishing tumor suppression of the immune response.

References

Ahmed S, Mineta T, Martuza RL et al. (1994) Antisense expression of protein kinase c-alpha inhibits the growth and tumorigenicity of human glioblastoma cells. Neurosurgery 35: 904–910

Andersen JK, Barber DA, Meaney CA et al. (1992) Gene transfer into mammalian CNS using herpes virus vectors: long term expression of bacterial lacZ in neurons using the neuron-specific enolase promoter. Hum Gene Ther 3:487–499

Badie B, Kramar MH, Lau L et al. (1998) Adenovirus-mediated p53 gene delivery potentiates the radiation-induced growth inhibition of experimental brain tumors. J Neurooncol 37:217–222

Bischoff JR, Kirn DH, William A et al. (1996) An Adenovirus mutant that replicates selectively in p53 deficient human tumor cells. Science 274:373–376

Blaese RM (1993) Treatment of severe combined immunodeficiency disease due to adenosine-deaminase deficiency with Cd34+ selected autologous peripherial blood cells transduced with a human ADA gene. Hum Gene Ther 4:521–527

Breakfield XO, Kramm CM, Chiocca EA, Pechan PA (1995) Herpes simplex vectors for tumor therpay. In: The Internet Book of Gene Therapy: Cancer Therapeutics. Sobol RE, Scanlon KJ, eds., Appleton and Large (Stamford CT), pp. 41–56

Calabretta B, Skorski T, Szzylik C. et al. (1993) Prospects for gene directed therapy with antisense oligodeoxynucleotides. Cancer Treat Rev 19:169–172

Chen SH, Shine HD, Goodman JC et al. (1994) Gene therapy for brain tumors:regression of experimental glioma by adenovirus mediated gene transfer in vivo. Proc Natl Acad Sci USA 91:3054–3057

Chiocca EA, Harsh G (1996) Gene transfer technology and its application to brain tumor therapy. The molecular basis of neurosurgical disease. William & Wilkins, Ed.Corey Raffel and Griffith R Harsh IV. pp 238–245..

Connors TA (1995) The choice of prodrugs for gene directed enzyme prodrug therapy of cancer. Gene Ther. 2:702–709

Dameron KM, Voipert OV, Tainsky MA et al. (1994) Control of angiogenesis in fibroblasts by p53 regulation of thrombospondin-1. Science 265:1582–1584

Dong Y, Wen P, Manome Y et al. (1996) In vivo replication-deficient adenovirus vector mediated transduction of the cytosine deaminase gene sensitizes glioma cells to 5-fluorocytosine. Hum Gene Ther 7:713–720

Dorigo O, Turla ST, Lebedeva S et al. (1998) Sensitization of rat glioblastoma mutiforme to cisplatin in vivo following restoration of wild type p53 function. J Neurosurg 88: 535–540

Dranoff G, Jaffee E, Lazenby A et al. (1993) Vaccination with irradiated tumor cells engineered to secrete murine granulocyte macrophage colony stimulating factor stimulate potent, specific, and long lasting antitumor immunity. Proc Natl Acad Sci USA 90:3539–3543

Fakhrai H, Dorigo O, Shawler DL et al. (1996) Eradication of established intracranial rat gliomas by transforming growth factor beta antisense therapy. Proc Natl Acad Sci USA 93:2909–2914

Fueyo J, Gomez-Manzano C, Puduvalli VK et al. (1998) Adenovirus- mediated p16 transfer to glioma cells induces G (1) arrest and protects from paclitaxel and topotecan: implications for therapy. International Journal of Oncology 12:665–669

Glick RP, Lichtor T, Kim TS et al. (1995) Fibroblasts genetically engineered to secrete cytokines suppress tumor growth and induce antitumor immunity to a murine glioma in vivo. Neurosurgery 36:548–555

Glorioso JC, Deluca NA, Fink DJ (1995) Development and application of herpes simplex virus vectors for human gene therapy. Annual Review of Microbiology 49:675–710

Gomez-Manzano C, Fueyo J, Kyritsis AP et al. (1996) Adenovirus-mediated transfer of p53 gene produces rapid and generalized death of human glioma cell via apoptosis. Cancer Res 56:694–699.

Halatsch ME, Schmidt U, Botefur I et al. (2000) Marked inhibition of glioblastoma target cell tumorigenicity in vitro by retrovirus-mediated transfer of a hairpin ribozyme against deletion-mutant epidermal growth factor receptor messager RNA. J Neurosurgery 92:297–305

Harada H, Nagagawa K, Iwata S et al. (1999) Restoration of wild type p16 down-regulates vascular endothelial growth factor expression and inhibits angiogenesis in human gliomas. Cancer Res 59:3783–3789

Harsh GR, Deisboeck TS, Louis DN et al. (2000) Thymidine kinase activation of ganciclovir in recurrent malignant gliomas: a gene marking and neuropathological study. J Neurosurgery 92:804–811

He TC, Zhou S, da Costa LT, Yu et al. (1998) A simplified system for generating recombinant adenoviruses. Proc Natl Acad Sci USA 95:2509–2514

Hsaio M, Tse V, Carmel J et al. (1997a) Intracavitary liposome-mediated p53 gene transfer into glioblastoma with endogenous wild-type p53 in vivo results in tumor suppression and long term survival. Biochem Biophys Res Commun 233:359–364

Hsaio M, Tse V, Carmel J et al. (1997b) Functional expression of human p21(waf1/CIP1) gene in rat glioma cells suppresses tumor growth in vivo and induces radiosensitivity. Biochem Biophys Res Commun 233:329–335

Hug P, Sleight RG (1994) Fusogenic virosomes prepared by partitioning of vesicular stomatitis virus G protein into preformed vesicles. J Biol Chem 269:4050–4056

Hung KS, Hong CY, Lee J et al. (2000) Expression of p16(INK4A) induces dominant suppression of glioblastoma growth in situ through necrosis and cell cycle arrest.Biochem Biophys Res Commun 260:718–725

Klatzmann D, Valery CA, Bensimon G et al. (1998)A phase 1/ 2 study of herpes simplex virus type 1 thymidine kinase suicide gene therapy for recurrent glioblastoma. Hum Gene Ther 9:2595–2604

Kramm CM, Chase M, Herrlinger U et al. (1997) Therapeutic efficiency and safety of a second-generation replication conditional HSV1 vector for brain tumor gene therapy. Hum Gene Ther 8:2057–2068

Laiu LM, Black KL, Prins RM et al. (1999) Treatment of intracranial gliomas with bone marrow-derived dendritic cells pulsed with tumor antigens. J Neurosurg 90:1115–1124

Laske DW, Youle RJ, Oldfield EH (1997) Tumor regression with regional distribution of target toxin TF-CRM 107 in patients with malignant brain tumors. Nat Med 3:1362–1368

Martuza RL, Malick A, Markert JM et al. (1991) Experimental therapy of human glioma by means of genetically engineered virus mutant. Science 252:854–856

Matsukado K, Inamura T, Nakano S et al. (1996) Enhanced tumor uptake of carboplatin and survival in glioma bearing rat by intracarotid infusion of bardykinin analog, RMP-7. Neurosurgery 39;125–133

Millauer B, Longhi MP, Plate KH et al. (1996) Dominant-negative inhibition of FLK-1 suppresses growth of many tumor types in vivo. Cancer Res 56:1615–1620

Nilaver G, Muldoon LL, Kroll RA et al. (1995) Delivery of herpesvirus and adenovirus to nude rat intracerebral tumors after osmotic blood brain barrier disruption. Pro Natl Acad Sci USA 92:9829–9833

OíReeilly MS, Holmgren L, Chen C et al. (1996) Angiostatin induces and sustains dormancy of human primary tumors in mice. Nat Med 2:689–692

Paulus W, Baur I, Boyce FM et al. (1996) Self contained tetracycline regulated retroviral vector system for gene delivery to mammalian cells. Journal of Virology 70:62–67

Perales JC, Ferkol T, Molas M et al. (1994) An evaluation of receptor-mediated gene transfer using synthetic DNA-ligand complexes. European Journal of Biochemistry 226:255–266

Pietsch T, Wiestler OD (1997) Molecular neuropathology of astrocytic brain tumors. J Neurooncol 35:211–222

Ram Z, Culver KW, Walbridge S et al. (1993) In situ retroviral-mediated gene transfer for the treatment of brain tumors in rats. Cancer Res53:83–88

Ram Z, Walbridge S, Shawker T et al. (1994) The effect of thymidine kinase transduction and ganciclovir therapy on tumor vasculature and growth of 9L gliomas in rats. J Neurosurg 81:256–260

Ram Z, Culver KW, Oshiro EM et al. (1997) Therapy of malignant brain tumors by intratumoral implantation of retrovirus vector producing cells. Nat Med 3, 3:1354–1361.

Saleh M, Stacker SA, Wilks AF (1996) Inhibition of growth of C6 glioma cells in vivo by expression of antisense vascular endothelial growth factor sequence. Cancer Res 56:393–401

Tamiya T, Wei MX, Chase M et al. (1995) Transgene inheritance and retroviral infection contribute to the efficiency of gene expression in solid tumors inoculated with retroviral vector producer cells. Gene Ther 2:531–538

Tenenbaum L, Darling JL, Hooghe-Peters E (1994) Adenovirus (AAV) as vector for gene transfer into glial cells of the human central nervous system. Gene Ther 1:580–585

Trojan J, Johnson TR, Rudin SD et al. (1993) Treatment and prevention of rat glioblastoma by C6 cells expressing antisense IGF-1 RNA. Science 259:94–97

Vogelbaum MA, Tong JXX, Higashikubo R et al. (1998) Transfection of C6 glioma cells with Bax gene and increased sensitivity to treatment of with cytosine arabinoside. J Neurosurgery 998;88:99–105

Zerrouqi A, Rixe O, Ghoumari AM et al. (1996) Liposomal delivery of the herpes simplex virus thymidine kinase gene in glioma: improvement cell sensitization to ganciclovir. Cancer Gene Ther 3:385–392

27 Radiation Therapy in the Management of Pediatric Brain Tumors

Robert S. Lavey

CONTENTS

27.1 Introduction

Tumors of the brain constitute 17% of all malignant tumors among children younger than 20 years of age in the United States, making them the most common solid neoplasm and the second most common malignancy in children after leukemia. The annual incidence is approximately 2.9 cases per 100,000 children per year, representing 2000 new cases in the United States annually. The incidence of childhood brain tumors sharply increased in the 1980s, coincident with the wide availability of magnetic resonance imaging, but was stable from 1986 to 1995 (GURNEY et al. 1996; RIES et al. 1999). Approximately 40% of children with brain tumors die of their disease (DUF-FNER et al. 1986). The 5-year relative survival for these tumors increased in the United States from 59% during 1975–1984 to 67% during 1985–1994 (RIES et al. 1999). The histologic distribution of childhood brain tumors, shown in Table 27.1, is markedly different from that seen in adults. The relative frequency of malignant central nervous system tumors among children under 20 years of age is:

astrocytomas 52%, primitive neuroectodermal tumors 21%, other gliomas 15%, ependymomas 9%, and others 3% (RIES et al. 1999). The supratentorial location predominates in infants as it does in adults, but infratentorial tumors constitute approximately half of all brain tumors in children 1–15 years of age. Radiation therapy is the mainstay of treatment of brain stem gliomas, and has an important role in the management of most other brain tumors. This chapter will discuss the role of radiation therapy in the management of the most common childhood brain tumors.

27.2 Radiation Therapy to the Brain in Children

Radiation therapy is generally delivered once per day, 5 days per week, in fractions of 180 cGy each. The number of fractions and total dose varies according to the tumor histology. In most cases, a cumulative dose of 4,500–5,940 cGy is given in 25–33 daily fractions over a period of 5–7 weeks. The treatment vol-

R. S. LAVEY, MD, MPH
Head, Radiation Oncology Program, Associate Professor, Department of Pediatrics and Radiation Oncology, University of Southern California, 4650 Sunset Boulevard, Mail Stop 54, Los Angeles, CA 90027-6016, USA

Table 27.1. Relative incidence of common brain tumors in children

Supratentorial tumors	49%	Infratentorial tumors	51%
Astrocytoma	23%	Medulloblastoma	20%
Malignant gliomas (anaplastic astrocytoma, glioblastoma multiforme)	6%	Astrocytoma	17%
Craniopharyngioma	6%	Brain stem glioma	8%
Embryonal tumors (PNET and others)	4%	Ependymoma	6%
Pineal region and germ cell tumors	3%		
Ependymoma	3%		
Oligodendroglioma	2%		
Other (meningioma, ganglioma, choroid plexus tumors, others)	2%		

ume includes the entire neuraxis (whole brain, spinal cord, and spinal nerve roots) for primitive neuroectodermal tumors, medulloblastoma, germinoma, and choroid plexus carcinoma. The target volume for other common brain tumors is the gross tumor with a 1- to 2-cm margin. Radiation fields are designed to minimize the volume of brain subjected to a high total dose and minimize the dose to such radiosensitive normal tissues as the lenses of the eyes, thyroid gland, and mucosa of the upper aerodigestive tract. The target volume is irradiated through multiple, custom-shaped fields each day to deliver a higher radiation dose to the target than to the surrounding normal tissues. Hyperfractionated, or twice daily, radiation has not been demonstrated to be beneficial for the treatment of any childhood brain tumor histology. To achieve adequate coverage of the target volume while minimizing radiation to surrounding normal tissues, the patient must be in the same position for each treatment, and must not alter position during the treatment. Brain irradiation is usually delivered in the supine position with a headrest under the neck and back of the head combined with a custom thermoplastic mask over the face or bite block molded to the maxillary teeth for immobilization and treatment field reproducibility. Craniospinal (neuraxis) irradiation is delivered in the prone position to permit visualization of the match line between the spinal and cranial fields along the posterior surface of the neck. Reproducible positioning in the prone position is aided by use of custom body and face cushions and a custom thermoplastic mask placed over the back of the head. The great majority of patients under the age of 6 years do not cooperate sufficiently to enable precise delivery of the radiation therapy. These children are sedated or anesthetized daily for treatment. Intravenous sedation is preferred to oral sedation as it is faster acting, requires a shorter recovery period, is more reliable, and requires less patient cooperation for administration.

The adverse effects of radiation therapy are classified according to time of onset. Early adverse effects occur during or within 1 month of the completion of treatment. If nausea, vomiting, fatigue, altered taste sensation, and anorexia do not occur during the first week of treatment, the patient will probably remain free of these symptoms. Hair loss within the radiation fields generally begins during the second or third week of therapy, and often becomes complete. Skin hyperpigmentation, erythema, dryness, and desquamation within the radiation fields generally occurs over the surfaces receiving high doses of radiation, becomes more pronounced toward the end of the course of treatment, and resolves starting in the second week following the completion of therapy. The pinnae and retroauricular skin surfaces tend to show the greatest radiation sensitivity. Diminished blood counts are generally seen with craniospinal irradiation, but not with irradiation of the brain alone. Craniospinal irradiation also commonly causes nausea, vomiting, and odynophagia. These early side effects generally completely resolve shortly after completion of radiation therapy with the exception of alopecia, which can be permanent in areas that are exposed to doses above 4000 cGy. Rare complications that may appear 1–2 months following completion of radiation therapy and persist for weeks to months are somnolence syndrome, consisting of lethargy, anorexia, and headache, and Lhermitte's sign in patients who have undergone craniospinal irradiation, a sensation of electric discharge down the spine and limbs on neck flexion.

The greatest concern related to brain irradiation of children is the development of late sequelae more than 6 months beyond the completion of therapy. The occurrence of all the late sequelae outlined in Table 27.2 increases in frequency and severity with increasing radiation dose and treatment volume. The severity of cognitive and learning deficits is inversely associated with patient age (GRILL et al. 1999; MULHERN et al. 1991, 1998; GOLDWEIN et al. 1996; MOORE et al. 1991; DENNIS et al. 1996). Due to unacceptable neuropsychologic sequelae, brain irradiation that would be indicated for tumors in children over 3 years of age is usually supplanted by chemotherapy in children less than 3 years old (SPUNBERG et al. 1981; SILBER et al. 1992; COPELAND et al. 1999). This chapter will discuss the treatment of children over the age of 3 years. Therapy for children younger than 3 years is discussed in Chap. 29. Irradiation of the pituitary gland can cause diminution of production of growth hormone, thyroid stimulating hormone, and gonadotropin starting 1–5 years after radiation therapy. Pituitary dysfunction should be expected after a dose above 3,000 cGy (SHALET 1982, 1993; NEWMAN et al. 1981; RICHARDS et al. 1976; DUFFNER et al. 1985; CONSTINE et al. 1993). Brain necrosis is a rare complication when radiation therapy is delivered using conventional fraction sizes to recommended dose limits. Symptoms include headache, personality change, seizures, lethargy, hemiparesis, nausea, and vomiting in addition to focal neurologic deficits, with onset 9–24 months after

Table 27.2. Childhood central nervous system toxicities from radiation (from PIZZO and POPLACK)

Syndrome	Cause	Incidence	Onset	Clinical manifestation	Outcome
Somnolence syndrome	Whole-brain RT	Increases with increasing doses of RT	4–8 weeks after RT	7–14 days of lethargy, malaise, nausea, vomiting, psychologic alterations	Resolves spontaneously
Radionecrosis	Dose >5,500 cGy or high fraction size	0.1–1% with conventional RT, common after stereotactic or interstitial RT	6 months to 3 years after RT	Focal neurologic dysfunction, seizures, obtundation, coma	Recovery after resection
Necrotizing leukoencephalopathy	High total dose or dose per fraction, potentiated by MTX	0.5–2.0% after 2,400 cGy RT alone; up to 55% with concomitant MTX	Usually 4–12 months after RT	Spasticity, ataxia, lethargy, dementia, pseudobulbar paresis	Stable or progressive
Mineralizing microangiopathy with dystrophic calcification	≥2,000 cGy RT	15–30% after 2,400 cGy		Usually none, TIA, headaches, seizures	Usually asymptomatic
Neuropsychologic damage	1,800 cGy	>50% after ≥2,400 cGy; Increased with younger age at treatment	1–3 years after RT	Cognitive deficits, learning deficits, behavioral abnormalities	Progressive
Endocrinologic dysfunction	>2,000 cGy to pituitary	75% after 3,600 cGy	1–5 years after RT	Growth failure, thyroid gonadotropin, deficiency	Static; requires hormonal replacement

treatment. Microangiopathy with dystrophic calcification is a common pathologic finding in patients treated with more than 1,800 cGy to the whole brain. It can be asymptomatic or manifest as headaches, seizures, transient ischemic events, and strokes (WRIGHT and BRESHAN 1976; RUDOLTZ et al. 1998). Moyamoya syndrome, a vasculopathy of the large vessels of the internal carotid artery in the circle of Willis, may occur after high-dose irradiation of the parasellar region and manifest as transient ischemic events and infarction (RAJAKULASINGAM et al. 1979; KESTLE et al. 1993). Diminution in cranial and spinal bone growth can occur after exposure to 1,000 cGy and should be expected after doses above 2,000 cGy (NEUHAUSER et al. 1952; SHALET et al. 1978; PROBERT et al. 1973; DENYS et al. 1998). Second neoplasms occur within the radiation field in at least 1% of patients. The majority of these tumors are high-grade gliomas, meningiomas, sarcomas, or thyroid carcinoma (DUFFNER et al. 1998; HAWKINS et al. 1987; LI et al. 1984; NEGLIA et al. 1991; TSANG et al. 1993; JANHOUN et al. 1990; PACKER et al. 1987; WALTER et al. 1998; RELLING et al. 1999).

27.3 Low-Grade Gliomas

Low-grade (WHO grade I–II) glioma tumors are a heterogeneous group of neoplasms. The most common histologies are astrocytomas or mixed astrocytoma-oligodendrogliomas in the supratentorium and pilocytic astrocytoma in the cerebellum. Reports differ as to whether the histologic subtype influences prognosis (POLLACK et al. 1995; HIRSCH et al. 1989; HAYOSTEK et al. 1993). Tumor location influences the extent of resection that is feasible. Among cerebellar astrocytomas, the presence of brain stem involvement is a poor prognostic factor (GEISSINGER and BUCY 1971; FERBERT 1985). Among supratentorial tumors, location is probably not a prognostic factor, independent of extent of resection and tumor grade. Patient age is not associated with prognosis within the pediatric population (PALMA and GUIDETTI 1985; SHIBAMOTO 1993). Most series suggest that pilocytic and oligodendroglial tumors have a better prognosis than the fibrillary and diffuse astrocytomas (POLLACK et al. 1995; SHAW et al. 1989;

HAYOSTEK et al. 1993; PALMA and GUIDETTI 1985; MEDBERY et al. 1988). Standard policy for diagnosis and treatment is maximum feasible surgical resection. Gross total excision for diagnosis and treatment is possible in the majority of tumors located in the cerebral hemispheres or cerebellum. Complete resection without adjuvant therapy is associated with 10-year survival rates of 70–90% for supratentorial tumors (POLLACK et al. 1995; HIRSCH et al. 1089; TIYAWORADUN et al. 1981; JANSS et al. 1995), and 90–100% for cerebellar tumors (GARCIA et al. 1989; LEIBEL et al. 1975). Given these high survival rates, the generally indolent natural history of low-grade astrocytomas, and the opportunity to perform a second resection if disease recurs, adjuvant postoperative radiation and chemotherapy are generally not used for completely resected low-grade gliomas.

There is much more controversy regarding postoperative treatment of incompletely resected astrocytomas. A prospective trial randomizing children with incompletely resected low-grade astrocytomas to observation vs radiation therapy conducted jointly by the Pediatric Oncology Group (POG) and Children's Cancer Group (CCG) was closed due to insufficient patient accrual. It is unlikely that another randomized trial to determine the role of postoperative radiation therapy for incompletely resected low-grade gliomas will be attempted. Postoperative involved field radiation therapy for incompletely resected supratentorial astrocytomas produced a 10-year progression-free survival of 80–90% in three series (POLLACK et al. 1995; SHAW et al. 1989; WALLNER et al. 1988). This was double the progression-free survival of incompletely resected patients not given postoperative radiation therapy in one institution, but did not translate into a significant benefit in overall survival (POLLACK et al. 1995). The age of the patient is an important factor in deciding whether to give postoperative radiation therapy. Younger children are more likely to be observed, with radiation therapy reserved until after a second incomplete resection for progressive disease. Arguments for the observation approach include the finding that a significant minority of incompletely resected tumors do not progress, tumors that do progress can be effectively treated by second resection and postoperative irradiation, and that the brain matures during the years between tumor resections, thereby decreasing the neuropsychologic sequelae of radiation therapy. An additional concern about use of radiation is the suggestion that it may be associated with late anaplastic transformation of low-grade tumors (POLLACK et al. 1995; DIRKSET et al. 1994). The rate of anaplastic degeneration of pilocytic astrocytomas, however, was noted to be no higher following surgery with postoperative radiation therapy than after surgery alone (KRIEGER et al. 1997). The rationale for immediate use of radiation therapy is that it decreases the likelihood of tumor progression and need for a second resection and that tumor growth or malignant degeneration may necessitate irradiation of a larger volume of brain. For tumors involving the optic nerves or optic chiasm causing visual deterioration, radiation therapy results in improved vision in 25–35% of children (TAO et al. 1997; JANSS et al. 1995; PACKER et al. 1983; HORWICH et al. 1985). Objective tumor reduction occurs in approximately 50% of children (FLETCHER et al. 1986; TAO et al. 1997). A CCG study opened in 1997 is investigating the efficacy of chemotherapy in place of radiation therapy for children less than 10 years old with progressive or incompletely resected tumors at high risk for causing neurologic impairment.

When radiation therapy is given for a low-grade astrocytoma, the volume selected is based on the finding that the vast majority of recurrences are local only. The target volume is usually defined by contrast-enhanced MRI scan with a 1–2-cm margin. For the unusual case with proven multifocal involvement or leptomeningeal dissemination, craniospinal irradiation is appropriate. Retrospective series indicate that radiation doses above 45–53 Gy result in better progression-free survival rates than lower radiation doses (SHAW et al. 1989, 1993; ALBRIGHT et al. 1985). A cumulative dose of 5,400–5,580 cGy is generally given over 6 weeks. The dose may be reduced to 5,040 cGy in children under 5 years of age.

27.4
High-Grade (Malignant) Gliomas

Approximately 85% of the high-grade (WHO grade III–IV) gliomas exclusive of brain stem glioma occur supratentorially. Survival in patients with high-grade astrocytomas is much lower than with low-grade astrocytomas, even among the minority whose tumor is grossly completely resected and despite the standard use of postoperative radiation therapy in patients above 3 years of age. A careful examination for evidence of metastatic disease is required prior to initiating radiation therapy. Leptomeningeal dissemination has been reported in 10–15% of children at diagnosis. Craniospinal irradiation to the whole spinal cord tolerance dose of 3,600 cGy is appropriate for children with disseminated disease. Tumor progression generally occurs locally prior to any evidence of metastatic spread. For tumors without evidence of metastases, the initial radiation field encompasses the contrast-enhancing lesion on preoperative MRI scan with a 2–3-cm margin. Most treatment protocols do not consider the area of signal abnormality consistent with edema that commonly surrounds these tumors as part of the tumor volume. The dose to the initial target volume is 4,500–5,400 cGy delivered over 5–6 weeks. This is followed by an additional dose to a boost volume including the preoperative enhancing lesion with a 1-cm margin to bring the cumulative dose to 5,940 cGy given over 6 1/2 weeks. The dose is limited by the tolerance of the normal brain. Despite maximum feasible surgical resection and postoperative irradiation, the 5-year overall survival of these patients is only 10–30% with a median duration of survival of 18–24 months (BLOOM et al. 1990; SPOSTO et al. 1987; DROPCHO et al. 1987). Long-term survival is only slightly better in grade III than in grade IV tumors, as shown in Table 27.3 (HEIDEMAN et al. 1997; FINLAY et al. 1995). Chemotherapy has not been shown to significantly improve survival (FINLAY et al. 1995). Techniques to increase the radiation dose to the tumor without exceeding normal tissue tolerance are being investigated in an attempt to improve patient survival. Multiple institutions have reported their experience with temporary implants of radioactive

Iodine-125 (GUTIN et al. 1985; VOGES et al. 1990; FORITANESI et al. 1995) or stereotactic radiosurgery (LOEFFLER et al. 1992). Additional experience is necessary to determine whether these or other techniques, such as dose escalation using conformal radiation therapy or radiosensitizers, are of benefit.

27.5
Brain Stem Gliomas

The clinical behavior of and treatment for brain stem gliomas is dependent upon the location and aggressiveness of the tumor. Of all brain stem tumors, 70–80% are of the diffusely infiltrating pontine glioma type. The diffusely infiltrating pontine tumors are diagnosed by MRI scan, and biopsy is unnecessary. Prognosis is not associated with their histologic grade. The standard treatment is involved field radiation therapy with dexamethasone to decrease the peritumoral inflammatory response and intracranial pressure. Dexamethasone is weaned over the course of radiation therapy as tolerated. Focal and dorsal exophytic tumors may be biopsied or partially resected. The dorsally exophytic tumors are generally pilocytic astrocytomas for which postoperative radiation therapy is not necessary even in cases of incomplete resection. Progression-free survival for the exophytic tumors after partial resection alone has

Table 27.3. Survival rate in high-grade pediatric astrocytomas according to therapy (from Pizzo and Poplack)

Treatment	Survival in years (%)				Reference
	1	2	3	5	
Surgery alone					
Grade IV	8		0		SHELINE 1977
Surgery+radiation	72	48	10–32	10–29	BLOOM et al. 1990; SPOSTO et al. 1989; DROPCHO et al. 1987
Grade III	74	56	50	0–44	MARCHESE et al. 1990; LEIBEL et al. 1975; SHELINE 1977
Grade IV	33–67	15–26		5–26	MARCHESE et al. 1990; LEIBEL et al. 1975; SHELINE 1977; DOHRMANN et al. 1985
Surgery+RT+CT	29–80			16–46	SPOSTO et al. 1989; FINLAY et al. 1995
Grade III				28	FINLAY et al. 1995
Grade IV				16	FINLAY et al. 1995

been reported to be 45–70% at 5–10 years (Hoffman et al. 1980; Pollack et al. 1993; Khatib et al. 1994; Heron et al. 1999). Leptomeningeal dissemination of dorsally exophytic tumors is rare. For tectal plate and dorsally exophytic tumors, progressive disease can usually be salvaged by involved field radiation therapy (Pollack et al. 1993; Stroink et al. 1986; Khatib et al. 1994; Heron et al. 1999).

The diffusely infiltrating pontine gliomas generally progress locally with subarachnoid seeding in 2–15% of cases (Packer et al. 1993; Mandell et al. 1999). Radiation therapy relieves the presenting neurologic symptoms and dependence on corticosteroids in most pontine glioma patients, but the respite from rapid local disease progression is temporary in 90% of cases. Chemotherapy, whether given concurrently with or following radiation therapy, has not been demonstrated to prolong survival. The initial radiation field should encompass the gross tumor as defined on MRI scan with a 2-cm margin to a total dose of 5,400–5,940 cGy over 6–6 1/2 weeks. Based on promising data from single institutions, POG performed a dose escalation trial to determine the optimal hyperfractionated, twice-daily radiation therapy regimen to test against the standard once-daily fractionation to 5,400 cGy (Freeman et al. 1993, 1996; Freeman 1996). The regimen with the best survival outcome, 117 cGy given twice daily to a total dose of 7,020 cGy, was tested in the randomized, phase III POG-9239 study. Adjuvant cisplatin chemotherapy was given to all 128 study patients. Clinical neurologic improvement during radiation therapy was reported for 95% of patients. Survival was equivalent in the two arms, 7% at 2 years and 4% at 3 years. The median time to disease progression was 5–6 months and median time to death was 8 months. Among patients with progressive disease, the initial site of progression was local only in 98% and local with subarachnoid seeding in 2% (Mandell et al. 1999). The POG findings are consistent with two single-arm CCG trials of hyperfractionated radiation therapy given to newly diagnosed pontine glioma patients in 100 cGy fractions twice daily. Among 53 children treated to a total dose of 7,200 cGy, overall survival was 14% at 2 years and 8% at 3 years. The median time to disease progression was 5.5 months, and median time to death was 9 months (Packer et al. 1993). Among 66 children treated to a total dose of 7,800 cGy, overall survival was 22% at 2 years and 11% at 3 years. The median time to disease progression was 8 months and median time to death was 10 months (Packer et al. 1994). Radiation dose escalation through the use of a stereotactic boost has also not

been successful in significantly prolonging median or long-term survival in preliminary reports.

27.6
Primitive Neuroectodermal Tumors Including Medulloblastoma

Primitive neuroectodermal tumors (PNET) may occur anywhere in the body within or outside the central nervous system. The most common location is in the cerebellum, where they are referred to as posterior fossa PNET or medulloblastoma. The incidence of leptomeningeal or subarachnoid dissemination is between 10 and 40% (Tomita et al. 1988; Albright et al. 1995; Geyer et al. 1994; Allen and Epstein 1982; Deutsch 1980). Extraneural dissemination, most commonly to bone, occurs in approximately 5% of patients (Kleinman et al. 1984; Tarbell et al. 1991; Evans et al. 1990; Campbell et al. 1984). The staging evaluation for PNET of the central nervous system includes cerebrospinal fluid cytology and MRI of the entire spine and brain. PNET is classified as high-risk if the primary tumor is located outside the posterior fossa, there is metastatic disease, or there is more than 1.5 cm^3 of residual disease on postoperative MRI scan. Posterior fossa tumors without dissemination that have been grossly resected (less than 1.5 cm^3 residual on postoperative MRI scan) are classified as average-risk. As extent of resection is a prognostic feature, maximum feasible resection is performed for diagnosis and treatment. Craniospinal irradiation is given starting 3–6 weeks following surgical resection. Traditional treatment for both average- and high-risk patients has included craniospinal radiation to a total dose of 3,500–3,600 cGy followed by a boost providing 5,400–5,580 cGy to the posterior fossa for medulloblastoma or the preoperative tumor volume with a 1-cm margin for supratentorial disease. Several retrospective series have reported a dose–response effect, with higher progression-free and overall survival rates noted among medulloblastoma patients treated to a cumulative posterior fossa dose greater than 5,000 cGy (Cumberlin et al. 1979; Chin and Maruyama 1981; Silverman and Simpson 1982; Khafaga et al. 1996), 5,200 cGy (Berry et al. 1981), or 5,300 cGy (Tarbell et al. 1991).

Postoperative radiation therapy for high-risk PNET is generally given according to the traditional protocol of 3,500–3,600 cGy to the entire neuraxis followed by a boost to the entire posterior fossa for a posterior fossa tumor or the preoperative tumor bed with a 1-cm margin for a supratentorial tumor to a total dose of 5,400–5,580 cGy over 6 weeks. Focal gross metastases in the spinal column are treated to a total dose of 5,040 cGy with a 2-cm margin. The dose to the gross disease in the spine is lower than in the brain to accommodate the tolerance of the spinal cord. Reported progression-free survival after radiation therapy alone in randomized cooperative group trials has ranged from 0–56%, partially due to different definitions of high-risk disease. Escalation of the radiation dose through hyperfractionated radiation has been shown to be feasible in single institution studies and the single-arm CCG-9931 trial, but has not resulted in improved patient survival. A retrospective study of 109 medulloblastoma patients treated at a single institution found no improvement in 5-year survival among the 32 children treated with 100 cGy twice daily to a total posterior fossa dose of 7,200 cGy (46%) compared to the 77 children treated with the conventional 180 cGy once daily to 5,400 cGy (51%) (WARA et al. 1999).

The high incidence and severity of cognitive deficits following 3,500–3,600 cGy to the entire brain has led to studies investigating whether the craniospinal irradiation dose can be reduced without sacrificing tumor control in average-risk PNET patients. A French multi-institutional trial assessed the efficacy of postoperative chemotherapy incorporating eight drugs in 1 day and high-dose methotrexate followed by posterior fossa and spinal irradiation for nondisseminated medulloblastoma. The omission of supratentorial irradiation resulted in a 4-year survival of 18%, with the supratentorium the initial site of recurrence in 56% of patients (BOUFFET et al. 1992). The International Society of Paediatric Oncology (SIOP) and German Society of Paediatric Oncology jointly conducted a double-randomization trial, in which 153 "low-risk" patients were randomized to receive a craniospinal dose of 3,500 or 2,500 cGy and postoperative radiation therapy alone or preceded

by a 6-week course of vincristine, procarbazine, and methotrexate. The 5-year progression-free survival was 68% in the conventional-dose arm compared to 55% in the reduced-dose arm (P=0.07). Among the 74 patients given preradiation chemotherapy, 5-year progression-free survival was markedly lower in the reduced craniospinal dose than the standard dose group (42% vs 75%, P=0.005). Progression-free survival did not differ significantly between the dose groups that received postoperative radiation therapy alone (60 vs 69%) (BAILEY et al. 1995).

The CCG and POG jointly conducted a trial in which 123 average-risk PNET patients were randomized to receive a craniospinal dose of 3,600 or 2,340 cGy. The boost dose to the posterior fossa was 5,400 cGy in both arms. The 5-year progression-free survival was 63% in the conventional-dose arm compared to 54% in the reduced-dose arm (P=0.06) (Table 27.4). The study was closed to patient accrual early due to the finding of a statistically significant increase in isolated neuraxis and total relapses in the reduced-dose group after a median follow-up of 16 months. Early closure of the study proved to be unfortunate, as with additional follow-up time the difference in progression-free survival between groups diminished to a trend not reaching statistical significance (DEUTSCH et al. 1996). Among the surviving patients, there was less chronic neuropsychologic toxicity in the group that received the 2,340 cGy craniospinal dose (MULHERN et al. 1998). The demonstrated reduction in toxicity provided a rationale for continuing to investigate the efficacy of reduced-dose craniospinal irradiation. The CCG conducted a single-arm pilot study evaluating the efficacy of 2,340 cGy craniospinal irradiation supplemented by concurrent weekly vincristine and followed by eight cycles of cisplatin, CCNU, and vincristine chemotherapy in 65 children with nondisseminated medulloblastoma. The 5-year progression-free survival was 79%, which is at least as good as obtained in prior CCG studies using 3,600 cGy craniospinal

Table 27.4. Average-risk medulloblastoma: Randomized cooperative group trials of craniospinal dose

Group	Patients	Craniospinal dose (Gy)	Posterior fossa dose (Gy)	Chemotherapy	5-year PFS	P value
SIOP	76	35	55	± PVM	68%	0.07
(BAILEY et al. 1995)		25	55	± PVM	55%	
POG/CCG	123	36	54	None	63%	0.06
(DEUTSCH et al. 1996)		23.4	54	None	54%	

PFS, progression-free survival; P, cisplatin; V, vincristine; M, methotrexate.

radiation alone (Packer et al. 1999). Given this encouraging result, the POG–CCG opened another joint randomized trial in 1994 comparing the efficacy and neuropsychologic toxicity of the pilot study regimen to 3,600 cGy craniospinal irradiation without chemotherapy. The posterior fossa was irradiated to a dose of 5,580 cGy in both treatment arms. The trial was closed in 1995 due to accrual of only 48 patients over 18 months, an insufficient number to answer the study questions. The current joint POG–CCG randomized protocol utilizes 2,340 cGy craniospinal irradiation with a boost dose of 5,580 cGy to the entire posterior fossa in both arms. Patients are randomized between two postradiation chemotherapy regimens. We will not learn how either of these regimens compares with giving 3,600 cGy craniospinal irradiation without chemotherapy.

In addition to craniospinal axis dose, a significant controversy in radiation therapy of medulloblastoma is the boost field volume. Currently, the inclusion of the entire posterior fossa must be considered the standard field. The necessity of boosting the entire posterior fossa rather than the tumor bed with a margin has been questioned (Fukunaga-Johnson et al. 1998). Institutions using a smaller boost field argue that the diminished field size may decrease the degree of ototoxicity and neuropsychologic deficits compared with full posterior fossa boost irradiation. It is unknown whether an increased incidence of failure within the posterior fossa will be seen with this approach. Until these data have been accumulated, a boost volume encompassing less than the entire posterior fossa must be considered experimental.

Several studies have been conducted to evaluate whether survival rates can be improved by the addition of chemotherapy to conventional-dose craniospinal irradiation. A CCG trial randomized 233 patients to radiation therapy with concurrent vincristine followed by eight cycles of CCNU, vincristine, and prednisone or radiation therapy alone (Table 27.5). The chemotherapy did not significantly improve 5-year progression-free (59% vs 50%) or overall survival (65% vs 65%) (Evans et al. 1990). In the SIOP I trial, 286 patients were randomized to radiation therapy with concurrent vincristine alone or followed by eight cycles of CCNU and vincristine. There was no significant difference in 5-year progression-free survival between treatment groups (42% vs 55%) (Tait et al. 1990). In both cooperative group studies, subgroup analysis suggested that maintenance chemotherapy following conventional-dose irradiation may be beneficial for medulloblastoma patients with high-risk characteristics. The combination of radiation with weekly vincristine followed by cisplatin, CCNU, and vincristine chemotherapy produced an 85% 5-year progression-free survival in a single-arm study conducted at five institutions in the United States. This trial included some patients who would currently be classified as average-risk. The subgroup of patients with metastatic disease had a 5-year progression-free survival of 67% (Packer et al. 1994). These results have led to the widespread use of combined radiation and chemotherapy for high-risk PNET, despite the lack of a randomized trial demonstrating the benefit of chemotherapy.

The potential value of giving chemotherapy prior to the start of radiation therapy has been assessed in several trials. The SIOP II trial randomized 364 patients to immediate postoperative radiation therapy

Table 27.5. Medulloblastoma: randomized cooperative group trials of postoperative radiation therapy (RT) alone vs postoperative radiation therapy and chemotherapy

Group	Patients	Treatment	5-year PFS	5-year OS
CCG (Evans et al. 1990)	233	RT Alone	50%	65%
		(RT+V) =>CVPred	59%	65%
SIOP I (Tait et al. 1990)	286	(RT+V)	42%	
		(RT+V) =>CV	55%	
SIOP II (Bailey et al. 1995)	244 Low-risk	RT alone	65%	
		PVM =>RT	59%	
	133 High-risk	RT =>VC	56%	
		PVM =>RT =>VC	53%	

RT+V, RT with weekly vincristine; Pred, prednisone; P, procarbazine; C, CCNU; V, vincristine; M, methotrexate; PFS, progression-free survival; OS, overall survival.

or a 6-week course of procarbazine, vincristine, and methotrexate prior to radiation therapy. Low-risk patients did not receive maintenance chemotherapy, while high-risk patients in both arms were given six cycles of vincristine and CCNU following radiation therapy. The preradiation chemotherapy did not improve 5-year progression-free survival overall (58% vs 60%, P=0.7) neither in the high-risk (56% vs 53%, P=0.7) nor low-risk subgroups (59% vs 65%) (BAILEY et al. 1995). A single-arm CCG study of preradiation chemotherapy followed by hyperfractionated radiation has shown a significant incidence of tumor progression during the 16-week course of neoadjuvant chemotherapy. In both the CCG and POG single-arm studies of neoadjuvant chemotherapy prior to craniospinal irradiation, disease progressed in a substantial proportion of patients during the neoadjuvant chemotherapy phase. An additional 25% of patients failed to undergo the course of standard radiation therapy (HEIDEMAN et al. 1995; HARTSELL et al. 1997; MOSIJCZUK et al. 1993). The POG-9031 trial randomized 226 patients to postoperative craniospinal irradiation and maintenance chemotherapy given alone or preceded by neoadjuvant chemotherapy. The 4-year progression-free survival was 62% with and 73% without preradiation chemotherapy. The SIOP III trial is again randomizing patients with nondisseminated medulloblastoma to conventional-dose craniospinal irradiation with or without preradiation chemotherapy. Given the negative results of previous trials, postoperative radiation therapy should be delayed for chemotherapy only in the setting of a clinical trial.

Conventional radiation therapy for PNET of the brain is 3,600 cGy to the entire neuraxis followed by a boost to give the local supratentorial primary site or the entire posterior fossa a dose of 5,400–5,580 cGy. Currently, either conventional-dose radiation thera-

py alone or reduced-dose craniospinal irradiation with concurrent and postradiation chemotherapy can be considered an acceptable treatment for average-risk PNET outside the study setting. High-risk PNET should be treated with conventional-dose radiation therapy. Single-arm studies and subgroup analyses of randomized trials suggest that concurrent and maintenance chemotherapy may improve survival for high-risk disease. Neoadjuvant chemotherapy and hyperfractionated radiation therapy have not been found to improve patient survival and should be considered experimental treatments.

27.7
Ependymomas

Ependymomas arise within or adjacent to the ependymal lining of the ventricular system of the brain. Two thirds occur in the posterior fossa along the linings of the fourth ventricle. Most series have found an association between survival and the extent of surgical resection. Five-year progression-free survival in retrospective series has been 0–35% for incompletely resected tumors compared with 51–82% after gross total resection (Table 27.6) (NAZAR et al. 1990; SUTTON et al. 1991; TOMITA et al. 1988; HEALEY et al. 1991; POLLACK et al. 1995; SCHIFFER et al. 1991; TIMMERMANN et al. 1999; MERCHANT et al. 1997).

Results in the literature differ as to whether ordinary or low-grade ependymomas have a better prognosis than those with anaplastic characteristics (CARRIE et al. 1995; KOVALIC et al. 1993; REZAI et al. 1996; ROUSSEAU et al. 1994; GOLDWEIN et al. 1990; POLLACK et al. 1995; SHAW et al. 1987; NAZAR et al. 1990). Infratentorial tumors have a better prognosis than supratentorial tumors in some series (MARKS

Table 27.6. Ependymoma: reported 5-year survival rates (%) after surgery and radiation therapy (from Pizzo and Poplack)

Overall	By grade		By location		Reference
	High	Low	Supratentorial	Infratentorial	
56*	65	40	46	59	ROUSSEAU et al. 1994
61*	29	71			SHAW et al. 1987
67*	75	67			WALLNER et al. 1986
				15	TOMITA et al. 1988
46	42	47	35	50	GOLDWEIN et al. 1990
51	36	67	48	53	VANUYTSEL et al. 1992
56			83	46	POLLACK et al. 1995

* Progression-free survival.

and ADLER et al. 1982; MERCHANT et al. 1997), but not in others (ROUSSEAU et al. 1993; TIMMERMANN et al. 1999). Tumor histology and location do not appear to be prognostic factors for outcome, independent of the extent of surgical resection.

Postoperative radiation therapy is standard treatment for all intracranial ependymomas in children over 3 years of age, regardless of the extent of resection. The value of postoperative radiation therapy is suggested by two retrospective single institution series. The investigators found 5-year overall survival to be 13% and 23% with resection alone compared to 45% and 63% with resection followed by radiation therapy (POLLACK et al. 1995; ROUSSEAU et al. 1994). Several retrospective series have reported that a radiation dose above 4,500 cGy to the primary tumor bed is associated with better local tumor control and/or overall survival (GOLDWEIN et al. 1990; SALAZAR et al. 1983; KOVALIC et al. 1993; MERCHANT et al. 1997; MARKS and ADLER 1982; GARRETT and SIMPSON 1983; KIM and FAYOS 1977). The recommended dose to the primary tumor bed is 5,400–5,940 cGy given over 6–6 1/2 weeks. Local relapse, usually as the only site of failure, occurs in the majority of subtotally resected patients despite the use of high-dose postoperative irradiation. The incidence of isolated distant recurrence is approximately 5% (GOLDWEIN et al. 1990; NAZAR et al. 1990; WALLNER et al. 1996; MERCHANT et al. 1997; TIMMERMANN et al. 1999). This failure pattern has led to pilot studies of local dose escalation through stereotactic radiosurgery (DUNBAR et al. 1994; AGGARWAL et al. 1997) or hyperfractionated radiation therapy (POG Cooperative Group Trial). Further experience will need to be gained to evaluate whether they increase local control and patient survival.

The incidence of subarachnoid seeding at diagnosis was under 10% in most retrospective series and in a recent POG trial (NAZAR et al. 1990; ROUSSEAU et al. 1994; GOLDWEIN et al. 1990; MERCHANT et al. 1997), but has been reported to be as high as 22% (POLLACK et al. 1995). Among patients with subarachnoid seeding, craniospinal irradiation to a total dose of 3,600 cGy followed by a boost to the sites of gross disease on presentation is indicated. For patients without evidence of disease dissemination on cerebrospinal fluid cytology and MRI scan, there is wide variation among radiation oncologists in initial treatment volume, from the preoperative tumor volume plus a 1-cm margin to full neuraxis irradiation. Some institutions give craniospinal irradiation for all infratentorial anaplastic posterior fossa ependymomas, based on reports of a 15–20% incidence of

subarachnoid seeding at the time of tumor recurrence (KIM and FAYOS 1977; BLOOM 1982). These series, however, included patients found to have disseminated disease only after uncontrolled or multiple local recurrences. Among infratentorial ependymomas, the incidence of subarachnoid dissemination at the time of initial failure was 0–9% (NAZAR et al. 1990; GOLDWEIN et al. 1990, 1991; TOMITA et al. 1988; VANUYSTEL et al. 1992). Several institutions have found no difference in spinal failure rate between patients given local compared to craniospinal irradiation (PAPADOPOULOS et al. 1990; NAZAR et al. 1990; GOLDWEIN et al. 1990; MERCHANT et al. 1997; CARRIE et al. 1995; TIMMERMANN et al. 1999; ROUSSEAU et al. 1993; SHAW et al. 1987; VANUYTSEL et al. 1991). The trend is therefore to limit radiation therapy to the cranium for any tumor that has not demonstrated leptomeningeal or subarachnoid seeding. Initial intracranial radiation volumes vary from the postoperative tumor bed with a 1–2-cm margin, to the preoperative tumor volume with a margin, the entire posterior fossa and upper cervical spine for infratentorial tumors, the entire ventricular system, or the whole brain. Regardless of the treatment volume employed, the vast majority of failures are within the initial tumor volume, and it is becoming common practice not to expand the radiation fields to encompass sites of potential subclinical disease.

27.8
Future Directions

A radiation dose–response relationship has been demonstrated in most types of pediatric brain tumor. The radiation dose recommended for each of the tumor types discussed above is greater than 5,000 cGy and limited by the tolerance of the surrounding normal brain tissue. Further dose escalation requires preferential dose delivery to the tumor over normal tissue. Investigations using various techniques to increase the dose delivered to the tumor without exceeding normal tissue tolerance, including proton beam, stereotactic, conformal, interstitial, and intensity modulated radiation therapy, are under way. In addition to allowing for dose escalation in older children, these techniques may permit the expanded use of local irradiation for infants and very young children, in whom tumor control rates are significantly below those in older children. Chemical agents that either sensitize tumor cells to radiation or protect normal cells from it are being routinely used with radiation therapy in the treatment of malignancies outside the central nervous system. The blood–brain barrier creates challenges to the development of radiosensitizers and radioprotectors for brain tumor therapy, but promising agents are currently being evaluated in clinical trials. Low tumor oxygenation, which is associated with radiation resistance in other malignancies, has been demonstrated to exist in human glial tumors. The efficacy of measures to enhance tumor oxygenation during radiation therapy is to be evaluated. Chemotherapy has provided less improvement in survival from brain tumors than from most extraneural malignancies. Almost half of children diagnosed with a brain tumor die from their disease. Major advances may be made from the development of cytotoxic or antiangiogenic agents that synergize with radiation. Several of the areas of investigation outlined above are anticipated to contribute to an improvement in prognosis for young brain tumor patients in the new decade.

References

Aggarwal R, Yeung D, Muhlbauer M, et al. (1997) Efficacy and feasibility of stereotactic radiosurgery in the primary management of unfavorable pediatric ependymoma. Radiother Oncol 43:269–273

Albright AL, Price RA, Guthkelch AN (1985) Diencephalic gliomas of children: a clinicopathologic study. Cancer 55:2789–2793

Albright AL, Wisoff JH, Zeltzer P, et al. (1995) Prognostic factors in children with supratentorial (nonpineal) primitive neuroectodermal tumors. Pediatr Neurosurg 22:1–7

Allen J, Epstein F (1982) Medulloblastoma and other primary malignant tumors of the CNS. J Neurosurg 57:446

Bailey CC, Gnekow A, Wellek S, Jones M, Round C, Brown J, Phillips A, Neidhardt MK (1995 Sep) Prospective randomised trial of chemotherapy given before radiotherapy in childhood medulloblastoma. International Society of Paediatric Oncology (SIOP) and the (German) Society of Paediatric Oncology (GPO): SIOP II. Medical & Pediatric Oncology 25(3):166–178

Berry MP, Jenkin RDT, Keen CW, Nair BD, Simpson WJ (1981 Jul) Radiation treatment for medulloblastoma. J Neurosurg 55:43–51

Bloom HJG (1982) Intracranial tumors: response and resistance to therapeutic endeavors. Int J Radiat Oncol Biol Phys 8:1083–1113

Bloom HJG, Glees J, Bell J (1990) The treatment and long-term prognosis of children with intracranial tumors: a study of 610 cases. Int J Radiat Oncol Biol Phys 18:723

Bouffet E, Bernard JL, Frappaz D, Gentet JC, Roche H, Tron P, Carrie C, Raybaud C, Joannard A, Lapras C, Choux M, Carton M, Aimard L, Philip T, Brunat-Mentigny M (1992

Mar) M4 protocol for cerebellar medulloblastoma: supratentorial radiotherapy may not be avoided. Int. J Radiation Oncology Biol Phys 24:79–85

Campbell A, Chan H, Becker L, et al. (1984) Extracranial metastasis in childhood primary tumors. Cancer 53:974

Carrie C, Mottolese C, Bouffet E, Negrier S, Bachelot TH, Lasset C, Helfre S, Guyotat J, Lapras CL, Brunat-Mentigny M (1995) Non-metastatic childhood ependymomas. Radiotherapy and Oncology 36:101–106

Chin HW, Maruyama Y (1981) Results of radiation treatment of cerebellar medulloblastoma. Int. J. Radiation Oncology Biol. Phys. 7:737–742

Constine LS, Woolf PD, Cann D, Mick G, McCormick K, Raubertas RF, Rubin P (1993 Jan) Hypothalamic-pituitary dysfunction after radiation for brain tumors. New Eng J of Med 328(2):87–94

Copeland DR, dMoor C, Moore III BD, Ater JL (1999 Nov) Neurocognitive development of children after a cerebellar tumor in infancy: a longitudinal study. Journal of Clinical Oncology 17(11):3476–3486

Cumberlin RL, Luk KH, Wara WM, et al (1979): Medulloblastoma. Treatment results and effect on normal tissues. Cancer 43:1014–1021

Dennis M, Spiegler BJ, Hetherington CR, Greenberg ML (1996) Neuropsychological sequelae of the treatment of children with medulloblastoma. J of Neuro-Oncology 29:91–101

Denys D, Kaste SC, Kun LE, Chaudhary MA, Bowman LC, Robbins KT (1998 Sep) The effects of radiation on craniofacial skeletal growth: a quantitative study. Int J of Pediatric Otorhinolaryngology 45(1):7–13

Deutsch M, Reigel D (1980) The value of myelography in the management of childhood medulloblastoma. Cancer 45:2194–2197

Deutsch M, Thomas PRM, Krischer J, Boyett JM, Albright L, Aronin P, Langston J, Allen JC, Packer RJ, Linggood R, Mulhern R, Stanley P, Stehbens JA, Duffner P, Kun L, Rorke L, Cherlow J, Freidman J, Finlay JL, Vietti T (1996) Results of a prospective randomized trial comparing standard dose neuraxis irradiation (3,600 cGy/20) with reduced neuraxis irradiation (2,340 cGy/13) inpatients with low-stage medulloblastoma. Pediatr Neurosurg 24:167–177

Dirks PB, Jay V, Becker LE, Drake JM, Humphreys RP, Hoffman HJ, Rutka JT (1994) Development of anaplastic changes in low-grade astrocytomas of childhood. Neurosurg 34:68–78

Dropcho EJ, Wisoff JH, Walker RW, et al. (1990) Supratentorial malignant gliomas in childhood: a review of fifty cases. Ann Neurol 22:355

Duffner PK, Cohen MR, Meyers MH, et al. (1986) Survival of children with brain tumors: SEER program1973–1980. Neurology 36:597–601

Duffner PK, Cohen ME, Voorhess ML, Mac Gillivray MH, Brecher ML, Panahon A, Gilani BB (1985) Long-term effects of cranial irradiaiton on endocrine function in children with brain tumors. Cancer 56:2189–2193

Duffner PK, Krischer JP, Horowitz ME, Cohen ME, Burger PC, Friedman HS, Kun LE, and the Pediatric Oncology Group (1998) Second malignancies in young children with primary brain tumors following treatment with prolonged postoperative chemotherapy and delayed irradiation: a pediatric oncolgy group study. Annals of Neurology 44(3):313–316

Dunbar SF, Tarbell NJ, Kooy HM, et al. (1994) Stereotactic radiotherapy for pediatric and adult brain tumors: preliminary report. Int J Radiat Oncol Biol Phys 30(3):531–539

Evans, AE, Jenkin RDT, Sposto R, Ortega JA, Wilson CB, Wara W, Ertel IJ, Kramer S, Chang CH, Leikin SL, Hammond GD (1990) Results of a prospective randomized trial of radiation therapy with and without CCNU, vincristine, and prednisone. J Neurosurg 72:572–582

Ferbert A, Gullotta F (1985) Remarks on the followup of cerebellar astrocytomas. J Neurol 232:134–136

Finlay JL, Boyett JM, Yates AJ, et al. (1995) Randomized phase III trial in childhood high-grade astrocytoma comparing vincristine, lomustine, and prednisone with the eight-drugs-in- 1-day regimen. J Clin Oncol 13:112–123

Fletcher WA, Imes RK, Hoyt WF (1986) Chiasmal gliomas: appearance and long-term changes demonstrated by computerized tomography. J Neurosurg 65:154–159

Fontanesi J, Muhlbauer M, Heideman RL, et al. (1995) High activity 1251 interstitial irradiation in the treatment of pediatric central nervous sy0 tumors: a pilot study. Pediatr Neurosug 22:289–298

Freeman CR (1996) Hyperfractionaed radiotherapy for diffuse intrinsic brain stem tumors in children. Pediatr Neurosurg 24:103–110

Freeman CR, Bourgouin PM, Sanford RA, et al. (1996) Long term survivors of childhood brain stem gliomas treated with hyperfractionated radiotherapy, clinical characteristics and treatment related toxicities. Cancer 77:555–562

Freeman CR, Krischer JP, Sanford RA, et al. (1993) Final results of a study of escalating doses of hyperfractionated radiotherapy in brain stem tumors in children. Int J Radiat Oncol Biol Phys 27:197–206

Fukunaga-Johnson N, Lee JH, Sandler HM, Robertosn P, McNeil E, Goldwein JW (1998) Patterns of failure following treatment for medulloblastoma: is it necessary to treat the entire posterior fossa? Int. J Radiation Oncology Biol. Phys. 42:143–146

Gajjar A, Sanford RA, Heideman R, Jenkins JJ, Walter A, Li Y, Langston JW, Muhlbauer M, Boyett JM, Kun LE (1997 Aug) Low-grade astrocytoma: a decade of experience at St. Jude Children's Research Hospital. Journal of Clinical Oncology 15(8):2792–2799

Garcia DM, Latifi HR, Simpson JR, et al. (1989) Astrocytomas of the cerebellum in children. J Neurosurg 71:661–664

Geissinger J, Bucy P (1971) Astrocytomas of the cerebellum in children: long term study. Arch Neurol 29:125

Geyer RJ, Zeltzer PM, Boyett JM, et al. (1994) Survival of infants with primitive neuroectodermal tumors or malignant ependymomas of the CNS treated with eight drugs in 1 day: a report from the Children's Cancer Group. J Clin Oncol 12:1607

Goldwein JW, Corn BW, Finlay JL, et al (1991) Is craniospinal irradiation required to cure children with malignant (anaplastic) intracranial ependymomas? Cancer 67:2766–2771

Goldwein JW, Leahy JM, Packer RJ, et al. (1990) Intracranial ependymomas in children. Int J Radiat Oncol Biol Phys 19:1497–1502

Goldwein JW, Radcliffe J, Johnson J, Moshang T, Packer RJ, Sutton LN, Rorke LB, D'Angio GJ (1996) Updated results of a pilot study of low dose craniospinal irradiation plus chemotherapy for children under five with cerebellar primitive neuroectodermal tumors (medulloblastoma). Intl J of Radiation Oncology Biol Phys 34(4):899–904

Grill J, Kieffer Renaux V, Bulteau C, Viguier D, Levy-Piebois C, Sainte-Rose C, Dellatolas G, Raquin MA, Jambaque I, Kalifa C (1999) Long-term intellectual outcome in children with posterior fossa tumors according to radiation doses and volumes. Int. J Radiation Oncology Biol Phys 45(1):137–145

Grovas AC, Boyett JM, Lindsley K, Rosenblum M, Yates AJ, Finlay J (1999) Treatment of children with medulloblastomas with reduced-dose craniospinal radiation therapy and adjuvant chemotherapy: a children's cancer group study. J Clin Oncol 17:2127–2136

Gurney JG, Davis S, Sverson RK, et al. (1996) Trends in cancer incidence among children in the U.S. Cancer 78:532–541

Gurney JG, Smith MA, Bunin GR (1999). In:Ries LAG, Smith MA, Gurney JG, Linet M, Tamra T, Young JL, Bunin GR (eds). Cancer incidence and survival among children and adolescents: United States SEER program 1975–1995, National Cancer Institute, SEER Program. NIH Pub. No. 99-4649. Bethesda, MD, pp. 51–63

Gutin PH, Edwards MSB, Wara WM, et al. (1985) Preliminary experience with 1251-brachytherapy of pediatric brain tumors. Pediatr Neurosurg 5:187–206

Hartsell WF, Gajjar A, Heideman RL, Langston JA, Sanford RA, Walter A, Jones D, Chen G, Kun LE (1997 Aug) Patterns of failure in children with medulloblastoma: effects of preirradiation chemotherapy. International Journal of Radiat Oncol Biol Phys 39(1):15–24

Hawkins MM, Draper GJ, Kingston JE (1987) Incidence of second primary tumors among childhood cancer survivors. Br J Cancer 56:339–347

Hayostek CJ, Shaw EG, Scheithauer B, et al. (1993) Astrocytomas of the cerebellum: a comparative clinicopathologic study. Cancer 72:856–869

Heideman RL, Kovnar EH, Kellie SJ, et al. (1995) Preirradiation chemotherapy with carboplatin and etoposide in newly diagnosed embryonal pediatric CNS tumors. J Clin Oncol 13:2247–2254

Heideman RL, Kuttesch J Jr., Gajjar AJ, Walter AW, Jenkins JJ, Li Y, Sanford RA, Kun LE (1997) Supratentorial malignant gliomas in childhood: a single institution perspective. Neurosurgery 80(3):497–504

Heron DE, Heideman RL, Langston J Parikh S, Mulhern RK, Jenkins JJ, Sanford RA, Kun LE (1999) Pediatric dorsally exophytic brain stem gliomas: radiologic and clinicopathologic correlation. Int. J. Radiat Oncol Biol Phys 45(suppl 3):234–235

Hirsh JF, Sainte Rose C, Pierre-Kahn A, et al. 1989) Benign astrocytic and oligodendrocytic tumors of the cerebral hemispheres in children. J Neurosurg 70:568–572

Hoffman HJ, Becker L, Craven MA (1980) A clinically and pathologically distinct group of benign brain stem gliomas. Neurosurg 7:243–248

Horwich A, Bloom HJG (1985) Optic gliomas: radiation therapy and prognosis. Int J Radiat Oncol Biol Phys 11:1067

Jannoun L, Bloom HJG (1989) Long-term psychological effects in children treated for intracranial tumors. Int. J Radiation Oncology Biol Phys 18:747–753

Janss AJ, Grundy R, Cnaan A, et al. (1995) Optic pathway and hypothalamic/chiasmatic gliomas in children younger than age 5 years with a 6-year follow-up. Cancer 75:1051–1059

Kestle JRW, Hoffman HJ, Mock AR (1993) Moyamoya phenomenon after radiation for optic glioma. J Neurosurg 79:32–35

Khafaga Y, Kandil AE, Jamshed A, Hassounah M, DeVol E, Gray AJ (1996) Treatment results for 149 medulloblastoma patients from one institution. I.J. Radiation Oncology Biol. Phys. 35(3):501–506

Khatib ZA, Heideman RL, Kovnar EH, Langston JA, Sanford RA, Douglas EC, Ochs J, Jenkins JJ, Fairclough DL, Greenwald C, et al. (1994) Predominance of pilocytic histology in dorsally exophytic brain stem tumors. Pediatric Neurosurgery 20(1):2–10

Kleinman G, Hochberg F, Richardson E 1984) Systemic metastases from medulloblastoma: report of two cases and review of the literature. Cancer 48:2296

Kovalic JJ, Flaris N, Grigsby, Pirkowski M, Simpson JR, Roth KA (1993) Intracranial ependymoma long term outcome, patterns of failure. J Neurooncol 15:125–131

Krieger MD, Gonzalez-Gomez I, Levy ML, et al. (1997) Recurrence patterns and anaplastic change in a long-term study of pilocytic astrocytomas. Pediatr Neurosurg 27:1–11

Leibel SA, Sheline GE, Wara WM, et al. (1975) The role of radiation therapy in the treatment of astrocytomas. Cancer 35:1551–1557

Li FP, Winston KR, Gimbrene K (1984) Followup of children with brain tumors. Cancer 54:135–138

Loeffler JS, Alexander E III, Shea WM, et al. (1992) Radiosurgery as part of the initial management of patients with malignant gliomas. J Clin Oncol 10:1379–1385

Mandell LR, Kadota R, Freeman C, Douglass EC, Fontanesi J, Cohen ME, Kovnar E, Burger P, Sanford RA, Kepner J, Friedman H, Kun LE (1999) There is no role for hyperfractionated radiotherapy in the management of children with newly diagnosed diffuse intrinsic brainstem tumors: results of a pediatric oncology group phase III trial comparing conventional vs. hyperfractionated radiotherapy. Int. J. Radiation Oncology Biol. Phys. 43(5):959–964

Marks JE, Adler SJ (1982) A comparative study of ependymomas by site of origin. Int J Radiat Oncol Biol Phys 8:37–43

Medbery CA, Straus KL, Steinberg SM (1988) Low-grade astrocytomas: treatment results and prognostic variables. Int J Radiat Oncol Biol Phys 15:837

Merchant TE, Haida T, Wang M-H, et al. (1997) Anaplastic ependymoma: treatment of pediatric patients with or without craniospinal radiation therapy. J Neurosurg 86:943–949

Moore IM, Kramer JH, Wara W, Halberg F, Ablin AR (1991 Nov) Cognitive function in children with leukemia. Cancer 68:1913–1917

Mosijezuk AD, Nigro MA, Thomas PRM, et al. (1993) Preradiation chemotherapy in advanced medulloblastoma: A Pediatric Oncology Group pilot study. Cancer 72:2755–2762

Mulhern RK, Fairclough D, Ochs J (1991) A prospective comparison of neuropsychologic performance of children surviving leukemia who received 18-Gy, 24-Gy, or no cranial irradiation. Journal of Clin Oncology 9(8):1348–1356

Mulhern RK, Kepner JL; Thomas PR, Armstrong FD, Friedman HS, Kun LE (1998) Neuropsychologic functioning of survivors of childhood medulloblastoma randomized to receive conventional or reduced-dose craniospinal irradiation: a pediatric oncology group study. Journal of Clinical Oncology 16:1723–1728

Nazar GB, Hoffman HJ, Becker LE, et al. (1990) Infratentorial ependymomas in chiildhood: prognostic factors and treatment. J Neurosurg 72:408–417

Neglia JP, Meadows AT, Robinson LL, et al. (1991) Second neoplasms after acute lymphoblastic leukemia in childhood. N Engl J Med 325:1330–1336

Neuhauser EBD, Wittenborg MH, Berman CZ, Cohen J (1952) Irradiation effects of roentgen therapy on the growing spine. Radiology 59(5):637–650

Newman CB, Levine LS, New MI (1981) Endocrine function in children with intrasellar and suprasellar neoplasms. Am J Dis Child 135:259–262

Packer RJ (1995) Early results of reduced-dose radiotherapy plus chemotherapy for children with non-disseminated medulloblastoma (MB): A Children's Cancer Group Stdy. Pediatr Neurosurg 55:518

Packer RJ, Boyett JM, Zimmerman RA, Albright AL, Kaplan AM, Rorke LB, Selch MT, Cherlow JM, Finlay JL, Ch B, Wara WM (1994) Outcome of children with brain stem gliomas after treatment with 7800 cGy of hyperfractionated radiotherapy. Cancer 74:1827–1834

Packer RJ, Boyett JM, Zimmerman RA, Rorke LB, Kaplan AM, Albright AL, Selch MT, Finlay JL, Ch B, Hammond GD, Wara WM (1993) Hyperfractionaed Radiation Therapy (72 Gy) for children with brain stem gliomas. Cancer 72:1414–1421

Packer RJ, Meadows AT, Rorke LB, et al. (1987) Long-term sequelae of cancer treatment on the central nervous system in childhood. Med Pediatric Oncology 15:241–253

Packer RJ, Savino PJ, Bilaniuk LT, et al. (1983) Chiasmatic gliomas of childhood: a reappraisal of natural history and effectiveness of cranial irradiation. Child's Brain 10:393–403

Packer RJ, Sutton LN, Elterman R, et al. (1994) Outcome for children with medulloblastoma treated with radiation and cisplatin, CCNU, and vincristine chemotherapy. J Neurosurg 81:690–698

Packer RJ, Zimmerman RA, Kaplan A, et al. (1993) Early cystic/necrotic changes after hyperfractionaed radiation therapy in children with brain stem gliomas. Data from the Children's Cancer Group. Cancer 71:2666–2674

Palma L, Guidetti B (1985) Cystic pilocytic astrocytomas of the cerebral hemispheres. J Neurosurg 62:811–815

Papadopoulos DP, Giri S, Evans RG (1990) Prognostic factors and management of intracranial ependymomas. Anticancer Research 10:689–692

Pizzo and Poplack, Eds. Principles and Practice of Pediatric Oncology, 3rd Edition, Philadelphia: Lippincott-Raven, 1997

Pollack IF, Gerszten PC, Martinez AJ, et al. (1995) Intracranial ependymomas of childhood: Long-term outcome and prognostic factors. Neurosurgery 37:655–667

Pollack IF, Hoffman HJ, Humphreys RP, et al. (1993) The long-term outcome after surgical treatment of dorsally exophytic brain-stem gliomas. J Neurosurg 78:859–863

Pollack IF, Claassen D, Al-Shboul Q, Janosky JE, Deutsch M (1995) Low-grade gliomas of the cerebral hemispheres in children: an analysis of 71 cases. J Neurosurg 82:536–547

Probert JC, Parker BR, Kaplan HS (1973) Growth retardation in children after megavoltage irradiation of the spine. Cancer 32:634–639

Rajakulasingam K, Cerullo LJ, Raimondi AJ (1979) Childhood moyamoya syndrome. Child's Brain 5:467–475

Relling MV, Rubnitz JE, Rivera GK, Boyett JM, Hancock ML, Felix CA, Kun LE, Walter AW, Evans WE, Pui CH (1999 Jul) High incidence of secondary brain tumor after radiotherapy and antimetabolites. Lancet 354:34–39

Rezai AR, Woo HH, Lee M, Cohen H, Zagzag D, Epstein FJ (1996) Disseminated ependymomas of the central nervous system. J Neurosurg 85:618–624

Richards GE, Wara WM, Grumbach MM, Kaplan SL, Sheline GE, Conte FA (1976) Delayed onset of hypopituitarism: sequelae of therapeutic irradiation of central nervous system, eye and middle ear tumors. The J of Pediatrics 89(4):553–559

Rousseau P, Habrand JL, Sarrazin D, et al. (1994) Treatment of intracranial ependymomas of children: review of a 15-year experience. Int J Radiat Oncol Biol Phys 28:381–386

Rudoltz MS, Regine WF, Langston JW, Sanford RA, Kovnar EH, Kun LE (1998) Multiple causes of cerebrovascular events in children with tumors of the parasellar region. Journal of Neuro-Oncology 37(3):251–261

Salazar OM, Casto-Vita M, Van Houtte D, et al. (1983) Improved survival in cases of intracranial ependymoma after radiation therapy: late report and recommendations. J Neurosurg 59:652–659

Shalet SM (1982) Growth and hormonal status of children treated for brain tumors. Child's Brain 9:284–293

Shalet SM (1993) Radiation and pituitary dysfunction. N Engl J Med 328:131–133

Shalet SM, Beardwell CG, Aarons BM, Pearson D, Morris Jones PH (1978) Growth impariment in children treated for brain tumours. Archives of Diseases in Childhood 53:491–494

Shaw EG, Scheithauer BW, Gilbertson DT, et al. (1989) Postoperative radiotherapy of supratentorial low-grade gliomas. Int J Radiat Oncol Biol Phys 16:663–668

Shaw EG, Scheithauer BW, O'Fallon JR (1993) Management of supratentorial low-grade gliomas. Oncology 7:97–107

Shibamoto Y, Kitakabu Y, Takahashi M, et al. (1993) Supratentorial low-grade astrocytoma. Cancer 72:190–195

Silber JH, Radcliffe J, Peckham V, Perilongo G, Kishnani P, Fridman M, Goldwin JW, Meadows AT (1992 Sep) J of Clin Oncology 10(9):1390–1396

Silverman CL, Simpson JR (1982) Cerebellar medulloblastoma: the importance of posterior fossa dose to survival and patterns of failure. Int. J. Radiation Oncology Biol. Phys. 8:1869–1876

Sposto R, Ertel IJ, Jenkin RD, et al. (1989) The effectiveness of chemotherapy for treatment of high rade astrocytoma in children: results of a randomized trial. A report from the Childrens Cancer Study Group. J Neurooncol 7:165–177

Spunberg JJ, Chang CH, Goldman M, Auricchio E, Bell JJ (1981) Quality of long-term survival following irradiation for intracranial tumors in children under the age of two. Int. J Radiation Oncology Biol Phys 7:727–736

Stroink AR, Hoffman HJ, Henrick EB, et al. (1986) Diagnosis and management of pediatric brain stem gliomas. J Neurosurg 65:745–750

Tait DM, Thornton-Jones H, Bloom HJ, Lemerle J, Morris-Jones P (1990) Adjuvant chemotherapy for medulloblastoma: the first multi-centre control trial of the International Society of Paediatric Oncology (SIOP I). European Journal of Cancer 26(4):464–469

Tao ML, Barnes PD, Billett AL, et al. (1997) Childhood optic chiasm gliomas: radiographic response following radiotherapy and long-term clinical outcome. Int J Radiat Oncol Biol Phys 39:579–587

Tarbell NJ, Loeffler JS, Silver B, et al. (1991) The change in patterns of relapse in medulloblastoma. Cancer 68:1600–1604

Timmermann B, Kortmann RD, Kuhl J, Meisner C, Bamberg M (1999) Combined postoperative irradiation and chemotherapy for anaplastic ependymoma in childhood: results of the german propective trials hit '88/'89 and HIT '91. Int J Radiat Oncol Biol Phys 45(suppl 3):185

Tiyaworabun S, Kazkaz S, Nicola N, et al. (1981) Supratentorial tumors in infants and children. In Voth D, Gutjahn P, Langmaid C(eds). Tumors of the nervous system in infancy and childhood. New York: Springer-Verlag 420

Tomita T, McLone DJ, Das L, et al. (1988) Benign ependymomas of the posterior fossa in children. Pediatr Neurosci 14:277

Tomita T, McLone DG, Yasue M (1988) Cerebral primitive neuroectodermal tumors in childhood. J Neurooncol 6:233–243

Tsang RW, Laperriere NJ, Simpson WJ, Brierley J, Panzarella T, Smyth HS (1993) Glioma arising after radiation therapy for pituitary adenoma. Cancer 72(7):2227–2233

Vanuytsel LJ, Bessell EM, Ashley SE, et al. (1992) Intracranial ependymoma: long-term results of a policy of surgery and radiotherapy. Int J Radiat Oncol Biol Phys 23:313–319

Vanuytsel LJ, Brada M (1991) The role of prophylactic spinal irradiation in localized intracranial ependymoma. Int. J Radiation Oncology Biol Phys 21:825–830

Voges J, Sturm V, Berthold F, et al. (1990) Interstitial irradiation of cerebral gliomas in childhood by permanently implanted 125 iodine-preliminary results. Klin Padiatr 202:270–274

Wallner KE, Gonzales M, Sheline GE (1988) Treatment results of juvenile pilocytic astrocytoma. J Neurosurg 69:171–176

Wallner KE, Wara WM, Sheline GE (1986) Intracranial ependymomas: results of treatment with partial or whole brain irradiation without spinal irradiation. Int J Radiat Oncol Biol Phys 12:1937–1941

Walter AW, Hancock ML, Pui CH, Hudson MM, Ochs JS, Rivera GK, Pratt CB, Boyett JM, Kun LE (1998) Secondary brain tumors in children treated for acute lymphoblastic leukemia at St Jude Children's Research Hospital. J Clin Oncol 16:3761–3767

Wara WM, Weil MD, Larson DA, Lamborn K, Edwards MS (1999) Hyperfractionated radiotherapy of medulloblastoma. Int J Radiat Oncol Biol Phys 45(suppl 3):212

Wright TL, Bresnan M (1976) Radiation-induced cerebrovascular disease in children. Neurology 26:540–543

28 Surgical Management of Pediatric Patients with CNS Tumors

Mark D. Krieger, J. Gordon McComb and Michael Levy

CONTENTS

28.1 Introduction

The role of surgical intervention in pediatric brain tumors has become more specific over the last two decades. Modern imaging modalities allow clear delineation of the lesion early in the patient's work-up. This detail improves both the efficacy and the safety of surgery. However, in most cases it does not obviate the need for surgery: tissue diagnosis is still required for treatment. Furthermore, the prognosis of many of these lesions is directly dependent on the degree of surgical resection. Thus, surgery remains central to the treatment of pediatric patients with brain tumors.

M. D. Krieger, MD; J.G. McComb, MD; M. Levy, MD
Childrens Hospital of Los Angeles, University of Southern California, Los Angeles, California, USA

28.2 General Principles

28.2.1 Objectives

Surgery plays three major roles in the treatment of CNS tumors in the young: (1) establishment of a tissue diagnosis; (2) total resection of the lesion with potential cure of the disease, where appropriate; and (3) alleviation of mass effect due either to the lesion itself or to noncommunicating hydrocephalus.

Tissue diagnosis remains an important goal in most cases. With the improvement in immunohistochemical stains, accurate diagnoses can be made with relatively small tissue samples. Tissue diagnosis is important for direction of further therapy. In most cases, when a benign histology is obtained, the surgeon can be directed towards continued resection for an attempt at cure. Even with some malignantly behaving tumors, continued surgery might be indicated based on the pathology results. Thus, intraoperative histological examination, usually done with frozen sections, has become the standard. Additional therapy, including radiation and chemotherapy, is then directed based on the pathology results.

In most cases in a pediatric population, tissue diagnosis is obtained by open biopsy. This is in contrast to adult tumor patients, where minimally invasive stereotactic biopsies are commonly performed (Chin et al. 1996). Several major reasons exist for this dichotomy. As will be discussed in more detail in subsequent sections, the prognosis of many pediatric brain tumors is dependent on the degree of resection. Thus, in most cases, a total resection has proven efficacy over a limited biopsy followed by adjuvant therapy. Secondly, many of these tumors occur in the posterior fossa, resulting in an obstruction to CSF flow and concomitant hydrocephalus. An open resection allows return of normal CSF dynamics, which cannot be achieved by a limited biopsy. Additionally, stereotactic biopsy is technically more difficult for posterior fossa masses. Lastly, a major advantage of stereotaxis is the avoidance of general anesthesia. While skilled pediatric anesthesiologists can provide adequate sedation to allow a stereotactic biopsy in the young, in many cases this advantage is lost.

Three major exceptions exist to the need for tissue diagnosis. Brainstem gliomas have a typical appearance on magnetic resonance imaging (MRI), which suggests the diagnosis with a high degree of accuracy (Fig. 28.1). Even a limited biopsy of this critical region can be accompanied by significant morbidity. Additionally, degree of resection of these lesions, in most cases, has not been shown to correlate with outcome. Thus, when the risks and the benefits are weighed, the decision usually is not to surgically address putative brainstem gliomas (EDWARDS and PRADOS 1987).

A second exception is putative germ cell tumors, most commonly seen in the pineal region (Fig. 28.2). In these cases, CSF markers, coupled with the appearance on MRI, can be highly suggestive of the diagnosis. If a radiosensitive germinoma is indicated, most treating physicians will proceed directly to a test dose of radiation without a tissue diagnosis. Contrarily, if a highly malignant germ cell tumor is indicated by the CSF studies and the imaging studies suggest diffuse spread, a tissue diagnosis might not be necessary before proceeding with alternative nonsurgical therapy.

A third circumstance where a surgically obtained tissue diagnosis might not be necessary is for recurrent or widely disseminated disease (Fig. 28.3). In these cases, various nonsurgical therapeutic strategies might be pursued without an attempt at resection of the primary mass, with or without CSF diagnosis.

As was previously mentioned, an additional goal of surgery is the alleviation of mass effect, either from the tumor mass itself or from hydrocephalus. Mass effect in children manifests itself differentially depending on the age of the child. In children greater than 18 months of age, the cranial sutures have fused. Thus, increased intracranial volume, due to hydrocephalus, a mass, or some combination of the two, is directly translated to a rise in intracranial pressure once compliance limits are reached. Symptoms might be indolent, consisting of a loss of developmental milestones or intellectual function, or more precipitous, including lethargy, nausea and vomit-

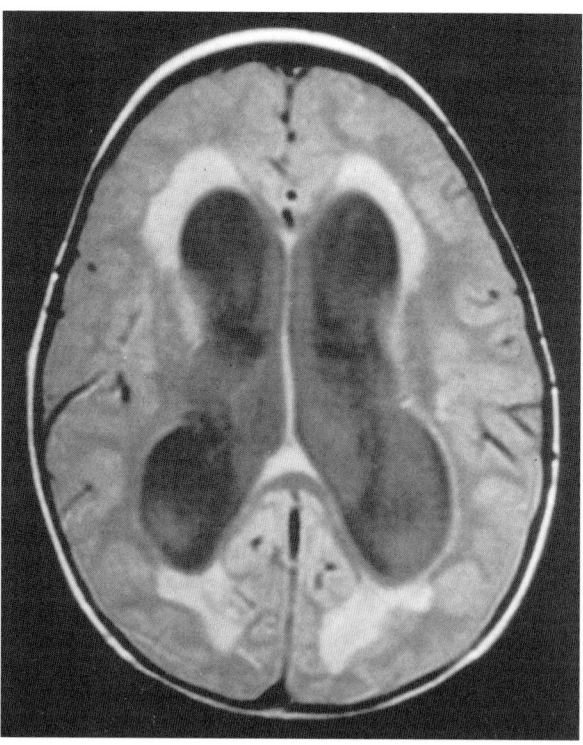

Fig. 28.1. Axial MRI of a patient with a posterior fossa PNET documenting associated hydrocephalus with evident transependymal edema

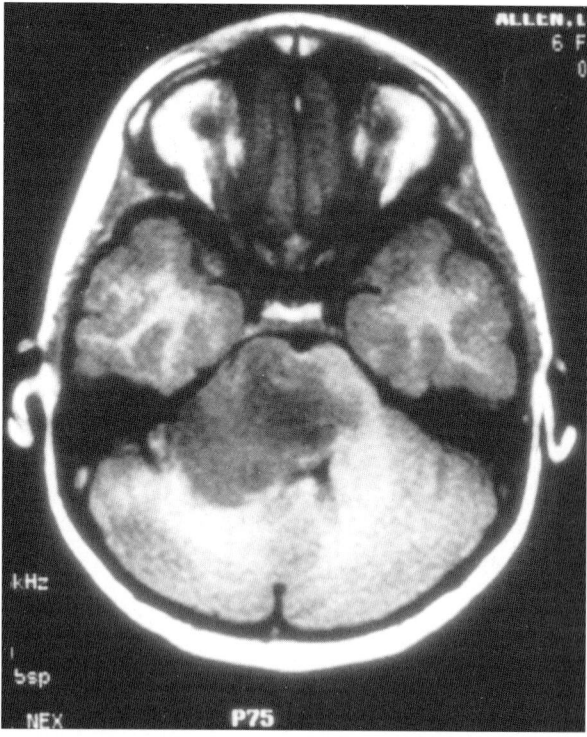

Fig. 28.2. T1-weighted axial MRI documenting a low-density lesion consistent with a brainstem glioma. Note the diffuse involvement of the brainstem, more so on the right than on the left side, in addition to slight effacement of the fourth ventricular chamber

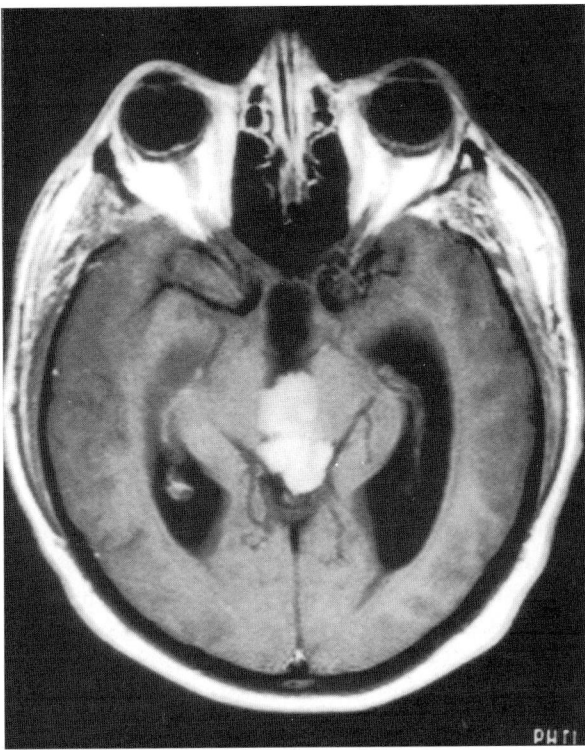

Fig. 28.3. T1-weighted post-contrast axial MRI study documenting the presence of a pineoblastoma involving the pineal region with extension and involvement of the posterior third ventricular chamber

ing, and progressive headaches. If left untreated, pressure buildup can result in herniation syndromes, coma, and death.

While these signs and symptoms may be seen in younger children, the clinical course is typically different. An expansion of the intracranial contents prior to the closure of the sutures more commonly does not result in a significant elevation of the intracranial pressure. Rather, small increases in pressure are translated into diastasis of the sutures, bulging of the fontanelle, and an expansion of the head circumference.

28.2.2
Preoperative Care

Preoperative care involves two goals: amelioration of presenting symptoms and surgical planning and preparation. The most important presenting symptoms which require address are elevated intracranial pressure and seizures. As was previously discussed, intracranial pressure elevation is usually due to some combination of tumor mass effect and hydrocephalus. The surest way to relieve these problems is to remove the mass. However, this is not always immediately feasible owing to the patient's status or logistical issues. Various temporizing measures can be used to lessen the effects of elevated intracranial pressure. Corticosteroids reduce vasogenic edema which accompanies tumors. Dexamethasone is the most commonly used agent for this purpose, although some prefer the lessened immune suppression seen with methylprednisolone. Osmotic diuretics, such as mannitol, can be used in conjunction with loop diuretics, such as furosemide, to further decrease acutely worsening cerebral edema.

Acute hydrocephalus obviously requires emergent management if intracranial pressure is high and herniation is imminent. Ventriculostomy placement can be lifesaving if used in this manner. However, care must be taken to place a ventriculostomy only when necessary. There is a suggestion that such a placement in the preoperative period may increase the likelihood that the patient will subsequently require a permanent shunt. Given the relative risk for shunt infection and failure, and the concomitant morbidity associated with these events, such a course is best avoided. Additionally, some argue that ventriculostomy placement introduces a risk of upward herniation prior to the resection of the tumor (EPSTEIN and MURALI 1978). For these reasons, the accepted practice is to place a ventriculostomy for hydrocephalus associated with major symptomatology. Permanent shunts are not placed prior to tumor resection.

Seizures are a relatively rare form of presentation for pediatric brain tumors. This fact most likely arises from the large incidence of posterior fossa tumors in children, which are not in epileptogenic cortex. However, supratentorial tumors can be associated with seizures. It is our practice to place the child on prophylactic seizure medications only when seizure activity exists with intracranial lesions upon admission.

Operative planning begins once the patient is medically stable. MRI with gadolinium enhancement has become the modality of choice for diagnosis and operative planning. MRI is particularly useful for imaging posterior fossa tumors, as there is less obstructive artifact from the bony landmarks in this region. MRI-compatible ventilators exist for the obtunded patient, or the young child who requires anesthesia for sedation during the examination. Imaging should involve the complete neuraxis, including the spine, especially when metastases are expected based on symptomatology or possible histology.

28.2.3
Operative Considerations

A full discussion of operative technique is beyond the scope of this chapter. However, recent advances in surgical technique have improved both the safety and the efficacy of surgery. Pediatric anesthesia has made great strides in recent years. New short-acting narcotics and paralytics allow close titration to effect. Close physiological monitoring also decreases morbidity. Intraoperative monitoring of evoked responses, brainstem function, and cranial nerves improves the safety of surgery. In addition, intraoperative cortical mapping of motor and speech enhances safety in the treatment of tumors involving eloquent cortex. Advances in the operating microscope allow improved illumination and magnification, aiding tumor resection while protecting normal brain. Frameless stereotaxy permits accurate and discrete localization in three-dimensional space, facilitating tumor resection. Unfortunately, frameless stereotaxy is not the panacea that one would assume owing to the fact the all reconstructions are based upon preoperative images. Tumor resection and brain shift may not be accurately displayed utilizing these systems. In addition, removal of only enhancing regions of tumor will still result in incomplete resection of malignant tumors. Instruments such as the Cavitron ultrasonic aspirator (CUSA) also greatly aid in tumor resection. Endoscopic techniques are effective in addressing intraventricular lesions in a minimally invasive fashion. Lastly, novel imaging techniques permit accurate depictions of the lesion, allowing improved pre- and intraoperative planning. Such techniques include MRI spectroscopy, positron emission tomography (PET) imaging, and computerized three-dimensional reconstructions.

Blood loss is always an important consideration in young children, whose blood volume is significantly less than that of adults. A widely used rule of thumb is that the average healthy individual has 60 cc of blood volume per kilogram. Twenty percent loss of blood volume results in shock. Thus, small children run a significant risk of cardiovascular collapse with even relatively small volumes of blood loss. Care must be taken to begin transfusion early in the course of a procedure when significant blood loss is expected. Blood must always be available for these cases.

Patient positioning is also an important consideration. Most pediatric tumors are located in the posterior fossa, necessitating a posterior fossa approach. While many adult neurosurgeons use the sitting position for these procedures, most pediatric neurosurgeons prefer either the prone position or, more commonly, the lateral decubitus position (McComb et al. 1997). Both of these positions lessen the chance of air embolism, and are generally more comfortable for the surgeon (Kobayashi 1983). For deep-seated midline lesions, such as those in the lateral ventricle, third ventricle, or pineal region, we prefer to use an interhemispheric approach. This approach avoids traversing normal cortex. Furthermore, it allows gravity to aid in retraction when combined with the lateral decubitus position.

28.2.4
Postoperative Care

Many of the preoperative issues persist into the postoperative period and must be addressed. Persistent cerebral edema can be managed with continued corticosteroids. An attempt should be made to taper these in the postoperative period. Ventricular drainage should be continued if hydrocephalus persists, or is threatened by persistent blood in the ventricular system. Given the progressive increased risk of infection, long-standing external drainage might need to be converted to an internalized ventriculoperitoneal shunt. Additionally a child's hematocrit, fluid balance, and serum electrolytes need to be followed closely in the postoperative period. The occurrence of SIADH or, much more commonly, cerebral salt wasting should always be anticipated in children.

An attempt should be made to quantify the degree of surgical resection in the postoperative period. MRI studies with and without intravenous gadolinium enhancement are most effective in this regard. Such studies should be performed within the first 48 h postoperatively to avoid enhancement associated with revascularization phenomena. These studies can then be used to direct subsequent therapy.

28.3
Primitive Neuroectodermal Tumors

Primitive neuroectodermal tumors (PNETs) of the posterior fossa are traditionally referred to as medulloblastomas (Fig. 28.4). These tumors account for approximately 30% of all childhood CNS tumors. Males are more commonly afflicted than females, and, although these tumors have been described in adults, the peak incidence is in the first decade (Russell and Rubinstein 1989).

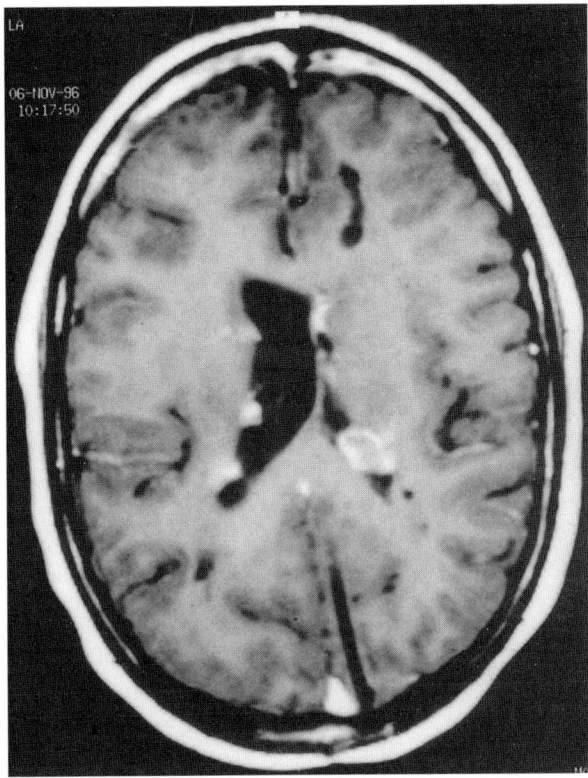

Fig. 28.4. T1-weighted axial MRI study documenting post-contrast enhancement of diffuse subependymal lesions metastatic from a primary PNET in the posterior fossa. Note the slight asymmetry of the ventricles and the left-sided shunt catheter

28.4
Astrocytomas

Astrocytomas represent a broad class of CNS neoplasms, originating from glial cells. Pilocytic astrocytomas are the most common type in children. These are classified as grade I by the World Health Organization's grading system (ZULCH 1979), and traditionally display a benign course. These tumors are classified based on their histology (Fig. 28.5). Although nuclear atypia and endothelial hyperplasia may occasionally be seen, these features do not herald a more ominous disease course; in fact, no prognostic information can be determined from any histological features of these tumors (HAYOSTEK et al. 1973). It should be noted that malignant progression has been documented in these tumors (KRIEGER et al. 1997).

Pilocytic astrocytomas are most commonly seen in the cerebellum, where they have also been called cerebellar astrocytomas or juvenile (pilocytic) astrocytomas. However, they also occur in the brainstem, cerebral hemispheres, hypothalamus, and anterior visual pathways (frequently associated with neurofibromatosis). There is no evidence that location influences the behavior of these tumors (WALLNER et al. 1988).

Surgical resection is the standard therapy for these lesions. A complete surgical resection is considered curative, with most studies citing survival rates of greater than 95% at 5 years (GILLES et al. 1995). However, resection may be limited when the tumor involves critical brain structures, such as the brainstem or optic chiasm/hypothalamic regions. In these cases, adjuvant therapy may be considered.

Nonpilocytic astrocytomas are also seen in children. As in adults, these range in malignancy from astrocytoma to anaplastic astrocytoma to glioblastoma multiforme. Unlike in adults, however, low-grade tumors are more common than high-grade ones.

Low-grade astrocytomas in children may have a better prognosis than in adults. In these cases, gross total resection may be sufficient, with adjuvant therapy indicated only for disease progression. In some series, 5-year progression-free survival can approach 95% after surgery alone (HIRSCH et al. 1989). Higher-grade tumors, however, carry a poor prognosis, and necessitate adjuvant therapy.

These lesions typically arise in the fourth ventricle. Given this location, they frequently present with hydrocephalus. The goals of up-front therapy are thus to relieve the hydrocephalus, obtain diagnostic tissue, and obtain maximal tumor resection. An attempt should be made to manage hydrocephalus without placement of a permanent CSF diversion. Early tumor removal with reconstitution of normal CSF pathways may be helpful in this regard. Various studies cite a less than 60% need for a permanent shunt if all cases are considered (ALBRIGHT 1989). Complete surgical resection is the goal. Initial studies which found statistically significant improved survival with resection greater than 90% have been borne out by subsequent practice (GEROSA 1981). All patients must be followed with serial MRI scans in the postoperative period to evaluate for residual or recurrent tumor (MENDEL et al. 1996). In all cases, spinal metastases should be searched for, and adjuvant therapy recommended.

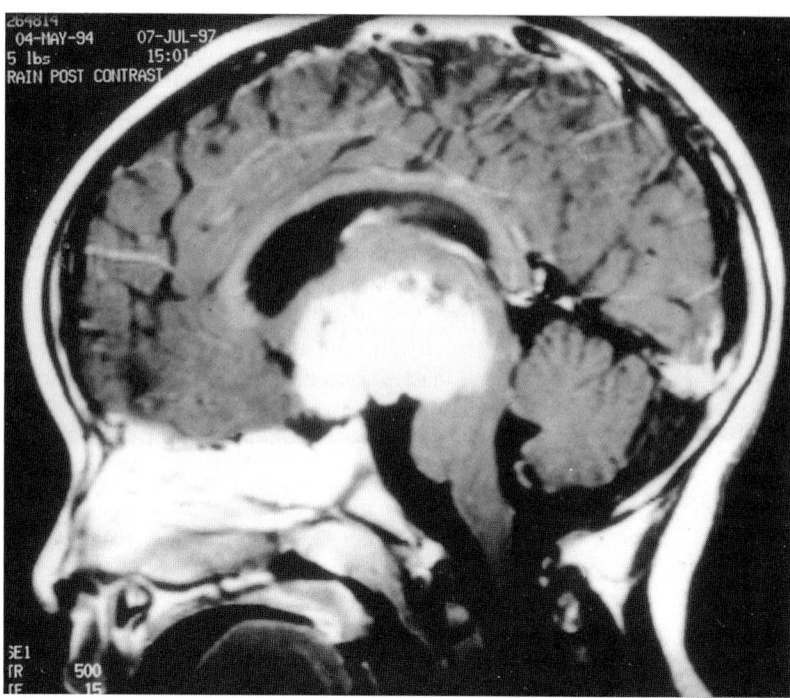

Fig. 28.5. T1-weighted post-contrast lateral MR image documenting marked enhancement of a large pilocytic astrocytoma involving the third ventricular chamber with marked compression of the mid brain

28.5
Ependymomas

Ependymomas are less common than either PNETs or astrocytomas in childhood. They represent approximately 10% of tumors in the young (Fig. 28.6). The peak age of incidence is at 5–6 years; they are rare tumors in patients older than 15 years (DOHRMANN et al. 1976).

Ependymomas arise from the ependymal cell layer, and thus are found in relation to the ventricular system. Rare cases may be entirely extraventricular, presumably arising from ependymal cell rests. These tumors are most commonly found in children in the posterior fossa; however, approximately one-third of ependymomas occur in the supratentorial compartment. These tumors may be solid or cystic, and form both rosettes and pseudorosettes. Anaplastic ependymomas display pleomorphism, necrosis, increased cellularity, and mitotic activity in addition to these typical features, and are found with increased frequency in the supratentorial compartment.

One particular problem inherent in the treatment of these tumors is their propensity for distal metastases, and spinal cord seeding in particular. Approximately 10% of intracranial ependymomas are associated with spinal cord seeding at some point in the disease course, although only 5% show such seeding at the time of diagnosis. Spinal cord metastases are more common with histologically high-grade tumors and with a posterior fossa primary site (LYONS et al. 1991)

Treatment must take into account the possibility of distant tumor spread. Surgery is the initial modality of choice as a means of diagnosis and, when appropriate, insuring CSF circulation. Complete resection is often impossible due to tumor invasion of the brainstem. Clinical significance can be obtained by gross total resection based on postoperative imaging studies (HELAY et al. 1991). However, surgery is not considered curative in itself and is usually followed by radiation therapy, as addressed elsewhere in this book.

Five-year survival rates are generally poor, ranging from 28% to 60% in various studies (GOLDWEIN et al. 1991; UNDJIAN et al. 1990). Young age, which might indicate a more malignant tumor and is often accompanied by limited or no radiation therapy, is associated with the poorest prognosis. Poor prognosis is also related to residual tumor burden postoperatively, distant metastases, and brain invasion. Histological grade and degree of surgical resection are controversial prognostic indicators.

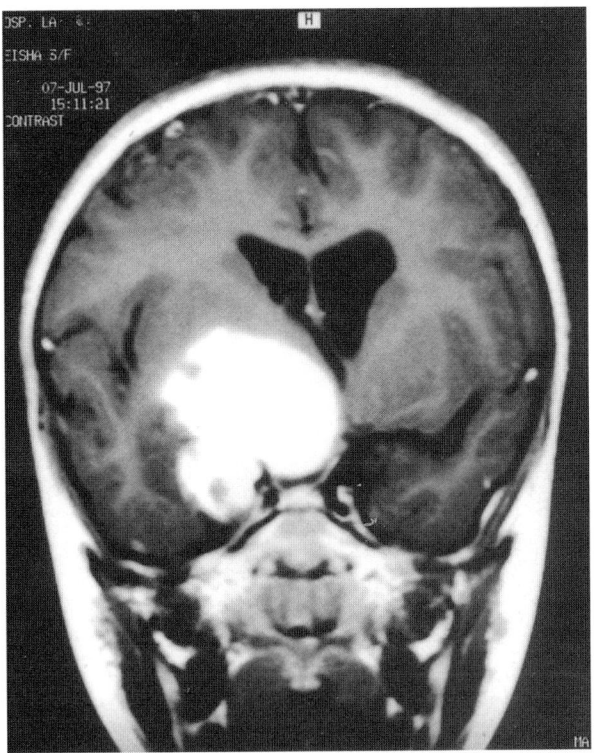

Fig. 28.6. T1-weighted post-contrast coronal MR image documenting a large temporal lobe astrocytoma. Note that this lesion is quite difficult to distinguish from a pilocytic astrocytoma. Note the marked shift of the third ventricular chamber and slight effacement of the lateral ventricular chamber on the right

28.6
Brainstem Gliomas

Brainstem tumors originate in the region between the diencephalon and the medulla. They typically occur at age 5–10 years, although they can be found in the very young as well as in adults. These tumors are typically astrocytic, and range from low- to high-grade histology. A small subgroup of these tumors is considered dorsally exophytic, with minimal brainstem involvement and a significant degree of extension into the fourth ventricle.

The general prognosis for these tumors is poor. Symptoms typically consist of cranial nerve abnormalities, disturbances of gait, and long tract signs. Hydrocephalus can be a relatively late finding. While the initial symptoms may be insidious, the course towards death is usually inexorable.

Surgery is of limited benefit. Some suggest the benefit of a biopsy to confirm the diagnosis, and rule out other treatable conditions (FRANK et al. 1988). However, the possibility of damage to this critical brain region weighs against its benefits. Additionally, limited biopsies can be of restricted value given the possibility of sampling error. In most cases, the imaging studies are all that is necessary for diagnosis.

Some do suggest surgery, however, for the so-called dorsally exophytic tumor. These tumors may have limited invasion of the brainstem, growing outward rather than inward. In these cases, long-term survival has been described with radical resection (EPSTEIN and WISOFF 1988).

28.7
Craniopharyngiomas

Craniopharyngiomas are histologically benign tumors which arise from retained elements of Rathke's pouch (Fig. 28.7). They are commonly seen in the late years of childhood. These tumors arise in the suprasellar region, and may extend into the third ventricle (see Chaps. 10 and 11).

Craniopharyngiomas come to clinical attention through elevation in intracranial pressure (due to

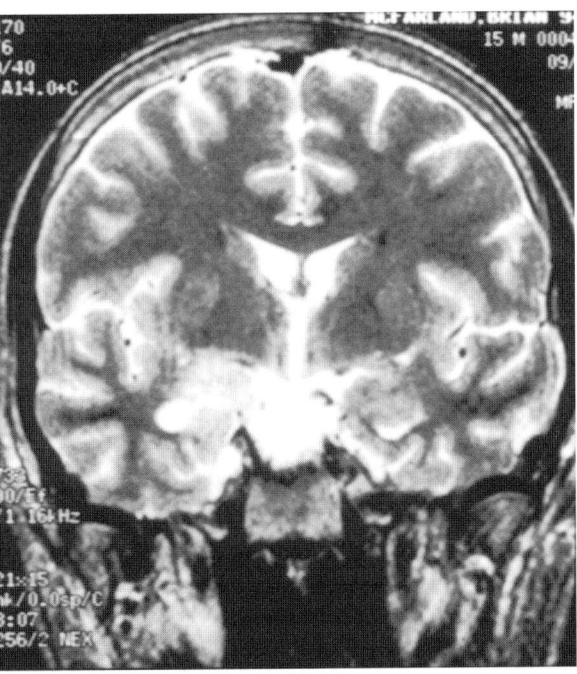

Fig. 28.7. T2-weighted coronal MR image documenting an anaplastic astrocytoma involving the mesial aspect of the temporal lobe on the right

mass effect or concomitant hydrocephalus), visual changes (due to pressure on the optic nerves/chiasm/or tract), or endocrine abnormalities. In children, these endocrine abnormalities usually consist of growth abnormalities, hypothyroidism, or diabetes insipidus.

Initial treatment consists of surgery. Complete resection is considered curative. However, the degree of resection is commonly limited by the adherence and invasive growth of these tumors within critical brain structures, particularly the hypothalamus and optic apparatus (LEVY et al. 1993; LEVY et al. 1997; LITOFSKY et al. 1993; APUZZO et al. 1991a,b). Postoperative endocrine compromise is common with aggressive surgical resection, and must be treated. In fact, endocrine dysfunction is common preoperatively as well, and must be assessed and treated to avoid complications with anesthesia. Many surgeons feel that an attempt at total surgical resection is unwarranted given the high rate of hypothalamic dysfunction seen, and advocate limited resection followed by radiation therapy. In some cases, these tumors contain a large cyst. When the symptomatology is related to the cyst, cyst aspiration can be effective. However, these cysts usually recur when the tumor is not extirpated, and consideration should be given to catheter placement for repeated cyst drainage. Some surgeons instill chemotherapeutic agents or radioactive elements into these cysts, resulting in cyst sclerosis and palliation in some cases.

28.8
Pineal Region Tumors

A heterogeneous group of tumors are found in the pineal region (Fig. 28.8). Broadly grouped, these include germinomas, nongerminoma germ cell tumors, and tumors of the pineal parenchyma. The incidence of these tumors varies greatly with geography. In particular, germinomas are extremely common in Japan, with a much lower incidence in the West (OI et al. 1992). These tumors are most commonly seen in adolescents, with a male predominance.

Germinomas are the most common tumor in the pineal region. These tumors, unlike germinomas in other regions of the CNS, are radiosensitive. Thus, the goal in their treatment is to make the diagnosis in as noninvasive a manner as possible and proceed with radiation. MRI studies can be suggestive, dis-

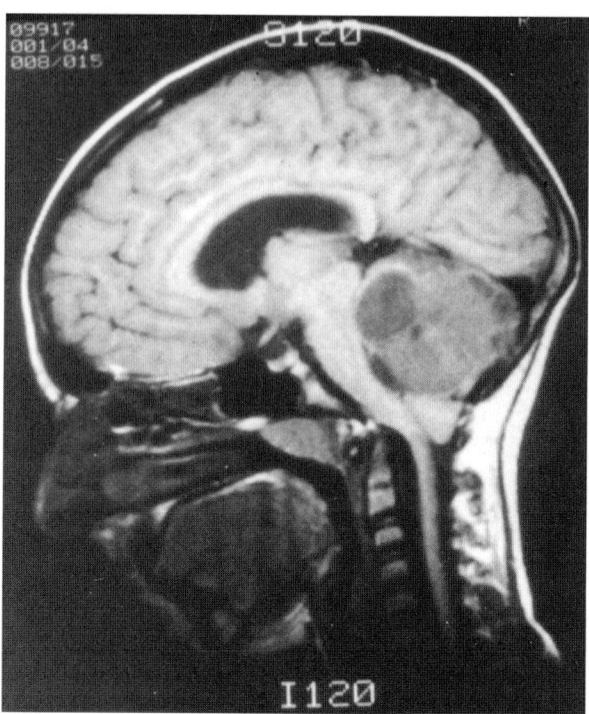

Fig. 28.8. T1-weighted pre-contrast lateral MRI study documenting a large posterior fossa astrocytoma

playing an evenly enhancing mass. Tumor markers, seen in the blood and CSF, are also helpful. Germinomas do not produce alpha-fetoprotein, distinguishing them from yolk cell tumors (such as endodermal sinus tumors and embryonal choriocarcinomas) and malignant teratomas. Germinomas can produce human chorionic gonadotrophin (HCG), particularly the beta subunit; however, levels are only modestly elevated (usually less than 100 mIU/ml), distinguishing them from choriocarcinomas (which evidence higher HCG levels).

Nongerminoma germ cell tumors are more rare than germinomas. This category includes relatively benign lesions such as dermoids, teratomas, and epidermoids. These lesions should be surgically resected when symptomatic. Less common lesions include choriocarcinomas, embryonal carcinomas, and endodermal sinus tumors. These are malignant, rapidly growing tumors which can metastasize outside of the CNS. Chemotherapy and radiation usually follow an attempt at surgical resection. Long-term survival is rare.

Tumors of the pineal body include pineocytomas and pineoblastomas. Pineoblastomas are histologically similar to PNETs, and carry a similar prognosis.

Pineocytomas are more commonly seen in adults, and rarely behave in an aggressive fashion. As with pineal cysts, treatment is predicated on the disease progression.

28.9
Choroid Plexus Tumors

Choroid plexus tumors are rare, representing less than 5% of all intracranial tumors in children (Fig. 28.9). In adults and older children, these tumors are seen more commonly in the fourth ventricle. However, in children they are usually seen in the lateral ventricles. The average age of onset is 9 months, with over half occurring before the age of 2 years (ALLEN et al. 1992)

Choroid plexus papillomas are benign lesions, with histology consistent with hyperplastic choroid plexus. They most commonly present with hydro-

cephalus, although it is a matter of some debate as to whether this is due to CSF overproduction (which has been shown to be as high as 5 times greater than normal) or decreased absorption (EISENBERG et al. 1974; MILHORAT et al. 1976; GUDEMAN et al. 1979). Choroid plexus carcinomas are rare lesions which can invade surrounding brain (Fig. 28.10). Both papillomas and carcinomas may seed the CSF, necessitating imaging of the complete neuraxis when this diagnosis is suspected.

The treatment of these lesions is surgical. Complete resection of a choroid plexus papilloma is curative, requiring no adjuvant therapy. The surgeon must acknowledge the vascularity of these lesions, and prepare for blood loss. Additionally, their deep location can make surgery a challenge. Choroid plexus carcinomas are rarely cured by surgery alone owing to their invasive nature. They do require subsequent therapy, as is discussed in subsequent chapters.

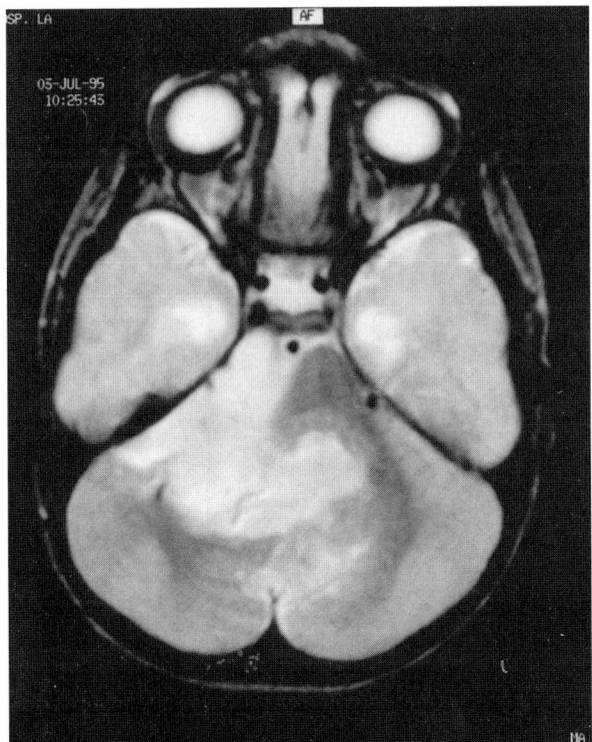

Fig. 28.9. T2-weighted axial MRI study documenting a large posterior fossa ependymoma. Note the significant involvement of the fourth ventricular chamber and extension of the tumor through the lateral foramen of Luschka with spread anterior to the pons, the tumor being adjacent to the basilar artery

28.10
Meningiomas

Meningiomas are relatively rare lesions in children. As in adults, complete resection is curative. However, meningiomas in children do have a tendency towards atypical behavior. They are larger than those seen in adults, and can show elements of sarcomatous change, with concomitant malignant behavior (DAVIDSON 1989). They also invade brain more frequently, and occasionally arise from ectopic cell rests, without a clear dural attachment. Complete surgical extirpation is the goal; residual tumor can be considered for radiation therapy.

28.11
Conclusions

Pediatric CNS tumors represent a heterogeneous class of tumors. In almost all of these cases, surgery plays a key role in the diagnosis and treatment. Degree of resection plays a large role in determining prognosis, and, in most cases, a total resection remains the goal. However, it must be kept in mind that surgery is only one facet of therapy for these lesions. A team approach is most effective, with new modalities offering significantly improved prognoses.

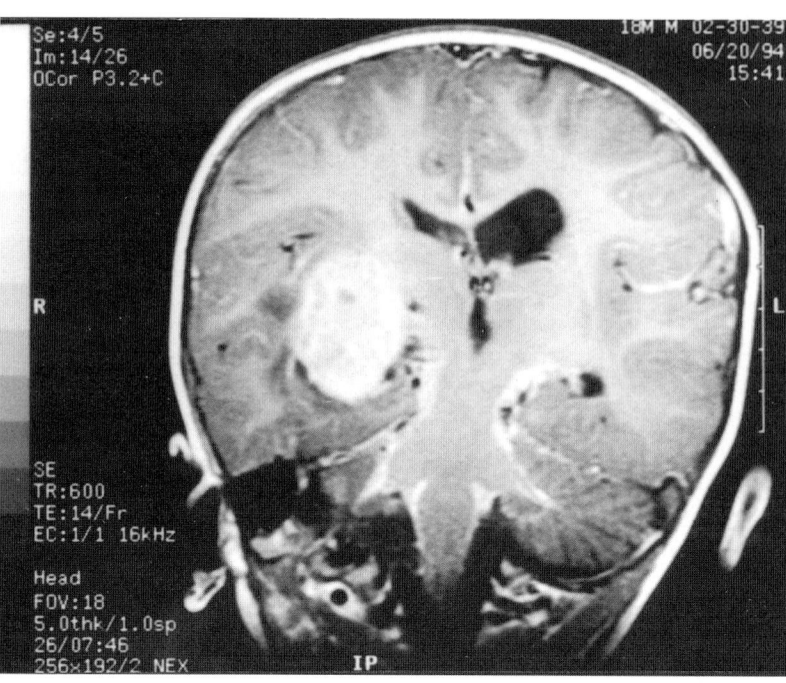

Fig. 28.10. T1-weighted coronal MR image documenting a choroid plexus carcinoma in a 2-year-old child. Note the significant enhancement and the presence in the right temporal horn

References

Albright AL (1989) Current neurosurgical treatment of medulloblastoma in children: A report from the Children's Cancer Group. Pediatric Neuroscience 15:276–282

Allen J, Wisoff J, Helson L, et al. (1992) Choroid plexus carcinoma: responses to chemotherapy alone in newly diagnosed young children. J Neurooncol 12:69–74

Apuzzo MLJ, Levy ML. (1991) Surgical management of craniopharyngioma and third ventricular tumors: Advances in Neurosurgery. Cont Neuro:17–26

Apuzzo MLJ, Levy ML, Tung H. (1991) Surgical strategies and technical methodologies in optimal management of craniopharyngioma and masses affecting the third ventricular chamber. Acta Neurochiurgica (suppl) 53:77–88

Chin L, Levy ML, Apuzzo MLJ. (1996) Principles of stereotactic surgery (ed) Youmans JR. Neurological Surgery. W.B. Saunders, Philadelphia, 767–785

Davidson GS, Hope JK. (1989): Meningeal tumors of childhood. Cancer 63:1205–1210

Dohrmann GJ, Farwell JR, Flannery JT. (1976) Ependymomas and ependymoblastomas in children. J Neurosurg 45:273–283

Edwards MS, Prados M. (1987) Current management of brain stem gliomas. Pediatr Neurosci 13: 309–315

Eisenberg HM, McComb JG, Lorenzo AV. (1974) Cerebrospinal fluid reproduction and hydrocephalus associated with choroid plexus papilloma. J Neurosurg 50:381–385

Epstein F, Murali R. (1978) Pediatric posterior fossa tumors: hazards of the "preoperative shunt." Neurosurgery 3:348–350

Epstein F, Wisoff JH. (1988) Intrinsic brain stem tumors in childhood: surgical indications. J Neurooncol 6:309–317

Frank F, Fabrizi AP, Frank-Ricci, Gaist G, Sedan R, Peragut JC. (1988) Stereotactic biopsy and treatment of brain stem lesions: combined study of 33 cases (Bologna-Marseille). Acta Neurochir 42:177–181

Gerosa MA, DiStefano E, Olivi A et al (1981) Multidisciplinary treatment of medulloblastoma: a 5-year experience with the SIOP trial. Child's Brain 8:107–118

Gilles FH, Sobel El, Tavare CJ, LevitonA, Hedley-Whyte ET, the Childhood Brain Tumor Consortium: (1995) Age-related changes in diagnosis, histological features, and survival in children with brain tumors: 1930–1979. Neurosurgery 37: 1056–1068

Goldwein JW, Leahy JM, Packer RJ, et al. (1990) Intracranial ependymomas in children. Int J Radiat Oncol biol Phys 19:1497–1502

Gudeman SK, Sullivan HG, Rosner MH, Becker DP. (1979) Surgical removal of bilateral papillomas of the choroid plexus of the lateral ventricles with resolution of hydrocephalus. J Neurosurg 50:677–681

Hayostek CJ, Shaw EG, Scheithauer B, O'Fallon JR, Weiland TL, Schomberg PJ, Kelly PJ, Ju TC: (1993) Astrocytomas of the cerebellum: A comparative clinicopathologic study of pilocytic and diffuse astrocytomas. Cancer 72:856–869

Healey EA, Barnes PD, Kupsky WJ, Scott RM, Sallan SE, Black PM, Tarbell NJ. (1991) The prognostic significance of postoperative residual tumor in ependymoma. Neurosurgery 28:666–671

Hirsch JF, Rose CS, Kahn AP, Pfister A, Hoppe-Hirsch E. (1989) Benign astrocytic and oligodendrocytic tumors of the cerebral hemispheres in children. J Neurosurg 70:568–572

Kobayashi S, Sugita K, Tanaka Y, Kyoshima K. (1983) Infratentorial approach to the pineal region in the prone position: Concorde position. J Neurosurg 58:141–143

Krieger MD, Gonzalez-Gomez I, Levy ML, McComb JG. (1997) Recurrence patterns and anaplastic change in a long-term study of pilocytic astrocytomas. Pediatr Neurosurg 27:1–11

Levy ML, Khoo L, McComb JG. (1997) Optimization of the operative corridor for the resection of craniopharyngiomas in children: the combined fronto-orbitozygomatic temporopolar approach. Neurosurg Focus 3: (6)

Levy ML, Litofsky NS, Apuzzo MLJ. (1993) Hypothalamic hypophyseal compromise attendant to craniopharyngioma management (ed) Apuzzo MLJ, Brain Surgery: Complication avoidance and management. Churchill, Livingston, New York. 319–338

Litofsky NS, Levy ML, Apuzzo MLJ. (1993) The spectrum of adverse sequelae in the surgical management of craniopharyngioma. (ed) Apuzzo MLJ, Brain Surgery: Complication avoidance and management. Churchill, Livingston, New York. 313–318

Lyons MK, Kelly PJ. (1991) Posterior fossa ependymomas: report of 30 cases and review of the literature. Neurosurgery 28:659–665

McComb JG, Levy ML, Apuzzo MLJ. (1997) Supratentorial interhemispheric approaches to the third ventricle. (ed) Apuzzo MLJ, Surgery of The Third Ventricle. Churchill, Livingston, New York.. 743–777

Mendel E, Raffel C, McComb JG, Gans W, Pikus H, Levy ML. (1996): Surveillance imaging in children with primitive neuroectodermal tumors. Neurosurgery 38:692–695

Milhorat TH, Davis DA, Hammock MK. (1976) Choroid plexus papilloma. II: Ultrastructure and ultracytochemical localization of Na-K-ATPase. Childs Brain 2:290–303

Oi S, Matsumoto S. (1992) Controversy pertaining to therapeutic modalities for tumors of the pineal region: a worldwide survey of different patient populations. Childs Nerv Syst; 8 (6):332–336

Russell DS, Rubinstein LJ 1989 Pathology of tumors of the nervous system, 5th Ed, Edward Arnold, London

Undjian S, Marinov M. Intracranial ependymomas in children. (1990) Childs Nerv Syst 6:131–134

Wallner KE, Gonzales MF, Edwards MSB, Wara WM, Sheline GE: (1988) Treatment results of juvenile pilocytic astrocytoma. J Neurosurg 69:171–176

Zulch KJ: Histological typing of tumors of the central nervous system. Geneva, World Health Organization, 1979

29 Chemotherapy in Pediatric Patients

Douglas J. Hyder

CONTENTS

29.1
Introduction

Brain tumors are now the most common malignancy affecting children and the proportion of cancer deaths due to central nervous system tumors has doubled in the last 25 years (BLEYER 1999). Use of adjuvant chemotherapy has facilitated outstanding improvement in progression-free survival (PFS) and overall survival (OS) for children with primitive neuroectodermal–posterior fossa medulloblastoma. In contrast, tumors affecting infants and children less than 3 years of age at diagnosis remain difficult to treat effectively with surgery and adjuvant chemotherapy, though recent studies demonstrate the utility of adjuvant chemotherapy as a means to delay radiation during the critical neurodevelopmental

D. J. HYDER, MD
Assistant Professor of Neurology and Pediatrics, University of Southern California, Childrens Hospital Los Angeles, 4650 Sunset Boulevard, Los Angeles, CA 90027, USA

window when radiation is associated with permanent neurocognitive sequelae. Other tumors, such as brainstem glioma and ependymoma, appear to be less sensitive or insensitive to the currently available chemotherapeutics.

This discussion focuses on chemotherapy clinical trials conducted during the last 20 years as a means to understand the current clinical studies and best available therapies. Emphasis is placed on the use of chemotherapy before first relapse since the prognosis for relapsed pediatric brain tumors remains poor and new chemotherapeutic trials accrue too rapidly to allow for a timely discussion.

29.2
Astrocytoma

Pediatric brain tumors arising from the glia – astrocytomas, oligodendrogliomas, and gangliogliomas – are conventionally lumped together in discussions of chemotherapy although it is likely that these tumors have distinct etiologies and responses to therapy. The World Health Organization (WHO) classification broadly classifies these tumors as low grade, anaplastic, and high grade, in contradistinction to the Daumas-Duport system widely used for adult brain tumors of glial origin (BROWN et al. 1998). This discussion is divided between the chemotherapy of pediatric low-grade astrocytomas and the treatment of high-grade gliomas.

29.2.1
Low-Grade Astrocytoma

Low-grade astrocytoma (LGA) is the most common brain tumor affecting children. About 450–500 LGA are diagnosed each year in the United States. The male-to-female ratio is about equal. Pediatric astrocytomas occur at all ages throughout the first 18 years, with peaks in incidence at 5 years and again at

13 years. About half of LGA are supratentorial; of these, half are hemispheric, and the other half are midline, diencephalic, or thalamic (REIS et al. 1999). Those with neurofibromatosis type 1 have an increased risk, as high as 5%–21%, of developing LGA involving the optic nerve or chiasm (COHEN and DUFFNER 1994). Conversely, about 50%–70% children with optic gliomas have NF-1. (PIERCE et al. 1990). Infratentorial astrocytomas involving the cerebellum are associated with a cyst in 80% of patients (GOL and MCKISSOCK 1959). These cerebellar tumors were recognized by Cushing to be curable if the mural nodule is completely resected (CUSHING 1931).

Symptoms of LGA are wide-ranging and dependent on the location of the tumor, but generally include headache and vomiting (SHIN and WEBSTER 1979). Hemispheric tumors can result in seizures or weakness, numbness, and incoordination. Optic chiasmatic tumors are associated with loss of visual acuity, changes in visual fields, hormonal dysfunction, and in children less than 3 years a severe weight loss despite good oral intake, called Russell's diencephalic syndrome (STARCESKI et al. 1990; RUSSELL 1980). Symptoms of cerebellar tumors are truncal or extremity incoordination, nystagmus, and symptoms related to increased intracranial pressure: morning headache, nausea, and vomiting.

Complete surgical resection is widely regarded as the best therapy for LGA. Cerebellar astrocytomas are usually cured with surgery alone. A complete surgical resection sometimes requires more than one procedure or approach. The results of Children's Cancer Group 9891 demonstrate that complete surgical resection is of benefit for LGA. The OS of children with these tumors is 95%, but if the tumor is not completely resected, the event-free survival (EFS) is only 75% (DHODAPKAR et al. 1999). Exceptions to surgical resection are when the patient has neurofibromatosis type 1 (the course is then more benign) and when the risk of permanent neurological dysfunction outweighs the potential gains of resection, such as in the case of thalamic tumors or tumors involving the speech and memory (LISTERNICK et al. 1999).

Chemotherapy has been extensively studied for the treatment of LGA. As a single agent, carboplatin used to treat progressive or recurrent LGA demonstrates prolonged disease stabilization between 2 and 68+ months (median 36+ months) (FRIEDMAN et al. 1992). Cyclophosphamide and, in a separate study, oral etoposide have also demonstrated efficacy against disseminated or recurrent LGA when used as single agents (MCCOWAGE et al. 1996; CHAMBERLAIN 1997).

Carboplatin and vincristine chemotherapy has demonstrated efficacy against recurrent or progressive LGA (PACKER et al. 1997). The most recent report reviews 78 children (mean age of 3 years) with newly diagnosed, progressive LGA. Overall, 56% of patients showed objective response to chemotherapy and PFS was 75% at 2 years and 68% at 3 years. There was no difference in PFS between those with NF-1 (15 patients) and those without NF. The only prognostic factor identified was age: children 5 years or younger at treatment had a better PFS (74%) than older children (39%).

The combination of thioguanine, procarbazine, CCNU, and vincristine (TPCV) is reported in two series. In a study of 16 children with LGA (median age 3.2 years) treated with TPCV after clinical or radiographic progression, 13 (81%) had either partial response or stabilization of disease (PETRONIO et al. 1991). The patients who failed chemotherapy were satisfactorily treated with radiation after relapse. Median time to tumor progression at publication had not been reached at 79 weeks. An update reported the use of TPCV in 42 patients with progressive LGA and demonstrated no patients with a complete response, but 15 (36%) with objective response and 25 (60%) with stabilization of disease. Median time to progression was 132 weeks, with 26 children suffering progressive disease (PRADOS et al. 1997).

Currently, the Children's Cancer Group is running a phase III study comparing carboplatin/vincristine and TPCV for children less than 10 years with progressive LGA. This study may help determine whether chemotherapy can effectively delay or obviate the need for radiation or extensive surgery. Considering the excellent OS, it may require many years to determine the effectiveness and long-term sequelae of these regimens.

29.2.2
High-Grade Glioma

In contrast to low-grade gliomas, high-grade gliomas (HGG) account for only about 10% of pediatric brain tumors; two-thirds of these tumors involve the cerebral hemispheres, 20% are diencephalic, and 15% are located in the posterior fossa including the brainstem. The median age at diagnosis is 9–10 years and there is no gender predilection (HEIDEMAN et al. 1997). Symptoms of HGG are wide-ranging, depend upon the location of the tumor, and similar to the symptoms of LGA. For the purposes of discussion, several histological types of tumor are frequently presented together. HGG includes anaplastic astrocytomas and glioblastoma multiforme, and other less common tumors such as high-grade oligodendroglioma and mixed high-grade oligoastrocytomas.

As is seen with adults, children with HGG present several therapeutic challenges since these are poorly circumscribed, invasive parenchymal tumors that may metastasize regionally or, in rare circumstances, to other sites in the body, are difficult to resect, and tend to recur even after optimum surgery and radiation.

Initial chemotherapy trials focused on nitrosoureas, paralleling adult studies (PHUPHANICH et al. 1984). Single-agent trials with platinum, procarbazine, cyclophosphamide, and etoposide have all led to occasional responses, but disappointing results overall (WALKER and ALLEN 1988; NEWTON et al. 1990; HEIDEMAN et al. 1995; ABRAHAMSEN et al. 1995; NEEDLE et al. 1997).

The combination of procarbazine, CCNU, and vincristine (PCV) remains the most widely used adjuvant regimen after surgery and radiation. LEVIN reported the use of PCV in 58 patients with recurrent or newly diagnosed HGG and demonstrated that 26% responded to therapy and an additional 35% had stabilization of disease (LEVIN et al. 1980). Better results were seen with the 19 patients not previously treated with another chemotherapy regimen: in this group, 42% responded to PCV and an additional 42% had stable disease. At the time of the report, 30% were alive without tumor progression at 1 year. The median time to progression was 26 weeks. CAIRNCROSS reported a dose-intensified PCV regimen used for 24 patients with anaplastic oligodendroglioma in which 75% of patients responded, 38% with complete responses (CAIRNCROSS et al. 1994).

Other combination chemotherapy regimens, such as MOPP (nitrogen mustard, vincristine, procarbazine, and prednisone), 7 drugs in 1 day (CCNU, vincristine, hydroxyurea, procarbazine, cisplatin, cytosine arabinoside, and DTIC), and cyclophosphamide and etoposide, have proven to be of limited efficacy (VAN EYS et al. 1988; PENDERGRASS et al. 1987; MISER et al 1989).

In a phase III adjuvant chemotherapy trial, CCG-943, the 8 in 1 regimen was compared with CCNU/vincristine (FINLAY et al. 1995). The 172 patients in the study had a 5-year PFS of 33% and 36% respectively on the two chemotherapy arms, a difference that was not statistically significant. Surgical resection was the most important factor influencing survival: 39% of patients with greater than 90% resection were progression-free survivors at 5 years, compared with 14% who had partial resection or less.

Trials of dose intensification with myeloablation and autologous stem cell transplant (ASCT) have been attempted. FINLAY reported use of etoposide (1500 mg/mg^2) and thiotepa (900 mg/m^2) in 43 patients with recurrent brain tumors, 18 of whom had HGG (FINLAY et al. 1996). Objective responses were seen in 4 (29%) of 14 evaluable patients. Five (28%) of 18 patients with minimal residual disease are progression-free survivors with follow-up between 39 and 59 months at the time of the report.

In 13 patients a combination of thiotepa (900 mg/m^2) and cyclophosphamide (6 g/m^2) used within a month of surgery then followed at day 60 with radiotherapy resulted in only one (8%) complete response and three (23%) partial responses (HEIDEMAN et al. 1993). The reported median OS was 14 months and the median PFS was 9 months.

Conventional surgery, radiation, and PCV chemotherapy remain the standard therapy. Several studies are currently underway to improve the outlook for patients with HGG. Ideas include better stratification of patients, dose intensification, the use of radiosensitizers, and newer agents such as anti-angiogenesis drugs. (POLLACK et al. 1999).

29.3
Primitive Neuroectodermal Tumors

29.3.1
Primitive Neuroectodermal Tumor – Posterior Fossa (PNET-PF)/Medulloblastoma

Medulloblastoma is one of the most common primary brain tumors affecting children (RIES 1999). Tremendous strides have been made in the treatment of medulloblastoma since it was first described by BAILEY and CUSHING (1925). About 300 children are diagnosed with medulloblastoma each year in the United States, and about 100 of them are considered average risk. For unclear reasons, the male-to-female ratio is approximately 3:2. The majority of low-risk patients are between 5 and 9 years old (RIES 1999). The most common presenting symptoms are headache, secondary to mass effect on the meninges or obstruction of cerebrospinal fluid (CSF) flow increasing intracranial pressure, incoordination, double vision, nausea, and vomiting (HEIDEMAN et al. 1997). Imaging the brain with computerized tomography (CT) or magnetic resonance imaging (MRI) demonstrates an inhomogeneously enhancing fourth ventricular mass, sometimes associated with enlarged lateral and third ventricles (ATLAS and LAVI 1996). Treatment begins with surgical resection. The goal of surgical resection is twofold: to safely remove as much tumor mass as possible and to establish, if necessary, CSF flow. Sometimes more than one surgical procedure is necessary to accomplish these goals.

Medulloblastoma can be locally invasive and may metastasize within the CSF, the neural axis (brain metastasis or spinal drop metastasis), or, rarely, elsewhere in the body (such as the bone marrow or abdominal cavity). Metastatic workup is determined by the individual patient's symptoms, but standard staging for all patients is a postoperative MRI of the brain to assess the extent of tumor resection and metastatic disease, MRI of the spine to look for metastatic disease, lumbar puncture to check CSF for tumor cells, and, if bone pain or an abnormal CBC is present, a bilateral bone marrow aspirate and biopsy. Although ideally staging is done prior to surgical resection, in many cases it is impractical and imprudent to delay surgery just to obtain staging tests.

Several outcome predictors have been identified by Chang (HARISIADIS and CHANG 1977). The Chang staging system (Table 29.1) is still commonly used, but with improvements in surgical instruments and technique, the preoperative size of the tumor (the T stage) does not, generally, have a significant impact on outcome. PNET-PF/medulloblastoma is currently divided into three risk categories: average risk, high risk, and infants. The average risk patient must be older than 3 years of age, have less than 1.5 cm^2 of residual tumor, and have no evidence of CSF or neural axis

metastatic disease (PACKER et al. 1986). Infants are considered to be patients younger than 3 years of age at diagnosis. High-risk patients, excluding infants, have greater than 1.5 cm^2 residual tumor after optimal safe resection, or metastatic disease. Although rare, medulloblastoma affecting adults over the age of 21 years are also considered high-risk cases.

Histologically, medulloblastoma is composed of sheets of small round cells that appear blue with hematoxylin/eosin staining. Immunohistochemistry is helpful in confirming the diagnosis; the usual positive markers are synaptophysin, cytokeratin, desmin, vimentin, neurofilament proteins, and occasionally glial fibrillary acid protein. Sometimes differentiation along neuronal or glial lines is present, but reports conflict as to the significance of this finding (GIANGASPERO et al. 1997).

It is generally considered that surgery alone will not cure even a completely resected medulloblastoma. In Cushing's 1930 series, only 1 patient out of 61 was alive at 3 years (CUSHING 1930). The need for adjuvant therapy was recognized and beginning around 1950, radiation of the entire neuraxis was used following surgical resection. Radiation therapy for medulloblastoma is discussed in detail in Chap. 27, but the recognition in the 1960s that chemotherapy was effective for other solid tumors led to the initial use of chemotherapy for medulloblastoma.

Initial reports of chemotherapy were published in the late 1960s with the use of intrathecal methotrexate and intravenous vincristine. In the early 1970s, the alkylating agents CCNU and BCNU gained favor because of their high lipid solubility, low molecular weight, and lack of ionization at physiological pH.

Table 29.1. Chang staging of medulloblastoma (from CHANG et al. 1969)

Stage	Definition
T1	Tumor <3 cm in diameter and limited to midline vermis, roof of fourth ventricle, and (less frequently) cerebellar hemispheres
T2	Tumor >3 cm in diameter, further invading one adjacent structure or partially filling fourth ventricle
T3a	Tumor invading two adjacent structures or completely filling fourth ventricle with extension into aqueduct of Sylvius, foramen of Magendie, or foramen of Luschka, thus producing marked internal hydrocephalus
T3b	Tumor arising from floor of fourth ventricle or brainstem and filling fourth ventricle
T4	Tumor further spreading through aqueduct of Sylvius to involve third ventricle of midbrain, or tumor extending to upper cervical cord
	Metastases
M0	No evidence of gross subarachnoid or hematogenous metastasis
M1	Microscopic tumor cells in cerebrospinal fluid
M2	Gross nodular seeding demonstrated in cerebellar, cerebral arachnoid space, or in third or lateral ventricles
M3	Gross nodular seeding in spinal subarachnoid space
M4	Extraneuronal metastasis

These chemotherapy trials failed to show an improvement in OS, but did suggest a positive result of chemotherapy. The standard of care through most of the 1980s remained surgery and radiation therapy for average risk medulloblastoma, resulting in about a 70% 3-year EFS.

The addition of cisplatin to the chemotherapy regimen was a breakthrough reported by PACKER et al. (1988). In this study, cisplatin, CCNU, and vincristine were administered to the high-risk patients after surgery and radiotherapy. Surprisingly, these high-risk patients did better than the low-risk patients who were treated without adjuvant chemotherapy. This study was quickly followed by reports demonstrating the effectiveness of this adjuvant chemotherapy regimen for average risk patients. Using vincristine during radiotherapy and eight cycles of adjuvant cisplatin, vincristine, and CCNU, average risk patients have a 90% 5-year EFS (PACKER et al. 1994).

Toxicities of the cisplatin, vincristine, and CCNU used for average risk medulloblastoma include fatigue, anorexia, weight loss, high-frequency hearing loss, anemia, thrombocytopenia, leukopenia, hypomagnesemia, constipation, and peripheral neuropathy. Renal dysfunction, liver dysfunction, and pulmonary fibrosis are less common but potential deleterious effects. About half of patients treated with this regimen will need the cisplatin dose to be reduced or eliminated because of hearing loss (PACKER et al. 1994).

Currently, Children's Cancer Group and Pediatric Oncology Group are sponsoring an intergroup phase III trial randomizing average risk PNET-PF/medulloblastoma patients to receive either adjuvant CCNU, cisplatin, and vincristine or cyclophosphamide, cisplatin, and vincristine.

29.3.2
Supratentorial and Pineal PNET

The treatment of high-risk medulloblastoma has not been as successful as treatment of average risk disease. High-risk disease is defined as greater than 1.5 cm^2 of residual tumor after surgery, disseminated disease at diagnosis, or non-posterior fossa location. Although absence of metastases at diagnosis and pineal involvement are independent predictors of better outcome, the 3-year PFS for supratentorial (45%) and pineal (61%) PNET is significantly worse than that for infratentorial PNET (>85%) (COHEN et al. 1995).

The efficacy of adjuvant chemotherapy for high-risk PNET was initially demonstrated by Packer, who

between 1975 and 1989 used adjuvant cisplatin, vincristine, and CCNU after surgical resection and radiation in selected high-risk patients (posterior fossa primary and age over 18 months at diagnosis, with either subtotal resection, metastatic disease at diagnosis, or brainstem involvement) and demonstrated that the entire cohort had a 5-year OS of 83%, and that patients with metastatic disease had a 5-year PFS of 67% (PACKER et al. 1994).

A group of 22 patients with supratentorial and pineal tumors treated with the same regimen were reviewed and the overall PFS was found to be 47% at 3 years and 37% at 5 years, demonstrating that patients in whom the tumor location is supratentorial or pineal do worse overall that patients with posterior fossa primary tumors (REDDY et al. 1998).

Three strategies are currently being studied to improve the efficacy of chemotherapy. The first approach is to use chemotherapy prior to radiation. The CCG 9931 trial that used five cycles of multi-agent chemotherapy prior to radiation resulted in 30% of patients suffering disease progression prior to radiation. Among those who completed the entire chemotherapy and radiation therapy protocol, the results were disappointing: patients with supratentorial PNET had a 60% 2-year EFS, those with metastatic disease at diagnosis had a 42% 2-year EFS, and those with incomplete primary resections had a 48% 2-year EFS (ALLEN et al. 1999). A similar strategy using cisplatin and etoposide either before or after radiation is currently being reviewed as POG 9031.

A second strategy to improve the efficacy of chemotherapy centering on dose intensification with autologous stem cell rescue is currently underway, based on treatment regimens developed for recurrent medulloblastoma. DUNKEL et al. (1998a) reported 23 patients with recurrent medulloblastoma who received high-dose carboplatin, thiotepa, and etoposide followed by autologous stem cell transplant. Among these patients, there were three (13%) toxic deaths and eight (35%) progression-free survivors at 3 years (DUNKEL et al. 1998a). Another report using thiotepa and busulfan in the conditioning regimen for recurrent medulloblastoma found a 50% EFS at 31 months (DUPUIS-GIROD et al. 1996).

The third strategy is to use chemotherapy during radiation. POG 9631 is investigating concurrent etoposide during radiation followed by adjuvant cisplatin, etoposide, cyclophosphamide, and vincristine, and CCG 99701 is attempting the use of concurrent carboplatin during radiation followed by one of two cyclophosphamide-based adjuvant regimens.

29.4
Infants and Children
Diagnosed Before Age 3 Years

Children who are diagnosed with a brain tumor before the age of 3 years account for about 20% of pediatric brain tumors and have a lower 5-year OS, ranging from 45% to 59%, than is seen in older children (RIES et al. 1999). Surgery alone is rarely curative for this group, and an attempt is made to avoid or delay radiation therapy because of the risk of poor long-term neurocognitive function (DUFFNER et al. 1993). Ependymomas and PNET are more commonly seen in this younger age group (REIS et al. 1999). Tumors such as teratomas and atypical teratoma/rhabdoid tumor are also seen more commonly in young children. Signs and symptoms of brain tumors in infants are macrocephaly, vomiting, eye movement abnormalities, loss of developmental milestones, lethargy, failure to thrive, and infrequently seizures (COHEN and DUFFNER 1994).

Chemotherapy is used in infants with brain tumors in an effort to supplement surgical resection while avoiding or delaying radiation therapy. The largest of these studies, using prolonged postoperative chemotherapy to defer radiation, was reported by DUFFNER et al. (1993). The phase II clinical trial, POG 8633, used cyclophosphamide and vincristine alternating with cisplatin and etoposide in 198 infants with malignant brain tumors. Children younger than 2 years of age received 24 months of chemotherapy followed by radiation therapy, while those between 2 and 3 years old received 12 months of chemotherapy and radiation therapy. At 2 years there was a 39% chemotherapy response rate and PFS of about 40%, demonstrating the ability to delay radiation therapy. In a recent follow-up, the authors reported the estimated risk of secondary malignancy 8 years after diagnosis to be 11% in their entire cohort, and almost 19% in children younger than 2 years of age (DUFFNER et al. 1998). Reasons suggested include a genetic predisposition to cancer and prolonged exposure to alkylating agents and etoposide with or without irradiation.

A Children's Cancer Group study (CCG 9921) using five courses of induction chemotherapy with either cyclophosphamide, cisplatin, etoposide, and vincristine or ifosfamide, carboplatin, etoposide, and vincristine and then eight cycles of maintenance chemotherapy with cyclophosphamide, etoposide, carboplatin, and vincristine enrolled 299 patients (GEYER et al. 1998). The study enrolled 102 (34%) infants with medulloblastoma, 59 (13%) with suprat-

entorial PNET, 76 (25%) with ependymoma, and 24 (8%) with high-grade gliomas. The PFS at 2 years for these groups was 30% for medulloblastoma, 34% for nonpineal supratentorial PNET, 9% for pineal PNET, and 31% for ependymoma. For the entire group, PFS and OS at 2 years were 29% and 53% respectively. In contrast to the Duffner study, radiation was reserved for patients with residual tumor after induction, metastatic tumor at diagnosis, or progressive disease. A small minority of patients reportedly received radiation therapy prior to disease progression.

High-dose chemotherapy with autologous stem cell transplant was reported in the treatment of children younger than 6 years of age who relapsed after conventional chemotherapy but had not received radiation therapy (GURUANGAN et al. 1998). One of the three chemotherapy regimens using thiotepa and etoposide-based protocols was used in 20 patients, followed by radiation therapy in patients with PNET (but not HGG). PFS of 50% is reported with median follow-up of 38 months after autologous stem cell transplant.

Newly diagnosed infants and children less than 6 years of age with malignant tumors were treated after maximal surgical resection with five cycles of vincristine, cisplatin, cyclophosphamide, and etoposide followed by myeloablative chemotherapy with carboplatin, thiotepa, and etoposide and then autologous bone marrow rescue (MASON et al. 1998). Radiation therapy was used in patients with residual tumor at consolidation or at tumor progression. Of the 62 children, 37 (60%) received induction and myeloablative chemotherapy. Radiation therapy was administered to 19 (31%) of these patients. Three-year EFS was 25% while OS was 40%.

Currently CCG study 99703 seeks to build on the experience with high-dose chemotherapy by both increasing the dose of chemotherapy and decreasing the interval between cycles using peripheral blood stem cells. In this study, only three cycles of cyclophosphamide, cisplatin, etoposide, and vincristine were used during induction preceded three cycles of thiotepa and carboplatin followed by peripheral blood stem cell support.

29.5
Brainstem Glioma

Brainstem glioma is one of the most challenging tumors affecting children. Since the tumor affects the brainstem, cortical cognitive functions remain largely intact while eye and facial movements, coordination, swallowing, and breathing gradually diminish. The tumor is usually not amenable to surgical resection, is temporarily delayed by radiation therapy, and is largely unresponsive to chemotherapy.

Brainstem glioma usually presents with headache, diplopia, difficulty in swallowing liquids, incoordination, and weakness. A careful neurological examination frequently reveals multiple cranial neuropathies. Functions of the cerebral cortex, such as visual acuity, language, and memory are usually normal. Sometimes, inappropriate affect, such as untimely laughter, is present. A careful skin examination, looking for café-au-lait macules and axillary freckling, and a slit lamp examination looking for Lisch nodules should be done to search for signs of neurofibromatosis type 1 (COHEN and DUFFNER 1994).

Imaging with CT or MRI reveals an enlarged pons, sometimes two or three times the normal size. The mass enhances with contrast. At times, blood or a fluid-filled cavity may be present within the mass. The differential diagnosis of a pontine mass is tumor, vascular malformation, infection, and sarcoidosis (ATLAS and LAVI 1996).

Radiation therapy is the most effective therapy for temporarily alleviating symptoms and delaying tumor growth. Doses generally used are 6–7 Gy without concomitant chemotherapy. Strategies to improve the effectiveness of chemotherapy, such as opening up the blood-brain barrier with RMP-7 and then administering carboplatin or using RSR-13 to improve oxygenation of the tumor tissue, are currently being studied.

Chemotherapy has been reported in multiple publications only to be of marginal benefit. Chamberlain reported the use of etoposide, a DNA topoisomerase II inhibitor, at a daily dose of 50 mg/m^2 daily for 3 weeks, followed by a 1-week rest (CHAMBERLAIN 1993). His cohort of 12 patients had all relapsed after radiation therapy, and five had also previously received nitrosourea-based chemotherapy. Six of the 12 patients demonstrated a radiographic response (one complete, three partial, and two stable disease) with a median duration of response of 8 months. Needle reported more disappointing results: of the three recurrent brain tumors treated with oral etoposide, only one had stabilization of disease (NEEDLE et al. 1997). There is no evidence to support the use of high-dose chemotherapy with autologous stem cell rescue for children with brainstem glioma (DUNKEL et al. 1998b).

In the patient with neurofibromatosis type 1, survival may be prolonged, even without treatment.

MOLLOY reports that brainstem glioma in those with neurofibromatosis type 1 may be a distinct clinical entity: of the 17 patients evaluated, 15 (88%) remained alive with median follow-up of 52 months, and 14 of these patients did not require adjuvant therapy (MOLLOY et al. 1995).

29.6
Ependymoma

Ependymomas account for 10%–12% of all childhood brain tumors. Two-thirds of ependymomas arise within the posterior fossa; the remainder are supratentorial. Although some ependymomas are considered histologically malignant, this has no demonstrated prognostic significance. Prognosis is related to extent of surgical resection and radiation therapy. Ependymomas that affect infants and children diagnosed before age 3 are not treated according to the infant protocols previously discussed.

Despite multiple attempts, there is little evidence to support the use of chemotherapy in children with ependymoma. BOUFFET and FOREMAN (1999) report in their meta-analysis that the response rate to single agents is 11% with less than 5% complete responses, cisplatin being the most active agent in phase II studies. Combination chemotherapy has a better response rate, approaching 26%, but only a 12% complete response rate. The current standard is to use surgery and radiation therapy for ependymomas in patients older than 3–5 years at diagnosis. Chemotherapy is reserved for experimental protocols and infants and children diagnosed before age 3 years.

29.7
Primary Central Nervous System Germ Cell Tumors

Primary CNS germ cell tumors are relatively uncommon in the United States, representing about 3% of all pediatric brain tumors. In Japan and Taiwan the incidence of these tumors approaches 9%–15% for unclear reasons (ROSENBLUM and NG 1997). Cell tumors can arise anywhere in the brain or spinal cord, but most commonly involve the pineal or suprasellar region. About two-thirds of these tumors are germinomas; the remainder, consisting of malignant teratomas, yolk sac tumors, embryonal carcinoma, and choriocarcinoma, are collectively called nongerminomatous germ cell tumors (NGGCT). The male-to-female ratio is 3:1 for pineal region germ cell tumors, but is 1:1 for suprasellar-based tumors. Approximately 90% of primary CNS germ cell tumors afflict children and adolescents less than 20 years of age. The peak incidence of these tumors is between 10 and 12 years.

Presenting symptoms depend on tumor location. Pineal region tumors usually present with headaches, nausea, and morning vomiting secondary to noncommunicating hydrocephalus, as well as ocular motor findings of Parinaud's syndrome: poor upward gaze, light-near dissociation of the pupillary light reflex, eyelid retraction making the eyes look too wide open, and sometimes retraction nystagmus. Suprasellar tumors may also present with headaches and signs of increased intracranial pressure, but often endocrinological dysfunction such as diabetes insipidus, precocious puberty, growth retardation, etc. brings the child or adolescent to medical attention. Optic field deficits are commonly found on examination; bitemporal hemianopsia is typical, but other visual field deficits may be found depending upon the relative pressure exerted by the tumor on the optic nerve, chiasm, or tract.

Diagnosis is usually accomplished with gadolinium-enhanced brain MRI. In children and adolescents with pineal or suprasellar region masses who are in the typical age range for germ cell tumors, serum and cerebrospinal fluid (if it can be safely obtained) markers should be tested. The most useful markers are α–fetoprotein (AFP, normally synthesized by yolk sac endoderm, fetal hepatocytes, and embryonic intestinal epithelium), b-HCG (normally secreted by syncytiotrophoblasts), and placental alkaline phosphatase (PLAP, made by syncytiotrophoblasts and primordial germ cells) (ROSENBLUM and NG 1997). Elevation of these markers is somewhat predictive of histology, as detailed in Table 29.2.

Table 29.2. Immunohistochemistry of CNS germ cell tumors (from ROSENBLUM and NG 1997)

	Placental alkaline phosphatase	α–Feto-protein	Human chorionic gonado-tropin
Germinoma	+	–	–
Teratoma	–	+/–	–
Yolk sac tumor	+	+	–
Embryonal carcinoma	+	–	–
Choriocarcinoma	+	–	+

Sometimes, surgery may be avoided when the patient has elevated markers, a typical clinical presentation, and an MRI consistent with a primary CNS germ cell tumor.

29.7.1
Germinoma

Germinomas are sensitive to both radiation therapy and chemotherapy. Standard therapy is radiation, as discussed in Chap. 27, resulting in long-term disease-free survival in excess of 80%–90% (WOLDEN et al. 1995).

With such high cure rates, chemotherapy has been evaluated as a way to decrease the potential risk of deleterious long-term radiation effects by decreasing the dose or volume of radiation necessary. Cyclophosphamide was one of the first medications to be tested in recurrent germ cell tumors (ALLEN et al. 1987). Allen et al. demonstrated that administration of two courses of cyclophosphamide prior to radiation therapy resulted in a complete response in seven of eight patients, allowing the radiation dose to be decreased. Due to concerns about the long-term effect of cyclophosphamide, other agents were subsequently tested. Carboplatin, used prior to radiation therapy, resulted in seven of ten patients achieving a complete response, but three of these patients required four doses of carboplatin to induce a complete response (ALLEN et al. 1994). Several European studies using multiagent platinum-based neoadjuvant chemotherapy combined with radiation doses ranging from 40 to 50 Gy to the primary site with 25–36 Gy to the craniospinal axis have demonstrated PFS rates comparable to those achieved with standard radiation without adjuvant chemotherapy (CALAMINUS et al. 1994). Recently, BUCKNER reported that seven of nine patients had a complete response to four cycles of neo-adjuvant cisplatin and etoposide (BUCKNER et al. 1999). Three of the six patients with local disease at diagnosis underwent reduced-dose local radiation to 30 Gy. All patients in this series have no evidence of disease with a median follow-up time of 4 years.

29.7.2
Nongerminomatous Germ Cell Tumors

Nongerminomatous germ cell tumors (NGGCT) are considerably less radiosensitive than germinomas and the prognosis following standard radiotherapy is poor, ranging between 20% and 45% (HOFFMAN et al 1991). Chemotherapy for primary CNS NGGCT initially mirrored treatment of non-CNS malignant germ cell tumors. Cisplatin, vinblastine, and bleomycin resulted in responses for both newly diagnosed and recurrent NGGCT, but the PFS was less than 40% (ITOMAYA et al. 1995; KIDA et al. 1986). Etoposide subsequently replaced vinblastine, and the combination of cisplatin, etoposide, and bleomycin, (PEB) is now standard for non-CNS germ cell tumors. Building on this backbone, ROBERTSON used four cycles of cisplatin and etoposide followed by radiation therapy and then further adjuvant chemotherapy with carboplatin, etoposide, bleomycin, and vincristine and demonstrated a 4-year PFS of 67% and OS of 74% (ROBERTSON et al. 1997). Ifosfamide and cyclophosphamide have also demonstrated efficacy in non-CNS germ cell tumors, in particular when there is an incomplete response to initial chemotherapy or relapse (MILLER et al. 1996).

The results of the German study MAKEI 89 using two cycles of PEB followed by biopsy or resection, standard radiation therapy, and then cisplatin, vinblastine, and ifosfamide demonstrated that 12 (80%) of 14 patients were event-free survivors with a median follow-up of 52 months (CALAMINUS et al. 1994). Particular emphasis in this article was placed on the dose of platinum: patients who received greater than 400 mg/m^2 of cumulative platinum in multiagent chemotherapy regimens combined with radiation therapy had an 86% 4-year actuarial survival compared with 56% for those who received a 200 mg/m^2 cumulative platinum dose.

High-dose chemotherapy has also been attempted to treat NGGCT. BALMACEDA et al. (1996) reported the use of high-dose carboplatin, etoposide, and bleomycin for four cycles without using radiotherapy in 26 patients with NGGCT; an initial complete response rate of 50% was achieved, but a high percentage of patients relapsed or had complications of chemotherapy, including five who died of chemotherapy-related causes.

29.8
Choroid Plexus Tumors

Choroid plexus tumors are rare tumors, accounting for about 4% of intracranial neoplasms in children (REIS et al. 1999). These tumors usually arise in the lateral, third, or fourth ventricle and frequently cause macrocephaly and signs and symptoms of increased intracranial pressure. Choroid plexus papillomas can be cured by surgical resection alone. In contrast, choroid plexus carcinomas (CPC) tend to invade adjacent neural tissue and may present with focal neurological signs in the absence of hydrocephalus. Histologically, CPC have an irregular papillary architecture and frequent mitotic figures.

Both, Packer, in a report of 11 children with CPC, and Duffner, in a report of eight infants with CPC, emphasize the importance of a complete surgical resection (PACKER et al. 1992; DUFFNER et al. 1995). In Packer's series four of the five children who were progression-free survivors had gross total surgical resections (GTR). Packer concluded from this that "there is little evidence to support radiation therapy or chemotherapy after a GTR." In Duffner's series three of the four children with GTR, treated with either postoperative chemotherapy alone or chemotherapy and radiation therapy, maintained disease control, supporting the importance of GTR.

Up to 30% of children with choroid plexus carcinomas tend to develop leptomeningeal metastases (DUFFNER 1995). In the presence of leptomeningeal metastases or partially resected CPC, the entire neuroaxis is frequently treated with radiation therapy. Since children with CPC tend to be younger than 3 years of age at diagnosis, the risks of radiation-induced intellectual deterioration, endocrinopathies, and spinal growth failure is a major concern (COHEN and DUFFNER 1994).

The contribution of adjuvant chemotherapy in the treatment of recurrent or incompletely resected CPC is unclear (GREENBERG 1999). Several small series have been reported, using various combinations of chemotherapy. At the time of initial diagnosis, (ALLEN et al. 1999) treated three patients with cisplatin, etoposide, vincristine, and cyclophosphamide followed by radiation, resulting in one survivor. Duffner reported on eight patients treated with cisplatin, etoposide, vincristine, and cyclophosphamide and radiation. Among the four who did not have GTR, there was only one progression-free survivor (DUFFNER et al. 1995). BERGER reported the French experience with 22 children with CPC and also found that all but one patient with incomplete surgery had tumor recurrence even though 17 of the children received postoperative chemotherapy (BERGER et al. 1998). A new approach has been reported by Souweidane: use of three courses of cisplatin, etoposide, vincristine, and cyclophosphamide preoperatively resulted in a 29.5% reduction in tumor volume, thereby permitting complete resection of a CPC in a 15-month-old patient who remains disease-free 31 months following diagnosis (SOUWEIDANE et al. 1999).

29.9
Conclusion

Unprecedented efforts are underway to improve the therapeutic efficacy of chemotherapy while decreasing the risk of long-term injury. Greater understanding of the molecular mechanisms responsible for tumor development and growth, better classification and identification of risk groups, clinical trials of new agents, and improved international cooperation will be necessary to achieve this goal.

References

Abrahamsen TG, Lange BJ, Packer RJ, et al. (1995) A phase I and II trial of dose-intensified cyclophosphamide and GM-CSF in pediatric malignant brain tumors. J Pediatr Hematol Oncol 17(2):134–139

Allen JC, Kim JH, Packer RJ (1987) Neoadjuvant chemotherapy for newly diagnosed germ-cell tumors of the central nervous system. J Neurosurg 67(1):65–70

Allen JC, DaRosso RC, Donahue B, Nirenberg A (1994) A phase II trial of preirradiation carboplatin in newly diagnosed germinoma of the central nervous system. Cancer 74(3):940–944

Allen JC, Prados M, Donahue B, et al. (1999) Preradiotherapy chemotherapy and hyperfractionated craniospinal radiotherapy for high-risk primitive neuroectodermal tumors: a preliminary report of CCG 9931

Atlas SW, Lavi E (1996) Intra-axial brain tumors. In: Atlas SW (ed) Magnetic Resonance Imaging of the Brain and Spine 2nd edn. Lippincott-Raven, Philadelphia, New York

Bailey P, Cushing H (1925) Medulloblastoma cerebelli: A common type of midcerebellar glioma of childhood. Arch Neurol Psychiatr 14:192–224

Balmaceda C, Heller G, Rosenblum M, et al. (1996) Chemotherapy without irradiation–a novel approach for newly diagnosed CNS germ cell tumors: results of an international cooperative trial. The First International Central Nervous System Germ Cell Tumor Study. J Clin Oncol 14(11):2908–2915

Berger C, Thiesse P, Lellouch-Tubiana A, et al. (1998) Choroid plexus carcinomas in childhood: clinical features and prognostic factors. Neurosurgery 42(3):470–475

Bleyer WA (1999) Epidemiologic impact of children with brain tumors. Childs Nerv Syst 15(11–12):758–763

Bouffet E, Foreman N (1999) Chemotherapy for intracranial ependymomas. Childs Nerv Syst 15(10):563–570

Brown WD, Gilles FH, Tavare CJ, et al. (1998) Prognostic limitations of the Daumas-Duport grading scheme in childhood supratentorial astroglial tumors. J Neuropathol Exp Neurol 57(11):1035–1040

Buckner JC, Peethambaram PP, Smithson WA, et al. (1999) Phase II trial of primary chemotherapy followed by reduced-dose radiation for CNS germ cell tumors. J Clin Oncol 17(3):933–940

Cairncross G, Macdonald D, Ludwin S, et al. (1994) Chemotherapy for anaplastic oligodendroglioma. National Cancer Institute of Canada Clinical Trials Group. J Clin Oncol 12(10):2013–2021

Calaminus G, Bamberg M, Baranzelli MC, et al. (1994) Intracranial germ cell tumors: a comprehensive update of the European data. Neuropediatrics 25(1):26–32

Chamberlain MC (1997) Recurrent cerebellar gliomas: salvage therapy with oral etoposide. J Child Neurol 12(3):200–204

Chamberlain MC (1993) Recurrent brainstem gliomas treated with oral VP-16 J Neurooncol 15(2):133–139

Chang CH, Houspian EM, Herber C, (1969) An operative staging system and a megavoltage radiotherapeutic technique for cerebellar medulloblastoma. Radiology 93:1351–1359

Cohen BH, Zeltzer PM, Boyett JM, et al. (1995) Prognostic factors and treatment results for supratentorial primitive neuroectodermal tumors in children using radiation and chemotherapy: a Childrens Cancer Group randomized trial. J Clin Oncol 13(7):1687–1696

Cohen ME, Duffner PK (1994) Brain Tumors in Children: principles of diagnosis and treatment 2nd edn. Raven Press, New York

Cushing H (1930) Experiences with the cerebellar medulloblastoma: a critical review of seventy-six cases. Acta Pathol Microbiol Scand 7:1–86

Cushing H (1931) Experiences with the cerebellar astrocytoma: a critical review of seventy-six cases. Surg Gyncecol Obstet 52:121–191

Dhadopkar K, Wisoff J, Sanford R, et al. (1999) Patterns of relapse and survival for newly diagnosed childhood low grade astrocytoma: initial results of CCG9891/POG9130. Med Ped Oncol 33(3):205

Duffner PK, Horowitz ME, Krischer JP, et al. (1993) Postoperative chemotherapy and delayed radiation in children less than three years of age with malignant brain tumors. N Engl J Med 328(24):1725–1731

Duffner PK, Krischer JP, Horowitz ME, et al. (1998) Second malignancies in young children with primary brain tumors following treatment with prolonged postoperative chemotherapy and delayed irradiation: a Pediatric Oncology Group study. Ann Neurol 44(3):313–316

Duffner PK, Kun LE, Burger PC, et al. (1995) Postoperative chemotherapy and delayed radiation in infants and very young children with choroid plexus carcinomas. The Pediatric Oncology Group. Pediatr Neurosurg 22(4):189–196

Dunkel IJ, Boyett JM, Rosenblum M, et al. (1998a) High-dose carboplatin, thiotepa, and etoposide with autologous stem-cell rescue for patients with recurrent medulloblastoma. Children's Cancer Group. J Clin Oncol 16(1):222–228

Dunkel IJ, Garvin JH Jr, Goldman S, et al. (1998b) High dose chemotherapy with autologous bone marrow rescue for children with diffuse pontine brainstem tumors. Children's Cancer Group. J Neurooncol 37(1):67–73

Dupuis-Girod S, Hartmann O, Benhamou E, et al. (1996) Will high dose chemotherapy followed by autologous bone marrow transplantation supplant cranio-spinal irradiation in young children treated for medulloblastoma? J Neurooncol 27(1):87–98

Finlay JL, Boyett JM, Yates AJ, et al. (1995) Randomized phase III trial in childhood high-grade astrocytoma comparing vincristine, lomustine, and prednisone with the eight-drugs-in-1-day regimen. Childrens Cancer Group. J Clin Oncol 13(1):112–123

Finlay JL, Goldman S, Wong MC, et al. (1996) Pilot study of high-dose thiotepa and etoposide with autologous bone marrow rescue in children and young adults with recurrent CNS tumors. The Children's Cancer Group. J Clin Oncol 14(9):2495–2503

Friedman HS, Krischer JP, Burger P, et al. (1992) Treatment of children with progressive or recurrent brain tumors with carboplatin or iproplatin: a Pediatric Oncology Group randomized phase II study. J Clin Oncol 10(2):249–256

Geyer R, Ater J, Axtell R, et al. (1998) Multiagent chemotherapy and deferred radiotherapy in infants with malignant brain tumors. 8th Internation Symposium on Pediatric Neuro-Oncology, Rome 6–9 May 1998, p. 41

Giangaspero F, Bigner SH, Giordana MT, et al. (1997) Medulloblastoma. In: Kleihues P, Cavenee WK (eds) Pathology and Genetics of Tumours of the Nervous System. International Agency for Research on Cancer, Lyon.

Gol A, McKissock W (1959) The cerebellar astrocytoma: a report of 98 verified cases. J Neurosurg 16:287–296

Greenberg ML (1999) Chemotherapy of choroid plexus carcinoma. Childs Nerv Syst 15(10):571–577

Guruangan S, Dunkel IJ, Goldman S, et al. (1998) Myeloablative chemotherapy with autologous bone marrow rescue in young children with recurrent malignant brain tumors. J Clin Oncol 16(7):2486–2493

Harisiadis L, Chang CH (1977) Medulloblastoma in children. A correlation between staging and results of treatment. Int J Radiat Oncol Biol Phys 2:833–841

Heideman RL, Douglass EC, Krance RA, et al. (1993) High-dose chemotherapy and autologous bone marrow rescue followed by interstitial and external-beam radiotherapy in newly diagnosed pediatric malignant gliomas. J Clin Oncol 11(8):1458–1465

Heideman RL, Douglass EC, Langston JA, et al. (1995) A phase II study of every other day high-dose ifosfamide in pediatric brain tumors: a Pediatric Oncology Group Study. J Neurooncol 25(1):77–84

Heideman RL, Packer RJ, Albright LA, et al. (1997) Tumors of the Central Nervous System. In: Pizzo PA, Poplack DG (eds) Principles and Practice of Pediatric Oncology 3rd edn. Lippincott-Raven, Philadelphia.

Hoffman HJ, Otsubo H, Hendrick EB, et al. (1991) Intracranial germ-cell tumors in children. J Neurosurg 74(4):545–551

Itoyama Y, Kochi M, Kuratsu J, et al. (1995) Treatment of intracranial nongerminomatous malignant germ cell tumors producing alpha-fetoprotein. Neurosurgery 36(3):459–464

Kida Y, Kobayashi T, Yoshida J, Kato K, Kageyama N (1986) Chemotherapy with cisplatin for AFP-secreting germ-cell tumors of the central nervous system. J Neurosurg 65(4):470–475

Levin VA, Edwards MS, Wright DC, et al. (1980) Modified procarbazine, CCNU, and vincristine (PCV 3) combination chemotherapy in the treatment of malignant brain tumors. Cancer Treat Rep 64(2–3):237–244

Listernick R, Charrow J, Gutmann DH (1999) Intracranial gliomas in neurofibromatosis type 1. Am J Med Genet 89(1):38–44

Mason WP, Grovas A, Halpern S, et al. (1998) Intensive chemotherapy and bone marrow rescue for young children with newly diagnosed malignant brain tumors. J Clin Oncol 16(1):210–221

McCowage G, Tien R, McLendon R, et al. (1996) Successful treatment of childhood pilocytic astrocytomas metastatic to the leptomeninges with high-dose cyclophosphamide. Med Pediatr Oncol 27(1):32–39

Miller K, Loehrer P, Einhorn L (1996) Salvage chemotherapy with vinblastine, ifosfamide and cisplatin in recurrent seminoma: long term follow up. Proc Am Soc Clin Oncol 15:24A

Miser J, Krailo M, Smithson W, et al. (1989) Treatment of children with recurrent brain tumors with ifosfamide, etoposide and mesna: results of a phase II Children's Cancer Group Study Group trial. Proc Annu Meet Am Soc Clin Oncol 8A328

Molloy PT, Bilaniuk LT, Vaughan SN, et al. (1995) Brainstem tumors in patients with neurofibromatosis type 1: a distinct clinical entity. Neurology 45(10):1897–1902

Needle MN, Molloy PT, Geyer JR, et al. (1997) Phase II study of daily oral etoposide in children with recurrent brain tumors and other solid tumors. Med Pediatr Oncol 29(1):28–32

Newton HB, Junck L, Bromberg J, et al. (1990) Procarbazine chemotherapy in the treatment of recurrent malignant astrocytomas after radiation and nitrosourea failure. Neurology 40(11):1743–1746

Packer RJ, Ater J, Allen J (1997) Carboplatin and vincristine chemotherapy for children with newly diagnosed progressive low-grade gliomas. J Neurosurg 86:747–754

Packer RJ, Perilongo G, Johnson D, et al. (1992) Choroid plexus carcinoma of childhood. Cancer 69(2):580–585

Packer RJ, Siegel KR, Sutton LN, et al. (1988) Efficacy of adjuvant chemotherapy for patients with poor-risk medulloblastoma: a preliminary report. Ann Neurol 24(4):503–508

Packer RJ, Sutton LN, D'Angio G, et al. (1986) Management of children with primitive neuroectodermal tumors of the posterior fossa/medulloblastoma. Pediatr Neurosci 12:272–282

Packer RJ, Sutton LN, Elterman R, et al (1994) Outcome for children with medulloblastoma treated with radiation, cisplatin, CCNU, and vincristine chemotherapy. J Neurosurg 81:690–698

Pendergrass TW, Milstein JM, Geyer JR, et al. (1987) Eight drugs in one day chemotherapy for brain tumors: experience in 107 children and rationale for preradiation chemotherapy. J Clin Oncol 5(8):1221–1231

Petronio J, Edwards MS, Prados M, et al (1991) Management of chiasmal and hypothalamic gliomas of infancy and childhood with chemotherapy. J Neurosurg 74(5):701–708

Phuphanich S, Edwards MSB, Levin VA, et al. (1984) Supratentorial malignant gliomas of childhood: results of treatment with radiation therapy and chemotherapy. J Neurosurg 60:495–499

Pierce SM, Barnes PD, Loeffler JS, et al. (1990) Definitive radiation therapy in the management of symptomatic patients with optic glioma. Survival and long-term effects. Cancer 65(1):45–52

Pollack IF, Boyett JM, Finlay JL (1999) Chemotherapy for high-grade gliomas of childhood. Childs Nerv Syst 15(10):529–544

Prados MD, Edwards MS, Rabbitt J, et al. (1997) Treatment of pediatric low-grade gliomas with a nitrosourea-based multiagent chemotherapy regimen. J Neurooncol 32(3):235–241

Reddy AT, Janss AJ, Packer RJ, et al. (1998) Outcome for Children with Supratentorial Primitive Neuroectodermal Tumors Treated with Surgery, Radiation and Chemotherapy. Ann Neurol 44(3):538

Reis LAG, Smith MA, Gurney JG et al. (1999) Cancer Incidence and Survival among Children and Adolescents: United States SEER Program 1975–1995, National Cancer Institute, SEER Program. NIH Pub. No. 99–4649. Bethesda

Robertson PL, DaRosso RC, Allen JC (1997) Improved prognosis of intracranial non-germinoma germ cell tumors with multimodality therapy. J Neurooncol 32(1):71–80

Rosenblum MK, Ng HK (1997) Germ cell tumors. In: Kleihues P, Cavenee WK (eds) Pathology and Genetics of Tumours of the Nervous System. International Agency for Research on Cancer, Lyon

Russell A (1980) A diencephalic syndrome of emaciation in infancy and childhood. Arch Dis Child 26:274

Shin KH, Webster JH (1979) Astrocytoma in children: a review of 79 cases 1960–1976. J Can Assoc Radiol 30:167–169

Souweidane MM, Johnson JH Jr, Lis E (1999) Volumetric reduction of a choroid plexus carcinoma using preoperative chemotherapy. J Neurooncol 43(2):167–171

Starceski PJ, Lee PA, Albright AL, et al. (1990) Hypothalamic hamartomas and sexual precocity. AJDC 144:225–228

van Eys J, Baram TZ, Cangir A, et al. (1988) Salvage chemotherapy for recurrent primary brain tumors in children. J Pediatr 113(3):601–606

Walker RW, Allen JC (1988) Cisplatin in the treatment of recurrent childhood primary brain tumors. J Clin Oncol 6(1):62–66

Wolden SL, Wara WM, Larson DA, et al. (1995) Radiation therapy for primary intracranial germ-cell tumors. Int J Radiat Oncol Biol Phys 32(4):943–949

30 Surgery for Primary and Metastatic Tumors of the Spine

Andrew T. Parsa, Barry D. Birch, Michael G. Kaiser and Paul C. McCormick

CONTENTS

A. T. Parsa, MD, PhD
Department of Neurological Surgery, Columbia Presbyterian Medical Center, College of Physicians and Surgeons of Columbia University, New York Presbyterian Hospital, 710 West 168th Street, New York, NY 10032, USA

B. D. Birch, MD
Department of Neurological Surgery, Columbia Presbyterian Medical Center, College of Physicians and Surgeons of Columbia University, New York Presbyterian Hospital, 710 West 168th Street, New York, NY 10032, USA

M. G. Kaiser, MD
Department of Neurological Surgery, Columbia Presbyterian Medical Center, College of Physicians and Surgeons of Columbia University, New York Presbyterian Hospital, 710 West 168th Street, New York, NY 10032, USA

P. C. McCormick, MD
Department of Neurological Surgery, Columbia Presbyterian Medical Center, College of Physicians and Surgeons of Columbia University, New York Presbyterian Hospital, 710 West 168th Street, New York, NY 10032, USA

30.1 Introduction

Elsberg's 1925 description of the surgical treatment of spinal-cord tumors is among the first extensive series on surgery of the spine (Elsberg 1925). The series illustrated the limitations at that time in delineating tumor size and location. These limitations were associated with long surgical procedures and a significant mortality rate. Prior to advances in microsurgical techniques, surgery of most spinal-cord tumors consisted of open biopsy and radiation therapy. Today, excellent results can be anticipated with all but the most malignant of spinal-cord tumors. This progress has been fostered by significant advances in disciplines that are essential to safe and efficacious surgery of the bony elements of the spine and the neural structures of the spinal-cord. In this chapter we present surgical considerations for patients with primary and metastatic tumors of the spine. Important advances and applications of radiation therapy for patients with spinal-cord tumors are discussed in the following chapter.

The diagnosis of spinal tumor is an important inclusion in the complete differential for any patient presenting with myelopathy, radiculopathy, neck or back pain. An expeditious and thorough work-up can quickly rule out a spinal tumor, while timely diagnosis can substantially improve the outcome for some patients with these lesions. Primary tumors that involve the spinal-cord or nerve-roots are similar in cellular type to intracranial tumors. They may arise from glial cells located within the parenchyma of the cord, Schwann cells of the nerve-roots, or meningeal cells covering the cord. Primary tumors which are unique to the spine can arise from the intraspinal vascular network, the sympathetic chain, or bony elements of the vertebral column. Metastatic spinal tumors can result from dissemination of a primary systemic cancer or, more rarely, from drop metastasis of primary intracranial lesions.

30.2
Pathology and Epidemiology

The location of the cell of origin of a spinal tumor has an important anatomical correlate that serves to guide diagnosis and treatment. Spinal tumors are classified according to location, into three major groups: intramedullary, intradural extramedullary, and extradural (MCCORMICK and FETELL 1996). Intramedullary tumors are typically derived from glial or ependymal cells that are found throughout the interstitium of the cord. Intradural extramedullary lesions include meningiomas derived from meningeal cells lining the surface of the cord. Extradural lesions are typically due to metastatic disease or schwannomas derived from the cells covering the nerve-roots. Occasionally, an extradural tumor extends through the intervertebral foramina, lying partially within and partially outside of the spinal-canal (dumb-bell or hourglass tumors).

The histological characteristics of different types of primary and secondary spinal tumors are similar to those of intracranial tumors. Intramedullary tumors are rare, accounting for only 5–10% of all spinal tumors. In contrast, the benign encapsulated tumors such as meningiomas and neurofibromas constitute between 55% and 65% of all primary spinal tumors. As a rule, intramedullary tumors are more common in children, and extramedullary tumors are more common in adults. The leading primary sites of metastatic tumors to the spine, in order of frequency, are lung, breast, and prostate (PERRIN 1992). However, several other systemic sites of spinal metastasis have been reported, including gastrointestinal tract (BROWN et al. 1999), lymphoma (DECHAMBENOIT et al. 1996), melanoma (BULLARD et al. 1981), kidney (GIEHL and KLUBA 1999, MAXWELL et al. 1999), sarcoma (SHAPIRO et al. 1999), and thyroid (GOLDSTEIN et al. 1988).

Tumors of the spinal-cord are much less frequent than intracranial tumors, with the overall prevalence approximating one spinal tumor for every four intracranial lesions (MCCORMICK and FETTELL 1996). When stratified for tumor type, this ratio of prevalence varies. For example, the intracranial:spinal ratio of astrocytomas is approximately 10:1, while the intracranial:spinal ratio of ependymomas can range from 3:1 to 20:1 depending upon the specific histological variant. Gender prevalence is equal except in the case of meningiomas which are more common in women, and ependymomas which are more common in men (MCCORMICK et al. 1990a, MCCORMICK and STEIN 1990a). Spinal tumors occur predominantly in young or middle-aged adults and are less common in childhood and old age. Although spinal tumors are more prevalent in the thoracic region, when the actual length of the various portions of the spinal-cord is taken into consideration, the distribution is relatively equal. Ependymomas may be either intramedullary or extramedullary. Ependymomas that originate at the conus (i.e., myxopapillary ependymomas) can be wholly or partially extramedullary at this site.

30.3
Intramedullary Tumors

30.3.1
Astrocytoma

About 3% of central nervous system (CNS) astrocytomas arise within the spinal-cord (McCormick and

Stein 1990a, Bourgouin et al. 1998). These tumors occur at any age but are most prevalent in the first three decades of life. They are also the most common pediatric intramedullary spinal-cord tumor, comprising about 90% of intramedullary tumors in patients of less than 10 years of age, and about 60% of adolescent intramedullary neoplasms (Innocenzi 1996). By about 30 years of age ependymomas become slightly more common than astrocytomas and increasingly predominate in the middle decades of life (McCormick et al. 1990b). In adults after the sixth decade of life, astrocytomas and ependymomas are encountered with about equal frequency. Nearly 60% of spinal astrocytomas occur in the cervical and cervicothoracic segments. A thoracic, lumbosacral, or conus medullaris location is less common. Filum terminale examples are rare. Spinal-cord astrocytomas represent a heterogeneous group with respect to histology, gross characteristics, and natural history (Innocenzi et al. 1997). These tumors include the low-grade fibrillary and pilocytic astrocytoma, malignant astrocytoma and glioblastoma, ganglioglioma, and the rare oligodendroglioma. About 90% of pediatric astrocytic tumors are benign. Most of these are fibrillary astrocytomas (Nadkarni and Rekate 1999). However, up to one-third represent juvenile pilocytic astrocytomas or gangliogliomas, which are both associated with a particularly indolent natural history. Malignant astrocytomas and glioblastomas account for about 10% of intramedullary astrocytomas. These lesions are characterized by a rapidly progressing clinical course, high incidence of cerebrospinal fluid tumor dissemination; and a poor patient survival rate (Sarabia et al. 1986, Ciappetta et al. 1991). Fibrillary astrocytomas prevail in the adult (Fig. 30.1), while juvenile pilocytic astrocytomas and gangliogliomas are rare and usually limited to early adulthood. The designation of a pilocytic astrocytoma in the adult usually reflects an abundance of pilocytic features which occur as secondary structures in an otherwise typical fibrillary astrocytoma (Rauhut et al. 1989). It is unclear whether these pilocytic features have an age-independent prognostic significance.

30.3.2
Ependymoma

Ependymomas are the most common intramedullary tumors in adults. They can occur at any time throughout life but are most common in the middle-adult years. Although the spinal-cord and filum terminale account for only 3% by weight of the CNS,

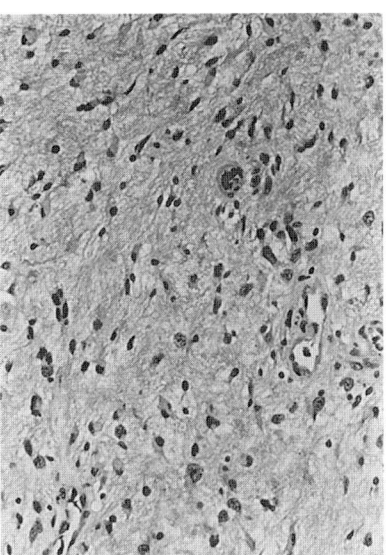

Fig. 30.1. Hematoxylin and eosin stained section, histopathology of fibrillary astrocytoma, demonstrates invasive tumor cells with mitotic activity

nearly half of all CNS ependymomas originate within the spinal-canal. The cervical region is the most common level of true intramedullary occurrence, however 40% of intradural ependymomas arise from the filum (McCormick et al. 1990b). For anatomical and surgical reasons, these lesions are generally considered to be extramedullary tumors.

A variety of histological ependymoma sub-types may be encountered. The cellular ependymoma is the most common (Fig. 30.2), but epithelial, tanacytic (fibrillar), sub-ependymoma, myxopapillary, or mixed examples also occur. Histological differentiation from astrocytoma may be difficult to see, but the presence of perivascular pseudorosettes or true rosettes establishes the diagnosis. Most spinal ependymomas are histologically benign, though necrosis and intratumoral hemorrhage are frequent (Yoshii et al. 1999). Although unencapsulated, these glial-derived tumors are usually well-circumscribed and do not infiltrate adjacent spinal-cord tissue. Recent attempts to correlate the expression of MIB-1 antigen with malignancy of ependymoma have been confounded by tumor heterogeneity (Ritter et al. 1998, Prayson 1999).

30.3.3
Hemangioblastoma

Hemangioblastomas are benign tumors of vascular origin which are sharply circumscribed but not en-

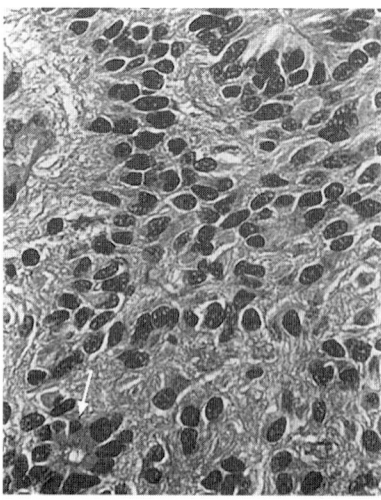

Fig. 30.2. Hematoxylin and eosin stained section, histopathology of cellular ependymoma, demonstrates characteristic rosette (*white arrow*) formed by homogeneous, darkly staining cells

capsulated. Almost all have a pial attachment and are dorsal or dorsolaterally located. They are distributed evenly throughout the spinal-cord but show a cervical predominance when they occur in association with the von Hippel-Lindau (VHL) syndrome (Neumann et al. 1995, Couch et al. 2000). Spinal hemangioblastomas account for 3–8% of intramedullary tumors and arise in any age-group, but are rare in early childhood (McCormick and Stein 1990a). Most patients present symptoms before the age of 40 years. Lesions are generally sporadic, but up to 25% of patients will have evidence of VHL. Patients with VHL tend to become symptomatic at an earlier age and occasionally have multiple tumors (Couch et al. 2000).

30.3.4
Miscellaneous Intramedullary Lesions

Metastases account for about 2% of intramedullary tumors. This low prevalence is probably due to the small size of the spinal-cord and its poor vascular accessibility to hematogenous tumor emboli (Connolly et al. 1996). Lung and breast are the most common sites for primary lesions. Melanocytoma, melanoma, fibrosarcoma, and myxoma have also been reported as intramedullary metastases (Connolly et al. 1996).

Other non-neoplastic entities can present as intramedullary spinal lesions (McCormick and Fetell 1996, McCormick and Stein 1990a). Vascular

malformations, particularly cavernous angiomas, may occur in the spinal-cord. Inclusion tumors and cysts are rarely intramedullary. Lipomas are the most common dysembryogenic lesion and account for about 1% of intramedullary masses. These are not true neoplasms but probably arise from inclusion of mesenchymal tissue within the spinal-cord itself. They typically enlarge and produce symptoms in early and middle adult years through increased fat disposition in metabolically normal fat cells. Lipomas are often considered to be juxtamedullary because they occupy a sub-pial location.

30.3.5
Genetic Syndromes and Mutations Associated with Intramedullary Spinal-Cord Tumors

30.3.5.1
Neurofibromatosis

The prevalence of certain intramedullary tumors in patients with genetic syndromes warrants consideration in formulating a differential diagnosis. There are two distinct types of neurofibroma (NF), each affecting cells derived embryologically from the neural crest. NF1 is a disease characterized by autosomal dominant inheritance with almost complete penetrance and variable expressivity. Approximately 50% of cases are new mutations with a 1 in 3,000 prevalence (Brill 1989, Roos and Muckway 1995). The NF1 gene is located on the long arm of chromosome 17 and codes for a neurofibromin guanosine triphosphatase-activating protein that influences cell proliferation and differentiation. Tumors associated with the NF1 syndrome include neurofibromas, malignant nerve-sheath tumors, optic-nerve gliomas, rhabdomyosarcomas, pheochromocytomas, and carcinoid tumors.

NF2 also segregates by autosomal dominant inheritance, with high penetrance. The NF2 gene is located on chromosome 22q12, with about 50% of reported cases representing new mutations (Kley et al. 1995). It is much less prevalent than is NF1, with a rate of 1 in 40,000. The NF2 gene-product encodes the protein "Merlin", which is a member of the ezrin-radixin-moesin protein family that links the cytoskeleton to the plasma membrane (Gusella et al. 1999). Neoplasms associated with NF2 include bilateral acoustic schwannomas, neurofibromas, ependymomas, gliomas, and meningiomas. There are two subtypes of NF2. The severe or "Wishart" form is characterized by early onset, rapid clinical progression, and multiple tumors. The mild or "Garner" form has a later onset, slower clinical progression, and fewer tumors.

In 1996, Lee and colleagues published a report of one of the largest series of studies of intramedullary spinal-cord tumors in patients with NF (LEE et al. 1996). Nine patients were described, including three patients with NF1, five patients with NF2 and one with "type uncertain". The predominant pathology associated with NF1 was astrocytoma (two low-grade and one anaplastic) while ependymoma was most closely associated with NF2 (four out of five patients). The reported incidence of intramedullary spinal-cord tumors in the NF population was approximately 19% (nine out of 48). This incidence may reflect referral patterns associated with highly specialized neurosurgical services. In 1997 Yagi and colleagues described a series of 44 patients presenting with intramedullary spinal-cord tumors, two of whom had NF1 (YAGI et al. 1997). In both cases the pathology of the lesion was astrocytoma (i.e., anaplastic astrocytoma and glioblastoma). Taken together, with selected case reports in the literature (EPSTEIN et al. 1992), these studies support the presumption that solitary intramedullary spinal-cord tumors in NF1 patients will most likely be astrocytomas. Similarly, it is reasonable to assume that an NF2 patient presenting with an intramedullary tumor will most likely have an ependymoma. However, NF2 patients have also been described with intramedullary schwannoma (LEE et al. 1996).

30.3.5.2
von Hippel-Lindau Disease

von Hippel-Lindau disease is an autosomal dominant disorder with 90% penetrance, attributable to loss of a tumor suppressor gene on chromosome 3p25–26 (KLEY et al. 1995, DECKER et al. 1996). Lesions associated with VHL include CNS hemangioblastoma, retinal angioma, renal cyst, renal cell carcinoma, pancreatic cyst, pheochromocytoma, and epidydimal cystadenoma (GLAVAC et al. 1996, RICHARD et al. 1998). VHL families can be grouped according to the presence or absence of pheochromocytomas (NEUMANN et al. 1995). Nearly all families with pheochromocytomas have missense mutations of the VHL gene. Hemangioblastomas are predominantly made up of endothelial cells and pericytes in a dense network of vascular channels, intermixed with lipid-laden stromal cells (RICHARD et al. 1998). Using tissue microdissection, Vortmeyer and colleagues have recently demonstrated

consistent loss of heterozygosity at the VHL gene locus in the stromal cells (VORTMEYER et al. 1997), implicating these cells in the pathogenesis of hemangioblastoma.

CNS hemangioblastoma occurs in both Type I (without pheochromocytoma) and Type II (with pheochromocytoma) VHL families. Sites of predilection are the posterior fossa (80%) and the cervical or lumbar regions of the spinal-cord (20%). Specific point mutations and deletions in the VHL gene have been characterized in both sporadic and VHL-related spinal hemangioblastoma (DECKER et al. 1996, KANNO et al. 1994, OBERSTRASS et al. 1996, OLSCHWANG et al. 1998). Hypermethylation of the VHL gene has also been implicated as a modality of inactivation (PROWSE et al. 1997). Several models of how VHL inactivation results in tumor formation have been proposed (RICHARD et al. 1998). The VHL tumor suppressor protein is known to inhibit transcription elongation through interaction with the elongin protein (STEBBINS et al. 1999). The VHL protein also suppresses vascular endothelial growth factor (VEGF) production (GNARRA et al. 1996). Loss of VHL protein function could cause VEGF up-regulation followed by angiogenesis.

30.3.5.3
Genetic Mutations in
Sporadic Intramedullary Astrocytomas

There are few published studies specifically examining the genetic mutations in sporadic intramedullary astrocytomas (IWATA et al. 1996). However, extensive work has been done on the pathogenic events causing intracerebral glioma. It is likely that some if not all of the genetic alterations described in intracerebral astrocytoma play a role in the progression of spinal astrocytoma. Three transitions have been studied as a paradigm for glioma progression: (1) astrocyte to astrocytoma, (2) astrocytoma to anaplastic astrocytoma, and (3) anaplastic astrocytoma to glioblastoma. In the first transition p53 mutations, chromosome 17p loss and chromosome 22q loss have been implicated (CHUNG et al. 1991, VON DEIMLING et al. 1992, LOUIS et al. 1993). Recently Rubio and colleagues have shown that the NF2 gene was not mutated in 30 astrocytomas examined, making it an unlikely candidate for the 22q locus lost during this transition (RUBIO et al. 1994). In the progression from astrocytoma to anaplastic astrocytoma, genetic defects include retinoblastoma gene mutations, chromosome 13q loss, P16 gene deletions, chromosome 9p loss, and chromosome 19q loss (VON DEIM-

LING et al. 1995). The transition from anaplastic astrocytoma to glioblastoma has been shown to involve chromosome 10 loss and EGF receptor gene amplification (LIU et al. 1997).

Several studies have identified the PTEN gene (also known as MMAC and TEP1) as one of the candidate chromosome 10 genes lost in glioblastoma (STECK et al. 1997, CHIARIELLO et al. 1998, BOSTROM et al. 1998, DUERR et al. 1998). The gene encodes a tyrosine phosphatase located at 10q23.3. The function of PTEN as a cellular phosphatase is consistent with the tumor suppressor label. Phosphatases act by turning off signaling pathways dependent upon phosphorylation (PARSONS 1998). When phosphatase activity is lost as a result of genetic mutation, signaling pathways can become activated constitutively, resulting in aberrant proliferation.

More specific description of genetic lesions in intramedullary spinal astrocytomas would require analysis of large cohorts of patients. This may prove difficult, due to the rarity of this disease process and the paucity of tumor that is resected once the diagnosis of astrocytoma is suspected. Unlike that from patients with intramedullary ependymoma, aggressive surgical resection of tumor from patients with intramedullary astrocytoma is currently of questionable long-term benefit (MCCORMICK and STEIN 1990).

30.3.5.4
Genetic Mutations in
Sporadic Intramedullary Ependymoma

The prognosis for patients with low-grade intramedullary ependymoma is excellent after aggressive surgical resection (MCCORMICK et al. 1990). Much of the work which characterizes genetic lesions in sporadic intramedullary ependymoma has focused on the NF2 gene. We have shown previously that five out of seven patients had mutations of the NF2 gene in their tumor (BIRCH et al. 1996). All of these mutations resulted in a truncated protein product and occurred in the region of the transcript that is functionally homologous to cytoskeletal proteins. Other groups have also shown NF2 mutations and loss of chromosome 22 in sporadic intramedullary spinal ependymoma, as well as loss of 17p (VON HAKEN et al. 1996).

A molecular distinction may exist between the events that lead up to a spinal ependymoma versus those that contribute to intracerebral tumor progression. In a recent study, Ebert and colleagues analyzed 62 ependymal tumors, including myxopapillary ependymomas, subependymomas, ependymomas, and anaplastic ependymoma (Ebert et al. 1999). They

showed informative allelic loss of 10q (five out of 56) and 22q (12 out of 54). Somatic mutations of NF2 were detected in six of the tumors examined and in each case the tumor was from a Grade II intramedullary ependymoma.

30.3.5.5
Genetic Mutations in
Other Intramedullary Tumors

The small number of cases associated with other types of sporadic tumors has limited the studies on their genetic makeup. These lesions include intramedullary neurocytoma (TATTER et al. 1994), primary intramedullary spinal-cord germinoma (ITOH et al. 1996), intramedullary non-Hodgkin's lymphoma (CARUSO et al. 1998), primary intramedullary primitive neuroectodermal tumor (PNET) of the spinal-cord (DEME et al. 1997), intramedullary subependymoma (JALLO et al. 1996), intramedullary neuroma (MELANCIA et al. 1996), intramedullary teratoma (HADER et al. 1999), and intramedullary lipoma (LEE et al. 1995).

30.4
Extramedullary Tumors

30.4.1
Meningioma

Meningiomas arise from arachnoid cap cells imbedded in dura near the nerve-root sleeve, reflecting their predominant lateral location and meningeal attachment. Other speculated cells of origin include fibroblasts associated with the dura or pia, which may account for occasional ventral or dorsal locations of these tumors. Meningiomas occur in all age groups, but the majority arise in individuals between the fifth and seventh decades of life (MCCORMICK et al. 1990). Seventy-five to 85% occur in women and about 80% are thoracic (KLEKAMP and SAMII 1996, GEZEN et al. 2000). The upper cervical region of the spine, and foramen magnum are also common sites (GUIDETTI and SPALLONE 1980). Here, meningiomas often occupy a ventral or ventrolateral position and may adhere to the vertebral artery near its intradural entry and initial intracranial course. Low cervical and lumbar meningiomas are infrequent. The majority of spinal meningiomas are entirely intradural, however about 10% may be both intradural and extradural, or entirely extradural. Meningiomas are generally solitary, but multiplicity can be observed in patients with neurofibromatosis. The overall incidence of multiplicity in the spine is 1 to 2% (CHAPARRO et al. 1993). The gross characteristics range from smooth and fibrous to the more frequent variegated, fleshy and friable appearance. Microscopic calcification may occur. The dural attachment is often broader than expected, but en plaque examples are unusual. Bony involvement does not occur in the spine because of the well-defined epidural space. Psammomatous meningioma is the most frequent histological subtype (Fig. 30.3).

30.4.2
Nerve-Sheath Tumor: Schwannoma and Neurofibroma

Nerve-sheath tumors are categorized as either schwannomas or neurofibromas. Although evidence from tissue culture, electron microscopy, and immunohistochemistry support a common Schwann cell origin of the neurofibroma and schwannoma, the morphologic heterogeneity of neurofibromas suggests participation of additional cell types, such as the perineural cell and fibroblast (McCormick et al. 1990). Neurofibromas and schwannomas merit separate consideration because of distinct demographic, histological, and biological characteristics. The histological appearance of neurofibromas consists of an abundance of fibrous tissue and the conspicuous presence of nerve fibers within the tumor stroma (Fig. 30.4). Grossly, the tumor produces fusiform enlargement of the involved nerve, which makes it impossible to distinguish between them. The presence of multiple neurofibromas establishes the diagnosis of neurofibromatosis, but this syndrome should be considered even in patients with solitary involvement. Schwannomas appear grossly as a smooth globoid mass, which does not produce enlargement of the nerve but is suspended eccentrically from it by a discrete attachment. The histological appearance consists of elongated bipolar cells with fusiform, darkly staining nuclei arranged in compact interlacing fascicles, which tend to palisade (Antoni-A pattern). A loosely arranged pattern of stellate-shaped cells (Antoni-B pattern) is less common (Fig. 30.5) (Sharma et al. 1990).

Nerve-sheath tumors account for about 25% of intradural spinal-cord tumors in adults (McCormick et al. 1990, Sharma et al. 1990). Most are solitary schwannomas, which occur throughout the spinal-canal. The fourth through sixth decades of life represent the peak incidence of occurrence, with men and women equally affected. The majority of nerve-sheath tumors arise from a dorsal nerve root, while ventral-root tumors are more commonly neurofibromas. Most nerve-sheath tumors are entirely intradural but 10–15% extend through the dural root sleeve as a dumb-bell tumor with both intradural and extradural components (Fig. 30.6) (McCormick 1996a,b). About 10% of nerve-sheath tumors are epidural or paraspinal in location. One

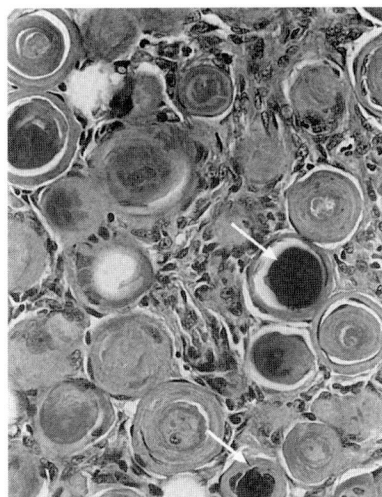
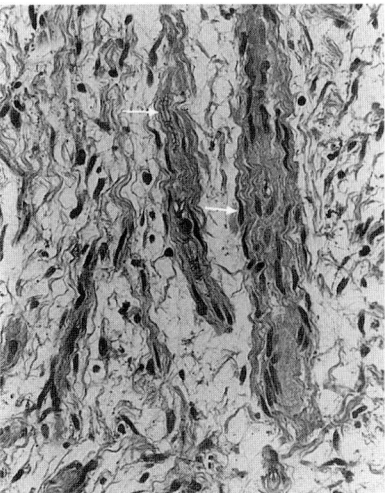
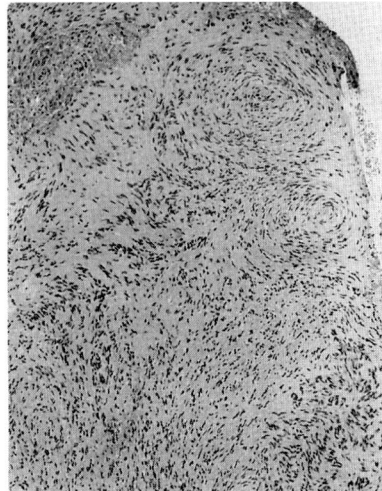

Fig. 30.3. Hematoxylin and eosin stained section, histopathology of psammomatous meningioma, demonstrates characteristic calcium deposits (*white arrows*) within the psammoma bodies

Fig. 30.4. Hematoxylin and eosin stained section, histopathology of neurofibroma, demonstrates loose reticular network, surrounding tumor (*white arrows*)

Fig. 30.5. Hematoxylin and eosin stained section, histopathology of schwannoma, demonstrates darkly staining tumor cells in whorls that can sometimes be mistaken for meningioma

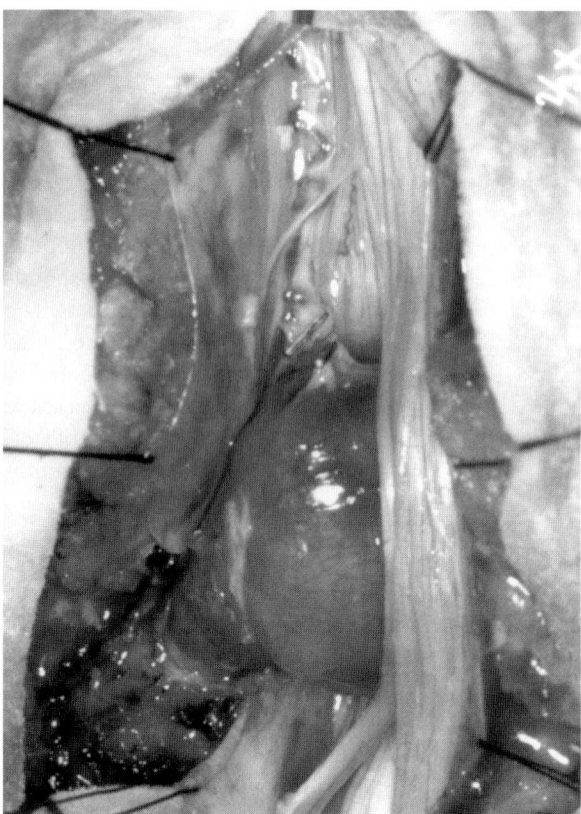

Fig. 30.6. Gross appearance of intraoperative dumb-bell tumor, demonstrating intradural component and extension of the nerve-root sleeve

percent are intramedullary and are believed to arise from the perivascular nerve-sheaths which accompany penetrating spinal-cord vessels. Centripetal growth of a nerve-sheath tumor may also result in subpial extension; this occurs most often with plexiform neurofibromas. In these cases both intramedullary and extramedullary tumor-components will be apparent. Brachial or lumbar plexus neurofibromas may extend centrally into the intradural space along multiple nerve-roots. Conversely, retrograde intraspinal extension of a paraspinal schwannoma usually remains epidural.

About 2.5% of intradural spinal nerve-sheath tumors are malignant (Sharma et al. 1989). At least one-half of these occur in patients with neurofibromatosis. Malignant nerve-sheath tumors carry a poor prognosis with patient-survival of generally less than one year. These tumors must be distinguished from the rare cellular schwannoma, which has aggressive histological features but is associated with a favorable prognosis (Deruz et al. 1993, Seppala and Haltia 1993).

30.4.3
Filum Terminale Ependymoma

Although filum ependymomas have been classified as intramedullary lesions by virtue of the neuroectodermal derivation of the filum terminale, it is appropriate to consider them with extramedullary tumors, from an anatomical and surgical perspective (Ferrante et al. 1992). About 40% of spinal-canal ependymomas arise within the filum terminale in its proximal intradural portion (McCormick and Fetell 1996, McCormick et al. 1990a). Astrocytoma, oligodendroglioma, and paraganglioma may also originate in the filum but are rare. Filum terminale ependymomas can occur at any time throughout life but are most common in the third to fifth decades, with men slightly more commonly affected than women. Filum ependymomas and cauda equina nerve-sheath tumors occur with about equal frequency (McCormick et al. 1990a).

Lesions are typically red, sausage-shaped growths with moderate vascularity (Fig. 30.7). Al-

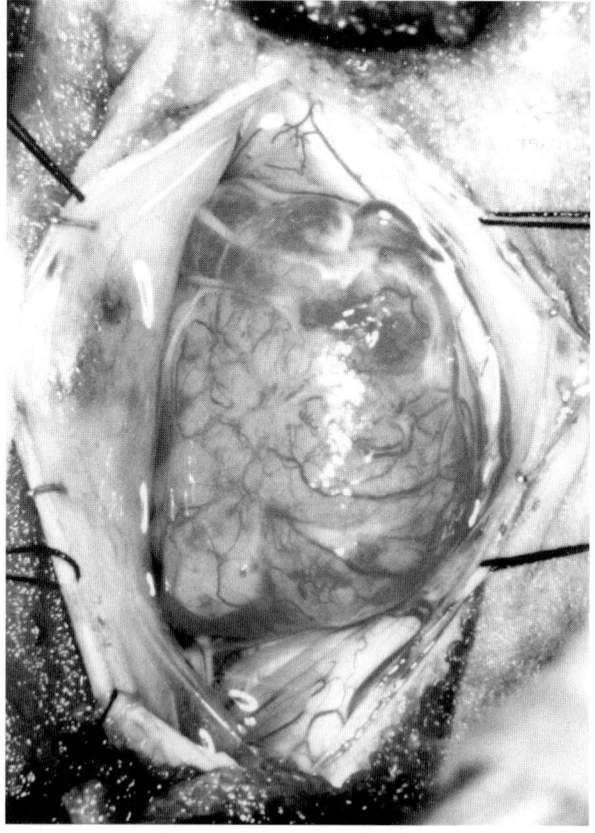

Fig. 30.7. Gross appearance of filum ependymomas can demonstrate unencapsulated but well-circumscribed lesions covered by arachnoid. Myxopapillary ependymoma is the most common histological type of tumor encountered in this region

though unencapsulated, they are usually well-circumscribed and may be covered by arachnoid. Myxopapillary ependymoma is the most common histological type encountered in filum terminale and cauda equina. The microscopic appearance consists of a papillary arrangement of cuboidal or columnar tumor cells surrounding a vascularized core of hyalinized and poorly cellular connective tissue. Nearly all filum ependymomas are histologically benign, but tend to be more aggressive in younger age-groups (ASAZUMA et al. 1999).

30.4.4
Miscellaneous Extramedullary Pathology

Extramedullary masses may be neoplastic or non-neoplastic. Dermoid, epidermoid, lipomas, teratomas, and neurenteric cysts are inclusion lesions which result from disordered embryogenesis McCORMICK and STEIN 1990b). They may occur throughout the spinal-canal but are more common in the thoracolumbar and lumbar regions of the spine, although intramedullary locations have also been reported. Associated anomalies such as cutaneous lesions, sinus tracts, occult anterior or posterior rachischisis, or split-cord malformations may be present. Inclusion tumors and cysts generally present as masses, but recurrent meningitis, tethered-cord syndrome, or congenital deformities may be the predominant clinical finding.

Paragangliomas are rare tumors of neural-crest origin, which may arise from the filum, terminale or cauda equina (KAMALIAN et al. 1987, FARO et al. 1997). These are benign, and usually non-functioning, tumors, which histologically resemble extra-adrenal paraganglia. They appear grossly as well-circumscribed vascular tumors and may be clinically and radiographically indistinguishable from filum terminale ependymomas. Identification of dense core neurosecretory granules, by electron microscopy, establishes the diagnosis. Complete removal can be accomplished in most cases. Cavernous malformations, hemangioblastomas, and ganglioneuromas may involve an intradural nerve-root and present as an extramedullary mass. These lesions may present clinically as a nerve-sheath tumor with early radicular symptoms.

Non-neoplastic lesions such as arachnoid cysts may present as extramedullary masses. These are most common in the thoracic region of the spine and are usually dorsal to the spinal-cord z. Herniated intervertebral discs have occasionally been reported to rupture the dura and present as an intradural, extramedullary mass (MCCORMICK and STEIN 1990b).

Inflammatory pathologies such as sarcoidosis, tuberculoma, or subdural empyema rarely present as intradural mass lesions. Although spinal carcinomatous meningitis frequently complicates systemic cancer, secondary metastatic mass lesions of the intradural, extramedullary compartment are rare. Malignant intracranial neoplasms which appose the subarachnoid space or ventricles are the most likely intracranial tumors to demonstrate cerebrospinal fluid (CSF) drop metastasis into the spinal subarachnoid space (BARLOON et al. 1987). Systemic cancer accesses the subarachnoid space either through direct dural-root sleeve penetration, or more commonly, hematogenously via the choroid plexus.

30.5
Extradural Tumors

The majority of epidural neoplasms are metastatic, with 66% of these disseminating from the breast, prostate, hematopoetic system, or lung (SARPEL et al. 1987, SUNDARESAN et al. 1995). Myelography of epidural lesions can reveal a characteristic saw-tooth pattern of partial to complete blockage, which, in conjunction with corroborating plain films and bone scans, constitutes a diagnosis of epidural metastasis. The general medical condition of the patient should influence the decision to treat epidural metastasis surgically. A scoring system employing various clinical parameters has been published in an attempt to advise neurosurgeons more uniformly (TOKUHASHI et al. 1990). The system rates patients according to six variables, including Karnofsky status and number of metastases. Patients who have low scores are unlikely to survive for more than 3 months postoperatively (Table 30.1). Those with high scores have a reasonable chance of surviving for more than a year postoperatively. In general, the surgical approach for re-

Table 30.1. Scoring system for preoperative evaluation of patients with metastatic spinal tumor: variables that relate to postoperative survival

Karnofsky rating
Number of extraspinal bony metastases
Number of metastases in the vertebral body
Presence of metastases to major organs
Primary site of cancer
Neurological status

moval of a spinal metastasis depends on the anterior or posterior location of the tumor.

The most common spinal tumors of middle-to-late adulthood are metastatic. These tumors are the result of hematogenous spread through the venous system of Batson's plexus into the vertebral elements of the spine. The vertebral body retains its red marrow longer than most other bony structures, and the microemboli of metastasis have a predilection for red marrow. As a result, the spine is the most common bony structure to acquire metastases. Metastatic tumors invade the epidural space and infiltrate the epidural fat from the surrounding bony spine. The dura can act to confine the metastatic tumor to the epidural compartment, with the thoracic region of the spine being more commonly involved than other regions.

The vertebral body and bony elements of the spine give rise to paravertebral tumors, which tend to both circumscribe the vertebral column and invade the epidural compartment. The paravertebral tumor often can be targeted for posterior percutaneous biopsy under computed tomography (CT) or fluoroscopic control, with a local anesthetic and sedation. With local anesthesia, inadvertent contact with the nerve-root can be immediately detected and avoided. Because 10% of spinal metastases present with no known primary tumor, biopsies can play an important role (MCCORMICK and FETELL 1996, MC-CORMICK 1994).

30.6
Spinal-Cord Syndromes and Clinical Neuroanatomy

The neurological symptoms associated with vertebral column abnormalities may result from a myelopathy, a radiculopathy, or a combination of both. Often, pain precludes any definitive neurological findings and prompts further neuroradiological investigation. An understanding of spinal-cord neuroanatomy and related cord syndromes allows the surgeon to recognize the need for neuroimaging within an appropriate region of interest.

30.6.1
Clinically Relevant Neuroanatomy

The cross-sectional anatomy of the spinal-cord consists of three funiculi, with one posterior and two anterolateral in location (Fig. 30.8). The lateral at-

tachments to the cord, of the dentate ligaments, define the anterior (ventral) and posterior (dorsal) halves of the spinal-cord. Motor symptoms are caused by damage to the descending corticospinal or pyramidal tract in the posterior portion of the anterolateral funiculus. Chronic disruption along this anatomical course causes upper motor-neuron (UMN) or long-tract findings that include a segmental level of paralysis or weakness, muscle atrophy, hyperactive deep-tendon reflexes, spasticity, a disturbance of fine movements, and a pathologic extensor response of the toes to plantar stimulation. Acute disruptions may evoke a flaccid paralysis or weakness that ultimately progresses to spasticity. In both acute and chronic disruptions, motor symptoms are ipsilateral to the pathology. Bilateral symptoms herald more diffuse spinal-cord involvement.

Lower motor-neuron (LMN) deficits can originate from the anterior horn cell, nerve-root, and any point along the peripheral nerve. LMN findings may occur jointly with a myelopathy and are otherwise associated with anterior horn-cell diseases, radiculopathies, and peripheral neuropathies. The clinical picture may overlap with pyramidal signs, but its distinguishing features include hypoactive or absent deep-tendon reflexes, decreased tone or flaccidity, fasciculations, and the absence of a pathologic extensor response of the toes. Within the descending motor tract, the cervical or arm axons are more centrally located, exiting through the ventral gray matter and ventral nerve-roots first. This is the anatomical basis of a central cord syndrome, which leaves the arms weaker than the legs.

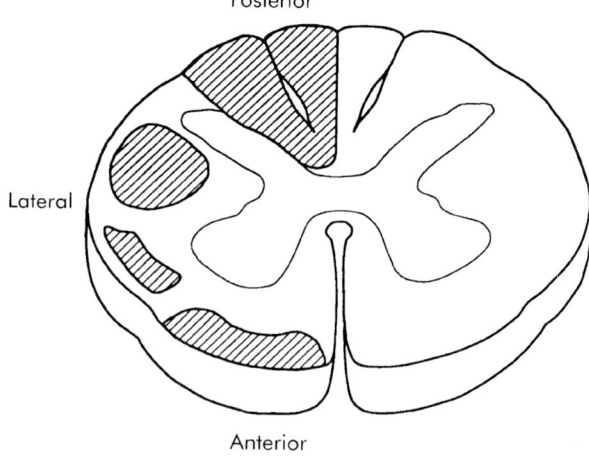

Fig.30.8. Cross-section of the spinal-cord, demonstrating the distribution of the major spinal tracts within the three funiculi

The ascending sensory nerves traverse the dorsal root ganglia and dorsal nerve-root to enter the dorsal-horn gray matter of the spinal-cord. A portion of these sensory fibers carry position, tactile (deep touch), and vibratory axons. They run directly to the ipsilateral half of the posterior funiculi or columns and ascend in the posterior portion of the cord. The remaining sensory fibers subserve pain (sharp, dull), temperature, and light-touch. These fibers synapse over several spinal levels in the dorsal horns before crossing to the opposite anterolateral funiculus, where they begin an ascent as the lateral spinothalamic tract. These tracts are located anterior to the dentate ligaments. In acute central cord injuries, the more centrally located cervical axons of the spinothalamic tract are disrupted. The remaining lateral axons account for the sacral sparing of perianal sensation.

Because pain and temperature synapses occur in the dorsal horns over several spinal levels, localization of a spinal-cord lesion can be approximated only to within three spinal segments. For localization, cord pathology is often dynamic and may ascend to include higher levels of motor, sensory, and autonomic dysfunction. It is crucial to define and follow the disparity between an osseous level of pathology shown radiographically and the actual neurological level of cord function. An ascending level of neurological loss should prompt a rapid reassessment of the patient's clinical status and vertebral alignment, and warrants reimaging of the cord itself. The crossing of pain and temperature axons through the central cord to the opposite side is an anatomical correlate for two neurological findings. Firstly, unilateral pain and temperature sensory levels or deficits are opposite the spinal-cord lesion. Secondly, central cord disruption impairs the sensation for pain and temperature axons, with preservation of posterior column sensory modalities. Clinically, the second finding constitutes a dissociated sensory disorder.

A myelopathy may impair motor, sensory, or autonomic function and can vary in severity. A partial or incomplete myelopathy will present as one of several major spinal-cord syndromes, each having a certain propensity for recovery, depending on the duration and extent of the spinal-cord insult.

30.6.2
Anterior-Cord Syndrome

The anterior-cord syndrome results from damage to the anterior two-thirds of the spinal-cord, which includes the anterior horn cells of the ventral gray mat-ter (LMN) and the axons or white-matter tracts of the anterolateral funiculi (UMN) (Fig. 30.9a). The anterior-cord syndrome occurs more commonly in the cervical region and is characterized by LMN-paralysis of the arms and UMN-paralysis of the legs. Below the level of injury there is motor paralysis with complete deficits of pain (sharp/dull), temperature, and light-touch sensory modalities. The partial myelopathy that presents as an anterior-cord syndrome is often due to ventral compression from retropulsed bone or disc, a flexion injury, or interruption of anterior spinal-artery blood flow. The variable sparing of the posterior columns accounts for residual tactile, vibration, and position sense in the lower extremities.

30.6.3
Central-Cord Syndrome

The central-cord syndrome is a common myelopathy (Fig. 30.9b). Acute central-cord syndromes are distinguished from chronic syndromes by the sacral sparing of pain (sharp/dull) and temperature sensory modalities, and by a more dense motor-weakness in the arms vs. the legs. In trauma, the acute central-cord syndrome presents with a central-cord contusion and/or hematoma (hematomyelia). This is often seen in the more rigid and spondylitic spines of older patients with extension injuries. Motor, sensory, and bladder functions have good prospects for recovery, with earlier improvements noted in the legs. Presen-

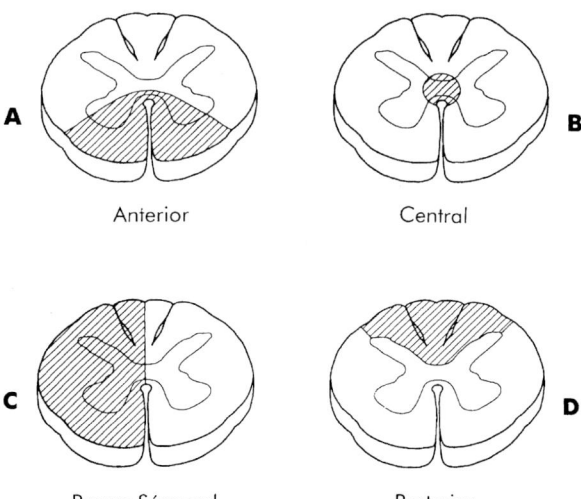

Fig. 30.9. Schematic representation of various cord lesions: Cross-section of the spinal-cord depicting distribution of injury for the major partial myelopathies relevant to surgical assessments

tations of a chronic central-cord syndrome can be caused by cysts, such as those in syringomyelia, or by intrinsic cord tumors. A dissociated sensory disorder, LMN-type flaccid paralysis, and muscle atrophy of the upper extremities are typically associated with a chronic central-cord syndrome. Progressive disruption of the dorsal horns accounts for the trophic disorders that may involve the arms and fingers.

A cord syrinx can present as an incomplete myelopathy and may extend rostrally to the medulla (syringobulbia) to impair various lower cranial-nerve functions, such as phonation and swallowing. It is not uncommon for abnormalities at the foramen magnum level to predispose patients to syringomyelia. This is frequently observed in the congenital Chiari malformations, which include a constricted volume in the posterior fossa, cerebellar tonsillar impaction, obliteration of local CSF cisterns, and abnormal local CSF dynamics. The concurrence of hydrocephalus and a rostral spinal-cord syrinx is termed hydromyelia and often responds to treatment of the hydrocephalus with ventriculoperitoneal shunting. Syringomyelia can also be the consequence of prior cord trauma, tumor, arachnoiditis, and compressive spondylosis.

30.6.4
Brown-Sequard Syndrome

The Brown-Sequard syndrome is less prevalent than the previously mentioned incomplete myelopathies (Fig. 30.9c). The lesion impairs one-half of the spinal-cord and spares the opposite half. Clinically, there is a UMN-paralysis and a loss of position sense ipsilateral to the lesion. This is consistent with unilateral disruption of both the corticospinal tract and the posterior columns, neither of which crosses during their course through the cord. Opposite the lesion, there is a level of sensory deficit for pain and temperature. Disruption of the spinothalamic tract impairs ascending pain and temperature axons, which have crossed from the side opposite the lesion. This syndrome may be observed with unilateral encroachment of epidural tumor through the neural foramina or intradural tumor from the nerve-root. Because of compression, a complete transverse myelopathy may supervene, with a worse prognosis for recovery. Penetrating or contusive injuries can impair one lateral half of the cervical or thoracic region of the cord to produce the Brown-Sequard presentation. The prognosis for motor recovery is better than that of other incomplete myelopathies but remains influ-

enced by the nature of the insult, rapidity of diagnosis, and, when appropriate, expeditious decompression.

30.6.5
Posterior-Cord Syndrome

For surgical considerations, the posterior-cord syndrome is a rare presentation of an incomplete myelopathy (Fig. 30.9d). A level of sensory loss for posterior column modalities coincides with preservation of motor function. Its rare occurrence limits the value of prognostic assessments. Of greater relevance is posterior column damage caused by disease not treated surgically, including multiple sclerosis, subacute combined degeneration (B12 deficiency), Friedreich's ataxia, tabes dorsalis, and pure sensory neuropathies. The latter may be observed in paraneoplastic syndromes and can be caused by the idiopathic synthesis of antibodies to the dorsal-root ganglia. The posterior column axons, within the dorsal-root ganglia, are the principal targets in pure sensory neuropathies.

Rarely, a dorsal extramedullary tumor may present as a posterior-cord syndrome. Disruption of posterior column function impairs position sense at the spinal-cord level and leads to an ataxic gait disturbance. The patient can partially compensate for this by using visual cues as cortical input to improve balance. During neurological examination, eye closure will exacerbate spinal ataxia and provoke more imbalance to indicate a positive Romberg's sign. Impaired position sense of the toes combined with a positive Romberg's sign localizes the cause of ataxia to a lesion in the spinal cord.

30.6.6
Conus and Cauda Equina Syndromes

Posterior to the T12 to L1 vertebral bodies, within the vertebral canal, the spinal-cord attenuates in diameter to form the conus medullaris. A lesion or injury at this level may produce impotence and a loss of bowel and bladder control. Any corticospinal (UMN) or motor lesion above the conus medullaris spares local lumbar and sacral bladder innervation. The result is a spastic bladder that will empty automatically or by reflex action at reduced volumes. An LMN lesion at or below the conus level (below L1) disrupts local lumbar and sacral innervation, leaving the bladder flaccid. The bladder's extent of neurological impairment can be accurately evaluated using cystometrics. Other physical findings of a conus medullaris syndrome include an anesthesia of the saddle region, reduced anal-sphincter tone during rectal examination, and variable sparing of the lower extremities. The prognosis for recovery of bowel and bladder control is poor. Below the T9 level, a greater percentage of the spinal cord is occupied by gray matter. Accordingly, there is a greater vulnerability to neurological morbidity during surgical manipulation or with the progression of a lesion caudal to T9.

Below L1 the conus medullaris or cord proper divides into the multiple lumbar and sacral nerve-roots of the cauda equina (L1- L5). The conus is anchored by a thin (2 mm) filum terminale that extends caudally through the cauda equina and the lumbar thecal sac. The sac ends at the mid-S1 vertebral level. UMN findings that are associated with the spinal-cord proper are not present in the cauda equina. Typical physical findings include variable LMN sensory and motor loss to the lower extremities, and sphincter disturbances.

30.7
Symptoms Associated with Specific Types of Spinal-Cord Tumors

Patients can experience neurological symptoms as a result of compromised spine stability, compression of nerve-roots and the cord proper, or interference with vasculature. Benign lesions generally present insidiously in the posterior region of the spine of children and young adults. Malignant neoplasms tend to occur in older patients, presenting as back pain that progresses to neurological deficit localized to the anterior structures of the spine (McCormick and Fetell 1996).

30.7.1
Primary Intramedullary Tumors

The symptoms of intramedullary tumors result from direct interference with the intrinsic structures of the spinal-cord. This can occur by means of intrinsic mass-effect and edema or by the development of a spinal syrinx. Primary intramedullary tumors usually extend over many spinal-cord segments, sometimes even the whole length of the spinal-cord. For this reason, as well as for the location of the lesion relative to spinal-cord tracts, the signs and symptoms of intramedullary tumors are more variable than those of extramedullary tumors (McCormick and Stein 1990a, Epstein and Wisoff 1987).

An intramedullary tumor that is restricted to one or two segments of the cord may present with a syndrome similar to that of an extramedullary tumor. More often, however, the intramedullary tumor involves several segments, with patterns of disassociated sensory loss attributable to dysfunction of crossing fibers. Pain may be an early manifestation if the dorsal-root entry zone is affected. The involvement of the crossing pain-fibers in the central portion of the cord may cause a pattern of pain and temperature loss only in the affected segments. Subsequently, the spinothalamic tracts can become affected as the tumor moves more peripherally. There is regional specificity associated with the clinical syndromes seen in patients with intramedullary tumors. In the thoracic and cervical regions of the cord, pain and temperature fibers from the sacral area lie near the external surface of the cord and may be initially uninvolved by an intramedullary tumor (i.e., sacral sparing). Involvement of the central gray matter leads to destruction of the anterior horn cells, with LMN weakness and atrophy in the appropriate segments. The clinical picture may be similar to that of syringomyelia, with sparing of pyramidal fibers (Madsen 1994).

Intramedullary lesions are often associated with cystic dilatation of the spinal-cord above or below the site of tumor (Li and HOLTAS 1991, SWEASEY et al. 1994). Symptoms associated with syrinx include dissociated sensory loss, cape-like distribution of dysesthetic pain, cervical or occipital pain, and LMN hand and arm weakness. Progression of these symptoms in a patient with an intramedullary lesion warrants reimaging and close follow-up with complete neurological examination.

30.7.2
Primary Extramedullary Tumors

Extramedullary tumors usually involve a few segments of the spinal-cord and cause specific clinical signs by focal compression of nerve-roots (McCORMICK et al. 1990a). Patients typically complain of radicular pain and paresthesias referable to a specific dorsal nerve root or group of roots. Sensory loss, weakness, and muscular wasting in the distribution of the affected roots soon follow this symptom pattern. Extramedullary tumors may progress to compromise the spinal-cord by mass compression of the cord, with complete loss of function below the level of the lesion. Compression of the spinal-cord first interrupts the functions of the pathways that lie at the periphery of the spinal-cord. As a result a constellation of early clinical signs that correlate with cord-compression include (1) spastic weakness below the lesion; (2) impairment of cutaneous and proprioceptive sensation below the lesion; (3) impaired control of the bladder and, to a lesser extent, of the rectum; and (4) increased tendon reflexes, extensor plantar responses, and loss of appropriate superficial abdominal reflexes (McCormick and Fetell 1996, McCormick 1994). If untreated, this syndrome may progress to signs and symptoms of complete transection of the spinal-cord, with wasting and atrophy of muscles at the level of the root lesion and, below the lesion, paraplegia or quadriplegia in flexion. The most common primary intradural tumors affecting the spinal-cord are neurofibromas, schwannomas, and meningiomas (McCormick and Stein 1990a).

30.7.3
Extramedullary Metastatic Tumors

Epidural spinal metastasis is a disorder of the vertebral column that can cause progressive neurological symptoms by extension into the spinal-canal (Constans et al. 1993). The advent of more effective adjuvant therapies has significantly increased the long-term survival of patients with primary cancers. This has resulted in a significant rise in the incidence of epidural spinal-cord compression. Currently 5 to 10% of all cancer patients experience cord-compression from an epidural lesion during the course of their disease (Wise et al. 1999). However, neither surgical extirpation nor radiation treatment of epidural tumor has been shown to prolong survival (Wise et al. 1999, Turgut et al. 1997).

Pain during recumbency (i.e., "nocturnal pain") is a sign of epidural tumor. Signs and symptoms of epidural spinal-cord compression can be easily overlooked in the patient with cancer, who is often wracked by asthenia and diffuse pain. The physician must respond to neck or back pain that is relentless and persists when the patient lies in bed, even if the pain is relieved by analgesics. Limb weakness, paresthesias in the distribution of a nerve-root, and bowel or bladder dysfunction are symptoms of a neurooncological emergency that requires prompt evaluation and treatment. Gait disorder secondary to sensory ataxia is a rare manifestation of cord-compression. The gait disturbance can occur without overt evidence of weakness, cutaneous sensory loss, or impaired proprioception. Spinocerebellar pathways have been

theorized to be involved in ataxia caused by compression of the cord (McCormick and Fetell 1996).

In more than half of reported cases, tumors causing epidural cord-compression arise from lung or breast. Greater than 80% of cases arise from primary tumors in lung, breast, gastrointestinal tract, prostate, melanoma, or lymphoma (Constans et al. 1983). Tumor can spread to the epidural space by (1) direct centripetal invasion from a paravertebral focus, entering through a nerve-root foramen; (2) hematogenous metastases to the vertebrae with extension from bone into epidural space; or (3) retrograde spread along Batson venous plexus. The most common route is through hematogenous spread. In approximately 85% of patients plain spine radiographs can be expected to demonstrate either lytic or blastic changes at the site of the lesion. Osteoblastic changes are common with myeloma, prostate carcinoma, and Hodgkin disease and occasionally are seen with breast cancer. Extradural tumors, particularly metastatic carcinoma and lymphoma may occlude spinal vessels. Hypoperfusion of the spinal-cord results in myelomalacia with signs and symptoms similar to those of severe intradural compression. The effect of compromising the vascular supply has regional specificity. Occlusion of the anterior spinal artery is better tolerated than other vascular tributaries of the spinal-cord. Symptoms of anterior spinal artery occlusion include focal LMN signs at the appropriate level, loss of pain and temperature sensation on both sides of the body, and some involvement of both pyramidal systems with UMN signs below the lesion. The posterior columns are generally spared.

30.7.4
Intramedullary Metastatic Tumors

In cancer patients with overt myelopathy and a normal myelogram, an intramedullary spinal-cord metastasis should be suspected. The most common tumors that cause intramedullary metastases are lung cancer or breast cancer (Connolly et al. 1996, Hashizume and Hirano 1983). In contrast to epidural cord-compression, plain radiographs of the spine are positive in only a quarter of these patients. The myelogram for these patients can be normal or can show cord enlargement, which is easily confirmed by CT. Intramedullary metastases are a sign of advanced metastatic disease. At autopsy up to 61% of patients with documented intramedullary metastases have multiple sites of cerebral or spinal lesions. Magnetic resonance imaging (MRI) is the best method for detection of intramedullary metastases. Reversal or stabilization of neurological signs depends on early diagnosis, however long-term survival after diagnosis is minimal (CONNOLLY et al. 1996).

30.8
Regional Syndromes of Spinal-Cord Tumors

The regional organization of the spinal-cord is an important consideration during the evaluation of patients with spinal tumors. Each segment of the spinal axis from the foramen magnum down to the conus has unique characteristics. Lesions can present with specific features attributable to neural elements in that region (McCormick and Fetell 1996).

30.8.1
Foramen Magnum Tumors

The clinical findings associated with foramen magnum lesions vary, depending upon the relative anterior, lateral, or posterior location of the pathology (GUIDETTI and SPALLONE 1980, YASUOKA et al. 1978, HONCH 1993, SAIRYO et al. 1997). In general, symptoms can include craniocervical pain localized to the neck and occiput that increases with head movement, as well as subjective feeling of weakness in the upper extremities. The phenomenon of "rotating paralysis" has been used to describe the sequential loss of function of ipsilateral upper extremity, ipsilateral lower extremity, and contralateral lower extremity, followed finally by the contralateral upper extremity. Definitive signs associated with foramen magnum lesions include dissociated sensory loss, loss of position and vibratory sense, greater in the upper extremities than in the lower extremities, spastic weakness of the extremities, and atrophy of the intrinsic muscles of the hands. Long-tract findings include brisk muscle stretch reflexes, loss of abdominal cutaneous reflexes, and a neurogenic bladder very late in the course of the disease. Ocular findings have been described, such as Horner's syndrome ipsilateral to the lesion, caused by compromise of cervical sympathetics, as well as downbeat nystagmus (YASUOKA et al. 1978).

Tumors in the region of the foramen magnum may extend into the posterior fossa or caudally into the cervical region. Involvement of primarily the twelfth, eleventh, and rarely the ninth and tenth lower cranial nerves causes specific syndromes. The most characteristic foramen magnum tumor is the ventrolateral meningioma. Growth of this tumor compresses the spinal-cord at the cervicomedullary junction to cause posterior column deficits with loss of position, vibratory, and light touch sensation more prominent in the arms than in the legs. There may be cutaneous sensory loss in distribution of C-2 or the occiput, with posterior cranial headache and high cervical pain. The progression of the sensory and motor symptoms may involve the limbs asymmetrically, whereas UMN signs can affect all four limbs.

30.8.2
Cervical Tumors

Patients with spinal tumors in the upper segments of the cervical region of the cord can present with pain or paresthesias in the occipital or cervical region, stiffness of the neck, as well as weakness and wasting of neck muscles. Below the lesion, there may be a spastic tetraplegia or hemiplegia and weakness of the ventrolateral region. Cutaneous sensation may be affected below the lesion with concurrent involvement of the descending trigeminal nucleus. In considering radicular symptoms associated with cervical tumors it should be noted that nerve-roots in the cervical region exit above the pedicle of the like-numbered vertebra. Anatomically the cervical nerve-root exits in close relation to the undersurface of the pedicle through the neural foramen. Characteristic findings associated with various cervical and upper thoracic levels are outlined in (Table 30.2).

30.8.3
Thoracic Tumors

Unlike the cervical or lumbar region of the cord, where motor dysfunction is easily discernable, the clinical localization of tumors in the thoracic region is facilitated more by sensory examination. It is difficult to determine the location of lesions in the upper half of the thoracic region of the cord by testing the strength of intercostal muscles. The Beevor sign, in which the umbilicus moves upward when the supine patient attempts to flex the head on the chest against resistance, can be used to localize lesions below T10. Abdominal skin reflexes are usually absent below the lesion.

Table 30.2. Characteristic findings associated with various cervical and upper thoracic levels that relate to postoperative survival

Root level	Clinical syndrome
C4	Paralysis of the diaphragm
C5	Atrophic paralysis of the deltoid, biceps, supinator longus, rhomboid, and spinalis muscles. The upper arms hang limply at the side. The sensory level extends to the outer surface of the arm. The biceps and supinator reflexes are lost
C6	Paralysis of triceps and wrist extensors. The fore arm is held semiflexed, and there is a partial wrist drop. The triceps reflex is lost. Sensory impairment extends to a line running down the middle of the arm slightly to the radial side
C7	Paralysis of the flexors of the wrist, and of the flexors and extensors of the fingers. Efforts to close the hands result in extension of the wrist and slight flexion of the fingers (preacher's hand). The sensory level is similar to that of the sixth cervical segment but slightly more to the ulnar side of the arm
C8	Atrophic paralysis of the small muscles of the hand with resulting clawhand (main-en-griffe). Horner's syndrome, unilateral or bilateral, results from lesions at this level, and is characterized by the triad of ptosis, small pupil (miosis), and loss of sweating on the face. Sensory loss extends to the inner aspect of the arm, and involves the fourth and fifth fingers and the ulnar aspect of the middle finger
T1	Lesions rarely cause motor symptoms because this nerve-root provides little functional innervation of the small hand muscles. Other signs of cervical tumors include nystagmus, especially with tumors in the upper segment. This condition is presumably due to damage to the descending portion of the median longitudinal fasciculus. Horner's syndrome may be found with intramedullary lesions in any portion of the cervical spinal-cord region if the descending sympathetic pathways are affected

30.8.4
Lumbar Tumors

The localization of a lumbar lesion can be easily deduced by the patient's root level of sensory loss and associated motor weakness. In the lumbar region, the nerve-root exits below and in close proximity to the pedicle of its like-numbered vertebra with the intervertebral disc space situated well below the pedicle. Tumors that compress only the first and second lumbar segments cause loss of the cremasteric reflexes. The abdominal reflexes are preserved while knee and ankle jerks are increased. If the tumor affects the third and fourth lumbar seg-

ments of the cord and does not involve the roots of the cauda equina, there is weakness of the quadriceps, loss of the patellar reflexes, and hyperactive Achilles reflexes. More commonly, lesions at this level also involve the cauda equina with resulting flaccid paralysis of the legs as well as loss of knee and ankle reflexes. If the spinal-cord and cauda equina are affected concurrently, there may be spastic paralysis of one leg, with increased ankle reflex ipsilaterally and flaccid paralysis with loss of reflexes contralaterally.

30.8.5
Tumors of the Conus and Cauda Equina

The initial symptom of tumors that involve the conus or cauda equina is pain in the back, rectal area, or both lower legs, often leading to a diagnosis of sciatica (Yoshii et al. 1999). Although the two regions are anatomically related there are several clinical features that can serve to distinguish conus lesions from cauda equina lesions (McCormick and Fetell 1996, McCormick et al. 1990a).

Spontaneous pain is rarely associated with conus lesions whereas it is usually the most prominent symptom in patients suffering from cauda equina lesions. The pain of a cauda equina lesion is severe, radicular in nature involving the perineum, thighs and legs, often asymmetrically. The pain of a conus lesion is usually bilateral and symmetric. Symmetric saddle anesthesia and dissociation mark the sensory deficit of a conus lesion secondary to compromise of crossing fibers. Patients with sensory deficits attributable to cauda equina lesions do not have dissociation, and often present with unilateral or asymmetric findings. Motor dysfunction is also symmetric for conus lesions and asymmetric for cauda equina lesions. Autonomic dysfunction such as bladder dysfunction and impotency is typically an early sign in patients with conus medullaris lesions whereas it is a late finding in patients with cauda equina lesions.

Patients with spinal tumors in the conus and cauda equina can have a combination of symptoms. As the tumor grows, there may be flaccid paralysis of the legs, atrophy of the leg muscles, and foot drop. Fasciculation may be seen in the atrophied muscles. Sensory loss may affect the perianal or saddle area as well as the remaining sacral and lumbar dermatomes. This loss may be slight, or it may be so severe that a trophic ulcer develops over the lumbosacral region, the buttocks, the hips, or heels.

Signs of raised intracranial pressure may be seen with ependymomas of this region if the CSF protein content is high.

30.9
Differential Diagnosis

Spinal tumors must be differentiated from other disorders of the spinal-cord. A complete differential list is extensive and can include the following: transverse myelitis, multiple sclerosis, syringomyelia, combined system disease, syphilis, anomalies of the cervical region of the spine and base of the skull, spondylosis, adhesive arachnoiditis, radiculitis of the cauda equina, hypertrophic arthritis, ruptured intervertebral discs, and vascular anomalies.

Multiple sclerosis, with a complete or incomplete transverse lesion of the cord, can usually be differentiated from spinal-cord tumors by the relapsing and remitting course. The signs and symptoms of lesions in more than one anatomical location, as well as evoked potential studies, cranial MRI, and presence of CSF oligoclonal bands are consistent with multiple sclerosis (MS). Acute transverse myelitis may occasionally enlarge the cord to simulate an intramedullary tumor (McCormick and Fetell 1996).

The differential diagnosis between syringomyelia and intramedullary tumors is complicated because intramedullary cysts are commonly associated with these tumors (Aoki 1991). Extramedullary tumors in the cervical region may give rise to localized pains and muscular atrophy in conjunction with a Brown-Sequard syndrome, producing a clinical picture similar to that of syringomyelia. The diagnosis of syringomyelia is likely when trophic disturbances are present.

The combination of atrophy of hand muscles and spastic weakness in the legs in ALS may suggest the diagnosis of a cervical cord tumor. Tumor is excluded by the normal sensory examination, the presence of fasciculation, or atrophy in leg muscles. Cervical spondylosis, with or without rupture of the intervertebral discs, may cause symptoms and signs of root irritation and compression of the spinal-cord. The osteoarthritis can be diagnosed by findings in plain radiographs, but this is so common in asymptomatic people that MRI may be necessary to determine whether there is spondylitic myelopathy or an extramedullary tumor.

Anomalies in the cervical region or at the base of the skull, such as platybasia or Klippel-Feil syndrome, are diagnosed by the characteristic radiographic findings. Occasionally arachnoiditis may interfere with the circulation in the cord, causing signs and symptoms of a transverse lesion. The CSF protein content is moderately elevated. Diagnosis is made by complete or partial arrest of the contrast column on myelography or by fragmentation of the material at the site of the lesion. Separation of the adhesions and removal of the thickened arachnoid by surgery have been of little benefit, with steroid therapy being equally ineffective (McCormick and Fetell 1996, McCormick and Stein 1990b).

Benign tumors of the spinal-cord are characterized by a slowly progressive course for many years. If a neurofibroma arises from a dorsal root, there may be years of radicular pain before the tumor is evident from other manifestations of growth. Intramedullary tumors are generally benign and slow-growing; they may attain enormous size (over the course of 6 to 8 years) before they are discovered. Conversely the sudden onset of a severe neurological disorder, with or without pain, is usually indicative of a malignant extradural tumor, such as metastatic carcinoma or lymphoma.

30.10
Radiographic Evaluation

The mainstay of radiographic diagnosis for all spinal-cord tumors is MRI (McCormick and Fetell 1996). MRI provides spatial and contrast resolution of neural structures which is unattainable by any other imaging modality. Plain X-rays have little role in the modern diagnosis of spinal-cord tumors as they do not image soft tissue adequately. However, the effects of intraspinal tumors on the vertebral elements are sometimes evident. Nerve-sheath tumors can cause enlargement the intervertebral foramina. Longstanding intramedullary lesions can produce erosion or scalloping of the posterior vertebral bodies and widening of the interpedicular interval. Myelography alone has a very limited role in the work-up of spinal-cord tumors. It is seldom performed without subsequent CT. Intradural extramedullary tumors typically produce rounded filling defects of the dye column on a plain myelogram. Intramedullary lesions characteristically cause focal widening of the spinal-cord shadow. CT and CT-myelography show greater enhancement of anatomical details than do plain X-rays and myelography. CT provides excellent visualization of osseous structures, but soft tissue detail is inferior to that of MRI.

For extramedullary tumors, CT-myelography provides excellent visualization of tumors arising in the
region of the neural foramen. Accompanying bony
changes are well-demonstrated. Intramedullary tumors are more difficult to demonstrate because they
are generally confined to the cord tissue. Although
widening of the cord may be seen with large lesions,
subtle ones may be missed. MRI with and without
intravenous contrast is the optimum initial radiographic examination for both tumor types.

30.10.1
Intramedullary Tumors

Most intramedullary tumors are isointense or slightly hypointense to the surrounding spinal-cord on
T1-weighted images (McCormick and Stein
1990a). Often, only subtle spinal-cord enlargement is

evident. T2-weighted images are more sensitive because most tumors are hyperintense to the spinal-
cord on these pulse sequences. T2-studies, however,
are not particularly specific and may not distinguish
the solid tumor from polar cysts. Nearly all intramedullary neoplasms will be enhanced on T1-
weighted contrast examinations.

30.10.1.1
Ependymoma

Ependymomas usually demonstrate uniform contrast enhancement and are symmetrically located
within the spinal-cord (Fig. 30.10). Polar cysts are
identified in the majority of cases, particularly with
cervical and cervicothoracic tumors. Heterogeneous
enhancement from intratumoral cysts or necrosis
can also be seen. In some cases, contrast enhancement of a cystic ependymoma may be minimal. In

a 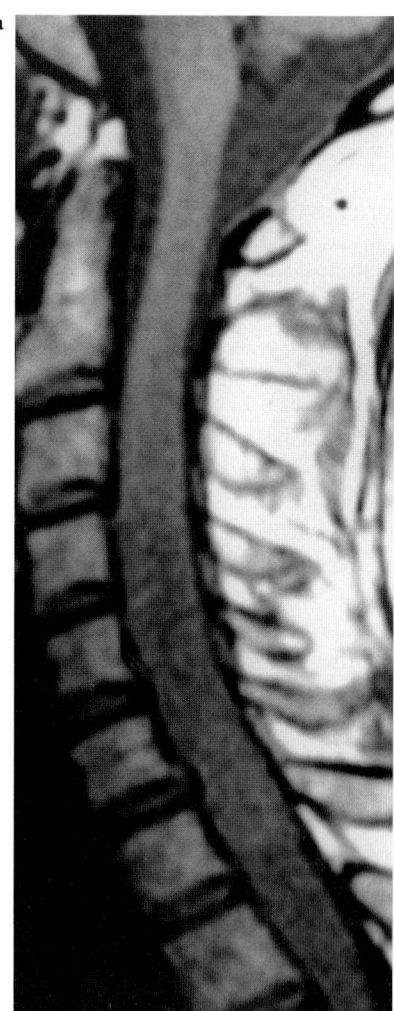 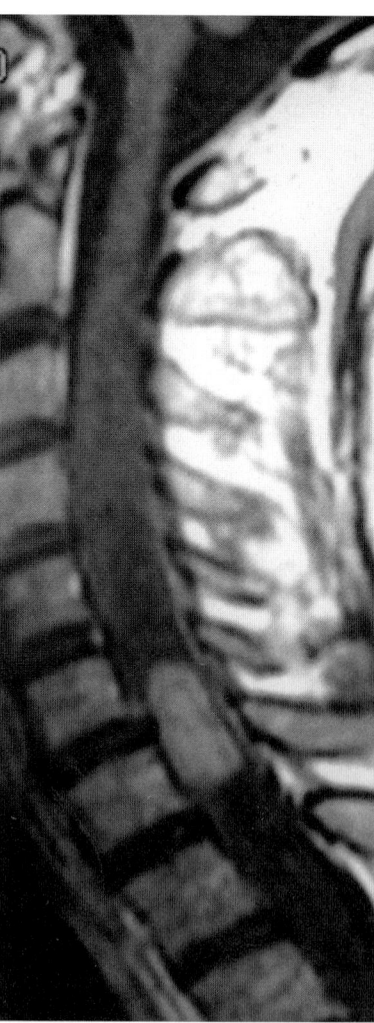 b

Fig. 30.10. T1-weighted MRI, **a** non-contrast and **b** contrast, demonstrates lesion with characteristics of intramedullary spinal ependymoma

these cases it is difficult to distinguish with certainty these tumors from intramedullary astrocytomas.

30.10.1.2
Astrocytoma

The MRI appearance of astrocytomas is variable. These tumors tend to be less well-defined than ependymomas on contrast enhanced MRI because of their irregular tumor margins. Contrast uptake may be minimal, uniform, or patchy (Fig. 30.11). Heterogeneous uptake is more commonly seen with astrocytomas because of intratumoral cysts or necrosis. Patchy, irregular tumor margins that extend over several spinal segments is also common.

30.10.1.3
Hemangioblastoma

Hemangioblastomas typically show marked and uniform contrast enhancement on MRI (Fig. 30.12). Vascular-flow voids may be seen on non-contrast images. Associated polar cysts are also common. Le-

sions rarely span more than one spinal segment. Despite characteristic MRI patterns, there is enough variability and overlap in appearance of intramedullary tumors to preclude competent histological diagnosis based on MRI characteristics alone.

30.10.2
Extramedullary Tumors

Lesion signal abnormalities, CSF capping, and spinal-cord or cauda equina displacement will identify most extramedullary masses on a technically adequate MRI study (McCormick et al. 1990a). The diagnosis of lipoma, neurenteric cysts, dermoid or epidermoid, arachnoid cysts, or vascular pathology may be established on the basis of imaging-characteristics alone (McCormick and Stein 1990b). Gadolinium-enhanced images markedly increase the sensitivity of MRI, particularly for small tumors. Most extramedullary tumors are isointense or slightly hypointense with respect to the spinal-cord on T1-weighted images. Nerve-sheath tumors are more

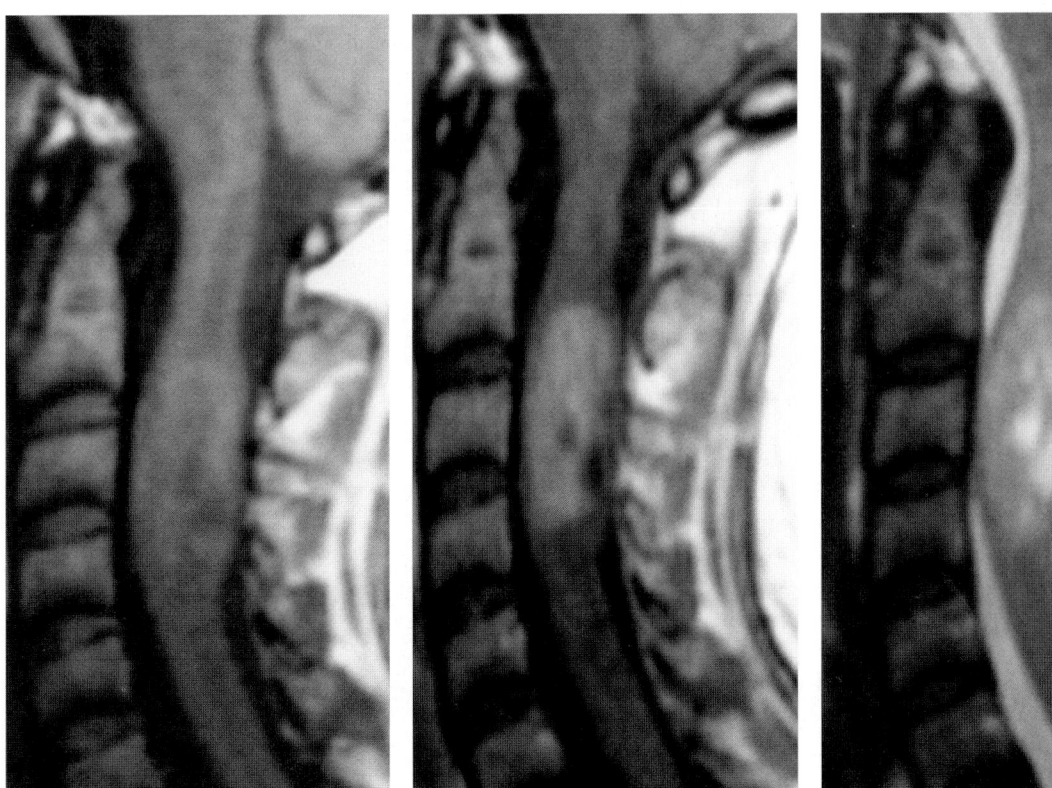
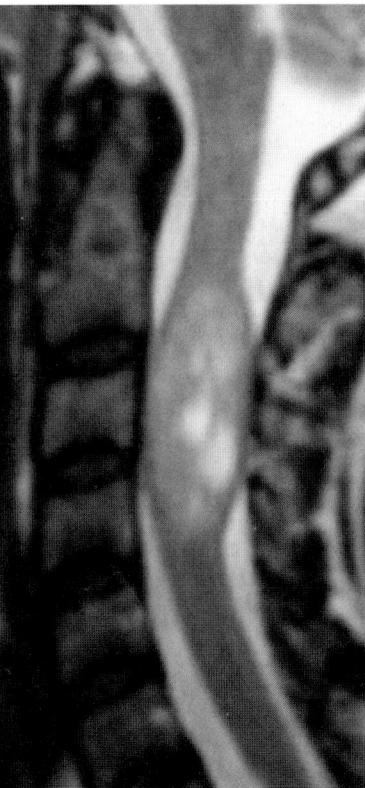

a   b,c

Fig. 30.11. T1-weighted MRI, **a** non-contrast and **b** contrast, demonstrates lesion with characteristics of intramedullary spinal astrocytoma, while **c** a T2-weighted image reveals cystic degeneration and blood products of variable ages

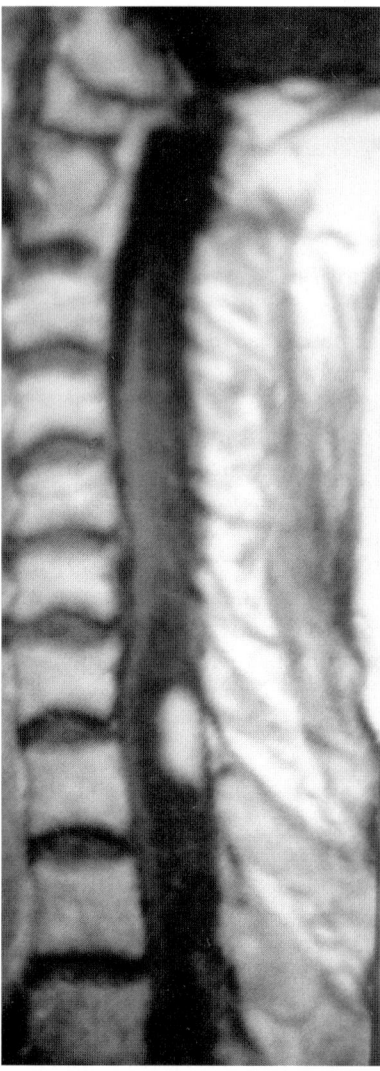

Fig. 30.12. T1-weighted MRI with contrast, demonstrates a cystic lesion with an enhancing mural nodule consistent with characteristics of intramedullary spinal hemangioblastoma

likely to be hyperintense relative to the spinal-cord than are meningiomas on T2-weighted images. Cauda equina tumors usually demonstrate increased signal intensity with respect to CSF on both T1 and T2 pulse sequences. Small cauda equina tumors are easily overlooked, however, on non-contrast scans.

Virtually all extramedullary spinal tumors demonstrate some degree of contrast enhancement. Meningiomas typically exhibit intense uniform enhancement, although non-enhancing calcifications or intratumoral cysts may be seen. Enhancement of the adjacent dura, a "dural tail", strongly supports the diagnosis of meningioma (Fig. 30.13). Although most nerve-sheath tumors and filum ependymomas

also demonstrate uniform contrast uptake, heterogeneous enhancement from intratumoral cysts, hemorrhage, or necrosis is frequent (Fig. 30.14).

30.11
Other Diagnostic Considerations

30.11.1
Cerebrospinal Fluid

When there is a complete subarachnoid block, the CSF is usually xanthochromic as a result of the high protein content. It may be only slightly yellow, or colorless if the subarachnoid block is incomplete. The cell count is usually normal, but a slight pleocytosis is found in about 30% of patients. Cell counts of between 25 and 100/mm^3 are found in about 15% of the patients with subarachnoid block secondary to spinal tumor. The protein content is increased in more than 95%. Values of over 100 mg/dl are present in 60% of the patients and values over 1,000 mg/dl are present in 5% and may, in rare cases, lead to

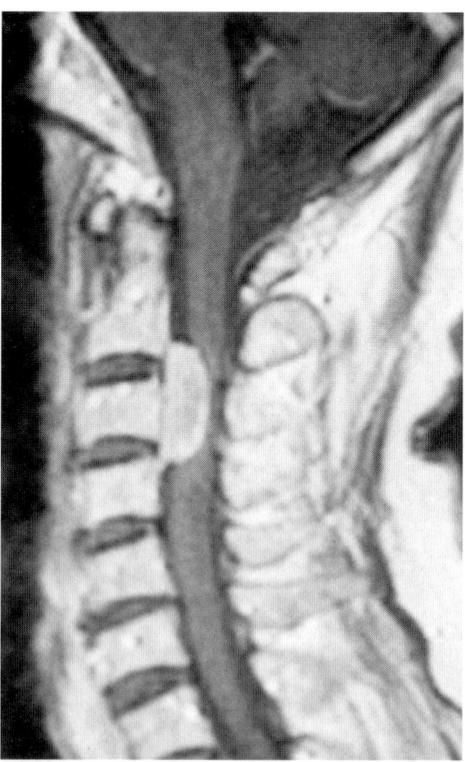

Fig. 30.13. T1-weighted MRI with contrast, demonstrates a homogeneously enhancing intradural extramedullary lesion consistent with characteristics of spinal meningioma

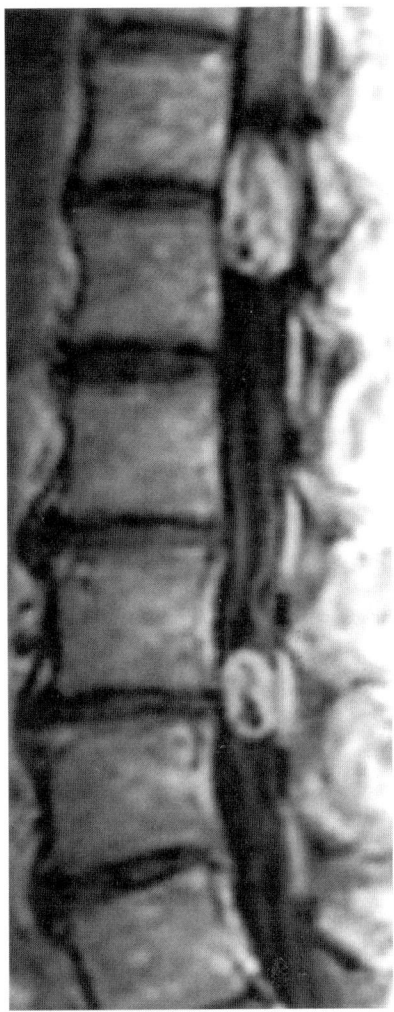

Fig. 30.14. T1-weighted MRI with contrast, demonstrates multiple lesions consistent with characteristics of spinal neurofibroma

communicating hydrocephalus. The glucose content is normal unless tumor of the meninges is present. Cytological evaluation of the CSF is useful when malignant tumors are suspected (McCormick and Fetell 1996).

30.11.2
Bone Scans

Radioisotope bone scans (Fig. 30.15) will show increased activity in the affected area of the spine in two-thirds of patients with metastatic disease. However this modality is actually less specific in predicting cord-compression than plain spine radiographs. The utility of bone scans in differentiating malignant

from non-malignant fractures is limited as well (An et al. 1995).

30.12
Management

Tissue diagnosis is necessary after clinical and radiographic evaluation reveal a lesion that is consistent with a spinal-cord tumor. The surgical objective for most spinal-cord tumors is gross total removal, and surgical planning must proceed accordingly. Immediately preoperatively, patients are given high-dose glucocorticoids and intravenous antibiotics. Most tumors are accessible with the patient in the prone position. For cervical lesions, stabilization of the head and neck, in pins, is necessary. Adequate exposure is crucial and is dictated by the location and extent of the lesion. Intraoperative monitoring with somatosensory evoked potentials (SSEP) and motor evoked potentials (MEP) should be routinely used. Intraoperative ultrasound is often useful to localize and detect the extent of intramedullary pathology. The extent of resection is guided by the anatomy of the lesion, intraoperative monitoring, the surgeon's

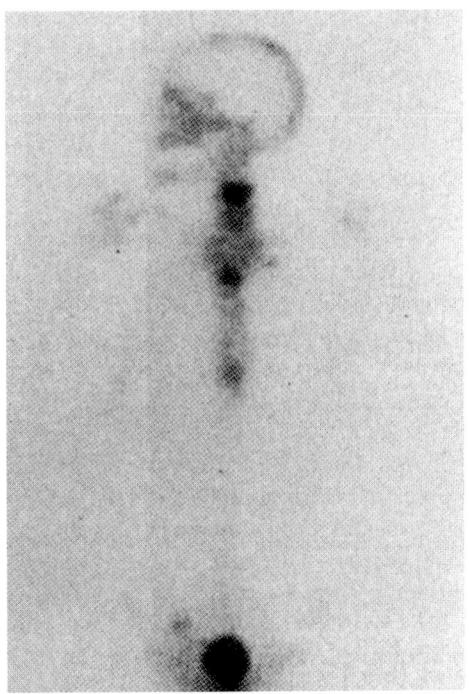

Fig. 30.15. Radioisotope bone scan of a patient with metastatic prostate cancer, demonstrates increased uptake of isotope in cervical region consistent with distal metastasis

experience, and the preliminary histological diagnosis on frozen sections of the lesion. A competent dural closure is essential to prevent CSF leaks. In the postoperative period, early mobilization and rehabilitation are encouraged while steroids are tapered. The debate over what constitutes appropriate adjuvant radiotherapy is on-going; and is addressed in the next chapter.

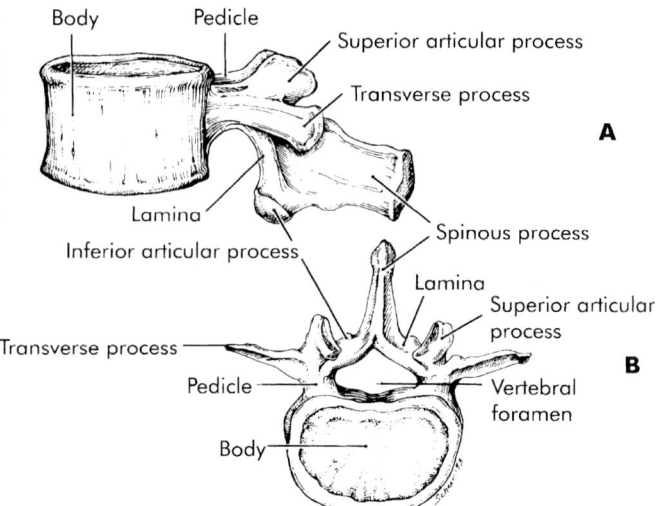

Fig. 30.16. Schematic of vertebral body, demonstrating pertinent surgical anatomy with lateral and axial views of a thoracic vertebra. In the lateral view, the lamina is obscured by both the transverse process and facets. The pedicle joins the vertebral body to the neural arch. In the axial view, the vertebral body, paired pedicles, transverse processes, facets, lamina, and spinous process are clearly demonstrated. These structures circumscribe the vertebral canal

30.13
Aspects of Neuroradiology Pertinent to Surgical Planning

30.13.1
Plain Film Assessment

Plain radiographs of the vertebral column remain essential to all cases despite substantial progress in spine-imaging techniques. The bony landmarks of the spine can have both local and remote responses to pathology affecting the spine, spinal-cord, or nerve-roots. Plain films allow a rapid review of bony landmarks and alignment. The anteroposterior (AP) projection can reveal an abnormal curvature of scoliosis that usually involves the thoracic part of the spine. Causes of scoliosis include neuromuscular imbalances of paraspinal muscle tone, unilateral irritation or pain, and structural abnormalities of the vertebral bodies and facets. The AP projection can also detect vertebral body abnormalities, erosion of the pedicles, and the presence of paraspinal masses.

With respect to neoplastic disease, the vertebral bodies often reveal specific patterns of bony destruction that suggest the aggressiveness of the tumor involved. A slowly expanding or benign lesion causes a regional or scalloping pattern of destruction. Conversely, a rapidly growing tumor produces a lytic or permeative pattern of bone destruction that may lead to vertebral body collapse. The pedicle adjoins the vertebral body to the posterior neural arch, which consists of the spinous process and paired laminae (Fig. 30.16). An AP projection may demonstrate pedicle erosion from either spinal-cord expansion or tumor emanating from the vertebral body itself. Widening of the vertebral canal occurs in response to chronic neoplastic or cystic expansions within or adjacent to the spinal-cord.

Lateral radiographic projections of the spine may be used to evaluate conditions involving malalignment or instability. A lateral plain film can demonstrate the anterior slipping of one vertebral body

over another. In the lumbosacral segments, this is referred to as a spondylolisthesis, and at other spinal levels this is often termed subluxation. Insidious instability occurs with an occult fracture or ligamentous failure. It can be accentuated by changes in head and body position or by dynamic fluoroscopy.

Oblique projections of the spine allow direct viewing of the foramina, through which nerve-roots must exit. Enlargement or constriction of foraminal outlets is caused by neoplasms involving the nerve-roots and degenerative vertebral changes, respectively (Fig. 30.17). These radiographic observations are often associated with the clinical findings of a radiculopathy. A loss of height or spontaneous fusion within the intervertebral disc space can be assessed and may relate to nerve-root and/or spinal-cord compression.

After the more global plain-film assessments, axial or horizontal radiographic slices with sagittal or vertical reconstruction can be obtained using CT. Through selective radiographic sectioning, CT scans elaborate any focal abnormalities evident on plain films. Three-dimensional spiral CT scans provide three dimensional multiplanar viewing of the vertebral column. Polytomography, although antiquated, retains its value in revealing fractures, extent of bone healing or fusion, and focal disruption of functional components of the vertebral column. Plain-film as-

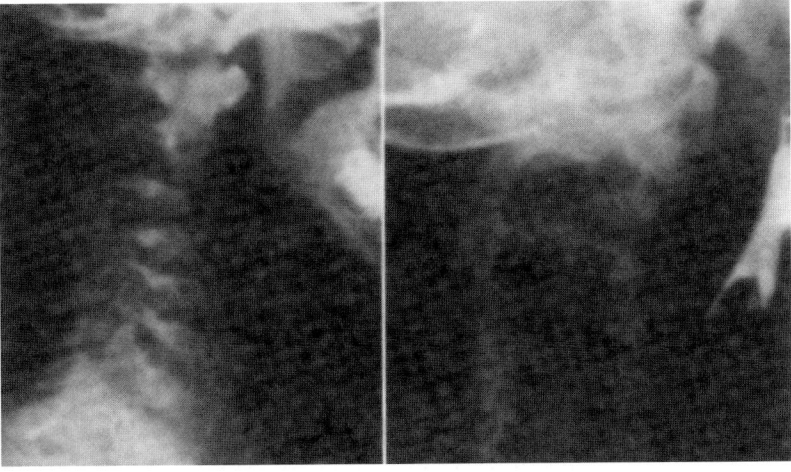

Fig. 30.17. Plain film demonstrating enlargement of foraminal outlets, from a lateral cervical radiograph of a child with neurofibromatosis, showing an enlarged neural foramina from C1 through C3

sessments of the targeted vertebral level fulfill a critical need for accurate intraoperative localization, using either anatomical landmarks or radio-opaque markers on the patient. Precise localization assures a direct approach, exposure of the pathology, and an overall economy of surgical efforts.

30.14
General Considerations for Surgery of the Spine

30.14.1
Stability

Good preoperative planning avoids an approach that has the possibility of iatrogenically destabilizing the spine. The vertebral spine and its ligamentous support can be divided into three columns of stability (Fig. 30.18). The anterior half of the vertebral body is part of the anterior column, which includes the anterior half of the intervertebral disc and the anterior longitudinal ligament. The middle column consists of the posterior half of the vertebral body and the intervertebral disc, with ligamentous support provided by the posterior longitudinal ligament. The posterior column includes the paired facets, which are superior and inferior to the pars interarticularis (pillars), the transverse and spinous processes, and the paired laminae. The capsule over the facet joints, intertransverse ligaments, interspinous ligaments, and ligamentum flavum are structures of ligamentous support specific to the posterior column (DENIS 1983). A normal spine remains stable unless two of the three columns have been disrupted.

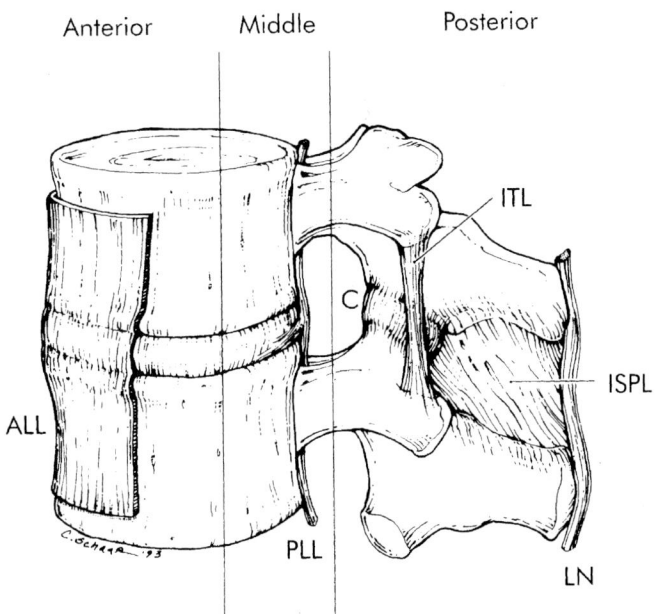

Fig. 30.18. Schematic illustration demonstrating that the spine and its ligamentous support can be divided into three columns of stability. Schematic representation of the vertebral columns with supportive ligamentous structures. Note that the three columns of stability are anterior, middle, and posterior. The anterior column includes the anterior longitudinal ligament (ALL) and the anterior annulus of the intravertebral disc space. The middle column includes the annulus of the posterior disc space and the posterior longitudinal ligament (PLL). The posterior column includes the capsular (C) attachments of the facet joint, intertransverse ligament (ITL), interspinous ligament (ISPL), and ligamentous nuchae (LN). Compromise of two of the columns of spinal stability imparts spinal instability

30.14.2
Posterior Approaches

30.14.2.1
Surgical Considerations

A posterior approach to the vertebral column typically requires that the patient be placed in a prone position. To avoid painful neck positions for the patient, the surgeon should assess the cervical range of motion preoperatively. Such an evaluation may reveal an incomplete range of motion, local neck pain, dysesthesia, or a sudden brief electric shock -like sensation radiating down the spine (Lhermitte's sign). Head positions that manifest any symptoms of discomfort are contraindicated intraoperatively. When there is doubt, the neck can remain in a neutral position, with the patient face-down while prone, and a cushioned horseshoe headrest used. The orbits require an occlusive covering. Pressure is to be avoided over the orbits and malar region of the face.

A preoperative and baseline electrophysiological study is advised if the patient is to be monitored intraoperatively. Data obtained during the preoperative assessment will assist the neurophysiologist or technician in configuring the optimal stimulus-response routine, given the site of spinal-cord deficit and the intended surgical approach. Sufficient electrical grounding for both electrocautery and neuromonitoring is obtained through the return pad of an electrocautery unit. To prevent the patient from conducting current between grounding sources, the surgeon confirms that no more than one grounding source is attached to the patient. In the operating-room, the location of cables and electronic instrumentation is configured to minimize AC (60 cycles) interference during electrophysiological neuromonitoring (PARSA and MILLER 2000).

It is advisable for the surgical team to determine the necessity of any additional venous access and arterial lines based on the medical condition of the patient, as well as the duration and nature of the procedure. Any substantial hemodynamic fluctuation after anesthetic induction may be exacerbated by prone positioning. Volume supplementation, vasoactive amines, central venous access, and arterial line monitoring serve to counteract possible repercussions of this hemodynamic fluctuation. Certain preoperative maneuvers can induce acute dysrhythmias and hypertension in patients with chronic paralysis from a complete cord lesion (autonomic hyperreflexia). Intubation, suctioning, prone positioning,

and bladder catheterization can each induce autonomic dysreflexia, the treatment of which requires optimum hemodynamic monitoring and the availability of sympatholytic agents. Patients with a high, complete cord lesion of greater than 1 week's duration may experience massive hyperkalemia after muscle relaxation with succinylcholine (PARSA and MILLER 2000). This is typically a result of extensive denervation and an abnormal response of the muscle-cell membrane to depolarizing agents. Compressive, thigh-length stockings help to counteract venous pooling in the lower extremities. In addition, segmental compression boots can be used since they also serve as a preventive measure for deep-venous thrombosis during long procedures. Bladder catheterization is indicated for most spinal procedures, and certainly for those involving cord manipulation. In addition, the use of epidural or intradural analgesics for control of early postoperative pain requires bladder catheterization (PARSA and MILLER 2000).

Any condition that reduces space in the cervical region of the spinal-canal precludes hyperextension of the neck during intubation. Patients with cervical spinal-canal impingement are best served by fiberoptic, laryngoscopic intubation while awake. Alternatively, having assessed neck mobility preoperatively, the anesthesiologist, in the presence of the surgeon, can conduct a simple laryngoscopic viewing with the cervical part of the spine in a neutral position. An obstructed view of the larynx, cervical instability, or radiographic evidence of cervical cord impingement, mandates fiberoptic intubation of a conscious patient with a locally anesthetized pharynx. An armored endotracheal (ET) tube will assure patency with any surgical positioning of the cervical spine. Given the difficulty associated with reintubating a patient in the prone position, the securing of the ET or nasotracheal (NT) tube is of paramount importance (PARSA and MILLER 2000).

30.14.2.2
Patient Positioning

Unimpeded head-side access to the posterior cervical part of the spine is facilitated by pin-fixation or the horseshoe headrest. The head is face-down and slightly flexed to expand both the interspinous and interlaminar spaces. The back of the neck faces the surgeon, parallel to the floor, and the patient's body is placed straight prone or in a semi-kneeling position. Both arms are pronated and secured by the patient's side to permit the surgeons to stand adjacent to the posterior neck. A footboard and restraining belt secure the patient for any necessary tilts of the operating-room table. Slight angulation of the body in a reverse Trendelenburg position, below the shoulder level, further reduces venous pressure in the cervical area of the spine. Proximal to sites of neural impingement, the epidural veins may remain compressed and engorged. Local epidural bleeding is usually controlled through low-wattage, bipolar electrocautery and hemostatic adjuvants. Under the microscope, even a minimal amount of bleeding will obscure the surgeon's view. Tilt can be altered to meet the needs of the surgeon and to suit the hemodynamic status of the patient.

Less commonly, posterior approaches to the cervical part of the spine are accomplished by placing the patient in a sitting position. There are several disadvantages to this, especially with regard to the fragile hemodynamic status of elderly patients with cardiac disease. In addition, this position increases the risk of air embolus, and limits the ability of the surgeon to tilt the operating-table during the course of the procedure (Parsa and Miller 2000). The principles of prone positioning remain consistent for all levels of the spine. The face-down, prone position is also optimal for posterior approaches to the cervicothoracic spinal region. At this level, avoidance of neck rotation helps to maintain midline alignment of the spinous processes. As in cervical posterior approaches, the arms remain at the patient's side. Thoracic and lumbar approaches are facilitated by moving the arms up into a semi-reaching position on arm boards. Each elbow is cushioned to prevent pressure-induced injury of the ulnar nerve at the olecranon. For the thoracic spinal area, the operating-table can be slightly flexed to optimize both the interspinous and interlaminar spaces.

Posterior approaches to the lumbar region of the spine benefit from specially equipped operating-tables. The prone patient can be flexed both at the hips and the knees after the head extension is removed (Fig. 30.19). The patient remains on cushioned bolsters and can assume a semi-kneeling to kneeling position, with the padded head extension now supporting the anterior tibial regions. In the kneeling position, the buttocks and lateral parts of the thighs are supported by extensions with cushioned plates. In the male patient, the scrotum remains free of any compression. This flexed position maintains abdominal relaxation, reduces traction on both the femoral and sciatic nerves, and opens the interspinous and interlaminar spaces. The weight-bearing points must be evenly distributed to avoid compressive injuries.

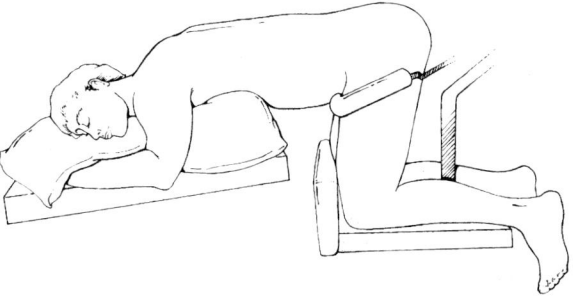

Fig. 30.19. Schematic illustration demonstrates positioning of prone patient in semi-kneeling position for posterior lumbar approach. Abdomen remains free of compression and weight is evenly distributed over well-cushioned anterior tibial surfaces. Cushioned support is provided for the anterior axillary regions and elbows

Some surgeons prefer the patient to be in a lateral decubitus position for posterior approaches to both the thoracic and lumbar regions of the spine (Fig. 30.20). An axillary roll between the patient and table permits unimpeded excursions of the chest with mechanical ventilation. Additional padding protects the weight-bearing points of the iliac crest, fibular head, and lateral malleolus. The arms are placed in front of the patient, with the up-side arm supported either by a pillow or a padded table extension. For disc removal, the patient's flank, on the dependent side, can be aligned above the flexion break of the table. Table flexion will elevate the adjacent flank and open the opposite side of the targeted disc space.

30.14.2.3
Operating Technique

In posterior approaches, a combination of radiographs and topographic examination allows appropriate placement of the incision. Lesions that are

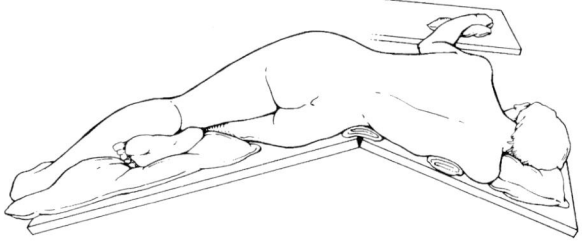

Fig. 30.20. Schematic illustration demonstrates lateral decubitus position for posterior approaches to the thoracic and lumbar spinal regions. Note the axillary roll on the dependent side, and padded protection of iliac crest, dependent fibular head, and lateral malleolus. The arm opposite the dependent side is supported by a cushioned Mayo stand

targeted by myelography should be marked, with a member of the surgical team confirming the aspect of the lesion (top, middle, or bottom) to which the marking refers. Radiographs are more useful surgically when they include the targeted lesion and a bony landmark that functions as a reference point for segmental counting. Coned-down views do not fulfill this purpose. In the operating-room, radiographic views are best displayed in the same orientation as the patient position.

Most posterior approaches are midline, with the initial surgical goal being the exposure of normal anatomy above and below any targeted lesion. On the patient, segmental counting of the spinous processes puts the surgeon in proximity to the target, and a needle is placed into the interspinous ligament with a cephalad angle. An image intensifier or plain X-ray locates the needle in reference to landmarks, which can include the foramen magnum for cervicothoracic localization in the lateral projection, the first rib for thoracic localization in the anteroposterior (AP) projection, and the top of the iliac crest and sacrum for thoracolumbar localization in the lateral projection. The needle is either on target or serves as a second reference from which an accurate incision can be made. Alternatively, when the surgical exposure incorporates known points of reference, the targeted level can be determined by segmental counting in the operative field. This is often the case for cervical and lumbar exposures with C2 as the first spinous process and S1 as the last.

When counting spinous processes, the surgeon can encounter anomalies that mandate radiographic imaging to confirm the segmental level. Sacralization of the L5 vertebra or lumbarization of the S1 vertebra and missing spinous processes can make accurate determination of the caudal cord level difficult. From 20% to 30% of the general population has spina bifida occulta within the lumbar region of the spine (PARSA and MILLER 2000). In spinal neoplasms, especially metastatic tumors, a whole vertebral body can be missing (Fig. 30.21).

During posterior approaches, the midline is incised to detach and mobilize the paraspinous muscles through a subperiosteal technique. Removal of the posterior neural arch in a piecemeal fashion is termed a laminectomy. Beneath the posterior neural arch is the ligamentum flavum (yellow ligament), which extends laterally to the facet. The epidural fat and veins lie between the ligamentum flavum and dura. For reconstructive purposes, multiple levels of the posterior neural arch can be elevated as one segment by drilling bilateral troughs in the lamina

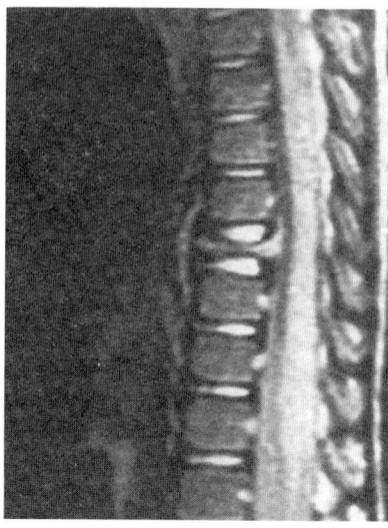

Fig. 30.21. MRI demonstrating nearly complete loss of vertebral body secondary to tumor, in the thoracic region of the spine, with pathological compression

(laminoplasty). This method preserves the interspinous and interlaminar ligaments of the mobilized segment (Fig. 30.22).

During intradural explorations and extradural nerve-root decompressions, laminectomies may require a more lateral exposure. This is accomplished by undercutting the medial one-third of the facet. The facet or apophyseal joints overlie the lateral recess, which contains the nerve-root and neural foramina. Ventral to the nerve-root and cord is the disc space.

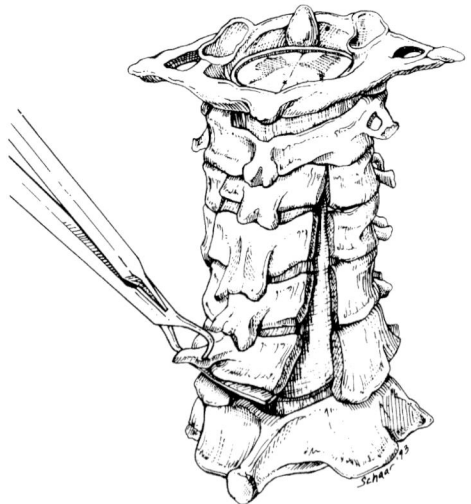

Fig. 30.22. Schematic illustration demonstrating the posterior cervical neural arch undergoing a laminoplasty for posterior exposure. This maneuver allows for reconstruction of the posterior neural arch after the completion of the procedure

A laminotomy is a partial resection of the laminae for two adjacent segmental levels. It provides access for disc removals and nerve-root decompressions. Extension of the laminotomy to the lateral recess with partial removal of the facet (facetectomy) is termed a foraminotomy. This procedure decompresses the nerve-root and provides access for posterior removal of a disc with lateral herniation in the cervical part of the spine. With extreme lateral retraction of the paraspinal muscles, the transverse process can be visualized lateral to the superior facet. The pedicle is anterior to the junction of the lamina, superior facet, and transverse process. The pedicle is the posterior entry point for transpedicular screwfixation. Removal of the lamina and superior facet permits a transpedicular approach to the vertebral body, with exposure of the lateral part of the spinalcord. Disruption of the posterior neural arch is compatible with retained spinal stability as long as the facets are preserved. The facets, facet capsule, and intertransverse ligament remain mostly intact for residual posterior column stability. Posterior approaches do not require instrumentation, provided that the anterior and middle columns of stability are intact.

30.14.3
Anterolateral Approaches

30.14.3.1
Anterior Atlantoaxial

At the atlantoaxial junction, the odontoid process may require a transoral resection to relieve or avert impingement of the cervicomedullary junction. Frequent indications include trauma, basilar impression, rheumatoid arthritis, and congenital dysgenesis of the odontoid process. Down's, Klippel-Feil and achondroplastic syndromes represent some congenital conditions with associated anomalies of the craniovertebral junction. More rarely, caudal extension of skull base tumors may require this approach (CROCKARD 1995).

Fiberoptic nasotracheal intubation with an armored cuffed tube is preferred. Tracheostomy is an option that may be advantageous, but the process of insertion requires intubation for airway control. The patient can remain in the supine position, with cranial fixation maintaining a neutral neck position. Skeletal traction can also be maintained in this position, to effect distraction. The traction lowers the tip of the odontoid process in relation to the clivus, and simplifies the surgical exposure. If traction is not

needed, some surgeons advocate a lateral position with a dependent axillary roll. The table can be put into a side-tilt away from the surgeon so that the patient is facing 45 degrees up toward the surgeon. This position allows the surgeon to sit, and after odontoid resection, the patient can be tilted in the opposite direction for posterior atlantooccipital fixation in a one-stage procedure, thus avoiding the hazardous movement of a patient with craniovertebral instability, to the prone position. Alternatively, most surgeons opt for posterior fixation as a second procedure, using external bracing or skeletal traction to maintain stability. The lateral position also pools secretions and blood on the dependent tonsillar pillar. Regardless of the position, radiographic confirmation of the odontoid process position should be obtained.

Before the transoral procedure takes place, the oral cavity is prepared and intravenous antibiotics are given. Steroid cream has been cited as effective for limiting postoperative swelling. The cream is applied to both the lips and tongue (KINGDOM et al. 1995). Intravenous steroids can also limit postoperative swelling. Unstable dentition must be protected and secured. A portion of the lateral part of the thigh should be prepared and draped, in case autogenous fascia lata is needed to cover an inadvertent CSF fistula. A transoral retractor is placed to retract both the mandible and tongue caudally. A self-retaining palatal extension allows the soft palate to be retracted up and laterally. The nasotracheal and nasogastric tubes are pushed laterally by the palatal extension. The posterior pharynx is inspected, and the midline must be identified through the bony tubercle of the anterior arch of C1. Midline location is particularly important in congenital craniovertebral anomalies, where there is often a component of atlantoaxial rotary luxation and hypoplasia of the odontoid process. The midline approach avoids contact with the lateral mass and the adjacent vertebral artery (Fig. 30.23).

With dural compression, neuromonitoring is advisable, but many surgeons rely exclusively on changes in spontaneous respiration, heart rate, and blood pressure. These changes should be immediate with excessive contact or pressure on the ventral brainstem. After the posterior pharyngeal incision, a microscope is used. The anterior arch of C1 is cleared of ligamentous attachments, which include the longus colli muscles and the anterior longitudinal ligament. Part of the clivus, basion, and anterior arch of C1 can be variably resected for adequate exposure and removal of the odontoid process. In

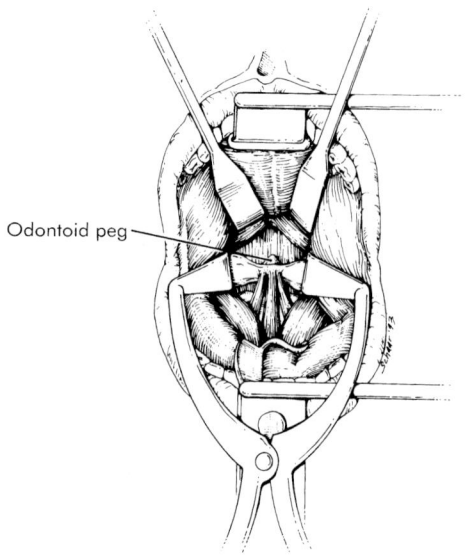

Odontoid peg

Fig. 30.23. Schematic illustration of the anterior, transoral approach to the odontoid process of C2. Note the anterior arch of C1 in front of the odontoid. Neural compression from the odontoid process can be approached in this manner

rheumatoid arthritis, there is often a pannus of inflammatory synovial tissue that requires debulking. Behind the odontoid process are the transverse ligament, posterior longitudinal ligament, and then dura. The odontoid tip contains suspensory ligaments that insert on the basion or clivus. An intraoperative X-ray can be used to substantiate the anatomy and degree of bony resection.

The patient should remain intubated after closure. This will prevent airway obstruction from oral and pharyngeal swelling. After 8 to 24 h, a lateral cervical spine X-ray can show the extent of prevertebral swelling before extubation. Early postoperative steroids can be maintained topically and intravenously for 2 days.

30.14.3.2
Anterior Cervical Approaches

The anterior cervical approach permits extensive access to levels ranging from C2 to C7. The approach is formally anterolateral and uses a bloodless, direct fascial plain within the anterior triangle of the neck. This approach can be applied to the rare tumor with an extensive ventral component in the cervical region. An advantage of the anterior cervical approach is that the patient remains supine with a near-neutral neck position after cautious intubation. The mandibular angle approximates the C3 level and requires

slight hyperextension of the neck to simplify access. A small roll behind the neck facilitates the exposure and supports the vertebral column. Other localizing landmarks include the hyoid bone for C4, cricoid cartilage for C5, the first tracheal ring for C6, and two fingerbreadths above the suprasternal notch for C7. A right-sided approach is more practicable for the right-handed surgeon, although the risk of injury to the recurrent laryngeal nerve is lower with a left-sided approach. The left side warrants consideration when the pathology is primarily on the left.

With single-level approaches, a horizontal incision heals with good cosmesis. However, an oblique medial sternocleidomastoid incision affords improved exposure for multilevel inspection, exerts less resistance to retraction, and is parallel to the surgical plane. The anterior approach retracts the carotid artery laterally, the esophagus and trachea medially, and the omohyoid muscle and recurrent laryngeal nerve inferiorly. The diagastric muscle and superior laryngeal and hypoglossal nerves are retracted superiorly. Careful retraction avoids distractive or perforation-type injuries to the non-muscular structures. Bradycardic responses may result from excessive carotid retraction or heightened carotid sinus sensitivity, and the surgeon should be alerted. Neuromonitoring is most important with multilevel, distractive fixation that changes the cervical curvature. Radiographic verification of the targeted vertebral level is mandatory, and an image intensifier may prove useful during the procedure. A sandbag is used to elevate the right anterior iliac crest as a donor site for autogenous graft. Within the disc space or vertebral body, excessive lateral or angulated drilling can injure the vertebral artery. Any bleeding should be controlled with light pressure and hemostatic adjuvants. After prolonged retraction or extensive bone work, the endotracheal tube can remain in place for 8 to 24h. This allows time to ascertain a stable, hemostatic wound site. Postoperative X-rays can check for appropriate alignment, dislodgment of a bone plug, tracheal deviation, and prevertebral swelling.

30.14.3.3
Anterolateral Approaches to
the Thoracic Spinal Region

The posterior laminectomy poses significant neurological risks with attempts to access or decompress anteriorly situated lesions of the thoracic vertebrae. Anterior access through a posterior laminectomy requires retraction of the thoracic region of the cord, and decompression constricts the posteriorly displaced cord at the rostral and caudal extents of the laminectomy. Either manipulation can lead to neurological deficit. For anteriorly situated vertebral tumors, anterolateral approaches have a superior outcome compared with radiotherapy alone or in combination with laminectomy, with the added advantage that stability of the posterior column remains intact (COOPER et al. 1993).

The intercostal transthoracic approach provides the most expansive exposure of the thoracic vertebrae with anterolateral viewing. Vertebral body resection, reconstruction, and anterior column instrumentation are best accomplished through this approach. Anterior epidural impingement from tumor, trauma, and infection can be directly decompressed without neural manipulation. Kyphotic deformities can be stabilized and/or corrected with distractive instrumentation. For degenerative disease, a centrally located disc or osteophyte is best viewed through the transthoracic approach.

Many patients with significant thoracic cord pathology will have concurrent conditions that adversely affect pulmonary function. Both paralysis and advanced spinal deformities require pulmonary assessment. A forced vital capacity of less than 1 l, an arterial blood-gas indicating elevated PCO_2 levels, and dyspnea are findings that may require postoperative mechanical ventilation, aggressive respiratory therapy, and early mobilization of the patient (Parsa and Miller 2000). Upper thoracic and cervical region cord deficits include neuromuscular compromise of intercostal thoracic excursions. The patient is left with diaphragmatic breathing and is prone to atelectasis and pneumonia. Tracheostomy may allow a more effective pulmonary care, avoid infectious complications, and hasten an end to full-time mechanical ventilatory support.

Transthoracic approaches require that the patient be placed in a lateral decubitus position. A double-lumen ET tube allows selective deflation of the lung, to optimize exposure of the thoracic vertebrae. During surgery, the collapsed lung is periodically reinflated to minimize atelectasis. A right-sided, intrapleural exposure of the upper thoracic vertebrae (T2–T5) avoids hindrance from the left carotid and subclavian arteries and aortic arch in the upper mediastinum. At the midthoracic levels (T5–T9), a left-sided approach takes advantage of the larger thoracic cavity. For further vertebral access, it is simpler to mobilize the segmental arteries and aorta on the left rather than the azygos vein and branches on the right. The intercostal incision circumscribes the rib

cage and should be made about two rib-levels above the targeted vertebrae. This is due to the downward obliquity of the rib cage. An axillary roll supports the dependent side and avoids protracted compression of neurovascular structures in the axilla, and flexion of the operating-table opens the contralateral disc spaces of the thoracic vertebrae. The up-side arm must be supported in a semi-reaching position to elevate the scapula away from the operating-site. A cross-table radiograph or fluoroscopy will yield an AP view of the chest for localization.

A left-sided approach avoids the liver and inferior vena cava when one is targeting the lower thoracic or thoracolumbar (T9–L2) levels. This approach requires an incision followed by repair of the diaphragm and incorporates a retroperitoneal approach to the vertebrae. The ureter elevates with the peritoneum. Routine preoperative angiography can be used to identify the dominant segmental artery of Adamkiewicz. Excluding angiography, several points help to avoid a vascular insult to the cord. Firstly, the paired segmental arteries of the aorta have excellent collateral circulation as they circumscribe each side of the vertebrae. Secondly, the least number of segmental vessels are ligated to access a vertebral body. Thirdly, segmental vessels are ligated in proximity to the aorta and left undisturbed when viewed as end-arteries in the neural foramen.

The resection of a vertebral body for neural decompression mandates replacement with a bony strut graft. Disruption of both the anterior and middle columns of stability requires anterior instrumentation (DENIS 1983). The exposed lateral surfaces of the vertebral bodies above and below the corpectomy site serve as fixation points for anterior instrumentation. Several fixation systems are available that include transverse insertions of paired cancellous screws with lateral plating for each vertebra (KAISER et al. 2000). Screw placement requires multiplanar fluoroscopic verification to assure optimum placement and to avoid vascular and neural injury. Unilateral, paired, and parallel rods can be attached to the screws, and aligned with the long-axis of the vertebral column. Cross-linkage fixation between the paired rods provides rotational stability. The instrumentation has versatility in configuring the amount of distraction and compression that is optimal to correct a spinal deformity. The long-term success of spinal instrumentation depends upon adequate bony fusion. The instrumentation allows early mobilization of the patient and provides an interval of stability pending bony fusion. Inadequate fusion ultimately leads to fatigue and failure of the instrumentation. Thoracolumbosacral orthosis (TLSO) is commonly used to supplement spinal stability with early mobilization. In cases with poor prospects for adequate fusion, such as those involving spinal metastases, corpectomy, or spinal instrumentation, acrylic polymers can be used as a substitute for strut grafts (KAISER et al. 2000).

30.14.4
Posterolateral Approaches to the Thoracic Spinal Region

As shown in Fig. 30.24, posterolateral approaches fall along a continuum that facilitates exposure of the ventral vertebral body (PARSA et al. 2000). The transpedicular approach has been well-described for use in thoracic disc disease (LEROUX et al. 1993) and can

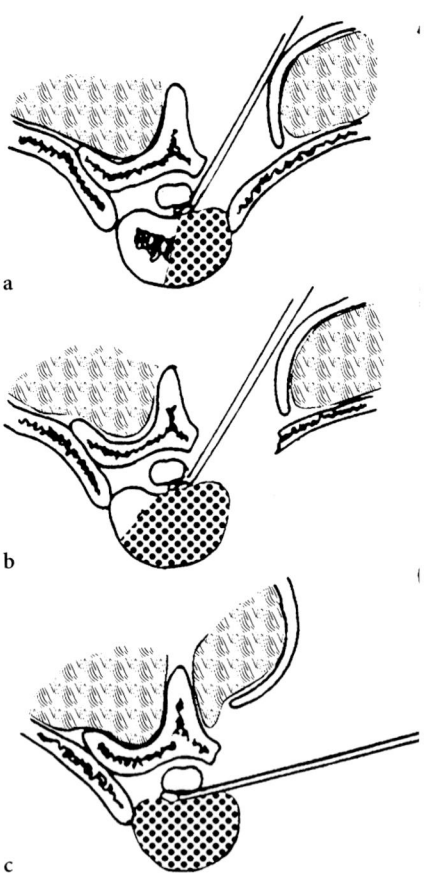

Fig. 30.24a–c. Schematic representation of posterolateral approaches, with diagram demonstrating the increasing ventral exposure obtained with the various approaches described in the text: **a** transpedicular approach, **b** costotransversectomy, and **c** lateral extracavitary approach. The main factor contributing to the difference in the ventral exposure is the lateral extent of rib resection

be useful for lesions within the ventral spinal canal that do not cross the midline. It can be used for the infrequent lesion that arises off the anterior aspect of the vertebral body, when access beyond the midline is not needed. The majority of chordomas and chondrosarcomas extensively involve the vertebral body, necessitating a more ventral exposure with the costotransversectomy (AHLGREN and HERKOWITZ 1995), or lateral extracavitary (MCCORMICK 1996a) approaches. The fourth through ninth vertebrae are the easiest to expose by means of a posterolateral thoracotomy. The diaphragm from the tenth thoracic rib to the first lumbar vertebrae typically obscures the thoracolumbar region of the spine.

30.14.5
Transpedicular Approach

After induction of general anesthesia the patient is placed in the prone position with appropriate padding to prevent pressure ulcerations. A neutral position is requisite for those patients with documented instability. The patient should be secured adequately to allow table rotation. Confirmation of the correct spinal level is achieved with intraoperative X-ray prior to prepping and draping.

The soft-tissue dissection is similar to that of a standard posterior approach extending laterally over the facet joint. A small laminotomy is performed with Kerrison rongeurs for identification of the pedicle, nerve-root, and neural foramen. Drilling is initiated through the posterior cortex of the pars interarticularis at its junction with the superior articular process. As more of the neural foramen is defined, care must be taken not to injure any of the neurovascular structures in its proximity. The pedicle is first drilled off internally, providing the surgeon with an external cortical rim of protection. When the remaining bone is sufficiently thin to allow easy removal, a pituitary forceps or rongeur can be used to extract the remaining cortical surface.

Once the pedicle has been resected, the vertebral body and disc space are identified. Partial corpectomy and discectomy provide a defect into which the tumor can be ventrally displaced with reverse-angled curettes. The tumor is then extracted with pituitary rongeurs and suction. Sacrifice of a thoracic nerve-root proximal to the dorsal root ganglion can usually be performed without significant sequelae. After tumor-removal and achievement of hemostasis, the question of placing graft material for stability must be addressed. Typically, if the majority of the vertebral body is intact after tumor resection, then stability is not a concern.

The transpedicular approach has been used extensively for thoracic disc disease without significant operative related morbidity (STILLERMAN et al. 1998). Surgical adjuncts such as specially designed curettes have been described to aid in this approach (LEROUX et al. 1993).

30.14.6
Costotransversectomy Approach

The costotransversectomy approach increases ventral exposure through resection of the proximal rib and displacement of the pleural contents. Intraoperative antero-posterior radiograph is used to identify the location of the tumor. The surgeon should be aware of individuals with normal anatomical variants including additional or missing ribs. The rib to be resected is based on the level of pathology. A preoperative spinal angiogram is valuable in identifying the Artery of Adamkiewiccz, to facilitate preservation of this important vascular structure.

Positioning options include the standard prone position or semiprone with one side of the chest elevated by 15 deg. We prefer a curvilinear incision, beginning and ending in the midline with its apex centered on the rib to be resected about 5–8 cm from midline. The superficial back muscles, the trapezius and latissimus dorsi, are transected with monopolar cautery in line with the skin incision and reflected medial. The appropriate rib is identified and the dorsal periosteum transected with monopolar cautery. The periosteum is then stripped from the dorsal, superior, and inferior surfaces of the rib with a periosteal elevator or Addison dissector. The ventral periosteum is then stripped with either an Addison dissector or a Doyne dissector. Extreme care should be taken during this maneuver so that the underlying pleura and inferior neurovascular bundle are not disturbed. The exposed rib is then resected medial to the rib angle, approximately 5 cm lateral to the rib head. The costotransverse and costovertebral joints are then disarticulated by sharply transecting the surrounding ligaments. The transverse process and rib head are then resected with rongeurs. The neurovascular bundle should be followed proximally into the intervertebral foramen. The pleura and lung are mobilized off the vertebral body, and retracted with a padded retractor blade. For retraction we use a table-mounted retractor, such as the Farley-Thompson retractor. Once the exposure is obtained, tu-

mor resection can commence. The necessity for surgical stabilization should be assessed at the end of tumor resection, based on the extent of vertebral body resection.

Once hemostasis has been achieved, the resection cavity is copiously irrigated with an antibiotic irrigation solution. The pleura should be inspected for tears; small tears can be repaired primarily. Chest-tube placement may be warranted for larger tears and associated air leaks. A layered closure with particular attention paid to adequate approximation of the muscular layer completes the operation.

30.14.7
Lateral Extracavitary Approach

Larson introduced the lateral extracavitary approach in 1976 as an extension of the costotransversectomy (LARSON et al. 1976). This approach increases the ventral exposure of the spine through a trajectory that is almost parallel to the posterior cortex of the vertebral body. This trajectory is obtained by resecting the rib at the rib angle, a more lateral point than in the costotransversectomy. The side of the exposure for a lateral extracavitary approach is ipsilateral to the most extensive part of the tumor. This approach consistently violates the radicular artery distal to its collateral branches and proximal to its spinal anastomosis. At most thoracic levels, the ligation of one or two such arteries is tolerable. Disruption of the radiculomedullary artery of Adamkiewicz must be avoided since sacrifice of this vessel places the cord at significant risk for infarction. Although the Artery of Adamkiewicz is located on the left in 80% of patients, spinal angiography may be warranted with a lower thoracic approach in order to identify its location. Preoperative identification of a significant radiculomedullary artery within the planned exposure may necessitate an alternative approach (i.e., lateral extracavitary approach from the opposite side or an anterolateral approach).

Once anesthesia has been induced the patient is positioned prone. A Mayfield head-holder for upper thoracic region tumors is sometimes desirable, whereas for mid and lower thoracic regions the arms can be outstretched on padded boards. A small bolster is placed under the patient opposite the point of surgical approach. This will enhance the ventral exposure when the operating-table is parallel to the floor, by placing the patient in a three-quarter prone position. For the initial exposure the operating-table is tilted toward the side of the tumor so the patient is in a true prone position. An intraoperative AP radiograph is obtained to identify the correct spinal level. A wide area of skin is prepped with betadine, and the skin infiltrated with a local anesthetic agent, such as lidocaine with epinephrine. The drapes are positioned in a rectangular fashion with at least 15 cm of lateral exposure on the surgical side.

A variety of skin incisions may be performed, including midline, semicircular, and paramedian incisions (Fig. 30.25). We employ a hockey-stick incision, since it requires a shorter length than a true midline incision, and is less apparent than a paramedian incision. The midline portion of the hockey-stick incision is centered over the tumor site. Adequate caudal exposure is needed prior to extending the incision laterally since this will limit the caudal extent of the exposure. The lateral limb of the incision is gently curved towards the side of the tumor, extending approximately 8 to 10 cm from the midline. The location of the thoracodorsal fascia, dorsal thoracic musculature, erector spinae muscles, and the dorsal part of the rib cage should be clearly delineated. The fascial investment of the longitudinal paraspinal muscles provides the plane of dissection for access to the lateral spinal compartment and ultimately the anterior paraspinal region. The midline incision is taken down through the subcutaneous tissue to the level of the spinous processes and thoracodorsal fascia. A routine subperiosteal dissection of the paraspinal muscles is performed with a Cobb dissector and monopolar cautery. The take-down is performed bilaterally if a more posterior exposure is required for instrumentation, otherwise a unilateral exposure is sufficient for paraspinal tumor resection. The lateral limb of the incision is opened by transecting the transversely oriented thoracic muscles (the latissimus dorsi, the trapezius, and the rhomboid muscles) in line with the skin incision. A myocutaneous flap is elevated laterally exposing the longitudinally oriented erector spinae musculature.

The paraspinal musculature runs in the trough created by the ribs, transverse process, facet joint and pedicle. The lateral margin of the erector spinae is identified and dissected medially to expose the underlying ribs. This dissection is then carried further over the facet joint eventually communicating with the posterior dissection. This mobilization of the erector spinae muscle allows access to the lateral spinal compartment. The longitudinal muscle mass is wrapped in a moist sponge to avoid desiccation and positioned medially or laterally, allowing the surgeon to work on either side. Complete dissection of the vertebral elements at a level above and below the tumor will insure adequate ventral exposure. The ventral and lateral rib surfaces are exposed with a Cobb elevator up to the vertebral body articulation. The surrounding soft tissue is dissected free in a subperiosteal fashion with a Doyne rib dissector (Fig. 30.26a,b). The exposed transverse process at the level of the tumor, along with 6 to 8 cm of the corresponding rib are then resected with a rib cutter and Lexel rongeur. The costotransverse and costovertebral joints are disarticulated and sharply transected. At the levels above and below, a portion of rib is also resected to enhance ventral exposure. Only 3 to 4 cm of rib are resected at these levels, to avoid a flail-chest deformity.

Once the rib and transverse processes have been removed, the neurovascular bundle is identified within the endothoracic fascia, deep in the intercostal musculature. The segmental nerves above and at the level of the tumor are dissected free and divided, with the proximal stump elevated medially toward the intervertebral foramen. Unlike at lumbar levels, the nerves at the thoracic levels can be sacrificed without a detectable deficit. Once the nerve is free, the parietal pleura is displaced ventrally to provide access to the anterior spinal compartment. The parietal pleura is maintained out of the operating-field with a table-mounted retractor system, such as the Farley-Thompson retractor system. A padded, wide retractor blade helps to avoid a pleural tear. At this point the operating-table is returned to a true prone position, enhancing the ventral visualization. With a Cobb elevator, the parietal pleura and diaphragm are bluntly dissected free from the ventrolateral aspect of the vertebral bodies. Sharp dissection may be required at the level of the disc space due to a more adherent connective

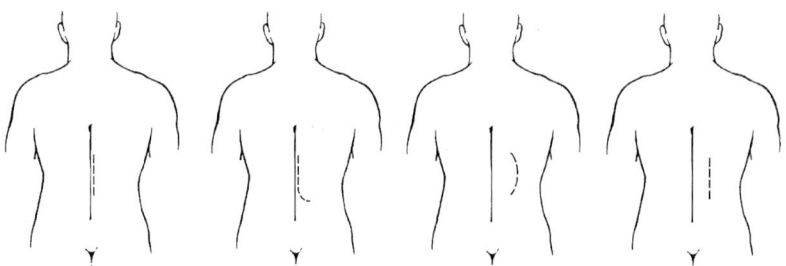

Fig. 30.25. Schematic illustration demonstrating a variety of skin incisions including midline, semicircular, and paramedian, that can be used for a lateral extracavitary approach

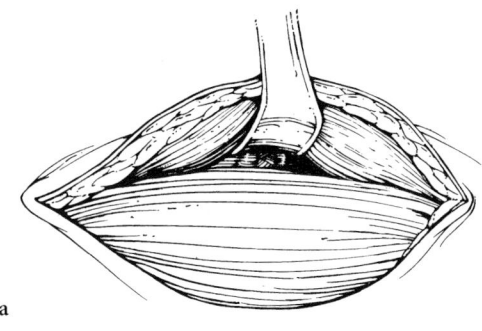

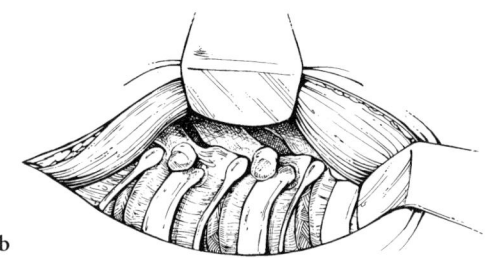

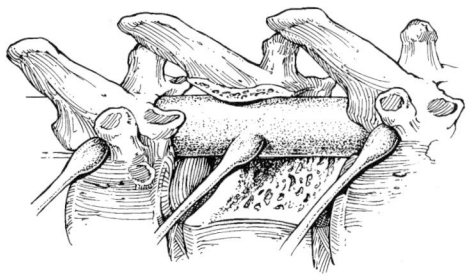

Fig. 30.27. Schematic illustration demonstrating exposure achieved with lateral extracavitary after rib removal and resection of a portion of the vertebral body

Fig. 30.26a, b. Schematic illustration demonstrating exposure achieved with lateral extracavitary approach. **a** Elevation of the myocutaneous flap reveals the underlying erector spinae muscles. Dissection along the lateral fascial plane of this muscle bundle will provide access to the lateral spinal elements. **b** Dissection of the surrounding soft tissue exposes the lateral vertebral body elements including the facet joints, pedicles, and ventrolateral portion of the vertebral bodies

tissue. If tumor is encountered within the lateral spinal compartment it is dissected from the pleura and surrounding fascia. If significantly large, the paraspinal portion of tumor must be resected to expose adequately the lateral vertebral body elements.

Once this dissection is complete, the vertebral body and lateral vertebral elements are exposed. With the use of either a high-speed drill or a Kerrison rongeur, the pedicle and facet joint are excised. Adequate irrigation is necessary during drilling to avoid excess heat build-up, which may damage the underlying dura. Once the lateral dural margin is exposed, the intervertebral disc at the involved level is resected prior to vertebral body excision. Disc material is typically extracted using a pituitary rongeur. Ventral decompression is subsequently achieved by drilling of the vertebral body (Fig. 30.27). Tumor extension or direct tumor-invasion will dictate the degree of vertebral body resection. A trough is initially drilled in the vertebral body, leaving a thin shelf of dorsal cortical bone in place. With the use of a reverse-angle curette, this remaining bone is delivered into the trough created. During this resection considerable blood-loss is possible due to

the proximity of the perineural venous plexus. Any bleeding should be controlled with Gelfoam and cautery, prior to tumor resection. The anesthesiologist should be made aware of this possibility, so that excessive blood-loss can be replaced with appropriate available blood products. Tumor within the ventral spinal canal can be delivered into the corpectomy site with the use of a reversed or down-angled curette. Resection of more than 50% is likely to lead to anterior column instability requiring stabilization with an interbody strut graft.

Once the tumor has been resected and hemostasis obtained, a spinal stabilization procedure can be performed. Typically, the anterior interbody strut graft is inserted prior to posterior instrumentation. If uninvolved with tumor, the sectioned rib provides an excellent source of graft material. Positioning the rib with the concave side directed dorsally assumes the natural kyphotic curvature of the thoracic part of the spine. Other non-autologous sources of support material such as methylmethacrylate and allograft may be preferable. Slots are drilled into the rostral and caudal vertebral bodies and the graft inserted. Ventral plating followed by dorsal instrumentation may then be inserted as deemed appropriate. The pleura are inspected for any air leaks. Minor leaks can be repaired primarily. Any significant leak mandates chest-tube placement for the immediate postoperative period. Once the pleura have been inspected and repaired the remainder of the wound is closed in layers.

The difficulty of the lateral extracavitary approach means that adequate surgical experience and a thorough understanding of the thoracic retropleural anatomy are essential for the avoidance of any significant pitfalls. The minimization of the abdominal pressure with appropriate positioning will decrease the amount of venous distension. Despite appropriate positioning, blood loss from the decompression of epidural venous channels and from the medullary bone may be considerable. Gelfoam and cautery are used to obtain hemostasis from the epidural bleeding. Although the entire exposure is extrapleural, the parietal pleura may be violated during the dissection. For small tears a primary closure is sufficient, however chest-tube drainage is necessary for larger tears associated with an air leak.

30.15
Operative Technique for Specific Spinal Tumors

30.15.1
Intramedullary Tumors

Intramedullary tumors are approached via standard laminectomy with the patient in the prone position. Although somatosensory-evoked potentials and direct motor-evoked potentials are routinely employed, only rarely do they influence surgical decisions or technique (McCormick and Stein 1990a). Laminoplasty is performed in pediatric patients, but does not guarantee long-term stability. The dura is opened in the midline and tented laterally to the muscle with suture, after which the operating microscope is brought into the field for the remainder of the operation. The arachnoid is sharply opened and the spinal-cord is inspected. The strategies for intramedullary tumor-removal depend upon the relationship of the tumor to the spinal-cord. Most tumors are totally intramedullary and are not apparent upon surface inspection. Intraoperative ultrasound may be used to localize and determine rostrocaudal tumor extent (Lunardi et al. 1994).

Tumors which do not present to the surface of the cord are best exposed through dorsal midline myelotomy. The myelotomy may be placed directly over an eccentrically located intramedullary tumor, which extends to the pial surface. A midline myelotomy is performed through the posterior median septum and should extend over the entire rostrocaudal extent of the tumor. The tumor is first encountered in the area of maximum cord enlargement. The dissection continues on the surface of the tumor until the entire rostrocaudal extent has been identified. Polar cysts, when present, are entered and drained. The technique of tumor-removal is determined by the surgical objective, tumor size, and gross and histological characteristics of the lesion. If no plane is apparent between tumor and surrounding spinal-cord,

then it is likely that an infiltrative neoplasm is present, and biopsy is obtained to establish a histological diagnosis. If an infiltrating or malignant astrocytoma is identified and is consistent with the intraoperative findings, further tumor-removal is not warranted. In most cases, however, a reasonably well-defined benign glial tumor will be present.

30.15.1.1
Ependymoma

Ependymomas have a smooth, reddish-gray, glistening tumor surface, which is sharply demarcated from the surrounding spinal-cord (Fig. 30.28). A variable vascular network crosses the tumor surface, distinguishing these tumors from astrocytomas, which rarely display such surface-characteristics. The plane between an ependymoma and surrounding spinal-cord is usually well-defined and easily developed. Large tumors may require internal decompression with an ultrasonic aspirator or laser. The tumor margins are then developed and feeding-arteries from the anterior spinal artery are easily identified, cauterized, and divided (McCormick et al. 1990b).

30.15.1.2
Astrocytoma

About one-third of adult patients have benign, infiltrative tumors without an identifiable tumor-mass. Biopsy for diagnosis is all that can be established in these patients. Dissection on the surface of an astrocytoma usually results in the development of laminated pseudo-planes (McCormick and Stein 1990a). Decompression is achieved with an ultrasonic aspirator or laser, and proceeds systematically from the center of the tumor, radially to the surface. Although a clean plane does not exist for the majority of astrocytomas, there is frequently a difference in the color of the tumor with respect to the spinal-cord (Fig. 30.29). Changes in motor sensory-evoked potentials or uncertainty of the interface between normal cord and tumor should prompt the surgeon to stop the resection.

30.15.1.3
Hemangioblastoma

Removal of hemangioblastomas is facilitated by excision of the pial attachment as part of the tumor-mass. Cauterization of the surface tumor-vessels is followed by a circumscribing incision around the pial base. The buried portion of the tumor within the spinal-cord is

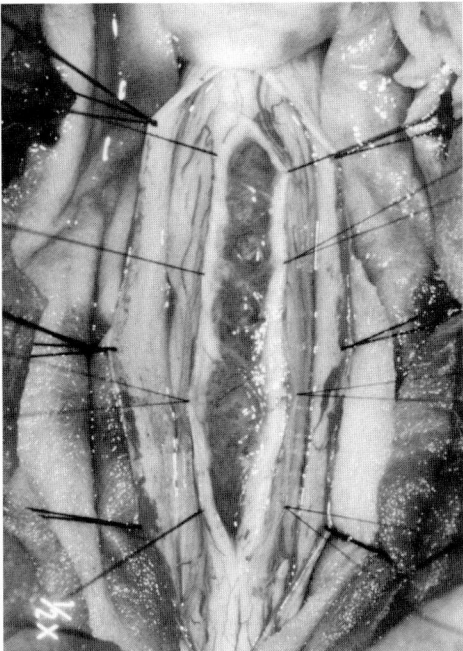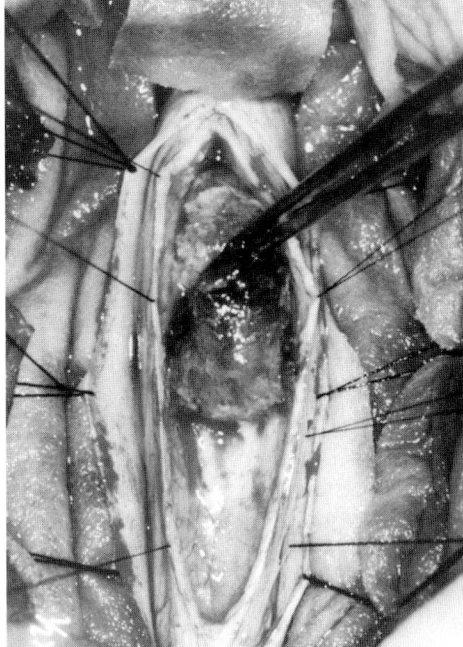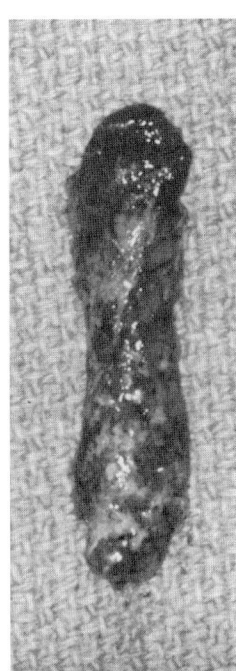

a,b   c

Fig. 30.28 Intraoperative photograph of ependymoma demonstrates **a** characteristic features of gross specimen, which can be removed with dissection along **b** a defined plane, resulting in **c** gross total resection of specimen

easily dissected and delivered with traction on the pial base. A small polar myelotomy may provide better visualization for larger tumors. Internal decompression cannot be performed with these neoplasms but cautery on the tumor surface usually shrinks it to a manageable size (McCormick 1994).

After the removal of an intramedullary tumor, the resection bed is inspected and any bleeding-points are controlled with warm saline solution or oxidized cotton. Closure of the myelotomy is not performed. The dura is usually closed primarily, although a dural patch graft may prevent dorsal tethering of the spinal-cord at the operating-site, which may be a potential cause of morbidity in the postoperative period. An autologous fascia lata or thoracodorsal fascia patch graft can be utilized. The remainder of the wound is closed in standard fashion. Meticulous closure techniques are especially important in re-operations or previously radiated cases, which present a high risk of postoperative CSF fistula. Early mobilization in the postoperative period is encouraged.

30.15.2
Extramedullary Tumors

The optimum treatment for intradural, extramedullary tumors is surgical excision. For nerve-sheath le-

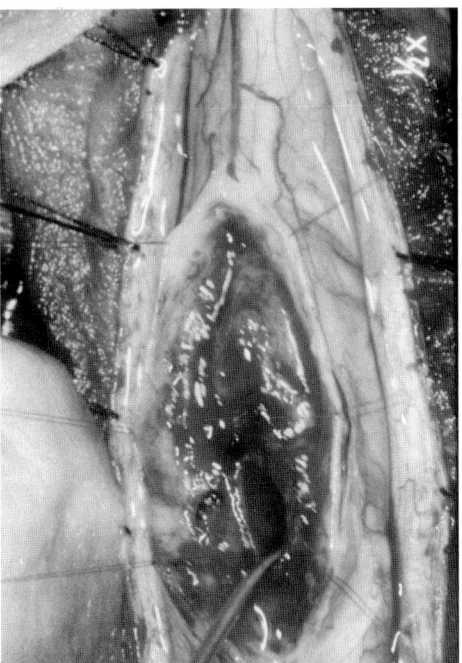

Fig. 30.29. Intraoperative photograph of astrocytoma demonstrates lack of a defined plane for dissection, making gross total resection impossible

sions, this can be accomplished in nearly all cases through a standard posterior laminectomy. Recurrences are rare when gross total removal has been achieved. Most nerve-sheath tumors are dorsal or dorsolateral to the spinal-cord and are easily seen after opening the dura (Fig. 30.30). Ventral tumors may require dentate ligament section to achieve adequate visualization. Lumbar tumors may be covered by the cauda equina or conus medullaris, and the nerve-roots must be separated, to give adequate visualization.

Posterior laminectomy provides acceptable exposure for spinal meningiomas in most cases. Unilateral laminectomy and facetectomy can be utilized for eccentrically located or ventral tumors. Large ventral tumors may also be approached satisfactorily through standard posterior exposures, because the tumors have already provided the necessary spinal-cord retraction. Suture retraction on a divided dentate ligament or non-critical dorsal root provides additional ventral exposure. Depression of the paraspinal muscle mass with table-mounted retractors further facilitates ventral access. Alternatively, a costotransversectomy or lateral extracavitary approach may be utilized for ventral thoracic tumors. The extreme lateral method is used when there is significant ventral tumor component above the foramen magnum (SEN and SEKHAR 1990, GILSACH 1991, BABU et al. 1994).

The role of surgery for filum terminale ependymoma depends on the size of the tumor and its rela-tionship to the surrounding roots of the cauda equina (McCORMICK et al. 1990a). Gross total en bloc resection should be attempted whenever possible. This can usually be accomplished for small and moderate size tumors, which remain well-circumscribed within the fibrous coverings of the filum terminale and easily separable from the cauda equina nerve-roots. A portion of uninvolved filum terminale generally is present between the tumor and spinal-cord. Amputation of the afferent and efferent filum segments is required for tumor removal. Internal decompression is not utilized for small and moderate size tumors because this may increase the risk of CSF dissemination. Recurrences following successful en bloc resection are rare.

Factors favoring surgical intervention for patients with spinal metastasis include rapid progression of neurological deficit, histological diagnosis of a radioresistant tumor, cord compression from bone fragments and/or malalignment, spinal instability, and failure of radiation therapy (PARSA and MILLER 2000). Patients with spinal metastases harbor the effects of chemotherapy, radiation therapy, tumor burden, and various inappropriate secretions of hormones from their tumors. They are often anemic, immunocompromised, osteoporotic, hypercalcemic, hypercoagulable, and deficient at wound-healing. A diligent preoperative evaluation is mandated, and the scope of the surgery must be concise and expeditious. In the case of progressive neurological deficit,

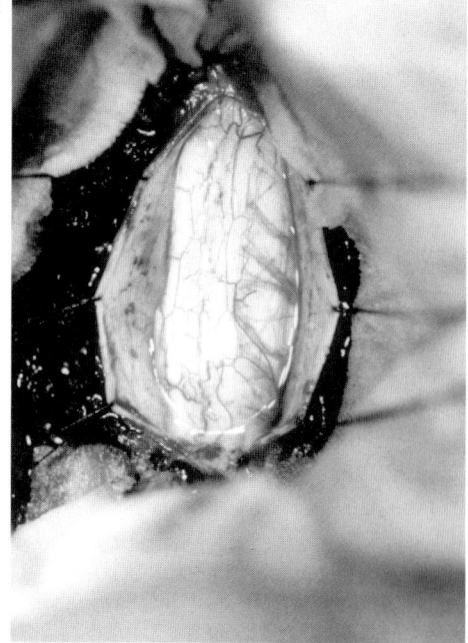 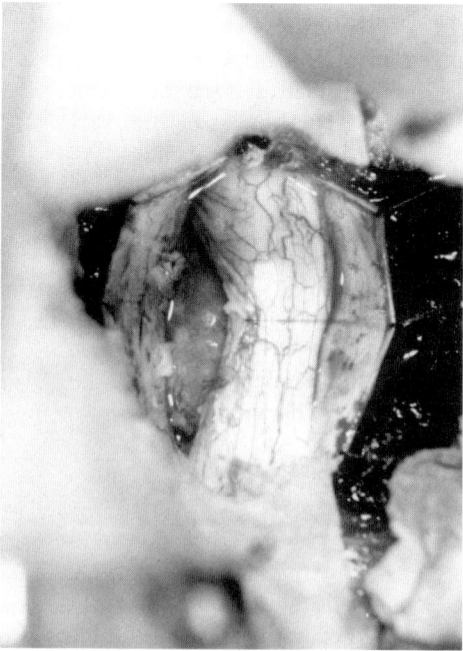

Fig. 30.30. Intraoperative photograph of nerve-sheath tumor demonstrates that **a** after initial exposure, the tumor may be obscured by the spinal-cord, requiring **b** manipulation to gain access

low-dose dexamethasone should be prescribed. There are no consistent data from clinical and prospectively controlled trials suggesting that high-dose dexamethasone is of any further benefit. For those spinal metastases known to be hypervascular, preoperative angiography and embolization are advisable. This preparation minimizes intraoperative blood-loss. As in all decompressive procedures of the spine, four units of packed red blood-cells should be available.

A decompressive laminectomy should extend at least one and often two levels above and below the tumor-induced cord compression. Resected bone should be sent for histopathological evaluation as it may harbor neoplasm. Resected bone cannot be used for reconstructive laminoplasty or as graft for fusion. Epidural tumor is debulked from the dorsum of the cord and the lateral gutters. Ideally, a decompressive procedure concludes with the surgeon observing epidural space above and below the formerly compressed segment, reappearance of epidural fat, and the possible resumption of cord pulsation. With posterolateral epidural tumor only, decompressive laminectomy is appropriate. Through MR, the stability of the anterior and middle columns can be scrutinized and may prompt a laminectomy followed by posterior spinal instrumentation.

The commonly involved thoracic spinal area benefits from the additional stability afforded by the rib cage. Most patients undergoing thoracic spinal surgery remain stable after laminectomy. Instability can be treated by insertion of pedicle screws in combination with plating and fusion.

30.15.2.1
Nerve-Sheath Tumors

The surgical exposure of nerve-sheath tumors depends on the specific anatomy of the lesion. Tumors that are small and strictly intradural, may be approached via posterior laminectomy. Ventrally located tumors may require facetectomy, transthoracic, or far lateral approaches. Once exposure is achieved, a plane of dissection directly on the tumor surface must be identified (McCormick 1996a,b). There is usually an arachnoid membrane tightly applied to the tumor surface. This is the fenestrated arachnoid layer which separately ensheathes each dorsal and ventral nerve-root within the subarachnoid space. This layer is sharply incised and reflected off the tumor surface. The tumor capsule is cauterized to diminish vascularity and to shrink tumor volume. Tumor removal requires identification and division

of the proximal and distal nerve-root tumor attachments, which may not be immediately apparent with large tumors. Internal decompression with a laser or ultrasonic aspirator is utilized in these cases. Sacrifice of the nerve-root of origin is usually required for tumor removal. Occasionally, some fascicles of the nerve-root may be preserved, especially with smaller tumors. It is usually possible, however, to preserve the corresponding intradural nerve-root because the fenestrated arachnoid sheaths allow anatomic separation of the dorsal and ventral nerve-roots to a point just distal to the dorsal root ganglion. In a typical case of a dorsal root tumor origin, for example, it is possible to preserve the ventral root which is tightly applied to the ventral tumor surface. Dumbbell extension through the root-sleeve, however, usually necessitates resection of the entire spinal nerve. This rarely causes significant deficit, even at the cervical and lumbar enlargements, because the function of the involved root has probably already been compensated for by adjacent roots. A very proximal tumor-origin may be partially embedded in the epipial tissue or may elevate the pia to occupy a subpial location. The tumor-cord interface may be difficult to develop in these cases and requires resection of a segment of pia to effect complete removal.

30.15.2.2
Meningioma

A variety of strategies can be utilized for removal of spinal meningiomas (McCormick et al. 1990a). Dorsal and dorsolateral lesions are delivered away from the spinal-cord with traction on the open dural margins, after which a circumscribing excision of the dural origin completes the removal. For lateral and ventral tumors, the arachnoid over the exposed portion of the tumor is incised and reflected so that the dissection may proceed directly on the tumor surface. The rostral and caudal tumor poles should be identified. Small cottonoid pledgets may be placed in the lateral canal gutters on either side of the tumor to minimize blood spillage into the subarachnoid space. The exposed tumor surface is then cauterized to diminish tumor vascularity, and to shrink the tumor mass.

Large tumors are bisected and debulked through a central trough. The tumor segment apposing the spinal-cord is then delivered into the resection cavity with gentle traction and surface dissection. The remaining dural-based tumor is amputated from the dural attachment. The attachment is then extensively coagulated. Alternatively, the dural base may be excised and replaced with a thoracodorsal fascia patch graft. All blood and debris are irrigated from the subarachnoid space with warm saline solution; subsequently, arachnoid adhesions which hold the cord in a deformed position are divided. These maneuvers may diminish the risk of postoperative complications such as spinal-cord tethering, arachnoiditis, delayed syrinx formation, and hydrocephalus, which occasionally complicate extramedullary tumor removal. Rarely, a spinal meningioma may extend through a dural nerve-root sleeve to present as a dumb bell tumor. The techniques for removal are similar to those already described for nerve-sheath tumors.

30.15.2.3
Filum Ependymoma

The exposure-procedure for resection of filum ependymomas is a standard posterior laminectomy over the involved levels. Removal consists of developing a clean arachnoid plane around the lesion and separating it from the involved nerve-roots (Fig, 30.31). Large filum. terminale ependymomas, however, can present significant problems with surgical resection. These tumors will have been present for many years, and present a risk of CSF tumor-dissemination. Unencapsulated pliable neoplasms may have insinuated among the roots and within the arachnoid sheaths of the cauda equina, compartmentalized by innumerable arachnoid septa. Filum ependymomas may also spread as contiguous tumor-sheaths along the arachnoid septa, which act as a scaffolding for surface growth. Dissemination into the CSF may occur because of the subarachnoid location. Tumor removal in these cases is necessarily piecemeal and will almost always be subtotal. Dense tumor attachments to the roots of the cauda equina present significant risks of postoperative deficits, because of the manipulation required for removal.

30.16
Treatment Outcomes

30.16.1
Intramedullary Tumors

The immediate results of surgery are related primarily to the patient's preoperative status, and the tumor location. In general, most patients note sensory loss in the early postoperative period, most likely as a result of the midline myelotomy. These complaints

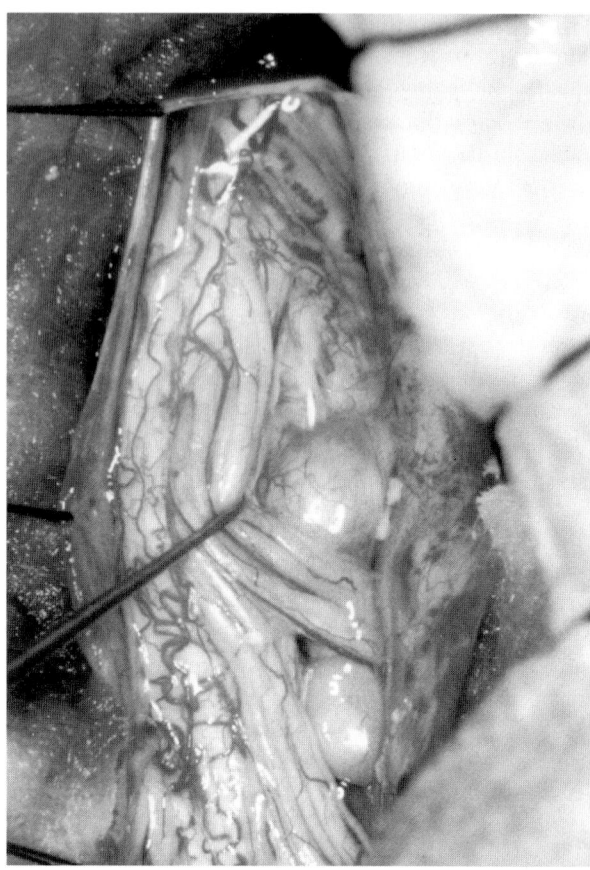

Fig. 30.31. Intraoperative photograph of filum ependymoma with overlying sacral nerve roots

are more subjective than objective, and can be significant even with little or no objective deficit. The sensory dysfunction tends to improve with time (McCormick and Stein 1990a). Additional surgical morbidity is directly related to the patient's preoperative status. Patients with significant or longstanding deficit rarely demonstrate any significant recovery and are more likely to worsen following surgery. Preservation, rather than restoration, of neurological function, is the appropriate goal for intramedullary tumor surgery. Those patients who are minimally symptomatic, have the potential for the greatest benefit and least morbidity of surgery for intramedullary tumors. This underscores the importance of early diagnosis and aggressive initial treatment prior to the onset of objective deficit. It is equally important in the follow-up period, since periodic MRI evaluation will most likely demonstrate evidence of tumor recurrence prior to clinical recurrence.

Long-term outcome and risk of recurrence are dependent primarily upon tumor histology, and are related to the completeness of the original resection. Malignant neoplasms are a notable exception to this generalization. It has become clear that gross total removal of benign intramedullary ependymomas consistently provides more long-term tumor control or cure than subtotal resection and radiation therapy (McCormick et al. 1990b, Asazuma et al. 1999, Epstein et al. 1993). Nevertheless, these tumors are friable and often quite adherent to the spinal-cord, which precludes microscopic total resection. Long-term follow-up with periodic clinical evaluation and gadolinium-enhanced MRI is mandatory, because of the continued risk of recurrence. Depending upon the patient's age and clinical circumstances, re-operation may be undertaken if tumor recurrence, on MRI, is clearly established. There is no evidence to support the efficacy of postoperative radiation following gross total complete resection.

30.16.1.1
Ependymoma

It is clear that total microsurgical removal alone is the optimal treatment for intramedullary spinal cord-ependymomas. In one series of 23 patients treated in this manner, with a mean follow-up time of 5 years, no definite clinical or radiographic evidence of tumor recurrence existed. The condition of seven of these patients was followed-up for more than 10 years (McCormick et al. 1990b). More recently, a cohort of 38 consecutive patients with intramedullary ependymoma was treated with surgery alone, and no adjuvant radiotherapy. Follow-up revealed no recurrences, and minimum morbidity (Epstein and Epstein 1982).

30.16.1.2
Astrocytoma

The treatment of intramedullary spinal-cord astrocytomas has been difficult to evaluate, because of the small sample-size and the biological variability. Age appears to be the most significant prognostic factor. Pediatric astrocytomas are associated with an indolent behavior that correlates with their predominantly benign histology (Epstein and Epstein 1981, 1982, Epstein 1986, 1990, Steinbok et al. 1992). Approximately 60% of patients below 21 years of age at diagnosis, are alive without recurrence 10 years after treatment, while only 40% of patients over the age of 21 at diagnosis are alive without recurrence 5 years following treatment (Steinbok et al. 1992). Astrocytomas in the adult are more aggressive, with

a higher incidence of malignant tumors and diminished survival (McCormick and Stein 1990a, Epstein et al. 1992). The optimum treatment for aggressive astrocytomas in adults remains to be determined. Selected studies from the literature suggest that increased survival correlates with extent of resection, in lower grade tumors, but not in high-grade tumors (McCormick and Stein 1990a, Epstein et al. 1992).

30.16.1.3
Hemangioblastoma

Hemangioblastomas are typically well-circumscribed, thus facilitating gross total removal, The risk of recurrence after complete resection is extremely rare. If there is concern that a total resection was not obtained, the patients' condition should be followed frequently, both clinically and by MRI. Symptom recurrence with evidence of residual or recurrent tumor is an indication for re-operation.

30.16.2
Extramedullary Tumors

The results of surgery for intradural extramedullary spinal-cord tumors are usually excellent. Neurological morbidity is typically less than 15%, with negligible mortality (McCormick et al. 1990a, McCormick and Stein 1990a). Complications are generally related to wound-healing and CSF leakage. As most of these patients will not have received radiation therapy, conservative management with lumbar drainage is sufficient management for CSF leak in most of these cases. Neurological complications are uncommon, and most often associated with manipulation of the cauda equina. Motor and sensory deficits typically improve postoperatively, with return of bladder function being variable. Improvement of preoperative deficits is typical and may be dramatic early in the postoperative period. Recovery is related to the duration and severity of the existing deficit and the age of the patient.

30.16.2.1
Nerve-Sheath Tumors

Total removal of neurofibromas and schwannomas which are not associated with neurofibromatosis is generally curative (McCormick 1994, 1996a,b). However, tumors with extensive paraspinal involvement, that are subtotally resected, have a definite propensity to recur. Deficits resulting from sacrifice of the involved nerve-roots are usually minor and well-tolerated. The condition of patients with multiple lesions from neurofibromatosis should be observed, with resection being reserved for progressive and symptomatic focal lesions.

30.16.2.2
Meningioma

Recurrence after total resection of spinal meningiomas is about 1% at 5 years and 6% at 14 years (McCORMICK et al. 1990a, GEZEN et al. 2000, McCORMICK 1994). Subtotally resected lesions have average recurrence rates of approximately 15%. The experience of the senior author is that dural resection versus coagulation apparently does not significantly affect recurrence. Meningiomas with extradural spread or en plaque lesions are more difficult to remove and tend to recur more frequently. These lesions also are associated with greater degrees of postoperative morbidity. These factors must be balanced when planning the extent of resection.

30.16.2.3
Filum Ependymoma

Neurological deterioration following removal of filum ependymomas is more frequent than that associated with nerve-sheath tumors and meningiomas. Lesions which involve the conus medullaris or are intimately adherent to many roots of the cauda equina, carry the highest risk of postoperative morbidity. Recurrence after gross total resection is rare, while subtotally removed lesions recur in approximately 20% of cases (McCormick et al. 1990a). Survival after total removal is almost 100%, while in the case of subtotally removed lesions, the condition of patients should be frequently followed by MRI.

30.17
Conclusion

Surgical considerations for the treatment of neurosurgical diseases of the spine and spinal-cord include evaluations that are performed before, during, and after the procedure. The progression starts with general preoperative diagnostics and includes the specific operative procedures to be used to treat the disease. In summary, treatment of intradural spinal-cord tumors remains a gratifying area of neurosur-

gery. Advances in imaging sensitivity, and the refinement of microsurgical skills have allowed removal alone to be viewed as definitive treatment in most cases. Early diagnosis and aggressive, definitive treatment can optimize the outcome of patients with these neoplasms.

References

Ahlgren BD, Herkowitz HN (1995) A modified posterolateral approach to the thoracic spine. J Spinal Disord 8: 69–75

Aithala GR, Sztriha L, Amirlak I, Devadas K, Ohlsson I (1999) Spinal arachnoid cyst with weakness in the limbs and abdominal pain. Pediatr Neurol 20: 155–156

An HS, Andreshak TG, Nguyen C, Williams A, Daniels D (1995) Can we distinguish between benign versus malignant compression fractures of the spine by magnetic resonance imaging? Spine 20: 1776–1782

Aoki N (1991) Syringomyelia secondary to congenital intraspinal lipoma. Surg Neurol 35: 360–365

Asazuma T, Toyama Y, Suzuki N, Fujimura Y, Hirabayshi K (1999) Ependymomas of the spinal cord and cauda equina: An analysis of 26 cases and a review of the literature. Spinal Cord 37: 753–759

Babu RP, Sekhar LN, Wright DC (1994) Extreme lateral transcondylar approach: technical improvements and lessons learned [see comments]. J Neurosurg 81: 49–59

Barloon TJ, Yuh WT, Yang CJ, Schultz D H (1987) Spinal subarachnoid tumor seeding from intracranial metastasis: MR findingsl. J Comput Assist Tomogr 11: 242–244

Birch BD, Johnson JP, Parsa A, Desai RD, Yoon JT, Lycette CA, Li YM, Bruce JN (1996) Frequent type 2 neurofibromatosis gene transcript mutations in sporadic intramedullary spinal cord ependymomas. Neurosurgery 39: 135–140

Bostrom J, Cobbers JM, Wolter M, Tabatabai G, Weber RG, Lichter P, Collins VP, Reifenberger G (1998) Mutation of the PTEN (MMAC1) tumor suppressor gene in a subset of glioblastomas but not in meningiomas with loss of chromosome arm 10q. Cancer Res 58: 29–33

Bourgouin PM, Lesage J, Fontaine S, Konan A, Roy D, Bard C, Del Carpio O'Donovan RA (1998) Pattern approach to the differential diagnosis of intramedullary spinal cord lesions on MR imaging. AJR Am J Roentgenol 170: 1645–1649

Brill C B (1989) Neurofibromatosis. Clinical overview. Clin Orthop 10–15

Brown PD, Stafford SL, Schild SE, Martenson JA, Schiff D (1999) Metastatic spinal cord compression in patients with colorectal cancer. J Neurooncol 44: 175–180

Bullard DE, Cox EB, Seigler HF (1981) Central nervous system metastases in malignant melanoma. Neurosurgery 8: 26–30

Caruso PA, Patel MR, Joseph J, Rachlin J (1998) Primary intramedullary lymphoma of the spinal cord mimicking cervical spondylotic myelopathy. AJR Am J Roentgenol. 171: 526–527

Chaparro MJ, Young RF, Smith M, Shen V, Choi, BH (1993) Multiple spinal meningiomas: a case of 47 distinct lesions in the absence of neurofibromatosis or identified chromosomal abnormality. Neurosurgery 32: 298–301; discussion 301–302

Chiariello E, Roz L, Albarosa R, Magnani I, Finocchiaro G (1998) PTEN/MMAC1 mutations in primary glioblastomas and short-term cultures of malignant gliomas. Oncogene 16: 541–545

Chung R, Whaley J, Kley N, Anderson K, Louis D, Menon A, Hettlich C, Freiman R, Hedley-Whyte ET, Martuza R, et al. (1991) TP53 gene mutations and 17p deletions in human astrocytomas. Genes Chromosomes Cancer 3: 323–331

Ciappetta P, Salvati M, Capoccia G, Artico M, Raco A, Fortuna A (1991) Spinal glioblastomas: report of seven cases and review of the literature. Neurosurgery 28: 302–306

Connolly ES Jr, Winfree CJ, McCormick PC, Cruz M, Stein BM (1996) Intramedullary spinal cord metastasis: report of three cases and review of the literature. Surg Neurol 46: 329–337; discussion 337–338

Constans JP, de Divitiis E, Donzelli R, Spaziante R, Meder JF, Haye C (1983) Spinal metastases with neurological manifestations. Review of 600 cases. J Neurosurg 59: 111–118

Cooper PR, Errico TJ, Martin R, Crawford B, DiBartolo T (1993) A systematic approach to spinal reconstruction after anterior decompression for neoplastic disease of the thoracic and lumbar spine [see comments]. Neurosurgery 32: 1–8

Couch V, Lindor NM, Karnes PS, Michels VV (2000) von Hippel-Lindau disease. Mayo Clin Proc 75: 265–272

Crockard H A (1995) Transoral surgery: some lessons learned. Br J Neurosurg 9: 283–293

Dechambenoit G, Piquemal M, Giordano C, Cournil C, Ba Zeze V, Santini JJ (1996) Spinal cord compression resulting from Burkitt's lymphoma in children. Childs Nerv Syst 12: 210–214

Decker HJ, Neuhaus C, Jauch A, Speicher M, Ried T, Bujard M, Brauch H, Storkel S, Stockle M, Seliger B, Huber C (1996) Detection of a germline mutation and somatic homozygous loss of the von Hippel-Lindau tumor-suppressor gene in a family with a de novo mutation. A combined genetic study, including cytogenetics PCR/SSCP, FISH, and CGH. Hum Genet 97: 770–776

Deme S, Ang LC, Skaf G, Rowed DW (1997) Primary intramedullary primitive neuroectodermal tumor of the spinal cord: case report and review of the literature. Neurosurgery 41: 1417–1420

Denis F (1983) The three column spine and its significance in the classification of acute thoracolumbar spine injuries. Spine 8: 817–831

Deruaz JP, Janzer RC, Costa J (1993) Cellular schwannomas of the intracranial and intraspinal compartment: morphological and immunological characteristics compared with classical benign schwannomas. J Neuropathol Exp Neurol 52: 114–118

Duerr EM, Rollbrocker B, Hayashi Y, Peters N, Meyer-Puttlitz B, Louis DN, Schramm J, Wiestler OD, Parsons R, Eng C, von Deimling A (1998) PTEN mutations in gliomas and glioneuronal tumors. Oncogene 16: 2259–2264

Ebert C, von Haken M, Meyer-Puttlitz B, Wiestler OD, Reifenberger G, Pietsch T, von Deimling A (1999) Molecular genetic analysis of ependymal tumors. NF2 mutations and chromosome 22q loss occur preferentially in intramedullary spinal ependymomas. Am J Pathol 155: 627–632

Elsberg C (1925) Tumors of the spinal cord and the symptoms of irritation and compression of the spinal cord and nerve roots: pathology, symptomatology, diagnosis and treatment, p. 206–239. New York: Paul B Hoeber

Epstein F (1986) Spinal cord astrocytomas of childhood. Adv Tech Stand Neurosurg 13: 135–169

Epstein F, Epstein N (1981) Surgical management of holocord intramedullary spinal cord astrocytomas in children. J Neurosurg 54: 829–832

Epstein F, Epstein N (1982) Surgical treatment of spinal cord astrocytomas of childhood. A series of 19 patients. J Neurosurg 57: 685–689

Epstein F, Wisoff J (1987) Intra-axial tumors of the cervicomedullary junction. J Neurosurg. 67: 483–487

Epstein FJ, Farmer JP (1990) Pediatric spinal cord tumor surgery. Neurosurg Clin N Am 1: 569–590

Epstein FJ, Farmer JP, Freed D (1992) Adult intramedullary astrocytomas of the spinal cord. J Neurosurg 77: 355–359

Epstein, FJ, Farmer JP, Freed D (1993) Adult intramedullary spinal cord ependymomas: the result of surgery in 38 patients. J Neurosurg 79: 204–209

Faro SH, Turtz AR, Koenigsberg RA, Mohamed FB, Chen CY, Stein H (1997) Paraganglioma of the cauda equina with associated intramedullary cyst: MR findings, AJNR Am J Neuroradiol 18: 1588–1590

Ferrante L, Mastronardi L, Celli P, Lunardi P, Acqui M, Fortuna A (1992) Intramedullary spinal cord ependymomas–a study of 45 cases with long-term follow-up. Acta Neurochir 119: 74–79

Gezen F, Kahraman S, Canakci Z, Beduk, A (2000) Review of 36 cases of spinal cord meningioma [In Process Citation]. Spine 25: 727–731

Giehl JP, Kluba T (1999) Metastatic spine disease in renal cell carcinoma–indication and results of surgery. Anticancer Res 19: 1619–1623

Gilsbach JM (1991) Extreme lateral approach to intradural lesions of the cervical spine and foramen magnum [letter; comment]. Neurosurgery 28: 779

Glavac D, Neumann HP, Wittke C, Jaenig H, Masek O, Streicher T, Pausch F, Engelhardt D, Plate KH, Hofler H, Chen F, Zbar B, Brauch H (1996) Mutations in the VHL tumor suppressor gene and associated lesions in families with von Hippel-Lindau disease from central Europe. Hum Genet 98: 271–280

Gnarra JR, Zhou S, Merrill MJ, Wagner JR, Krumm A, Papavassiliou E, Oldfield EH, Klausner RD, Linehan WM (1996) Post-transcriptional regulation of vascular endothelial growth factor mRNA by the product of the VHL tumor suppressor gene. Proc Natl Acad Sci U S 93:10589–10594

Goldstein SI, Kaufman D, Abati AD(1988) Metastatic thyroid carcinoma presenting as distal spinal cord compression. Ann Otol Rhinol Laryngol 97: 393–396

Guidetti B, Spallone A (1980) Benign extramedullary tumors of the foramen magnum. Surg Neurol 13: 9–17

Gusella JF, Ramesh V, MacCollin M, Jacoby LB (1999) Merlin: the neurofibromatosis 2 tumor suppressor. Biochim Biophys Acta 1423: M29–36

Hader WJ, Steinbok P, Poskitt K, Hendson G (1999) Intramedullary spinal teratoma and diastematomyelia. Case report and review of the literature. Pediatr Neurosurg 30: 140–145

Hashizume Y, Hirano A (1983) Intramedullary spinal cord metastasis. Pathologic findings in five autopsy cases. Acta Neuropathol 61: 214–218

Honch GW (1993) Spinal cord and foramen magnum tumors. Semin Neurol 13: 337–342

Innocenzi G, Raco A, Cantore G, Raimondi AJ (1996) Intramedullary astrocytomas and ependymomas in the pediatric age group: a retrospective study. Childs Nerv Syst 12: 776–780

Innocenzi G, Salvati M, Cervoni L, Delfini R, Cantore G (1997) Prognostic factors in intramedullary astrocytomas. Clin Neurol Neurosurg 99: 1–5

Itoh Y, Mineura K, Sasajima H, Kowada M (1996) Intramedullary spinal cord germinoma: case report and review of the literature. Neurosurgery 38: 187–190; discussion 190–191

Iwata K, Nakagawa H, Hashizume Y (1996) Significance of MIB-1, PCNA indices, and p53 protein over-expression in intramedullary tumors of the spinal cord. Noshuyo Byori 13: 73–78

Jallo GI, Zagzag D, Epstein F (1996) Intramedullary subependymoma of the spinal cord [see comments]. Neurosurgery 38: 251–257

Kaiser M, Parsa A, McCormick P (2000) Anterior thoracic instrumentation. In: V. Sonntag (ed.) Youmann's Neurological Surgery. New York: Saunders

Kamalian N, Abbassioun K, Amirjamshidi A, Shams-Shahrabadi M (1987) Paraganglioma of the filum terminale internum. Report of a case and review of the literature. J Neurol 235: 56–59

Kanno H, Kondo K, Ito S, Yamamoto I, Fujii S, Torigoe S, Sakai N, Hosaka M, Shuin T, Yao M (1994) Somatic mutations of the von Hippel-Lindau tumor suppressor gene in sporadic central nervous system hemangioblastomas. Cancer Res 54: 4845–4847

Kingdom TT, Nockels RP, Kaplan MJ (1995) Transoral-transpharyngeal approach to the craniocervical junction. Otolaryngol Head Neck Surg 113: 393–400

Klekamp J, Samii M (1996) Surgical results of spinal meningiomas. Acta Neurochir Suppl 65: 77–81

Kley N, Whaley J, Seizinger BR (1995) Neurofibromatosis type 2 and von Hippel-Lindau disease: from gene cloning to function. Glia 15: 297–307

Larson SJ, Holst RA, Hemmy DC, Sances A, Jr, (1976) Lateral extracavitary approach to traumatic lesions of the thoracic and lumbar spine. J Neurosurg 45: 628–637

Le Roux PD, Haglund MM, Harris AB (1993) Thoracic disc disease: experience with the transpedicular approach in twenty consecutive patients. Neurosurgery 33:58–66

Lee M, Rezai AR, Abbott R, Coelho DH, Epstein FJ (1995) Intramedullary spinal cord lipomas. J Neurosurg 82: 394–400

Lee M, Rezai AR, Freed D, Epstein FJ (1996) Intramedullary spinal cord tumors in neurofibromatosis. Neurosurgery 38: 32–37

Li MH, Holtas S (1991) MR imaging of spinal intramedullary tumors. Acta Radiol 32: 505–513

Liu W, James CD, Frederick L, Alderete BE, Jenkins RB (1997) PTEN/MMAC1 mutations and EGFR amplification in glioblastomas. Cancer Res 57: 5254–5257

Louis DN, von Deimling A, Chung RY, Rubio MP, Whaley JM, Eibl RH, Ohgaki H, Wiestler OD, Thor AD, Seizinger BR (1993) Comparative study of p53 gene and protein alterations in human astrocytic tumors. J Neuropathol Exp Neurol 52: 31–38

Lunardi P, Acqui M, Ferrante L, Fortuna A (1994) The role of intraoperative ultrasound imaging in the surgical removal of intramedullary cavernous angiomas, Neurosurgery. 34: 520–523; discussion 523

Madsen PW, 3rd, Yezierski RP, Holets VR (1994) Syringomyelia: clinical observations and experimental studies. J Neurotrauma 11: 241–254

Maxwell M, Borges LF, Zervas NT (1999) Renal cell carcinoma: a rare source of cauda equina metastasis. Case report. J Neurosurg 90: 129–132

McCormick P, Fetell M(1996) Spinal Cord Tumors. In: L. Rowland (ed.) Merrits Textbook of Neurology. New York: Lippincott Williams

McCormick PC (1994) Anatomic principles of intradural spinal surgery. Clin Neurosurg 41: 204–223

McCormick PC (1996a) Surgical management of dumbbell and paraspinal tumors of the thoracic and lumbar spine. Neurosurgery 38: 67–74; discussion 74–75

McCormick PC (1996b) Surgical management of dumbbell tumors of the cervical spine, Neurosurgery 38: 294–300

McCormick PC, Post KD, Stein BM (1990a) Intradural extramedullary tumors in adults. Neurosurg Clin N Am 1: 591–608

McCormick PC, Stein BM (1990a) Intramedullary tumors in adults. Neurosurg Clin N Am 1: 609–630

McCormick PC, Stein BM (1990b) Miscellaneous intradural pathology. Neurosurg Clin N Am 1: 687–699

McCormick PC, Torres R, Post KD, Stein BM (1990b) Intramedullary ependymoma of the spinal cord. J Neurosurg 72: 523–532

Melancia JL, Pimentel JC, Conceicao I, Antunes JL (1996) Intramedullary neuroma of the cervical spinal cord: case report. Neurosurgery 39: 594–598

Nadkarni TD, Rekate HL (1999) Pediatric intramedullary spinal cord tumors. Critical review of the literature. Childs Nerv Syst 15: 17–28

Neumann HP, Lips CJ, Hsia YE, Zbar B (1995) Von Hippel-Lindau syndrome. Brain Pathol. 5: 181–193

Oberstrass J, Reifenberger G, Reifenberger J, Wechsler W, Collins VP (1996) Mutation of the Von Hippel-Lindau tumour suppressor gene in capillary haemangioblastomas of the central nervous system. J Pathol. 179: 151–156

Olschwang S, Richard S, Boisson C, Giraud S, Laurent-Puig P, Resche F, Thomas G (1998) Germline mutation profile of the VHL gene in von Hippel-Lindau disease and in sporadic hemangioblastoma. Hum Mutat 12: 424–430

Parsa A, Kaiser M, McCormick P (2000) Posterolateral Approaches To The Thoracic Spine. In: G. e. a. Harsh (ed.) Chordoma and Chondrosarcoma. New York: Thieme

Parsa A, Miller J (2000) Neurosurgical Diseases of the Spine and Spinal Cord: Surgical Considerations (Chapter 27). In: J. Cottrell and D. Smith (eds.), Anesthesia and Neurosurgery, pp. (In Press). Philadelphia: Mosby

Parsons R (1998) Phosphatases and tumorigenesis. Curr Opin Oncol 10: 88–91

Perrin RG (1992) Metastatic tumors of the axial spine. Curr Opin Oncol 4:525–532

Prayson RA (1999) Clinicopathologic study of 61 patients with ependymoma including MIB-1 immunohistochemistry. Ann Diagn Pathol 3: 11–18

Prowse AH, Webster AR, Richards FM, Richard S, Olschwang S, Resche F, Affara NA, Maher ER (1997) Somatic inactivation of the VHL gene in Von Hippel-Lindau disease tumors [see comments]. Am J Hum Genet 60: 765–771

Rauhut F, Reinhardt V, Budach V, Wiedemayer H, Nau HE (1989) Intramedullary pilocytic astrocytomas–a clinical and morphological study after combined surgical and photon or neutron therapy. Neurosurg Rev 12: 309–313

Richard S, Campello C, Taillandier L, Parker F, Resche F (1998) Haemangioblastoma of the central nervous system in von Hippel-Lindau disease. French VHL Study Group. J Intern Med 243: 547–553

Ritter AM, Hess KR, McLendon RE, Langford LA (1998) Ependymomas: MIB-1 proliferation index and survival. J Neurooncol 40: 51–57

Roos KL, Muckway M (1995) Neurofibromatosis. Dermatol Clin 13: 105–111

Rubio MP, Correa KM, Ramesh V, MacCollin MM, Jacoby LB, von Deimling A, Gusella JF, Louis DN (1994) Analysis of the neurofibromatosis 2 gene in human ependymomas and astrocytomas. Cancer Res 54: 45–47

Sairyo K, Henmi T, Endo H (1997) Foramen magnum schwannoma with an unusual clinical presentation: case report. Spinal Cord 35: 554–556

Sarabia M, Millan JM, Escudero L, Cabello A, Lobato RD (1986) Intracranial seeding from an intramedullary malignant astrocytoma. Surg Neurol 26: 573–576

Sarpel S, Sarpel G, Yu E, Hyder S, Kaufman B, Hindo W, Ezdinli E (1987) Early diagnosis of spinal-epidural metastasis by magnetic resonance imaging. Cancer 59: 1112–1116

Sen CN, Sekhar LN (1990) An extreme lateral approach to intradural lesions of the cervical spine and foramen magnum [see comments]. Neurosurgery 27: 197–204

Seppala MT, Haltia MJ (1993) Spinal malignant nerve-sheath tumor or cellular schwannoma? A striking difference in prognosis. J Neurosurg 79: 528–532

Shapiro S, Scott J, Kaufman K (1999) Metastatic cardiac angiosarcoma of the cervical spine. Case report. Spine 24: 1156–1158

Sharma BS, Banerjee AK, Kak VK (1989) Malignant schwannoma of brachial plexus presenting as spinal cord compression. Neurochirurgia (Stuttg) 32: 189–191

Sharma S, Sarkar C, Mathur M, Dinda AK, Roy S (1990) Benign nerve sheath tumors: a light microscopic, electron microscopic and immunohistochemical study of 102 cases. Pathology 22: 191–195

Stebbins CE, Kaelin WG, Jr, Pavletich NP (1999) Structure of the VHL-ElonginC-ElonginB complex: implications for VHL tumor suppressor function. Science 284: 455–461

Steck PA, Pershouse MA, Jasser SA, Yung WK, Lin H, Ligon AH, Langford LA, Baumgard ML, Hattier T, Davis T, Frye C, Hu R, Swedlund B, Teng DH, Tavtigian SV (1997) Identification of a candidate tumour suppressor gene, MMAC1, at chromosome 10q23.3 that is mutated in multiple advanced cancers, Nat Genet. 15: 356–362

Steinbok P, Cochrane DD, Poskitt K (1992) Intramedullary spinal cord tumors in children, Neurosurg Clin N Am. 3: 931–945

Stillerman CB, Chen TC, Couldwell WT, Zhang W, Weiss MH (1998) Experience in the surgical management of 82 symptomatic herniated thoracic discs and review of the literature. J Neurosurg 88: 623–633

Sundaresan N, Sachdev VP, Holland JF, Moore F, Sung M, Paciucci PA, Wu LT, Kelligher K, Hough L (1995) Surgical treatment of spinal cord compression from epidural metastasis. J Clin Oncol 13: 2330–2335

Sweasey TA, Brunberg JA, McKeever PE, Sandler HM, Chandler WF (1994) Cystic cervical intramedullary ependymoma with previous intracyst hemorrhage. Magnetic resonance imaging at 1.5T. J Neuroimaging 4: 111–113

Tatter SB, Borges LF, Louis DN (1994) Central neurocytomas of the cervical spinal cord. Report of two cases [published erratum appears in J Neurosurg 1995 Apr;82(4):706], J Neurosurg 81: 288–293

Tokuhashi Y, Matsuzaki H, Toriyama S, Kawano H, Ohsaka S (1990) Scoring system for the preoperative evaluation of metastatic spine tumor prognosis. Spine 15: 1110–1113

Turgut M, Gul B, Girgin O, Taskin Y (1997) Role of surgical treatment in 70 patients with vertebral metastasis causing cord or root compression, Arch Orthop Trauma Surg. 116: 415–419

von Deimling A, Eibl RH, Ohgaki H, Louis DN, von Ammon K, Petersen I, Kleihues P, Chung RY, Wiestler OD, Seizinger BR (1992) p53 mutations are associated with 17p allelic loss in grade II and grade III astrocytoma. Cancer Res 52: 2987–2990

von Deimling A, Louis DN, Wiestler OD (1995) Molecular pathways in the formation of gliomas, Glia. 15: 328–338

von Haken MS, White EC, Daneshvar-Shyesther L, Sih S, Choi E, Kalra R, Cogen PH (1996) Molecular genetic analysis of chromosome arm 17p and chromosome arm 22q DNA sequences in sporadic pediatric ependymomas. Genes Chromosomes Cancer 17: 37–44

Vortmeyer AO, Gnarra JR, Emmert-Buck MR, Katz D, Linehan WM, Oldfield EH, Zhuang Z (1997) von Hippel-Lindau gene deletion detected in the stromal cell component of a cerebellar hemangioblastoma associated with von Hippel-Lindau disease. Hum Pathol 28: 540–543

Wise JJ, Fischgrund JS, Herkowitz HN, Montgomery D, Kurz LT (1951) Complication, survival rates, and risk factors of surgery for metastatic disease of the spine. Spine 24: 1943–1951

Yagi T, Ohata K, Haque M, Hakuba A (1997) Intramedullary spinal cord tumour associated with neurofibromatosis type 1. Acta Neurochir 139: 1055–1060

Yasuoka S, Okazaki H, Daube JR, MacCarty CS (1978) Foramen magnum tumors. Analysis of 57 cases of benign extramedullary tumors. J Neurosurg 49: 828–838

Yoshii S, Shimizu K, Ido K, Nakamura T (1999) Ependymoma of the spinal cord and the cauda equina region. J Spinal Disord 12: 157–161

31 Radiotherapy for Tumors of the Spine

Zbigniew Petrovich, Mark Liker and Gabor Jozsef

CONTENTS

31.1
Introduction

Primary tumors of the spinal cord are very uncommon neoplasms representing from 4% to 15% of all CNS tumors (Chun et al. 1990; Farwell et al. 1977; McCormick and Stein 1996). Ependymomas and astrocytomas account for nearly 90% of all spinal cord tumors, most of the remainder being meningiomas and schwannomas (Linstadt et al. 1989; Whitaker et al. 1991). Owing to the relative rarity of these tumors, their behavior and management are infrequently reported in the literature. Metastatic

Z. Petrovich, MD
Professor of Radiation Oncology and Urology, Chairman, Department of Radiation Oncology, USC School of Medicine, 1441 Eastlake Ave., G34, Los Angeles, CA 90033, USA
M. Liker, MD
Senior Resident, Department of Neurosurgery, USC School of Medicine, 1200 North State Street, Room 5046, Los Angeles, CA 90033, USA
G. Jozsef, MD
Assistant Professor, USC School of Medicine, 1441 Eastlake Ave., G34, Los Angeles, CA 90033, USA

lesions to the spine are much more common than the primary neoplasms. It has been estimated that in the United States approximately 18,000 new patients with symptomatic spinal metastasis are diagnosed each year and about 10% of patients with solid tumors develop spinal metastasis during the course of their disease (Slatkin and Posner 1983; Black 1979; Barron et al. 1959; Young et al. 1980). Nearly all patients presenting with spinal metastasis have epidural space disease; intramedullary spinal cord metastases are very rare, with about 100 patients being reported in the literature (Edelson et al. 1972; Posner 1977).

Surgery and radiation therapy, alone or in combination, are the fundamental tools in the treatment of neoplastic diseases of the spine. Radiotherapy is frequently used as the only treatment modality in selected patients with primary tumors of the spine and in a majority of patients with metastatic lesions (Young et al. 1980; Sundaresan et al. 1991). In certain tumors, postoperative radiotherapy has been shown to be effective in prolonging survival and improving outcome following surgery. In recent years, following the introduction of 3-D conformal radiotherapy, stereotactic radiosurgery, and particle beam radiotherapy, there has been a considerable increase in the indications for radiotherapy in patients with early primary and metastatic lesions, which would have previously been considered for an open neurosurgical procedure (Hamilton et al. 1995; Hamilton et al. 1996; Isacsson 1997).

It is expected that better systemic therapy for solid tumors will result in a longer patient survival, allowing for the development of CNS metastasis in a greater number of patients. Modern imaging modalities, particularly magnetic resonance imaging (MRI), permit diagnosis in patients with early symptoms or no symptoms of spinal metastases or primary spinal cord tumors. Such patients may be expected to have a more effective treatment, resulting in a better survival and a more optimal quality of life than were obtained in the past.

31.2
Primary Tumors

Primary tumors of the spinal cord and meninges are very uncommon neoplasms, with about 2700 new cases diagnosed annually (LENHARD 1996). Published reports describe a relatively small number of patients treated in various medical centers using different treatment protocols. Frequently, the extent of surgical resection is also variable and it may range from a biopsy only to a total gross tumor removal. Some patients receive postoperative radiotherapy with the use of different doses and treatment techniques and vaguely defined treatment indications. Additionally, as would be expected, there is variation in tumor size, site, and histology. Histology and tumor grade are known to be important prognostic parameters for extramedullary and intramedullary neoplasms. All these factors make evaluation of therapy outcomes based on published reports very difficult, and interpretations should be made with caution. Ependymoma and astrocytoma are the most frequently seen primary lesions, with the former being twice as common in some reports but of equal frequency to astrocytomas in other series (LINSTADT et al. 1988; KOPELSON et al. 1980; GARCIA 1985; WALDRON et al. 1993; SCHWADE et al. 1978) (Table 31.1). Primary CNS tumors may metastasize via the cerebrospinal fluid (CSF) pathways, with extraneural spread being rare but documented in meningioma and high-grade astrocytoma. The primary mode of spread for spinal tumors, however, is direct extension. So-called drop metastatic lesions or leptomeningeal seeding from CNS sites generally occur in the subarachnoid space and rest on the surface of the spinal cord or cauda equina. Lymphatic metastases are also rare, as are intramedullary metastases of primary CNS lesions (WONG et al. 1990; ZUMPANO 1978).

31.2.1
Ependymoma

In contrast to intracranial ependymoma, which occurs primarily in children, the peak incidence of spinal ependymoma is in the fourth decade of life and it is the most common primary spinal tumor in adults (KARLSON and BRADY 1987; WALDRON et al. 1993; MICHALSKI and GARCIA 1997). These tumors tend to grow slowly and cause symptoms due to local tumor progression. Ependymoma may involve a considerable length of the spine. Tumor location in the spine was reported in a study of 58 patients (WHITAKER et al. 1991). The most frequent site of tumor involvement was the cauda equina, in 24 (41%) patients, followed by the conus medullaris in 14 (24%) and the thoracic and cervical spine in 10 (17%) patients each. Treatment usually consists in

Table 31.1. Primary tumors of the spine (modified from Michalski and Garcia 1997)

Site	% Incidence	Histology	Comments
Extradural	<5	Meningioma	10% of spinal meningiomas
Intradural-extramedullary	70	Schwannoma	45% of lesions at this site, favors Th. spine
		Meningioma	<40% of lesions at this site, favors Th. spine
		Caudal ependymoma	60% of spinal ependymomas, favors L-S spine
		Vascular malformations	<10% of lesions at this site
		Teratoma, dermoid	10% of tumors at this site
		Squamous cell ca.	Favors sacrococcygeal region
		Lipoma	Uncommon, subpial
Intradural-intramedullary	30	Ependymoma	<40% of spinal ependymomas
		Astrocytoma	<45% of tumors at this site
		Oligodendroglioma	15% of tumors at this site
		Vascular malformations	Uncommon
		Teratoma	Uncommon
		Hemangioma	Uncommon

Th., Thoracic; L-S, lumbosacral

an attempt at surgical excision with or without adjuvant irradiation.

A report from Princess Margaret Hospital on the management of 59 patients with ependymoma is of interest (WALDRON et al. 1993). There were 36 male and 23 female patients with a median age of 37 years (range 8–66 years) and a median follow-up of nearly 11 years. Symptoms at diagnosis were pain in 75%, sensory deficit in 71%, and motor dysfunction in 68%. Functional status was classified into three groups: (1) minimal neurological impairment, present in 49%; (2) moderate neurological impairment, present in 36%; and (3) severe impairment, present in 17%. All patients had a histologically confirmed diagnosis of ependymoma, with three subtypes being identified as follows: (1) cellular, present in 32 (54%); (2) myxopapillary, present in 16 (12%); and (3) anaplastic, present in four (7%). In the remaining seven patients (12%) the histological subtype was not identified. All patients were initially treated surgically, with gross total tumor resection in 16 (27%), partial resection in 38 (64%), and a biopsy only in five (9%).

Radiotherapy to the tumor bed with proximal and distal normal tissue margins of several centimeters was given to 41 (69%) patients while the craniospinal axis with boost to the tumor bed was used in the remaining 18 (31%) patients. Radiation dose to the tumor site in 23 patients was 50 Gy in 25 equal daily fractions, with a few additional patients receiving <50 Gy or >50 Gy. The craniospinal axis was treated to up to 36 Gy in 10–25 fractions with a subsequent boost dose to the tumor bed. Nearly all study patients were treated with a 6-MV photon beam. The 5- and 10-year actuarial survival was 83% and 75%, respectively. The 5- and 10-year actuarial disease-free survival (DFS) was 83% and 83%, respectively. Of the 59 study patients, 11(19%) died of ependymoma. In four (7%) death was due to other causes. Following radiotherapy 11 (19%) patients had a treatment failure, including six with in-field recurrence, three with in-field and remote recurrence, and two with remote recurrence alone. Of the nine important tumor- and treatment-related parameters examined in univariate analysis, only tumor grade was predictive of treatment outcome (P=0.001). The authors recommended a postoperative course of irradiation in patients with spinal ependymoma as it results in an excellent long-term overall and disease-free survival.

The use of postoperative radiotherapy in patients with spinal ependymoma was evaluated in a study of 58 patients treated in the Royal Marsden Hospital in London, England. Basically, this study confirmed the findings of the Princess Margaret Hospital group

that tumor grade is the only significant independent prognostic factor for survival (P<0.005) (WHITAKER et al 1991). To a large extent similar outcomes in patients with ependymomas were observed by other investigators (CHUN et al. 1990; LINSTADT et al. 1989, 1998; WHITAKER et al. 1991; KOPELSON et al. 1980; GARCIA 1985; READ 1984). Studies on the relationship between grade of ependymoma and prognosis, however, remain equivocal (VIJAYAKUMAR et al. 1988; WHITAKER et al. 1991; WALDRON et al. 1993). Similarly, some investigators have recommended minimal surgery followed by postoperative irradiation while others have recommended more radical surgery without radiotherapy (COOPER 1989; COOPER and EPSTEIN 1985; GREENWOOD 1963; DI MARCO et al. 1988; FISHER and MANSUY 1980; WEN et al. 1991; LINSTADT et al. 1989; McCORMICK et al. 1990; WOOD et al. 1954; BROTCHI et al. 1991). Based on review of the literature and our experience we recommend maximal safe tumor resection followed by involved-field radiotherapy consisting of about 55 Gy given at 1.8-Gy daily increments. This approach provides the best obtainable incidence of local tumor control and survival (SCHILD et al. 1998; STUBEN et al. 1997; WEN et al. 1991; McLAUGHLIN et al. 1998; SHAW et al. 1986).

31.2.2
Astrocytoma

Astrocytoma is the second most common spinal cord neoplasm in adults while it is the most common spinal tumor in children (EPSTEIN and EPSTEIN 1982; ALLEN et al. 1998). The other important difference between pediatric and adult patients is in the use of chemotherapy, which is an important treatment modality in childhood but has not been particularly effective in adult patients. Astrocytoma usually shows slow tumor progression with gradually increasing symptoms. This tumor may involve a considerable length of the spinal cord. In a study of 24 patients with astrocytoma, thoracic cord was involved most frequently and the number of involved segments ranged from 1 to 29 with a median of 3 (ABDEL-WAHAB et al. 1999).

A number of published reports have examined the importance of various prognostic factors. These studies have shown a good correlation between patient age, degree of neurological disability, tumor location, duration of symptoms, extent of resection, tumor histology, tumor grade, and prognosis (GARCIA 1985; GARRET and SIMPSON 1983; ILGREN et al.

1984; McCormick et al. 1990; Peschel et al. 1983; Sgouros et al. 1996; Mork and Loken 1977; Shaw et al. 1986; Sonneland et al. 1985; Whitaker et al. 1991). Based on the above reports, it has been clearly established that the extent of surgical resection is an important factor influencing survival. Complete resection clearly provides a better survival than a partial resection or biopsy only, even in those patients in whom optimal postoperative irradiation is given (Sonneland et al. 1985; Whitaker et al. 1991). Unfortunately, complete resection of intramedullary glioma may only be accomplished in a small minority of patients (Cooper et al. 1989; Vijayakumar et al. 1988). Patients with low-grade astrocytoma of the spinal cord have a relatively good prognosis when surgical resection is combined with radiotherapy in properly selected cases. Those with high-grade tumors, however, have a poor prognosis (Kopelson and Lingwood 1982; Cohen et al. 1989). Most patients who fail the treatment show tumor recurrence primarily within the radiation portals and such a recurrence is a cause of death in 82% of patients (Garcia 1985).

Based on a review of the literature in patients with spinal cord astrocytoma we recommend maximal safe (compatible with a good neurological function) surgical resection to be followed by a planned course of external beam radiotherapy. There is good evidence suggesting the need for a radiation dose of about 55 Gy, given at 1.8-Gy daily increments. Careful treatment planning using MRI and computerized tomography (CT) and the use of devices to immobilize the patient for radiotherapy are required in order to maintain good position reproducibility for each treatment. For low-grade astrocytoma we use about 10-mm proximal and distal normal tissue margins as determined on an imaging study. This margin is increased to about 20 mm in those with grade III or IV lesions.

31.2.3
Meningioma

Meningioma is the most common nonglial tumor of the spine and represents about 10% of all primary spinal lesions (Schiebe et al. 1997; Maier et al. 1992). More than 90% of spinal meningiomas are considered benign, with <10% reported as anaplastic or malignant (Russel and Rubenstein 1989; Dolmann and Berry 1981). Spinal meningioma primarily (80%) affects the thoracic spine and is uncommon in the lumbosacral spine. This disease is most common (80%) among middle-aged women

(Levy et al 1982; Linstadt et al 1989). Benign meningioma tends to grow slowly, with symptoms caused by the spinal cord or nerve root compression. On the other hand malignant meningioma is characterized by rapid tumor growth causing symptoms due to compression and invasion into the neighboring neural elements. Early tumor recurrence in spite of applied therapy is very common, leading to rapid tumor progression and death. Tumor spread through the CNS pathway and outside of the CNS has been occasionally reported (Russel and Rubinstein 1989; Levy et al. 1982; Linstad et al. 1989). The treatment of choice for patients with benign meningioma is surgical resection, which is likely to control this disease in most patients who have a complete resection. In patients who have residual disease or cannot undergo surgery, local radiotherapy to about 54 Gy is an effective treatment in preventing tumor progression (Goldsmith et al. 1992). Meningioma regression following radiotherapy is not commonly observed. Presently available treatment for malignant meningioma, which may include surgery, radiotherapy, and chemotherapy, is not very effective.

31.2.4
Nerve Sheath Tumors

This group is represented by schwannoma and neurofibroma characterized by their common origin from Schwann cells (McCormick and Stein 1996). Schwannomas are nearly evenly distributed throughout the spine, being least common in the sacrum. This disease affects middle-aged males and females with equal frequency. Nearly 90% of schwannomas are intradural and they tend to have a long natural history. Successful surgical removal is the treatment of choice, with radiation therapy reserved for postsurgical recurrences or those patients who cannot undergo surgery.

31.2.5
Other Tumors

Arteriovenous and cavernous malformations are uncommon lesions of the spinal cord. Their treatment consists of surgery alone, with radiotherapy having only a minor role in the management. Hemangioma, hemangioblastoma, and neurofibroma are encountered in the context of the neurocutaneous syndromes, such as von Hippel-Lindau disease and neurofibromatosis I or II, and thus are more common in the pediatric population, however, these lesions are also seen in adults. These lesions tend to grow by slow local expansion. Radiotherapy again has a minor role in the management of these patients.

Other tumors which are primarily intradural-extramedullary include dermoid, epidermoid tumors, and lipoma. All of these tumors are very rare. Their progression appears slow and treatment consists of surgery. A number of extradural tumors are seen, with most being metastatic, and they will be discussed below. Bone tumors such as osteogenic sarcoma, chondroma, chondrosarcoma, chordoma, and Ewing sarcoma commonly spread into the spinal canal. Similarly, lymphoma, neuroblastoma, fibrosarcoma, and other soft tissue sarcomas may spread into the spinal canal. The behavior and treatment outcome in the above-listed tumors are highly variable and depend on: histology, tumor grade, tumor location, tumor volume, length of the spine involved, and patient age. Surgery again is the primary treatment, with adjuvant radiotherapy and/or chemotherapy used for some selected lesions. Chordoma and sarcoma of the spinal axis are particularly difficult tumors to treat surgically, owing to anatomical considerations and infiltrative tumor potential (FULLER and BLOOM 1988). Surgery is unlikely to result in complete resection owing to frequently present bone invasion, extension along nerve roots, and wide soft tissue involvement (CHETIYAWARDANA 1984; DEWAR and DUNCAN 1985; HIGINBOTHAM et al. 1967). Spinal chordoma usually presents in the sacral spine (RICH et al. 1985). The management of these patients with chordoma requires the use of careful radiation treatment planning and radiation dose >60 Gy in order to minimize the probability of tumor recurrence. Long-term tumor control is expected in a high proportion of patients treated postoperatively with radiotherapy (PEARLMAN and FRIEDMAN 1970; REDDY et al. 1981). In view of the need to deliver relatively high radiation doses to a well-defined target volume, consideration should be given in selected patients with chordoma to the use of particle beam radiotherapy (SHOENTHALER et al. 1993). High-grade sarcomas are usually managed with an aggressive multidisciplinary therapeutic approach. On the other hand, low-grade sarcomas are less likely to be widespread and surgical resection with or without local radiotherapy may be warranted; such treatment is expected to result in tumor control in a majority of patients.

All sarcomas require relatively high (>65 Gy) radiation doses in order to achieve a high probability of tumor control. This unfortunately is frequently impossible owing to the limited local tissue (spinal cord and nerve roots) tolerance to radiation.

31.3
Metastatic Tumors

Metastatic tumors are about 8 times as common as the primary lesions of the spine and their incidence is increasing (SLATKIN and POSNER 1983; BLACK 1979; BARRON et al. 1959; YOUNG et al. 1980). This increase in the incidence is probably related to advances in therapy resulting in a longer survival in many patients with solid tumors. It has been estimated that between 5% and 10% of patients with solid tumors develop spinal metastases during the course of their disease (SLATKIN and POSNER 1983; BLACK 1979; DESFORGES 1992). Nearly all spinal metastases are extradural, with intramedullary involvement alone being very rare (HASHIZUME et al. 1983; BARRON et al. 1959; EDELSON et al. 1972). The primary mode of spread to the spine is via the hematogenous route, although in some tumors such as renal cell carcinoma or superior sulcus carcinoma, direct extension from the primary site is not uncommon (CONNOLLY et al. 1996; CONSTANS et al. 1983; HASHIZUME et al. 1983). Most (85%) patients with spinal metastases have their disease initially in the vertebral body or pedicles, with secondary tumor spread into the epidural space and usually anterior or lateral compression of the spinal cord or nerve roots (BARRON et al. 1959; GILBERT et al. 1978). The remaining 15% of patients have the spine secondarily involved from the neighboring tumor-involved lymph nodes or as a result of direct invasion from a primary lesion such as is the case in a few patients with renal cell carcinoma or superior sulcus tumor.

The incidence of spinal metastases in published series varies widely depending to a large extent on the prevalence of a given primary tumor in a reporting medical center. Generally, tumors of the breast, lung, prostate, and gastrointestinal tract, melanoma, renal cell carcinoma, lymphoma, and multiple myeloma are the most common neoplasms reported with spread into the spine (BARRON et al. 1959; YOUNG et al. 1980; HELWEG-LARSEN et al. 1997; SORENSEN et al. 1990; DESFORGES 1992). In a large study reported from Denmark, lung and prostate cancers were the most frequent primary sites responsible for spinal cord compression, accounting for 19% and 18% of cases, respectively (Table 31.2) (SORENSEN et al. 1990). A similar distribution of primary sites in spinal metastases was reported in study of 153 patients (HELWEG-LARSEN et al. 1997). The thoracic spine was the most frequent (67%) segment of the spine to be involved by metastatic disease, followed by the lumbosacral and cervical spine with 29% and 4%, respectively (HELWEG-LARSEN et al. 1997). Most patients with epidural metastases are initially asymptomatic, with localized pain being the most frequent symptom. Spinal pain, particularly with radicular signs, in a patient with a diagnosis of cancer should alert physicians managing such a patient to a probability of spinal metastases. MRI of the spine should be promptly ordered and treatment given upon diagnosis of this manifestation of metastatic disease. In one report on 127 patients, progression of neurological deficit was studied and all patients ultimately had an autopsy (BARRON et al. 1959). Thirty percent of patients developed paraplegia within 1 week of onset of symptoms while four (3%) patients with slowly progressing paraparesis developed paraplegia and incontinence within 24 hours. The above study clearly validates the need for expeditious treatment in patients with symptomatic spinal lesions.

31.3.1
External Beam Radiotherapy

Primary surgical management in patients with spinal metastases is discussed in Chap. 30. An important nonrandomized study on the treatment of 345 patients with spinal compression syndrome was reported from Denmark (SORENSEN et al. 1990). There were 226 (66%) male and 119 (34%) female patients

Table 31.2. The frequency of spinal compression by primary site in a study of 345 patients

Primary site	No.	%
Lung	66	19
Prostate	61	18
Breast	44	13
Kidney	35	10
Miscellaneous	34	10
Lymphoma	30	9
Myeloma	16	5
Gastrointestinal	12	4
Melanoma	7	2
Leukemia	1	<1
Unknown	39	11
Total	345	100

with a median age of 63 years and an age range from 14 to 84 years. Upon diagnosis, 108 (31%) patients had normal bowel and bladder function, 74 (22%) had mild dysfunction, 159 (46%) had severe dysfunction, and in 4 (1%) bowel and bladder function was not evaluated. Of the 345 patients, 16 (5%) had no motor signs or symptoms, 115 (33%) were ambulatory with moderate motor deficit, 165 (48%) were paraplegic, and 48 (14%) patients were classified as paralytic. Patients were treated with radiotherapy alone [n=149 (43%)], laminectomy alone [n=105 (30%)] or laminectomy followed by postoperative radiotherapy within 5–8 days [n=91 (26%)]. Due to the nonrandomized nature of this study and a lack of reported criteria for inclusion to a given treatment arm, treatment outcomes are difficult to compare between the three treatment groups. Treatment results primarily depended on the degree of neurological dysfunction at diagnosis. A total of 79% of ambulatory patients retained their walking ability following the treatment, while only 21% of paraplegic and 6% of paralytic patients were able to walk after the treatment.

Patients treated with laminectomy followed by radiotherapy did better than those treated with laminectomy alone or radiotherapy alone. These results need to be interpreted with caution as they may represent selection bias.

Treatment results in 29 patients with spinal metastases were evaluated in a prospective randomized trial (YOUNG et al. 1980). Of these 29 patients, 16 (55%) were treated with laminectomy followed by radiotherapy (group I) while 13 (45%) received radiotherapy alone (group II). All patients received corticosteroid therapy. Treatment in both groups was given within 2 h of diagnosis based on an imaging study. Radiotherapy in group I consisted of 30 Gy given in 3-Gy daily fractions while in group II it consisted of 12 Gy at 4 Gy a day followed by 18 Gy given at 2.7 Gy daily. Radiation beams and techniques (except for radiation doses) were the same. No significant difference in treatment outcomes, including survival, the degree of pain control, improvement in ambulation, and sphincter control, was noted between these two treatment groups. It is of importance to note that there was excellent pain control in both treatment groups, with an incidence of 88% in group I and 92% in group II. Similar treatment outcomes were reported in other studies (SUNDARESAN et al. 1991; SLATKIN and POSNER 1983; POSNER 1977; BYRNE 1992; GREENBERG et al. 1980). There is a general agreement that treatment outcome depends on neurological status of patients at diagnosis and that radiotherapy alone is an excellent treatment in most patients with spinal compression syndrome (LEVIOV et al. 1993; SORENSEN et al. 1990; KIM et al. 1990; MARANZANO et al. 1992).

An interesting treatment protocol with the use of radiotherapy for epidural compression was recommended in a study of 83 patients (GREENBERG et al. 1980). The treatment program consisted of high doses of dexamethasone followed by a course of external beam radiotherapy. Spinal irradiation was begun with 15 Gy given in three equal fractions of 5 Gy each. This was followed by a 4-day rest period and continued irradiation to an additional dose of 30 Gy in 3-Gy daily fractions. Of the 83 study patients, 47 (53%) were ambulatory after the treatment course. These data are similar to those reported by other investigators who used a more conventional fractionation schedule.

At USC, patients who present with a rapid onset of neurological deficit are treated with surgery to be followed by planned local external beam radiotherapy initiated within 10 days of surgery. Radiation doses depend on tumor histology. As an example, patients with metastatic breast carcinoma will receive 30 Gy at 3 Gy per fraction while those with renal cell carcinoma receive 50 Gy at 2 Gy per fraction. Patients who are not a good surgical risk and who present with rapidly progressing signs and symptoms are treated with dexamethasone and local external beam radiotherapy. They receive 16 Gy at 4 Gy per fraction to be followed by 26 Gy at 2 Gy per fraction.

31.3.2
Particle Beam Radiotherapy

An important study with the use of charged particle radiotherapy was reported by the group from University of California Lawrence Berkeley Laboratory (CASTRO et al. 1989). A total of 47 patients with circumferential or nearly circumferential tumors of the brainstem and spinal cord were treated with charged particle beams. The following lesions were treated in this study: chordoma, $n=15$ (32%); chondrosarcoma, $n=12$ (26%); other sarcomas, $n=9$ (19%); metastasis, $n=5$ (11%); and other lesions, $n=6$ (13%). Of the 47 patients, 14 (30%) had postsurgical recurrences, including five (11%) who also received external beam radiotherapy. Follow-up ranged from 6 to 90 months with a median of 20 months. Careful patient immobilization technique was used in order to assure treatment accuracy and reproducibility. Tumor dose ranged from 60 to 75 GyE (mean dose 67 GyE) with

a daily dose of 2 GyE, given 4 times per week. The dose was defined to the 90% isodose line. Relative biological effectiveness (RBE) was 1.8 for helium beam and 4.5 for the neon beam. Local tumor control was obtained in 29 (62%) patients and the median survival was 58 months. Local failure was reported in 18 (38%) patients, six (33%) of whom were treated for recurrent tumor. Severe toxicity was noted in six (13%) patients and included two spinal cord injuries, one brain stem injury, one brachial plexus injury, and two cases of severe skin changes. Of the six patients with severe toxicity, three (50%) had prior conventional external beam radiotherapy.

The same group from Lawrence Berkeley Laboratory reported excellent treatment outcomes obtained in 52 patients with perispinal tumors that are known to respond poorly to external beam radiotherapy (NOWAKOWSKI et al. 1991). These lesions included chordoma and chondrosarcoma, $n=24$ (46%); other sarcomas, $n=14$ (27%); and other tumors, $n=14$ (27%). Patients received a median dose of 70 GyE. For the 36 (69%) previously untreated patients, local tumor control was obtained in 21 (58%) and the 3-year survival was 61%. Of the 16 (31%) previously treated patients, seven (44%) had local tumor control and the 3-year actuarial survival was 51%. As expected, tumor volume was an important factor predicting local control. Severe toxicity was reported in six (11%) study patients. In a subsequent report in 14 sacral chordoma patients who received their treatment with helium or neon beam, the overall 5-year actuarial survival was 85% and the 5-year incidence of local control was 55% (SCHOENTHALER et al. 1993). A dosimetric advantage with the use of proton beam in patients with spinal lesions was clearly demonstrated by the group from Uppsala, Sweden (ISACSSON et al. 1997). It is apparent that charged particle beam radiotherapy is an important treatment in properly selected patients with spinal and brain stem tumors. A major problem with wide use of charged particle beam radiotherapy in clinical practice is the extremely high cost of these centers.

31.3.3
Brachytherapy

A group from Memorial Sloan-Kettering Medical Center reported on the use of brachytherapy in 35 patients who had a prior gross total tumor removal (ARMSTRONG et al. 1991). Brachytherapy was used to prevent local tumor recurrence and to minimize the probability of spinal cord and/or nerve root toxicity, which could be expected from the use of high-dose external beam radiotherapy. Metastatic lung cancer was the most frequent diagnosis ($n=18$, 51%) while sarcoma and other tumors were next in frequency ($n=8$, 23%, and $n=7$, 20%), respectively. Removable iridium-192 implants were employed in 21 (60%) patients, delivering 30 Gy to the periphery of the volume of interest. A single-plane implant technique was used in these patients. The remaining 14 (40%) patients received permanent iodine-123 implants, delivering a total of 125 Gy to the periphery of a designated volume of interest. Local control was recorded in 18 (51%) patients and there was no significant toxicity in spite of the use of prior external beam irradiation in 21 (60%) patients. It appears that this treatment technique, while feasible and well tolerated, has little to add to contemporary external beam irradiation.

31.4
Stereotactic Radiosurgery

Physical principles of stereotactic radiosurgery are extensively discussed in Chaps. 5, 6, and 19. Stereotactic radiosurgery for properly selected intracranial targets has become a well-established and indispensable treatment modality in the management of numerous patients. There have been many attempts to adapt stereotactic technique to permit safe treatment of selected patients with limited spinal primary or metastatic tumors (MACIUNAS et al. 1994). Reported studies from the University of Arizona actually describe a minimal degree of morbidity and evidence of radiographic regression of tumor (HAMILTON et al. 1995, 1996; TAKACS and HAMILTON 1999). Patients were treated with the use of a specially designed stereotactic frame and a modified linear accelerator. Reconstructed images formed the basis to devise a treatment plan. A single dose of 8–10 Gy defined to the 80% isodose line was used to treat the nine study patients. Multiple isocenters were used to treat these patients. In all cases, the neoplasms, comprising three metastatic sarcomas and six metastatic carcinomas, were treated with chemotherapy and were felt to be unresponsive to conventional radiotherapy. The outcomes of this study, however, need to be interpreted with caution since it involved a small number of patients and a relatively short follow-up period (HAMILTON et al. 1996). The main problems with full implementation of stereotactic spinal radiosurgery include (1) position uncertainty, and (2)

complexity of this procedure, with the need for a highly qualified radiation oncology faculty and staff.

At USC a spinal stereotactic radiosurgery program began in 1993 with the development of a custom-designed stereotactic board and associated noninvasive immobilization system. The necessary computer software was developed and was completely phased-in in early 1996. The first two patients to be treated had symptomatic lesions involving the Vth lumbar vertebra. The diagnosis was metastatic melanoma in the first and metastatic renal cell carcinoma in the second. Both of these patients had undergone a prior course of palliative radiotherapy consisting of 40 and 45 Gy, respectively. They presented with an intractable pain problem and were treated with the use of multiple fixed fields with the 20-MV photon beam (PETROVICH et al. 1999). The resulting 80% isodose line was U-shaped, treating the tumor-invaded area with relative sparing of the critical central part containing the cauda equina. Both of these patients responded to the treatment well, with pain controlled for several months, until death due to widely disseminated metastatic disease. At the present time we use multiple (12–18) fixed fields or multiple arcs or a combination of both. Stereotactic radiosurgery of the spine is a time-consuming procedure with several hours required for imaging, treatment planning, and verification simulation. In addition treatment itself may take as long as 1 h. Patients selected for this treatment include those with symptomatic tumor involvement of a single vertebral level. We still use a total dose of 20–25 Gy, defined to the 80% isodose line and given in four to five fractions. The dose to the spinal cord is limited to 20% of dose maximum.

A U-shaped isodose surface can be created with a field arrangement, shown in Figs. 31.1 and 31.2. The isocenter is set approximately at the center of the spinal cord. Two posterior fields irradiate the spine partially, to the left of the spinal cord. Five oblique and lateral fields on the patient's right and left at 30° intervals from the posterior field deliver the dose to the right and left parts of the spine, respectively, as viewed from the direction of each beam. The spinal cord, therefore, never receives direct radiation from any of the treatment fields. For the anterior, oblique, and lateral fields, the 20-MV photon beam was used to achieve a better dose distribution. The posterior oblique and posterior fields, being closer to the target volume, were treated using the 6-MV photon beam. The dose contribution of each field is adjusted empirically to obtain the desired U-shaped dose distribution with

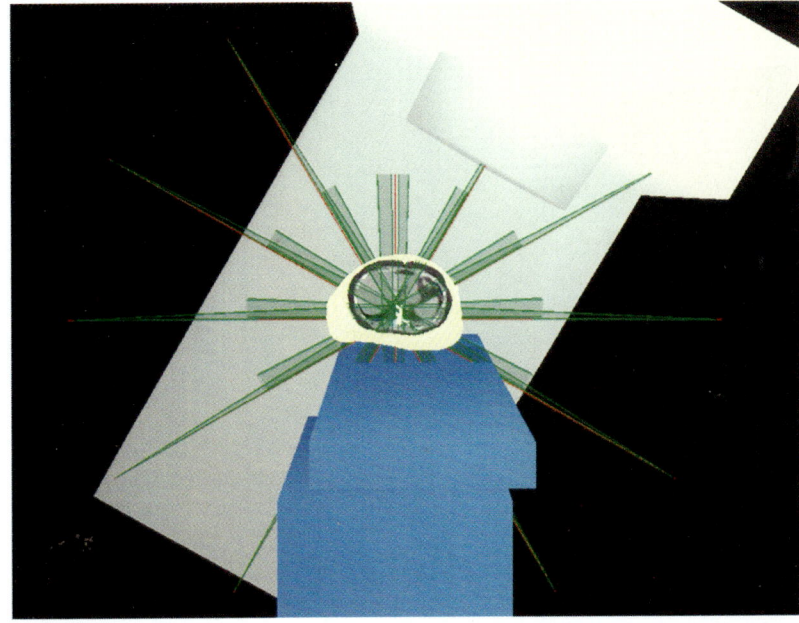

Fig. 31.1. Field arrangement to achieve a U-shaped dose distribution, excluding the spinal cord from the high-dose region. The anterior oblique and two lateral fields are treated with the 20-MV photon beam while the posterior and posterior oblique fields are treated with the 6-MV photon beam. Preferential weighting is given to the posterior and posterior oblique fields

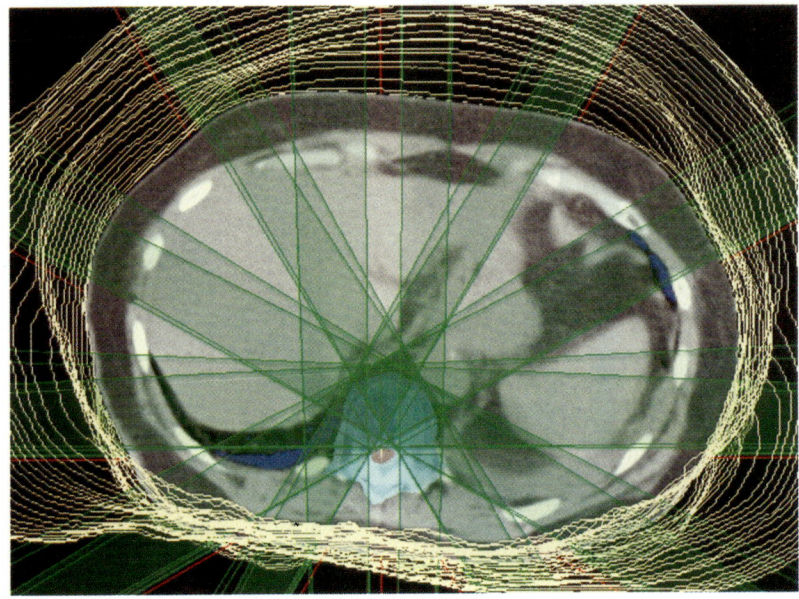

Fig. 31.2. Magnified view of Fig. 31.1. The selective blocking of the fields clearly demonstrates no direct radiation beam crossing the spinal cord

the highest isodose surface. In the case shown in Figs. 31.3 and 31.4, the 70% isodose line (relative to dose maximum) shows the desired shape. The ratio of doses delivered by the treatment fields (weight factors) are approximately 4:3:1 for the posterior, posterior-oblique, and anterior-oblique and lateral fields, respectively.

A similar 12-field arrangement was used to form a ring-shaped isodose surface as shown in Figs. 31.5 and 31.6. The posterior fields are the same; the oblique fields, however, alternatively irradiate the left or right side of the spine, while the spinal cord is always blocked. Because of the symmetry of this arrangement and the desired shape of the isodose surface, equal weights can be applied, and for all fields the 20-MV photon beam was used. This plan resulted in the dose distribution shown in Figs. 31.7 and 31.8.

Based on our limited experience, much more developmental work needs to be done to obtain the same level of sophistication in the spine as has been achieved with cranial content stereotactic radiosurgery.

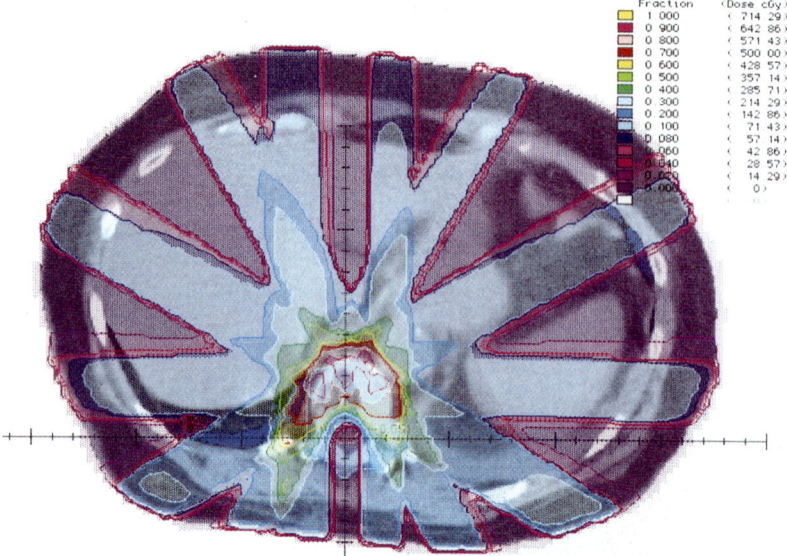

Fig. 31.3. The desired U-shaped dose distribution in the transverse plane. The dose was prescribed to the 70% isodose line (*red*) of the dose maximum

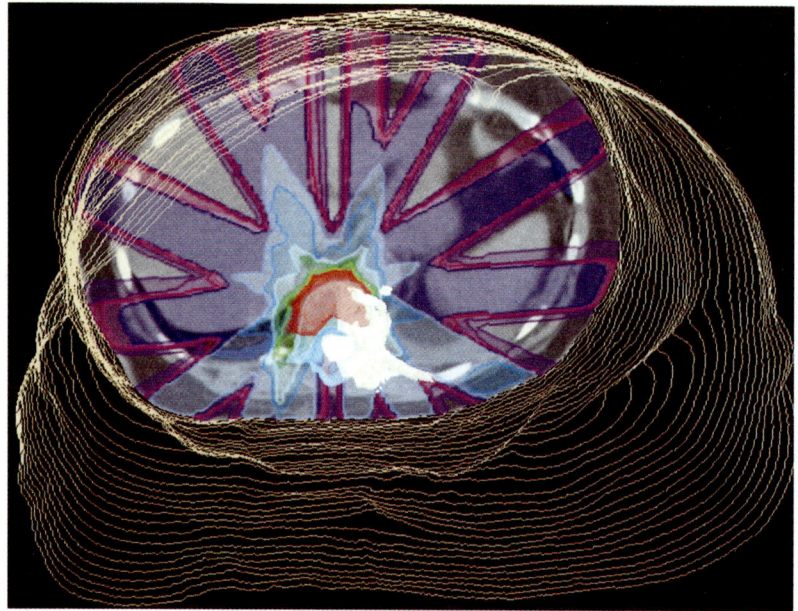

Fig. 31.4. 3-D view of the U-shaped dose distribution

An important new technological development is the Cyber knife, which was designed at Stanford University and is presently utilized at five medical centers. It incorporates a robotic arm-affixed specially designed linear accelerator using noninvasive image-guided localization of the lesion. A detailed description of frameless stereotaxy and its application is provided in Chap. 20. This development heralds a potential new modality in the treatment of primary and metastatic lesions of the spinal axis. Frameless stereotactic radiosurgery may well be the future of this important treatment modality.

31.5
Radiation Tolerance of the Spinal Cord

Chronic progressive radiation myelopathy or radiation myelitis is alternatively known as radiation myelitis (REAGAN et al. 1968). It is an irreversible process without known effective treatment (SCHULTHEISS et al. 1986). The syndrome begins approximately 6–15 months following completion of irradiation. The posterior columns are initially affected, as the patient describes paresthesias and other sensory disturbances. Symptoms progress over

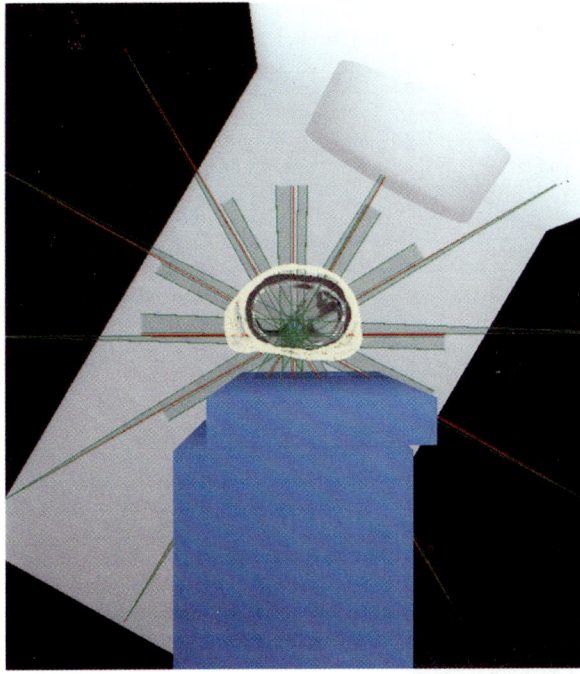

Fig. 31.5. Field arrangement to achieve a ring-shaped dose distribution around the spinal cord. All fields were treated with the 20-MV photon beam. Nearly equal weight is given to all fields

the next 1–6 months as multiple spinal tracts become involved. Plateau of symptoms may occur but a high rate of mortality has been documented due to intercurrent infection (PALLIS et al. 1961; PHILLIPS and BUSCHKE 1969).

The first to describe a set of four patients with transverse myelitis following radiation treatment of the cervical spine was AHLBOM (1941). Since then a number of studies have attempted to define the maximum tolerated radiation dose, initially believed to be in the range of 35–43 Gy (BAEKMARK 1975; BODEN 1948; KIM and FAYOS 1981). Regarding the size of the radiation fraction, most studies indicate that the optimal tolerated daily dose to the spinal cord is 2 Gy or less (BAEKMARK 1975; JEREMIC et al. 1991; KOPELSON 1982; MARCUS and MILLION 1990; SCHULTHEISS 1990). Others have investigated the relationship between the volume treated and the incidence of myelitis. An important study identified practically no risk of myelopathy in patients receiving a dose of 55 Gy in 27 fractions given in 37 days (ABBATUCCI et al. 1978). Severe complications are nearly certain in those receiving a dose >70 Gy in 35 fractions over a period of 49 days. The same study determined the importance of length of the spinal cord irradiated. The safe treatment was felt to limit radiation dose to 50 Gy in 25 daily fractions to three to five vertebral bodies.

Spinal cord and nerve roots are the dose-limiting structures in the treatment of spinal axis tumors, although it is believed that the cauda equina may be

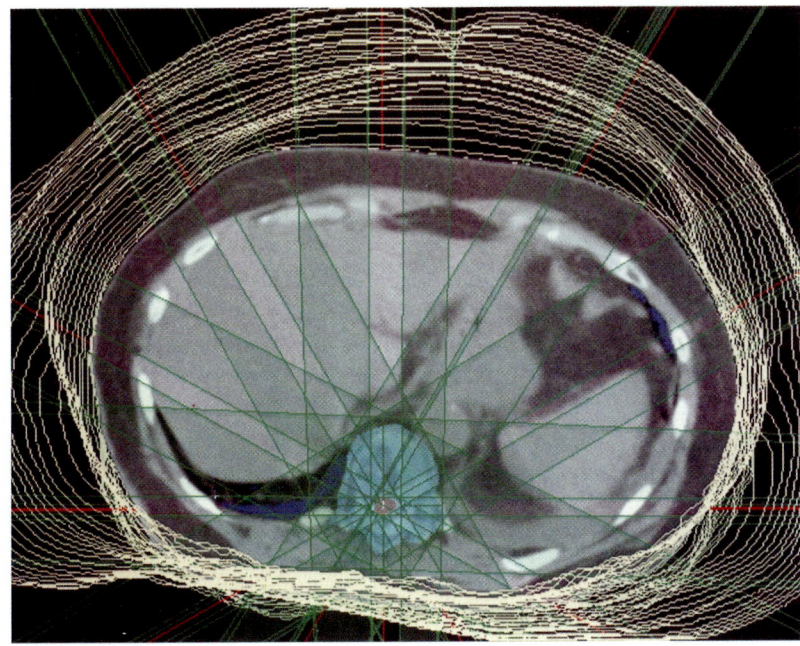

Fig. 31.6. Magnified view of Fig. 31.5. The selective blocking of each field clearly shows a good protection of the spinal cord

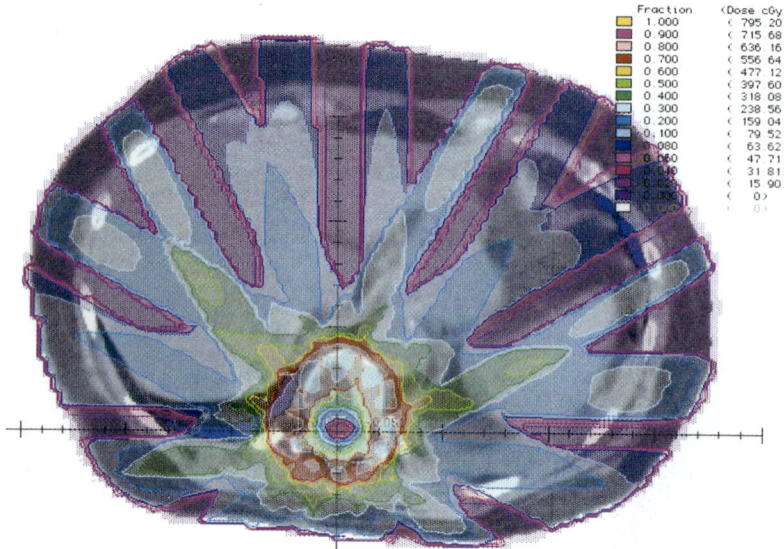

Fig. 31.7. Ring-shaped dose distribution in the transverse plane. The dose was prescribed to the 70% isodose line (*red*)

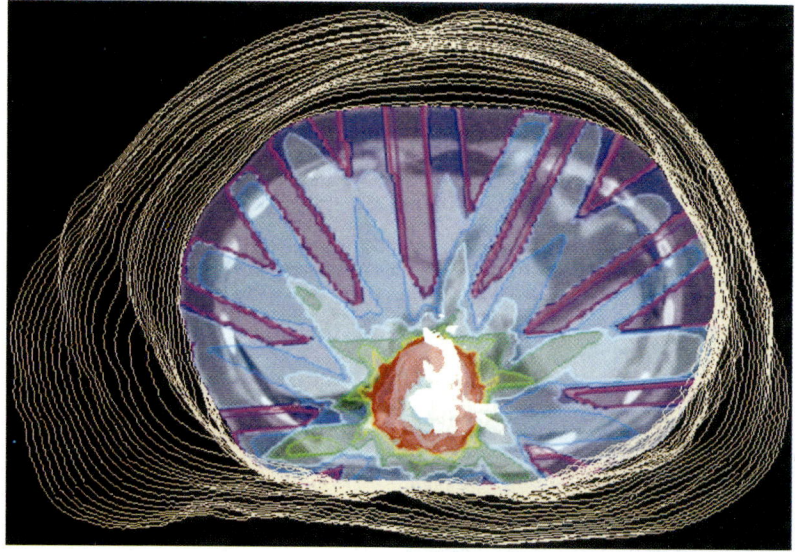

Fig. 31.8. 3-D view of the ring-shaped dose distribution

somewhat more resistant to radiation than the spinal cord. It has been reported that the thoracic cord is more sensitive to radiation injury than the cervical cord, although variations in technique may deliver different radiation doses that could account for the discrepancy in ascribed sensitivity (WARA et al. 1975; SHELINE et al. 1970).

The majority of the studies cited above involve radiation given to the normal spinal cord. Vascular changes, edema, or compression may alter neural structures in association with a contiguous enlarging mass. Investigating this hypothesis, three studies found similar rates of radiation myelitis among pa-

tients treated with radiation for various spinal axis lesions. Combining and summarizing the findings, only one patient of a total of 94 (1%) suffered from radiation myelitis following treatment doses ranging from 40 to 55 Gy in standard fractions (JEREMIC et al. 1991; KOPELSON 1982; MARCUS and MILLION 1990; SCHULTHEISS 1990). Thus, "abnormal" neural tissue does not appear to be more sensitive to radiation exposure than "normal" tissue.

At the present time, with advances in imaging and a wide availability of sophisticated computer software, there is no need to exceed the normal tissue tolerance while treating tumors of the spinal axis.

31.6
Conclusion

Rapid advances in imaging modalities and the development of faster computers have allowed for major improvement in the management of patients with many spinal lesions, including metastases. Better imaging has assisted in earlier and more accurate diagnosis and the timely application of appropriate treatment. Advances in neurosurgery and radiation therapy permit many lesions of the spinal axis to be treated while preserving good quality of life. Improved stereotactic techniques will allow more efficient treatment of many patients with early spinal lesions. The important new technological development of frameless stereotaxy will undoubtedly dominate the field of spinal therapeutics in the years to come.

References

Abbatucci JS, Delozier T, and Quint R, et al. (1978) Radiation myelopathy of the cervical spinal cord: time, dose and volume factors. Int J Radiat Oncol Biol Phys 4:239–248

Ahlbom HE (1941) The results of radiotherapy of hypopharyngeal cancer at the Radiumhemmet, Stockholm, 1930–1939. Acta Radiol (Oncol) 22:155–171

Abdel-Wahab M, Corn B, Wolfson A et al. (1999) Prognostic factors and survival in patients with spinal cord gliomas after radiation therapy. Am J Clin Oncol 22: 344–351

Allen JC, Aviner S, Yates AJ et al. (1998) Treatment of high-grade spinal cord astrocytoma of childhood with "8-in-1" chemotherapy and radiotherapy: A pilot study of CCG-945. J Neurosurg 88: 15–220

Armstrong JG, Fass DE, Bains M, et al. (1991) Paraspinal tumors: Techniques and results of brachytherapy. Int J Radiat Oncol Biol Phys 20: 87–790

Baekmark UB (1975) Neurological complications after irradiation of the cervical spinal cord for malignant tumor of the head and neck. Acta Radiat Ther Phys Biol 14:33–41

Barron KD, Hirano A, Araki S, Terry RD (1959) Experiences with metastatic neoplasms involving the spinal cord. Neurology 9:91–106

Black P (1979) Spinal metastasis: current status and recommended guidelines for management. Neurosurg 5:726–746

Boden G (1948) Radiation myelitis of the cervical spinal cord. Br J Radiol 21:464–469

Brotchi J, Dewitte O, Levivier M et al. (1991) A survey of 65 tumors within the spinal cord: Surgical results and the importance of preoperative magnetic resonance imaging. Neurosurg 29:651–657

Byrne TN (1992) Spinal cord compression from epidural metastases. New Eng J Med 327:614–619

Castro JR, Collier JM, Petti PL et al. (1989) Charged particle beam radiotherapy for lesions encircling the brain stem or spinal cord. Int J Radiat Oncol Biol Phys 17:477–484

Chetiyawardana AD (1984) Chordoma: Results of treatment. Clinical Radiology 35:629–632

Chun HC, Schmidt-Ullrich RK, Wolfson A, et al. (1990) External beam radiotherapy for primary spinal cord tumors. J Neuro-Onc 9: 211–217

Cohen AR, Wisoff JH, and Epstein F (1989) Malignant astrocytomas of the spinal cord. J Neurosurg 70:50–54

Connolly ES Jr, Winfree CJ, McCormick PC, et al. (1996) Intramedullary spinal cord metastasis: report of three cases and review of the literature. Surgical Neurology 46:329–337

Constans JP, de Divitiis E, Donzelli R, et al. (1983) Spinal metastases with neurological manifestations. Review of 600 cases. J Neurosurg 59:111–118

Cooper PR (1989) Outcome after operative treatment of intramedullary spinal cord tumours in adults: Intermediate and long-term results in 51 patients. Neurosurg 25:855–859

Cooper PR and Epstein F (1985) Radical resection of intramedullary spinal cord in adults. Recent experience in 29 patients. J Neurosurg 63:492–499

Desforges JF (1992) Spinal cord compression from epidural metastases. New Engl J Med 327:614–619

Dewar JA and Duncan W (1985) A retrospective study of the role of radiotherapy in the treatment of soft-tissue sarcoma. Clin Radiol 36:629–632

Di Marco A, Griso C, Pradella R, et al. (1988) Postoperative management of primary spinal cord ependymomas. Acta Oncol 27:371–375

Dolmann SI, Berry K (1981) Malignant meningioma: clinical and pathological features. J Neurosurg 5:929–934

Edelson RN, Deck MDF, Posner JB (1972) Intramedullary spinal cord metastases. Neurol 22:1222–1231

Farwell JR, Dohrmann GJ, Flannery JT (1977) Central nervous system tumors in children. Cancer 40:3123–3132

Fischer G and Mansuy L (1980) Total removal of intramedullary ependymomas: follow-up study of 16 cases. Surg Neurol 14:243–249

Fuller DB, Bloom JG (1988) Radiotherapy for chordoma.. Int J Radiat Oncol Biol Phys 15:331–339

Garcia DM (1985) Primary spinal cord tumors treated with surgery and postoperative irradiation. Int J Radiat Oncol Biol Phys 11:1933–1939

Garrett PG and Simpson WJK (1983) Ependymomas: results of radiation treatment. Int J Radiat Oncol Biol Phys 9:1121–1124

Gilbert RW, Kim JH, and Posner JB (1978) Epidural spinal cord compression from metastatic tumor: diagnosis and treatment. Ann Neurol 3:40–51

Goldsmith BJ, Wara WM, Wilson CB, et al (1992) Post-operative external beam irradiation for sub-totally resected meningioma.. Int J Radiat Oncol Biol Phys 24: 126–127

Greenberg HS, Kim JH, Posner JB (1980) Epidural spinal cord compression from metastatic tumor: Results with a new treatment protocol. Ann Neurol 8:361–366

Greenwood J Jr (1963) Intramedullary tumors of the spinal cord. A follow-up study after total surgical removal. J Neurosurg 20:665–668

Hamilton AJ, Lulu BA, Fosmire H, et al. (1995) Preliminary clinical experience with linear accelerator-based spinal stereotactic radiosurgery. Neurosurg 36:311–319

Hamilton AJ, Lulu BA, Fosmire H, et al. (1996) LINAC-based spinal stereotactic radiosurgery. Stereo Funct Neurosurg 66:1–9

Hashizume Y and Hirano A, (1983) Intramedullary spinal cord metastasis. Pathologic findings in five autopsy cases. Acta Neuropathologica. 61(3–4):214–218

Helweg-Larsen S, Johnsen A et al. (1997) Radiologic features compared to clinical findings in a prospective study of 153 patients with metastatic spinal cord compression treated by radiotherapy. Acta Neurochir (Wien) 139: 105–111

Higinbotham NL, Phillips RF, Farr HW, et al. (1967) Chordoma – thirty-five year study at Memorial Hospital. Cancer 20:1841–1850

Ilgren EB, Stiller CA, Hughes JT, et al. (1984) Ependymomas: A clinical and pathological study. Part II – Survival features. Clin Neuropathol 3:122–127

Isacsson U, Hagberg H, Johansson KA, Montelius A (1997) Potential advantages of protons over conventional radiation beams for paraspinal tumours. Radiother Oncol 45:63–70

Jeremic B, Djuric L and Mijatovic L (1991) Incidence of radiation myelitis of the cervical spinal cord at doses of 5500 cGy or greater. Cancer 68:2138–2141

Karlson UL, Brady LW (1987) Tumors of the spinal cord and canal. In: Principles and practice of radiation oncology. Perez CA, Brady LW (Eds.), Philadelphia, PA, Lippincott Co, pp. 437–452

Kim RY, Spencer SA, Meredith RF, et al. (1990) Extradural spinal cord compression: analysis of factors determining functional prognosis – prospective study. Radiology 176:276–282

Kim YH and Fayos JV (1981) Radiation tolerance of the cervical spinal cord. Radiology 139:473–478

Kopelson G (1982) Radiation tolerance of spinal cord previously damaged by tumor and operation: Long-term neurologic improvement and time-dose-volume relationships after irradiation of intraspinal gliomas. Int J Radiat Oncol Biol Phys 8:925–929

Kopelson G, Linggood RM (1982) Intramedullary spinal cord astrocytoma versus glioblastoma: The prognostic importance of histologic grade. Cancer 50: 732–735

Kopelson G, Linggood RM, Kleinman GM et al. (1980) Management of intramedullary spinal cord tumors. Radiology 135:473–479

Landmann C, Hunig R, Gratzl O (1992) The role of laminectomy in the combined treatment of metastatic spinal cord compression. Int J Radiat Oncol Biol Phys 24:627–631

Lenhard RE,Jr. (1996) Cancer statistics: A measure of progress. CA Cancer J Clin 46: 3–27

Leviov M, Dale J, Stein M (1993) The management of metastatic spinal cord compression: A radiotherapeutic success ceiling. Int J Radiat Oncol Biol Phys 27:231–234

Levy W, Bay J, Dohn D (1982) Spinal cord meningioma.. J Neurosurg 57: 804–809

Linstadt DE (1998) Spinal cord tumors. In: Leibel SA and Phillips TL (eds) Textbook of Radiation Oncology. W.B. Saunders Company, Philadelphia pp 401–414

Linstadt DE, Wara WM, Leibel SA et al. (1989) Postoperative radiotherapy of primary spinal cord tumors. Int J Radiat Oncol Biol Phys 16:1397–1403

Maciunas RJ, Galloway RL, Jr., Latimer JW (1994) The application accuracy of stereotactic frames. Neurosurg 35:682–695

Maier H, Ofner D, Hittmair A et al. (1992) Classic, atypical and anaplastic meningioma: Three histological subtypes of clinical relevance. Neurosurg 77:616–623

Maranzano E, Latini P, Checcaglini F, et al. (1992) Radiation therapy of spinal cord compression caused by breast cancer: Report of a prospective trial. Int J. Radiat Oncol Biol Phys 24:301–306

Marcus RB and Million RR (1990) The incidence of myelitis after irradiation of the cervical spinal cord. Int J Radiat Oncol Biol Phys 19:3–8

McCormick PC, Torres R, Post KD, et al. (1990) Intramedullary ependymoma of the spinal cord. J Neurosurg 72:523–532

McCormick PC, Stein BM (1996) Intramedullary tumors in adults. In: Neurological surgery, 4th Ed., Youman JR Ed., Saunders WB, Philadelphia, pp. 3102–3120

McLaughlin MP, Marcus RB, Buatti JM et al (1998) Ependymoma: Results, prognostic factors and treatment recommendations. Int J Radiat Oncol Biol Phys 40:845–850

Michalski JM, Garcia DM (1997) Spinal canal. In: Principles and practice of radiation oncology. Perez CA, Brady LW (Eds.) 3rd Ed Lippincott-Raven, Philadelphia, pp. 849–866

Mork SJ and Loken AC (1977) Ependymoma. A follow-up study of 101 cases. Cancer 40:907–915

Nowakowski VA, Castro JR, Petti PL, et al. (1991) Charged particle radiotherapy of paraspinal tumors. Int J Radiat Oncol Biol Phys 22:295–303

Pallis Ca, Louis S, and Morgan RL (1961) Radiation myelopathy. Brain 84:460–479

Pearlman AW and Friedman M (1970) Radical radiation therapy of chordoma.. Am J Roentgenol 108:333–341

Peschel RE, Kapp DS, Cardinale F, et al. (1983) Ependymomas of the spinal cord. Int J Radiat Oncol Biol Phys 9:1093–1096

Petrovich Z, Jozsef G, Yu C, Zee CS (1999) The role of radiotherapy in the management of patients with renal cell carcinoma. In: Petrovich Z, Baert L, Brady LW (Eds.) Carcinoma of the kidney and testis, and rare urologic malignancies. Innovations in management, Springer, Berlin, pp131–148

Philips TL and Buschke F (1969) Radiation tolerance of the thoracic spinal cord. Am J Roentgenol 105:659–664

Posner JB (1977) Management of central nervous system metastases. Sem Oncol 4:81–91

Read G (1984) The treatment of ependymoma of the brain or spinal canal by radiotherapy: A report of 79 cases. Clin Radiol 35:163–166

Reagan TJ, Thomas JE, and Colby MY Jr (1968) Chronic progressive radiation myelopathy. It's clinical aspects and differential diagnosis. JAMA 203:106–110

Reddy EK, Mansfield CM, Hartman GV, et al. (1981) Chordoma.. Int J Radiat Oncol Biol Phys 7:1709–1711

Rich TA, Schiller A, Suit HD, et al. (1985) Clinical and pathological review of 48 cases of chordoma.. Cancer 56:182–187

Russel DS, Rubenstein LJ (1989) Pathology of tumors of the central nervous system, 5th Ed., Edward Arnold, London, pp 452–506

Schiebe ME, Hoffman W, Kortmann RD, Bamberg M (1996) Radiotherapy in recurrent malignant meningiomas with multiple spinal manifestations. Acta Oncol 36: 88–90

Schild SE, Nisi K, Scheithauer BW et al. (1998) The results of radiotherapy for ependymomas: The Mayo Clinic experience. Int J Radiat Oncol Biol Phys 42: 953–958

Schoenthaler R, Castro JR, Petti PL, et al. (1993) Charged particle irradiation of sacral chordomas. Int J Radiat Oncol Biol Phys 26: 291–298

Schultheiss TE (1990) Spinal cord radiation "tolerance": doctrine versus data. Int J Radiat Oncol Biol Phys 19:219–221

Schultheiss TE, Stephens LC and Peters LJ (1986) Survival in radiation myelopathy. Int J Radiat Oncol Biol Phys 12:1765–1769

Schwade JG, Wara WM, Sheline GE, et al. (1978) Management of primary spinal cord tumors. Int J Radiat Oncol Biol Phys 4:389–393

Sgouros S. Malluci CL. Jackowski A. (1996) Spinal ependymomas–the value of postoperative radiotherapy for residual disease control. Br J of Neurosurg 10:559–66

Shaw EG, Evans RG, Scheithauer BW, et al. (1986) Radiotherapeutic management of adult intraspinal ependymomas. Int J Radiat Oncol Biol Phys 12:323–327

Sheline GE, Wara WM, Smith V (1980) Therapeutic irradiation and brain injury. Int J Radiat Oncol Biol Phys 6:1215–1228

Slatkin NE, Posner JB (1983) Management of spinal epidural metastases. Clin Neurosurg 30:698–716

Sonneland PRL, Scheithauer BW, Onofrio BM (1985) Myxopapillary ependymoma. A clinicopathologic and immunocytochemical study of 77 cases. Cancer 56:883–893

Sorensen PS, Borgesen SE, Rasmusson B (1989) Metastatic epidural spinal cord compression. Cancer 65:1502–1508

Stuben G, Stuschke M, Kroll M, et al. (1997) Postoperative radiotherapy of spinal and intracranial ependymomas: analysis of prognostic factors. Radiother Oncol 45: 3–10

Sundaresan N, Digiancinto GV, Hughes JE, et al (1991) Treatment of neoplastic spinal cord compression: Results of a prospective study. Neurosurgery 29:645–650

Takacs I, Hamilton AJ (1999) Extracranial stereotactic radiosurgery. Applications for the spine and beyond. Neurosurg Clin North Am 10:257–270

Turner S, Marosszeky B, Timms I, et al. (1993) Malignant spinal cord compression: A prospective evaluation. Int J Radiat Oncol Biol Phys 26:141–146

Vijayakumar S, Estes M, Hardy RW, et al. (1988) Ependymoma of the spinal cord and cauda equina: a Review. Cleve Clin J Med 55: 163–170

Waldron JN, Laperriere NJ, Jaakkimainen L, et al. (1993) Spinal cord ependymomas: A retrospective analysis of 59 cases. Int. J. Radiat Oncol Biol Phys 27:223–229

Wara WM, Phillips TL, Sheline GE, et al. (1975) Radiation tolerance of the spinal cord. Cancer 35:1558–1562

Wen B-C, Hussey DH, Hitchon PW, et al. (1991) The role of radiation therapy in the management of ependymomas of the spinal cord. Int J Radiat Biol Phys 20:781–786

Whitaker SJ, Bessell EM, Ashley SE, et al. (1991) Postoperative radiotherapy in the management of spinal cord ependymoma.. J Neurosurg 74:720–728

Wong DA, Fornasier VL, and MacNab I (1990) Spinal metastases: The obvious, the occult, and the imposters. Spine 15:1–4

Wood EH, Berne AS, Tavaras JM (1954) the value of radiation therapy in the management of intrinsic tumors of the spinal cord. Radiology 63:11–24

Young RF, Post EM, King GA (1980) Treatment of spinal epidural metastases: Randomized prospective comparison of laminectomy and radiotherapy. J Neurosurg 53:741–748

Zumpano BJ (1978) Spinal intramedullary metastatic medulloblastoma. Case report. J Neurosurg 48:632–635

32 Management of Rare Central Nervous System Tumors

GERY HSU and RAYMOND SAWAYA

CONTENTS

32.1
Introduction

The management of rare central nervous system (CNS) tumors varies greatly, depending upon several key factors. The location of the tumor may be the most important consideration in the management, specifically the neurosurgical management, of any intracranial lesion. The location, of course, determines what neurological deficits a patient may have and the degree of resectability of the tumor. For instance, a tumor involving the basal ganglia is managed in a fashion completely different from that of a similar tumor found in the anterior frontal lobe. The histological behavior of the tumor is also very important. Does the tumor invade surrounding tissue, or does it merely displace it? Does it engulf important structures such as normal blood vessels and cranial nerves, or is it well encapsulated? What is the tumor's natural history?

G. HSU, MD
Department of Neurosurgery, Baylor College of Medicine, Houston, Texas, USA
R. SAWAYA, MD
Department of Neurosurgery, The University of Texas, M.D. Anderson Cancer Center, Houston, Texas, USA

Other factors are also important in the management of these tumors and include:

I.   Patient issues
     A. Risk
     B. Expected benefit
II. Personal physician experience
     A. Previous similar cases
     B. Existing literature
III. Available neurosurgical instrumentation
     A. Image-guidance systems
     B. Intraoperative monitoring/mapping
     C. Stereotactic capabilities
     D. Endoscopic capabilities
IV. Available adjuvant therapy
     A. Chemotherapy
     B. Radiation therapy
1.   External beam radiation
2.   Stereotactic radiosurgery
3.   Frameless stereotactic radiosurgery

Because of the multitude of factors involved in the management of rare CNS tumors, providing a step-by-step guide and proclaiming a standard of care is not possible. In general, maximum excision with minimal neurological sequelae is the first step in management. With recent advances in intraoperative neurosurgical equipment and techniques, achievement of these initial goals is realized more frequently. Gross total resection can be achieved safely even in cases with tumors involving eloquent areas of the brain (SAWAYA et al. 1998). Tumor control is the next step. Advances in chemotherapy, and in radiotherapy including stereotactic and frameless stereotactic radiosurgery, continue to show the effectiveness of these important modalities.

These rapidly evolving options available to physicians will be likely to change patient care. Thus, a case by case approach to management is preferred. In this chapter, various rare CNS tumors are grouped according to their common location of occurrence. This arrangement is preferred because these groups tend to share the same or similar neurosurgical options. These groups are sub-classified according to general histological characteristics.

32.2
Parenchymal Tumors

Parenchymal tumors usually present with signs of cortical dysfunction or mass effect. Seizure activity, gradual alterations in mentation, unilateral weakness, speech difficulties are common among the myriad of possibilities. Uncommon are cranial nerve deficits, bilateral weakness, and acute changes in mentation. The effects of a parenchymal mass lesion may be due to destruction of normal brain or irritation of the surrounding brain from either mass effect or edema. Usually, the symptoms of such a mass can be lessened with dexamethasone, given by mouth or intravenously. This allows for adequate work up to be completed prior to surgical intervention of any kind. Large parenchymal tumors may require angiography and even embolization prior to operative excision. Other masses may require stereotactic planning. Infrequently, parenchymal tumors may require acute surgical intervention. These cases are usually secondary to tumor hemorrhage, and the physicians involved may not have the luxury of time to obtain all desired tests.

Surgical considerations for parenchymal tumors focus on the approach and preservation of surrounding brain tissue. Placement of the incision is simplified with the use of image-guidance systems based on preoperative MRI. Standard "horseshoe" flaps are the most common for scalp opening. Masses in the frontal lobes may require bicoronal or three-quarter coronal incisions to avoid unsightly scars of the forehead. Linear or "S" incisions may also be employed; however, these are not recommended for deeper parenchymal tumors since the self-retaining retractors and the retracted scalp may impede reach. Dangers during craniotomy include contusion of underlying brain tissue and damage to various sinuses, complications accompanied by significant morbidity. Tumors which are located near or in the motor cortex are more safely approached after intraoperative cortical mapping. Awake-craniotomy, an undertaking that requires complete unison of the entire surgical team and patient, may be considered in patients with lesions near the speech areas.

32.2.1
Tumors of Unknown or Glial Origin

32.2.1.1
Pleomorphic Xanthoastrocytoma

Pleomorphic xanthoastrocytoma (PXA) is a rare glioma marked by a distinct radiographic pattern, and as its name suggests, cellular pleomorphism and xanthomatous change. It is thought to arise from subpial astrocytes, and long-term survival is expected despite the pleomorphic features (Kepes et al. 1979). This generally benign lesion is found mainly in the temporal lobes of young adults, though the frontal lobes are a common site as well. Eccentric and multicentric lesions have been reported (Zarate and Sampaolesi 1999; Haga et al. 1996; Glasser et al. 1995; Herpers et al. 1994; Wasdahl et al. 1994; Mascalchi et al. 1994). The lesions characteristically are cystic with a superficial solid mural nodule usually directly adjacent to the meninges. However, atypical radiographic features have been reported (Pierallini et al. 1999). Although considered benign, PXAs have been reported to show malignant transformation (Prayson and Morris 1998; Tonn et al. 1997; Whittle et al. 1989; Weldon-Linne et al. 1983), which is estimated to occur in 10 to 25% of cases. Local recurrence as well as leptomeningeal or neuraxial dissemination has been reported as well (Glasser et al. 1995).

32.2.1.1.1
CLINICAL FEATURES
Patients are usually young adults who present with seizures or headaches or symptoms of increased intracranial pressure. It affects men and women equally, with an average age of diagnosis in the late twenties (GIANNINI et al. 1999). The tumor is found in the temporal lobe in 50% of patients (Fig. 32.1).

32.2.1.1.2
HISTOLOGICAL FEATURES
Though the tumor nodule appears to be distinct from the adjacent brain tissue, microscopic examination often shows parenchymal infiltration in deeper areas. The characteristic microscopic findings show considerable pleomorphism and cellularity, but with a distinct lack of mitotic figures, necrosis, and neovascularity. Cases in which increased mitotic activity is seen are associated with a much worse prognosis than the typical PXA (Macaulay et al. 1993). Cases of mixed PXA-ganglioglioma features have recently been reported (Perry et al. 1997; Furuta et al. 1992; Lindboe et al. 1992). These tumors have a

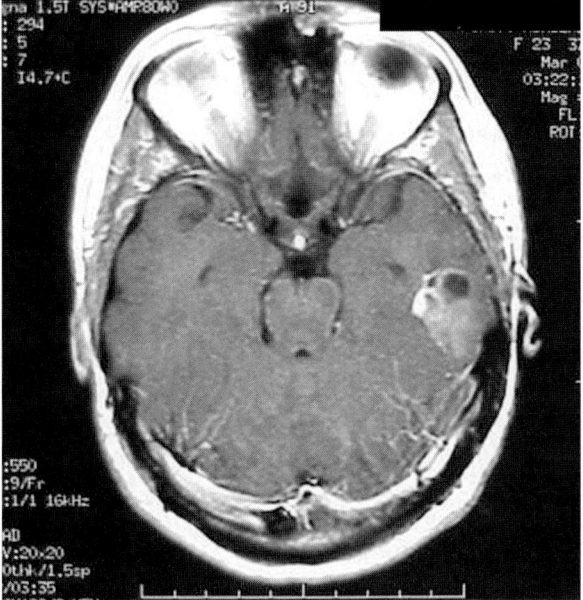

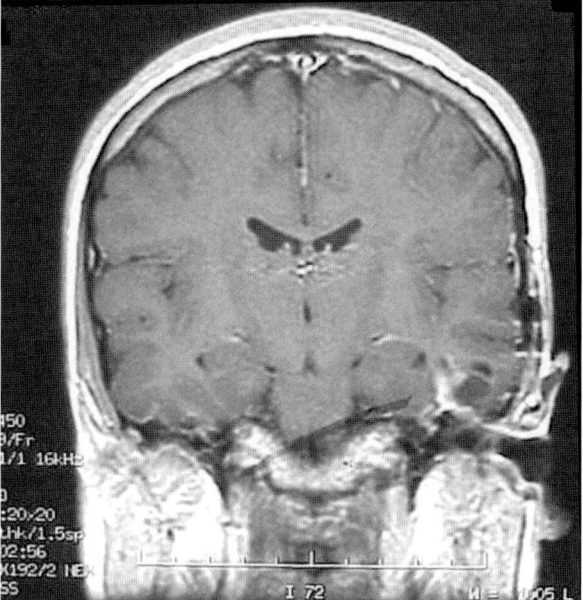

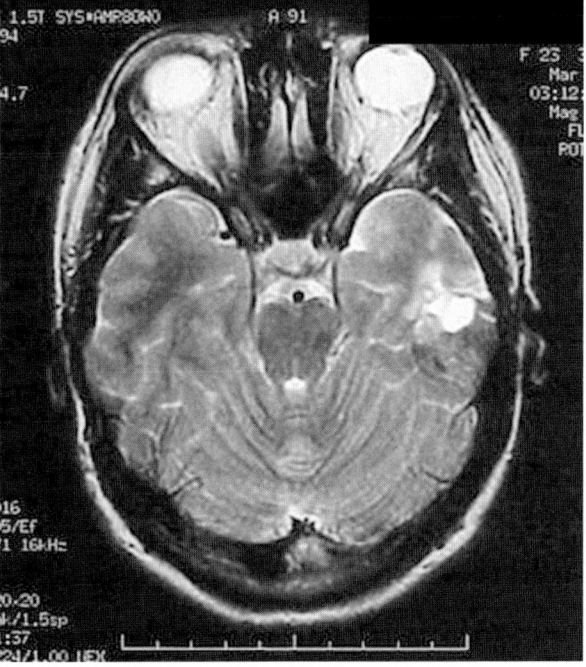

Fig. 32.1a–c. Pleomorphic xanthoastrocytoma. **a** Axial T1WI with gadolinium shows a left temporal cystic mass with mixed enhancement. **b** Coronal T1WI with gadolinium shows the same lesion. **c** T2WI exhibits the cyst component well

natural history more consistent with the glial component of the lesion (Lindboe et al. 1992). Immunohistological features include positivity for GFAP and S-100 protein.

32.2.1.1.3
TREATMENT

Surgical excision. A craniotomy is performed for gross total excision of the mural nodule and decompression of the cyst.

32.2.1.1.4
ADJUVANT THERAPY

For cases where gross total excision is achieved, radiation therapy is indicated for local recurrence and leptomeningeal spread only. Radiation therapy is given in cases where subtotal excision is achieved. Chemotherapy is also used in cases with subtotal excision, but not as frequently as is XRT (Giannini et al. 1999).

32.2.1.2
Gliomatosis Cerebri

Gliomatosis cerebri is a rare process characterized by diffuse proliferation of neoplastic glial cells affecting significant portions of white and gray matter of one or both hemispheres, without a focal mass. Instead, diffuse enlargement of the affected brain tissue is seen, including a characteristic thickening of the corpus callosum. The cerebellum and brainstem have also been reported to be sites of involvement. This disease is associated with a poor prognosis (Ross et al. 1991; PONCE et al. 1998). Mean survival time has been estimated to be 38 months in a series of 16 cases with post-operative radiation.

32.2.1.2.1
CLINICAL PRESENTATION AND
RADIOGRAPHIC STUDIES

Patients commonly present with mental status change, headache, seizures, or motor deficits. Symptoms of increased intracranial pressure may also be seen.

MRI characteristics include enlargement of affected regions of the brain, common corpus callosum and basal ganglial involvement, and involvement of at least two lobes. No contrast enhancement is seen (DEL CARPIO-O'DONOVAN et al. 1996). T2 images revealed diffuse high-signal intensity in the cerebral hemispheres; T1 images showed the involved brain to be iso- or hypointense compared with normal brain (SHIN et al. 1993).

CT is inadequate to evaluate cases of gliomatosis cerebri (SHIN et al. 1993). Fig. 32.2 demonstrates typical imaging features of gliomatosis cerebri.

32.2.1.2.2
HISTOLOGY

This is a diffusely infiltrative process that generally spares the normal parenchyma. The neoplastic cells tend to have little cytoplasm, and nuclei that may vary in appearance from small and round to oval and elongated. These neoplastic cells tend to collect around normal parenchyma such as vessels and normal neurons, forming secondary structures. Mitoses are infrequent, and necrosis should not be seen. The presence of necrosis would place a lesion in a higher grade, changing the diagnosis.

Some authors believe that gliomatosis cerebri should not be regarded as a separate entity but as a diffusely infiltrating low-grade glioma (FALLENTIN et al. 1997). Transformation into radiographically more circumscribed masses with histologically more

malignant features has also been seen (KANNUKI et al. 1998).

32.2.1.2.3
TREATMENT

No adjuvant therapy has been shown to increase survival, though radiation therapy has shown limited success in isolated cases (KANNUKI et al. 1998; COZAD et al. 1996; Ross et al. 1991). Steroids may be helpful acutely. There is no surgical procedure that has been shown to help survival; however, open or stereotactic biopsy should be performed for tissue diagnosis (ONAL et al. 1996; Ross et al. 1991). Gross total excision is not an option secondary to the large regions involved and the relative preservation of host tissue.

32.2.1.3
Hemangioblastoma

Hemangioblastoma is a benign tumor of unknown origin. It is thought to arise from the endothelium of cranial vessels. These tumors represent 1% of all brain tumors and about 10% of posterior fossa masses in adults, second only to metastases, and tend to occur in male adults in their 4th decade or later. Hemangioblastomas have been associated with von Hippel-Lindau syndrome, a neurocutaneous syndrome associated with chromosome-3. Patients with this disease tend to have hemangioblastomas of the brain and spine, retinal angiomas, and renal cell carcinomas.

32.2.1.3.1
CLINICAL PRESENTATION

Patients can present with many different symptoms, depending on the location of the tumor. In the posterior fossa, the most common location, patients may exhibit symptoms of hydrocephalus, headache, or incoordination. Rare lesions may occur in the supratentorial compartment. Cases associated with von Hippel-Lindau syndrome may have spinal cord involvement.

These tumors classically form cystic structures with an enhancing mural nodule. However, they may also be solid, or cystic without a mural nodule. The vascularity of these tumors lends for strong enhancement with contrast (Fig. 32.3). Hydrocephalus may also be found in cases involving the posterior fossa, where the aqueduct of Sylvius is obstructed, halting the flow of cerebral spinal fluid from the third to fourth ventricle.

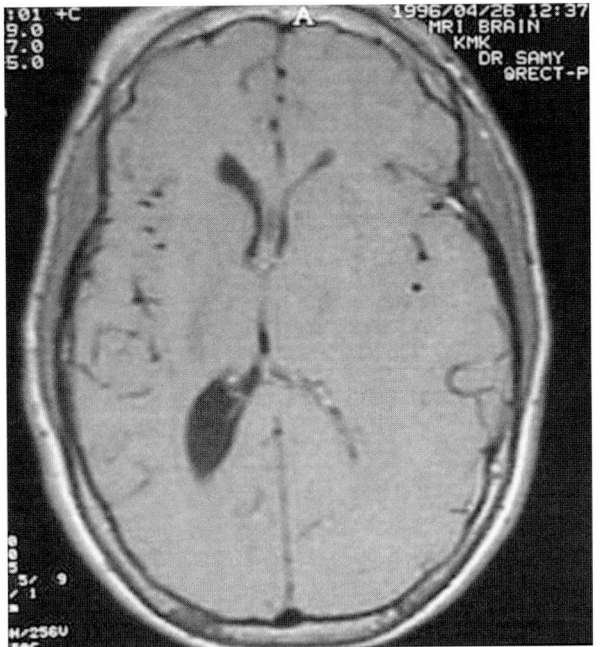
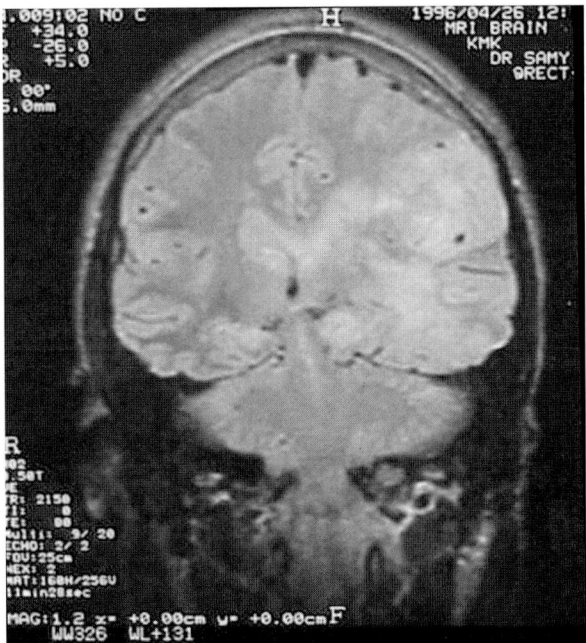
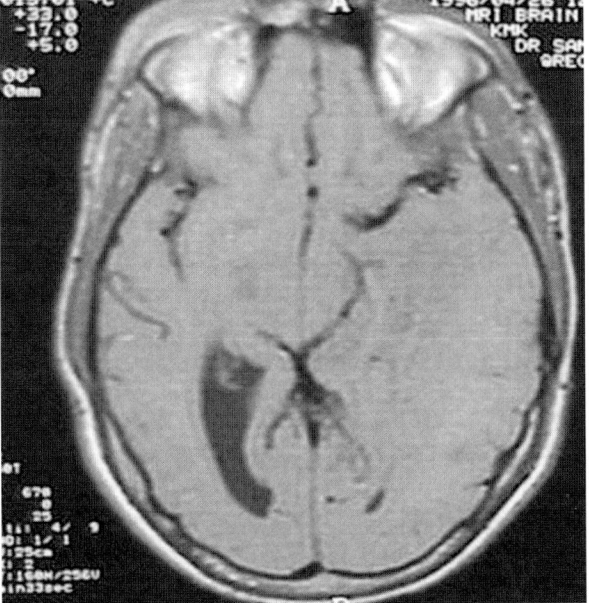

Fig. 32.2a–c. Gliomatosis cerebri. Left hemispheric fullness compared with the right is evident on all images presented. **a**, **b** Note the lack of enhancement. **c** FLAIR shows the extent of the tumor

32.2.1.3.2
HISTOLOGICAL FEATURES
Hemangioblastomas can vary microscopically from being highly cellular to paucicellular. Highly vascular, these tumors appear reddish grossly. A slight yellow tint may be found secondary to the tumors' varying lipid content. Specimens high in lipid exhibit clear cytoplasmic vacuoles on permanent section due to the loss of lipid during tissue processing. Hemangioblastomas also contain mast cells, unusual for an intrace-

rebral tumor. Nuclei may vary considerably. Mitoses are rare if present, and necrosis is absent.

32.2.1.3.3
TREATMENT
Surgical excision of these tumors is usually curative. Treatment of the cyst wall depends on the enhancement pattern. In general, if the cyst wall does not enhance, only the cyst needs decompression with removal of the mural nodule. However,

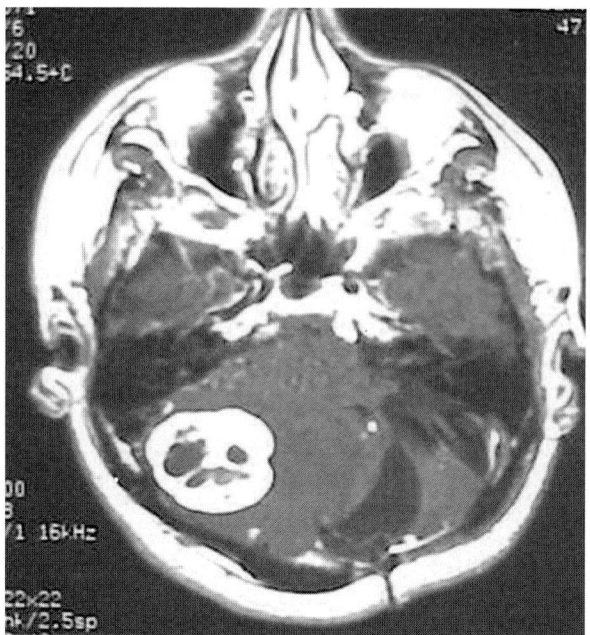

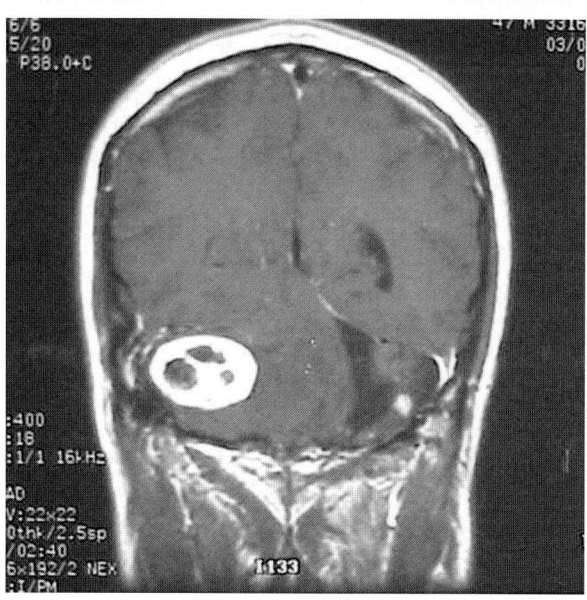

Fig. 32.3a,b. Hemangioblastoma in a patient with known von Hippel-Lindau disease. Patient had a previous left-sided sub-occipital craniectomy for removal of a hemangioblastoma. Both **a** coronal and **b** axial images are with contrast

should the cyst wall enhance, then effort should be made to clear the walls of any suspicious tissue. Though rare, shunting of ventricular fluid may be necessary.

Gamma knife radiosurgery (GKR) has been employed for treatment of this tumor (NIEMELA et al. 1996; CHANDLER and FRIEDMAN 1994). However, surgical excision is still considered to be the stan-

dard treatment. GKR may be more useful in cases where a solid tumor is located in an inaccessible area (PAN et al. 1998), or for patients with extremely high surgical risk. Linear accelerator-based radiosurgery has also had early promising results and may be a reasonable alternative for patients with multiple lesions (CHANG et al. 1998).

32.2.1.4
Hemangiopericytoma

Hemangiopericytoma is a rare tumor of aggressive nature that arises from the perivascular pericytes. Though cortical vessels have pericytes as well, hemangiopericytomas arise from those of the meninges. These highly cellular tumors are attached to the dura and are frequently, in the preoperative stage, mistaken for meningiomas. Unlike meningiomas, there is no gender predilection. These tumors usually occur in adults (McDonald 1999).

32.2.1.4.1
CLINICAL PRESENTATION
Patients may present with seizure, or symptoms of increased intracranial pressure. Focal weakness of one side of the body can also be frequently seen.

Radiographically, these tumors appear more aggressive than meningiomas and are highly vascular, enhancing strongly on both CT and MRI. These tumors can also cause destructive lesions of overlying bone. Angiographic studies reveal extreme vascularity with recruitment from both dural and parenchymal arteries (Fig. 32.4).

32.2.1.4.2
HISTOLOGICAL FEATURES
These tumors tend to be attached to dura, lobulated, and hypervascular. They can be pink to gray in color. Microscopically, these tumors are highly cellular and have a characteristic slit-like pattern formed from vessels referred to as a "staghorn" pattern. Mitosis is almost always found. Necrosis can be seen as well. Psammoma bodies and calcification are not found. These tumors are positive for vimentin, but negative for epithelial membrane antigen (EMA), features which clearly differentiate these tumors from meningiomas.

32.2.1.4.3
SURGICAL TREATMENT
Complete surgical excision is the goal of therapy (GALANIS et al. 1998). The key issue in excising these tumors is the minimization of blood loss. Preoperative embolization of the tumor should be employed if

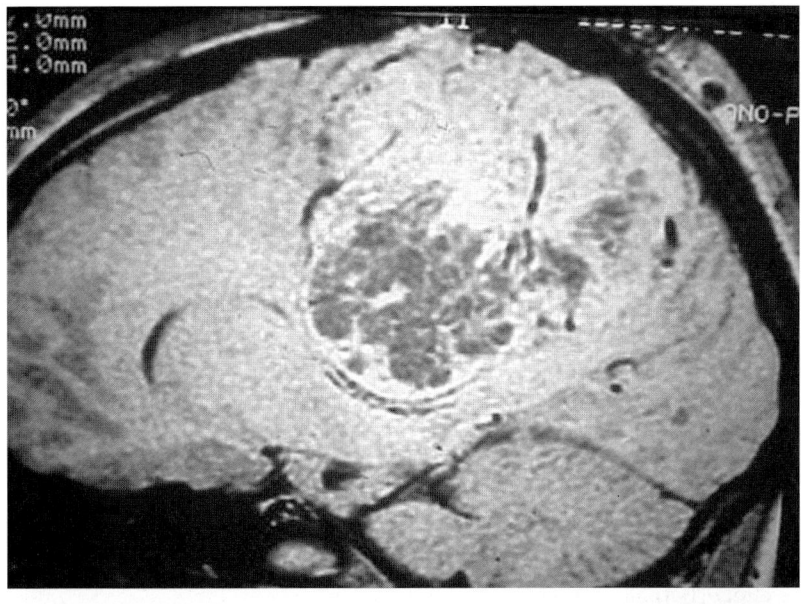

a

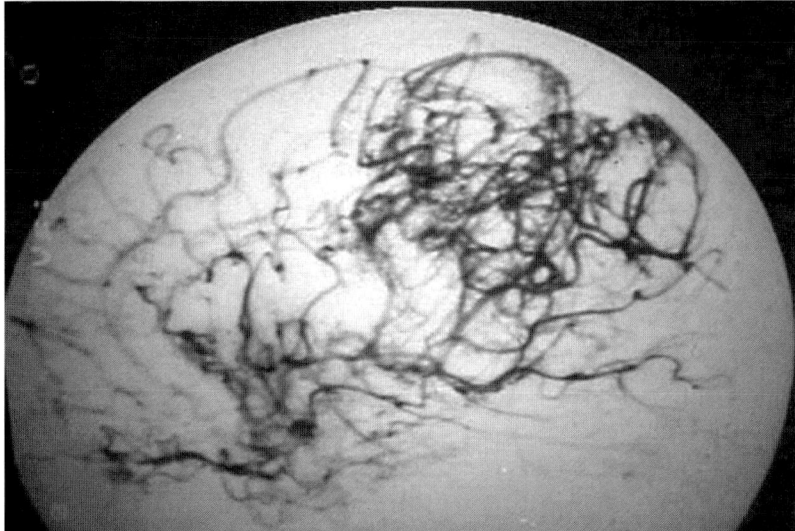

b

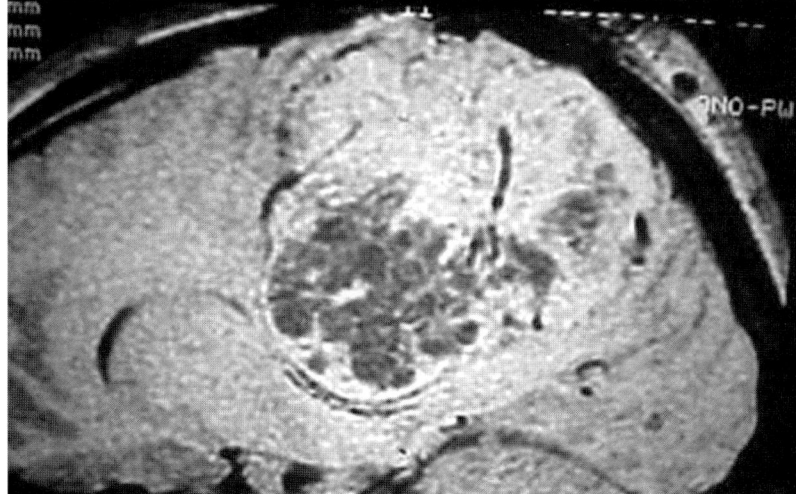

c

Fig. 32.4a,b. Hemangiopericytoma. **a** Sagittal MRI shows a large mass lesion with heterogeneous features. **b** Angiography shows dural and parenchymal vascular supply

available. This can significantly reduce the number and flow of arterial feeders. During surgery, significant blood loss should be treated promptly with transfusions, since profuse, continuous bleeding is a possibility until the entire tumor has been excised. Involved dura and bone should not be replaced. Dural patching using various available products can be performed. Bony defects can be filled with split calvarial grafting, cranial plating, or methylmethacrylate polymer grafting.

32.2.1.4.4
ADJUVANT THERAPY

Because of a high rate of local and distant recurrence and spread, postoperative radiotherapy is usually recommended, especially if the resection is incomplete. XRT has been shown to delay time of recurrence, but has not been shown to affect mortality. Chemotherapy can also be employed, but has had little effect (GALANIS et al 1998). Linear accelerator radiosurgery has been used to treat recurrent hemangiopericytomas (KOCHER et al 1998), and GKR has been found to be useful for small and medium-sized recurrent intracranial hemangiopericytomas (COFFEY et al 1993).

32.2.2
Tumors of Neuronal or Mixed Neuronal-Glial Origin

32.2.2.1
Ganglioglioma

Gangliogliomas, as the name suggests, are tumors of mixed neuronal and glial elements. Most of these cases are histologically of low grade. However, recurrences after gross total excision are common (LANG et al. 1993). Uncommon cases of malignant behavior have been reported, a behavior attributed to the high-grade nature of the glial component of the tumor. Indeed, specimens that display anaplastic features have a worse outcome (HAKIM et al. 1997; SASAKI et al. 1996). These tumors are frequently found in the temporal lobe (60%), are said to be cystic (50%), and are associated with seizure disorders. However, they can be found in all locations of the neuraxis, including the spinal cord.

These tumors equally affect male and female sufferers, and have an affinity for the young. The average age of patients with this tumor type is about 20 years. The average age of adults with this tumor is about 34 years.

32.2.2.1.1
CLINICAL PRESENTATION

Seizure disorder is a common presenting symptom, especially in tumors of the temporal lobe. Symptoms of increased intracranial pressure are also common. Calcification is rare. Contrast studies, either CT or MRI, tend to show a variably enhancing mass lesion with frequent associated cystic structures with or without mural enhancement. The majority of these lesions are supratentorial and the most common location in this sector is the temporal lobe. The radiographic characteristics of this tumor are difficult to differentiate from juvenile pilocytic astrocytomas (JPA), PXA, and primitive neuroectodermal tumors (PNETs) of the temporal lobe. Definitive diagnosis can be made only by histological confirmation (Fig. 32.5).

32.2.2.1.2
HISTOLOGICAL FEATURES

The histological characteristics of gangliogliomas are varied. The abnormality may be only paucicellular stroma with few groups of abnormal neurons or clusters of various neurons, lymphocytes, and ganglion cells. These ganglion cells can frequently resemble normal neurons, but without the regular arrangement within the cortical stroma.

With the advent of immunohistochemical testing, the diagnosis of these tumors has been facilitated, with the neuronal components displaying synaptophysin and the glial portions showing GFAP staining.

32.2.2.1.3
SURGICAL TREATMENT

Gross total excision is the treatment of choice. Due to the favorable cortical location of these tumors, this can usually be achieved. Tumors of the medial temporal lobe, especially on the left side, may benefit from image-guidance systems to facilitate tumor identification and excision. When speech areas are involved or are nearby, awake-craniotomies can be employed to test speech during excision. Cortical stimulation can also be used during such a procedure, to determine what tissue cannot be safely resected. Intraoperative ultrasound can also be used. Future advances with intraoperative MRI are expected to greatly facilitate surgery on medial temporal lobe tumors as well as other locations, regardless of histological diagnosis.

32.2.2.1.4
ADJUVANT THERAPY

Radiotherapy is generally not considered as a treatment for these tumors, unless there is an exceptional

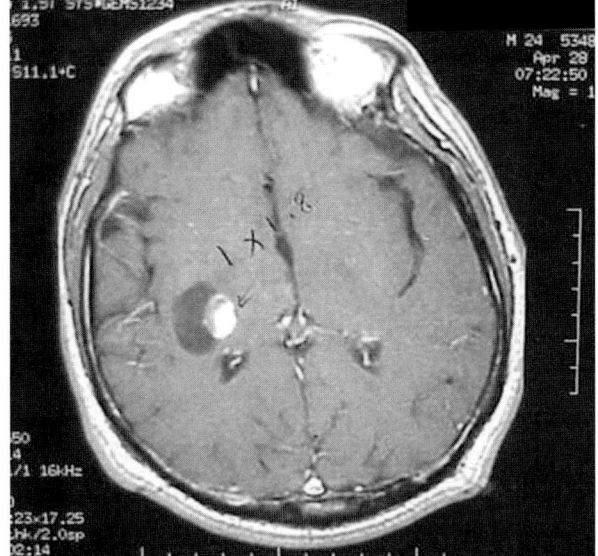

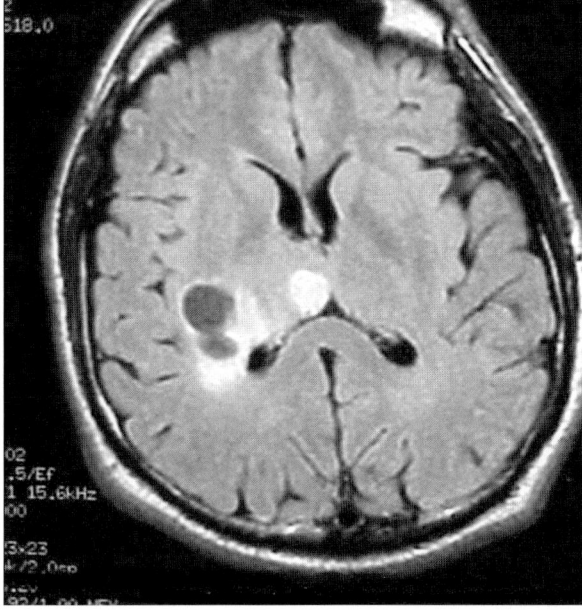

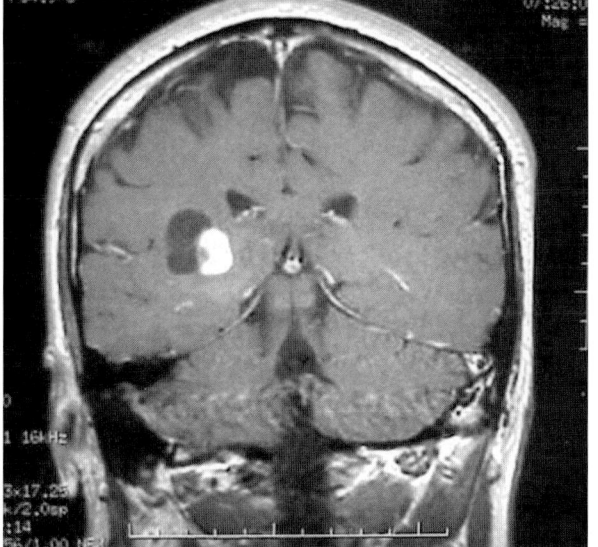

Fig. 32.5a–c. Ganglioglioma. **a** Axial and **c** coronal T1WI with gadolinium show an insular cystic lesion with mural nodule. **b** FLAIR shows thalamic involvement

case with particular malignant behavior (SASAKI et al. 1996). Such cases have been reported, possibly representing malignant transformation (MITTLER et al. 1999; JAY et al. 1994). Cases in which gross total excision is achieved requires only observation (KROUWER et al. 1993).

32.2.2.2
Lhermitte-Duclos Disease

Lhermitte-Duclos disease technically is a nonneoplastic hypertrophic process of the cerebellum. However, its unusual characteristics and rarity merit brief discussion. Also called dysplastic cerebellar gangliocytoma, this tumor-like process

involves expansion of cerebellar folia, usually of one cerebellar hemisphere, secondary to the hypertrophy of neurons in the internal granular layer. This disease process has been associated with Cowden's syndrome, otherwise known as multiple hamartoma syndrome (Koch et al. 1999). Linked to chromosome 10q, this neurocutaneous syndrome is characterized by hamartomas of the skin, breast, thyroid, oral mucosa, and intestines (Nelen et al. 1996).

32.2.2.2.1
CLINICAL PRESENTATION
Patients usually present as children or young adults with symptoms of increased intracranial pressure

or hydrocephalus (RAINOV et al. 1995; SIDDIQI and FEHLINGS 1994). Cerebellar dysfunction is the exception, not the rule. Currently, symptomatic treatment employing decompressive surgery is the only option for this disease. Syrinx has been reported in association with this disease (MARCUS et al. 1996). Postoperative prognosis is usually favorable, considering the indolent nature of this disease process.

Radiographic features are: CT: nonspecific cerebellar mass, non-enhancing (ASHLEY et al, 1990). MRI: hypointense on T1 and characteristic stripes of increased signal-intensity in T2-weighted images, without contrast enhancement (WOLANSKY et al. 1996; ASHLEY et al. 1990). Some cases of contrast enhancement have been reported (ORTIZ et al. 1995; AWWAD et al. 1995). The characteristic T2-weighted image stripes, coined "tiger stripes", may allow for strong preoperative suspicions of this disease (CARTER et al. 1989; REEDER et al. 1998; KULKANTRAKORN et al. 1997) (Fig. 32.6).

32.2.2.2.2
HISTOLOGICAL FEATURES
Macroscopic inspection reveals hypertrophic folia. Microscopic evaluation reveals changes in the internal granular layer. The resident granular cells are replaced by large neurons with vesicular nuclei and prominent nucleoli. These cells, larger and more uniform than those found in gliomas, are arranged haphazardly. Absence of polymorphism and multinuclearity is also found. Few if any mitotic figures are seen. Immunohistochemically, the abnormal neurons stain for synaptophysin.

32.2.2.2.3
TREATMENT
Gross total decompressive surgery is the treatment of choice (MILBOUW et al. 1988; LEECH et al. 1977). However, due to the poor demarcation of the disease margins, subtotal resection is sometimes the only possibility. Placement of a ventriculostomy may also be necessary. The surgery is commonly performed with the patient in the prone position, through a suboccipital craniectomy. Areas of obvious folia hypertrophy are resected. Postoperative problems may include hydrocephalus, pseudomeningocele, and cerebral spinal fluid leak.

Periodic follow-up with MRI is indicated. Recurrence has been reported after gross total excision. Chemotherapy and radiation therapies have not been employed to treat this disease process.

32.3
Ventricular and Periventricular Tumors

Ventricular tumors pose a challenge quite different from that of parenchymal lesions. Patients may present with acute symptoms, such as altered mental status or seizure activity, or chronic symptoms, such as headache or mild incoordination. The symptoms may be due to local mass effect such as compression of the cerebellum or brain stem, or may develop secondary to hydrocephalus. In cases in which hydrocephalus is an acute issue, emergent surgical intervention may be necessary prior to the complete evaluation of the lesion. Certainly, the management of ventricular region masses has changed recently with the advent of neuroendoscopic technology and improved microsurgical techniques.

Surgical considerations include the issues of acute and permanent cerebral spinal fluid (CSF) shunting and the surgical approach. Obviously, patients who present with acute symptoms of hydrocephalus deserve urgent CSF shunting. Ventriculostomy and placement of a ventriculoperitoneal shunt have been standard treatment options. Recent advances in neuroendoscopic technology have added another option. An endoscopic approach to masses allows for biopsy and third ventriculostomy during the same surgical sitting. Also, should an attempted third ventriculostomy not succeed, a ventriculostomy can be easily placed. Multiple approaches to the various ventricles have been described, and these approaches are beyond the scope of this chapter.

32.3.1
Tumors of Non-Neuronal or Glial Origin

32.3.1.1
Ependymoma

Ependymomas are neoplasms of the ependymal lining, represent about 1–2% of all intracranial tumors and about 5% of all primary brain tumors. They commonly occur in children, but are also found, rarely, in adults. They arise throughout the entire CNS; always where there is an ependymal surface. In adults, the fourth ventricle is the most common location, and the third ventricle is rarely a reported site (Oppenheim et al. 1994). Ectopic tumors and extraneural metastases have been reported, but are exceedingly rare (Newton et al. 1992). Most intracranial ependymomas occur in children, and most spinal ependymomas occur in adults.

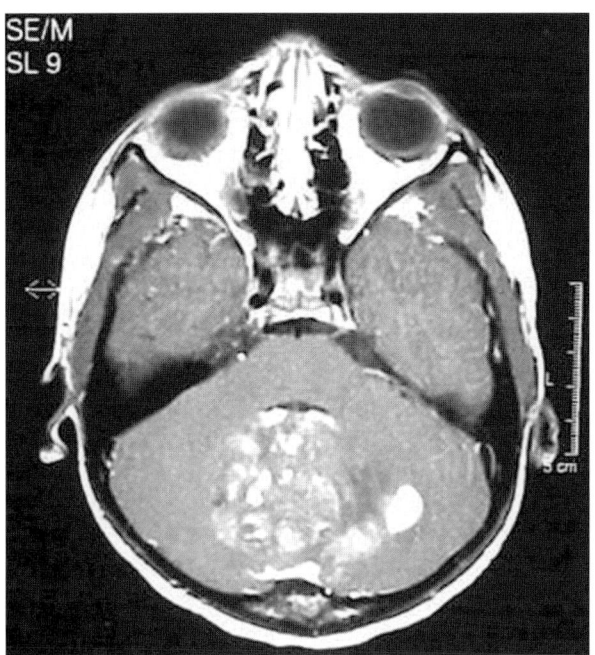

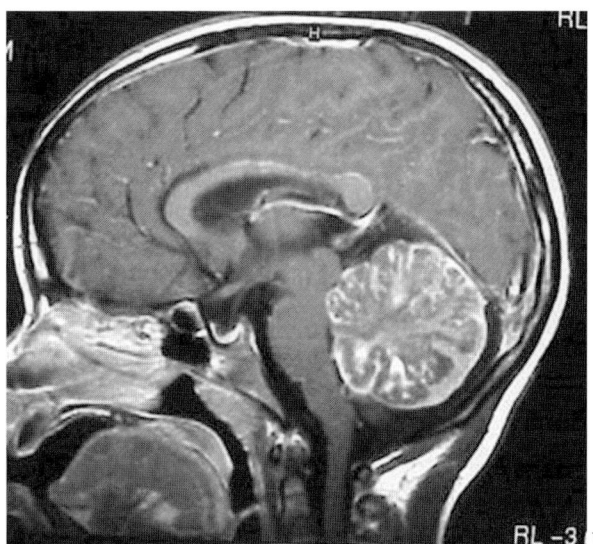

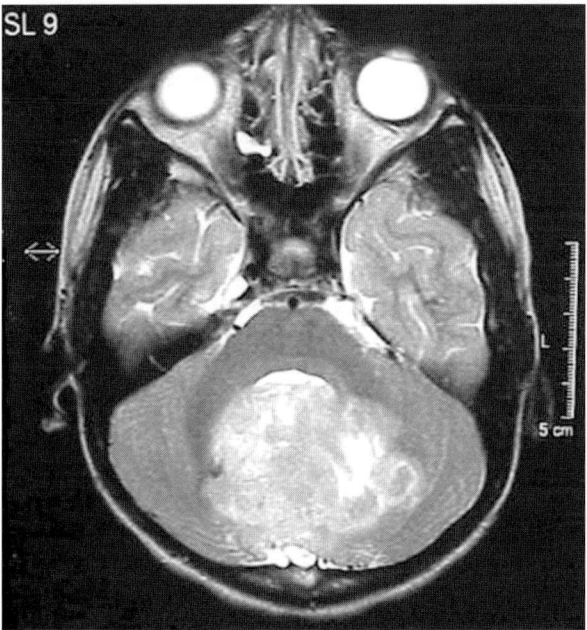

Fig. 32.6a,b. Lhermitte-Duclos disease. **a** Axial T1WI with gadolinium shows a discrete heterogeneous mass. **b** Sagittal T1WI with contrast reveals a more diffuse enlargement of the cerebellar folia. **c** T2WI does not show the classic "tiger stripes," commocly seen in this uncommon condition

32.3.1.1.1

CLINICAL PRESENTATION

Patients may present with symptoms of increased intracranial pressure or of hydrocephalus, acute or compensated. Cranial nerve deficits can also be seen, due to the proximity of these tumors to the brain stem when these tumors occur in the fourth ventricle (Fig. 32.7).

MRI reveals a lobulated tumor, frequently intraventricular or periventricular, that is discrete and enhances with contrast. It tends to be hypo- or isointense on T1WI and hyperintense on T2WI. The tumor classically has a plastic appearance, filling the shape of the involved ventricular spaces. These tumors tend to displace rather than invade brain tissue.

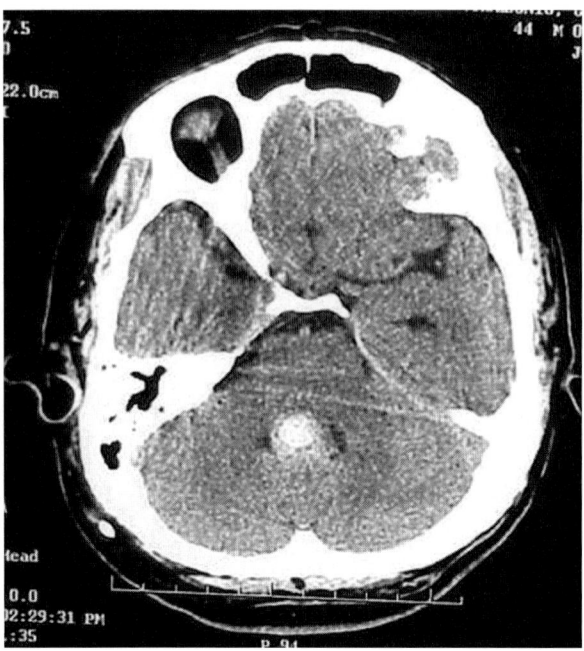

Fig. 32.7. Ependymoma. Axial NCECT shows a discreet hyperdense mass in the fourth ventricle

CT: The tumors are usually isodense and are frequently large, cystic, calcified, and periventricular (FURIE and PROVENZALE 1995). Greater than 50% will show calcification, a characteristic uncommon with medulloblastomas (PNETs).

32.3.1.1.2
HISTOLOGICAL FEATURES
True ependymal rosettes and perivascular pseudorosettes are seen on microscopic evaluation. However, the latter is a more frequent and important diagnostic feature. Tumors with two or more of the following: mitotic figures, hypercellularity, vascular proliferation, necrosis, are more likely to behave aggressively (Prayson 1999).

32.3.1.1.3
SURGICAL TREATMENT
Gross total excision is the goal of surgery and can often be achieved now with the advent of advanced microsurgical equipment and techniques, and intraoperative image-guidance systems. When total excision cannot be achieved, elective second-look surgery has been proposed as a reasonable option (Foreman et al. 1997). Suboccipital craniectomy is performed for fourth-ventricular tumors. Many patients with tumors in this location will also require ventriculoperitoneal shunting. Peritoneal metastasis

has been reported, but is exceedingly rare. Local recurrence has historically been the rule, but gross total excision has been reported to result in cure on an increasingly more frequent basis. Together with adjuvant therapy, long-term survival is now common in a tumor previously regarded as rapidly fatal.

32.3.1.1.4
ADJUVANT THERAPY
Focal radiotherapy is recommended after resection of the tumor, regardless of the extent of the resection. Less than 5% of ependymomas disseminate through the CSF. In such unfortunate cases, a combination of radiation to the entire neuraxis and chemotherapy has been used to extend survival. Local recurrence is treated with further surgery, stereotactic radiosurgery, or chemotherapy.

32.3.1.2
Subependymoma

Subependymomas are benign tumors associated with the ventricular system and its lining. The exact incidence of these tumors is unknown because of their extremely indolent nature, with few such lesions actually requiring surgical attention. This tumor is included here, not only because of its rarity, but also because of the rarity for necessary surgical intervention. Indeed, most of these tumors are noted in the postmortem. They are sporadic in nature but rare familial occurrences have been reported (RYKEN et al. 1994; CLARENBACH et al. 1979).

32.3.1.2.1
CLINICAL PRESENTATION
Most of these lesions never cause symptoms. A rare lateral ventricular tumor may cause hydrocephalus if large enough or if in close proximity to the foramen of Monro (IQBAL and SUTCLIFFE 1994). In the fourth ventricle, these tumors may compress the brain stem and cause cranial nerve deficits, weakness, incoordination, or hydrocephalus. Sudden deaths have been reported (RYDER et al. 1986), but these are rare.

CT shows these lesions to be hypo- to isodense to brain parenchyma (LOBATO et al. 1986). Calcification can be seen, especially in tumors of the fourth ventricle (CHIECHI et al. 1995). Minimal to no enhancement should be present. An intraventricular location is typical (STEVENS et al. 1984).

On MRI, the tumors are homogeneously hypo- to isointense on T1WI, and hyperintense on T2WI (SPOTO et al. 1990). Also, subependymomas tend to have little or no associated edema and have little or no contrast enhancement (HOEFFEL et al. 1995). These tumors may be difficult to differentiate from ependymomas on radiographic characteristics alone (Fig. 32.8). A tissue sample is required for definitive diagnosis.

32.3.1.2.2
HISTOLOGICAL FEATURES

A paucicellular glial neoplasm with a fibrillary stroma is commonly seen. Mitosis can be seen in half of all specimens of subependymomas, despite the indolent nature of the tumor, and is not related to prognosis or survival (Lombardi et al. 1991). Microcystic changes can also be seen. Neovascularity, necrosis, pseudorosettes, and true rosettes should not be seen.

32.3.1.2.3
SURGICAL TREATMENT

Surgical excision of these tumors is limited to symptomatic cases. Tumors of the fourth ventricle may be difficult to resect completely (JOOMA et al. 1985). Shunting may be required in some cases. For lesions associated with the foramen of Monro, endoscopic biopsy followed by ventriculoperitoneal shunting may be a good option in some patients.

32.3.1.2.4
ADJUVANT THERAPY

Adjuvant therapy is not employed for subependymomas, except in cases of symptomatic residual or recurrent tumor (LOMBARDI et al. 1991). Anaplastic

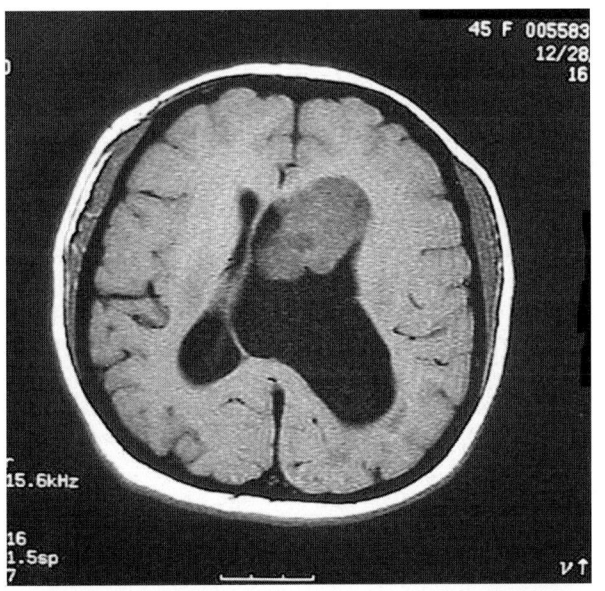
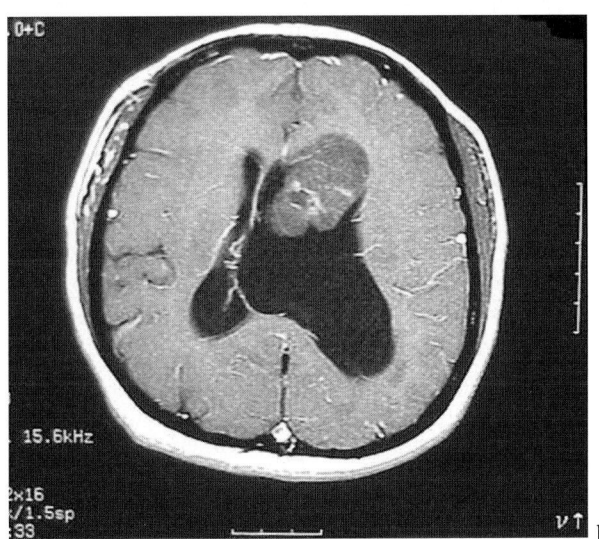
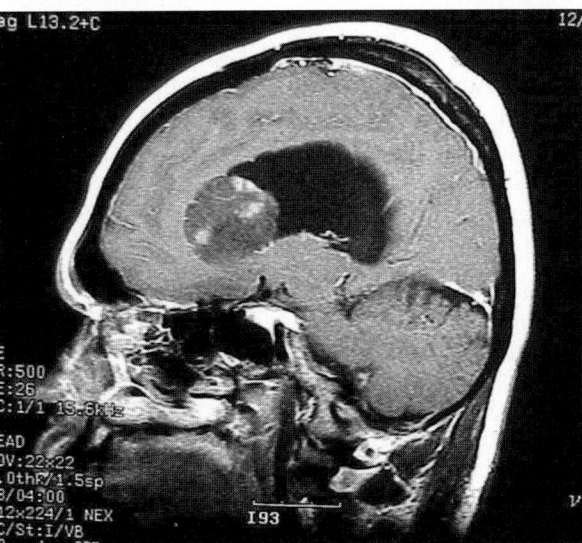

Fig. 32.8a–d. Subependymoma. a–c Various T1WI with (b,c) and without (a) gadolinium; d FLAIR. Note the dilated left lateral ventricle due to obstruction of the foramen of Monro

transformation has not been reported. However, highly vascularized tumors have been reported (LINDBOE et al. 1992). Also, patients with mixed features of ependymoma have a higher mortality rate and should be treated more aggressively with adjuvant therapy (SCHEITHAUER 1978).

32.3.1.3
Choroid Plexus Tumors

Choroid plexus tumors include the choroid plexus papilloma and carcinoma. These tumors tend to occur in children before the age of 5 years. However, adult cases have also been reported. These tumors account for about 10–20% of intracranial tumors in patients under the age of 1 year, but represent only about 3% of all pediatric brain tumors. In adults, they represent 0.5% of all brain tumors. These tumors tend to occur in the lateral ventricle, in children, with the left side more often affected than the right. In adults, the fourth ventricle is the most common site of involvement. Isolated case reports have reported occurrence in the third ventricle, where no choroid plexus exists (NAKANO et al. 1997; COSTA et al. 1997; SHUTO et al. 1995). CPA tumors have also been reported (TASDEMIROGLU et al. 1996; CHAN et al. 1983). Symptoms of hydrocephalus usually present patients to medical attention. The hydrocephalus can be caused by obstruction of CSF efflux from the ventricular system, overproduction of CSF (CASEY and VRIES 1989), or less likely, by decreased CSF absorption.

Radiographic studies include: CT: These heterogeneous lobulated lesions tend to be hyperdense and may be calcified. Intense enhancement is found. Vasogenic edema is sometimes found surrounding the carcinomas, suggesting stromal invasion. MRI: These well-demarcated tumors are hypo- to isointense on T1 and T2, and enhance intensely (Fig. 32.9).

Histologically, the tumors resemble normal choroid plexus, having numerous frond-like papillae composed of columnar or cuboidal epithelium.

32.3.1.3.1
SURGICAL TREATMENT
Complete surgical excision of these tumors is the goal of any operative procedure. Access to the lateral ventricles can be attained transcortically or interhemispherically if the lesion is medially located. Access to the fourth ventricle can be attained via a suboccipital craniotomy and retraction of the cerebellum. Sometimes, the inferior portion of the vermis is split to allow visualization of the rostral-most portion of the fourth ventricle. As with any surgery involving a mass affecting the ventricular system, a shunting procedure may be necessary either in the acute perioperative stage or even permanently. Preoperative shunting has been performed to treat hydrocephalus prior to surgical excision (RAIMONDI and TOMITA 1981). This procedure, once common, is no longer the usual surgical tactic. The fears of upward herniation and peritoneal seeding, coupled with a possible shunt infection, and the possibility that the patient may be shunt-independent postoperatively, have led surgeons to perform third ventriculostomies, or to leave external ventricular drainage devices after tumor excision. In patients with external drainage, the need for permanent shunting is evaluated during the postoperative course.

32.3.1.3.2
ADJUVANT THERAPY
Radiation therapy or chemotherapy is not considered postoperatively in patients with choroid plexus papilloma (CPP) and total excisional surgery. Some authors believe that radiation therapy is indicated for subtotal excision (Sharma et al. 1994). Radiation following recurrence of CPP is better-accepted (McGirr et al. 1988). Also, radiosurgery has been used to treat CPPs in difficult-to-access regions of the brain (Duke et al. 1997); however, total surgical excision of a CPP is generally considered to be a cure (Pencalet et al. 1998). The use of adjuvant therapy is considered in cases of choroid plexus carcinoma (CPC). Chemotherapy has been used after surgical excision of CPC, whether total or partial, and has been found to reduce the rate of tumor recurrence (Pencalet et al. 1998). However, the amount of excision of CPC has been found to be the prominent factor in prognosis and recurrence (Berger et al. 1998; Packer et al. 1992). Postoperative chemotherapy and delayed radiation have been found to produce long-term survival in children with less than a gross total excision of CPC (Duffner et al. 1995). Radiotherapy has also been used, but is not given to infants under a certain age, because of the ill- effects of radiation on the development of the brain (Carpenter et al. 1982).

32.3.1.4
Colloid Cyst

Colloid cysts are histologically benign masses associated frequently with the anterior third ventricle. This endodermally derived structure is lined with epithelium and is commonly found in the anterosuperior portion of the third ventricle, with an attach-

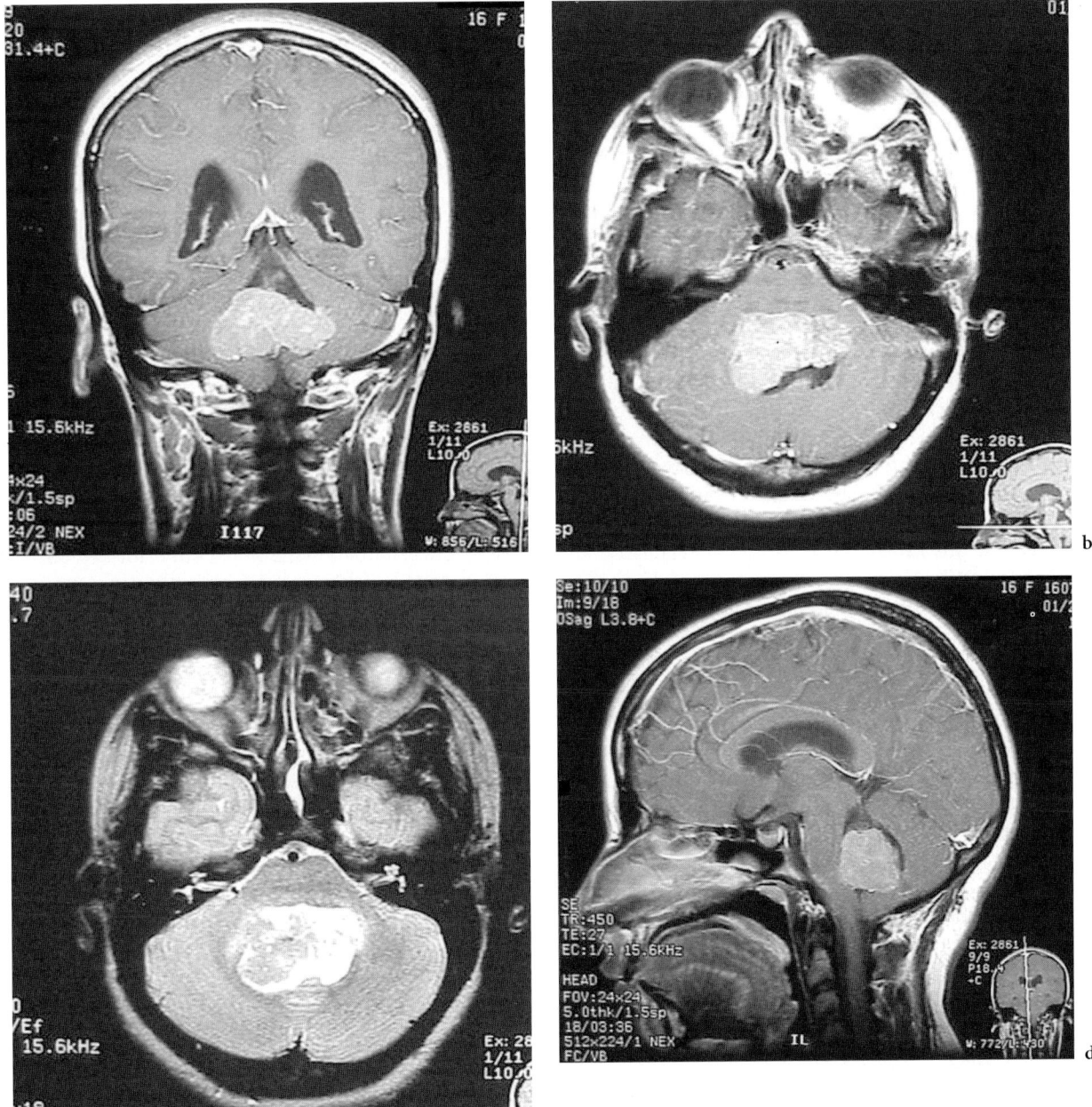

Fig. 32.9a-d. Choroid plexus papilloma. Axial, coronal and sagittal images demonstrate this tumor very well. The fourth ventricle is the most common location for this tumor in the adult. Note the relationship of the tumor to the floor of the ventricle

ment between the columns of the fornices (Lach et al. 1993). These cysts, however, may be found elsewhere in the brain, including the parenchyma, other ventricles, and the subarachnoid space (Muller et al. 1999). Colloid cysts contain dense, viscous fluid with varying other deposits such as CSF, hemosiderin, cholesterol, and various ions. They are almost entirely found sporadically in adults, but familial cases have been reported (Akins et al. 1996) as have pediatric cases (Macdonald et al. 1994).

32.3.1.4.1
CLINICAL PRESENTATION
Colloid cysts are known to cause hydrocephalus by blocking the foramina of Monro, due to their strategic location. The blockage may be intermittent as the

cyst falls in and out of position like a ball-valve. Intermittent headaches are the usual complaint. Well-heeded are the reports of sudden death in patients with colloid cysts with acute hydrocephalus (ARONICA et al. 1998; BUTTNER et al. 1997). Recent experience suggests that sudden death may not be as common as previously thought.

CT appearance of colloid cysts in the absence of frank hydrocephalus may be subtle. The cysts may range in size from mere millimeters to over a centimeter in diameter. Small cysts may be missed because of too great an interval between images. Others may be missed because they may be isodense in comparison with the associated ventricular spaces. MRI identification of colloid cysts is based more on the shape and location, and less on signal-intensity. Usually, any round cystic structure in the anterosuperior third ventricle is expected to be a colloid cyst. On T1, colloid cysts may range from low to high intensity. The same variances are noted on T2 studies. Peripheral enhancement of colloid cysts may occur; solid enhancement suggests another diagnosis (Fig. 32.10).

32.3.1.4.2
SURGICAL TREATMENT

The decision to excise these lesions surgically has long been made, upon discovery. Due to the purported risk of sudden death, few patients refuse surgical intervention. However, smaller cysts found incidentally which are asymptomatic, may no longer be sure surgical candidates, especially in patients with poor expected survival from other medical illnesses. The risk of surgery and the expected benefits, or in this case, the expected reduction of the chance of neurological catastrophe, should be clearly defined prior to surgical excision of this slow-growing benign lesion. Pollock and Huston (1999) have suggested that asymptomatic colloid cysts can be safely watched with serial neuroimaging, with surgical intervention only with cyst enlargement or with the development of symptoms or hydrocephalus.

Open surgical excision of this lesion is usually performed via an interhemispheric transcallosal approach (MATHIESEN et al. 1997; APUZZO et al. 1982). Access via the lateral ventricle can also be utilized via a transcortical approach. The approach selected depends upon each specific case, with each method having both advantages and disadvantages. The transcallosal approach provides for excellent exposure, but requires the cutting of a portion of the corpus callosum, which may manifest postoperatively as difficulties with short-term memory. Intraoperative risks include damage to the superior sagittal sinus, anterior cerebral artery distribution strokes, and intraventricular hemorrhage. The transcortical approach is implemented by first performing a frontal craniotomy in the non-dominant hemisphere. A cortisectomy is performed in the frontal lobe using the same trajectory as if to perform a ventriculostomy. This point can be determined grossly by using surface markings. One centimeter anterior to the coronal suture and 2.5 cm lateral to the sagittal suture will grossly estimate the proper placement of the cortisectomy. The cortex is then spread or resected to reach the frontal horn of the lateral ventricle. Once within the ventricle, self-retaining retractors

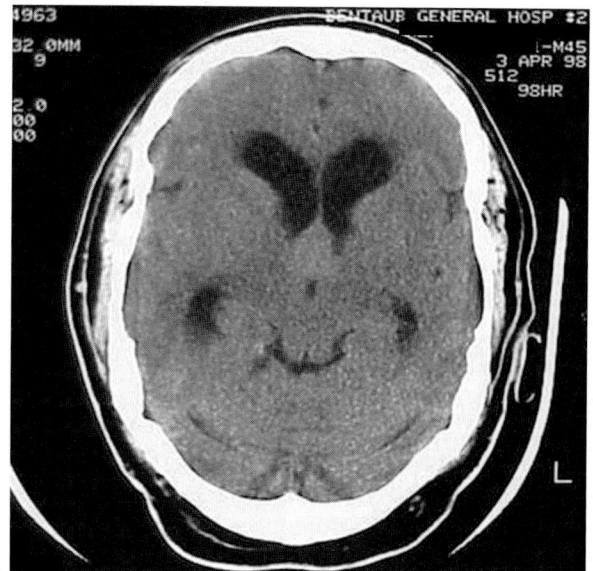

a

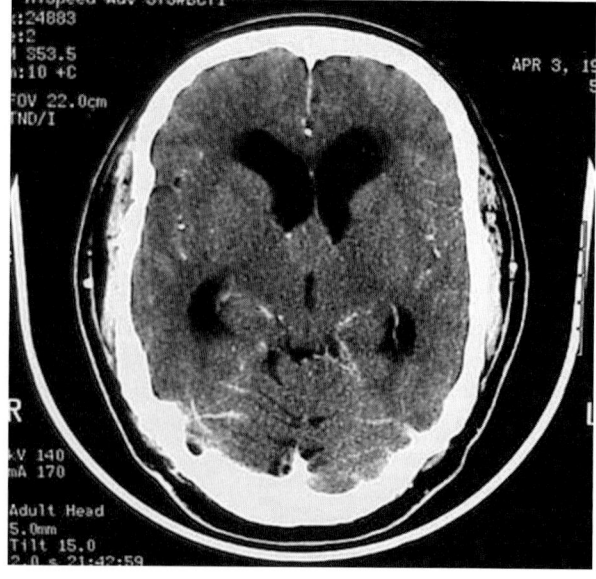

b

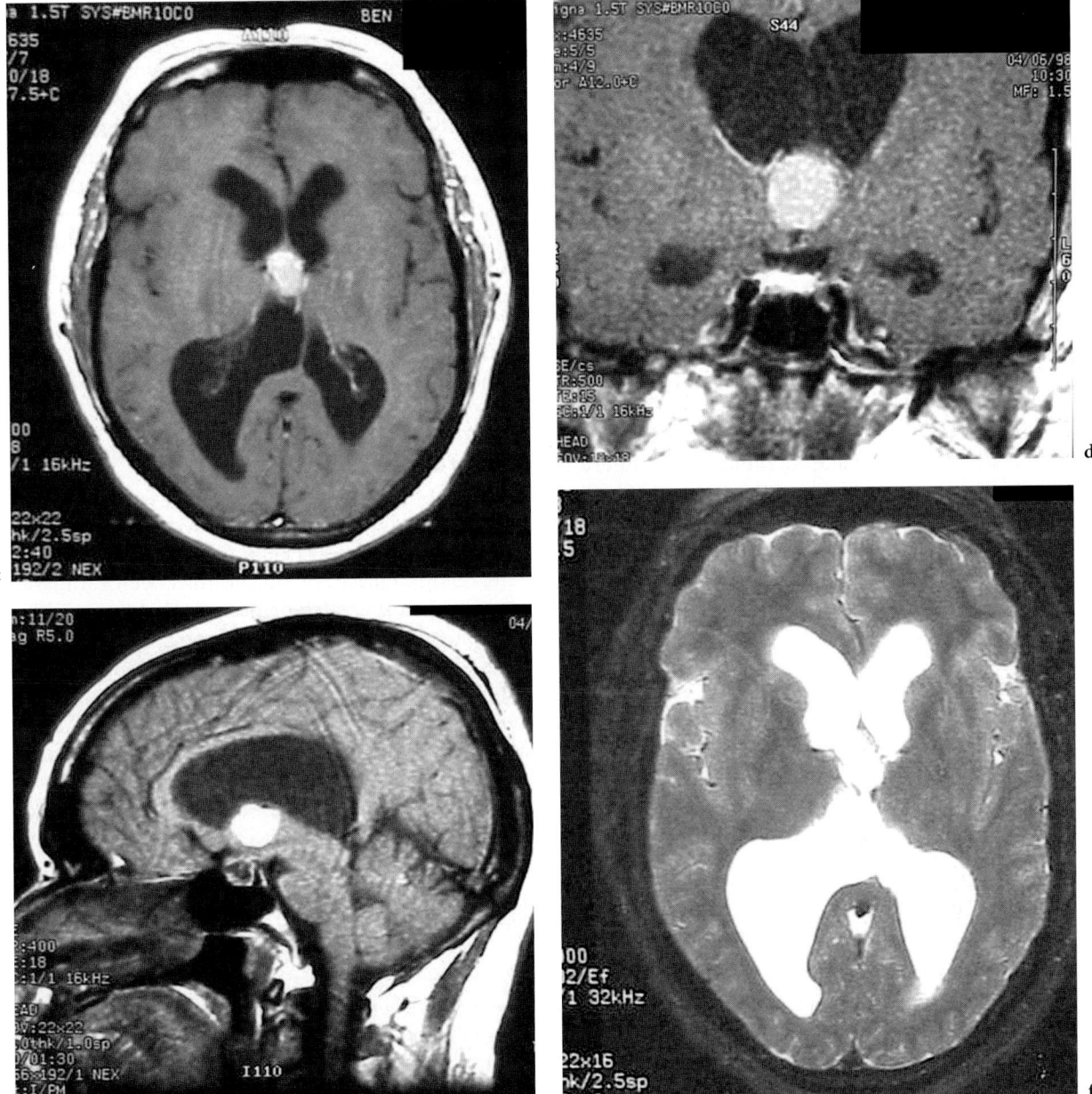

Fig. 32.10a–f. Colloid cyst, **a, b** Lesion appears to be grossly isodense to brain on axial NCE and CECT. **c, d** T1WI with gadolinium are not significantly different from **e** non-enhanced studies. **f** T2WI

are used to maintain visualization of the lateral ventricular structures. The colloid cyst should then be seen through the foramen of Monro, and is thereby resected. Disadvantages to this approach include the necessity to dissect through normal brain tissue. The largest advantage is that there is little risk for short-term memory loss.

Stereotactic aspiration and variations of stereotactic treatments have also been employed for the treatment of colloid cysts with excellent results (APUZZO et al. 1984; RIVAS and LOBATO 1985; KONDZIOLKA and LUNSFORD 1991; KUMAR et al. 1998; CABBELL and ROSS 1996; ABERNATHEY et al. 1989; HALL and LUNSFORD 1987; MOHADJER et al. 1987). However, aspiration alone has been associated with recurrent colloid accumulation, persistent symptoms, and failure to achieve decompression (MATHIESEN et al. 1993).

Recently, neuroendoscopic approaches have been reported to be successful in the complete excision of colloid cysts (Abdou and Cohen 1998; Decq et al. 1998; Gaab and Schoeder 1998; King et al. 1999; Lewis et al. 1994). Through a frontal burrhole, an endoscope is placed transcortically into the non-dominant side lateral ventricle. The third ventricle is then accessed through the foramen of Monro. The endoscopic approach to colloid cysts has advantages over stereotactic methods, including giving the surgeon the ability to excise the entire cyst, the ability to control intraoperative intraventricular hemorrhage if any, and the ability to perform third ventriculostomy at the same operation. Advantages of endoscopy over open craniotomy include smaller risk of memory deficits, less invasive surgery, and shorter recovery time. The main drawback to endoscopic surgery is that it is difficult to perform in the absence of hydrocephalus. Though a new procedure with few long-term results, endoscopic resection appears already to be a strong alternative to the classic open transcallosal approach, and may replace stereotactic methods as the minimally invasive surgery of choice. Further improvement in technology and a growing number of neurosurgeons trained and experienced in the use of such instruments, suggest that open craniotomy for the treatment of colloid cysts may be indicated only in the absence of hydrocephalus.

32.3.1.5
Chordoid Glioma

A recently described entity, chordoid glioma is a tumor associated with the third ventricle. Only about 15 cases have been reported in the literature. Clinically, this tumor is unusual in that it has been most frequently associated with middle-aged women. It also has characteristic radiological findings including its peculiar location in the third ventricle, strong enhancement, and occasional cystic component (Tonami et al. 2000). Figure 32.11 demonstrates a typical example of chordoid glioma of the third ventricle. Surgically, the tumor tends to have discrete margins and has little tendency to infiltrate surrounding brain parenchyma. Histologically, chordoid gliomas are striking for their slight resemblance to chordomas, having clusters of epitheloid cells with abundant cytoplasm and uniform nuclei; intermixed are lymphocytes are plasma cells (Brat et al. 1998). Immunohistochemically, the cells are strongly positive for GFAP and vimentin (Reifenberger et al. 1999), and negative for EMA (Vajtai et al. 1999). There is no evidence for neuronal differentiation.

The natural history of this tumor is yet unknown. In the largest series (Brat et al., 1998), eight patients were reported, with gross total excision performed in two cases. Two patients with subtotal resection died within 3 years of surgery. The remaining patients have no disease, stable disease, or were lost to follow-up. There are no published reports of the use of adjuvant therapy, but radiotherapy should probably be considered in subtotal resections and recurrent disease.

32.3.2
Tumors of Neuronal Origin

32.3.2.1
Central Neurocytoma

Central neurocytoma, a recently described tumor of neuronal origin, has generally been considered a rare, benign entity. This tumor has been estimated to comprise 0.1% of all primary brain tumors, characteristically sporadically occurring in young adults from 20–40 years old; however, cases in more elderly patients have been reported (Ferreol et al. 1989). Previously to its designation, this tumor was likely to have been diagnosed as an intraventricular oligodendroglioma; however, with the advent of modern staining techniques, these tumors were found to be separate entities, differentiating along neuronal lines. Central neurocytomas classically are ventricular tumors closely associated with the septum pellucidum and the foramen of Monro. Other locations including the posterior fossa and the spinal axis have also been reported, though rarely (Enam et al. 1997; Tatter et al. 1994). Malignant behavior, recurrence, and dissemination have been reported recently, suggesting that this tumor may occasionally not be as benign as previously thought (Eng et al. 1997; Kim et al. 1996; Yasargil et al. 1992). A report of differentiation into ganglioglioma has also been made (Schweitzer and Davies 1997).

Patients tend to present with symptoms of hydrocephalus secondary to the blockage of CSF flow from the lateral ventricles (Fig. 32.12). Headaches, nausea, and vomiting are common.

Radiographic findings are follows:

MRI: heterogeneous signal, to isointense to gray matter on T1 with moderate to strong contrast enhancement (Wichmann et al. 1991).

CT: calcifications may be present in about 50% of cases.

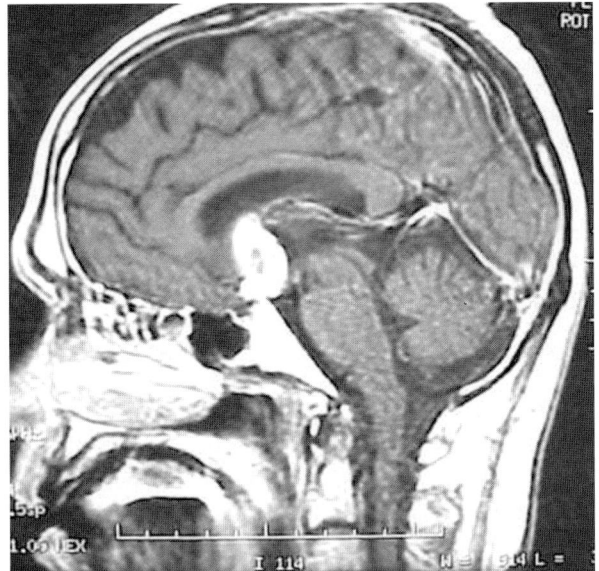

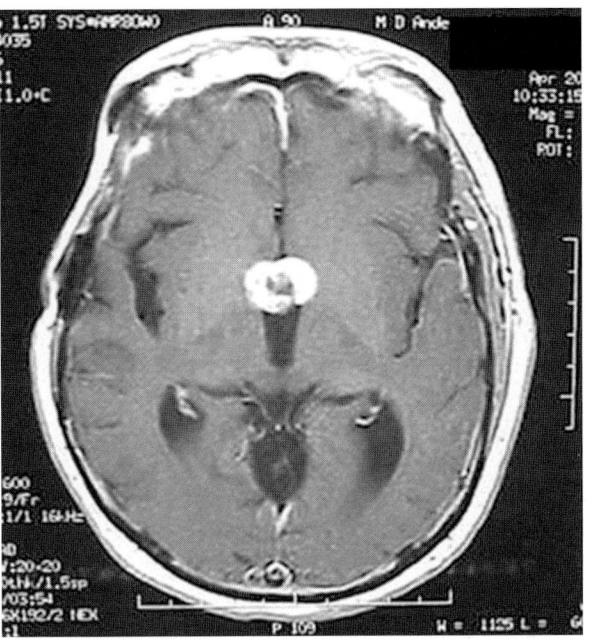

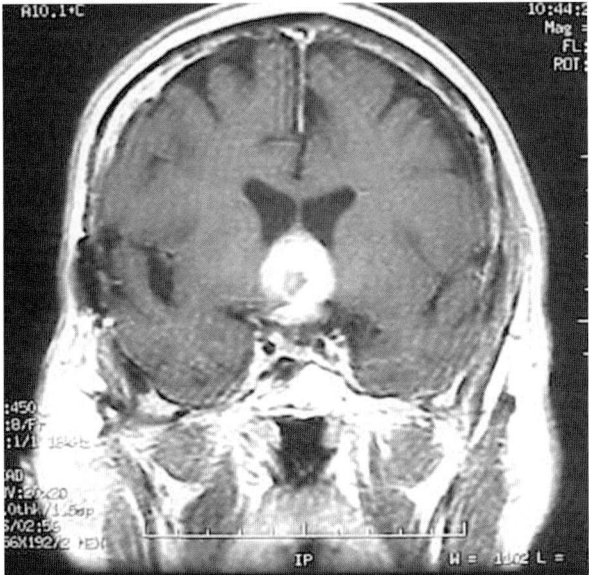

Fig. 32.11a–c. - Chordoid glioma. These post-contrast T1WI show intense enhancement of the third ventricular mass with a central necrotic region. This patient was unusual in that he was male

32.3.2.1.1
HISTOLOGICAL FINDINGS

Central neurocytomas are well-circumscribed tumors, usually grayish in color. The tumor is comprised of small monotonous blue cells with prominent areas of perivascular zones of fibrillarity. Artifactual perinuclear halo formation can also be seen, mimicking oligodendroglioma. Multinucleation and pleomorphism are absent and mitoses are rare, if at all seen. The nuclei exhibit small nucleoli and fine chromatin.

Immunohistochemical features show synaptophysin reactivity in the perivascular fibrillar zones as being the rule. GFAP reactivity is limited to few scattered reactive astrocytes.

32.3.2.1.2
TREATMENT

Surgical treatment is preferred The classic tumor, associated with the septum pellucidum and foramen of Monro, can usually be excised completely via a transcallosal approach. Alternatively, a transcortical-transventricular approach may be employed. Endoscopic excision through this method may also be considered. The classic transcallosal technique is described briefly. A variety of relatively small frontal incisions may be employed for a midline frontal craniotomy situated over the coronal suture. Generally, two-thirds of the craniotomy is placed anterior to the coronal suture. This placement is a result of a

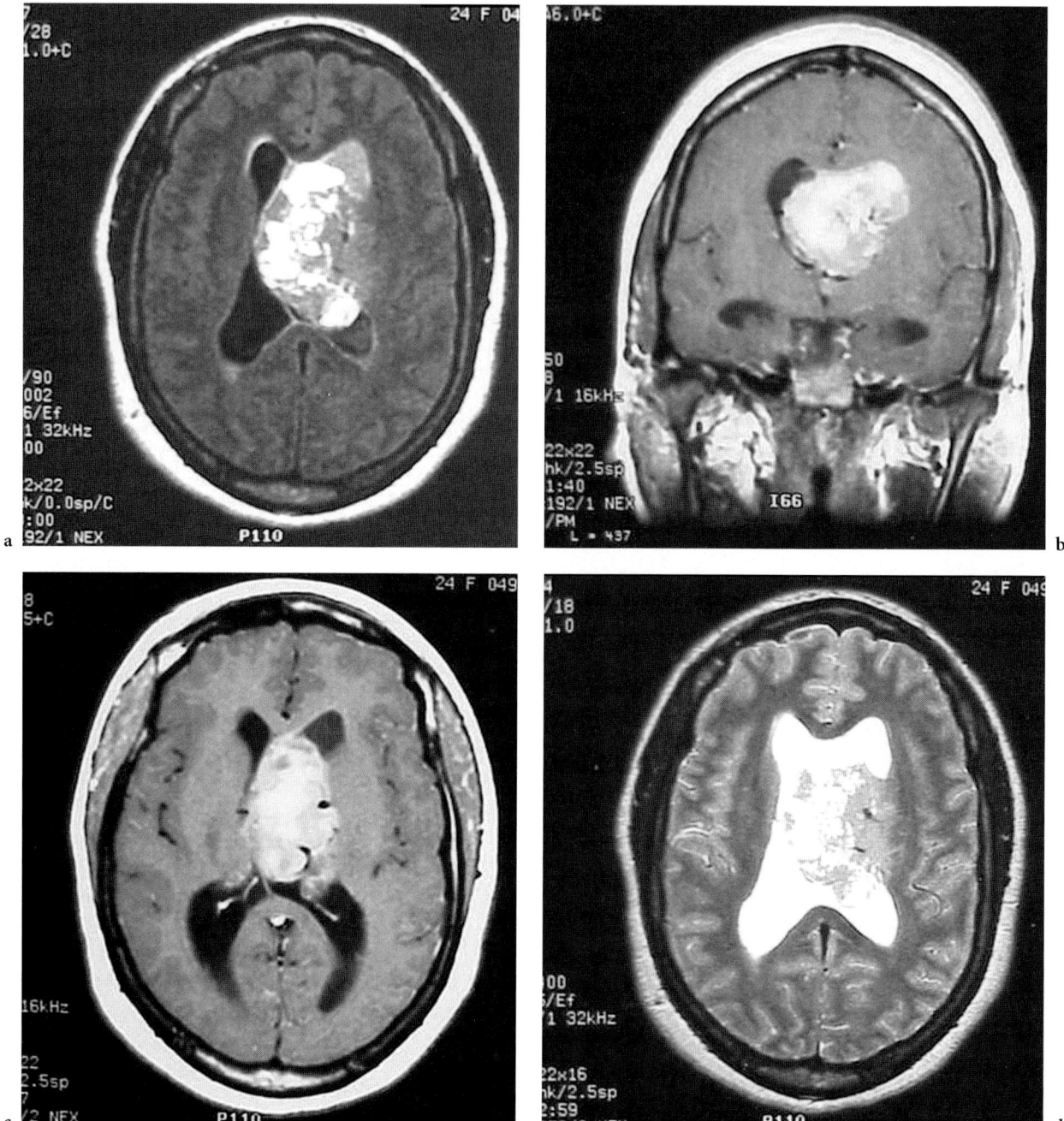

Fig. 32.12a–d. Central neurocytoma. **a** FLAIR, **b, c** T1WI with gadolinium, and **d** T2WI show a large heterogeneous lesion with mild associated hydrocephalus. **c** Note the flow voids; these vessels were not associated with the tumor and were spared during surgery

compromise between appropriate exposure and acceptable neurological deficits secondary to the callosotomy. A more-posterior location for the surgical exposure may lead to unacceptable neurological sequelae, and a more-anterior exposure may compromise the surgery itself. Care is taken to preserve bridging veins to the superior sagittal sinus and of course,

the sinus itself. Self-retaining retractors are used to expose the corpus callosum. The anterior cerebral arteries are identified and protected. After the callosotomy is performed, the tumor is easily identified and differentiated from brain and choroid plexus. The well-circumscribed tumor may be removed by a variety of methods, but usually can be easily removed using a combination of the suction catheter and the bipolar cautery. The ventricular system is carefully irrigated after tumor removal to minimize retained ventricular blood. Residual blood clot may complicate the postoperative sequence. During the surgery, a ventriculostomy is usually placed after the excision of the tumor to control postoperative hydrocephalus if present. The ventriculostomy may be left open to drainage at a certain level or placed to monitor, and drained only if the intracranial pressure exceeds a certain reading. Should continued CSF drainage via the ventriculostomy be necessary, the patient may require conversion to a more permanent shunting system. An excessive or poorly placed callosotomy may result in deficits in short term memory.

Chemotherapy has not been used to treat this tumor. Radiation therapy may be used in rare cases of recurrence, dissemination, and malignancy. Unfortunately, there are no data regarding adjuvant therapy in treating central neurocytomas at this time.

32.3.3
Pineal Region Tumors

Pineal region tumors, representing about 1% of all brain tumors, are an interesting group of neoplasms. More commonly found in children, they can also be found in adults, though rarely. There is also a male preponderance (Cho et al. 1998). Tumors derived from the pineal gland, including pineocytomas and pineoblastomas are uncommon. The most frequently diagnosed type is the germ-cell tumor, including the germinomas, (Fig. 32.13) teratomas, yolk-sac tumors, and choriocarcinoma. Germinomas are most common, followed by teratomas (Fig. 32.14). Because of the wide range of tumor-type in this region of the brain, definitive histological diagnosis is of great importance in determining the treatment plan.

The pineal area represents a challenging zone to access, for the neurosurgeon. Complete resection of a tumor in this region is difficult to achieve. Certainly, an attempt to obtain complete resection comes with great risks, no matter what approach is employed, due to the central location of the region and its important and delicate constituents. Historically, the morbidity associated with surgery in this area showed that the best survival rate was found in patients who were shunted and received radiation only (Abay et al. 1981). Others opted for trial radiotherapy. With the advent of new microsurgical tools and techniques as well as image-guidance systems, however, a push to maximally resect these tumors was renewed (Edwards et al. 1988). Again though, neurosurgery in this area seems to be evolving towards minimal invasion and minimum risk. Frequently, if the diagnosis of a tumor sensitive to adjuvant therapy can be made from spinal fluid markers or from a tissue biopsy, chemotherapy and radiotherapy are then employed as the mainstay of the treatment of these tumors. Further neurosurgical involvement may only include a shunting procedure should these patients so require. However, some neurosurgeons believe that extensive resection of these tumors still purports to a better prognosis (Edwards et al. 1988).

Alpha-fetoprotein (yolk sac tumor or embryonal carcinoma) and beta HCG (embryonal carcinoma or choriocarcinoma) have been shown to be useful in the diagnosis of pineal tumors. Germinomas and teratomas do not produce markers. Serum level of bHCG seems to correlate positively with germ-cell tumor growth and regression. However, the absence of elevated serum markers does not exclude germ-cell tumors. Detection of these markers in the CSF may obviate the need for tissue diagnosis (Choi et al. 1998); however, since morbidity for tissue diagnosis in these tumors is now lower, due to improved microsurgical techniques, biopsy at the very least has been suggested for all patients (Edwards et al. 1988; Kang et al. 1998; Linggood and Chapman 1992; Baumgartner and Edwards 1992). Access to CSF, however, is often limited because of the hydrocephalus that frequently accompanies tumors in this region (compression of the Aqueduct of Sylvius, preventing efflux of CSF from the third to fourth ventricle). Lumbar puncture in patients with obstructive hydrocephalus is contraindicated for the possibility of downward herniation of the brain. No consensus on the proper management of pineal tumors exists. Minimal invasive surgery via stereotactic biopsy or endoscopic biopsy has been suggested to be a reasonable first surgery in all cases of pineal tumors (Oi 1998; Dempsey and Lunsford 1992).

32.3.3.1
Clinical Presentation

A myriad of symptoms is possible in tumors of the pineal region. Symptoms of increased intracranial pressure from hydrocephalus are common when the aqueduct of Sylvius is compromised. Symptoms may include headache, lethargy, nausea, vomiting, or irritability. Clinically, patients may have papilledema on fundoscopic examination. Compression of the midbrain may result in a classic Parinaud's syndrome.

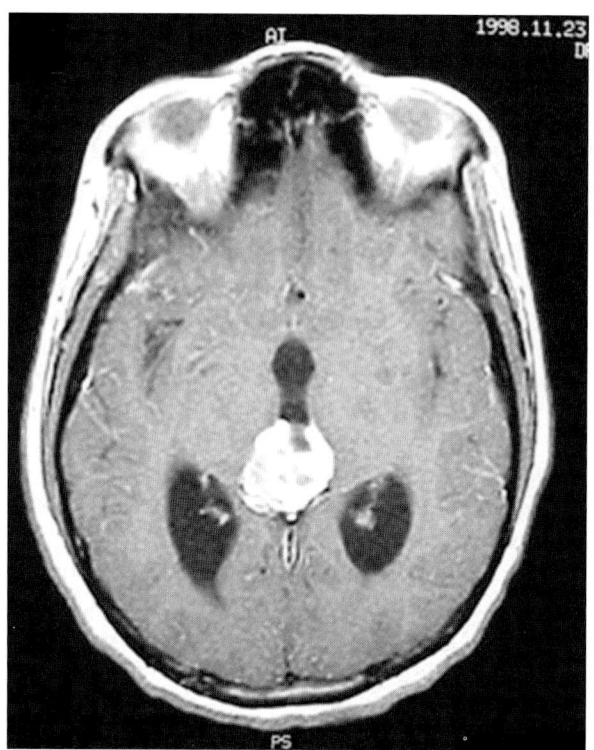

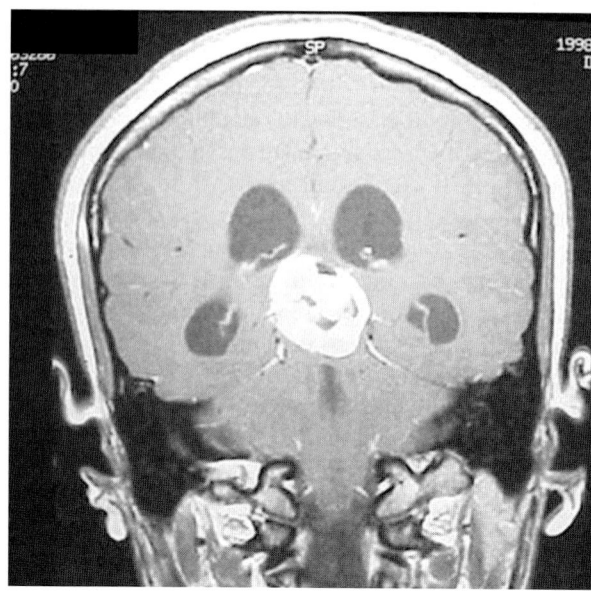

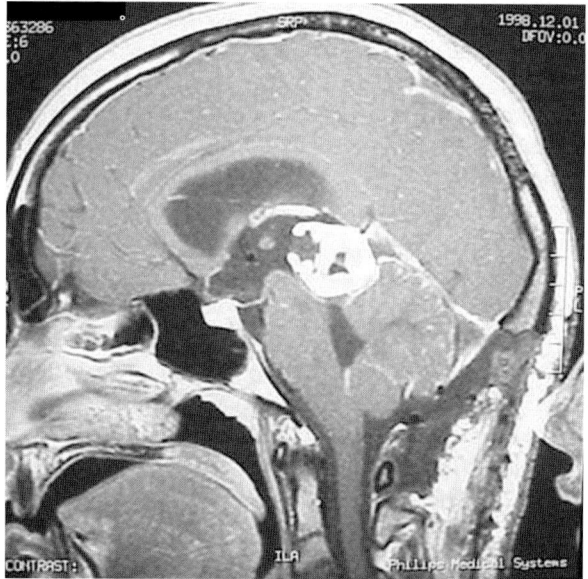

Fig. 32.13a–c. Germinoma of the pineal region. **a** axial, **b** sagittal and **c** coronal MR images. All images are with gadolinium. Patient underwent neuroendoscopic surgery. Her tumor was biopsied and a third ventriculostomy was performed through a right frontal burrhole

32.3.3.2
Radiological Studies

The radiographic appearance of these tumors is greatly varied. Though MRI has been useful in identifying pineal tumors and their relationship to surrounding anatomy, no definitive patterns of enhancement or imaging can obviate the necessity for tissue diagnosis, particularly important in this region due to the wide range of pathologies possible and their widely differing treatment protocols.

Consistencies in CT or MRI imaging for these tumors include the presence of hydrocephalus, posterior third ventricular mass, and often effacement of the brain stem (Fig. 32.13). Venous phase cerebral angiogram may show displacement of the deep venous systems.

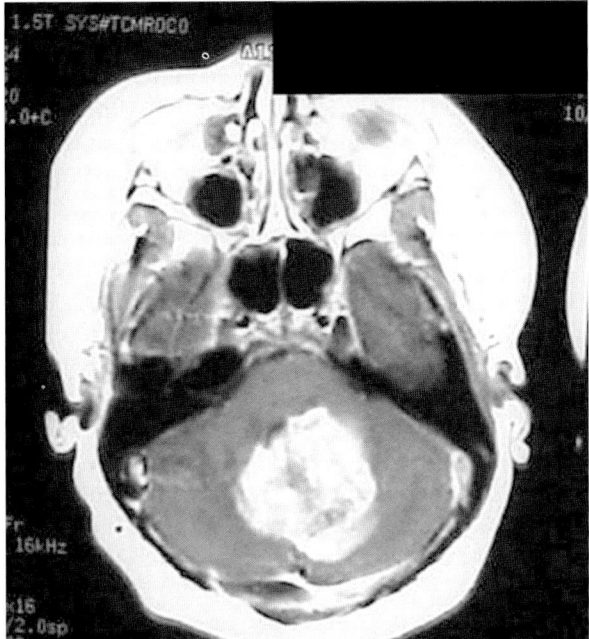

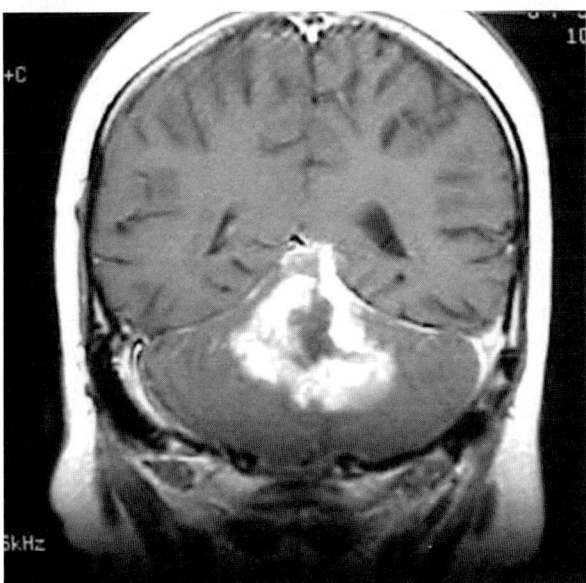

Fig. 32.14a,b. Axial and coronal images with gadolinium in a patient with malignant teratoma of the pineal region. This strongly enhancing tumor reveals a necrotic central zone

32.3.3.3
Surgical Treatment

Indications for surgery include the need for tissue diagnosis and tumor debulking. The extent of surgical excision completed depends heavily upon two factors: the histological type of tumor and the surgeon. Certainly, in tumors such as germinomas that respond so well to chemotherapy, minimal surgical

risk should be taken. That is, once tissue diagnosis of a pure germinoma is made, further resection is contraindicated (Sawamura et al. 1997; Hoffman et al. 1991). Most data regarding pineal region tumors are based on child- studies, given the far higher incidence of these tumors in this age group (Hoffman et al. 1991; Edwards et al. 1988; Drummond and Rosenfeld 1999). For other tumors, the risk involved in further resection of the tumor mass should be carefully compared with the expected benefits. Since individual surgical experience and skill may vary, there may be a discrepancy, from surgeon to surgeon, in the management of tumors in the pineal region.

There are many surgical options available. For tissue diagnosis, open biopsy allows for the gathering of larger specimens, and also decreases possible sampling error. Open biopsy can be performed by craniotomy and approaches may be supracerebellar, transtentorial, or interhemispheric. The first two methods, which are achieved with the patient in the sitting position, are the most common ones (Fukui et al. 1998). In the last approach, the patient is usually positioned prone. A combined supra- and infratentorial transsinus approach is sometimes needed for large pineal region tumors (Ziyal et al. 1998). All of these techniques have their advantages and disadvantages; however, they are all highly invasive and come with high risk. The risks involve air embolus (in the sitting position), damage to deep venous structures, damage to the cerebellum, bleeding in the pineal region, and general risks involved with extended procedures. A reduction of surgical risk may be realized by image-guided surgical systems (Saenz et al. 1998). Intraoperative MRI may replace image-guidance systems; however, this technology is still under investigation in limited centers. The high risk involved has increased interest in less invasive procedures for tissue diagnosis. Stereotactic biopsy may be considered. Some authors previously suggested that the management of all pineal region tumors should begin with stereotactic biopsy (Dempsey and Lunsford 1992). However, because of the proximity of the pineal region tumors to the ventricles and deep venous structures, the decrease in risk versus an open procedure is dubious. In experienced hands, this procedure may nevertheless be an acceptable alternative (Kreth et al. 1996; Popovic and Kelly 1993; Dempsey and Lunsford 1992). Also, the samples obtained are uniformly small and may often be nondiagnostic. Endoscopic biopsy is an increasingly popular route for biopsy, found to be effective in both tissue diagnosis, obtaining CSF for marker analysis, and the treatment of hydrocephalus (Ellenbogen and Moores 1997; Gaab and Schoeder 1998). Indeed, the days of trial radiotherapy are probably over (Baumgartner and Edwards 1992). Here, surgeons create a burrhole in the frontal region and introduce an endoscope into the lateral ventricle transcortically. The endoscope is then directed under direct vision through the foramen of Monroe into the third ventricle, from where it is aimed posteriorly to the back of the third ventricle, where pineal region tumors can frequently be seen bulging into the ventricle. Biopsies are then obtained through the endoscope. Though the specimens are small, positive visual confirmation of the biopsy site is ensured. Minor bleeding from the biopsy site or sites can be controlled either with cautery or extensive irrigation. Furthermore, a frontal ventriculostomy can be left in the same transcortical tract used for the endoscope, if CSF shunting is deemed necessary. An alternative to external shunting is the third ventriculostomy. This is a procedure that is also achieved through an endoscopic approach and can be completed during endoscopic biopsy of the pineal tumor. In this procedure, the floor of the third ventricle is fenestrated using a balloon catheter between the infundibular recess and the mammillary bodies. This fenestration creates a communication between the blocked ventricular system and the prepontine cistern, and typically remains open due to constant CSF flow and pressure. Failure of third ventriculostomies probably represents a communicating type with the defect at the level of the arachnoid granulations. The advantage of third ventriculostomy is that it mainly avoids the possible complications of standard ventriculoperitoneal shunting, such as failure or infection. Also, third ventriculostomy avoids the risk of extraneural metastasis to the peritoneum from the shunting of seeded CSF, occasionally reported (Apuzzo et al. 1982). The risk of third ventriculostomy is bleeding. Slight hemorrhage from the fenestrated ventricular floor can be easily controlled with extensive irrigation via the endoscope. However, damage to vessels in the prepontine, namely the basilar artery and its branches, can cause extensive uncontrollable bleeding. Bleeding in this area carries with it a poor prognosis.

32.3.3.4
Adjuvant Therapy

Adjuvant therapy plays a large role in the treatment of pineal region tumors, since complete surgical excision is not usually possible. Fortunately, the most common of these tumors, the germinoma, is extremely sensitive to radiation, with many treatment centers reporting a complete cure rate of 100%. Teratomas are more difficult to treat, because of their low incidence and the incomplete understanding of their natural history (SHAFFREY et al. 1996). Pineocytomas and pineoblastomas (Fig. 32.15) are treated with surgical excision, then XRT for residual tumor. Greater than 50 Gy are recommended in this setting (SCHILD et al. 1993). Pineocytomas, which are cystic and calcified, have a good prognosis after surgical removal (VAQUERO et al. 1990). Chemotherapy should also be considered in patients with pineoblastoma; however, because of the rarity of these tumors and related literature, its usefulness is unclear.

Some authors believe that chemotherapy is reasonable for all germinoma patients with ventriculoperitoneal shunts for possible seeding of the peritoneal space (ONO et al. 1994; SMITH et al. 1991). This risk, though, is considered small, since the incidence of such seeding is exceedingly rare.

Some authors suggest that pretreatment with chemotherapy, for patients with positive markers is indicated (HERMANN et al. 1994; USHIO et al. 1999). Once serum marker levels are normalized, debulking of the tumor is performed, followed by radiotherapy (HERMANN et al. 1994). Neoadjuvant chemotherapy using various combinations in conjunction with radiotherapy has been used to treat patients with highly malignant pineal tumors (GHIM et al. 1993; ALLEN et al. 1987; KURISAKA et al. 1998; MATSUTANI et al. 1998). However, a consensus treatment standard does not exist for non-germinomatous malignant pineal region tumors.

Intracranial germinomas are known to be extremely sensitive to radiation therapy, with most authors reporting complete recovery in the majority or all cases (FRANZINI et al. 1998; HUH et al. 1996). Prophylactic craniospinal irradiation is also a reasonable option for patients with positive CSF cytology. Placement of radioactive seeds (192-iridium) into pineal tumors has also been explored, though incompletely.

32.4
Dural-Based Tumors

Patients with dural-based tumors present with symptoms of mass effect. Compression of the adjacent brain tissue may cause cortical dysfunction or seizure activity. Larger lesions may cause alterations in mental status.

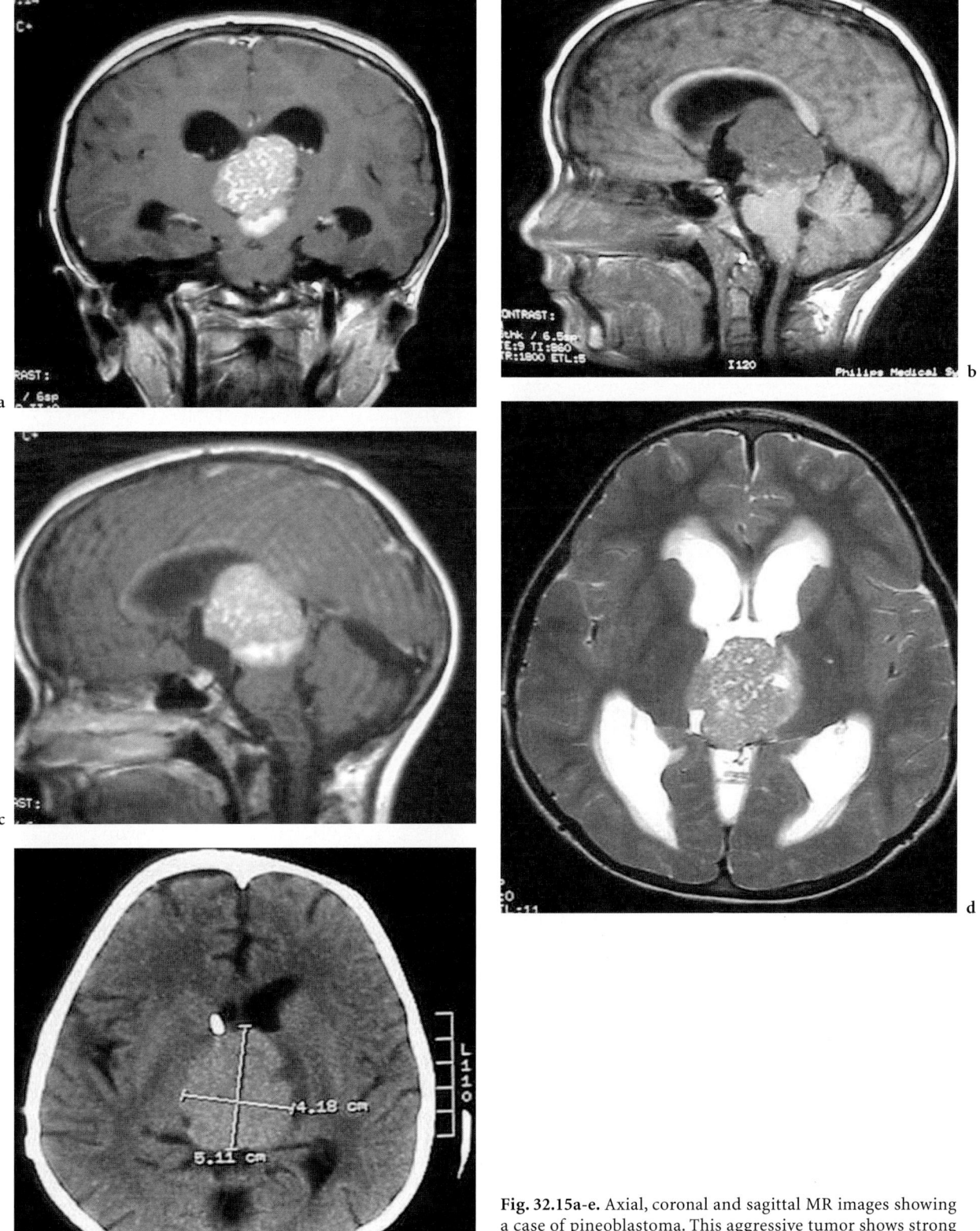

Fig. 32.15a-e. Axial, coronal and sagittal MR images showing a case of pineoblastoma. This aggressive tumor shows strong enhancement. The patient underwent multimodality management, which included chemotherapy and external beam irradiation

Surgical considerations include management of the dura. Intraoperatively, if the dura appears abnormal, it should be resected or at least biopsied. A dural graft can be implanted or taken from the pericranium.

32.4.1
Intracranial Rosai-Dorfman Disease

Also known as sinus histiocytosis, this disease is a rare idiopathic histoproliferative disease affecting the lymph nodes. Recently described, this disease is characterized by systemic lymphadenopathy. Occasionally, intracranial involvement without evidence of disease elsewhere in the body, has been encountered. Many lobes of the brain have been affected, without any definite pattern (Gaetani et al. 2000; Udono et al. 1999; Huang et al. 1998; Deodhare et al. 1998; Kim et al. 1995). Suprasellar location and presentation with diabetes insipidus have also been reported (Woodcock et al. 1999; Kelly et al. 1999). Spinal lesions have also been cited (Kelly et al. 1999). Because of the lesions' usual proximity to dura, and also because of their customary strong enhancement with contrast, these intracranial tumors are commonly thought to be meningiomas in the preoperative stages (Fig. 32.16). Tissue samples are necessary for definitive diagnosis. The surgical approach de-

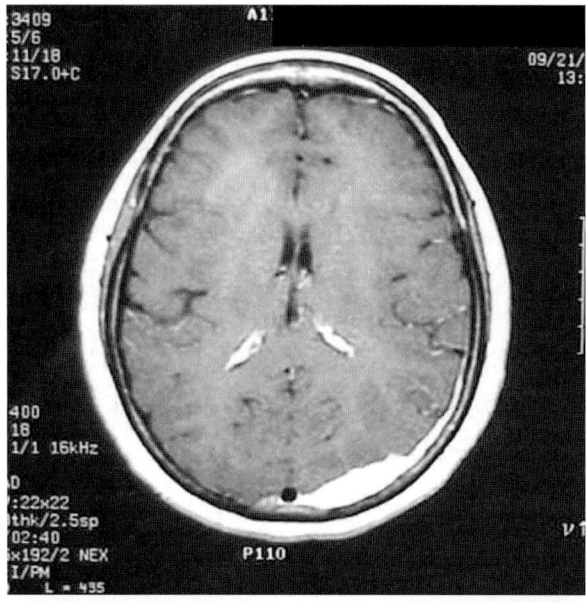

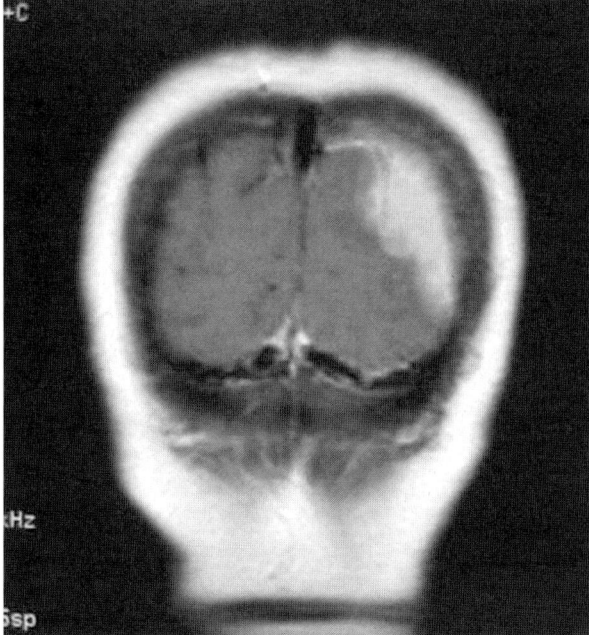

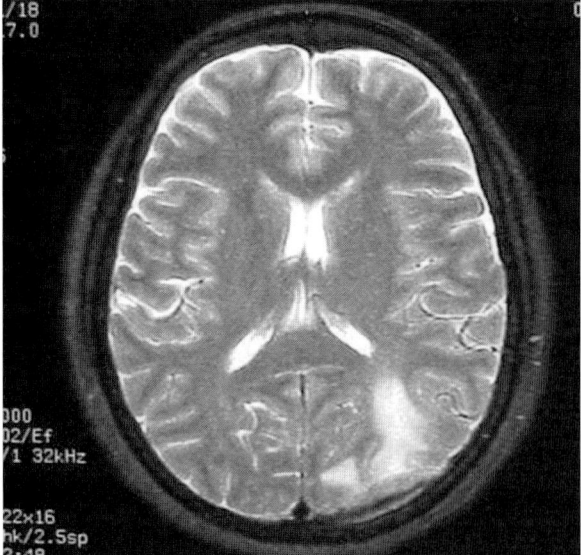

Fig. 32.16a–c. Rosai-Dorfman disease. **a** Axial and **b** coronal T1WI. Preoperatively, this lesion was thought to be an enplaque meningioma. Intraoperatively, there was no suspicion of unusual pathology until results of frozen sections were reported. **c** T2WI shows local edema

pends upon the location of the tumor. No difficulty has been reported in the surgical excision of these tumors. Their natural history appears to be benign; after surgical excision, there is no known risk of recurrence (Gaetani et al. 2000). There is no experience with adjuvant therapy.

32.4.1.1
Histology

Many inflammatory cells are present, mostly mature histiocytes. Immunohistochemical staining reveals strong positivity for S-100, CD-68 antigen, and vimentin (GAETANI et al. 2000). Emperipolesis (intracytoplasmic lymphocytes and monocytes) is characteristic of this disease.

32.5
Conclusion

The goals of management of rare CNS tumors are no different from those of more common malignancies. As physicians, we strive to delay mortality, maintain neurological function, and preserve quality of life. Secondary to their infrequent nature, rare CNS tumors are often treated with management plans borrowed from proven and accepted treatments of common CNS tumors. The advent of additional options and technical advances, in surgery and adjuvant therapy, are likely to alter the care of patients with rare brain tumors. Certainly though, each patient will remain an individual, and the exact management will be based upon many factors unique to the case. This fact, together with the expanding options and resources of today's medical world, and the paucity of related literature, will ensure that decision-making in the treatment of rare CNS tumors will remain challenging.

References

Abay EO 2d, Laws ER Jr, Grado GL, et al. (1981) Pineal tumors in children and adolescents. Treatment by CSF shunting and radiotherapy. J Neurosurg 55:889–895

Abdou MS, Cohen AR (1998) Endoscopic treatment of colloid cysts of the third ventricle. Technical note and review of the literature. J Neurosurg 89:1062–1068

Abernathey CD, Davis DH, Kelly PJ (1989) Treatment of colloid cysts of the third ventricle by stereotaxic microsurgical laser craniotomy. J Neurosurg 70:525–529

Allen JC, Kim JH, Packer RJ (1987) Neoadjuvant chemotherapy for newly diagnosed germ-cell tumors of the central nervous system. J Neurosurg 67:65–70

Akins PT, Roberts R, Coxe WS, et al. (1996) Familial colloid cysts of the third ventricle: case report and review of associated conditions. Neurosurgery 38:392–395

Apuzzo ML, Chikovani OK, Gott PS, et al. (1982) Transcallosal, interfornical approaches for lesions affecting the third ventricle: surgical considerations and consequences. Neurosurgery 10:547–554

Apuzzo ML, Chandrasoma PT, Zelman V, et al. (1984) Computed tomographic guidance stereotaxis is the management of lesions of the third ventricular region. Neurosurgery 15:502–508

Aronica PA, Ahdab-Barmada M, Rozin L, et al. (1998) Sudden death in an adolescent boy due to a colloid cyst of the third ventricle. Am J Forensic Med Pathol 19:119–122

Ashley DG, Zee CS, Chandrasoma PT, et al. (1990) Lhermitte-Duclos disease: CT and MR findings. J Comput Assist Tomogr 14:984–987

Awwad EE, Levy E, Martin DS, et al. (1995) Atypical appearance of Lhermitte-Duclos disease with contrast enhancement. Am J Neuroradiol 16:1719–1720

Baumgartner JE, Edwards MS (1992) Pineal tumors. Neurosurg Clin N Am 3:853–862

Berger C, Thiesse P, Lellouch-Tubiana A, et al. (1998) Choroid pleus carcinomas in childhood: clinical features and prognostic factors. Neurosurgery 42:470–475

Brat DJ, Scheithauer BW, Staugaitis SM, et al. (1998) Third ventricular chordoid glioma: a distinct clinicopathologic entity. J Neuropathol Exp Neurol 57:283–290

Buttner A, Winkler PA, Eisenmenger W, et al. (1997) Colloid cysts of the third ventricle with fatal outcome: a report of two cases and review of the literature. Int J Legal Med 110:260–266

Cabbell KL, Ross DA (1996) Stereotactic microsurgical craniotomy for the treatment of third ventricular colloid cysts. Neurosurgery 38:301–307

Carpenter DB, Michelsen WJ, Hays AP (1982) Carcinoma of the choroid plexus. Case report. J Neurosurg 56:722–727

Carter JE, Merren MD, Swann KW (1989) Preoperative diagnosis of Lhermitte-Duclos disease by magnetic resonance imaging. Case report. J Neurosurg 70:135–137

Casey KF, Vries JK (1989) Cerebral fluid overproduction in the absence of tumor or villous hypertrophy of the choroid plexus. Childs Nerv Syst 5:332–334

Chan RC, Thompson GB, Durity FA (1983) Primary choroid plexus papilloma of the cerebellopontine angle. Neurosurgery 12:334–336

Chandler HC Jr., Friedman WA (1994) Radiosurgical treatment of a hemangioblastoma: case report. Neurosurgery 34:353–355

Chang SD, Meisel JA, Hancock SL, et al. (1998) Treatment of hemangioblastomas in von Hippel-Lindau disease with linear accelerator-based radiosurgery. Neurosurgery 43:28–34

Chiechi MV, Smirniotopoulos JG, Jones RV (1995) Intracranial subependymomas: CT and MR imaging features in 24 cases. Am J Roentgenol 165:1245–1250

Cho BK, Wang KC, Nam DH, et al. (1998) Pineal tumors: experience with 48 cases over 10 years. Childs nerv Syst 14:53–58

Choi JU, Kim DS, Chung SS, et al. (1998) Treatment of germ cell tumors in the pineal region. Childs Nerv Syst 14:41–48

Clarenbach P, Kleihues P, Metzel E, et al. (1979) Simultaneous clinical manisfestation of subependymoma of the fourth ventricle in identical twins. Case report. J Neurosurg 50:655–659

Coffey RJ, Cascino TL, Shaw EG (1993) Radiosurgical treatment of recurrent hemangiopericytomas of the meninges: preliminary results. J Neurosurg 78:903–908

Costa JM, Ley L, Claramunt E, et al. (1997) Choroid plexus papillomas of the III ventricle in infants. Report of three cases. Childs Nerv Syst 13:244–249

Cozad SC, Townsend P, Morantz RA, et al. (1996) Gliomatosis cerebri. Results with radiation therapy. Cancer 78:1789–1793

Decq P, Le Guerinel C, Brugieres P, et al. (1998) Endoscopic management of colloid cysts. Neurosurgery 43:1288–1294

del Carpio-O'Donovan R, Korah I, Salazar A, et al. (1996) Gliomatosis cerebri. Radiology 198:831–835

Dempsey PK, Lunsford LD (1992) Stereotactic radiosurgery for pineal region tumors. Neurosurg Clin N Am 3:245–253

Deodhare SS, Ang LC, Billbao JM, et al. (1998) Isolated intracranial involvement in Rosai-Dorfman disease: a report of two cases and review of the literature. Arch Pathol Lab Med 122:161–165

Drummond KJ, Rosenfeld JV (1999) Pineal region tumours in childhood. A 30-year experience. Childs Nerv Syst 15:119–126

Duffner PK, Kun LE, Burger PC, et al. (1995) Postoperative chemotherapy and delayed radiation in infants and very young children with choroid plexus carcinomas. The Pediatric Oncology Group. Pediatr Neurosurg 22:189–196

Duke BJ, Kindt GW, Breeze RE (1997) Pineal region choroid plexus papilloma treated with stereotactic radiotherapy: a case study. Comput Aided Surg 2:135–138

Edwards MS, Hudgins RJ, Wilson CB, et al. (1988) Pineal region tumors in children. J Neurosurg 68:689–697

Ellenbogen RG, Moores LE (1997) Endoscopic management of a pineal and suprasellar germinoma with associated hydrocephalus: technical case report. Minim Invasive Neurosurg 40:13–15

Enam SA, Rosenblum ML, Ho KL (1997) Neurocytoma in the cerebellum. Case report. J Neurosurg 87:100–102

Eng DY, DeMonte F, Ginsberg L, et al. (1997) Craniospinal dissemination of central neurocytoma. Report of two cases. J Neurosurg 86:547–552

Fallentin E, Skriver E, Herning M, et al. (1997) Gliomatosis cerebri– an appropriate diagnosis? Cases reports. Acta Radiol 38:381–390

Ferreol E, Sawaya R, de Courten-Myers GM (1989) Primary cerebral neuroblastoma (neurocytoma) in adults. J Neurooncol 7:121–128

Foreman NK, Love S, Gill SS, et al. (1997) Second-look surgery for incompletely resected fourth ventricle ependymomas: technical case report. Neurosurgery 40:856–860

Franzini A, Leocata F, Servello D, et al. (1998) Long-term follow-up of germinoma after stereotactic biopsy and brain radiotherapy: a cell kinetics study. J Neurol 245:593–597

Fukui M, Natori Y, Matsushima T, et al. (1998) Operative approaches to the pineal region. Childs Nerv Syst 14:49–52

Furie DM, Provenzale JM (1995) Supratentorial ependymomas and subependymomas: CT and MR appearance. J Comput Assist Tomogr 19:518–526

Furuta A, Takahashi H, Ikuta F, et al. (1992) Temporal lobe tumor demonstrating ganglioglioma and pleomorphic xanthoastrocytoma components. Case report. J Neurosurg 77:143–147

Gaab MR, Schroeder HW (1998) Neuroendoscopic approach to intraventricular lesions. J Neurosurg 88:496–505

Gaetani P, Tancioni F, Di Rocco M, et al. (2000) Isolated cerebellar involvement in Rosai-Dorfman disease: case report. Neurosurgery 46:479–481

Galanis E, Buckner JC, Scheithauer BW, et al. (1998) Management of recurrent meningeal hemangiopericytoma. Cancer 82:1915–1920

Ghim TT, Davis P, Seo JJ, et al. (1993) Response to neoadjuvant chemotherapy in children with pineoblastoma. Cancer 72:1795–1800

Giannini C, Scheithauer BW, Burger PC, et al. (1999) Pleomorphic xanthoastrocytoma: what do we really know about it? Cancer 85:2033–2045

Glasser RS, Rojiani AM, Mickle JP, et al. (1995) Delayed occurrence of cerebellar pleomorphic xanthoastrocytoma after supratentorial pleomorphic xantroastrocytoma removal. Case report. J Neurosurg 82:116–118

Haga S, Morioka T, Nishio S, et al. (1996) Multicentric pleomorphic xanthoastrocytomas: case report. Neurosurgery 38:1242–1244

Hakim R, Loeffler JS, Anthony DC, et al. (1997) Gangliogliomas in adults. Cancer 79:127–131

Hall WA, Lunsford LD (1987) Changing concepts in the treatment of colloid cysts. An 11-year experience in the CT era. J Neurosurg 66:186–191

Herpers MJ, Freling G, Beuls EA (1994) Pleomorphic xanthoastrocytoma in the spinal cord. Case report. J Neurosurg 80:564–569

Herrmann HD, Westphal M, Winkler K, et al. (1994) Treatment of nongerminomatous germ-cell tumors of the pineal region. Neurosurgery 34:524–529

Hoeffel C, Boukobza M, Polivka M, et al. (1995) MR manifestations of subependymomas. Am J Neuroradiol 16:2121–2129

Hoffman HJ, Otsubo H, Hendrick EB, et al. (1991) Intracranial germ-cell tumors in children. J Neurosurgery 74:545–551

Huang HY, Huang CC, Lui CC, et al. (1998) Isolated intracranial Rosai-Dorfman disease: case report and literature review. Pathol Int 48:396–402

Huh SJ, Shin KH, Kim IH, et al. (1996) Radiotherapy of intracranial germinomas. Radiother Oncol 38:19–23

Iqbal Z, Sutcliffe JC. (1994) Subependymoma of the lateral ventricle: case report and literature review. Br J Neurosurg 8:83–85

Jay V, Squire J, Becker LE, et al. (1994) Malignant transformation in a ganglioglioma with anaplastic neuronal and astrocytic components. Report of a case with flow cytometric and cytogenetic analysis. Cancer 73:2862–2868

Jooma R, Torrens MJ, Bradshaw J, et al. (1985) Subependymomas of the fourth ventricle. Surgical treatment in 12 cases. J Neurosurg 62:508–512

Kang JK, Jeun SS, Hong YK, et al. (1998) Experience with pineal region tumors. Childs Nerv Syst 14:63–68

Kannuki S, Hirose T, Horiguchi H, et al. (1998) Gliomatosis with secondary glioblastoma formation: report of two cases. Brain Tumor Pathol 15:111–116

Kelly WF, Bradey N, Scoones D, et al. (1999) Rosai-Dorfman disease presenting as a pituitary tumour. Clin Endocrinol 50:133–137

Kepes JJ, Rubinstein LJ, Eng LF (1979) Pleomorphic xanthoastrocytoma: a distinctive meningocerebral glioma of young subjects with relatively favorable prognosis. A study of 12 cases. Cancer 44:1839–1852

Kim DG, Kim JS, Chi JG, et al. (1996) Central neurocytoma: proliferative potential and biological behavior. J Neurosurg 84:742–747

Kim M, Provias J, Bernstein M (1995) Rosai-Dorfman disease mimicking multiple meningioma: case report. Neurosurgery 36:1185–1187

King WA, Ultman JS, Frazee JG, et al. (1999) Endoscopic resection of colloid cysts: surgical considerations using the rigid endoscope. Neurosurgery 44:1103–1109

Koch R, Scholz M, Nelen MR, et al. (1999) Lhermitte-Duclos disease as a component of Cowden's syndrome. Case report and review of the literature. J Neurosurg 90:776–779

Kocher M, Voges J, Staar S, et al. (1998) Linear accelerator radiosurgery for recurrent malignant tumors of the skull base. Am J Clin Oncol 21:18–22

Kondziolka D, Lunsford LD (1991) Stereotactic management of colloid cysts: factors predicting success. J Neurosurg 75:45–51

Kreth FW, Schatz CR, Pagenstecher, et al. (1996) Stereotactic management of lesions of the pineal region. Neurosurgery 39:280–289

Krouwer HG, Davis RL, McDermott MW, et al. (1993) Gangliogliomas: a clinicopathologic study of 25 cases and review of the literature. J Neurooncol 17:139–154

Kulkantrakorn K, Awaad EE, Levy B, et al. (1997) MRI in Lhermitte-Duclos disease. Neurology 48:725–731

Kumar K, Kelly M, Toth C, et al. (1998) Stereotactic cyst wall disruption and aspiration of colloid cysts of the third ventricle. Stereotact Funct Neurosurg 71:145–152

Kurisaka M, Arisawa M, Mori T, et al. (1998) Combination chemotherapy (cisplatin, vinblastin) and low-dose irradiation in the treatment of pineal parenchymal cell tumors. Childs Nerv Syst 14:564–569

Lach B, Scheithauer BW, Gregor A, et al. (1993) Colloid cyst of the third ventricle. A comparative immunohistochemical study of neuraxis cysts and choroid plexus epithelium. J Neurosurg 78:101–111

Lang FF, Epstein FJ, Ransohoff J, et al. (1993) Central nervous system gangliogliomas. Clinical outcome. J Neurosurg 79:867–873.

Leech RW, Christoferson LA, Gilvertson RL, et al. (1977) Dysplastic gangliocytoma (Lhermitte-Duclos disease) of the cerebellum. Case report. J Neurosurg 47:609:612

Lewis AI, Crone KR, Taha J, et al. (1994) Surgical resection of third ventricle colloid cyst. Preliminary results comparing transcollosal microsurgery with endoscopy. J Neurosurg 81:174–178

Lindboe CF, Cappelen J, Kepes JJ (1992) Pleomorphic xanthoastrocytoma as a component of a cerebellar ganglioglioma: case report. Neurosurgery 31:353–355

Lindboe CF, Stolt-Nielson A, Dale LG (1992) Hemorrhage in a highly vascularized subependymoma of the septum pellucidum: case report. Neurosurgery 31:741–745

Linggood RM, Chapman PH (1992) Pineal tumors. J Neurooncol 12:85–91

Lobato RD, Sarabia M, Castro S, et al. (1986) Symptomatic subependymoma: report of four new cases studies with computed tomography and review of the literature. Neurosurgery 19:594–598

Lombardi D, Scheithauer BW, Meyer FB, et al. (1991) Symp-

tomatic subependymoma: a clinicopathological and flow cytometric study. J Neurosurg 75:583–588

Macaulay RJ, Jay V, Hoffman HJ, et al. (1993) Increased mitotic activity as a negative prognostic indicator in pleomorphic xanthoastrocytoma. Case report. J Neurosurg 79:761–768

Macdonald RL, Humphreys RP, Rutka JT, et al. (1994) Colloid cysts in children. Pediatr Neurosurg 20:169–177

Marcus CD, Galeon M, Peruzzi P, et al. (1996) Lhermitte-Duclos disease associated with syringomyelia. Neuroradiology 38:529–531

Mascalchi M, Muscas GC, Galli C, et al. (1994) MRI of pleomorphic xanthoastrocytoma: case report. Neuroradiology 36:446–447

Mathiesen T, Grane P, Lindquist C, et al. (1993) High recurrence rate following aspiration of colloid cysts in the third ventricle. J Neurosurg 78:748–752

Mathiesen T, Grane P, Lindgren L, et al. (1997) Third ventricle colloid cysts: a consecutive 12-year series. J Neurosurg 86:5–12

Matsutani M, Sano K, Takakura K, et al. (1998) Combined treatment with chemotherapy and radiation for intracranial germ cell tumors. Childs Nerv Syst 14:59–62

McDonald JV (1999) Intraventricular hemangiopericytoma. J Neurosurg 91:167

McGirr SJ, Ebersold MJ, Scheithauer, et al. (1988) Choroid plexus papillomas: long-term follow-up results in a surgically treated series. J Neurosurg 69:843–849

Milbouw G, Born JD, Martin D, et al. (1988) Clinical and radiological aspects of dysplastic gangliocytoma (Lhermitte-Duclos disease): a report of two cases with review of the literature. Neurosurgery 22:124–128

Mittler MA, Walters BC, Fried AH, et al. (1999) Malignant glial tumor arising from the site of a previous Hamartoma/ Ganglioglioma: coincidence or malignant transformation? Pediatr Neurosurg 30:132–134

Mohadjer M, Teshmar E, Mundinger F, et al (1987) CT-stereotactic drainage of colloid cysts in the foramen of Monro and the third ventricle. J Neurosurg 67:220–223

Muller A, Buttner A, Weis S (1999) Rare occurrence of intracerebellar colloid cyst. Case report. J Neurosurg 91:128–131

Nakano I, Kondo A, Iwasaki K, et al. (1997) Choroid plexus papilloma in the posterior third ventricle: case report. Neurosurgery 40:1279–1282

Nelen MR, Padberg, Peeters EA, et al. (1996) Localization of the gene for Cowden disease to chromosome 10q22–23. Nat Genet 13:114–116

Newton HB, Henson J, Walker RW, et al. (1992) Extraneural metastases in ependymoma. J Neurooncol 14:135–142

Niemela M, Lim YJ, Soderman M, et al. (1996) Gamma knife radiosurgery in 11 hemangioblastomas. J Neurosurg 85:591–596

Oi S (1998) Recent advances and radical differences in therapeutic strategy to the pineal region tumor. Childs Nerv Syst 14:33–35

Onal C, Bayindir C, Siraneci R, et al. (1996) A serial CT scan and MRI verification of diffuse cerebrospinal gliomatosis: a case report with stereotactic diagnosis and radiological confirmation. Pediatr Neurosurg 25:94–99

Ono N, Isobe I, Uki J, et al. (1994) Recurrence of primary intracranial germinomas after complete response with radiotherapy: recurrence patterns and therapy. Neurosurgery 35:615–620

Oppenheim JS, Strauss RC, Mormino J, et al. (1994) Ependymomas of the third ventricle. Neurosurgery 37:350–352

Ortiz O, Bloomfield S, Schochet S (1995) Vascular contrast enhancement in Lhermitte-Duclos disease: case report. Neuroradiology 37:545–548

Packer RJ, Perilongo G, Johnson D, et al. (1992) Choroid plexus carcinoma of childhood. Cancer 69:580–585

Pan L, Wang EM, Wang BJ, et al. (1998) Gamma knife radiosurgery for hemangioblastomas. Stereotact Funct Neurosurg 70:179–186

Pencalet P, Sante-Rose C, Lellouch-Tubiana, et al. (1998) Papillomas and carcinomas of the choroid plexus in children. J Neurosurg 88:521–528

Perry A, Giannini C, Scheithauer BW, et al. (1997) Composite pleomorphic xanthoastrocytoma and ganglioglioma: report of four cases and review of the literature. Am J Surg Pathol 21:763–771

Pierallini A, Bonamini M, De Stefano, et al. (1999) Pleomorphic xanthoastrocytoma with CT and MRI appearance of meningioma. Neuroradiology 41:30–34

Pollock BE, Huston J 3rd (1999) Natural history of asymptomatic colloid cysts of the third ventricle. J Neurosurg 91:364–369

Ponce P, Alverez-Santullano MV, Otermin E, et al. (1998) Gliomatosis cerebri: findings with computed tomography and magnetic resonance imaging. Eur J Radiol 28:226–229

Popovic EA, Kelly PJ (1993) Stereotactic procedures of the pineal region. Mayo Clin Proc 68:965–970

Prayson RA, Morris HH 3rd (1998) Anaplastic pleomorphic xanthroastrocytoma. Arch Pathol Lab Med 122:1082–1086

Prayson RA (1999) Clinicopathologic study of 61 patients with ependymoma including MIB-1 immunohistochemistry. Ann Diagn Pathol 3:11–18

Raimondi AJ, Tomita T (1981) Hydrocephalus and infratentorial tumors. Incidence, clinical picture, and treatment. J Neurosurg 55:174–182

Rainov NG, Holzhausen HJ, Burkert W (1995) Dysplastic gangliocytoma of the cerebellum (Lhermitte-Duclos disease). Clin Neurol Neurosurg 97:175–180

Reeder RF, Saunders RF, Roberts DW, et al. (1988) Magnetic resonance imaging in the diagnosis and treatment of Lhermitte-Duclos disease (dysplastic gangliocytoma of the cerebellum). Neurosurgery 23:240–245

Reifenberger G, Weber T, Weber RG (1999) Chordoid glioma of the third ventricle: immunohistochemical and molecular genetic characterization of a novel tumor entity. Brain Pathol 9:617–626

Rivas JJ, Lobato RD (1985) CT-assisted stereotactic aspiration of colloid cysts of the third ventricle. J Neurosurg 62:238–242

Ross IB, Robitaille Y, Villemure JG, et al. (1991) Diagnosis and management of gliomatosis cerebri: recent trends. Surg Neurol 36:431–440

Ryder JW, Kleinschmidt-DeMasters BK, Keller TS, et al. (1986) Sudden deterioration and death in patients with benign tumors of the third ventrilce area. J Neurosurg 64:216–223

Ryken TC, Robinson RA, VanGilder JC (1994) Familial occurrence of subependymoma. Report of two cases. J Neurosurg 80:1108–1111

Saenz A, Zamorano L, Matter A, et al. (1998) Interactive image guided surgery of the pineal region. Minim Invasive Neurosurg 41:27–30

Sasaki A, Hirato J, Nakazato Y, et al. (1996) Recurrent anaplastic ganglioglioma: pathological characterization of tumor cells. Case report. J Neurosurg 84:1055–1059

Sawamura Y, de Tribolet N, Ishii N, et al. (1997) Management of primary intracranial germinomas: diagnostic surgery or radical resection? J Neurosurg 87:262–266

Sawaya R, Hammoud M, Schoppa D, et al. (1998) Neurosurgical outcomes in a modern series of 400 craniotomies for treatment of parenchymal tumors. Neurosurgery 42:1044–1055

Scheithauer BW (1978) Symtomatic subependymoma. Report of 21 cases with review of the literature. J Neurosurg 49:689–696

Schild SE, Scheithauer BW, Schomberg PJ, et al. (1993) Pineal parenchymal tumors. Clinical, pathologic, and therapeutic aspects. Cancer 72:870–880

Schweitzer JB, Davies KG (1997) Differentiating central neurocytoma. Case report. J Neurosurg 86:543–546

Shaffrey ME, Lanzino G, Lopes MB, et al. (1996) Maturation of intracranial immature teratomas. Report of two cases. J Neurosurg 85:672–676

Sharma R, Rout D, Gupta AK, et al. (1994) Choroid plexus papillomas. Br J Neurosurg 8:169–177

Shin YM, Chang KH, Han MH, et al. (1993) Gliomatosis cerebri: comparison of MRI and CT features. Am J Roentgenol 161:859–862

Shuto T, Sekido K, Ohtsubo Y, et al. (1995) Choroid plexus papilloma of the III ventricle in an infant. Childs Nerv Syst 11:664–666

Siddiqi SN, Fehlings MG. (1994) Lhermitte-Duclos disease mimicking adult-onset aqueductal stenosis. Case report. J Neurosurg 80:1095–1098

Smith DB, Newlands ES, Begent RH, et al. (1991) Optimum management of pineal germ cell tumours. Clin Oncol 3:96–99

Spoto GP, Press GA, Hesselink JR, et al. (1990) Intracranial ependymoma and subependymoma: MR manisfestations. Am J Neuroradiol 11:83–91

Stevens JM, Kendall BE, Love S (1984) Radiological features of subependymoma with emphasis on computed tomography. Neuroradiology 26:223–228

Tasdemiroglu E, Awh MH, Walsh JW (1996) MRI of cerebellopontine angle choroid plexus papilloma. Neuroradiology 38:38–40

Tatter SB, Borges LF, Louis DN (1994) Central neurocytoma of the cervical spinal cord. Report of two cases. J Neurosurg 81:288–293

Tonami H, Kamehiro M, Oguchi M, et al. (2000) Chordoid glioma of the third ventricle: CT and MR findings. J Comput Assist Tomogr 24:336–338

Tonn JC, Paulus W, Warmuth-Metz M, et al. (1997) Pleomorphic xanthoastrocytoma: report of six cases with special consideration of diagnostic and therapeutic pitfalls. Surg Neurol 47:162–169

Udono H, Fukuyama K, Okamoto H, et al. (1999) Rosai-Dorfman disease presenting multiple intracranial lesions with unique findings on magnetic resonance imaging. Case report. J Neurosurg 91:335–339

Ushio Y, Kochi M, Kuratsu J, et al. (1999) Preliminary observations for a new treatment in children with primary intracranial yolk sac tumor or embryonal carcinoma. Report of 5 cases. J Neurosurg 90:133–137

Vajtai I, Varga Z, Scheithauer BW, et al (1999) Chordoid glioma of the third ventricle: confirmatory report of a new entity. Hum Pathol 30:723–726

Vaquero J, Ramiro J, Martinez R, et al. (1990) Clinicopathologic experience with pineocytomas: report of five surgically treated cases. Neurosurgery 27:612–618

Wasdahl DA, Scheithauer BW, Andrews BT, et al. (1994) Cerebellar pleomorphic xanthoastrocytoma: case report. Neurosurgery 35:947–950

Weldon-Linne CM, Victor TA, Groothuis DR, et al. (1983) Pleomorphic xanthoastrocytoma. Ultrastructural and immunohistochemical study of a case with a rapidly fatal outcome following surgery. Cancer 52:2055–2063

Whittle IR, Gordon A, Misra BK, et al. (1989) Pleomorphic xanthoastrocytoma. Report of four cases. J Neurosurg 70:463–468

Wichmann W, Schubiger O, von Deimling A, et al. (1991) Neuroradiology of central neurocytoma. Neuroradiology 33:143–148

Wolansky LJ, Malantic GP, Heary R, et al. (1996) Preoperative MRI diagnosis of Lhermitte-Duclos disease: case report with associated enlarged vessel and syrinx. Surg Neurol 45:470–475

Woodcock RJ Jr, Mandell JW, Lipper MH, et al. (1999) Sinus histiocytosis (Rosai-Dorfman disease) of the suprasellar region: MR imaging findings– a case report. Radiology 213:808–810

Yasargil MG, von Ammon K, von Deimling A, et al. (1992) Central neurocytoma: histological variants and therapeutic approaches. J Neurosurg 76:32–37

Zarate JO, Sampaolesi R (1999) Pleomorphic xanthroastocytoma of the retina. Am J Surg Pathol 23:79–81

Ziyal IM, Sekhar LN, Salas E, et al. (1998) Combined supra/infratentorial-transsinus approach to large pineal region tumors. J Neurosurg 88:1050–1057

33 Toxicity of Therapy and Quality of Life in Patients Treated for CNS Tumors

Silvia C. Formenti and Zbigniew Petrovich

CONTENTS

33.1 Introduction

Quality of life is a complex and difficult-to-define concept with physical, spiritual, and psychosocial components. This concept is directly dependent on the health status of an individual and closely related to the subjective perception of well-being. During the past decade substantial efforts have been made to find measurable parameters of "health-related quality of life" (HRQOL) and to define a standardized health status instrument. Different quality of life studies based on patient self-assessment reports (MACKWORTH et al. 1992) or using multiple instruments (TAPHOORN et al. 1992) have been used for this purpose.

It is well known that a diagnosis of cancer has a multifactorial impact on the quality of life of patients.

S. C. FORMENTI, MD
Associate Professor, USC Keck School of Medicine, Department of Radiation Oncology, 1441 Eastlake Avenue, Los Angeles, CA 90033, USA
Z. PETROVICH, MD
Professor and Chairman, Department of Radiation Oncology, USC Keck School of Medicine, 1441 Eastlake Avenue, Room G356, Los Angeles, CA 90033, USA

The anatomical site of tumor is almost always associated with general and specific symptoms that directly impact on the quality of life of an individual. These symptoms are an expression of both the direct effects of the tumor and those derived from therapy. This chapter focuses on issues relevant to quality of life of patients with primary and metastatic CNS tumors.

33.2 Incidence

It has been estimated that in the United States up to 170,000 patients per year develop metastatic brain lesions (PATCHELL 1995; O'NEILL et al. 1994) and about 17,000 patients per year are diagnosed with primary brain tumors (NEWTON 1984; BLACK 1991; LANDIS et al. 1999). The incidence of primary CNS tumors is age related, with the first peak occurring between 0 and 4 years of age, the second peak between 15 and 24 years, and the third peak between 65 and 79 years. (See Chaps. 1 and 2 for details on the epidemiology of CNS tumors.) In childhood, brain tumors represent the second most common malignancy. Primary CNS tumors are much less common among adults. More than half of adult brain tumors are, however, malignant with poor survival rates. The median survival in patients with primary malignant brain tumors ranges from 12 to 30 months, and it is 6 months or less in patients with brain metastasis (PATCHELL 1995; O'NEIL et al. 1994; BLACK 1991).

Primary and metastatic CNS tumors have different influences on patients' quality of life in the different age groups. The anatomical site of tumor involvement is associated with a specific neurological deficit, which may produce disability dramatically affecting quality of life. The severity of symptoms and signs experienced by patients with CNS tumors to a large extent also depends on the tumor progression rate and the phase of the disease process. Additionally, any form of therapy for CNS tumors is rarely devoid of acute or long-term side-effects that affect quality of life. The complexity of interaction of the above multiple factors needs to be assessed when measuring quality of life in these patients.

The factors most frequently considered in assessing quality of life issues include:

1. Age at diagnosis of symptoms
2. Anatomical location of the tumor in the brain or spinal cord
3. Tumor aggressiveness and the degree of surrounding edema
4. Treatment modality or modalities used in the management of patient
5. Phase in the course of disease

Table 33.1. SOMA for CNS (modified from RUBIN et al. 1997)

Subjective	Objective	Management	Analytic
Headache/ somnolence	Neurological deficits	Anticonvulsive therapy	MRI
			CT
Memory loss	Cognitive function	Steroids	MRS
Intellectual competence	Mood and personality changes	Sedatives	PET
Functional competence	Seizures		CSF analysis

33.3
Instruments Available to Measure Treatment Toxicity

Because of the narrow therapeutic ratio in the management of CNS tumors, accurate reports on and measurement of treatment toxicity are particularly relevant. Since long-term survivors are most likely to develop toxicity with potential implications for quality of life, detailed description of late toxicity is imperative in all reports describing treatment outcomes. A recent National Cancer Institute (NCI) Consensus Conference has introduced the SOMA classification for late toxicity representing subjective and objective signs and symptoms, management methods, and analytic laboratory and imaging procedures (Overgaard and Bartelink 1995; Rubin 1995).

This classification system allows description, for each treated organ, of the manifestations of late injuries due to treatment administered, with LENT representing late effects on normal tissue. The following steps describe the general process for LENT diagnosis:

1. Clinical detection
2. Time course of events
3. Dose/time/volume
4. Chemical biological modifier
5. Radiological imaging
6. Laboratory tests
7. Differential diagnosis
8. Pathologic diagnosis
9. Management
10. Follow-up

Table 33.1 summarizes the SOMA classification as applied to CNS toxicity.

33.4
Treatment Complications

33.4.1
External Beam Radiotherapy

In the process of classifying treatment toxicity it is useful to separately describe radiation effects, chemotherapy effects, and effects due to their combination. Early effects of brain irradiation usually consist of temporary exacerbation of preexisting signs and symptoms of CNS tumor. These complications are rarely severe, infrequently of clinical significance, and have low impact on the quality of life of treated patients (SHELINE et al. 1980). Complications of clinical relevance are those occurring from several weeks to many months following completion of cranial irradiation. The most severe late effect of brain irradiation is necrosis. Several experimental models have proven its dependence on the volume of brain irradiated. Approximately 1%–5% of patients treated with whole brain irradiation to a dose of 55–60 Gy, given over a period of 6 weeks, develop brain necrosis. In about 75% of patients who develop brain necrosis, it becomes evident within 3 years of radiotherapy (MARKS et al. 1981; SHELINE et al. 1980). Most importantly, radiation fraction size has been shown to be a major determinant of whole brain irradiation toxicity (SHELINE et al. 1980). This was well demonstrated in an important study in which a single dose of radiation of 10 Gy was given to the brain for the treatment of metastatic disease. This treatment resulted within 48 h in a 7% incidence of mortality (HINDO et al. 1970). In view of the above data, it is imperative to treat brain lesions using the smallest possible target volume and to keep the daily dose of radiation to 2

Gy in patients in whom long-term survival is expected and 3 Gy in those treated with a palliative intent only. Whole brain irradiation should only be considered when the use of more selective radiation treatment is clearly inappropriate (LEVINE et al. 1999).

33.4.2
Stereotactic Radiosurgery

It has been well established that a combination of large CNS volume and large radiation fractions is associated with severe morbidity. Data on the tolerance of small brain volumes treated usually with a single or with a few large radiation fractions is rapidly accruing from the experience with stereotactic radiosurgery (SRS) used in the management of vascular brain lesions and benign and malignant brain tumors. This treatment is usually very well tolerated, effective, and compatible with good quality of life (LEVINE et al. 1999; JOSEPH et al. 1996; SHRIEVE et al. 1995; MEHTA et al. 1995). Acute toxicity of SRS was reported to occur in about 30% of 78 study patients by WERNER-WASIK et al. (1999). This acute toxicity depended on radiation dose, volume of tissue treated, and anatomical site included in the high-dose region. In a study of 100 SRS-treated patients with brain metastases, 14% developed acute treatment toxicity, 6% had subacute toxicity, and 4% had late toxicity with one patient death due to brain necrosis (SHIAU et al. 1997). In a study of 120 patients treated with SRS for brain metastases, late toxicity manifested by focal brain necrosis was reported in 20 (17%) patients (JOSEPH et al. 1996). Quality of life issues are of importance in planning treatment strategy for patients with recurrent glioblastoma multiforme (GBM). Of the 32 patients treated with interstitial implantation, 44% required a reoperation, while among the 86 SRS-treated patients the incidence of reoperation was 22% (SHRIEVE et al. 1995). Both groups of patients had similar survival rates. Based on the above data, one would prefer to use SRS rather than interstitial implantation in the management of patients with recurrent GBM. In many patients who present with solitary metastatic lesions in the brain, the use of SRS would be preferable to whole brain irradiation (LEVINE et al. 1999; MEHTA et al. 1997; ALEXANDER et al. 1995).

It is of interest to compare the experience with SRS in a few medical centers. The reported incidence of focal brain necrosis requiring craniotomy varies widely, from a low of less than 5% at University of Southern California to a high of up to 40% in other published reports (Levine et al. 1999; Chen et al. 2000; Joseph et al. 1996; Shiau et al. 1997; Shrieve et al. 1995; Alexander et al. 1995). It is not readily apparent why these differences in the incidence of focal necrosis exist. They do not seem to be related to radiation dose, target volume, or histological diagnosis.

Caution needs to be exercised in the evaluation of late toxicity in patients treated with SRS for brain metastasis and in those with malignant gliomas. Median survival in this patient population is limited and there may not be enough time to see expression of late injury in a substantial proportion of patients. Therefore, it is of interest to assess the risk of late injury in patients treated with SRS for acoustic neuromas and meningiomas. In a report on SRS treatment of 162 patients with acoustic neuromas, 98% of patients did not require resection and at 5 years post-treatment, 79% had normal facial function, 73% had normal trigeminal nerve function, and 51% had no change in hearing (Kondziolka et al. 1998). Those data showed an excellent treatment tolerance and patients were able to maintain a good quality of life throughout the period of follow-up. Similar good outcomes were noted in 88 patients treated with SRS for skull base meningiomas (Morita et al. 1999). No visual impairment was noted, and in nine (10%) patients with new trigeminal nerve neuropathy the problem was clearly dose related and to a large extent preventable.

33.4.3
Chemotherapy

Most chemotherapeutic agents used in the management of CNS tumors are known to be associated with a risk of cerebral encephalopathy (SHULTHEISS et al. 1995) (Table 33.2).

The onset of encephalopathy is particularly dramatic in children, and it is in this age group that most experience has been acquired with the use of chemo-radiotherapy combinations. Over the past 30 years important toxicity data have been obtained through careful monitoring and reporting of toxicity by pediatric oncologists. This work has demonstrated the pitfalls of sequencing or combining the two treatment modalities. The best illustration of this problem in sequencing therapy is in the use of radiation and methotrexate. Radiation impairment of the blood-brain barrier affects its permeability to the drug, with consequent damage and necrosis (Griffin

Table 33.2. Antineoplastic agents associated with cerebral encephalopathy

Antimetabolites	Alkylating agents	Plant alkaloids	BMT drugs	Miscellaneous
High-dose methotrexate	Cisplatin	Vincristine	Nitrogen mustard	Mitotane
5-FU (with allopurinol)	Ifosfamide		VP-16 (etoposide)	Misonidazole
Cytarabine (Ara-C)	BCNU (carmustine)		Procarbazine	L-Asparaginase
Fludarabine	Spiromustine			
PALA				

BMT, Bone marrow transplantation; PALA, L-aspartic acid *N*-(phosphonoacetyl disodium)

et al. 1977). Scheduling radiation therapy after methotrexate can prevent the development of this toxic effect. Further important toxicity data derived from the pediatric population concern the long-term effect of treatment on neurocognitive skills and emotional dysfunction. Table 33.3 summarizes some of the reported experience on this subject.

Of interest is a study which demonstrated similar incidence of late toxicity among irradiated and nonirradiated children with medulloblastoma or primary cerebellar astrocytoma (LEBARON et al. 1988). When patients are managed with a multimodality approach, the specific contribution of radiation to neurocognitive deficits remains impossible to assess.

33.4.4
Surgery

Surgery is frequently the most important initial modality used in the management of almost all primary brain tumors. The role of surgery includes:

1. To obtain a tissue sample to establish a diagnosis
2. To remove tumor bulk and possibly to prolong life
3. To enhance the efficacy of adjuvant treatment(s)

It is well documented that any surgical intervention in brain tumors, such as biopsy or total or subtotal resection, can induce new or exacerbate the preexistent neurological symptoms. This occurs for instance in 5%–10% of patients operated on for malignant astrocytomas. Owing to the infiltrative nature of these tumors, they are most likely to develop postoperative edema (Rosenblum 1990). Other complications of surgery which may occur include infections and bleeding.

33.4.5
Multimodality Therapy

The infiltrative and aggressive nature of GBM and anaplastic astrocytomas makes a true "total resec-

Table 33.3. Neurocognitive effects of radiation therapy to the brain

Series	Tumor	No. of patients	Radiation therapy dose (Gy)	Outcome
HIRSCH et al. 1979	Medulloblastoma	28	35 WB/55 PF	12% had IQs>90, 31% <70; 93% had behavioral disturbances
DANOFF et al. 1982	Several	38	40–65	17% had IQs<70, 56% >90; 37% had emotional difficulties
DUFFNER et al. 1985	Posterior fossa	10	26–40	40% had IQs<70, 20%>90; 4 of 5 with IQs>80 were learning disabled
KUN et al. 1983	Several	26	40–58 WB/ 50–55 local	8 of 15 who underwent surgery and irradiation had IQs<90; serial testing in 10 showed improvement in 2, stability in 5, and further deterioration in 3
PACKER et al. 1987	Medulloblastoma	28	35–40 WB/ 50–55 PF	Mean IQ, 96 (range 50–120)

WB, Whole brain; PF, posterior fossa boost

tion" of these tumors impossible to obtain (HOCH-BERG and PRUITT 1980). The standard treatment in patients with malignant gliomas, including surgery and radiotherapy, results in a relatively limited median survival. Considerable efforts have been made to find efficacious chemotherapeutic regimens capable of improving survival when used in combination with surgery and radiotherapy. Some chloroethylnitrosoureas (carmustine, lomustine, nimustine, etc.) and procarbazine have been shown to be able to cross the blood-brain barrier and display activity in brain tumors (LEVIN 1985; LEVIN 1986; LEVIN and WILSON 1981; KUMAR et al. 1974). In a meta-analysis an improved survival was demonstrated in patients with malignant gliomas treated with chemotherapy (FINE et al. 1993). Most of the studies analyzed used chemotherapy with a single-agent nitrosourea and radiotherapy, and the outcomes were compared with those in patients who only received radiotherapy. These results need careful evaluation in the context of toxicity and effect on quality of life. In fact, an increase in the median survival from 9.4 to 12 months in the adjuvant chemotherapy group was associated with the well-known toxicity of nitrosoureas, which included myelosuppression, nausea, and vomiting. Patients treated with higher doses of these drugs develop hepatotoxicity and progressive subacute encephalopathy associated with areas of coagulation necrosis in the brain (BURGER et al. 1981).

Subsequent studies suggested that the nitrosourea-based drug combinations may be more efficacious than nitrosourea used as a single agent. Particularly postradiation regimens with procarbazine (BCNU) and vincristine (PCV) were promising in the subset of patients with anaplastic astrocytomas and oligodendrogliomas (LEVIN et al. 1990; CAIRNCROSS et al. 1994; MASON et al. 1996). It is of interest to note the results of a study on the relative benefits of chemotherapy with BCNU versus PCV following 60 Gy radiation/oral hydroxyurea, based on reanalysis of the data from the Northern California Oncology Group protocol 6G61 (LEVIN et al. 1990). The protocol was closed in February 1983 and the data were reviewed in December 1988. Patients randomized into this trial had been diagnosed with GBM and anaplastic astrocytoma. (AA). A total of 63 patients were treated with BCNU alone (GBM, $n=30$; AA, $n=33$) and 64 patients were treated with PCV combination (GBM, $n=31$; AA, $n=33$). The authors found that the differences between BCNU and PCV therapy were significant only for patients with anaplastic astrocytomas, in whom PCV produced a two-

fold increase in time to tumor progression and survival at the 50th and 25th percentiles.

Another study compared the outcomes in 76 GBM patients and 72 patients with anaplastic astrocytomas treated with BCNU or the PCV combination after radiation therapy (60 Gy)/oral hydroxyurea (LEVIN et al. 1985). In patients with Karnofsky performance scores of 70–100, PCV was of greater benefit than BCNU for GBM ($P=0.15$) and for anaplastic astrocytomas ($P=0.13$). In GBM patients the 25th percentile times to progression were 70 weeks with PCV and 40 weeks with BCNU, whereas median time to progression in anaplastic astrocytoma was 123 weeks with PCV and 77 weeks with BCNU. The PCV toxicity included myelosuppression, nausea, vomiting, anorexia, weight loss, skin rash, fever, hepatotoxicity, and peripheral neuropathy. The use of the "intensive PCV," compared with the "standard PCV" developed by LEVIN et al. (1980), is correlated with more pronounced side-effects and encephalopathy, possibly procarbazine related. The outcomes have been shown to be only slightly better ($P=0.056$) compared with traditional PVC (CAIRNCROSS et al. 1994; SALGADO et al. 1996).

Most of the available chemotherapeutic agents can be toxic to the CNS when administered at high doses or when given with regional delivery (WEISS et al. 1974). A recent study showed the spectrum of neurological complications that occurred in 92 patients, primarily children, with recurrent malignant brain tumors or brain tumors resistant to conventional therapy who had undergone high-dose chemotherapy and autologous bone marrow rescue (KRAMER et al. 1997). The agents used in that report were: thiotepa, etoposide, nitrosourea, and carboplatinum. Neurological complications were observed in 50 patients (54%) and included encephalopathies with or without hallucinations or coma, seizures, headaches, and ataxia-tremor-dysarthria. Acute side-effects were often reversible. They mostly occurred with drug infusion and it was impossible to distinguish whether they were due to the toxic effect of antineoplastic agents, to antiemetic drugs, or to the dysmetabolic state of the treated patients. Only a few patients were found to develop delayed neurological complications unrelated to disease progression, presumably because no patient in this series was treated with total body irradiation. A review of treatment toxicity in 57 children who underwent autologous bone marrow rescue and were treated with a preparative therapy consisting of total body irradiation and systemic chemotherapy is of interest (WIZNITZER et al. 1984). These authors found neuropsychological dysfunctions in four of five long-term survivors. In 14 (24%) of 19 patients who had postmortem examinations, CNS abnormalities were detected, including cerebral atrophy (LEVIN and WILSON 1981). Similarly, other bone marrow transplant series have shown delayed neurological side-effects such as leukoencephalopathy with intellectual changes, memory alterations, motor abnormalities, and cerebellar dysfunction, with no correlation with the use of radiation therapy (PATCHELL et al. 1985; SNIDER et al. 1994; DAVIS and PATCHELL 1988).

Concomitant radiotherapy has been shown to enhance the toxicity of chemotherapy (DEANGELIS and SHAPIRO 1991). Intrathecal and intravenous use of methotrexate during prophylactic cranial irradiation in children affected by acute lymphoblastic leukemia represents an important example of brain toxicity derived from combined modality therapy. In these patients radiation doses of 24 Gy, normally well tolerated, were found in 45% of patients to be associated with severe delayed neurological complications, mineralizing microangiopathy and necrotizing leukoencephalopathy (BLEYER and GRIFFIN 1980). As a consequence of this toxicity methotrexate is currently administrated before radiotherapy.

To overcome the relatively limited results obtained with the use of systemic chemotherapy, intrathecal chemotherapy has been investigated. The agents used for the intrathecal administration have included methotrexate, thiotepa, and cytarabine. While this regional chemotherapy administration is associated with a low systemic toxicity and high CSF drug levels, it also increases CNS morbidity. Brain toxicity ranges from reversible fever and chills to permanent leukoencephalopathy and myelitis.

As previously discussed, treatment toxicity and its impact on quality of life is sometimes age-specific. A report on the treatment of 31 patients affected by primary CNS lymphoma is of interest (DEANGELIS et al. 1992). Patients were treated with whole brain irradiation followed by systemic methotrexate, 1 g/m^2, delivered by an Ommaya catheter. In this study the combination of radiation and chemotherapy was associated with a higher risk of late treatment-related toxicity ($P<0.0001$) in the subset of patients >60 years old. Significant late side-effects were noted in 69% of patients older than 60 years of age but in only 6% of patients <50 years of age. Late treatment toxicity consisted of progressive dementia, gate ataxia, urinary incontinence, and significant decline in Karnofsky performance score, requiring custodial care in a few cases (ABREY et al. 1998).

Another technique of regional drug delivery is through the intraarterial administration of chemotherapeutic agent via carotid or vertebral arteries (IAC). The first trials using intraarterial high doses of BCNU and cisplatin resulted in an unacceptable level of neurotoxicity, which included blindness due to retinal vasculitis, seizures, and death (FEUN et al. 1984; STEWART et al. 1984). In a recently reported study 168 patients affected by primary and metastatic brain tumors were treated with intraarterial cisplatin/etoposide with either concomitant or subsequent radiotherapy (TFAYLI et al. 1999). The dose of cisplatin was substantially reduced compared with the former studies and resulted in a lower incidence of toxicity. Complications consisted of mild nausea and vomiting in 14% of patients. The only patient who developed leukomalacia had received previous radiotherapy.

33.5
Instruments to Measure Quality of Life: the Need for Self-assessment

Unfortunately, limited evidence exists with regard to the best tools to assess quality of life among CNS tumor patients. Most studies are limited by a small sample size and heterogeneity of brain tumor location and histology, making interpretation of the results very difficult. Further longitudinal studies to develop a common instrument to measure health-related quality of life in this patient population are justified by the potential identification of modifiable impairments.

The level of observed functional impairment induced by brain tumors can be easily measured by health professionals using instruments like the Karnofsky performance status (KPS; KARNOFSKY et al. 1948) or Eastern Cooperative Oncology Group (ECOG) performance status. These instruments have been shown to be very useful in the pretreatment decision-making process. They have also been proved to correlate well with survival. In patients with gliomas the KPS has also been widely used to make a rough determination of a patient's quality of life (SACHSENHEIMER et al. 1993; KLEINBERG et al. 1993; TROJANOWSKI et al. 1989; LEIBEL et al. 1989; SCERRATI et al. 1994). In the above studies, performance status and length of survival have often been the two main measures of outcome used in clinical research.

Quality of life remains a mainly subjective issue. Health-related quality of life is defined as the best possible physical and emotional state compatible with a medical condition. It may vary among patients with similar level of health depending on the subjective perception of the disease process. A study was conducted on 200 adult patients with primary brain tumors who had undergone surgery and radiotherapy, with the majority also receiving chemotherapy (MACKWORTH et al. 1992). Patients were requested to complete a multidimensional questionnaire on the status of their health using the model developed by the European Organization for the Research and Treatment of Cancer (EORTC) (AARONSON et al. 1987). This questionnaire included items reflecting multiple aspects of satisfactory quality of life as follows:

1. High energy level
2. Enjoyment of leisure time
3. Normal cognitive ability
4. Good social life
5. Congenial work environment
6. Satisfactory sex life
7. Freedom from depression
8. A sense of well-being
9. Strong memory skills

During the same day on which the patient completed the questionnaire, a physician blinded to the result of the patient self-assessment examined the patient. The physician then assigned an appropriate KPS score on the basis of his/her examination. The aim of the study was to define the relative importance of the different dimensions of quality of life in brain tumor patients and at the same time to compare these findings with the KPS scores. In 66% of patients with a KPS of 90–100, a poor correlation was demonstrated between the KPS and the self-reported quality of life scores. Those with a KPS of 90–100 represented a group of relatively healthy patients and KPS was found to be inadequate to give a representative picture of quality of life. It is apparent that KPS is focused on self-care, daily activity, evidence of disease, and ability to work, but it does not explore the emotional or cognitive state of the patient. For instance it lacks sensitivity to depression, considered a critical clinical factor. In contrast, the incidence of survival at 1 year was well predicted by KPS.

Another study measured the overall burden of morbidity by using the Health Utilities Index mark 2 and mark 3 (HUI2 and HUI3) (WHITTON et al. 1997). These indices are based on seven and eight domains

of health, with three to five levels of function for each domain in HUI2 and five to six levels in HUI3. The method calculates a single summary score of quality of life. When applied to 50 brain tumor patients, the investigators found that the total amount of morbidity reported by the self-administered questionnaires greatly exceeded the reduction in performance status calculated by the KPS. Furthermore, unexpected problems were detected such as pain, which was reported by nearly 50% of the study patients. The study concluded that at least some of the detected impairments, like pain, once identified, could be modifiable.

Ultimately the use of a modular approach with multidimensional quality of life instruments has become the state of the art in this field (AARONSON et al. 1988; WEITZNER et al. 1995a; OSOBA et al. 1997). The EORTC has recently published new guidelines adopted for the modular approach to quality of life in cancer clinical trials (SPRANGERS et al. 1998). The core of the instrument is represented by the EORTC-QOL-C30, which encompasses numerous issues relevant to the majority of patients with cancer. The addition of subscale (modules) specifically designed for different tumor sites or histological diagnoses enriches this core.

33.6
Neurocognitive Function

Neurocognitive disorders such as dementia, psychotic disorders, and mood and personality changes are common among patients with CNS tumors (PASSIK et al. 1994). A recent study has shown that up to 41% of patients with brain tumors have cognitive disorders (MASSIE et al. 1991). Therefore, it is of importance to include routine neurocognitive tests in the assessment of patients with brain tumors (WEITZNER and MEYERS 1997). These tests often allow distinction between organic causes, due to a direct effect of tumor in the brain, and other causes such as those resulting from side-effects of therapy. Problems like major depression and apathy have to be recognized and treated as appropriate with antidepressant and stimulant therapy, respectively (WEITZNER et al. 1995b). The quality of life issues of those patients can be enormously improved by the judicious use of psychopharmacology, psychotherapy, and rehabilitation.

It is to be noted that self-report quality of life questionnaires and neurocognitive tests are applicable only to moderately compromised individuals. A large subgroup of patients is so functionally impaired, because of physical and/or cognitive deficits, that they are unable to complete the questionnaires. An interesting approach to this problem was recommended in a recently published report, which included proxies to document the patient's quality of life (SNEEUW et al. 1997). Quality of life was measured by EORTC-QOL-C30 with the use of a specific module for brain tumors, referred to as QOL-BCM (AARONSON et al. 1993; SPRANGERS et al. 1993; OSOBA et al. 1996). The study was based on 103 sets of patients affected by high-grade gliomas and patients' proxies. Approximately 60% of the study patient and proxy responses were in good agreement. The relevant discrepancies were noted in the most impaired patients, with lower level of agreement and more biased ratings. Patients with significant cognitive deficits, who needed more help from proxies, were rated by significant others as having a lower quality of life than that assessed by the patients themselves. Paradoxically, the use of significant others seemed to be less reliable among those who most needed to have proxies to complete the questionnaires.

Recent studies have focused on the quality of life of children who are survivors of brain tumors. In fact long-term survivors of pediatric brain tumors present a wide range of physical, cognitive, and psychological sequelae due to the tumor itself or to antitumor therapy (MOSTOW et al. 1991; LANNERING et al. 1990). All of these studies have used the Health Utility Index (HUI) developed at McMaster University of Canada (FEENY et al. 1989). In a study conducted in the United Kingdom the greatest burden of morbidity in the 30 patients examined was reported for emotion and cognition (each affected in more than 50%) and for pain (present in approximately one-third) (GLASER et al. 1999). These results were confirmed in a study using the HUI modified mark 2 (HUI2) and mark 3 (HUI3) on a population of 44 patients (BARR et al. 1999). In that report two-thirds of children presented with deficit of cognition and one-third had pain. The study investigators noted the global performance status reduction in children who had undergone radiation therapy before the age of 5 years. The utility scores were inversely related to the volume of tissue irradiated. In these two studies, children, parents, or health professionals, depending on the particular situation, filled in the questionnaires. FOREMAN et al. (1999) used a modification of HUI2, with two sections added, describing the social involvement with peers and the cosmetic appearance, in a group of 52 survivors of brain tumors. In this trial the patients' mothers were requested to complete the questionnaire in order to obtain a more homogeneous sample. The findings of the study showed the global health status index to be lower than in the previously surveyed survivors of leukemia or other childhood cancers. In fact only 33% of these patients had normal social activities for their age, 23% presented physical stigmata impossible to disguise, and 19% lamented pain from headache or craniotomy scars.

33.7
Conclusion

Patients affected by brain tumor face the problems resulting from the presence of the lesion in a particular anatomical site of CNS, as well as the effects of different treatment modalities used in their management. To distinguish the impact of these factors on quality of life remains a crucial ethical issue, which may help to narrow treatment choices in a given patient. An accurate assessment of side-effects of administered therapy is mandatory to assure that the treatment does not produce more injury to patients than the disease process itself.

In this very difficult decision-making process, access to an accurate health-related quality of life measure instrument, ideally based on patients' self-reports as a central source of information, is extremely useful. Due to the recognition of the importance of issues pertinent to quality of life, all published reports on the management of patients with CNS tumors should be required to add relevant details on early and late treatment toxicity. A consensus should be established among neurooncologists as to the use of common and easy-to-reproduce indices to measure quality of life of patients treated for CNS tumors.

References

Aaronson NK, Ahmedzai S, Bergman B, et al. (1993) The European Organization for Research and Treatment of Cancer QLQ-C30: a quality of life instrument for use in international clinical trials in oncology. J Natl Cancer Inst 85: 365–376

Aaronson NK, Bakker W, Stewart AL, et al. (1987) Multi-dimensional approach to the measurements of quality of life in lung cancer clinical trials. In: Aaronson NK, Beckmann JH (eds) The quality of life of cancer patients. Raven Press, New York, pp 63–82

Aaronson NK, Bullinger M, Ahmedzai S (1988) A modular approach to quality-of-life assessment in cancer clinical trials. Recent Results Cancer Res 111: 231–249

Abrey LE, DeAngelis ML, Yahalom J (1998) Long-term survival in primary CNS lymphoma. J Clin Oncol 16: 859–863

Alexander E, Moriarty TM, Davis RB, et al. (1995) Stereotactic radiosurgery for definitive, noninvasive treatment of brain metastases. J Natl Cancer Inst 87: 34–40

Barr RD, Simpson T, Whitton A, et al. (1999) Health-related quality of life in survivors of tumors of the central nervous system in childhood: a preference-based approach to measurement in a cross-sectional study. Eur J Cancer 35: 248–255

Black PM (1991) Brain tumors. Second of two parts. N Engl J Med 324: 1555–1564

Bleyer WA, Griffin TW (1980) White matter necrosis, mineralizing microangiopathy, and intellectual abilities in survivors of childhood leukemia. In: Gilbert HA, Kagan AR (eds) Radiation damage to the nervous system. Raven Press, New York, p 155

Burger PC, Kamenar E, Schold CS (1981) Encephalomyelopathy following high-dose BCNU therapy. Cancer 48: 1318–1327

Cairncross JG, Macdonald D, Ludwin S, et al. (1994) Chemotherapy for anaplastic oligodendroglioma. J Clin Oncol 12: 2013–2021

Chen JCT, Petrovich Z, ODay S, et al. (2000) Stereotactic radiosurgery in the treatment of metastatic disease to the brain. Neurosurg (In press)

Constine LS (1998) Tumors in children in cure with preservation of function and aesthetics. In: Wilson JF, (ed) Syllabus: A categorical course in radiation therapy. RSNA, Oak Brook, IL, pp 75–91

Danoff BF, Cowchock FS, Marquette C, et al. (1982) Assessment of the long-term effects of primary radiation therapy for brain tumors in children. Cancer 49: 1580–1586

Davis DG, Patchell RA (1988) Neurologic complications of bone marrow transplantation. Neurol Clin 6: 377–387

DeAngelis LM, Shapiro WR (1991) Drug/radiation interactions and central nervous system injury. In: Gutin PH, Leibel SA, Sheline GE, (eds) Radiation injury to the nervous system. Raven Press, New York, p 361

DeAngelis LM, Yahalom J, Thaler HT, et al. (1992) Combined modality treatment for primary CNS lymphoma. J Clin Oncol 10: 635–643

Duffner PK, Cohen ME, Thomas PR, et al. (1985) The long term effects of cranial irradiation on the central nervous system. Cancer (Suppl) 56: 1841–1846

Feeny D, Furlong W, Barr RD, et al. (1992) A comprehensive multiattribute system for classifying the health status of survivors of childhood cancer. J Clin Oncol 10: 923–928

Feun LG, Wallace S, Yung WK, et al. (1984) Phase I trial of intracarotid BCNU and cisplatin in patients with malignant intracerebral tumors. Cancer Drug Deliv 1: 239–245

Fine HA, Dear KB, Loeffler JS, et al. (1993) Meta-analysis of radiation therapy with and without adjuvant chemotherapy for malignant gliomas in adults. Cancer 71: 2585–2597

Foreman NK, Faestel PM, Pearson J, et al. (1999) Health status in 52 long-term survivors of pediatric brain tumors. J Neurooncol 41: 47–53

Glaser AW, Furlong W, Walker DA, et al. (1999) Applicability of the Health Utilities Index to a population of childhood survivors of central nervous system tumours in the U.K. Eur J Cancer 35: 256–261

Griffin TW, Rasey JS, Bleyer WA (1977) The effect of photon irradiation on blood-brain barrier permeability to methotrexate in mice. Cancer 40: 1109–1111

Hindo WA, De Trana FA, Lee MS, et al. (1970) Large dose increment irradiation in treatment of cerebral metastases. Cancer 26: 138–141

Hirsch JF, Renier D, Czernichow P, et al. (1979) Medulloblastoma in childhood. Survival and functional results. Acta Neurochir 48: 1–15

Hochberg FH, Pruitt A (1980) Assumptions in the radiotherapy of glioblastoma. Neurology 30: 907–911

Joseph J, Adler JR, Cox RS, et al. (1996) Linear accelerator-based stereotactic radiosurgery for brain metastases: the influence of number of lesions on survival. J Clin Oncol 14: 1085–1092

Karnofsky DA, Abelman WH, Craver LF (1948) The use of nitrogen mustards in palliative treatment of carcinoma. Cancer 1: 634–656

Kleinberg L, Wallner K, Malkin MG (1993) Good performance status of long-term disease-free survivors of intracranial gliomas. Int J Radiat Oncol Biol Phys 26: 129–133

Kramer ED, Packer RJ, Ginsberg J, et al. (1997) Acute neurologic dysfunction associated with high-dose chemotherapy and autologous bone marrow rescue for primary malignant brain tumors. Pediatr Neurosurg 27: 230–237

Kun LE, Mulhern RK, Crisco JJ (1983) Quality of life in children treated for brain tumors. Intellectual, emotional and academic function. J Neurosurg 58: 1–6

Landis SH, Murray T, Bolden S, et al. (1999) Cancer statistics, 1999. Ca Cancer J Clin 49: 8–31

Lannering B, Marky I, Lundberg A, et al. (1990) Long-term sequelae after pediatric brain tumors: their effect on disability and quality of life. Med Pediatr Oncol 18: 304–310

Lavine SD, Petrovich Z, Cohen-Gadol MD, et al. (1999) Gamma knife radiosurgery for metastatic melanoma: an analysis of survival, outcome, and complications. Neurosurg 44: 59–66

LeBaron S, Zeltzer PM, Zeltzer LK, et al. (1988) Assessment of quality of survival in children with medulloblastoma and cerebellar astrocytoma. Cancer 64: 1215–1222

Leibel SA, Gutin PH, Wara WM, et al. (1989) Survival and quality of life after interstitial implantation of removable high-activity iodine-125 sources for the treatment of patients with recurrent malignant gliomas. Int J Radiat Oncol Biol Phys 17: 1129–1139

Levin VA (1985) Chemotherapy of primary brain tumors. Neurol Clin 3: 855–866

Levin VA (1986) Pharmacokinetics and CNS chemotherapy. In: Hellmann K, Carter SK (eds) Fundamentals of cancer chemotherapy. McGraw-Hill, New York, p 28

Levin VA, Wilson CB (1981) Clinical characteristics of cancer in brain and spinal cord. In: Crook ST, Prestayko A (eds) Cancer and chemotherapy: introduction to neoplasia and antineoplastic chemotherapy. Academic Press, New York, p 167

Levin VA, Edwards MS, Wright DC, et al. (1980) Modified procarbazine, CCNU, and vincristine (PCV3) combination chemotherapy in treatment of malignant brain tumors. Cancer Treat Rep 64: 237–244

Levin VA, Wara WM, Davis RL, et al. (1985) Phase III comparison of BCNU and the combination of procarbazine, CCNU, and vincristine administered after radiotherapy with hydroxyurea for malignant gliomas. J Neurosurg 63: 218–223

Levin VA, Silver P, Hannigan J, et al. (1990) Superiority of post-radiotherapy adjuvant chemotherapy with CCNU, procarbazine, and vincristine (PCV) over BCNU for anaplastic gliomas: NCOG 6G61 final report. Int J Radiat Oncol Biol Phys 18: 311–324

Mackworth N, Fobair P, Prados MD (1992) Quality of life self-reports from 200 brain tumor patients: comparisons with Karnofsky performance scores. J Neurooncol 14: 243–253

Marks JE, Baglan RJ, Prassad SC, et al. (1981) Cerebral radionecrosis: incidence and risk in relation to dose, time, fraction and volume. Int J Radiat Oncol Biol Phys 7: 243–252

Mason WP, Krol GS, DeAngelis LM (1996) Low-grade oligodendroglioma responds to chemotherapy. Neurology 46: 203–207

Massie MJ, Breitbart W, Butler R (1991) Psychiatric diagnoses and neuropsychological evaluation of patients with neurooncologic illness. In: Neuro-Oncology IV: Recent Developments in the Management of Neuro-Oncologic Illnesses [syllabus of the postgraduate course]. Sloan-Kettering Cancer Center, New York

Mehta M, Noyes W, Craig B, et al. (1997) A cost-effectiveness and cost-utility analysis of radiosurgery vs resection for single-brain metastases. Int J Radiat Oncol Biol Phys 39: 445–454

Mostow EN, Byrne J, Connelly RR, et al. (1991) Quality of life in long-term survivors of CNS tumors of childhood and adolescence. J Clin Oncol 9: 592–599

Newton HB (1994) Primary brain tumors: review of etiology, diagnosis and treatment. Am Fam Physician 49: 787–797

ONeill BP, Buckner JC, Coffey RJ, et al. (1994) Brain metastatic lesions. Mayo Clin Proc 69: 1062–1068

<refereOsoba A, Aaronson NK, Muller MJ, et al. (1996) The development and psychometric validation of a brain cancer quality-of-life questionnaire for use in combination with general cancer-specific questionnaires. Qual Life Res 5: 139–150

Osoba D, Aaronson NK, Muller M, et al. (1997) Effect of neurological dysfunction on health-related quality of life in patients with high-grade glioma. J Neurooncol 34: 263–278

Overgaard J, Bartelink H (1995) Late effects consensus conference: RTOG/EORTC. Radiother Oncol 35:1–82

Packer RJ, Meadows AT, Rorke LB, et al. (1987) Long-term sequelae of cancer treatment on the central nervous system in childhood. Med Pediatr Oncol 15: 241–253

Passik SD, Malkin MG, Breitbart WS, et al. (1994) Psychiatric and psychosocial aspects of neurooncology. J Psychosocial Oncol 12: 101–122

Patchell RA (1995) Metastatic brain tumors. Neurol Clin 13: 915–925

Patchell RA, White CL, Clark AW, et al. (1985) Neurologic complications of bone marrow transplantation. Neurology 35: 300–306

Rosenblum ML (1990) General surgical principles, alternatives and limitations. Neurosurg Clin N Am 1: 19–36

Rubin P (1995) Special issue: late effects of normal tissues (LENT) consensus conference, including RTOG/EORTC SOMA scales, San Francisco, California August 26–28, 1992 Int J Radiat Oncol Biol Phys 31: 1035–1360

Rubin P, Constine LS, Williams JP (1997) Late effects of cancer treatment: radiation and drug toxicity. In: Perez CA, Brady LW (eds) Principles and practice of radiation oncology. Lippincott-Raven, 3rd Ed, pp 155–211

Sachsenheimer W, Piotrowski W, Bimmler T (1992) Quality of life in patients with intracranial tumors on the basis of Karnofsky's performance status. J Neurooncol 13: 177–181

Salgado D, Costa I, Pimentel T, et al. (1996) PCV for anaplastic oligodendroglioma [abstract]. J Neurooncol 30: 150

Scerrati M, Montemaggi P, Iacoangeli M, et al. (1994) Interstitial brachytherapy for low-grade cerebral gliomas: analysis of results in a series of 36 cases. Acta Neurochir 131: 97–105

Sheline GE, Wara WM, Smith V (1980) Therapeutic irradiation and brain injury. Int J Radiat Oncol Biol Phys 6: 1215–1228

Shiau CY, Sneed PK, Shu HKG, et al. (1997) Radiosurgery for brain metastases:relationship of dose and pattern of enhancement to local control. Int J Radiat Oncol Biol Phys 37: 375–383

Shrieve DC, Alexander E, Wen PY, et al. (1995) Comparison of stereotactic radiosurgery and brachytherapy in the treatment of recurrent glioblastoma multiforme. Neurosurg 36: 275–284

Shultheiss TE, Kun LE, Ang KK, et al. (1995) Radiation response of the central nervous system. Int J Radiat Oncol Biol Phys 31: 1093–1012

Sneeuw KC, Aaronson NK, Osoba D, et al. (1997) The use of significant others as proxy raters of the quality of life of patients with brain cancer. Med Care 35: 490–506

Snider S, Bashir R, Bierman P (1994) Neurologic complications after high-dose chemotherapy and autologous bone marrow transplantation for Hodgkin's disease. Neurology 44: 681–684

Sprangers MA, Cull A, Bjordal K, et al. (1993) The European Organization for Research and Treatment of Cancer approach to quality of life assessment: guidelines for developing questionnaires. Qual Life Res 2: 287–295

Sprangers MA, Cull A, Groenvold M, et al. (1998) The European Organization for Research and Treatment of Cancer approach to developing questionnaire modules: an update and overview. EORTC Quality of Life Study Group. Qual Life Res 7: 291–300

Stewart DJ, Grahovac Z, Benoit B, et al. (1984) Intracarotid chemotherapy with a combination of 1,3-bis(2-chloroethyl)-1-nitrosourea (BCNU), cis-diaminedichloroplatinum (cisplatin), and 4'-O-demethyl-1-O-(4,6-O-2-thenylidene-beta-D-glucopyranosyl) epipodophyllotoxin (VM-26) in the treatment of primary and metastatic brain tumors. Neurosurgery 15: 828–833

Taphoorn MJ, Heimans JJ, Snoek FJ, et al. (1992) Assessment of quality of life in patients treated for low-grade glioma: a preliminary report. J Neurol Neurosurg Psychiatry 55: 372–376

Tfayli A, Hentschel P, Madajewicz S, et al. (1999) Toxicities related to intraarterial infusion of cisplatin and etoposide in patients with brain tumors. J Neurooncol 42: 73–77

Trojanowski T, Peszynski J, Turowski K, et al. (1989) Quality of survival of patients with brain gliomas treated with postoperative CCNU and radiation therapy. J Neurosurg 70: 18–23

Vasantha Kumar AR, Renaudin J, Wilson CB, et al. (1974) Procarbazine hydrochloride in the treatment of brain tumors. J Neurosurg 40: 365–371

Weiss HD, Walker MD, Wiernik PH (1974) Neurotoxicity of commonly used antineoplastic agents. N Engl J Med 291: 127–133

Weitzner MA, Meyers CA (1997) Cognitive functioning and quality of life in malignant glioma patients: a review of the literature. Psychooncology 6: 169–177

Weitzner MA, Meyers CA, Gelke CK, et al. (1995a) The Functional Assessment of Cancer Therapy (FACT) Scale Development of a brain subscale and revalidation of the general version (FACT-G) in patients with primary brain tumors. Cancer 75: 1151–1161

Weitzner MA, Meyers CA, Valentine AD (1995b) Methylphenidate in the treatment of neurobehavioral slowing associated with cancer and cancer treatment. J Neuropsychiatry Clin Neurosci 7: 347–350

Werner-Wasik M, Rudoler S, Preston PE, et al. (1999) Immediate side effects of stereotactic radiotherapy and radiosurgery. Int J Radiat Oncol Biol Phys 43: 299–304

Whitton AC, Rhydderch H, Furlong W, et al. (1997) Self-reported comprehensive health status of adult brain tumor patients using the Health Utilities Index. Cancer 80: 258–265

Wiznitzer M, Packer RJ, August CS, et al. (1984) Neurological complications of bone marrow transplantation in childhood. Ann Neurol 16: 569–576

34 Complexity of Nursing in Patients Undergoing Treatment for CNS Tumors

Evangeline M. Thomson

CONTENTS

34.1
Introduction

Patients with tumors of the central nervous system (CNS) present an array of complex clinical issues for the neuroscience nurse. Nurses play a critical role during the treatment and long-term care of these patients. Dealing with patients harboring CNS tumors requires a high level of nursing expertise and a great deal of compassion and understanding.

E. M. Thomson, RN, MBA, CNRN, CCRC
Los Angeles County-University of Southern California Medical Center, 1200 N. State Street, Suite 5046, Los Angeles, CA 90033, USA

Patients with these diagnoses are impacted far beyond their physical presentation. The nurse, using the assessment skills of both the patient and their family, assists them to cope with changes in their condition and suggests methods to help improve their quality of life throughout the illness. The nurse needs to be fully knowledgeable in neurological assessment, CNS tumors, and treatment options and their implications, and to be able to apply the knowledge to each individual patient.

Tumors may be classified as primary or metastatic. Specifics of nursing care depend on the location and type of tumor. When caring for patients with metastatic lesions as a complication of primary cancer, nurses should consult an oncological nursing text for specific nursing management and interventions that should be integrated into the nursing care plan.

This chapter will provide an overview of the specialized nursing management required during diagnosis, surgery, radiation, and chemotherapy. Nursing issues related to quality of life and hospice care will also be addressed. The emphasis of the chapter will be on brain tumors since they constitute the majority of CNS tumors. Primarily adult care and treatments will be addressed. Spinal cord tumors and tumors unique to children will also be covered but in less detail.

34.2
Neurological Assessment

The basic key to neuroscience nursing is thorough understanding of neurological assessment. The nurse should begin assessing the patient immediately upon presentation, and conduct a baseline assessment of vital and neurological signs. When admitting the patient, a nursing admission history and complete physical assessment of all systems will provide a comprehensive database for planning nursing care. The neurological assessment focuses on selected critical components that are likely to change as well as those that provide an overview of the patient's general condition. The frequency and extent of the assessment depend on the stability of the patient and the underlying pathology. Doctor's orders stipulate frequency of neurological vital signs, but nurses need to use their independent clinical judgement to assess the patient more frequently when indicated. A minimal neurological assessment usually includes checking level of consciousness, pupillary signs, and motor function. The nurse should decide what other parameters, if any, should be added while monitoring the patient. For example, when taking care of patients with skull base tumors or other tumors that may cause cranial nerve findings, examination of specific cranial nerves may be added to the neurological evaluation. Patients with large pituitary tumors may require checking of visual fields. Patients harboring spinal cord tumors will need assessment of sensory and motor levels to identify the highest level of function. The nurse utilizes highly developed assessment skills and clinical reasoning to plan nursing care. The initial nursing database provides continuity of care as the patient moves through various levels of care during their hospitalization. When a patient is transferred, the nurse must be sure that all charting is fully documented and a complete report given. The receiving nurse must review prior status of the patient and make his or her own assessment as soon as the patient arrives.

34.3
Diagnosis

There is no classical presentation for CNS tumors. The signs and symptoms vary depending on the location, size, and type of tumor. Brain tumor patients frequently present with alterations of consciousness, cognitive dysfunction, headaches, seizures, and/or vomiting. Localizing signs and papilledema may also cause patients to seek care. Generally, spinal cord tumors are identified due to pain and/or weakness.

When a tumor is suspected, neuroradiological imaging studies are ordered. The imaging study of choice for tumor diagnosis today is magnetic resonance imaging (MRI). Computed tomography (CT) remains a commonly used modality for initial patient evaluation. There is limited use of magnetic resonance angiography (MRA) and conventional angiography to define vascularity of tumors. Prior to surgery a few selected patients may undergo embolization to facilitate surgical resection or venous sampling to better localize small pituitary tumors.

A major role of the nurse is to provide information about the diagnostic tests. The nurse should provide a detailed explanation of the procedure, emphasizing what the patient should expect and what is required of them. Patients having imaging procedures need to be instructed not to move during the procedure. If the patient has decreased cognition, the explanation must be simple and repeated several times. If the patient is unable to comply, sedation may be required. The family should also be educated regarding the diagnostic tests. Nurses must answer all questions for involved parties with regard to expectations during the imaging study.

Patients and families are often aware that the purpose of the study is to rule out a tumor. They are often fearful, anxious, and needing emotional support. Compassionate nurses offer support by answering questions and calmly providing information about the procedure.

Having a nurse present while the patient is being informed of the diagnosis is a key feature in helping patients gain control of their illness (McKivengin and Daubenmire 1994). After presentation of diagnosis, the physician will discuss treatment options. The nurse can then clarify and re-enforce the information that the physician has presented. The nurse incorporates this information and specialized knowledge of the CNS tumor and its treatment to develop a patient family teaching plan. Frequently, physicians spend very little time with the patient; therefore the task of informing and teaching patients is left to the nurse. These patients deserve compassionate and timely answers to their questions.

34.4
Treatment Options

The three major modalities used in treatment of CNS tumors are surgery, irradiation, and chemotherapy. Surgery remains the primary treatment, especially with benign tumors, because complete resection offers the best chance of cure. Many tumors cannot be totally removed, so a surgical debulking is done to establish a tissue diagnosis and possibly improve the patient's symptoms. A stereotactic biopsy of an intracranial lesion may be performed when surgical resection is not possible or does not offer any therapeutic advantage. Conventional radiation therapy, brachytherapy, radiosurgery, and chemotherapy may also be used to treat CNS tumors, in any combination. Treatment decisions are based on location of tumor, type and size of tumor, symptomatology, and the general condition and age of the patient.

34.4.1
Surgery

34.4.1.1
Preoperative Care

When surgery is the elected treatment, preoperative teaching begins. The experienced nurse uses the history and ongoing assessment of physical and psychosocial issues to plan nursing care. Physical care will depend on the deficits exhibited by the patient and the treatments they receive.

Patients undergoing intracranial surgery have many fears. These include fear of dying, disability, loss of independence, loss of mental abilities, personality changes, and the effect the illness and treatment will have on significant family members. The preoperative teaching should provide information about what is happening and what can be expected, thereby lessening fear and anxiety.

Prior to any teaching, the nurse assesses the patient's memory and comprehension abilities. Procedures can then be demonstrated. Questions should be encouraged and learning should be evaluated by having the patient do return demonstrations and state what was taught in his or her own words. Patients with moderate or slight cognitive deficits require modifications during teaching, such as use of simple words and visual aids. If severe deficits are present, the family must be taught. Also, family members should be encouraged to take care of themselves with sufficient rest and nutrition during this critical time.

The advent of diagnosis-related groupings (DRGs) and the determination of need for preoperative days by Health Maintenance Organization (HMO) and/or insurance companies have drastically altered the number of days that patients may be admitted for procedures. Since patients are admitted early on the morning of their surgery, many institutions utilize a nurse-run preoperative clinic to prepare patients for surgical procedures. Patients are often admitted at 6:00 A.M. and are in the operating room by 7:30 A.M. When the decision to perform surgery or an outpatient procedure is made, outpatients are seen in the preoperative clinic 1 or 2 days prior to the procedure. During this clinic visit each patient is fully evaluated by an anesthesiologist. The nurse assesses the com-

plete patient, not just their neurological status. Laboratory work is drawn, including a complete blood count, a prothrombin time, and an electrolyte panel. Urine is analyzed, women of child-bearing age undergo a pregnancy test, and chest radiography is performed (if not done within the last 6 months). An electrocardiogram is performed if the patient is over 40 years of age, obese, has a history of drug abuse, or has cardiac problems. The nurse assesses compliance with the prescribed medication regimen. Patients taking anticonvulsant medication(s) also have a serum drug level drawn. Any abnormalities in the preoperative workup are reported to the neurosurgeon.

The neurosurgeon ideally has discussed the procedure at length with the patient and family. Preoperative teaching now becomes the responsibility of the nurse in the clinic setting. The nurse instructs each patient not to eat or drink anything after midnight before the procedure. Patients who are taking antiseizure medication or cardiac medications are instructed to take them in the early morning with a sip of water on the day of the procedure. Time should be allotted for each patient to ask questions and receive information about the procedure as well as the disease process in relation to symptoms that they are experiencing. Frequently, the nurse also contacts the patient after discharge by telephone. Since the same nurse provides preoperative instruction and postoperative follow-up, a close, trusting relationship is frequently formed (see Table 34.1 for several common nursing diagnoses and interventions).

34.4.1.2
Perioperative Care

As with all operations, when the patient arrives in the operating room nurses quickly assess the patient, check the consent, and make certain all necessary preoperative procedures have been completed. Nursing interactions are done in a calm, supportive way which reassures the patient. The nurse attaches necessary monitoring equipment and the neuroanesthesiologist begins intravenous induction of anesthesia. After the patient loses consciousness, the remaining monitoring devices and lines are placed. For all cranial surgeries a Foley catheter is inserted. The nurse assists with positioning of the patient according to the physician's directions. Since many surgical procedures for CNS tumor resection may be lengthy, careful padding of pressure areas must be accomplished. It is essential that the room setup be completed prior to the start of surgery. The nurse should be familiar with the neurosurgeon's preferences and

Table 34.1. Preoperative plan of nursing care for surgically treated patients with CNS tumors

Nursing diagnosis	Nursing interventions	Expected outcomes
Knowledge deficit related to surgery and outcome	Institute preoperative teaching	Patient and family demonstrate understanding of reason for surgery, care that will be given, and the anticipated outcome of surgery
	Assess learning needs of patient regarding: Probable diagnosis Purpose of surgery Reinforce explanations given by others Provide personal patient instruction about surgery including: Personnel who will be present Sedation that will be administered Potential sensations prior to anesthesia	
Fear and anxiety secondary to upcoming surgery and diagnosis	Encourage expression of concerns and fears regarding surgery and the seriousness of disease Correct any misconceptions Provide emotional support Provide information about disease process in relationship to symptoms	Decreased signs and symptoms of fear and anxiety

the appropriate instrumentation needs, including operating microscope, for each case. The scrub nurse or surgical technician should be fully knowledgeable of neurosurgical procedures, techniques, and instruments. For cranial surgery a headrest or stereotactic frame is placed. Throughout surgery, the neuroanesthesiologist, surgeon, and nurse monitor the patient for movement and changes in vital signs and oxygenation. All nursing personnel need to be familiar with emergency procedures. If surgery is performed utilizing the sitting position, observation for air emboli must be vigilant and all members of the surgical team must be ready and aware of their role in treatment if air emboli occur.

If a surgical procedure is especially long, or takes considerably longer than was estimated preoperatively, the family should be kept updated on the progress of the case and status of the patient. A nurse may speak with the family in the waiting room on advisement of the physician.

After surgery anesthesia may be reversed in the operating room, the recovery room, or the neurosurgical intensive care unit (ICU). The nurse or designated operating room representative contacts the recovery area and informs the receiving unit of what equipment is needed, gives a report on the status of the patient, and lets the unit know when to expect the patient.

Upon completion of the surgery, the patient is transferred to the appropriate recovery area. The anesthesiologist and operating room nurse accompany the patient to the receiving unit and give the necessary reports to the receiving nurses. The surgeon speaks with the family in the waiting room, informing them how surgery went, if any complications occurred, and what they should expect to see when they visit the patient.

34.4.1.3
Postoperative Care

After surgery, the patient is taken either to the recovery room or the neuroscience ICU. Generally patients remain in the ICU for 24–72 h until their condition is stable. The anesthesia is reversed and the patient is awakened. The patient's respiratory and hemodynamic status is assessed immediately upon arrival. The patient may be intubated on a ventilator or in the process of being weaned from a ventilator. Arterial blood gases assist with evaluation of gas exchange. Nurses apply monitoring equipment as needed. The nurse completes a postoperative baseline neurological nursing assessment and reviews the physician's orders. During the early postoperative period frequent hemodynamic monitoring continues. Neurological signs are assessed frequently for changes and trends providing early recognition of increased intracranial pressure or other complications. When making this assessment it is important for the ICU nurses to have knowledge of the patients' preoperative status. In addition, the nurse monitors electrolyte levels and input and output carefully.

Nursing care also includes concern for the comfort of the patient. Patients are assessed for headache or pain and medicated accordingly. Following certain craniotomies, swelling of the eye or eyes and face may occur. Ice packs may be applied. The patient and family should be informed that this is not unusual and that the swelling will gradually decrease.

Nurses observe the head dressing for evidence of blood or cerebrospinal fluid (CSF) drainage. When the head dressing has been removed, nurses monitor the incision for redness, drainage, or signs of wound infection. As with all postoperative patients, general nursing assessment for nutrition, constipation, positioning, safety, and discharge planning are necessary responsibilities.

Positioning of the head of bed (HOB) depends on the specific surgical procedure and the preference of the physician. The doctor's order sheet should be reviewed for HOB restrictions. If there are any position restrictions, a sign should be posted above the patient's head where all caregivers can see it, as well as in the kardex.

Careful assessment by the nurse allows prevention and early recognition of complications. Common complications following craniotomy include hemorrhage, hypotension, cardiac arrhythmias, increased intracranial pressure, cerebral edema, respiratory problems, gastrointestinal bleeding, hydrocephalus, seizures, CSF leak, meningitis, wound infection, and thrombophlebitis. Neurological, hemodynamic, and physical assessment assists the nurse in identifying these problems should they occur (Table 34.2).

In the following sections a few specific intracranial procedures and tumor types that present specific challenges to the neuroscience nurse are discussed.

34.5
Pituitary Tumors

Pituitary tumors are classified according to the type of hormone they secrete. The most commonly seen pituitary tumors are classified as nonfunctional because they produce symptoms as a result of pressure on adjacent structures and cause no endocrine ab-

normalities. The most commonly seen functional pituitary tumor is a prolactinoma (60%–70%), followed by growth hormone-secreting tumors (10%–15%). Other tumors secrete adrenocorticotropic hormone (ACTH), thyroid-stimulating hormone (TSH), follicle-stimulating hormone (FSH), and luteinizing hormone (LH) (HICKEY and ARMSTRONG 1997). Treatment options include surgery, radiation, and drug therapy used either separately or in combination when necessary.

34.5.1
Prolactinomas

The nursing care for prolactinoma patients who are treated medically focuses on education. The patient must be taught to understand the implications of their endocrine abnormalities as well as symptoms of tumor regrowth. Signs of growth of the tumor include amenorrhea, galactorrhea, impotence, increasing prolactin levels, and decreasing visual fields, if the tumor is large. When patients are treated with bromocriptine, the side-effects of the drug should be explained. Primarily these include hypotension, headache, nausea, and/or vomiting. If adverse effects, such as vomiting, cause the patient to be unable to take the medication, the dose should be reduced to a very small initial amount (i.e. one-half of a 2.5-mg tablet each day) and gradually increased. Most prolactin levels will decrease when patients take 10 mg/day or less of bromocriptine. Patients may also be treated with the longer-acting form, cabergoline.

If female patients undergo surgical treatment, they must understand that fertility is a benefit of the surgery, although not all patients will be able to become pregnant following surgery.

34.5.2
Growth Hormone-Secreting Tumors

Patients exhibiting signs of acromegaly may be treated with octreotide given by subcutaneous injection three times a day. However, the cost of this medication is extremely high. Patients should be taught how to give the injection to themselves and the importance of managing the acromegaly. If medical management is not acceptable, surgery becomes the treatment of choice. These patients frequently also have hypertension, diabetes, and atherosclerotic cardiovascular disease. Nurses play an important role in

Table 34.2. Postoperative plan of nursing care for surgically treated patients with CNS tumors. Pulmonary and hemodynamic status are monitored closely by the nurse, as with any postoperative patient. The following interventions summarize several neuro-specific nursing interventions

Nursing diagnosis	Nursing interventions	Expected outcomes

Increased intracranial pressure due to edema, manipulation or bleeding	Document baseline neurological status
	Monitor NVS at regular intervals, including:
	  Level of consciousness
	  Pupillary equality and reactivity to light and accommodation
	  Ability to move all extremities and move eyes in all directions
	Elevate HOB as ordered and maintain head/neck alignment
		Early recognition of increased intracranial pressure to allow timely intervention

Pain related to intra-cranial surgery	Assess for degree of discomfort Medicate for pain Elevate HOB Encourage rest in a quiet environment Provide mouth care and lip gel frequently as needed	Minimal postoperative discomfort, patient will appear comfortable

Potential for seizures due to intracranial tumor and/or manipulation of brain during surgery	Observe for seizure activity
	Administer anticonvulsants as ordered
	If seizure occurs:
	  Maintain airway
	  Suction PRN
	  Protect patient from injury
	  Administer STAT medications per orders
	Observe for effectiveness and side-effects of anticonvulsant medications including:
	  Nystagmus and visual disturbances
	  Ataxia and/or syncope
	  Nausea and vomiting
	  Rash
	  Confusion
	  Monitor drug levels
		Seizure activity is eliminated or controlled

Potential for infection related to operation	Assess dressing or incision for increasing blood or CSF drainage
	Observe for signs and symptoms of infection:
	  Temperature elevation
	  Increased WBC count
	  Lethargy
	  Nuchal rigidity
	Use strict aseptic technique when managing wound or dressing
		Early detection of infection

NVS, Neurological vital signs; HOB, head of bed

teaching and managing these illnesses as well. Treatment for the acromegaly must be aggressive, since the condition ultimately threatens the life of the patient. Often a combination of medical, surgical, and radiation therapy is required.

34.5.3
ACTH-Secreting Tumors

Patients with these, usually small pituitary tumors present with signs of Cushing's disease. These signs include central obesity, hypertension, hirsutism, fatigue, easy bruisability, abdominal striae, moon face, dorsal fat pad, and often depression or other mental changes. In 80% of cases, the etiology of the hypercorticalism is an ACTH-secreting tumor. The treatment of choice is transsphenoidal exploration of the pituitary, since there is no satisfactory long-term medical treatment of Cushing's disease. Some patients may require inferior petrosal sinus sampling to help identify the laterality of the tumor. The nurse will assist the neuroradiologist during these procedures and must educate the patient on what to expect during the procedure.

34.5.4
Nonfunctioning Pituitary Tumors

These tumors are the most common of all pituitary tumors and frequently present with visual loss. Since there are no endocrine symptoms, the nurse must educate the patient in the importance of frequent visual field testing and the treatment that is chosen for the tumor.

34.5.5
Surgical Treatment

Most patients will undergo transsphenoidal resection of the tumor, allowing normal preservation of pituitary gland function. Those with extremely large tumors may require a transcranial approach. When patients are managed surgically, preoperative and postoperative teaching from the nurse is essential. The following discussion refers to the transsphenoidal approach.

Preoperative teaching includes detailed explanation of the surgical route, discussion of standard care in immediate postoperative period, and instruction in mouth breathing, since nostrils will be packed postoperatively. The importance of not sneezing, blowing the nose, or coughing must be emphasized. The nurse instructs the patient to report excessive swallowing, increased thirst, and/or large amounts of urinary output. Frequently intravenous glucocorticoids are given. Following surgery this is gradually tapered over several days.

After surgery, the HOB should be elevated at least 30°. Neurological vital signs are checked frequently, as are gross visual fields. Humidified oxygen may be administered through a face tent for patient comfort. The nurse observes the moustache dressing and changes it as necessary. Nurses remind patients to keep their hands off the dressing and packing and not to sneeze or blow their nose. A small amount of drainage may occur. However, if there is a constant drip of clear fluid, nurses should collect it and check to see if it is CSF. Careful and frequent oral care is imperative since the patient will be mouth breathing. Care should be taken not to irritate the incision. A toothbrush should not be used the first few days postoperatively. Nurses monitor fluid intake and output carefully.

The nurse must assess the patient for commonly occurring postoperative complications. These are CSF leak and diabetes insipidus. If lumbar punctures are necessary, the nurse assists the physician and patient during the procedure. CSF leaks may close spontaneously or require a second surgical procedure to stop the leak. Postoperatively, diabetes insipidus may develop and it is usually transient. Signs of this entity include urinary output greater than 300 cc for two consecutive hours and a specific gravity of less than 1.002, along with excessive thirst. If this occurs, serum and urinary osmolarity and serum sodium should be measured. In diabetes insipidus the serum osmolarity increases to greater than 300 mOsm/l and serum sodium elevates above 150 mEq/l. The urine osmolarity decreases to less than 200 mOsm/l. If the patient can take enough oral and intravenous fluids to prevent dehydration, no medical treatment is necessary. If diabetes insipidus requires treatment, desmopressin acetate (DDAVP) is given subcutaneously or intranasally. The action of this drug lasts 18–36 h, which in most cases allows the condition to resolve. If longer treatment is required, DDAVP nasal spray may be continued at home. Nurses must instruct patients how to use the spray correctly.

34.5.6
Radiation Therapy

When tumors are partially resected, and medical treatment is unsuccessful or not available, selected patients will require irradiation to their residual tumor. Some patients receive external beam therapy to their residual tumor and other selected patients may undergo radiosurgery primarily or secondarily.

34.5.7
Acoustic Neuromas

Acoustic neuromas are benign, usually slow-growing tumors arising from the eighth cranial nerve. Surgery is the best treatment option for most patients because it is the only option that has an excellent chance of curing the lesion. Several surgical approaches may be used, including suboccipital, middle fossa or retrosigmoid, and the frequently used translabyrinthine approach. Advantages of the last-mentioned approach are the better visualization of the facial nerve and direct approach to the cerebellopontine angle. With this approach chances of facial nerve preservation are better, as is the chance of total removal. The disadvantage to this approach is loss of hearing on the affected side. Postoperatively patients may experience vertigo, facial weakness, and eye problems such as inability to close the eye completely and persistent dryness (Foote and Holcombe 1994).

Nurses can prepare the patient for some of the more likely postoperative complications at a preoperative teaching consultation. Alterations in living environment can be made prior to hospitalization. Safety can be promoted through preparation for possible balance problems. Throw rugs and clutter can be removed. A night light placed in the bathroom and adaptations for showering such as a plastic chair and a hand-held shower spray might be helpful. The family and patient must be warned of possible facial asymmetry and informed that often these changes resolve with time.

Postoperatively, dizziness, imbalance, and nausea can be major problems. Medication should be administered as ordered. Nurses assess the abdomen or thigh wound if a fat graft was taken. The patient's safety is always a major concern for the nurse. When ambulating, the nurse encourages the patient to look at a distant point, not down, to maintain balance, and to increase the length of ambulation daily. Damage to the facial nerve may cause decreased tear production and facial movement. The nurse assesses the patient's eye closure and dryness immediately after surgery. If necessary, artificial tears and/or lacrilube ointment are applied frequently. A moisture chamber should be worn over the eye at all times to protect from corneal abrasion. At night the eye may be taped shut, thus providing double protection. If drooping of the mouth occurs, the nurse encourages the use of straws. Since some patients have difficulty opening their mouths, liquid or soft foods may be given for several days with progression to foods requiring more chewing. Since hearing will be lost on the affected side, the telephone and television speaker should be positioned on the unaffected side.

After discharge patients should be reminded that fatigue heightens dizziness, nausea, and balance problems, so rest periods should be encouraged. The facial drooping usually improves, but until it does, the nurse instructs the patient and the patient's family to utilize straws when the patient is drinking. The nurse also instructs the patient that extra care must be taken when applying makeup or shaving the face.

34.5.8
Stereotactic Biopsy

Many brain tumor patients undergo stereotactic biopsy to establish diagnosis. Fear and anxiety surround the patient and family as ultimate prognosis is unknown when the lesion is found. Once the patient arrives in the operating room, the nurse continues to educate and support the patient. The procedure is again outlined and questions answered. Local anesthesia and mild/conscious sedation is given. A stereotactic frame is placed and a CT or MRI scan is performed. The neurosurgeon, nurse, and neuroanesthesiologist accompany the patient to CT or MRI scan and return to the operating room with the patient. The correct trajectory and the coordinates of the target site are computed. During the procedure the operating room nurse is constantly alert for possible complications such as seizure activity or vomiting, although these rarely occur. Since the patient is awake, frequent reassurance should be provided, either verbally or by a touch from the circulating nurse. After the neurosurgeon has obtained adequate biopsy specimens, the cannula is withdrawn, the incision closed, and the base ring removed. Following completion of the procedure, the patient is transported to the imaging center, where a postbiopsy scan is performed to assess targeting accuracy and identify any postbiopsy hemorrhage that may be present.

During the immediate postoperative period, the nurse assesses the patient's neurological status frequently. Often neurological vital signs are taken every 15 min for 2 h, then every hour for 2 h, and then every 4 h. The patient is observed for the development of complications, including intracranial bleeding (manifested by nausea and vomiting and increasing headache or change in level of consciousness). Most patients experience an uneventful postoperative course and are discharged the next morning. At the time of discharge, patients are usually able to function as they did when they were admitted. Generally they have minimal or no pain. Patients and the families must be taught signs and symptoms of complications that would require medical attention. These include increasing neurological deficits, signs of infection, and increasing pain.

At discharge the final results of the biopsy are not generally available. Since follow-up treatment is decided according to the results of the procedure, many questions arise regarding posthospitalization plans. Discharge planning by the nurse includes the patient and significant others, as well as all members of the health care team. Appointments for follow-up and directions regarding medications are thoroughly explained and given in writing. Nursing personnel provide the patient with the names of the physician and nursing area with phone numbers to call if problems occur.

34.6
Radiation Therapy

Radiation therapy plays a major role in the treatment of primary and metastatic CNS tumors. It may be used either alone or in combination with surgery, as well as chemotherapy. The neuroscience nurse must have an understanding of the concepts involved to treat the tumor with radiation to either cure the tumor or merely control its growth. While the radiation oncologist and their associates are developing the treatment plan, the nurse's role is primarily patient and family teaching. Along with the physicians, the neuroscience nurse provides the patients with a full explanation of the treatment and the potential side-effects. The nurse discusses the patient's concerns and fears and is available to answer questions. Nursing assists the patients with communicating information to appropriate team members. As the radiation consult begins, the nurse must assure the patient of continued follow-up throughout and beyond the radiation treatment period.

34.6.1
External Beam Radiotherapy

Nursing care of patients with CNS tumors receiving irradiation includes patient and family teaching, monitoring, and assisting with management of side-effects and psychological support. There are complex quality of life issues that are specific to brain tumor patients. During the radiation period, most patients will come in daily (Monday to Friday) for fractionated treatments for a period of 5–6 weeks. A close and supportive relationship will develop between patients and their family members with the radiation oncology nurse.

Patients diagnosed with malignant CNS tumors often exhibit a surprising passivity. Often they use denial to protect themselves. Frequently they are docile and express few negative reactions when told that they need radiation treatment. To improve the quality of care, rapport between health care providers and the patient must be established early in the treatment phase. Prior to beginning the irradiation a pretreatment meeting is held with the radiation oncologist. Ideally nursing is present to meet the patient and their significant family members. This creates a sense of the team approach, which is required for treatment of CNS tumors. Nurses play an essential role in understanding the patient's underlying fears and concerns. The nurse, having knowledge of the tumor type and what the patient may expect during irradiation, conveys concern and warmth to the patient and their family. Nurses anticipate the patient's difficulties in following the treatment regimens, and communicate information in a manner that promotes the patient's cooperation. In many radiation therapy centers, nurses complete an initial patient/family assessment to obtain baseline information, identify potential problems, and develop a preliminary plan of care. Often the amount of information is too lengthy and overwhelming to be covered in an initial session with an already anxious patient and family. Teaching is an ongoing process that continues throughout the treatment period and beyond. Much nursing time is spent reinforcing, reviewing, and clarifying information previously discussed. Prior to the start of treatment the nurse answers any questions the patient and/or family members have. They must be informed fully regarding the radiation schedule and what to expect during treatment. The schedule should be given in writing.

Most brain radiation therapy simulations take less than 1 h. The nurse informs the patient of what to expect. Colored marks or tattoos will be placed on the patient's face and head to mark the radiation portals. The nurses instruct the patient not to wash off the ink marks or attempt to redraw them.

Side-effects to radiation therapy can be divided into three groups: acute, early delayed, and late delayed (BUCHOLTZ 1997) (Table 34.3). Acute reactions occur during the radiation treatment period. These include increased cerebral edema, which may be manifested in headache, nausea and vomiting, and neurological changes, fatigue, alopecia (limited to areas transited by beam), skin irritation, and inflammation of the ear. Cerebral edema is lessened if patients are on an adequate dose of steroids prior to beginning the irradiation. Nurses inform patients

Table 34.3. Side-effects of radiation therapy to the brain

Acute – occur during treatment and immediately after:
    Cerebral edema
    Fatigue
    Alopecia
    Skin reactions – scalp
Subacute or early delayed – 1–6 months after treatment:
    Fatigue
    Somnolence
Late delayed effects – greater than 6 months after treatment:
    Radiation necrosis
    Cognitive changes
    Decreased hormone production
    White matter changes
    Radiation-induced neoplasms

---

that hair loss will begin approximately 2–4 weeks after the first treatment. It may or may not grow back. Skin care is important. Patients may be given Sween cream if the scalp becomes red or dry and flaky. Nurses instruct patients to apply it to the red scaly scalp areas twice a day – after the treatment and before bed. Nurses also instruct patients to report blistering or open or draining scalp wounds to the nurse or physician and not to use home remedies as these may interfere with the treatment. The hair may be washed once a week with baby shampoo for the first 2 weeks, but after that the hair and scalp should only be washed with warm water and patted dry with a soft towel. The treated area should be exposed to air as much as possible, but not to dramatic temperature changes and direct heat. Direct sunlight should be avoided. The nurse may suggest the wearing of a scarf or hat during treatment. A wig may be worn approximately 1 month after completion of the treatment as desired. If the radiation field is near the ear, patients should be informed that hearing may decrease. Most of these precautions must be followed during the radiation treatment and for approximately 1 month after the treatment is completed. At the 1-month post-treatment check-up with the radiation oncologist the patients should be informed of what restrictions are still necessary.

The nurse in radiation oncology monitors the patient for side-effects of the brain irradiation as well as side-effects of the drugs commonly used by brain tumor patients. Teaching patients regarding these side-effects is a nursing responsibility. During treatment the nurse assesses the skin at the radiation site, since the skin may become red and easily injured. The nurse carefully assesses neurological functioning. Neurological deficits may develop and steroid doses may need to be increased. Dexamethasone

may cause an increase in appetite, elevated glucose levels, increased urination, fluid retention, leg cramps, and mood changes. While taking dexamethasone, patients are usually maintained on a histamine blocker to prevent gastrointestinal irritation. If neurological status remains unchanged, the doctor will decrease the amount of medication slowly over time. The nurse makes sure that the patient understands the directions and knows not to stop the dexamethasone abruptly. The nurse also reviews the side-effects of anticonvulsant medications with the patient and assesses the patient for compliance with the drug regimen and any problems that may occur.

If the patient experiences nausea and/or vomiting, antiemetic medications should be administered. The nurse must make sure that medications for home treatment are prescribed. The patient may become anorexic. If this occurs, the nurse instructs the patient to eat small, frequent portions of easily digested, bland foods. Proper nutrition may improve overall health and perhaps assist the patient to tolerate the treatment better. The nurse also monitors the weekly complete blood count, paying close attention to the white cell count and the platelet count.

Fatigue is a commonly occurring side-effect of radiation therapy that often begins in the late course of treatment. The nurse teaches the patient that the fatigue is not weakness or progression of disease, but instead an anticipated side-effect. The nurse may assist the patient to analyze their lifestyle and make changes to conserve energy. The patient should be instructed to set up schedules that allow sufficient time for rest in between activities.

34.6.2
Stereotactic Radiosurgery

Selected CNS tumor patients undergo stereotactic radiosurgery as primary or adjunctive treatment. This treatment is frequently used for recurrent gliomas and cerebral metastatic lesions as well as craniopharyngiomas, pituitary adenomas, acoustic neuromas, and meningiomas. The objective of radiosurgery is to deliver a finely focused radiation beam precisely to the tumor without harming surrounding normal tissue (see Sect. 6.19). Several machines are currently available to provide this treatment. These include (1) gamma knife, (2) linear accelerator, and (3) proton beam (Luxton et al. 1993).

The radiosurgery nurse prepares the patient both physically and emotionally for the treatment. Patient and family education is essential throughout the procedure. Time must be allowed to answer all questions comprehensively and accurately, which will decrease patient anxiety. As well as educating the patient and family, the radiosurgery nurse also educates the nursing staff who will care for the patient immediately following treatment. Nurses must understand the potential problems and complications that may occur.

Patient preparation begins when the radiosurgery option is presented. After the referral is made to the radiosurgery center, the nurse contacts the patient to obtain more information and to explain the entire procedure. The patient is instructed not to eat or drink anything after midnight the night prior to the procedure. They are also instructed to wash their hair and face before arriving at the hospital and to not wear make-up or hair spray. The nurse assesses the patient's understanding of these directions. Routine preoperative laboratory work is done a few days prior to the procedure or when the patient is admitted on the morning of the procedure. Patient safety and understanding of the procedure are the radiosurgery nurse's primary goals.

Upon admission for the procedure, the nurse obtains a baseline neurological assessment and vital signs. An intravenous access line is inserted. Extra doses of anticonvulsants or corticosteroids may be given per physician orders, since postprocedural seizures and brain swelling have been reported (LUNSFORD et al. 1989; FINE and FLAMM 1985). In order to lessen the chance of increased seizures, therapeutic or above levels of anticonvulsants should be established prior to radiosurgery. In adults radiosurgery is generally done under local anesthesia and mild sedation, while in children and neurologically impaired, uncooperative adults it is done under general anesthesia. The remainder of this discussion will be applicable to adult radiosurgery.

The first step of the procedure is application of a frame to the head. The nurse sets up the equipment and assists the doctor with sterile insertion of pins. Then the nurse accompanies the patient to either the CT or the MRI suite for baseline scanning and coordinate identification. The patient is then returned to the radiosurgery suite. Family may be allowed to visit in between steps. When the physicist and neurosurgeon have complete appropriate calculations for dosing, the patient is placed inside the unit and given the treatment. While positioning the patient, bony prominences are padded to prevent skin breakdown. During the procedure the nurse monitors the patient frequently. The patient is assessed for nausea and vomiting since the patient's head cannot be moved. Patients are instructed to notify the nurse if nausea

occurs. Also patients are observed for seizure activity.

Upon completion of the treatment, the stereotactic frame is removed. The nurse applies antibacterial ointment to the pin sites and covers them with a Band-Aid. The patient is transferred to the recovery room, neuroscience unit, or day surgery unit for continued monitoring as per institutional protocol. Possible but uncommon complications following treatment include seizure activity, headache, nausea, vomiting, and increased neurological deficits. Medications for these complications are given as needed. Diet and activity are progressed as tolerated.

Most patients are discharged home on the evening of the procedure. The nurse gives discharge and follow-up instructions to the patient and family. Patients are taught to look for redness, swelling, or drainage at pin sites. The day after discharge, Band-Aids may be removed and normal hygiene procedures may continue (i.e., bathing or washing hair). Patients are instructed to continue taking their routine medications (anticonvulsants and corticosteroids), and medication may be given as necessary for pain following the procedure. All patient and family questions are answered and follow-up phone numbers and appointments given in writing prior to discharge.

34.6.3
Brachytherapy

Brachytherapy utilizes the placement of radiation sources directly into tumors or near tumors. The technique delivers a relatively high dose to the tumor while minimizing the effect of radiation on surrounding normal tissues in selected tumor patients. With the advent of radiosurgery and other treatments, the use of brachytherapy has declined. The treatment may be used as part of initial tumor management or at the time of recurrence. Modern brachytherapy utilizes stereotactic targeting, cross-sectional imaging, and computerized dosimetry. Preoperatively, the nurse informs the patient of what to expect during the procedure. Brachytherapy is usually done with local anesthesia. The patient has a stereotactic frame placed and a CT scan is obtained. An appropriate seed placement and radiation dose are computed. The neurosurgeon places catheters in the tumor, typically through twist drill holes. Inner catheters are placed with the selected number of radioactive seeds. Finally the patient returns to CT scan to check placement of seeds and to determine the length of time the seeds will need to remain in the patient to deliver a defined dose to the edge of the tumor. Commonly used isotopes in brachytherapy for brain tumors include iodine-125, iridium-192, phosphorus-32, rhenium-186, and yttrium-90 (Laperriere 2000). The procedure may also be done in combination with hyperthermia. This has been shown to increase the cellular response to the radiation (Sneed 2000). In this procedure temperature probes are inserted into the tumor and the tumor is heated to approximately 40°C 30 min before and after the brachytherapy.

34.6.4
Guidelines for Radiation Safety

Radiation implants have always provoked fear in nurses and other health care workers. Since this fear may be transmitted to the patient, it can negatively influence patient care. Prior to beginning a program with brachytherapy for CNS tumors, the entire nursing staff must be educated with basic knowledge of radiation biology and radiation implants. They must be given the information needed to care for these patients safely without any danger to themselves (STRICKIN 1994).

To decrease the amount of radiation exposure, nurses working with interstitial implants must adhere to three general principles. The first is time. The shorter the time the nurse is exposed to the radiation source, the less radiation will be absorbed. A general recommendation is to limit direct nursing care to 30 min for every 8-h shift (Dunne-Daly 1994). The second and quite well understood concept by nurses is distance. The intensity of radiation decreases as the distance from the source increases. The following rule can be used to calculate exposure: amount of radiation exposure at 1 m from the radioactive source + distance squared = the amount of radiation exposure at any distance from the source + distance squared (Bucholtz 1997). Lastly, shielding may decrease radiation exposure for nursing personnel. When used properly, lead shields decrease radiation exposure. However, they may also provide nurses with a false feeling of security. The importance of maximizing distance and minimizing time cannot be overly stressed. If nurses utilize these concepts, they can provide complete patient care while protecting themselves with or without shielding.

Law requires personal monitoring devices for health care providers working around radiation. These devices simply record the amount of radiation exposure. The institution radiation safety officers must carefully monitor the exposure rates.

34.7
Chemotherapy

The limited use of chemotherapy in brain tumors is probably related to the inability of drugs to cross the blood-brain barrier. However, some chemotherapeutic agents such as the nitrosoureas, cisplatin, and procarbazine have been shown to be able to enter the brain (see Chap. 24). Various combinations of drugs and administration routes have been investigated, including intra-arterial chemotherapy, systemic delivery by mouth or intravenously, interstitial administration, biodegradable polymers, blood-brain barrier disruption, bone marrow transplantation, and immunotherapy. Intravenous chemotherapeutic drugs are usually administered in an area of the hospital dedicated to chemotherapy infusions. The nurses are certified in line placement and monitoring of the infusion. Assessment for complications is continual. Nurses must recognize the signs and symptoms of complications and know how to manage them. Physicians should be readily available if complications do occur.

Nurses play an essential role in education of patient and family during chemotherapy treatments. The nurse must know what drugs are being administered and the related common side-effects. The nurse relays and reinforces this information to the patient and family. The most common side-effects of chemotherapy are nausea, vomiting, diarrhea, stomatitis, anorexia, alopecia, and bone marrow suppression (Hickey and Armstrong 1997). The bone marrow suppression is a serious side-effect and patients are instructed when this is most likely to occur and which precautions are necessary. Patients may experience anemia and should be taught to eat a diet high in iron and to take multivitamins. Neutropenia lessens the immune response and a fatal infection could occur. Patients should be taught to maintain a clean healthy lifestyle through frequent handwashing, washing all fresh foods well, and avoiding crowds and sick people. Safety issues should be emphasized to avoid injuries that could result in open wounds and possible infection. As mentioned above, most other side-effects involve the digestive system. Patients should be taught oral hygiene and inspection techniques. They should be advised to inform the nurse or physician if oral lesions appear. They must also be taught how to treat oral lesions and how to decrease the discomfort of such lesions. Lastly nurses make sure that patients have access to antinausea medicines when necessary. Preventing nausea and vomiting increases compliance with chemotherapy. Usual interventions to prevent constipation and diarrhea should be taught since these side-effects can cause anal skin breakdown in the anal area and a life-threatening infection.

Prognosis for patients with recurrent primary gliomas is poor (SHAPIRO 1986). Various chemotherapeutic agents and methods of administration have been reported. Standard chemotherapy for high-grade astrocytomas utilizes the nitrosourea drug, BCNU, given in combination with radiation therapy. Reported response rates are 10%–40% (FINE et al. 1993). Also procarbazine treatment is recognized as standard treatment for recurrent glial tumors. Combinations of Procarbazine, lomustine (CCNU), and vincristine have been used to treat anaplastic astrocytomas and oligodendrogliomas.

The Karnofsky Performance Status (KPS) is the most widely used physician-rated outcome measure in the brain tumor literature (MEYERS 1992) (Table 34.4). Patients with a good performance status prior to chemotherapy seem to have improved response rates to treatment (WAYNE et al. 1992).

Brain metastases are not routinely treated with chemotherapy since effectiveness is limited (SITTON 1998). Chemotherapy, however, is a primary treatment for leptomeningeal metastases, malignant disease found in the leptomeninges and CSF (CHAMBERLAIN 1994). Chemotherapy can be placed directly into the CSF with agents such as methotrexate, cytarabine, and thiotepa. These drugs can be injected directly into the CSF by lumbar puncture or ventricular devices, thus allowing high concentrations of the drug at the site of the tumor without excessive systemic toxicity. Careful nursing assessment is required to identify signs and symptoms of hydrocephalus or other neurological deficits. During administration of the drug, the nurse assists the physician and supports the patient. The physician will have explained the procedure to the patient and the nurse reinforces the information and may give more detail when necessary.

Metastases to the spine may be treated with chemotherapy when adult patients have chemosensitive cancer and are not able to undergo surgery or radiation therapy. Chemotherapy is frequently administered to children with spinal metastases because irradiation causes increased risks of growth abnormalities and secondary cancers.

34.8
Spinal Cord Tumors

Spinal cord tumors may be either primary, arising from the tissues that press on or invade the spinal cord or surrounding meninges, or secondary, i.e., metastatic lesions from other parts of the body, usually lung, breast, prostate, colon, or uterine. Primary spinal cord tumors constitute approximately 10%–15% of primary CNS tumors. There is no gender predilection and the tumors usually affect 20- to 50-year-olds. Rarely are spinal cord tumors seen in patients younger than 10 years or in the elderly (SIMEONE 1990).

Primary spinal cord tumor patients commonly present with axial spinal pain, which frequently has been present for 3–6 months. The most frequently seen presenting sign of a metastatic spinal cord tumor is localized back pain and radicular pain. This typically progresses to localized tenderness over the affected vertebra, muscle weakness, and sensory deficits. Most metastatic lesions affect the lower thoracic spine. Often rapid-onset paraplegia, urinary retention, and severe pain bring the patient to the emergency room.

Diagnosis of spinal cord tumor is made using a history, physical examination, and a contrast-enhanced MRI scan. Nurses may need to explain the MRI procedure to the patient. Due to the unexplained loss of lower extremity functioning, the patient's anxiety level is high. Nurses should answer all questions from the patient and family in a calm manner with a competent attitude.

The primary treatment goal for spinal cord tumor patients is to preserve neurological function. If any spinal instability is suspected, the patient must be immobilized in spinal precautions. The neuroscience nurse, understanding the complexities of the spinal cord functions, maintains the immobilization until surgical stabilization can be undertaken or stability determined. A combined surgical, medical, and radiological approach is required for treatment. Edema is often present around the tumor, so high-dose corticosteroids are administered and then tapered.

Table 34.4. Karnofsky Performance Scale

100	Normal; no complaints, no evidence of disease
90	Able to carry on normal activity; minor symptoms
80	Normal activity with effort; some symptoms
70	Cares for self; unable to carry on normal activity
60	Requires occasional assistance; cares for most needs
50	Requires considerable assistance and frequent medical care
40	Disabled; requires special assistance and care
30	Severely disabled; hospitalized, death not imminent
20	Very sick; active supportive treatment needed
10	Moribund; fatal processes are rapidly progressing
0	Dead

As previously discussed in brain tumor nursing care, patient teaching and education are essential while caring for spinal cord tumor patients. Patients treated with surgery or radiation therapy require full explanations of procedures and treatments. Patients who undergo surgical resection require nursing care for laminectomy patients. Nurses must obtain vital signs and a baseline neurological assessment. The key areas of assessment include pain, motor and sensory deficits, and bowel and bladder functioning.

The quality, location, and type of pain should be documented. Any change in pain or circumstances that exacerbate pain should be noted. Nurses monitor pain at least every 4 h and administer analgesics as ordered, prior to escalation of pain. Teaching the patient techniques for pain control is beneficial. These include relaxation, imagery, and distraction activities. Physical comfort measures including repositioning at least every 2 h, while maintaining proper body alignment. Massage may also lessen a patient's pain.

Motor and sensory functioning should be assessed. Each side of the body should be checked separately and findings compared. Sensory modalities including light touch, pinprick (pain), and position sense should be checked with the patient's eyes closed, beginning at the feet and working upward. The highest level of sensation should be recorded. Muscle strength and tone should also be tested as well as deep tendon reflexes and coordination. If the patient is ambulatory, gait should be assessed, noting any spasticity or abnormal movement. Physical and occupational therapy should be consulted as early as possible.

Evaluation of bowel and bladder function requires determination of the normal frequency of bowel and bladder evacuation. Assessment should be made for change in bowel patterns, and the abdomen auscultated in all four quadrants for bowel sounds and distention. Urinary retention and/or inability to void are commonly seen in spinal cord tumor patients. This places the patient at high risk for urinary tract infection. An intermittent catheterization schedule should be established as soon as possible when indicated. It is important to teach the patient how to catheterize themselves and the necessary procedures to prevent urinary tract infections.

When the patient's deficits have stabilized, those with more complete injuries to the cord require many nursing interventions. Complete nursing care interventions for these patients are beyond the scope of this chapter.

Prognosis varies greatly, depending on the type of tumor and the neurological deficits present. Each patient requires evaluation to identify individual re-habilitation needs. Many patients with neurological deficits will benefit from a short-term in-patient rehabilitation program.

34.9
Tumors in Children

Central nervous system tumors are the most common solid tumors in children. Over 60% of childhood CNS tumors are located in the posterior fossa (see Chap. 27). These tumors include medulloblastoma, cerebellar astrocytomas, fourth ventricle ependymomas, and brainstem gliomas. The most common tumor is a medulloblastoma, also called primitive neuroectodermal tumor (PNET), which may seed along the neuraxis and outside the nervous system (Friedman et al. 1991; Kirk et al. 1995). Supratentorial tumors include low- and high-grade astrocytomas, hypothalamic and optic pathway tumors, and craniopharyngiomas. MRI is the best diagnostic test for CNS tumors. As in adults, treatment modalities include surgery, radiation, and chemotherapy. The survival rates for children are higher than in adults. Some CNS tumors can be cured using advanced surgical techniques alone. Radiation is part of the standard care for many pediatric tumors but as children are living longer with their tumors the neurotoxic and extraneural toxic effects of radiation are becoming apparent. Late side-effects may include decreased growth and cognitive impairments when very young children are irradiated (Archibald et al. 1994; Friedman et al. 1991; Shiminski-Maher and Shields 1995). It is now common practice to avoid or minimize the use of cranial and spinal irradiation in children, or to at least delay it until the child is older. Chemotherapy has become standard in treating many pediatric CNS tumor patients. Adjuvant chemotherapy is now used to defer or replace radiation therapy in very young children (<3 years of age), and to reduce the amount of radiotherapy in older children. High-dose chemotherapy followed by stem cell or autologous bone marrow rescue is also being used with good outcomes in several high-grade tumors. Children treated at cancer centers with expertise in pediatric neuro-oncology have a better prognosis than children treated in the community (Stewart and Cohen 1998).

Long-term side-effects of CNS tumors and their treatments include decreased intellect, decreased growth hormone resulting in short stature, and increased chance of second malignancy (Albright 1993; Moore 1995; Tomita 1992).

When a child is diagnosed with a CNS tumor a family-centered nursing approach must be taken in which all information that the physician gives is clarified and reinforced by the nurse. Nurses need to be fully informed regarding treatment and prognosis. A close relationship with a compassionate nurse can support the child and family throughout this difficult time. Nursing monitors the child for neurological changes and any intellectual, endocrinological, and oncogenic late effects of the treatment. Appropriate referrals to rehabilitative services and special schooling when needed must be initiated. Nursing assists with coordinating the long-term care of these patients. A complete discussion of nursing care for these children is beyond the scope of this chapter.

34.10
Nurses' Role in Discharge Planning

Preparing the patient for discharge is a major nursing responsibility. Discharge planning varies according to the type of tumor (benign vs malignant), the procedure that was done (stereotactic biopsy, craniotomy or laminectomy with tumor resection), and the amount of neurological deficits that the patient exhibits. Individual discharge planning with identification of rehabilitation needs is based upon the nurses' ongoing assessment of the patient, as well as the assessment of other members of the health care team (i.e., physical therapist, occupational therapist, speech therapist, and social worker). Family support and resources are also addressed. During the hospitalization the family may have participated in basic patient care and activities of daily living routines. These family members are more prepared to take the patient home. Patients and their families must be helped to set realistic goals. Depending on the type of surgery, amount of deficits, and prognosis, the patient and/or family may be required to make major decisions about discharge facilities and treatment choices. Patients may be discharged home, to subacute nursing units, to nursing homes, or to rehabilitation centers.

34.11
Quality Of Life Issues

Quality of life (QOL) issues include the physical, social, and psychological dimensions of the illness experience (KING et al. 1997). When the nurse assesses QOL, they should evaluate the impact the tumor diagnosis has had on work-related activities, activities of daily living, support systems, outlook, and mood. This is an overall assessment that requires an open, intimate relationship with the patient, which the nurse will have developed while caring for the patient. Patients often appreciate talking to the nurse, since they often think doctors are too busy to listen. Nurses have diverse knowledge and skills and are able to make appropriate referrals when needed. QOL issues should be discussed early in the treatment period, not only when there are no further options for the patient. Relatively early in the course of the illness, it is helpful to raise these issues for discussion. It must be anticipated that those with malignant brain tumors will be less and less able to contribute to the decision-making process as the illness progresses.

It is important to remember that tumor patients and their families need to talk. Whether the tumor is benign or malignant, a CNS tumor patient and the family need to express their fears and concerns and have their questions answered in a calm, patient manner. This job frequently is designated to the nurse. A compassionate, knowledgeable nurse can do much to allay patient and family anxiety. Although answers are not always what the patients want to hear, they do want to know the truth. Helping the patient and their families communicate their concerns with each other is beneficial. When a patient's cognitive level is decreased, frequently the most support is given to the caregivers.

Patients and their families should be encouraged to gain all the information available on their type of tumor and its treatment. Phone numbers and Internet access to organizations providing this information should be given to the patients. Nurses need to have contact information readily available. The following list contains several of the available resource organizations:

- American Brain Tumor Association, 2720 River Road, Suite 146, Des Plaines, IL 60018, (847) 827-9910
- National Brain Tumor Foundation, 785 Market Street, Suite 1600, San Francisco, CA 94103, (800) 934-CURE
- Brain Tumor Foundation of Canada, 650 Waterloo Street, Suite 100, London, Ontario N6B 2R4, (519) 642-7755
- The Brain Tumor Society, 124 Watertown Street, Suite 3H, Watertown, MA 02472, (617) 924-9997
- The Brain Tumor Foundation for Children, Inc., 1835 Savoy Drive, Suite 316, Atlanta, GA 30341, (770) 458-555
- American Cancer Society, (800) 227-2345

Also brain tumor and cancer support groups may be presented and contact phone numbers given. Social workers and neuropsychologists may also be beneficial. Access to information on clinical trials should also be made readily available.

A fully informed patient may elect for all possible treatments or no treatment at all. After having all options explained completely, the decision is theirs. Some terminal patients may be referred to hospice, where supportive, compassionate care will continue.

When the tumor cannot be cured and the patient approaches a terminal state, the goals of therapy usually become limited to comfort measures, including relief of pain, agitation, and respiratory distress. Seizures must be controlled and fever managed. Management of the symptoms at the end of life becomes more complex for the nurse, as alterations in consciousness and difficulty swallowing can make the use of medication difficult. Many times this care can be provided at home with the help of hospice services. Most hospice organizations have an associated pharmacy which is able to compound necessary medications into liquid or suppository forms. Alternate routes for pain and seizure medications are also available. Hospice organizations provide an essential service to the patients and their families through nursing and emotional support for the aspects of grieving and death. Involvement of hospice should be obtained long before the patient reaches a terminal stage, even if only for introductory purposes. This helps the patient and family to develop a realistic and practical view of what to expect and what types of support are available. Diligence in managing symptoms at the end of life comforts the patient and assists caregivers in coping with the impending loss of a loved one.

34.12
Clinical Trials

Evaluation of new treatments for malignant gliomas continues. The neuroscience research nurse plays a pivotal role in ensuring the smooth running of a successful clinical trial by being present and involved in each step of the research study. Research nurses must be fully knowledgeable in Federal Drug Administration (FDA) regulations, hospital and Institutional Review Board (IRB) policies, and the clinical protocol itself. The research nurse compiles prestudy documents and maintains study files.

When preclinical studies indicate that a drug may be effective and can be safely administered to human subjects, clinical trials begin. Clinical studies are divided into four phases (Table 34.5). Most studies for CNS tumors are multicenter and usually phase II or III studies. High-grade gliomas have had the emphasis of chemotherapy trials due to the high incidence rate and aggressive nature of the tumors.

Prior to initiation of a clinical trial the protocol must be submitted to and approved by the IRB. After approval of the study, the research nurse must in-service all nursing areas where patients will receive care. Many trials are conducted on an outpatient basis and the research nurse is the main patient contact. Other trials involve admission of patients to General Clinical Research Centers (GCRCs) or day admission units for chemotherapy. Some trials involve surgery, which require few to several days of hospitalization. Nurses in all involved areas need to understand the purpose of the study, the protocol, and all required nursing responsibilities. The nurses must understand when to contact the research nurse or principal investigator and have contact numbers readily available

When entering patients into a clinical trial, all inclusion–exclusion criteria must be met. Frequently nurses may assist in identifying patients for studies. The physician will obtain informed consent. The nurse should be present while this information is provided by a physician to the study patient. Following this, the nurse can reinforce the information the doctor has presented and explain in even more detail what the patient should expect during participation in the clinical trial. Patient and family teaching and education are essential to improve compliance with all required procedures. Throughout the trial, the nurse is often the patient's primary contact person. The nurse coordinates the subsequent activities of the investigators and subjects. The nurse sees that all requirements of the trial are met, with correct documentation and successful collection of data. The research nurse is in constant contact with the physician (principal investigator), drug or device company, or clinical research organization (CRO) and the IRB.

The research nurse must be present and involved in each step of the clinical trial procedure. All studies must be performed to Good Clinical Practices (GCPs) as established by the FDA. All serious adverse events (SAEs) must be reported to the sponsor or CRO within 24 h, as well as to the IRB. It is essential that the research nurse know all regulatory deadlines.

Table 34.5. Types of clinical studies

Phase I	Initial studies to evaluate safety of the drug and to determine what the safe dose is
Phase II	Studies to determine the efficacy of the drug and to better define the dose
Phase III	A randomized study comparing the drug to an existing standard treatment
Phase IV	Postmarketing surveillance studies and other special trials designed to further detail the safety and efficacy of the drug

34.13
Conclusion

The neuroscience nurse plays a pivotal role in the care and treatment of CNS tumor patients. The nurse works collaboratively with physicians and other health care team members to provide optimal patient care management. Due to frequent advances in CNS tumor treatment and rapid technological changes, the professional nurse can no longer depend only on his/her basic training. The increasingly complex base of knowledge required for neuroscience nurses reflects this progress. When caring for CNS tumor patients, ongoing education and acquisition of new skills are required. A knowledgeable, up to date neuroscience nurse, using a high level of critical thinking skills is an effective member of the health care team.

The impact of CNS tumors is often overwhelming and has far-reaching implications for patients and families. A major nursing responsibility is patient and family teaching. CNS tumor patients face a complex and often confusing array of procedures that must be fully explained in terms they comprehend. The functional losses may include decreased cognition and progressive physical disabilities. Throughout the continuum of care, the neuroscience nurse provides ongoing assessment, care, education, and support. These responsibilities continue well beyond the hospital setting, as the patient either recovers or requires increasing levels of nursing care.

References

Albright I (1993) Pediatric brain tumors. Cancer J Clin 43:272–288

Archibald YM, Lunn D, Ruttan LA et al. (1994) Cognitive functioning in long-term survivors of high-grade gliomas. J Neurosurg 80:247–253

Bucholtz JD (1997) Central Nervous System, Tumors. In: Dow KH, Bucholtz JD, Iwamoto RR et al (eds) Nursing Care in Radiation Oncology (2nd ed). W.B. Saunders Company, Philadelphia, pp 136–151

Chamberlain MC (1994) New approaches to and current treatment of leptomeningeal metastases. Curr Opin Neurol 7:492–500

Dunne-Daly C (1994) Brachytherapy. Cancer Nurs 17(4):355–364

Fine HA, Dean KBG, Loeffler JS et al. (1993) Meta-analysis of radiation therapy with and without adjuvant chemotherapy for malignant gliomas in adults. Cancer 71:2582–2597

Foote AW, Holcombe J (1994) Acoustic neuroma: suggestions for helping the patient adapt after translabyrinthine surgery. J Neurosci Nurs 26:162–165

Friedman HS, Horowitz M, Oakes WJ et al. (1991) Tumors of the central nervous system. Improvement in outcome through a multimodality approach. Pediatr Clin North Am 38:381–391

Hickey JV, Armstrong T (1997) Brain Tumors. In: Hickey SR (ed) The clinical practice of neurological and neurosurgical nursing 4th ed. Lippincott Williams & Wilkins, Hagerstown pp 501–526

King C, Haberman M, Berry D et al. (1997) Quality of life and the cancer experience: the state-of-the-knowledge. Oncol Nurs For 24:27–41

Kirk EA, Howard VC, Scott CA (1995) Description of posterior fossa syndrome in children after posterior fossa brain tumor surgery. J Pediatr Oncol Nurs 12:181–187

La Perriere NJ (2000) Brachytherapy. In: Bernstein M, Berger MS (eds). Neuro-Oncology: The Essentials. Thieme Publishers Inc, New York pp 198–204

Lunsford LD, Flickinger J, Lindner G et al. (1989) Stereotactic radiosurgery of the brain using the first United States 201 cobalt-60 source gamma knife. Neurosurg 24(2):151–159

Luxton G, Petrovich Z, Jozsef G et al. (1993) Stereotactic radiosurgery: principles and comparison of treatment methods. Neurosurg 32:241–259

McKivengin MJ, Daubenmire MJ (1994) The healing process of presence. J Holist Nurs 12(1):65–81

Meyers CA (1992) Quality of life of brain tumor patients. In: Bernstein M, Berger MS (eds). Neuro-Oncology The Essentials. Thieme Publishers Inc, New York pp 466–472

Moore IM (1995) Central nervous system toxicity of cancer therapy in children. J Pediatr Oncol Nurs 12:203–210

Shapiro WR (1986) Therapy of adult malignant brain tumors. Sem Oncol 13:38–45

Shiminski-Maher T, Shields M (1995) Pediatric brain tumors: diagnosis and management. J Pediatr Oncol Nurs 12:188–198

Simeone FA (1990) Spinal cord tumors in adults. In J.R.Youmans (ed). Neurological Surgery (3rd ed.) W.B. Saunders Company, Philadelphia pp 3531–3547

Sitton E (1998) Central nervous system metastases. Sem Oncol Nurs 14(3):210–219

Sneed PK (2000) Hyperthermia. In: Bernstein M, Berger MS (eds). Neuro-Oncology The Essentials. Thieme Publishers Inc, New York pp 218–224

Steiner L, Lindquist CH (1985) Radiosurgery in cerebral arteriovenous malformations. In: Fine JM, Flamm ES (eds) Cerebrovascular Surgery Vol IV. Spring-Verlag, Berlin, pp 1181-

Stewart ES, Cohen DG (1998) Central nervous system tumors in children. Sem Oncol Nurs 14(1):34–42

Strickin L (1994) Strategies for overcoming nurses' fears of radiation exposure. Cancer Nurs 2(4):275–279

Tomita T (1992) Long-term effects of treatment for childhood brain tumors. Pediatr Neuro-Oncol 3(4):959–971

Wayne K, Hannisdal MD, Ole N et al. (1992) Combined intra-arterial and systemic chemotherapy for recurrent malignant brain tumors. Neurosurg 30(2): 223–227

Subject Index

List of Contributors

Roscoe Atkinson, MD
Assistant Professor, Clinical Medicine
Pathology and Neurology
University of Southern California
Keck School of Medicine
McKibben Annex 346
2011 Zonal Avenue
Los Angeles, CA 90033
USA

John R. Adler, Jr., MD
Professor and Director of Radiosurgery
and Stereotactic Neurosurgery
Departments of Neurosurgery and Radiation Oncology
Stanford University School of Medicine
300 Pasteur Dr.
Stanford, CA 94305
USA

Arun P. Amar, MD
Department of Neurological Surgery
Children's Hospital of Los Angeles
University of Southern California
Keck School of Medicine
1300 North Vermont, Suite 906
Los Angeles, CA 90033
USA

Michael L.J. Apuzzo, MD
Edwin M. Todd/Trent H. Wells, Jr.
Professor of Neurological Surgery
and Professor of Radiation Oncology
University of Southern California
Keck School of Medicine
Los Angeles, CA 90033
USA

Michael Bamberg, MD
Professor, Department of Radiotherapy
Eberhard-Karls-Universität
Hoppe-Seyler-Strasse 3
72076 Tubingen
Germany

Anna Bettini, MD
Research Fellow
Departments of Radiation Oncology and Medicine
University of Southern California School of Medicine
1441 Eastlake Avenue
Los Angeles, CA 90033
USA

Barry D. Birch, MD
Department of Neurological Surgery
Columbia Presbyterian Medical Center
College of Physicians and Surgeons of Columbia University
New York Presbyterian Hospital
710 West 168th Street
New York, NY
USA

Luther W. Brady, MD
Hylda Cohn/American Cancer Society
Professor of Clinical Oncology, and Professor
Department of Radiation Oncology
Hahnemann University Hospital
Broad & Vine Sts., Mail Stop 200
Philadelphia, PA 19102
USA

Steven D. Chang, MD
Cerebrovascular Surgery Fellow
Department of Neurosurgery
Stanford University School of Medicine
300 Pasteur Dr.
Stanford, CA 94305
USA

Joseph Chen, MD, PhD
Fellow, Department of Neurosurgery
University of Southern California School of Medicine
1441 Eastlake Avenue
Los Angeles, CA 90033
USA

Reiner Class, PhD
Assistant Professor, Department of Radiation Oncology
Director, Flow Cytometry Core Laboratory
MCP Hahnemann University, MS 102
Broad and Vine Streets
Philadelphia, PA 19102
USA

Peter Conti, MD
Professor of Radiology, Director of Neuroradiology
Division of Neuroradiology and PET Imaging
University of Southern California School of Medicine
1200 North State Street, Room 5139
Los Angeles, CA 90033
USA

Jennifer L. Daigle, SB
Graduate Student Researcher
Roy E. Coats Research Laboratories
and Department of Radiation Oncology
University of California, Los Angeles
10833 LeConte Avenue
Los Angeles, CA 90095-1714
USA

J. Diaz Day, MD
Director, Neurological Surgery
House Neurological and Skull Base Surgery Associates
House Ear Clinic, Inc.
2100 W. 3rd St.
Los Angeles, CA 90057
USA

Barbara Dykes
Research Associate, Division Medical Oncology
John Wayne Cancer Institute at Saint John's Hospital
2001 Santa Monica Blvd., Suite 560W
Santa Monia, CA 90404
USA

Jeremy Flagel, BS
Medical Student
University of Southern California
Keck School of Medicine
1200 North State Street, Suite 5046
Los Angeles, CA 90033-0804
USA

Silvia C. Formenti, MD
Associate Professor
Departments of Radiation Oncology and Medicine
University of Southern California
Keck School of Medicine
1441 Eastlake Avenue
Los Angeles, CA 90033-0804
USA

Rick A. Freidman, MD
Neuro-otologist
House Ear Clinic, Inc.
2100 W. 3rd St.
Los Angeles, CA 90057
USA

Bernard George, MD
Professor and Chief of Service
Department of Neurosurgery, Hôpital Lariboisière
Publique de Paris
2 rue Ambroise Paré
75010 Paris
France

Sanjay Ghosh, MD
Department of Neurological Surgery
University of Southern California School of Medicine
1200 North State Street, Room 5046
Los Angeles, CA 90033
USA

Steven L. Giannotta, MD
Professor, Department of Neurological Surgery
University of Southern California School of Medicine
1200 North State Street, Room 5046
Los Angeles, CA 90033
USA

John L. Go, MD
Division of Neuroradiology and PET Imaging
University of Southern California School of Medicine
1200 North State Street, Room 5139
Los Angeles, CA 90033
USA

Anca-Ligia Grosu, MD
Department of Radiotherapy
Klinikum Rechts der Isar
Technische Universität Munich
Ismaninger Strasse 22
81675 Munich
Germany

Griff Harsh, MD, MBA
Professor, Department of Neurosurgery
Stanford University, School of Medicine
300 Pasteur Drive, Edwards Building, R227
Stanford, CA 94305-5327
USA

Gery Hsu, MD
Department of Neurosurgery
Baylor Colloege of Medicine
Houston, Texas
USA

David Huang, MD
Senior Resident, Department of Radiation Oncology
University of Southern California School of Medicine
1441 Eastlake Avenue G34
Los Angeles, CA 90033
USA

Douglas J. Hyder, MD
Assistant Director of Brain Tumor Program
Assistant Professor of Neurology and Pediatrics
Children's Hospital of Los Angeles
4650 Sunset Blvd., M.S. 54
Los Angeles, CA 90027
USA

Branislav Jeremic, MD
Department of Radiotherapy
Eberhard-Karls-Universität
Hoppe-Seyler-Strasse 3
72076 Tübingen
Germany

Gabor Jozsef, PhD
Assistant Professor, Department of Radiation Oncology
University of Southern California Keck School of Medicine
1441 Eastlake Avenue, Room G350
Los Angeles, CA 90033-0804
USA

Michael G. Kaiser, MD
Department of Neurological Surgery
Columbia Presbyterian Medical Center
College of Physicians and Surgeons of Columbia University
New York Presbyterian Hospital
710 West 168th Street
New York, NY
USA

Larry T. Khoo, MD
Clinical Instructor, Department of Neurosurgery
University of Southern California
Keck School of Medicine
1200 North State Street, Suite 5046
Los Angeles, CA 90033-0804
USA

Paul Kim, MD
Division of Neuroradiology and PET Imaging
University of Southern California
School of Medicine
1200 North State Street, Room 5139
Los Angeles, CA 90033
USA

Martin Kocher, MD
Department of Radiotherapy
University of Cologne
Joseph-Stelzmann-Strasse 9
50924 Köln
Germany

Rolf Dieter Kortmann, MD
Department of Radiotherapy
Eberhard-Karls-Universität
Hoppe-Seyler-Strasse 3
72076 Tübingen
Germany

Mark D. Krieger, MD
Division of Pediatric Neurosurgery
Children's Hospital of Los Angeles
University of Southern California
Keck School of Medicine
1300 North Vermont, Suite 906
Los Angeles, CA 90027
USA

John E. Lahaniatis, MD
Department of Radiation Oncology
Hahnemann University Hospital
Broad & Vine Sts., Mail Stop 200
Philadelphia, PA 19102
USA

Robert S. Lavey, MD, MPH
Head, Radiation Oncology Program
Associate Professor
Department of Pediatrics and Radiation Oncology
University of Southern California
4650 Sunset Boulevard, Mail Stop #54
Los Angeles, CA 90027-6016
USA

Michael L. Levy, MD
Assistant Professor
Division of Pediatric Neurosurgery
Children's Hospital of Los Angeles
University of Southern California Keck School of Medicine
1300 North Vermont, Suite 906
Los Angeles, CA 90027
USA

Mark Liker, MD
Clinical Instructor, Department of Neurosurgery
University of Southern California Keck School of Medicine
1200 North State Street, Suite 5046
Los Angeles, CA 90033-0804
USA

David P. Martin, MD
Clinical Assistant Professor, Department of Neurosurgery
Stanford University School of Medicine
300 Pasteur Dr.
Stanford, CA 94305
USA

William H. McBride, DSc
Professor and Director
Roy E. Coats Research Laboratories
and Department of Radiation Oncology
University of California, Los Angeles
10833 LeConte Avenue
Los Angeles, CA 90095-1714
USA

J. Gordon McComb, MD
Professor, Department of Pediatrics
Division of Pediatric Neurosurgery
Children's Hospital of Los Angeles
University of Southern California Keck School of Medicine
1300 North Vermont, Suite 906
Los Angeles, CA 90027
USA

Paul C. McCormick, MD
Neurological Institute
710 West 168th Street
New York, NY 10032-2603
USA

Curtis T. Miyamoto, MD
Associate Professor and Clinical Service Chief
Department of Radiation Oncology
The Brain Tumor Center, M.S. 200
MCP Hahnemann University
216 North Broad Street
Philadelphia, PA 1902-1192
USA

Michael Molls, MD, PhD
Professor, Direktor, Klinik und Poliklinik für
Strahlentherapie und Radiologische Onkologie
Klinikum rechts der Isar der Technischen Universität München
Ismaninger Strasse 22
81675 Munich
Germany

ROLF-PETER MÜLLER, MD
Professor, Department of Radiotherapy
University of Cologne
Joseph-Stelzmann-Strasse 9
50924 Köln
Germany

MARTIN J. MURPHY, PhD
Radiation Physicist
Department of Radiation Oncology
Stanford University School of Medicine
300 Pasteur Dr.
Stanford, CA 94305
USA

STEVEN O'DAY, MD
Associate Director, Medical Oncology
John Wayne Cancer Institute at Saint John's Hospital
2001 Santa Monica Blvd., Suite 560W
Santa Monia, CA 90404
USA

ANDREW T. PARSA, MD, PhD
Department of Neurological Surgery
Columbia Presbyterian Medical Center
College of Physicians and Surgeons of Columbia University
New York Presbyterian Hospital
710 West 168th Street
New York, NY
USA

ZBIGNIEW PETROVICH, MD, FACR
Professor and Chairman
Department of Radiation Oncology
University of Southern California Keck School of Medicine
1441 Eastlake Avenue, Room G356
Los Angeles, CA 90033-0804
USA

SUSAN PRESTON-MARTIN, PhD
Professor, Department of Preventive Medicine
University of Southern California
Keck School of Medicine
1441 Eastlake Avenue, MS #44,
Los Angeles, CA 90089
USA

MICHAEL SALCMAN, MD
Head, Division of Neurological Surgery
Sinai Hospital
9101 Franklin Square Drive, Suite 310
Baltimore, MD 21237-3928
USA

RAYMOND SAWAYA, MD
Professor and Chairman
M.D. Anderson Cancer Center
Department of Neurosurgery
1515 Holcombe Blvd., Box 064
Houston, TX 77030
USA

MICHAEL SELCH, MD
Professor of Radiation Oncology
University of California Los Angeles
200 Medical Plaza
Suite B265
Los Angeles, CA 90095
USA

EVANGELINE M. THOMSON, RN, MBA, CNRN, CCRC
Los Angeles County-University of Southern California
Medical Center
1200 North State Street, Room 5046
Los Angeles, CA 90033
USA

VICTOR C.-K. TSE, MD, PhD
Assistant Professor, Department of Neurosurgery
Stanford University, School of Medicine
300 Pasteur Drive, Boswell Building, A301
Stanford, CA 94305-5327
USA

JÜRGEN VOGES, MD
Department of Stereotactic and Functional Neurosurgery
University of Cologne
Joseph-Stelzmann-Strasse 9
50931 Köln
Germany

MARTIN H. WEISS, MD,
Professor and Chairman, Department of Neurological Surgery
USC School of Medicine
LAC+USC Medical Center
1200 North State Street, Room 5046
Los Angeles, CA 90033
USA

H. RODNEY WITHERS, MD, DSc
Professor and Chairman
Laboratories and Department of Radiation Oncology
University of California Los Angeles
10833 LeConte Avenue
Los Angeles, CA 90095-1714
USA

CHENG YU, PhD
Assistant Professor, Department of Radiation Oncology,
University of Southern California
School of Medicine
1441 Eastlake Avenue
Los Angeles, CA 90033
USA

CHI-SHING ZEE, MD
Professor of Radiology, Director of Neuroradiology
Division of Neuroradiology and PET Imaging
University of Southern California
School of Medicine
1200 North State Street, Room 5139
Los Angeles, CA 90033
USA

MEDICAL RADIOLOGY
Diagnostic Imaging and Radiation Oncology

Titles in the series already published

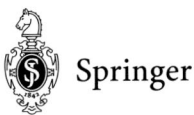 Springer

MEDICAL RADIOLOGY
Diagnostic Imaging and Radiation Oncology

Titles in the series already published

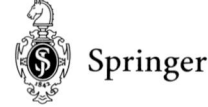

Springer

Printing and Binding: Stürtz AG, Würzburg